CHILD
DEVELOPMENT

CHILD DEVELOPMENT

Fifteenth Edition

JOHN W. SANTROCK
University of Texas at Dallas

KIRBY DEATER-DECKARD
University of Massachusetts Amherst

JENNIFER E. LANSFORD
Duke University

CHILD DEVELOPMENT, FIFTEENTH EDITION

Published by McGraw-Hill Education, 2 Penn Plaza, New York, NY 10121. Copyright © 2021 by
McGraw-Hill Education. All rights reserved. Printed in the United States of America. Previous editions
© 2014, 2011, and 2009. No part of this publication may be reproduced or distributed in any form or
by any means, or stored in a database or retrieval system, without the prior written consent of
McGraw-Hill Education, including, but not limited to, in any network or other electronic storage or
transmission, or broadcast for distance learning.

Some ancillaries, including electronic and print components, may not be available to customers outside the
United States.

This book is printed on acid-free paper.

1 2 3 4 5 6 7 8 9 LWI 24 23 22 21 20

ISBN 978-1-260-24591-2 (bound edition)
MHID 1-260-24591-8 (bound edition)
ISBN 978-1-260-42571-0 (loose-leaf edition)
MHID 1-260-42571-1 (loose-leaf edition)

Senior Portfolio Manager: *Ryan Treat*
Product Development Manager: *Dawn Groundwater*
Marketing Manager: *Olivia Kaiser, AJ Laferrera*
Content Project Managers: *Mary E. Powers* (Core), *Jodi Banowetz* (Assessment)
Buyer: *Sandy Ludovissy*
Design: *David W. Hash*
Content Licensing Specialist: *Carrie Burger*
Cover Image: *Chinnapong/Shutterstock*
Compositor: *Aptara®, Inc.*

All credits appearing on page or at the end of the book are considered to be an extension of the copyright
page.

Library of Congress Cataloging-in-Publication Data

Names: Santrock, John W., author. | Deater-Deckard, Kirby D., author. |
    Lansford, Jennifer E., author.
Title: Child development / John W. Santrock, Kirby Deater-Deckard, Jennifer
    E. Lansford.
Description: Fifteenth edition. | New York, NY : McGraw-Hill Education,
    [2021] | Includes bibliographical references and index.
Identifiers: LCCN 2019033986 (print) | LCCN 2019033987 (ebook) |
    ISBN 9781260245912 (hardcover) | ISBN 9781260425710 (spiral bound) |
    ISBN 9781260425741 (ebook) | ISBN 9781260425772 (ebook other)
Subjects: LCSH: Child development. | Child psychology.
Classification: LCC RJ131 .S264 2021 (print) | LCC RJ131 (ebook) | DDC
    618.92/89—dc23
LC record available at https://lccn.loc.gov/2019033986
LC ebook record available at https://lccn.loc.gov/2019033987

The Internet addresses listed in the text were accurate at the time of publication. The inclusion of a website
does not indicate an endorsement by the authors or McGraw-Hill Education, and McGraw-Hill Education
does not guarantee the accuracy of the information presented at these sites.

mheducation.com/highered

Dedication

*With special appreciation to my mother,
Ruth Santrock, and my father, John Santrock.*

—John W. Santrock

*I am dedicating this edition to all of the wonderful
"kids" in my family who continue to teach me about human
development—my daughters Anna and Elly, eleven nieces
and nephews, and two great-nieces.*

—Kirby Deater-Deckard

*I gratefully acknowledge my parents, David and Maxine Kuehn,
my husband, Chris Lansford, and our children, Katherine and Nick,
who have guided my development and given me insights into theirs.*

—Jennifer E. Lansford

brief contents

contents

SECTION 1   THE NATURE OF CHILD DEVELOPMENT   1

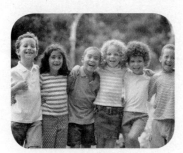

Ariel Skelley/Blend Images LLC

SECTION 2   BIOLOGICAL PROCESSES, PHYSICAL DEVELOPMENT, AND PERCEPTUAL DEVELOPMENT   42

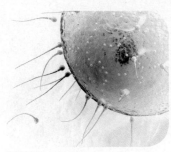

MedicalRF.com/Getty Images

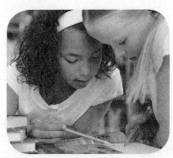

SECTION 4   SOCIOEMOTIONAL DEVELOPMENT   270

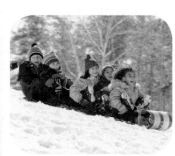

Ariel Skelley/Blend Images/Getty Images

SECTION 5   SOCIAL CONTEXTS OF DEVELOPMENT   379

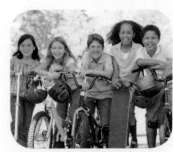

Monkey Business Images/Getty Images

Mc Graw Hill connect McGraw-Hill Education Psychology APA Documentation Style Guide

about the authors

John W. Santrock

John Santrock received his Ph.D. from the University of Minnesota in 1973. He taught at the University of Charleston and the University of Georgia before joining the program in Psychology in the School of Behavioral and Brain Sciences at the University of Texas at Dallas, where he currently teaches a number of undergraduate courses and has received the University's Effective Teaching Award.

John has been a member of the editorial boards of *Child Development* and *Developmental Psychology*. His research on father custody is widely cited and used in expert witness testimony to promote flexibility and alternative considerations in custody disputes. He also has conducted research on children's self-control. John has authored these exceptional McGraw-Hill texts: *Psychology* (7th edition), *Children* (14th edition), *Adolescence* (17th edition), *Life-Span Development* (17th edition), *A Topical Approach to Life-Span Development* (10th edition), and *Educational Psychology* (6th edition).

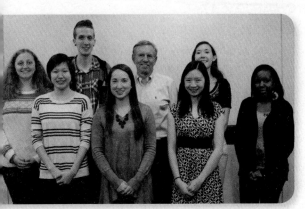

John Santrock (back row middle) with recipients of the Santrock Travel Scholarship Award in developmental psychology. Created by Dr. Santrock, this annual award provides undergraduate students with the opportunity to attend a professional meeting. A number of the students shown here attended the meeting of the Society for Research in Child Development.
Courtesy of Joanna Kain Gentsch, Ph.D.

For many years, John was involved in tennis as a player, teaching professional, and a coach of professional tennis players. As an undergraduate, he was a member of the University of Miami (FL) tennis team that still holds the record for most consecutive wins (137) in any NCAA Division I sport. John has been married for four decades to his wife, Mary Jo, who created and directed the first middle school program for children with learning disabilities and behavioral disorders in the Clarke County Schools in Athens, Georgia, when she was a professor at the University of Georgia. More recently, Mary Jo has worked as a Realtor. He has two daughters—Tracy and Jennifer—both of whom are Realtors after long careers in technology marketing and medical sales, respectively. In 2016, Jennifer became only the fifth female to have been inducted into the SMU Sports Hall of Fame. He has one granddaughter, Jordan, age 25, who completed her master's degree from the Cox School of Business at SMU and currently works for Ernst & Young, and two grandsons—the Belluci brothers: Alex, age 14, and Luke, age 13. In the last decade, John also has spent time painting expressionist art.

Kirby Deater-Deckard

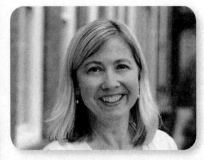

Courtesy of Michael McDermott

Kirby Deater-Deckard is a Professor in the Department of Psychological and Brain Sciences at the University of Massachusetts Amherst, where he serves as graduate program leader in developmental science, and neuroscience and behavior. He also is a Fellow of the Association for Psychological Science and director of the Healthy Development Initiative in Springfield, Massachusetts. He earned his Ph.D. in Developmental Psychology from the University of Virginia in 1994. Dr. Deater-Deckard has authored more than 200 publications that focus on the biological and environmental influences in the development of individual differences in social-emotional and cognitive outcomes in childhood and adolescence. The emphasis of his recent work is on parenting and inter-generational transmission of self-regulation (e.g., executive function, emotion regulation) that uses behavioral, cognitive neuroscience, and genetic research methods. He is principal or co-investigator on several longitudinal studies funded by the National Institutes of Health and the US-Israel Binational Science Foundation. Dr. Deater-Deckard serves as a consulting investigator on several longitudinal research project teams around the globe and is a scientific review panelist for the Institute of Education Sciences (US Department of Education). He is co-editor of the book series, *Frontiers in Developmental Science* (Taylor & Francis), and serves on editorial boards for journals in developmental and family sciences. Dr. Deater-Deckard's wife, Keirsten, is a community volunteer, and they have two daughters, Anna, age 22, and Elly, age 15.

Jennifer E. Lansford

Courtesy of Erika Hanzely-Layko

Jennifer E. Lansford is a Research Professor at the Sanford School of Public Policy and Faculty Fellow of the Center for Child and Family Policy at Duke University. She earned her Ph.D. in Developmental Psychology from the University of Michigan in 2000. Dr. Lansford has authored more than 200 publications that focus on the development of aggression and other behavior problems during childhood and adolescence, with particular attention to how parent, peer, and cultural factors contribute to or protect against these problems. Dr. Lansford leads the Parenting Across Cultures Project, a longitudinal study of mothers, fathers, and children from nine countries (China, Colombia, Italy, Jordan, Kenya, Philippines, Sweden, Thailand, and the United States). In addition, Dr. Lansford has consulted for UNICEF on the evaluation of parenting programs in several low- and middle-income countries and on the development of a set of international standards for parenting programs. She serves in editorial roles on several academic journals and has served in a number of national and international leadership roles, including chairing the U.S. National Institutes of Health Psychosocial Development, Risk and Prevention Study Section; chairing the U.S. National Committee for Psychological Science of the National Academies of Sciences, Engineering, and Medicine; chairing the Society for Research in Child Development International Affairs Committee; and serving on the Secretariat of the International Consortium for Developmental Science Societies. Dr. Lansford's husband, Chris, is a surgeon who specializes in head and neck cancer. They have two children: Katherine, age 16, and Nick, age 13.

expert consultants

Child development has become an enormous, complex field, and no single author, or even several authors, can possibly keep up with all of the rapidly changing content in the many different areas of child development. To solve this problem, the authors have sought the input of leading experts about content in a number of areas of child development. The experts provided detailed evaluations and recommendations in their area(s) of expertise.

The following individuals are among those who served as expert consultants for one or more of the previous editions of this text:

Celia Brownell	Susan Harter	Catherine McBride
Steven Ceci	Nancy Hazen	David Moore
Dante Cicchetti	Diane Hughes	Herb Pick
Cynthia Garcia Coll	Scott Johnson	Carolyn Saarni
W. Andrew Collins	Rachel Keen	Dale Schunk
John Colombo	Claire Kopp	Robert Siegler
Tiffany Field	Deanna Kuhn	Janet Spence
Mary Gauvain	Jeffrey Lachman	Robert J. Sternberg
Hill Goldsmith	Debbie Laible	Ross Thompson
Joan Grusec	Michael Lamb	Lawrence Walker
Daniel Hart	Michael Lewis	

Following are the biographies of the expert consultants for the fifteenth edition of this text, who (like the expert consultants for the previous editions) literally represent a Who's Who *in the field of child development.*

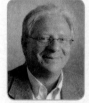

Courtesy of John Colombo

John Colombo   John Colombo is a leading expert on cognitive development during infancy and early childhood. He obtained his Ph.D. in Psychology at the State University of New York at Buffalo, and held faculty positions at Canisius College, Niagara University, and Youngstown State University before moving to the University of Kansas in the early 1980s. He is currently a Professor of Psychology and Director of the Schiefelbusch Institute for Life Span Studies at the University of Kansas. His research interests focus on the developmental cognitive neuroscience of attention and learning, with a special focus on early individual differences in these areas and how they relate to the typical and atypical development of cognitive and intellectual functioning. Dr. Colombo is the author/editor of six books, more than 115 peer-reviewed articles, and over 20 book chapters. He has also served on numerous editorial boards for journals in developmental psychology, including two terms as an associate editor for *Child Development*, and editor of the journal *Infancy.*

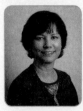

Courtesy of Rina Eiden

Rina Eiden   Rina D. Eiden is a leading expert on the development of children of substance-using parents. She obtained her Ph.D. from the University of Maryland and is currently Senior Research Scientist in the Department of Psychology, University at Buffalo, State University of New York. Her studies, many of which follow cohorts of children across multiple years, seek to understand the developmental mechanisms, such as infant-parent attachment, self-regulation, and individual differences in children's autonomic and stress reactivity, which explain the association between parental risk factors and children's developmental outcomes. Her work also examines the developmental processes in children that promote resilience in the face of risk; implications of these issues for early intervention or prevention programs for at-risk children; and preventive interventions with substance-using parents. She has been an Associate Editor of *Psychology of Addictive Behaviors* and on the editorial boards of several major developmental and addiction journals. She is a Division 50 Fellow of the American Psychological Association. Dr. Eiden's work has been published in leading research journals such as *Child Development, Developmental Psychology, Developmental Psychobiology, Psychology of Addictive Behaviors, Nicotine and Tobacco Research,* and *Neurotoxicology and Teratology.*

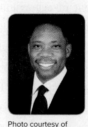

Photo courtesy of Lauren H. Adams

James Graham   James A. Graham is a leading expert on the community aspects of ethnicity, culture, and development. He obtained his undergraduate degree from Miami University and received masters and doctoral degrees in developmental psychology from the University of Memphis. Dr. Graham's current position is Professor of Psychology, The College of New Jersey (TCNJ). His research addresses the social-cognitive aspects of relationships between group and dyadic levels across developmental periods in community-based settings. Three interdependent dimensions of his research program examine (1) populations that are typically understudied, conceptually limited, and methodologically constrained; (2) development of empathy and prosocial behavior with peer groups and friends; and (3) developmental science in the context of community-engaged research partnerships. Currently, he is Coordinator of the Developmental Specialization in Psychology at TCNJ. For a decade, Dr. Graham taught graduate courses in psychology and education in Johannesburg, South Africa, through TCNJ's

Graduate Summer Global Program. He is the co-author of *The African American Child: Development and Challenges* (2nd ed.) and *Children of Incarcerated Parents: Theoretical, Developmental, and Clinical Issues.* Dr. Graham has presented his work at a variety of international and national conferences and has published articles in a wide range of journals, including *Social Development, Child Study Journal, Behavior Modification, Journal of Multicultural Counseling and Development,* and *American Journal of Evaluation.*

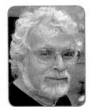

Courtesy of Stacey Napoli

Michael Lewis

Michael Lewis is widely recognized as one of the world's leading experts on children's socioemotional development. He currently is University Distinguished Professor of Pediatrics and Psychiatry, and Director of the Institute for the Study of Child Development, at Rutgers Robert Wood Johnson Medical School. Dr. Lewis also is Professor of Psychology, Education, Biomedical Engineering, and Social Work at Rutgers University, and serves on the Executive Committee of the Cognitive Science Center. He has written and edited more than 35 books including *Social Cognition and the Acquisition of Self* (1979), *Children's Emotions and Moods* (1983), *Handbook of Emotions* (1993, 2000, 2008, 2016), which was awarded the 1995 Choice Magazine's Outstanding Academic Book Award, *Shame, The Exposed Self* (1992), and *Altering Fate: Why The Past Does Not Predict The Future* (1997), which was a finalist for the 1998 Eleanor Maccoby Book Award. Dr. Lewis also edited *The Cambridge Handbook of Environment in Human Development* (2012), *Gender Differences in Prenatal Substance Exposure* (2012), and the third edition of the *Handbook of Developmental Psychopathology* (2014). His most recent book, *The Rise of Consciousness and the Development of Emotional Life* (Guilford Press, 2014), won the William James Book Award from the American Psychological Association. In addition, Dr. Lewis has had more than 350 articles and chapters published in professional journals and scholarly texts. Among his honors, Dr. Lewis is a Fellow of the New York Academy of Sciences, American Psychological Association, and the American Association of the Advancement of Science, as well as the Japan Society for the Promotion of Science. Dr. Lewis received the 2009 Urie Bronfenbrenner Award for Lifetime Contribution to Developmental Psychology in the Service of Science and Society from the American Psychological Association, as well as the 2012 Hedi Levenback Pioneer Award from The New York Zero-to-Three Network. The Society for Research in Child Development awarded him the 2013 Distinguished Scientific Contributions to Child Development award, in recognition of Professor Lewis's lifetime contribution to the scientific body of knowledge and understanding of children's development. In 2018, the International Congress of Infant Studies (ICIS) awarded Dr. Lewis an inaugural Distinguished Contribution Award.

Courtesy of Craig T. Salling

Virginia Marchman

Virginia Marchman is a leading expert on children's language development. She currently is a Research Associate at the Stanford University Language Learning Laboratory. Dr. Marchman obtained her Ph.D. at the University of California–Berkeley. Her main research areas are language development, language disorders, and early childhood development. Dr. Marchman's specific interests focus on individual differences in typically-developing and late-talking children, as well as lexical and grammatical development in monolingual and bilingual learners. Her studies have incorporated a variety of experimental methods as well as computational approaches and naturalistic observation. Dr. Marchman has worked extensively with the MacArthur-Bates Communicative Development Inventories (CDI), developing the CDI Scoring program and serving on the MacArthur-Bates CDI Advisory Board. She has been a consulting editor for *Journal of Speech, Language, and Hearing Research,* and *Child Development.* Dr. Marchman's most recent work involves the development of real-time spoken language understanding using the "looking-while-listening" task in typically-developing and at-risk children. Current studies explore links between children's language processing skill, early learning environments, and individual differences in monolingual and bilingual English-Spanish learners from diverse backgrounds.

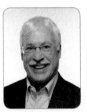

Courtesy of Karl Rosengren

Karl Rosengren

Karl S. Rosengren is an expert on children's cognitive and motor development. He obtained his Ph.D. from the Institute of Child Development at the University of Minnesota. He is currently a professor in the Brain and Cognitive Sciences Department and the Clinical and Social Sciences in Psychology at the University of Rochester, having previously been a professor at the University of Wisconsin-Madison, the University of Michigan, the University of Illinois at Urbana-Champaign, and Northwestern University. In the area of cognitive development, his research focuses on how children learn about events in the world and how they separate fantasy from reality. His most recent work in this area has focused on children's understanding of death and how parents in the United States and Mexico socialize children with respect to death. In the area of motor development, his research has focused on the development of balance and gait, as well as the development of children's drawing. Dr. Rosengren is a Fellow of the Association for Psychological Science. He has edited two books and is a co-author of a research methods textbook. Dr. Rosengren has published over 100 research articles and his work has been published in leading research journals, such as *Child Development, Psychological Science,* and *Science.*

Connecting *Research* and *Results*

Child Development connects current research and real-world applications. Through an integrated, personalized digital learning program, students gain the insight they need to study smarter and improve performance.

McGraw-Hill Education's **Connect** is a digital assignment and assessment platform that strengthens the link between faculty, students, and course work, helping everyone accomplish more in less time. *Connect for Child Development* includes assignable and assessable videos, quizzes, exercises, and interactivities, all associated with learning objectives. Interactive assignments and videos allow students to experience and apply their understanding of psychology to the world with fun and stimulating activities.

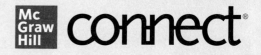

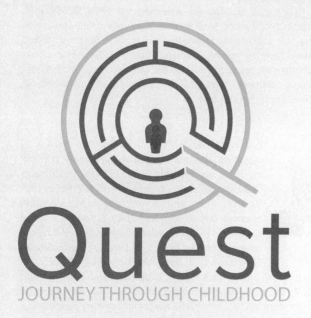

Apply Concepts and Theory in an Experiential Learning Environment

An engaging and innovative learning game, **Quest: Journey through Childhood** provides students with opportunities to apply content from their human development curriculum to real-life scenarios. Students play unique characters who range in age and make decisions that apply key concepts and theories for each age as they negotiate events in an array of authentic environments. Additionally, as students analyze real-world behaviors and contexts, they are exposed to different cultures and intersecting biological, cognitive, and socioemotional processes. Each quest has layered replayability, allowing students to make new choices each time they play–or offering different students in the same class different experiences. Fresh possibilities and outcomes shine light on the complexity of and variations in real human development. This new experiential learning game includes follow-up questions, assignable in Connect and auto-graded, to reach a higher level of critical thinking.

Real People, Real World, Real Life

At the higher end of Bloom's taxonomy (analyze, evaluate, create), the McGraw-Hill Education **Milestones** video series is an observational tool that allows students to experience life as it unfolds, from infancy to emerging adulthood. This ground-breaking, longitudinal video series tracks the development of real children as they progress through the early stages of physical, social, and emotional development in their first few weeks, months, and years of life. Assignable and assessable within Connect for Child Development, Milestones also includes interviews with adolescents and adults to reflect development throughout the entire life span.

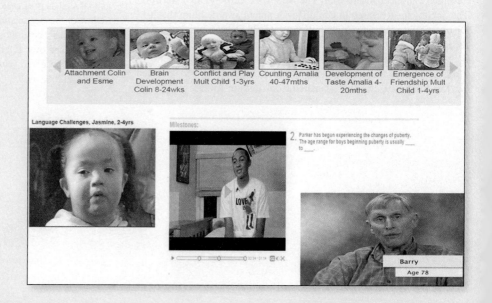

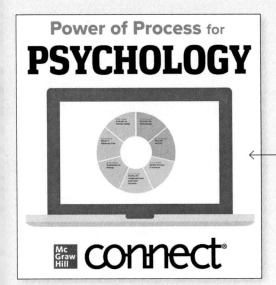

Power of Process for PSYCHOLOGY

Mc Graw Hill **connect**®

Prepare Students for Higher-Level Thinking

Also at the higher end of Bloom's taxonomy, **Power of Process** for Psychology helps students improve critical thinking skills and allows instructors to assess these skills efficiently and effectively in an online environment. Available through Connect, pre-loaded journal articles are available for instructors to assign. Using a scaffolded framework such as understanding, synthesizing, and analyzing, Power of Process moves students toward higher-level thinking and analysis.

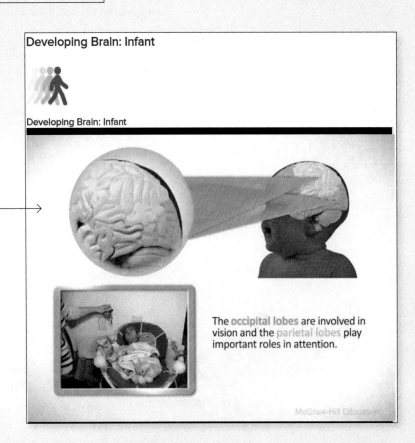

Developing Brain: Infant

Developing Brain: Infant

The occipital lobes are involved in vision and the parietal lobes play important roles in attention.

McGraw-Hill Education

Inform and Engage on Psychological Concepts

At the lower end of Bloom's taxonomy, students are introduced to **Concept Clips**—the dynamic, colorful graphics and stimulating animations that break down some of psychology's most difficult concepts in a step-by-step manner, engaging students and aiding in retention. They are assignable and assessable in Connect or can be used as a jumping-off point in class. Accompanied by audio narration, Concept Clips cover topics such as object permanence and conservation, as well as theories and theorists like Bandura's social cognitive theory, Vygotsky's sociocultural theory, Buss's evolutionary theory, and Kuhl's language development theory.

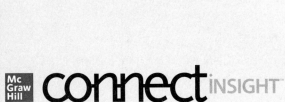

Mc Graw Hill **connect**INSIGHT™

Powerful Reporting

Whether a class is face-to-face, hybrid, or entirely online, Connect for Child Development provides tools and analytics to reduce the amount of time instructors need to administer their courses. Easy-to-use course management tools allow instructors to spend less time administering and more time teaching, while easy-to-use reporting features allow students to monitor their progress and optimize their study time.

- **Connect Insight** is a one-of-a-kind visual analytics dashboard—available for both instructors and students—that provides at-a-glance information regarding student performance.

- The **At-Risk Student Report** provides instructors with one-click access to a dashboard that identifies students who are at risk of dropping out of the course due to low engagement levels.

- The **Category Analysis Report** details student performance relative to specific learning objectives and goals, including APA outcomes and levels of Bloom's taxonomy.

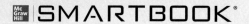
SMARTBOOK®

Better Data, Smarter Revision, Improved Results

McGraw-Hill Education's **SmartBook** helps students distinguish the concepts they know from the concepts they don't, while pinpointing the concepts they are about to forget. SmartBook's real-time reports help both students and instructors identify the concepts that require more attention, making study sessions and class time more efficient.

SmartBook is optimized for mobile and tablet use and is accessible for students with disabilities. Content-wise, measurable and observable learning objectives help improve student outcomes. SmartBook personalizes learning to individual student needs, continually adapting to pinpoint knowledge gaps and focus learning on topics that need the most attention. Study time is more productive and, as a result, students are better prepared for class and coursework. For instructors, SmartBook tracks student progress and provides insights that can help guide teaching strategies.

Online Instructor Resources

The resources listed here accompany *Child Development*, Fifteenth Edition. Please contact your McGraw-Hill representative for details concerning the availability of these and other valuable materials that can help you design and enhance your course.

Instructor's Manual   Broken down by chapter, this resource provides chapter outlines, suggested lecture topics, classroom activities and demonstrations, suggested student research projects, essay questions, and critical thinking questions.

Test Bank and Computerized Test Bank   This comprehensive Test Bank includes more than 1,500 multiple-choice and approximately 75 essay questions. Organized by chapter, the questions are designed to test factual, applied, and conceptual understanding.

Test Builder   New to this edition and available within Connect, Test Builder is a cloud-based tool that enables instructors to format tests that can be printed or administered within a Learning Management System. Test Builder offers a modern, streamlined interface for easy content configuration that matches course needs, without requiring a download. Test Builder enables instructors to:

*   Access all Test Bank content from a particular title
*   Easily pinpoint the most relevant content through robust filtering options
*   Manipulate the order of questions or scramble questions and/or answers
*   Pin questions to a specific location within a test
*   Determine your preferred treatment of algorithmic questions
*   Choose the layout and spacing
*   Add instructions and configure default settings

PowerPoint Slides   The PowerPoint presentations, now WCAG compliant, highlight the key points of the chapter and include supporting visuals. All of the slides can be modified to meet individual needs.

preface

Making Connections . . . From the Classroom to *Child Development* to You

The material in *Child Development* has been shaped by thousands of students taking countless undergraduate developmental courses across four decades. These students have consistently said that when instructors highlight the connections among the different aspects of children's development, they can more readily understand the concepts, theories, and research presented in the course. As a result, *Child Development* has focused on providing a systematic, integrative approach that helps students make these connections in their learning and practice. This new edition continues that philosophy with the addition of Dr. Kirby Deater-Deckard of the University of Massachusetts Amherst and Dr. Jennifer Lansford of Duke University to the author team, who are recognized as leading researchers and educators in the field and have served as Expert Consultants for many editions of this successful Life-Span franchise. This combined experience has influenced the main goals for the text, as follows:

1. **Connecting with today's students** Helping students learn about child development more effectively

2. **Connecting research to what we know about children's development** Providing students with the best and most recent *theory and research* in the world today about each of the periods of child development

3. **Connecting topical and developmental processes** Guiding students in making *developmental connections* across different points in child development

4. **Connecting development to real life** Helping students understand ways to *apply* content about child development to the real world and improve people's lives, and to motivate students to think deeply about *their own personal journey through life* and better understand who they were, are, and will be

Connecting with Today's Students

Development courses are challenging because of the amount of material often covered. To help today's students focus on the key ideas, the Learning Goals system in *Child Development* provides extensive learning connections throughout the chapters. The learning system connects the chapter-opening outline, learning goals for the chapter, mini-chapter maps that open each main section of the chapter, *Review, Connect, and Reflect* at the end of each main section, and the chapter summary at the end of each chapter.

The learning system keeps the key ideas in front of the student from the beginning to the end of the chapter. The main headings of each chapter correspond to the learning goals, which are presented in the chapter-opening spread. Mini-chapter maps that link up with the learning goals are presented at the beginning of each major section in the chapter.

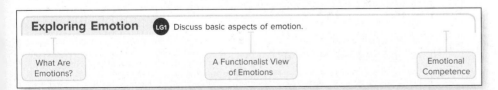

Then, at the end of each main section of a chapter, the learning goal is repeated in *Review, Connect, and Reflect,* which prompts students to review the key topics in the section, connect these topics to existing knowledge, and relate what they learned to their own personal journey through life. *Reach Your Learning Goals,* at the end of the chapter, guides students through the bulleted chapter review, connecting with the chapter outline/learning goals at the beginning of the chapter and the *Review, Connect, and Reflect* material at the end of each major section.

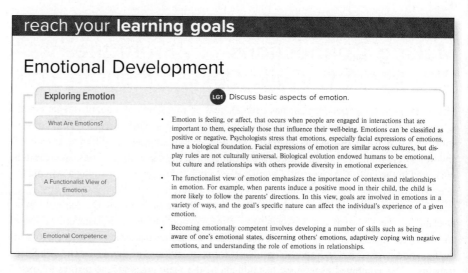

reach your **learning goals**

Emotional Development

Exploring Emotion	**LG1** Discuss basic aspects of emotion.
What Are Emotions?	• Emotion is feeling, or affect, that occurs when people are engaged in interactions that are important to them, especially those that influence their well-being. Emotions can be classified as positive or negative. Psychologists stress that emotions, especially facial expressions of emotions, have a biological foundation. Facial expressions of emotion are similar across cultures, but display rules are not culturally universal. Biological evolution endowed humans to be emotional, but culture and relationships with others provide diversity in emotional experiences.
A Functionalist View of Emotions	• The functionalist view of emotion emphasizes the importance of contexts and relationships in emotion. For example, when parents induce a positive mood in their child, the child is more likely to follow the parents' directions. In this view, goals are involved in emotions in a variety of ways, and the goal's specific nature can affect the individual's experience of a given emotion.
Emotional Competence	• Becoming emotionally competent involves developing a number of skills such as being aware of one's emotional states, discerning others' emotions, adaptively coping with negative emotions, and understanding the role of emotions in relationships.

Connecting Research to What We Know About Children's Development

It is critical to include the most up-to-date research available. As with previous editions, we continue to look closely at specific areas of research, involve experts in related fields, and update research throughout. **Connecting Through Research** describes a study or program to illustrate how research in child development is conducted and how it influences

connecting through research

How Does Theory of Mind Differ in Children with Autism?

Approximately 1 in 59 children is estimated to have some sort of autism spectrum disorder (National Autism Association, 2019). Autism can usually be diagnosed by the age of 3 years, and sometimes earlier. Children with autism show a number of behaviors different from typically developing children their age, including deficits in social interaction and communication as well as repetitive behaviors or interests. They often show indifference toward others, in many instances preferring to be alone and showing more interest in objects than people. It now is accepted that autism is linked to genetic and brain abnormalities (Tremblay & Jiang, 2019). Children and adults with autism have difficulty in social interactions. These deficits are generally greater than deficits in children the same mental age with intellectual disability (Greenberg & others, 2018). Researchers have found that children with autism have difficulty in developing a theory of mind, especially in understanding others' beliefs and emotions (Fletcher-Watson & Happé, 2019). Although children with autism tend to do poorly when reasoning on false-belief tasks, they can perform much better on reasoning tasks requiring an understanding of physical causality. Individuals with autism might have difficulty in understanding others' beliefs and emotions not solely because of theory of mind deficits but also due to other aspects of cognition such as problems in focusing attention, eye gaze, face recognition, memory, language impairment, or some general intellectual impairment (Boucher, 2017).

In relation to theory of mind, however, it is important to consider the effects of individual variations in the abilities of children with autism. Children with autism are not a homogeneous group, and some have less severe social and communication problems than others. Thus, it is not surprising that children who have less severe forms of autism do better than those who have more severe forms of the disorder on some theory of mind tasks (Jones & others, 2018). A further important consideration in

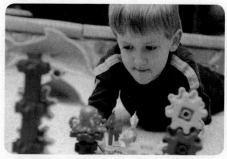

A young boy with autism. *What are some characteristics of children who are autistic? What are some deficits in their theory of mind?*
Robin Nelson/PhotoEdit

thinking about autism and theory of mind is that children with autism might have difficulty in understanding others' beliefs and emotions not solely due to theory of mind deficits but to other aspects of cognition such as problems in focusing attention or some general intellectual impairment. For instance, weaknesses in executive function may be related to the problems experienced by those with autism in performing theory of mind tasks. Other theories have pointed out that typically developing individuals process information by extracting the big picture, whereas those with autism process information in a very detailed, almost obsessive way. It may be that in autism, a number of different but related deficits lead to social cognitive deficits (Moseley & Pulvermueller, 2018; Rajendran & Mitchell, 2007).

our understanding of the discipline. Topics range from "Do Children Conceived Through In Vitro Fertilization Show Significantly Different Outcomes in Childhood and Adolescence?" to "How Can We Study Newborns' Perception?" to "What Are the Perspective Taking and Moral Motivation of Bullies, Bully-Victims, Victims, and Prosocial Children?".

The tradition of obtaining detailed, extensive input from leading experts in different areas of child development also continues in this edition. Biographies and photographs of the leading experts in the field of child development appear on pages xvi–xvii. Finally, the research discussions have been updated in every period and topic in order to keep *Child Development* as current as possible. To that end, there are more than 1,300 citations from 2017, 2018, and 2019 in this new edition.

Connecting Topical and Developmental Processes

Too often we forget or fail to notice the many connections from one point in child development to another. Thus, several features have been designed to help students connect topics across the processes and periods of child development:

1. *Developmental Connections,* which appears multiple times in the margins of each chapter, points students to where the topic is discussed in a previous, current, or subsequent chapter. This feature highlights links across development *and* connections among biological, cognitive, and socioemotional processes. The key developmental processes are typically discussed in isolation from each other, and so students often fail to see their connections. Included in *Developmental Connections* is a brief description of the backward or forward connection.

2. A *Connect* question appears in self-reviews—*Review, Connect, and Reflect*—at the end of each main section in a chapter so students can practice making connections among topics.

Connecting Development to Real Life

In addition to helping students make research and developmental connections, *Child Development* shows the important connections among the concepts discussed and the real world. Real-life connections are explicitly made in the chapter-opening vignette, in *Caring Connections, Connecting with Diversity,* and *Connecting with Careers.*

Each chapter begins with a story designed to increase students' interest and motivation to read the chapter. *Caring Connections* provides applied information about parenting, education, or health and well-being in relation to topics ranging from "From Waterbirth to Music Therapy" to "Parents, Coaches, and Children's Sports" to "Guiding Children's Creativity."

developmental **connection**

Nature and Nurture

In the epigenetic view, development is an ongoing, bidirectional interchange between heredity and the environment. Connect to "Biological Beginnings."

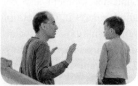
Child Development puts a strong emphasis on diversity. For a number of editions, this text has benefited from the involvement of one or more leading experts on diversity to ensure that it provides students with current, accurate, sensitive information related to diversity in children's development.

Although diversity is discussed throughout this edition, the chapter "Culture and Diversity" includes extensive material on the subject with substantial research updates. Further, a feature called **Connecting with Diversity** appears throughout the text, focusing on a diversity topic related to the material at that point in the chapter. Topics range from "The Increased Diversity of Adopted Children and Adoptive Parents" to "Cultural Variations in Guiding Infants' Motor Development" to "The Contexts of Ethnic Identity Development."

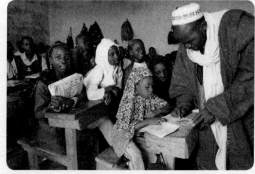

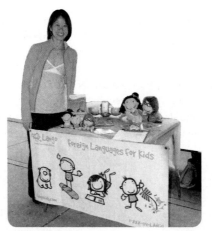
Connecting with Careers profiles careers ranging from genetic counselor to toy designer to supervisor of gifted and talented education, all of which require knowledge of child development. The careers highlighted extend from the Careers Appendix, which provides a comprehensive overview of careers to show students where knowledge of child development could lead them.

Finally, part of applying knowledge of child development to the real world is understanding its impact on oneself. Students should be motivated to think deeply about their own journey through life. *Reflect: Your Own Personal Journey of Life* prompts in the end-of-section review ask students to reflect on some aspect of the discussion in the section they have just read and connect it to their own life. For example, related to a discussion of the early-later experience issue in development, students are asked,

Can you identify an early experience that you believe contributed in important ways to your development?

Can you identify a recent or current (later) experience that you think had (is having) a strong influence on your development?

Content Revisions

A significant reason that *Child Development* has been successfully used by instructors for edition after edition is the painstaking effort and review that goes into making sure the text provides the latest research on all topic areas discussed in the classroom. This new edition is no exception, with more than 1,300 citations from 2017, 2018, and 2019.

New research and content that has especially been updated and expanded in this new edition focus on the following topics: cultural factors, including expanded coverage of international research; biological factors and their interaction with environments and experiences (e.g., genetics, brain functioning); gender similarities and differences, including gender identity; digital technology (e.g., Internet, social media, and screen time); and family socioeconomic and demographic factors (e.g., poverty rates, family structures). Following is a sample of the many chapter-by-chapter changes that were made in this new edition of *Child Development*.

Chapter 1: Introduction

- New and updated "Connecting with Careers" boxes highlighting the child and adolescent clinical psychology work of Dr. Gustavo Medrano, and research and administration work on gender and women's development by Dr. Pam Reid
- Expanded and updated consideration of major topics and controversies in child development research and policy
- Updated definitions and descriptions of sociocultural factors in children's lives that affect their development (such as family socioeconomic status, gender, and race/ethnicity) (Craig, Rucker, & Richeson, 2018; Desmet, Ortuño-Ortin, & Wacziarg, 2017)
- New theory and research studies addressing children's and families' resilience in the face of chronic and acute stressors (Masten & Cicchetti, 2016)
- Up-to-date and expanded consideration of the data on poverty rates for children in multiple countries (OECD, 2018; US Census Bureau, 2017)
- Updates on research addressing periods of development (e.g., childhood, adolescence) and cohort effects, including consideration of distinct features of the "Millennials Generation" (Bornstein, 2018; Frey, 2018)
- Contemporary framing of "Nature" and "Nurture" as co-contributing and interacting factors in child development
- Updated treatment of the major theoretical foundations in children's social-emotional and cognitive development (Bandura, 2018; Hayes & others, 2017; Veraksa & Sheridan, 2018)
- Recent research describing advanced brain-imaging techniques using functional magnetic resonance imaging and other physiological methods (Li & others, 2019)
- Up-to-date sources and information on diversity of children and adolescents in the United States (US Census Bureau, 2017; Yip, 2018)

Chapter 2: Biological Beginnings

- New anthropological research from current hunter-gatherer societies, such as the Hadza in Tanzania, suggesting that mothers' and grandmothers' foraging supplies the large majority of families' caloric intake (Hawkes, 2017), which has implications for understanding why social orientation and cooperation are so central to our species

- Updated estimates that humans have approximately 43,000 genes (Pertea & others, 2018)
- Updated prevalence rates for chromosomal and gene-linked abnormalities
- New statistics on the percentage of births in the United States resulting from in vitro fertilization
- Research showing that twins born through in vitro fertilization, compared to twins born through natural conception, are at slightly higher risk of low birth weight, prematurity, and adverse neonatal outcomes suggesting that additional prenatal care and attention following birth may be needed for twins born through assisted reproductive technology (Wang & others, 2018)
- A longitudinal study to compare children conceived through assisted reproductive technologies with demographically-matched, spontaneously-conceived children, finding no significant differences in mental health problems through age 18 (Klausen & others, 2017)
- Updated descriptions of cross-ethnic adoptions
- A review of studies of children living in orphanages in the Russian Federation compared to children adopted within the Russian Federation or in the United States to compare outcomes of children adopted at different ages and describe an intervention that focused on improving caregiver-child interactions in orphanages (McCall & others, 2018)
- New information on open versus closed adoptions and on adoptions by gay men and lesbian women (Brodzinsky & Goldberg, 2016)
- A new study showing that identical twins are more similar to one another on measures of conduct problems than are fraternal twins, suggesting the importance of heredity in conduct problems (Saunders & others, 2018)
- Longitudinal studies suggesting that earlier in development, parenting or other environmental effects are stronger than these effects are later in development (Lansford & others, 2018)
- Research suggesting the importance of child characteristics in eliciting particular types of environmental inputs (Hadd & Rodgers, 2017)
- Additional theories that characterize gene × environment interactions, including the diathesis-stress or dual-risk model and the biological sensitivity to context or differential susceptibility model

Chapter 3: Prenatal Development and Birth

- The latest information about the structure and function of the placenta and umbilical cord in prenatal development (Kallol & others, 2018; Sebastiani & others, 2018)

- Updated research on prenatal organogenesis with particular attention to neuronal, spine, and brain development (Arck & others, 2018; Hadders-Algra, 2018) and teratogen effects at specific stages of development (Chudley, 2017; Teratology Society, 2017)

- Up-to-date coverage of the effects of fetal exposure to alcohol and other legal substances such as prescription medications, nicotine, and caffeine (Campagne, 2018; Leviton, 2018; Nguyen & others, 2017)

- New research and theory about the short-term and long-term effects of fetal exposure to illicit drugs such as cocaine and methamphetamine (Kwiatkowski & others, 2018; Lowell & Mayes, 2019)

- Updated research on pregnant women's chronic infections and illnesses, including HIV infection and diabetes (Freemark, 2018; UNICEF, 2017), and maternal factors such as age, diet, and stress (Fedock & Alvarez, 2018; Taminga & others, 2018)

- Latest research on paternal environmental toxin exposure effects on the fetus through the sperm cells (Oldereid & others, 2018; L. Wang & others, 2018)

- Updated and expanded consideration of global efforts to improve and enhance prenatal care of mothers and their babies (Hetherington & others, 2018; Moller & others, 2017), and the latest outcomes of the prenatal intervention program CenteringPregnancy (Grant & others, 2018)

- Up-to-date statistics and information about the use of midwives and doulas in labor and delivery (McLeish & Redshaw, 2018; Weisband & others, 2018)

- Updated research and practice guidelines for childbirth methods for improving infant health and reducing pain and injury to the mother and baby (Capogna & others, 2018; Charles, 2018; Martin & others, 2018)

- The latest research and benchmark information for the APGAR, NBAS, and NNNS newborn assessment tools for determining newborn health and functioning levels at birth (Ojodu & others, 2017; Provenzi & others, 2018)

- Updated information about the rates of preterm and low birth weight births in multiple diverse countries (OECD, 2018), and the short-term and long-term effects of these risk factors (Boghossian & others, 2018; Martin & others, 2018)

- Recent research on the mothers' postnatal period adjustment and functioning, including physical changes (e.g., sleep, energy) (Lillis & others, 2018) and mood shifts (e.g., depression) (Olin & others, 2017)

Chapter 4: Physical Development and Health

- Updated information on the height and weight of children around the world related to nutrition (UNICEF, 2018)

- Research on trajectories of body image for individuals' perceptions of their own appearance, weight, and attributions related to their bodies that are related to gender, identity, and psychological functioning (Nelson & others, 2018)

- A new study that compared children and young adults who had brain damage in the left hemisphere (where language functions are generally controlled) to children and young adults without brain damage, finding that in more than 80 percent of the individuals with damage to the left hemisphere of their brain, the right hemisphere dominated the language functions usually controlled by the left side of the brain (Chilosi & others, 2017)

- Research on how myelination is related to breast feeding and verbal and nonverbal cognitive abilities (Deoni & others, 2018)

- Studies of how brain structure and patterns of connectivity in the brain are associated with aggressive behavior (Saxbe & others, 2018)

- A study of how hippocampal volume and parental cultural socialization are both predictive of academic achievement and behavioral adjustment for Mexican-American adolescents (Qu & others, 2018)

- Research demonstrating that less disrupted infant sleep is predicted by mothers' emotional availability at bedtime as well as less household chaos, suggesting that better-regulated infant sleep is promoted by feelings of safety and security (Whitesell & others, 2018)

- Infant sleep problems have been related to a range of family difficulties, including marital conflict, and are reduced by sensitive caregiving from both mothers and fathers (El-Sheikh & Kelly, 2017)

- A study showing that infant sleep problems can be a source of marital discord, as mothers and fathers who disagree about how to respond to infants' nighttime wakings perceive themselves as having lower quality co-parenting relationships (Reader, Teti, & Cleveland, 2017)

- Updated data on prevalence and risk factors for sudden infant death syndrome (SIDS)

- Data showing that shorter sleep duration at age 12 predicted a greater likelihood of heavy alcohol use and marijuana use later in adolescence (Miller, Janssen, & Jackson, 2017)

- Studies showing that sleep problems in childhood predict subsequent problems with emotional regulation and attention, which in turn predict future sleep problems in a cycle that perpetuates over time (Williams & others, 2017)

- A review of research studies concluding that inadequate sleep during childhood is related to impairments in brain structures and functions (Dutil & others, 2018)

- A study in which Mexican-American adolescents completed nightly sleep diaries for two weeks at the age of 15 and then again about a year later, finding that the amount of sleep associated with the best mental health (in terms of less anxiety and depression and fewer behavior problems) was about one hour more than the amount of sleep associated with having the highest grades, suggesting complex trade-offs in different aspects of adjustment related to sleep (Fuligni & others, 2018)

- Recommendations from the American Academy of Sleep Medicine that school boards and educational institutions implement start times no earlier than 8:30 a.m. in middle and high schools because adolescents who attend schools with later start times get more sleep and have better school performance, better physical and mental health, and engage in less risky behavior, such as unsafe driving (Watson & others, 2017)
- Updated statistics from the Centers for Disease Control and Prevention regarding the leading causes of childhood deaths and childhood lead exposure
- Updates on other serious childhood health problems, including HIV/AIDS and cancer
- A national study of Americans indicating that by 6 months, 37% of infants were already consuming snacks and that by the age of 12 months, 25% of daily energy intake was from snacks (Deming & others, 2017)
- Data suggesting that infants and young children are consuming more junk food and fewer fruits and vegetables than recommended by nutrition experts; for example, 25% of 6- to 11-month-olds and 20% of 12- to 23-month-olds consumed no vegetables over the course of the study period in a national sample of Americans (Miles & Siega-Riz, 2017)
- Updated data on breast feeding and obesity
- Several studies in different countries demonstrating the benefits of nutrition supplements to physical growth and cognitive and psychosocial development (Ip & others, 2017)
- A study showing that preschool children's physical activity is enhanced by participating in sports and play with parents but that less than 1 percent of time that mothers and young children spend together is in moderate to vigorous physical activity (Dlugonski, DuBose, & Rider, 2017)
- Interventions finding that even brief interruptions in sedentary behavior (with 3 minutes of moderate-intensity walking every 30 minutes across 3 hours) improve glucose metabolism and are a promising strategy for reducing metabolic risk in overweight and obese children (Broadney & others, 2018)

Chapter 5: Motor, Sensory, and Perceptual Development

- Updated research and theory regarding "Dynamic Systems" viewpoints of motor, sensory, and perceptual development (Dineva & Schöner, 2018; Lee & others, 2018)
- Expansion of research regarding international and cross-cultural comparisons of motor, sensory, and perceptual development from infancy through early childhood, showing patterns of similarity as well as cultural differences in development and childrearing behaviors (Adolph, Hoch, & Cole, 2018; Ertem & others, 2018; Haga & others, 2018; Otsuka, 2017)
- Recent research on the developmental progression of infant reflexes and early brain development (Gieysztor & others, 2018)
- Up-to-date research on development of motor control of the head and trunk during early infancy, and subsequent upright walking (Adolph & Hoch, 2018; Hadders-Algra, 2018; Hallemans & others, 2018)
- Update of the research and theory on individual differences in motor skills in childhood and adolescence and links with physical fitness, athleticism, and health (Walton-Fisette & Wuest, 2018; Weedon & others, 2018)
- Latest research on fine motor development and progression of skills in infancy and early childhood, such as grasping, manipulating, and holding objects (Corbetta & others, 2018)
- Recent research and theory on the "Ecological Perspective" on perceptual development in infancy, including coverage of research methods for studying perceptual skills and development (Adolph & Hoch, 2018; Plumert, 2018)
- Update of research on key behaviors for visual attention that are used to measure sensation and perception development in infancy and toddlerhood, including preference, habituation/dishabituation, orienting, and eye tracking paradigms (Addabbo & others, 2018; Shultz, Klin, & Jones, 2018; Slone & others, 2018)
- Inclusion of recent theory and research reviews documenting that even very young infants' perception of the world is coherent, patterned, and informative, rather than chaotic and "all noise" (Maurer & Lewis, 2018; Vogelsang & others, 2018)
- Current understanding of newborns' and young infants' capacities to perceive and understand human faces from early in life, even before visual acuity has fully developed (Sugden & Marquis, 2017)
- Update of research demonstrating the rapid developmental emergence in infancy of perception of the constancy of physical properties of objects (Chen, Sperandio, & Goodale, 2018)
- Recent research and theory on young infants' (by 2 months) capacity to understand that an object remains whole and constant even when occluded by another object (Johnson, 2019)
- Up-to-date coverage of perceptual development beyond infancy into toddlerhood and early childhood, including depth perception and understanding of the physical properties of objects and the world, such as gravity (Johnson & Hannon, 2015; Palmquist, Keen, & Jaswal, 2018)
- Inclusion of the latest research using brain imaging of fetuses, showing how they sense and how their brains' process auditory information as early hearing capacity develops in the womb (Draganova & others, 2018)

- Update on developmental outcomes for children with serious chronic inner ear infections (Klopp-Dutote & others, 2018) and for deaf or hard-of-hearing infants and children who receive cochlear implants at various points in their development (Lavelli & others, 2018; Percy-Smith & others, 2018)

- The latest research on how fetuses learn and develop preferences for certain tastes in the womb, and on the developmental emergence of preference for salty tastes (Liem, 2017; Podzimek & others, 2018)

- Up-to-date theory and research evidence on the development of "Intermodal Perception"—how infants integrate information from various sensory sources in ways that help them better understand and learn about the world (Bahrick, Todd, & Soska, 2018; Bremner & Spence, 2017)

- Update of research on critical and sensitive periods in visual perception development based on studies of infants who have cataracts removed at different points in development (Maurer, 2017; Maurer & Lewis 2018)

Chapter 6: Cognitive Developmental Approaches

- An updated description of parameters that affect whether infants make A-not-B errors, such as when only the hands and arms rather than the full body of an experimenter are visible, 9-month-old infants are less likely to make A-not-B errors, suggesting that part of the error is due to infants' imitation of body movements (Boyer & others, 2017)

- A description of the methodology of infant looking-time studies that have been designed to test infants' expectations of how physical objects and people will behave

- New studies of infants' expectations regarding the physical world (Hespos & others, 2016)

- A new study in which 4-month-old infants were more surprised by a video in which a stranger ignored rather than comforted an infant (Jin & others, 2018)

- A description of new neuroimaging techniques and measures of psychophysiology that have been used to assess infants' cognitive development (Ellis & Turk-Browne, 2018)

- A description of how improvements in fine motor control and working memory contribute to increased realism with age in children's drawings (Morra & Panesi, 2017)

- Data suggesting that by the time children enter preschool, they ask an average of 76 questions per hour seeking information, and by the age of 5 their questions are well-formulated to elicit information children need to learn new concepts (Kurkul & Corriveau, 2018)

- Studies showing that adolescents who score low on perceptions of risks are more likely to engage in a given behavior than are adolescents who perceive the behavior as more risky; for example, misuse of opioids is higher among adolescents who do not perceive opioid use as risky (Voepel-Lewis & others, 2018)

- Findings that adolescents who face traumatic experiences that disrupt their sense of psychological invulnerability are more at risk of developing depression, anxiety, and other mental health problems (Chen & others, 2017)

- Contemporary interventions that target spatial visualization skills capitalizing on the potential of training to improve children's performance in early math skills (Hawes & others, 2017)

- Caution that taking a procedure, such as a standard Piagetian task, and applying it in a new cultural context in which the materials and even manner of an adult questioning a child about a problem to which the adult already knows the answer may be quite unusual and can lead children to respond in ways that do not reflect knowledge they hold in situations that are closer to their lived experiences (Rogoff, Dahl, & Callanan, 2018)

- Findings that preschoolers who use private speech are better able to regulate their behaviors and internalize new information (Day & Smith, 2019)

- A description of flipped classrooms in which student-centered learning activities, such as team problem-solving, are prioritized over teacher-centered delivery of information as a contemporary approach based on Vygotsky's theory (Lo, Hew, & Chen, 2017)

- An updated study of students in schools randomly assigned to use the Tools of the Mind curriculum compared to students in control schools that did not use the Tools of the Mind curriculum (Blair & Raver, 2014)

Chapter 7: Information Processing

- Updates to the research and thinking behind theories about the development of information processing across childhood and adolescence (Bjorklund & Casey, 2017; Siegler, 2016)

- Elaboration of international research on processing speed and learning capacities in reading and related academic skills (Kail, Lervåg, & Hulme, 2016), in a wide variety of languages (Tibi & Kirby, 2018)

- The latest knowledge about ways in which neuronal and brain development, along with learning through experience, support growth in processing speed and capacity (Battista & others, 2018; Oyefiade & others, 2018)

- Up-to-date research and theory regarding the definitions for different types of attention: selective, divided, sustained, and executive (Isbell & others, 2017; Rueda, 2017)

- Updated research on the development of orienting and emergence of sustained attention in infancy (Lewis & others, 2017)

- New research showing that parents notice how their behavior interacts with their infant's habituation and dishabituation as the baby moves on to explore other novel things (Deák & others, 2018)

- Updates on studies and theory regarding joint attention between caregivers and infants—how joint attention functions and develops, and how it relates to later growth in cognitive skills (Hakuno & others, 2018; Leith, Yuell, & Pike, 2018; Mundy, 2018)

- Updated review of research about "screen time" in early childhood and its potentially deleterious effects on children's development (Anderson & Subrahmanyam, 2017)
- Newer evidence regarding the developmental growth of attentional control across early and middle childhood, reflecting learning and brain development (Jiang & others, 2018; Rueda, 2018)
- The latest research on the growth of attentional control and its links with academic functioning in adolescence (Kim-Spoon & others, 2019), as well as adolescent multitasking and distracted behavior involving smartphones and social media (Li & others, 2018; Toh & others, 2019)
- Updated coverage of theories of working memory and its links with executive attention and other cognitive capacities (Baddeley, 2018; Camos & Barrouillet, 2018), and on competing theories of how memories are encoded and stored in childhood and beyond (Camos & others, 2018; Gobet, 2018; Kiraly & others, 2017)
- New research indicating that families play a key role in sharing stories that become part of children's developing memories, and cultural factors can influence this process (Reese & others, 2017)
- Updates on the research and interpretation of suggestibility and children's false memories (Ceci, Hritz, & Royer, 2017; Otgaar & others, 2018)
- Up-to-date research on how infants learn to categorize information and objects as they rapidly learn about the world across the first and second years of life (Poulin-Dubois & Pauen, 2017; Ware, 2017)
- The latest research on executive function and its development across childhood, its connections to achievement skills and other aspects of cognition, and limitations to how "trainable" executive function may be (Duckworth & others, 2019; Friedman & Miyake, 2017; Kassai & others, 2019; McDermott & Fox, 2018)
- Updated information about "mindfulness" and how teaching it can enhance self-regulation and both academic and social-emotional skills in school (Carsley, Khoury, & Heath, 2018; Sheinman & others, 2018)
- Newest research on the growth of scientific reasoning, and use of analogies and other strategies in middle childhood (Geurten & others, 2018; Whitaker & others, 2018)
- Coverage of the latest evidence on continuing changes in information processing capacities and strategies across adolescence, including critical thinking and decision making (Reyna, 2018; Steinberg & others, 2018)
- Up-to-date research and theory about "metacognition" across childhood and adolescence—how it develops, whether and how it can be improved, and the role it plays in learning, problem solving, and academic skill growth (Bjorklund & Causey, 2017; de Boer & others, 2018)
- The newest research on "theory of mind" and its development in childhood, and deficits in theory of mind as a key aspect of autism spectrum disorder and other developmental disorders (Boucher, 2017; Burge, 2018; Fletcher-Watson & Happé, 2019; Tomasello, 2018)
- Updated information about the prevalence of autism in the U.S. (National Autism Association, 2019)

Chapter 8: Intelligence

- A description of how, if IQ scores are misused, they have the potential to lead to self-fulfilling processes if teachers and others provide more learning opportunities to students with a high IQ, and IQ is then further bolstered by enhanced learning opportunities (Murdock-Perriera & Sedlacek, 2018)
- Addition of a new section on entity versus incremental theories of intelligence
- A description of how interventions to improve emotional intelligence that focus on teaching children how to regulate emotions more effectively have been found to reduce anger and other negative emotions as well as physical and verbal aggression (Castillo-Gualda & others, 2018)
- A study demonstrating that for adolescents who have been cyberbullied, higher emotional intelligence plays a protective role in reducing suicidal ideation and low self-esteem that are otherwise associated with being bullied (Extremera & others, 2018)
- New critiques of the concept of emotional intelligence and challenges in assessing it (Fiori & Vesely-Maillefer, 2018)
- An updated review of studies of brain structure and function in relation to intelligence, relying on new brain-imaging studies suggesting that more intelligent children are able to process information more efficiently across different brain regions (Khundrakpam & others, 2017)
- Recent work in neuroscience suggesting that as much as 80% of the variance in general intelligence can be explained by the speed with which individuals process information, which leads to more efficient communication among brain regions responsible for attention, working memory, and long-term storage (Schubert & others, 2017)
- Updates on genetic and environmental contributions to intelligence to include genome-wide association studies, a method that looks at individuals' entire genome in relation to observed traits, which have identified polygenic scores that integrate thousands of genetic sequences that contribute to intelligence (Plomin & von Stumm, 2018)
- Data showing that factors such as prenatal and postnatal nutrition are related to intelligence (Freitas-Vilela & others, 2018), and have been proposed as explanations for historical changes in intelligence test scores (Bratsberg & Rogeberg, 2018)
- A meta-analysis of 42 data sets including over 600,000 participants showing that each additional year of formal education raised IQ scores by 1 to 5 points, even taking into account that people with a higher propensity for intelligence stay in school longer (Ritchie & Tucker-Drob, 2018)

- Data from Khartoum, Sudan, showing changes in IQ that could be attributed to the implementation of compulsory schooling (Dutton & others, 2018)
- An update on age 30 outcomes associated with the Abecedarian Project (Ramey, 2018)
- Attention to how individuals can demonstrate intellectual skills in different ways in different cultural contexts; for example, children in an Inuit community in Canada performed poorly in traditional classrooms but were able to navigate for long distances between villages in the Arctic during winter with no visible landmarks (Sternberg, 2017) and Kenyan children who performed poorly in school were able to administer hundreds of herbal treatments for illnesses, suggesting that intelligence encompasses a broader array of intellectual abilities than those captured in traditional tests (Sternberg, 2017)
- Added cautions regarding comparing different demographic groups on intelligence tests
- An update of studies finding that measures of intelligence in infancy are correlated with measures of intelligence later in childhood (Muentener & others, 2018)
- New information on stability and change in intelligence from infancy through adolescence
- Results from neuroimaging studies related to intelligence

Chapter 9: Language Development

- Updated studies on the functions of infants' pointing in relation to shared attention and language development, including a study showing that when 18-month-olds pointed at novel objects in an experiment and were provided with labels for the objects, they were less likely to persist in pointing than if the experimenter did not label the objects, suggesting that infants were pointing to obtain information (Lucca & Wilbourn, 2019)
- A new study showing how 8-month-olds are able to use features of words to parse them when embedded in sentences (Karaman & Hay, 2018)
- Research showing that infants as young as 4 months old can understand that specific words refer to specific body parts when their parents touch their bodies while saying words referring to the body parts (Tincoff & others, 2018)
- Additional information on language acquisition in a variety of languages, including reasons that children learning to speak Asian languages may have a proportionally larger repertoire of verbs than English language learners
- Acknowledgement of variability in the ages at which infants reach language milestones, depending on factors such as socioeconomic status and other environmental inputs as well as infants' abilities such as sustained attention (Brooks, Flynn, & Ober, 2018)
- Updated references regarding fast mapping, including that fast mapping may have more to do with knowing what a word refers to in the immediate environment rather than truly learning the word because children can rarely recall the

words they have apparently learned in a fast mapping context (McMurray, Horst, & Samuelson, 2012)
- A revised and updated section on how early family environments contribute to language development
- Addition of studies using structural and functional MRI to examine the brains of 4- to 6-year-old children that have shown that children who engage in more conversational turns have different white matter properties and engage in tasks differently from children who hear fewer conversational turns (Romeo & others, 2018)
- A new study showing that the amount of talk that children hear between 18 to 24 months is correlated with language and cognitive outcomes in adolescence (Gilkerson & others, 2018)
- A description of how recent studies of language make use of LENA recording technology, which is a small digital audio-recorder that is worn by the child in specialized clothing and records all speech that is "near and clear" to the child over the course of up to 16 hours to provide a comprehensive picture of the talk that young children hear
- A study using the LENA device demonstrating that meaningful differences in the amount of talk that children hear as a function of SES is present as early as 18 months (Fernald, Marchman, & Weisleder, 2013)
- Updated research on how linguistic input when parents read to toddlers predicts language and literacy outcomes in elementary school, even controlling for parents' other linguistic input, perhaps in part because vocabulary is more diverse and syntax more complex in reading than everyday conversation (Demir-Lira & others, 2018)
- A new study showing that mothers' responsiveness and linguistic input during a shared picturebook reading task at 18 months predicted children's pre-academic skills at the age of 4.5 years (Wade & others, 2018)
- More attention to learning to read in a different language, such as that phonological awareness is less important for early reading development in languages that use characters, such as Chinese, rather than alphabets (Ruan & others, 2018)
- Addition of longitudinal research showing that vocabulary at 19 months predicted reading comprehension at 12 years (Suggate & others, 2018)
- An updated perspective on phonics versus whole language approaches to reading instruction
- New research on bilingualism and second-language acquisition
- A study demonstrating that vocabulary size in bilingual children is related to a number of factors, including metalinguistic awareness and whether they have a preference for one language over the other (Altman, Goldstein, & Armon-Lotem, 2018)
- Research showing that bilingualism has been found to narrow gaps in executive functioning and self-regulation otherwise found between children from higher versus lower socioeconomic backgrounds (Hartanto, Toh, & Yang, 2018)

- Research studies comparing English-only versus dual-language programs in which dual-language programs have shown benefits for students' academic achievement above and beyond students' proficiency in English (MacSwan & others, 2017)
- Addition of brain-imaging studies showing that language depends on networks connecting different regions of the brain (Alemi & others, 2018)
- Inclusion of an experimental study showing how children's language acquisition benefits from adults' undivided attention. When mothers were asked to teach their 2-year-old two new words in a laboratory setting, children did not learn the new word in a condition that was interrupted by a cell phone call placed by the experimenter but did learn the new word in the uninterrupted condition, even though the mothers said the new words the same number of times in both conditions (Reed, Hirsh-Pasek, & Golinkoff, 2017).

Chapter 10: Emotional Development

- Addition of a meta-analysis of 22 studies finding that when parents talked with young children more about mental states, children had a better understanding of emotions (Tompkins & others, 2018)
- A study showing that infants as young as 4 months expect unfamiliar adults to respond to a crying baby (Jin & others, 2018)
- Neuroscience additions including that infant crying elicits neuropsychological responses in mothers and that mothers who are better able to regulate their own emotional responses to their infants' cries are able to respond to infants in more sensitive ways (Firk & others, 2018)
- A longitudinal study following infants from the age of 10 to 18 months finding that infants with mothers who engaged in sensitive caregiving showed better emotion regulation and took longer to become distressed; maternal sensitivity was especially important for infants who showed low or medium levels of sustained attention, suggesting that infants who do not have the internal resources to regulate their emotions especially benefit from external supports (Frick & others, 2018)
- Research showing that when mothers are physiologically aroused and emotionally dysregulated in caregiving situations that are distressing to infants, infants are less likely to develop secure attachment relationships and are more at risk for developing behavior problems (Leerkes & others, 2017)
- A study showing that parents' use of different discipline strategies to invoke shame differs across cultural contexts and is especially common in China (Fung, Li, & Lam, 2017)
- Description of an intervention in which toddlers either participated in conversations about emotions or not after listening to emotion-based stories, finding that toddlers who participated in the conversations about emotions showed more prosocial behavior following the intervention than did toddlers who did not participate in the emotion conversations (Ornaghi & others, 2017)

- A description of three mechanisms accounting for how parents influence children's emotions: children's observations of their parents' emotions and emotion regulation, emotion-related parenting practices, and the family's emotional climate (Morris & others, 2017)
- Studies showing that the pattern of emotion socialization children receive from both mothers and fathers is related to children's social competence and behavior problems (Miller-Slough & others, 2018)
- Research demonstrating that mothers' knowledge about what comforts their children predicts children's ability to cope with distressing situations on their own (Sherman, Grusec, & Almas, 2017)
- An update on studies of children's coping with stress, including a study that found that a year after the 2015 earthquake in Nepal, 51% of children continued to have moderate to severe PTSD symptoms, which were stronger for younger than older children (Acharya, Bhatta, & Assannangkornchai, 2018)
- An acknowledgement that all children benefit from high-quality early child care more than low-quality childcare, but childcare quality is especially important for children with a difficult temperament (Johnson, Finch, & Phillips, 2018)
- A study showing that better effortful control at the age of 54 months predicted less externalizing behavior from kindergarten to sixth grade, which was partly accounted for by having fewer conflicts with teachers over that developmental period (Crockett & others, 2018)
- Addition of a study comparing toddler temperament in Chile, Poland, South Korea, and the United States, revealing several differences that might be consistent with cultural values; for example, toddlers in South Korea scored highest on effortful control (Krassner & others, 2017)
- A meta-analysis of 84 studies finding that, compared with children with an easy temperament, children with a more difficult temperament were more vulnerable to negative parenting but also benefited more from positive parenting (Slagt & others, 2016)
- A study that found that attending publicly-funded preschool programs can be especially beneficial for improving school readiness and reducing behavior problems for low-income children with difficult temperaments (Johnson, Finch, & Phillips, 2018)
- Research demonstrating that infants' autonomic nervous system activity changes reliably during both the still face and recovery period using the still-face paradigm (Jones-Mason & others, 2018)
- A new study showing that in the second year of life, infants become more sophisticated in understanding whether adults' emotions are specific to individual attitudes or provide more generalizable information (Hoehl & Striano, 2018)
- A meta-analytic review finding that early attachment predicted social competence with peers, internalizing behaviors such as anxiety, and externalizing behaviors such as aggression (Groh & others, 2017)

- Data suggesting that children can be highly resilient and adaptive, even in the face of wide variations in parenting and other environmental contexts (Masten, 2018)
- Research showing that during middle childhood, children who are securely attached to their parents are better at regulating their emotions (Movahed Abtahi & Kerns, 2017) and that secure attachment during middle childhood predicts better school adaptation, social competence with peers, and self-esteem, and fewer behavioral problems (Brumariu & others, 2018)
- Brain-imaging studies that have revealed connections among infants' cues such as crying, mothers' responses, and brain activity (Esposito & others, 2017)
- Updated research on fathers as caregivers, including data showing that when fathers are actively involved as caregivers, children are more likely to interact in similar ways with fathers and mothers (McHale & Sirotkin, 2019)
- Updated statistics on childcare arrangements and barriers to childcare
- New studies on links between early childcare arrangements and later developmental outcomes

Chapter 11: The Self and Identity

- Updated research about the development of self-recognition and understanding in infancy and the second year of life (Davoodi, Nelson, & Blake, 2018; Filippetti & Tsakiris, 2018), across the preschool years of early childhood (Starmans, 2017), middle childhood, and adolescence (Harter, 2015; Killen, Rutland, & Yip, 2016)
- New research and theory about the development of understanding of others' minds and intentions, including evidence that even young children may be less "egocentric" in their thinking than previously understood (Fizke & others, 2017; Quintanilla, Giménez-Dasí, & Gaviria, 2018), and that young children are able to establish and understand joint obligations and commitments to their peers by the time they begin school (Kachel & Tomasello, 2019)
- Updating of knowledge about how empathy and understanding of generosity toward others (publicly and privately) develop across middle childhood and into adolescence (Hein & others, 2018; Heyman & others, 2016)
- New evidence that understanding and empathy toward others continues to develop across adolescence, and includes recognition of the distinction between experiences of people in vulnerable groups in society (e.g., racial and gender discrimination; Seider & others, 2019)
- Up-to-date research about age-group and individual differences in self-concept and self-esteem in childhood and adolescence—how these develop, and how they are linked with healthy functioning and well-being as well as emotional and behavioral problems (Becht & others, 2017; Kadir, Yeung, & Diallo, 2018; Paxton & Damiano, 2017; Reed-Fitzke, 2019)

- Latest research and theory about the co-development of global self-concept and domain-specific (e.g., physical, academic) self-concept and competencies (Cvencek & others, 2018; Harter, 2015; Nagai & others, 2018)
- Description of the largest meta-analysis of self-esteem ever completed, including over 160,000 participants from around the world and showing that self-esteem increases over childhood and again in early adulthood, with stable and small increases across adulthood into old age (Orth, Erol, & Luciano, 2018)
- Consideration of the cross-cultural/global phenomenon in many cultures of extending adolescence beyond the teenage years due to increasing demands on advanced education and training—and, the implications of this for development of independence (Stetka, 2017)
- Updated research and theory regarding identity development and commitment in adolescence (Meeus, 2019) and the transition to adulthood (Murray & Arnett, 2019), and updated coverage of the use of the "narrative approach" to studying and defining the identity development processes (Fivush, 2019; McLean & Lilgendahl, 2019)
- Updating of the research evidence regarding the role of family, peer, and romantic relationships in identity development (Cooper & Seginer, 2018), including description of cross-cultural evidence for links between secure attachment relationships with parents in adolescence and healthy identity development (Sugimura & others, 2018), and the important role of peers and partners in identity development (Kerpelman & Pittman, 2018; Strudwick-Alexander, 2017)
- New research and theory regarding ethnic identity development in multiple cultural contexts, examining the role of family, peers, minority status, and other correlated factors that contribute to this important aspect of identity in childhood, adolescence, and adulthood (Cooper & Seginer, 2018; Feliciano & Rumbaut, 2018; Vietze & others, 2018) and the importance of positive ethnic identity to optimal developmental outcomes (Umaña-Taylor & others, 2018)
- The latest research on how children's beliefs about their capacity to learn and improve in their skills through practice and hard work (that is, having an "incremental" theory of intelligence and learning) is linked with better learning outcomes (Gunderson & others, 2018)
- Expansion of coverage of research examining cultural similarities and differences in the values placed on self-esteem in childhood, reflected in parents' and children's attitudes and practices around one's own growth and supporting the growth of others in their family, school, and community (Becker & others, 2014; Miller & Cho, 2018)
- Updating of research on Erikson's theory, with newer theories about the continuous process of identity development across childhood, adolescence, and adulthood (Crocetti, 2017)

Chapter 12: Gender

- A study showing that mothers' gender role attitudes were not related to their 2-year-olds' gender-typed appearance, but 2-year-olds' own ability to recognize and use gender labels was related to their gender-typed appearance, suggesting that children are aware of gender from a very early age and motivated to adhere to gender stereotypes by dressing in traditionally masculine or feminine ways (Halim & others, 2018)

- A study demonstrating that sex-typed toy play predicted sex-typed behaviors five years later, regardless of whether children were being reared by lesbian, gay, or heterosexual parents (Li, Kung, & Hines, 2017)

- An update on studies of congenital adrenal hyperplasia

- A review of 184 studies that included 1.6 million students from 21 countries showing that despite the increase in single-sex education, the highest quality studies showed that same-sex education did not provide benefits compared to mixed-sex education (Pahlke & others, 2014)

- Addition of a review of 135 studies finding that in both laboratory settings and in everyday life, exposure to media portrayals that sexually objectify women are related to men's and women's views of women as being less competent and less moral and to more tolerance of sexual violence against women (Ward, 2016)

- Studies of how adolescent girls internalize sexualized images from the media, increasing their likelihood of wearing sexualized clothing and feeling shame about their bodies (McKenney & Bigler, 2016)

- An analysis of whether gender stereotypes changed between the early 1980s and 2014 in the United States, indicating that males' and females' descriptions of typical traits, role behaviors, occupations, and physical characteristics that men and women would have were as stereotyped in 2014 as in the 1980s (Haines, Deaux, & Lofaro, 2016)

- An analysis of how, at a societal level, there is evidence that men and women in countries higher in gender equality (as indicated by education, representation at high levels of government, and the like) have less stereotypical gender roles within the family and that children interact more similarly with their mothers and fathers (Bartel & others, 2018)

- A study of eighth-grade students in 36 countries showing that, in every country, girls had more egalitarian attitudes about gender roles than boys did and that girls had the most egalitarian gender attitudes in countries with higher levels of societal gender equality (Dotti Sani & Quaranta, 2017)

- Data on how gender stereotyping changes with development (Brannon, 2017) and over historical time (Miller & others, 2018)

- Updated studies on gender and the brain

- Updated statistics on gender and education, such as dropout rates and college attendance (National Center for Education Statistics, 2018)

- An analysis of recorded conversations between same-sex and mixed-sex pairs of undergraduates, finding several gender differences in self-disclosure and negotiation (Leaper, 2019)

- A description of changes over historical time in students' reports of their femininity, masculinity, and androgyny (Donnelly & Twenge, 2017)

- Addition of a section on gender identity encompassing children's understanding of themselves in terms of cultural construals of what it means to be male or female

- New studies of socially transitioned transgender children who refer to themselves using pronouns of the gender with which they identify rather than their sex at birth but with no hormonal or surgical interventions involved (Olson & Gülgöz, 2018)

- Consideration of prejudice, discrimination, bullying, family rejection, and lack of self-acceptance as concerns for transgender children (Adelson, Stroeh, & Ng, 2016) and the importance of family support for transgender children's mental health (Olson & others, 2016)

- A study demonstrating that girls are more likely than boys to notice when bullying is occurring, react with empathy, and intervene (Jenkins & Nickerson, 2019)

- International data on gender equality in education

Chapter 13: Moral Development

- Presentation of the latest research on empathy and the role of emotion in moral judgement and thinking (Decety, Meidenbauer, & Cowell, 2018; Malti & others, 2017)

- New research and theory regarding Smetana's social cognitive domain theory of moral development, noting the latest empirical evidence and interpretations of domains of thinking that influence morality (Dahl & Killen, 2018; Jambon & Smetana, 2018)

- Coverage of the most recent empirical and theoretical work by Ross Thompson and Grazyna Kochanska regarding conscience, moral development, and the role of parenting and parent-child relationships in their growth (Kim & Kochanska, 2017; Thompson, 2015)

- Updating of literature regarding Haidt's theory that, in contrast to Kohlberg's theory, moral thinking is usually an intuitive "gut reaction" that begins with rapid judgments of others rather than with slower strategic reasoning that happens afterwards (Graham & Valdesolo, 2017; Haidt, 2017)

- Coverage of the latest research regarding adolescent civic and community engagement and volunteering conducted in the United States, Chile, and elsewhere, showing that internal motivation and consistent support from family, school, and community for such engagement are key aspects (Henderson, Brown, & Pancer, 2019; Kim & Morgül, 2017; Martínez & others, 2019)

- Inclusion of findings from a large comprehensive study of cheating motivation and behavior among high school students in Stockholm, Sweden, showing that cheating was least common in schools that had a culture emphasizing fairness and honesty, and in which administrators and teachers were engaged with the students (Ramberg & Modin, 2019)

- Updated research evidence regarding the development of understanding of fairness and equality across early and middle childhood, with cross-cultural differences in some patterns of when such beliefs about fairness and equal treatment emerge depending on the culture's value placed on individualism and collectivism (Huppert & others, 2019)

- Update on the results from an ongoing longitudinal study in the United States tracking adolescents' gratitude toward others, showing that increases in gratitude over time were linked with lower levels of antisocial behaviors, higher levels of prosocial behaviors, and better well-being (Bono & others, 2019)

- Inclusion of the latest evidence and theory about the development of antisocial behavior patterns and disorders (e.g., conduct disorder) in childhood and adolescence, including family, peer, and school risk and protective factors as well as approaches to treatment (Allen & others, 2018; Frietag & others, 2018; Henderson, Hogue, & Dauber, 2019; McCoy & others, 2019; Mohan & Ray, 2019)

- Updating of the prevalence of juvenile arrests and incarceration rates for males and females in the United States (Hockenberry, 2019)

- Expansion on the latest information about U.S. and international laws and policies regarding incarceration and capital punishment of minors, and the uneven enforcement of such laws around the globe (DPIC, 2019)

- Up-to-date international research evidence showing that supportive, authoritative parenting environments that include monitoring of older children's and adolescents' whereabouts and activities, is a key aspect of decreasing risk for growth in delinquent behaviors across a wide range of contexts (Deater-Deckard & others, 2019; Nkuba, Hermenau, & Hecker, 2019; Ruiz-Hernández & others, 2019)

- Recently published evidence from several large longitudinal studies showing the important role that deficits in self-regulation (including poorer emotion regulation and executive functioning) play across adolescence and into adulthood, in the growth and maintenance of delinquency and other antisocial behaviors (Bekbolatkyzy & others, 2019; Nikulina & Widom, 2019)

- Updating of research evidence regarding religious engagement, participation, and identity among adolescents and young adults around the globe, showing steady levels in equatorial and southern hemisphere regions but continuing decreases in northern hemisphere regions including the United States (Pew Research Center, 2018; Sugimura & others, 2019)

Chapter 14: Families

- Updates to research regarding mutual synchrony and reciprocity in parent-child face-to-face interaction, including evidence on similar patterns in multiple cultures (Kuchirko, Tafuro, & Tamis-LeMonda, 2017), and the role of brain activity in both interaction partners (Leong & others, 2017)

- Recent advances in theory regarding bidirectional socialization and reciprocal influences of parents and children on each other in family processes (Fiese, Jones, & Saltsman, 2018; Grusec, 2017)

- Updated information about the connections between parents' marital satisfaction and parenting, parent-child relationships, and child adjustment and functioning in families (Berryhill & others, 2016; Knopp & others, 2017)

- Updated overview of the changing rates of adolescent pregnancy and delayed childbirth (including childlessness) into middle age for different groups of women (Beal, Crockett, & Peugh, 2016; Martinez, G. M., & others, 2018; Mathews & Hamilton, 2016)

- Addition of evidence that national-level economic recessions around the globe have been linked to increases in problems in family functioning (Brooks-Gunn, Schneider, & Waldfogel, 2013; Solantaus, Leinonen, & Punamäki, 2004; UNICEF, 2014)

- Updated evidence for an increase in the prevalence of grandparents raising their grandchildren because the parents are not able or willing to fulfill their role (Hayslip, Fruhauf, & Dolbin-MacNab, 2017)

- Reference to recent research and theory about the impact of social and cultural changes in family structures and activities, such as the rapid rise of the use of the Internet and digital technologies in families (Blumberg & Brooks, 2017) and the ongoing shifts in family structures around the globe due to economic and demographic changes (e.g., divorce, remarriage, relocation) (Ganong & Coleman, 2017)

- Recent research pointing to the many areas of adaptation and change required in families as adults transition to parenthood, including the interconnected effects of challenges in the new parenting role and changes in the parenting couples' satisfaction and conflict (Carlson & van Orman, 2017; Maas & others, 2018; Newkirk, Perry-Jenkins, & Sayer, 2017)

- Updating of research regarding the shift from coregulation between parent and child in early childhood, toward more autonomy and self-regulation across middle childhood, as part of the family socialization process (Koehn & Kerns 2017)

- Updated information about the role of parents as "managers" of the household and their children's activities, experiences, and lives (Beckmeyer & Russell, 2018)

- Recent research on parental monitoring of older children and adolescents—how levels of monitoring depend in part on individual differences in youths' willingness to share and disclose information to their parents (Chan, Brown, & von Bank, 2015), and links between monitoring and academic and behavioral functioning in a variety of cultural and ethnic groups (Degol & others, 2017; Jeynes, 2017)

- Expanded and updated coverage of the literature on Baumrind's (2013) parenting styles of authoritarian and authoritative parenting, and links with child and adolescent adjustment and functioning in a variety of cultural contexts including China, which has the largest national population of adolescents in the world (Larzelere, Morris & Harrist, 2013; Prevoo & Tamis-Lemonda, 2017; Zhang & others, 2017)

- Updated international research regarding gradual decreases in the use of harsh physical and verbal punishment in families, reflecting cultural changes in childrearing attitudes and practices as well as shifts in social policy (Alampay & others, 2017; Lansford & others, 2017; Pinquart, 2017)

- Recent research on the role of coparenting—parents working together in a coordinated way, to most effectively monitor and socialize their children and adolescents in ways that are consistent with the couples' and family's values and practices (Padilla & others, 2017; Young, Riggs, & Kaminski, 2017)

- Updates on the definitions and prevalence of various types of child abuse and maltreatment in the United States (Child Welfare Information Gateway, 2016; U.S. Dept. of Health and Human Services, 2016), and international evidence regarding interrelated risks for abuse such as parents' stress and substance use (Laslett & others, 2017)

- New research documenting the impact of child maltreatment on child and adolescent mental and physical health, and educational and economic outcomes (Jaffee, 2017; Kaufman-Parks & others, 2017)

- Evidence from a recent study showing some ethnic group variations in the link between parental granting of autonomy and independence (and less reliance on psychological control) of adolescents, and lower levels of teen emotional and behavioral problems (Eagleton, Williams, & Merten, 2016)

- Results of a meta-analysis suggesting that the well-established gender difference in autonomy granting in adolescence that favors greater independence for males may be smaller and inconsistent across studies (Endendijk & others, 2016)

- Up-to-date research on first and second generation adolescent immigrants in the United States, and the distinct opportunities and challenges in development for these youth who face acculturation stress within and outside of their family and school contexts (Gassman-Pines & Skinner, 2018; Titzmann & Gniewosz, 2017)

- The latest research on the features and effects of sibling relationship processes spanning from warmth to conflict, how these connect with other relationships (including peers), cross-cultural similarities and differences, and how interventions can be effective in improving sibling relationships when help is needed (Hughes, McHarg, & White, 2018; Smorti & Ponti, 2018; Tucker & Finkelhor, 2017)

- Updating of research, theory, and interpretation of findings around relative birth order (that is, comparisons of first, second, and later born siblings) and comparisons between singletons and children with siblings, suggesting that the effects are quite small and inconsistent (Rohrer, Egloff, & Schmukle, 2015; Yang & others, 2017)

- Newer research evidence (including inclusion of international studies) regarding effects or lack of effects on child development, of maternal employment and mother-father

co-management of work-family conflicts and demands (Lightbody & Williamson, 2017; Lombardi & Coley, 2017; Shockley & others, 2017)

- Updated information about rates and trends of parental divorce in the United States and other countries, and links between divorce and parenting as well as child and adolescent adjustment following the divorce (Davies, Martin, & Cummings, 2018; OECD, 2016; Sands, Thompson, & Gaysina, 2017)

- Newest information on laws regarding gay marriage and on research and theory regarding youth in gay and lesbian parent families in the United States and other countries, indicating few differences in family functioning or developmental outcomes compared to children raised in heterosexual-parent households (Golombok, 2017)

Chapter 15: Peers

- The latest research on the role of positive, supportive peer relationships in children's social-emotional, academic, cognitive, and physical health and functioning in childhood and adolescence (Bassett, 2019; Thomas, Connor, & Scott, 2018; Thompson, 2019; Voltmer & von Salisch, 2017)

- Evidence from ten longitudinal studies indicating strong and consistent links between positive, supportive parent-child relationships with better peer relationships and youth developmental outcomes (Walters, 2019)

- Up-to-date description of the dimensions and sub-types of peer acceptance and rejection and their correlates (Ladd & others, 2017; McDonald & Asher, 2018; Rytioja, Lappalainen, & Savolainen, 2019; Xhang & others, 2018)

- Results of a large international survey of adolescents' self-reported stress in their relationships with parents and peers, showing international and cultural-group distinctions in relationship stressors and only modest gender differences (Persike & Seiffge-Krenke, 2016)

- Updates to research and theory regarding the importance of play of all kinds for younger and older children—its role in supporting overall development and functioning, as well as specific skill-building in facets of communication and language, academic competencies, and social-emotional assets (Ariel, 2019; Germeroth & others, 2019; Lillard, 2018; Neuman, 2019; Theodotou, 2019)

- Research, theory, and parenting/educator recommendations on imaginative or pretend play in early childhood, its role in cognitive and social-emotional development, and how it can be encouraged to create imaginative play groups for children in formal and informal learning settings (Breathnach, Danby, & O'Gorman, 2018; Lillard & Taggart, 2019; Riede & others, 2018; Tunçgenç & Cohen, 2018)

- Latest research on the rates of digital game play and developmental changes across childhood and adolescence in the United States (Pew Research Center, 2018a)

- Recent evidence on the importance of intimacy in close friendships in adolescence (Laninga-Wijnen & others, 2019) and regarding gender differences in children and adolescents' attitudes and norms around sharing of feelings and other disclosures toward their same-sex friends (Carlucci & others, 2018; Dunbar, 2018; Pollastri & others, 2018; Rose & others, 2016)

- Updating and expansion of coverage of international research evidence regarding prevalence of bullying and peer victimization throughout countries on every continent, and the most recent data on prevalence among children and adolescents in the United States (Chen & others, 2017; Lebrun-Harris & others, 2018)

- Description of the latest evidence for anti-bullying prevention and intervention programs in multiple countries, showing that schoolwide programs can be effectively implemented and reduce rates of victimization while also improving school climate in positive ways (Divecha & Brackett, 2019; Huang & others, 2019; Olweus, Limber, & Breivik, 2019; Smith, 2019)

- Up-to-date coverage of the prevalence of same- and opposite-sex friendships in childhood and adolescence in the United States, and how a culturally premature emphasis on opposite-sex relationships in early adolescence increases risk for a host of delinquent behavioral outcomes (Grard & others, 2018; Weger & others, 2019; Wilson & Jamison, 2019)

- Newer research indicating developmental increases then decreases (peaking at about 15 years of age) in adolescents' conformity with peer group standards and norms, and growth in independent value judgements in the transition to early adulthood (Closson, Hart, & Hogg, 2017; Goliath & Pretorius, 2016)

- Updated research on groups and cliques, and the important role that membership plays in socialization, identity formation and development, and maladjustment in adolescence (Ellis & Zarbatany, 2017; Jordan & others, 2019; Moran & others, 2017; Schwartz & others, 2017)

- Recent evidence and theory regarding the developmental importance and role of romantic relationships in adolescence and emergent adulthood, and how early initiation of such relationships can increase risk for sexually transmitted diseases and teen pregnancy (Birnbaum & Ries, 2019; Low & Shortt, 2017; van de Bongardt & others, 2015)

- Updated research regarding opposite-sex and same-sex attraction, relationships, and sexual contact in adolescence and emergent adulthood in the United States and other countries, and information about cultural differences in attitudes about gay, lesbian, and bisexual youth (Flores & others, 2018; Kaestle, 2019; Rosario, 2019)

- Expanded coverage of research on the links between supportive parent-adolescent relationships and positive romantic relationship formation and functioning in adolescence, in multiple cultural groups and for same-sex and opposite-sex relationships (Feinstein & others, 2018; Viejo & others, 2018)

- Research noting the strong connection between romantic partner conflict and jealousy in adolescence, and subsequent intimate partner violence in late adolescence and emergent adulthood (Collibee, Furman, & Shoop, 2019)

- Updated description of research on socioeconomic and cultural contexts in the United States and other countries, and how these context differences are related to differences in adolescents' attitudes and behaviors involved in dating, sex, and gender role and expression (De Meyer & others, 2017; Stein & others, 2018; Taggart & others, 2018; Twenge & Park, 2019)

Chapter 16: Schools and Achievement

- An update on legislation guiding public education in the United States, including information on the Common Core State Standards Initiative (2019)

- New international comparisons among students in different countries based on scores in math, science, and other subjects (McFarland & others, 2018)

- Updated studies of the effects of Head Start and Early Head Start (Paschall, Mastergeorge, & Ayoub, 2019)

- A meta-analysis of 107 studies finding that self-esteem and motivation variables decreased over the course of schooling, with the sharpest declines for intrinsic motivation, math, and language academic self-concepts, mastery achievement goals, and performance-approach achievement goals (Scherrer & Preckel, 2019)

- Studies suggesting that students' academic motivation and engagement often drop during school transitions, especially if students perceive themselves as lacking control and efficacy to meet new academic challenges (Anderson & others, 2019) but that school transitions are less stressful for students who have relationships with teachers characterized by high levels of warmth and low levels of conflict (Hughes & Cao, 2018)

- Information on the role of peers and parents in helping students handle school transitions (Fite & others, 2019)

- A longitudinal study in 26 middle schools in the United States showing that over two-thirds of friendships were either gained or lost in the first year of middle school and that greater instability in friendships was predictive of less school engagement and lower grades (Lessard & Juvonen, 2018)

- New data on early childhood education in low- and middle-income countries and how the Sustainable Development Goals guiding the international agenda through 2030 call for universal access to at least one year of preschool for all children globally (UNICEF, 2019)

- Updated school dropout rates by gender and ethnicity

- A description of interventions that have been developed to prevent students from dropping out of high school

- An update of effective approaches that can be used to improve educational outcomes of students with learning disabilities (Alquraini & Rao, 2019)

- A meta-analysis of 11 studies suggesting that ADHD symptoms, hyperactivity, inattention, executive functioning, and on-task behavior of children with ADHD can be improved through yoga, mindfulness, and meditation (Chimiklis & others, 2018)

- An update on educational settings in which students with disabilities are served (National Center for Education Statistics, 2018)
- Description of an experiment in which children were provided with either positive or negative feedback delivered in either a controlling or autonomy-supportive way that found that children were most intrinsically motivated to complete a similar task in the future and persisted longer in the face of challenges when adults had provided positive feedback delivered in an autonomy-supportive way on their prior activities (Mabbe & others, 2018)
- A study of how high school teachers promote motivation in the classroom (Patall & others, 2018)
- Studies regarding self-efficacy, school performance, and career aspirations
- Information on how students', teachers', and parents' expectations are all important to consider in relation to students' motivation and achievement. If teachers or parents have high expectations for students' success in school, these high expectations can serve as a buffer when students' own expectations fall short (Wigfield & Gladstone, 2019).
- Update on how the racial climate of the school as well as teachers' ethnic diversity and cultural competence have implications for biases and expectations encountered by students, which in turn affect students' achievement (Whaley, 2018)

Chapter 17: Culture and Diversity

- Updated definition and description of theories about culture and cross-cultural group similarities and differences in children's developmental outcomes and their family, peer, and school contexts (Bornstein & Lansford, 2018; Molitor & Hsu, 2019; White, Nair, & Bradley, 2018)
- Description of a study of Mexican 8- to 10-year-olds' peer interactions during game play, showing higher levels and distinct types of collaborative and cooperative behaviors among rural indigenous youth compared to urban youth (Correa-Chavez, Mangione, & Mejia-Arauz, 2016)
- Expanded treatment of the distinction between individualism and collectivism in cultures (Oyserman, 2017), and updated research and theory indicating individual and family-level variations in both dimensions *within* cultures and emphasis on the potential effects of globalization and technology on these cultural values (Greenfield, 2018; Vignoles & others, 2016)
- Updated research and theory regarding neighborhood contexts and socioeconomic differences between neighborhoods, along with related factors (e.g., parenting environments, school quality, crime, and safety), and their influences on developmental outcomes in childhood and adolescence (Manduca & Sampson, 2019; Owens & Candipan, 2019; Ramdahl & others, 2018)
- Up-to-date information about the link between growing up in a low-socioeconomic status family and neighborhood and

having more mental and behavioral health problems and poorer school achievement outcomes in childhood and adolescence (Reiss & others, 2019; Rivenbark & others, 2019)

- Newer research on Suniya Luthar's theory and earlier evidence for certain types of mental and behavioral health problems among youth from affluent families and neighborhoods (Ebbert, Kumar, & Luthar, 2019; Luthar, Small, & Ciciolla, 2018)
- Updated data on poverty rates for children younger than 18 years old in the United States and the world, and the strong associations between income disparities and race/ethnicity in the United States (Children's Defense Fund, 2017; Duncan, Kalil, & Ziol-Guest, 2017)
- Latest evidence indicating the short-term and long-lasting links between growing up in poverty and greater challenges in youth developmental outcomes, spanning mental, behavioral, psychological, and biological measures, such as school failure, depression, antisocial behavior, and stress (Kim, Evans, & others, 2018; McLoyd, Jocson, & Williams, 2016; Pryor & others, 2019; Reiss & others, 2019)
- Updates on two-generation antipoverty programs with families designed to reduce poverty and its negative effects on family functioning and children's development (Sommer & others, 2018)
- New information about the landmark peer mentoring program "Quantum Opportunities Program" to reduce multigenerational poverty that has now been expanded nationally (www.eisenhowerfoundation.org/qop)
- Up-to-date data regarding recent and projected growth of ethnic minority groups in the United States and other countries, including youth who have emigrated between countries (Frey, 2019; Zhou & Gonzales, 2019)
- The latest research and theory regarding the unique risks, as well as distinct strengths, of immigrant families and youth and their developmental outcomes and overall healthy functioning in their new countries (i.e., risk model, paradox model) (Brady & Stevens, 2019; Marks & Garcia-Coll, 2018)
- Updated research on "bicultural" orientation of immigrant youth and their parents and grandparents, as children and adolescents develop and grow while seeking to maintain aspects of their new culture and their native culture (Schwartz & others, 2019; Shen, Kim, & Benner, 2019) while also nurturing pride in their ethnicity and awareness of discrimination (Liu, Simpkins, & Lin, 2018)
- Recent research indicating the likely effects of stress on mental and behavioral health in adolescence arising from ethnic and racial discrimination of ethnic minority youth (Lo & others, 2017; Stein & others, 2016)
- New information about recent trends in digital technology and Internet access and use among children and teenagers in the United States, other industrialized nations, and emerging economy nations around the world (Pew Research Center, 2018a, b)
- Updated research and interpretation of evidence indicating fewer effects of digital technology use on cognitive development

compared to more and consistent effects on mental and behavioral health and wellness in childhood and adolescence (Blumberg & others, 2019; Twenge & Campbell, 2019)

- New evidence indicating likely connections between more extensive "screen time" and subsequent higher levels of poorer sleep and diet, weight gain and poorer fitness, and lower academic engagement in adolescence (LeBourgeois & others, 2017; Simonato & others, 2018)

- Updates to research on some of the risks that children and adolescents are exposed to through frequent and prolonged time spent on the Internet, ranging from exposure to sexual and violent content that is not age appropriate, to victimization by cyberbullying, to distracted multitasking or cyber-slacking (Flanigan & Kiewra, 2018; Rosa & others, 2019; Selkie, Fales, & Moreno, 2016)

- The latest research and recommendations on what parents can do to help guide children's and adolescents' online time and activities, in ways that can reduce risk of exposure to harmful content and experiences, and increase beneficial learning from exposure to enriching content and experiences (Fardouly & others, 2018; Van Petegem & others, 2019; Vanwesenbeeck & others, 2018)

acknowledgments

We very much appreciate the support and guidance provided by many people at McGraw-Hill. Ryan Treat, Senior Portfolio Manager for Psychology, has provided excellent guidance, vision, and direction for this edition. Vicki Malinee provided considerable expertise in coordinating many aspects of the editorial process. Janet Tilden again did an outstanding job as the text's copy editor. Mary Powers did a terrific job in coordinating the text's production. Dawn Groundwater, Product Development Manager, did excellent work on various aspects of the development, technology, and learning systems. Thanks also to A.J. Laferrera and Olivia Kaiser for their extensive and outstanding work in marketing *Child Development*. And Jennifer Blankenship again has provided excellent choices of new photographs. We also wish to thank Sophie Sharp and Anna Deater-Deckard, who assisted with library literature research.

QUEST: JOURNEY THROUGH CHILDHOOD BOARD OF ADVISORS AND SUBJECT MATTER EXPERTS

Admiration and appreciation go to the following experts who have devoted a significant portion of their time and expertise to creating the first of its kind learning game for Developmental Psychology: Cheri Kittrell, State College of Florida; Brandy Young, Cypress College; Becky Howell, Forsyth Technical College; Gabby Principe, College of Charleston; Karen Schrier Shaenfield, Marist College; Steven Prunier, Ivy Tech; Amy Kolak, College of Charleston; Kathleen Hughes Stellmach, Pasco-Hernando State College; Lisa Fozio-Thielk, Waubonsee Community College; Tricia Wessel-Blaski, University of Wisconsin-Milwaukee, Washington County; Margot Underwood, Joliet Junior College; Claire Rubman, Suffolk County Community College; Alissa Knowles, University of California-Irvine; Cortney Simmons, University of California-Irvine; Kelli Dunlap; Level Access-WCAG Accessibility Partners.

EXPERT CONSULTANTS

As each new edition is developed, we consult with leading experts in their respective areas of life-span development. Their invaluable feedback ensures that the latest research, knowledge, and perspectives are presented. Their willingness to devote their time and expertise to this endeavor is greatly appreciated. The Expert Consultants who contributed to this edition can be found on pages xvi–xvii.

REVIEWERS

A special debt of gratitude goes to the reviewers who have provided detailed feedback on *Child Development* over the years.

Kristine Anthis, *Southern Connecticut State University;* **Brein K. Ashdown**, *St. Louis University;* **Ruth L. Ault**, *Davidson College;* **Mary Ballard**, *Appalachian State University;* **William H. Barber**, *Midwestern State University;* **Marjorie M. Battaglia**, *George Mason University;* **Jann Belcher**, *Utah Valley State College;* **Wayne Benenson**, *Illinois State University;* **Michael Bergmire**, *Jefferson College;* **David Bernhardt**, *Carleton University;* **Kathryn Norcross Black**, *Purdue University;* **Elain Blakemore**, *Indiana University;* **Susan Bland**, *Niagara County Community College;* **Bryan Bolea**, *Grand Valley State University;* **Amy Booth**, *Northwestern University;* **Marc Bornstein**, *National Institute of Child Health and Human Development;* **Teresa Bossert-Braasch**, *McHenry County College;* **Megan E. Bradley**, *Frostburg State University;* **Albert Bramante**, *Union County College;* **Jo Ann Burnside**, *Richard J Daley College;* **Catherine Caldwell-Harris**, *Boston University;* **Maureen Callahan**, *Webster University;* **Victoria Candelora**, *Brevard Community College;* **Gustavo Carlo**, *University of Nebraska;* **D. Bruce Carter**, *Syracuse University;* **Elaine Cassel**, *Marymount University, Lord Fairfax Community College;* **Lisa Caya**, *University of Wisconsin—LaCrosse;* **Steven Ceci**, *Cornell University;* **Theodore Chandler**, *Kent State University;* **Dante Cicchetti**, *University of Rochester;* **Audrey E. Clark**, *California State University, Northridge;* **Debra E. Clark**, *SUNY—Cortland;* **Robert Cohen**, *The University of Memphis;* **John D. Coie**, *Duke University;* **Cynthia Garcia Coll**, *Wellesley College;* **W. Andrew Collins**, *University of Minnesota;* **Robert C. Coon**, *Louisiana State University;* **Roger W. Coulson**, *Iowa State University;* **William Curry**, *Wesleyan College;* **Fred Danner**, *University of Kentucky;* **Darlene DeMarie**, *University of South Florida;* **Marlene DeVoe**, *Saint Cloud State University;* **Denise M. DeZolt**, *Kent State University;* **K. Laurie Dickson**, *Northern Arizona University;* **Daniel D. DiSalvi**, *Kean College;* **Ruth Doyle**, *Casper College;* **Diane C. Draper**, *Iowa State University;* **Sean Duffy**, *Rutgers University;* **Jerry Dusek**, *Syracuse University;* **Beverly Brown Dupré**, *Southern University at New Orleans;* **Glen Elder, Jr.**, *University of North Carolina;* **Claire Etaugh**, *Bradley University;* **Karen Falcone**, *San Joaquin Delta College;* **Dennis T. Farrell**, *Luzerne County Community College;* **Saul Feinman**, *University of Wyoming;* **Gary Feng**, *Duke University;* **Tiffany Field**, *University of Miami;* **Oney Fitzpatrick, Jr.**, *Lamar University;* **Jane Goins Flanagan**, *Lamar University;* **Kate Fogarty**, *University of Florida—Gainesville;* **L. Sidney Fox**, *California State University—Long Beach;* **Janet Frick**, *University of Georgia;* **Douglas Frye**, *University of Virginia;* **Dale Fryxell**, *Chamainde University;* **Janet A. Fuller**, *Mansfield University;* **Irma Galejs**, *Iowa State University;* **Mary Gauvain**, *University of California, Riverside;* **Eugene Geist**, *Ohio University;* **John Gibbs**, *Ohio State University;* **Colleen Gift**, *Highland Community College;* **Margaret S. Gill**, *Kutztown University;* **Beverly Goldfield**, *Rhode Island College;* **Hill Goldsmith**, *University of Wisconsin—Madison;* **Cynthia Graber**, *Columbia University;* **Stephen B. Graves**, *University of South Florida;* **Donald E. Guenther**, *Kent State University;* **Julia Guttmann**, *Iowa Wesleyan College;* **Renee Ha**, *University of Washington;* **Robert A. Haaf**, *University of Toledo;* **Craig Hart**, *Brigham Young University;* **Susan Harter**, *University of Denver;* **Robin Harwood**, *Texas Tech University;* **Elizabeth Hasson**, *Westchester University;* **Rebecca Heikkinen**, *Kent State University;* **Joyce Hemphill**,

University of Wisconsin; **Shirley-Anne Hensch,** University of Wisconsin; **Stanley Henson,** Arkansas Technical University; **Alice Honig,** Syracuse University; **Cynthia Hudley,** University of California–Santa Barbara; **Diane Hughes,** New York University; **Stephen Hupp,** Southern Illinois University–Edwardsville; **Vera John-Steiner,** University of New Mexico; **Helen L. Johnson,** Queens College; **Kathy E. Johnson,** Indiana University–Purdue University, Indianapolis; **Seth Kalichman,** Loyola University; **Kenneth Kallio,** SUNY–Geneseo; **Maria Kalpidou,** Assumption College; **Daniel W. Kee,** California State University–Fullerton; **Christy Kimpo,** University of Washington; **Melvyn B. King,** SUNY–Cortland; **Claire Kopp,** UCLA; **Deanna Kuhn,** Columbia University; **John Kulig,** Northern Illinois University; **Janice Kupersmidt,** University of North Carolina; **Michael Lamb,** National Institute of Child Health and Human Development; **Daniel K. Lapsley,** University of Notre Dame; **Michael Lewis,** Rutgers University; **David B. Liberman,** University of Houston; **Robert Lickliter,** Florida International University; **Hsin-Hui Lin,** University of Houston–Victoria; **Marianna Footo Linz,** Marshall University; **Gretchen S. Lovas,** Susquehanna University; **Pamela Ludemann,** Framingham State College; **Kevin MacDonald,** California State University–Long Beach; **Virginia A. Marchman,** University of Texas at Dallas; **Saramma T. Mathew,** Troy State University; **Barbara McCombs,** University of Denver; **Dottie McCrossen,** University of Ottawa; **Sheryll Mennicke,** Concordia College, St. Paul; **Carolyn Meyer,** Lake Sumter Community College; **Dalton Miller-Jones,** NE Foundation for Children; **Marilyn Moore,** Illinois State University; **Carrie Mori,** Boise State University; **Brad Morris,** Grand Valley State University; **Winnie Mucherah,** Ball State University; **John P. Murray,** Kansas State University; **Dara Musher-Eizenman,** Bowling Green State University; **José E. Nanes,** University of Minnesota; **Sherry J. Neal,** Oklahoma City Community College; **Larry Nucci,** University of Illinois at Chicago; **Daniel J. O'Neill,** Briston Community College; **Randall E. Osborne,** Southwest Texas State University; **Margaret Owen,** University of Texas at Dallas; **Robert Pasnak,** George Mason University; **Barbara Aldis Patton,** University of Houston–Victoria; **Judy Payne,** Murray State University; **Elizabeth Pemberton,** University of Delaware; **Herb Pick,** University of Minnesota; **Kathy Lee Pillow,** Arkansas State University, Beebe; **Nan Ratner,** University of Maryland; **Brenda Reimer,** Southern Missouri State University; **John Reiser,** Vanderbilt University; **Cynthia Rickert,** Dominican College; **Cosby Steele Rogers,** Virginia Polytechnic Institute and State University; **Kimberly A. Gordon Rouse,** Ohio State University; **Jaynati Roy,** Southern Connecticut State University; **Kenneth Rubin,** University of Maryland; **Donna Ruiz,** University of Cincinnati; **Alan Russell,** Flinders University; **Carolyn Saarni,** Sonoma State University; **Douglas B. Sawin,** University of Texas, Austin; **Krista Schoenfeld,** Colby Community College; **Ed Scholwinski,** Southwest Texas State University; **Dale Schunk,** Purdue University; **Bill M. Seay,** Louisiana State University; **Matthew J. Sharps,** California State University, Fresno; **Marilyn Shea,** University of Maine, Farmington; **Susan Shonk,** SUNY–College of Brockport; **Susan Siaw,** California Polytechnic Institute–Pomona; **Robert Siegler,** Carnegie Mellon University; **Evelyn D. Silva,** Cosumnes River College; **Mildred D. Similton,** Pfeiffer University; **Dorothy Justus Sluss,** Virginia Polytechnic Institute and State University; **Janet Spence,** University of Texas–Austin; **Melanie Spence,** University of Texas–Dallas; **Richard Sprott,** California State University, East Bay; **Robert J. Sternberg,** Tufts University; **Mark S. Strauss,** University of Pittsburgh; **Margaret Szewczyk,** University of Chicago; **Ross Thompson,** University of California–Davis; **Donna J. Tyler Thompson,** Midland College; **Marion K. Underwood,** University of Texas–Dallas; **Margot Underwood,** College of DuPage; **Cherie Valeithian,** Kent State University; **Jaan Valsiner,** Clark University; **Robin Yaure,** Pennsylvania State–Mont Alto; **Kourtney Valliancourt,** New Mexico State University; **Elizabeth Vera,** Loyola University–Chicago; **Lawrence Walker,** University of British Columbia; **Kimberlee L. Whaley,** Ohio State University; **Belinda M. Wholeben,** Northern Illinois University; **Frederic Wynn,** County College of Morris.

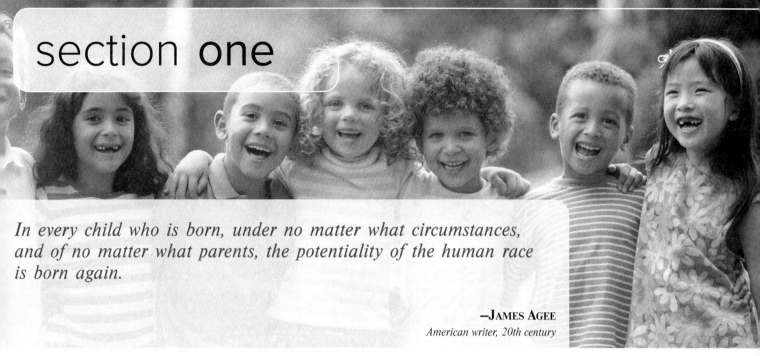

In every child who is born, under no matter what circumstances, and of no matter what parents, the potentiality of the human race is born again.

—JAMES AGEE
American writer, 20th century

The Nature of Child Development

Examining the shape of childhood allows us to understand it better. Every childhood is distinct, the first chapter of a new biography in the world. *Child Development* is about children's development, its universal features, its individual variations, its nature during the twenty-first century. It is about the rhythm and meaning of children's lives, about turning mystery into understanding, and about weaving together a portrait of who each of us was, is, and will be. In Section 1, you will read one chapter: "Introduction."

INTRODUCTION

chapter outline

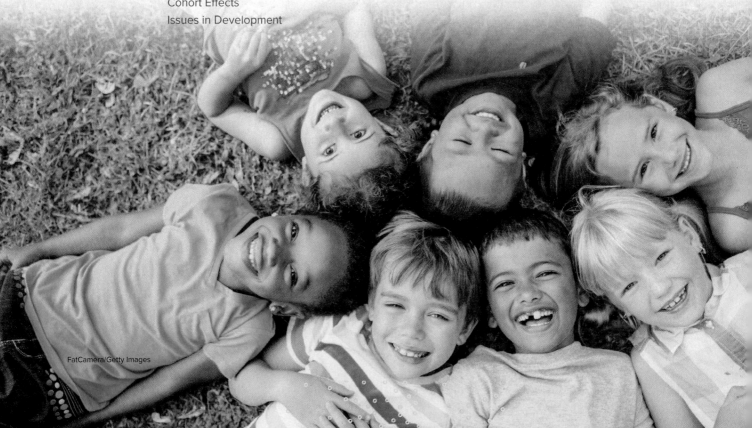

FatCamera/Getty Images

Ted Kaczynski sprinted through high school, not bothering with his junior year and making only passing efforts at social contact. Off to Harvard at age 16, Kaczynski was a loner during his college years. One of his roommates at Harvard said that he avoided people by quickly shuffling by them and slamming the door behind him. After obtaining his Ph.D. in mathematics at the University of Michigan, Kaczynski became a professor at the University of California at Berkeley. His colleagues there remember him as hiding from social circumstances—no friends, no allies, no networking.

After several years at Berkeley, Kaczynski resigned and moved to a rural area of Montana, where he lived as a hermit in a crude shack for 25 years. Town residents described him as a bearded eccentric. Kaczynski traced his own difficulties to growing up as a genius in a kid's body and sticking out like a sore thumb in his surroundings as a child. In 1996, he was arrested and charged as the notorious Unabomber, America's most wanted killer. Over the course of 17 years, Kaczynski had sent 16 mail bombs that left 23 people wounded or maimed and 3 people dead. In 1998, he pleaded guilty to the offenses and was sentenced to life in prison.

A decade before Kaczynski mailed his first bomb, Alice Walker spent her days battling racism in Mississippi. She had recently won her first writing fellowship, but rather than use the money to follow her dream of moving to Senegal, Africa, she put herself into the heart and heat of the civil rights movement. Walker had grown up knowing the brutal effects of poverty and racism. Born in 1944, she was the eighth child of Georgia sharecroppers who earned $300 a year. When Walker was 8, her brother accidentally shot her in the left eye with a BB gun. Since her parents had no car, it took them a week to get her to a hospital. By the time she received medical care, she was blind in that eye, and it had developed a disfiguring layer of scar tissue. Despite the counts against her, Walker overcame pain and anger and went on to win a Pulitzer Prize for her book *The Color Purple*. She became not only a novelist but also an essayist, a poet, a short-story writer, and a social activist.

What leads one individual, so full of promise, to commit brutal acts of violence and another to turn poverty and trauma into a rich literary harvest? If you have ever wondered why people turn out the way they do, you have asked yourself the central question we will explore in this edition.

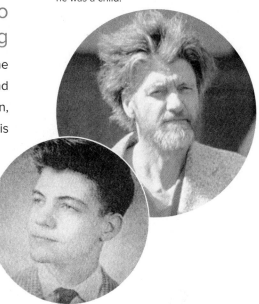

Ted Kaczynski, the convicted Unabomber, traced his difficulties to growing up as a genius in a kid's body and not fitting in when he was a child.

Ted Kaczynski, about age 15–16.

(*top*): Seanna O'Sullivan; (*bottom*): WBBM-TV/AFP/Getty Images

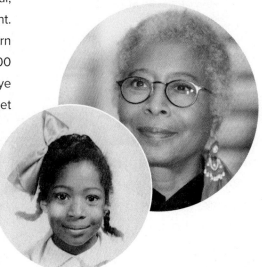

Alice Walker won the Pulitzer Prize for her book *The Color Purple*. Like the characters in her book, Walker overcame pain and anger to triumph and celebrate the human spirit.

Alice Walker, about age 8.

(*top*): Monica Morgan/WireImage/Getty Images; (*bottom*): Courtesy of Alice Walker

preview

Why study children? Perhaps you are or will be a parent or teacher, and responsibility for children is or will be a part of your everyday life. The more you learn about children and the way researchers study them, the better you can guide them. Perhaps you hope to gain an understanding of your own history—as an infant, as a child, and as an adolescent. Perhaps you accidentally came across the course description and found it intriguing. Whatever your reasons, you will discover that the study of child development is provocative, intriguing, and informative. In this first chapter, we will explore historical views and the modern study of child development, consider why caring for children is so important, examine the nature of development, and outline how science helps us to understand it.

Caring for Children Identify five areas in which children's lives need to be improved, and explain the roles of resilience and social policy in children's development.

> Improving the Lives of Children

> Resilience, Social Policy, and Children's Development

What do we mean when we speak of an individual's development? **Development** is the pattern of change that begins at conception and continues through the life span. Most development involves growth, although it also includes decline. Anywhere you turn today, the development of children captures public attention.

Caring for children is an important theme of this text. To understand why caring for children is so important, we will explore why it is beneficial to study children's development, identify some areas in which children's lives need to be improved, and explore the roles of resilience and social policy in children's development.

IMPROVING THE LIVES OF CHILDREN

If you were to read the headlines in any newsfeed or magazine, you might see information like this: "Political Views May Be Written in the Genes," "Mother Accused of Tossing Children into Bay," "Gender Gap Widens," and "FDA Warns About ADHD Drug." Researchers are examining these and many other topics of contemporary concern. The roles that health and well-being, parenting, education, and cultural contexts play in child development, as well as how social policy is related to these issues, are a particular focus of this edition.

Health and Well-Being   Does a pregnant woman endanger her fetus if she has a few beers a week? How does a poor diet affect a child's behaviors and learning skills? Are children less physically active today than in the past? What roles do parents and peers play in whether adolescents abuse drugs? Throughout this edition, we will discuss many questions like these regarding psychological and physical health and well-being.

Health professionals today recognize the power of lifestyles and psychological factors in children's health and well-being (Asarnow & others, 2017). In every chapter, issues of health and well-being are integrated into our discussion.

Clinical psychologists are among the health professionals who help people improve their well-being. In *Connecting with Careers,* you can read about clinical psychologist Gustavo Medrano, who helps adolescents with problems. The Careers Appendix following this chapter describes the education and training required to become a clinical psychologist or to pursue other careers in child development.

Parenting   Are young children harmed if both parents work outside the home? Does spanking have negative consequences for a child's development? Is parental divorce damaging to children's mental health? Do the gender and sexual orientation of parents affect children's development? The answers to potentially controversial questions like these

Children are the legacy we leave for the time we will not live to see.

—ARISTOTLE
Greek philosopher, 4th century B.C.

We reach backward to our parents and forward to our children to a future we will never see, but about which we need to care.

—CARL JUNG
Swiss psychoanalyst, 20th century

development The pattern of movement or change that begins at conception and continues through the life span.

Gustavo Medrano, Clinical Psychologist

Gustavo Medrano specializes in helping children, adolescents, and adults of all ages improve their lives when they have problems involving depression, anxiety, emotion regulation, chronic health conditions, and life transitions. He works individually with clients and also provides therapy for couples and families. As a native Spanish speaker, he also provides bicultural and bilingual therapy for clients.

Dr. Medrano is a faculty member at the Family Institute at Northwestern University in Evanston, Illinois. He obtained his undergraduate degree in psychology at Northwestern and then became a high school teacher through Teach for America, a program where participants spend at least two years teaching in a high-poverty area. He received his master's and doctoral degrees in clinical psychology at the University of Wisconsin–Milwaukee. As a faculty member at Northwestern, he does clinical therapy with clients and conducts research focusing on how family experiences, especially parenting, influence children's and adolescents' ability to cope with chronic pain and other challenges.

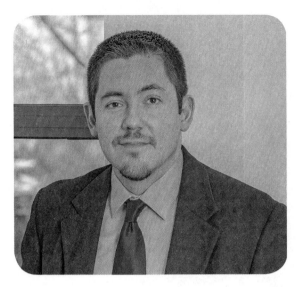

Gustavo Medrano, clinical psychologist, provides therapy for children, adolescents, and adults. His bilingual background and skills help him to work effectively with Latino clients.
Avis Mandel Pictures

For more information about what clinical psychologists do, see the Careers in Child Development appendix that directly follows this chapter.

reflect pressures on the contemporary family (Fiese, 2018). We'll examine these questions and others in order to understand factors that influence parents' lives and their effectiveness in raising their children. Another major emphasis in this edition is the ways in which parents and other adults make a positive difference in children's lives.

You might already be a parent or plan to become one someday. You understand the importance of rearing your children, because they are the future of our society and world. "Good parenting" takes time and effort. If you plan to become a parent, commit yourself day after day, week after week, month after month, and year after year to providing your children with a warm, supportive, safe, and stimulating environment that will make them feel secure and allow them to reach their full potential as human beings. The poster on this page that states "Children learn to love when they are loved" reflects this important goal.

Understanding the nature of children's development can help you become a better parent (Grusec & others, 2013). Many parents learn parenting practices from their parents. Unfortunately, when parenting practices and child-care strategies are passed from one generation to the next, both desirable and undesirable ones are usually perpetuated. This edition and your instructor's lectures in this course can help you become more knowledgeable about children's development. This will help you understand your own upbringing and decide which practices you should continue or abandon.

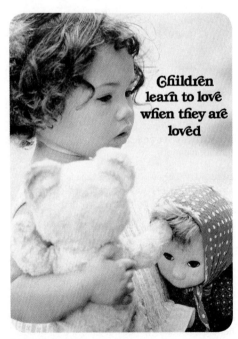

Children learn to love when they are loved

Robert Maust/Photo Agora

Education   There is widespread agreement that society needs to continuously improve education for all children (Darling-Hammond, 2018; McCombs, 2013). There are many questions involved in improving schools: Are U.S. schools teaching children to be ethical and moral individuals? How are schools faring with teaching, reading, writing, and calculating? Should there be more accountability in schools, with adequacy of student learning and teaching examined using assessments and other data? Should schools challenge students more? Should schools focus only on developing children's knowledge and cognitive

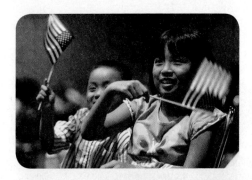

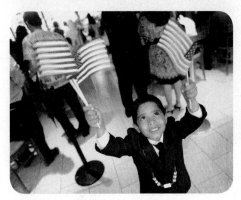

(*Top*) These two Korean-born children on the day they became U.S. citizens represent the dramatic increase in the percentage of ethnic minority children in the United States. (*Bottom*) Inderjeet Poolust, 5, from India celebrates being one of 27 schoolchildren who recently became U.S. citizens at an induction ceremony in Queens, New York.
Zuma Press Inc./Alamy Stock Photo; Debbie Egan-Chin/NY Daily News Archive/Getty Images

context The settings, influenced by historical, economic, social, and cultural factors, in which development occurs.

culture The behavior patterns, beliefs, and all other products of a group that are passed on from generation to generation.

cross-cultural studies Comparisons of one culture with one or more other cultures. These provide information about the degree to which children's development is similar, or universal, across cultures, and the degree to which it is culture-specific.

ethnicity A characteristic based on cultural heritage, nationality, race, religion, and language.

socioeconomic status (SES) Categorization based on a person's occupational, educational, and economic characteristics.

gender The characteristics of people as males and females.

skills, or should they pay more attention to the whole child and consider the child's socioemotional and physical development as well? In this text, we will examine such questions about the state of education in the United States and consider recent research on solutions to educational challenges.

Sociocultural Contexts and Diversity   Health and well-being, parenting, and education—like development itself—are all shaped by their sociocultural context (Bennett, 2012; Gauvain, 2013). The term **context** refers to the settings in which development occurs. These settings are influenced by historical, economic, social, and cultural factors (Gauvain, 2013; Legare & Harris, 2016). Four contexts that we address in this edition are culture, ethnicity, socioeconomic status, and gender.

Culture encompasses the behavior patterns, beliefs, and all other products of a specific group of people that are passed on from generation to generation. Culture results from the interaction of people over many years (Gauvain, 2013). A cultural group can be as large as the United States or as small as a single rural Appalachian town. Whatever its size, the group's culture influences the behavior of its members. **Cross-cultural studies** compare aspects of two or more cultures. The comparison measures the degree to which development is similar, or universal, across cultures, or is instead culture-specific (Lansford & others, 2016; Mistry, Contreras, & Dutta, 2013).

Ethnicity (the word *ethnic* comes from the Greek word for "nation") is rooted in cultural heritage, nationality, race, religion, and language. African Americans, Latinos and Latinas, Asian Americans, Native Americans, Polish Americans, and Italian Americans are a few examples of ethnic groups in the United States. Diversity exists within each ethnic group (Desmet, Ortuño-Ortin, & Wacziarg, 2017), contradicting commonly held stereotypes. Of particular concern is the discrimination and prejudice experienced by ethnic minority youth (Benner, 2017).

Socioeconomic status (SES) refers to a person's position within society based on occupational, educational, and economic characteristics. Socioeconomic status implies certain inequalities. Generally, members of a society have (1) occupations that vary in prestige, with some individuals having more access than others to higher-status occupations; (2) different levels of educational attainment, with some individuals having more access than others to advanced education; (3) different economic resources; and (4) different levels of power to influence a community's institutions. These differences in SES produce unequal opportunities (Doob, 2015).

Gender is another key dimension of children's development. **Gender** refers to the characteristics of people as males and females. Few aspects of our development are more central to our identity and social relationships than gender (Hyde & Else-Quest, 2017; Leaper, 2013). How you view yourself, your relationships with other people, your life, and your goals are shaped to a great extent by your gender and how your culture defines gender roles (Wood & Eagly, 2015).

In the United States, the sociocultural context is continuously becoming more and more diverse (Craig, Rucker, & Richeson, 2018). The U.S. population includes a greater variety of cultures and ethnic groups than ever before. This changing demographic tapestry promises not only the richness that diversity produces but also difficult challenges in extending the American dream to all individuals (Schaefer, 2015). We will discuss sociocultural contexts and diversity in each chapter. In addition, *Connecting with Diversity*, which highlights an issue related to diversity, appears in every chapter. The *Connecting with Diversity* interlude on the next page focuses on gender, families, and children's development around the world.

RESILIENCE, SOCIAL POLICY, AND CHILDREN'S DEVELOPMENT

Some children develop confidence in their abilities despite negative stereotypes about their gender or their ethnic group, and some children triumph over poverty or other adversities. They show *resilience*. Think back to the chapter-opening story about Alice Walker. In spite

Gender, Families, and Children's Development

Around the world, the experiences of female children and adolescents continue to be quite different from those of males (Mistry, Contreras, & Dutta, 2013; UNICEF, 2012). For example, one analysis that is still relevant today found that a higher percentage of girls than boys around the world have never had any education (UNICEF, 2004) (see Figure 1). The countries with the fewest females being educated are in Africa, where girls and women in some areas receive no education at all. Canada, the United States, and Russia have the highest percentages of educated women. In developing countries, 67 percent of women over the age of 25 (compared with 50 percent of men) have never been to school. At the beginning of the twenty-first century, 80 million more boys than girls were in primary and secondary educational settings around the world (United Nations, 2002).

A special cross-cultural concern is the educational and psychological conditions of females around the world (UNICEF, 2012). Inadequate educational opportunities, violence, and mental health issues are just some of the problems faced by many females.

In many countries, adolescent females have less freedom to pursue a variety of careers and engage in various leisure acts than males (Helgeson, 2009; UNICEF, 2012). Gender differences in sexual expression are widespread, especially in India, Southeast Asia, Latin America, and Arab countries, where there are far more restrictions on the sexual activity of adolescent females than males. In certain areas around the world, these gender differences do appear to be narrowing over time. In some countries, educational and career opportunities for women are expanding, and in some parts of the world control over adolescent girls' romantic and sexual relationships is weakening. However, in many countries females still experience considerable discrimination, and much work is needed to bridge the gap between the rights of males and females.

Consider Dhaka, Bangladesh, where sewers overflow, garbage rots in the streets, and children are undernourished. Nearly two-thirds of the young women in Bangladesh get married before they are 18. Doly Akter, age 17, who lives in a slum in Dhaka, created an organization supported by UNICEF in which girls go door-to-door to monitor the hygiene habits of households in their neighborhood. The girls' monitoring has led to improved hygiene and health in the families. Also, the organization Doly formed has managed to stop several child marriages by meeting with parents and convincing them that early marriage is not in their daughter's best interests. When talking with parents in their neighborhoods, the girls in the organization emphasize how staying in school will improve their daughter's future. Doly says the girls in her organization are far more aware of their rights than their mothers were (UNICEF, 2007).

What health and well-being, parenting, and educational problems and interventions have affected the development of females worldwide?

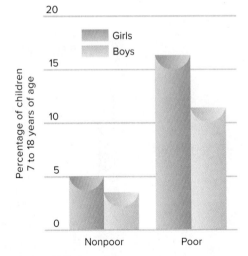

FIGURE 1

PERCENTAGE OF CHILDREN 7 TO 18 YEARS OF AGE AROUND THE WORLD WHO HAVE NEVER BEEN TO SCHOOL OF ANY KIND. When UNICEF (2004) surveyed the education that children around the world are receiving, it found that far more girls than boys receive no formal schooling at all.

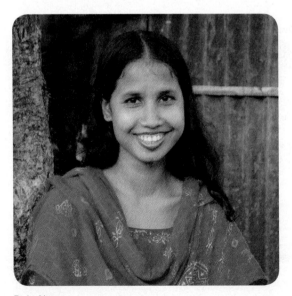

Doly Akter
Naser Siddique/UNICEF Bangladesh

developmental **connection**

Peers

Peers especially play an important role in gender development during childhood. Connect to "Gender."

developmental **connection**

Socioeconomic Status

An increasing number of studies show that positive outcomes can be achieved by intervening in the lives of children experiencing poverty conditions. Connect to "Culture and Diversity."

Ah! What would the world be to us
If the children were no more?
We should dread the desert
behind us
Worse than the dark before.

—Henry Wadsworth Longfellow

American poet, 19th century

social policy A government's course of action designed to promote the welfare of its citizens.

of racism, poverty, low socioeconomic status, and a disfiguring eye injury, she went on to become a successful author and champion for equality.

Are there certain characteristics that make children like Alice Walker resilient? Are there other characteristics that make children lash out against society, like Ted Kaczynski, who became a killer despite his intelligence and education? Extensive research on this topic (Masten & Cicchetti, 2016) concludes that a number of individual factors, such as good self-control and intellectual functioning, influence resiliency. In addition, as Figure 2 shows, resources within and outside of resilient children's families tend to show certain features. For example, resilient children are likely to have a close relationship to a caring parent figure and bonds to caring adults outside the family.

Should governments also take action to improve the contexts of children's development and aid their resilience? **Social policy** is a government's course of action designed to promote the welfare of its citizens. The shape and scope of social policy related to children are tied to the political and economic system. The values held by citizens and elected officials, the nation's economic strengths and weaknesses, and partisan politics all influence the policy agenda.

Out of concern that policy makers are doing too little to protect the well-being of children, researchers increasingly are undertaking studies that they hope will lead to wise and effective decision making about social policy around the world (Yousafzai & others, 2018). Children who grow up in poverty represent a special concern, because of the lifelong effects on development. In 2016, 18 percent of U.S. children and adolescents were living in families with household incomes below the federal poverty line, with African American and Latino or Latina families with children and adolescents having especially high rates of poverty (27 to 30 percent) (U.S. Census Bureau, 2017a). These poverty rates for all children are slightly below the 50-year peak of 22.7 percent of all children in 1993. As indicated in Figure 3, one classic study found that a higher percentage of U.S. children in poor families than in middle-income families were exposed to family turmoil, separation from a parent, violence, crowding, excessive noise, and poor housing (Evans & English, 2002). One recent study revealed that the years children spend living in poverty, when household chaos and family conflict are also present, are linked with hormonal measures of stress (Doom & others, 2018).

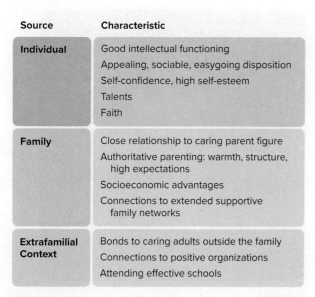

FIGURE 2

CHARACTERISTICS OF RESILIENT CHILDREN AND THEIR CONTEXTS

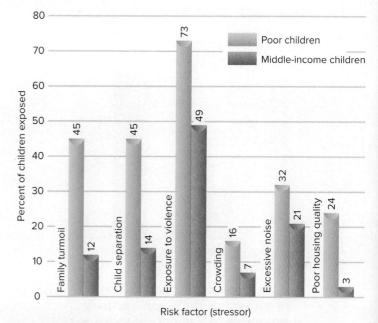

FIGURE 3

EXPOSURE TO SIX STRESSORS AMONG POOR AND MIDDLE-INCOME CHILDREN. One study analyzed the exposure to six stressors among poor children and middle-income children (Evans & English, 2002). Poor children were much more likely to face each of these stressors.

The U.S. figure of 18 percent of children living in poverty in 2016 is much higher than those from other industrialized nations. The average is 13 percent among the 36 members of the Organization for Economic Cooperation and Development, ranging from 3 percent in Denmark to 33 percent in China (OECD, 2018).

What can we do to lessen the effect of these stressors on children and those who care for them? Strategies for improving the lives of children include improving social policy for families (Doob, 2015; Duncan & others, 2012). In the United States, the national government, state governments, and city governments all play a role in influencing the well-being of children. When families fail or seriously endanger a child's well-being, governments often step in to help.

At the national and state levels, policymakers for decades have debated whether helping poor parents ends up helping their children as well. Researchers are providing some answers by examining the effects of specific policies (Sherman & Mitchell, 2017). For example, the Minnesota Family Investment Program (MFIP) was designed in the 1990s primarily to influence the behavior of adults—specifically, to move adults off income assistance into paid employment. A key element of the program was that it guaranteed that adults participating in the program would receive more income if they worked than if they did not. When the adults' income rose, how did that affect their children?

A study of the effects of MFIP found that increases in the incomes of working poor parents were linked with benefits for their children (Gennetian & Miller, 2002). The MFIP was one of many similar interventions and studies. These have shown that increasing family income sometimes does not have an effect, but often it does. These effects are reflected in decreases in children's exposure to risks to their development (for example, abuse, maternal depression), and increases in positive influences on their development (for example, safety, cognitive stimulation, sensitive parenting) (Cooper & Stewart, 2017).

A recent large-scale effort to help children escape from poverty is the *Ascend* two-generation education intervention being conducted by the Aspen Institute (2018). The focus of the intervention emphasizes education (increasing postsecondary education for mothers and improving the quality of their children's early childhood education), economic support (housing, transportation, financial education, health insurance, and food assistance), and social capital (peer support including friends and neighbors; participation in community and faith-based organizations; school and work contacts).

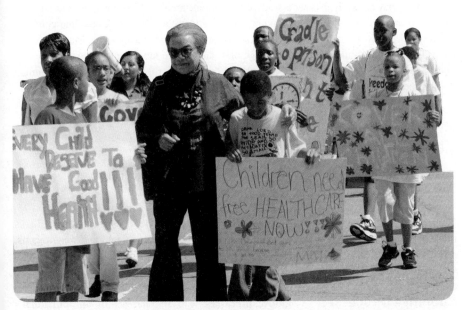

Marian Wright Edelman, president of the Children's Defense Fund (shown here interacting with young children), has been a tireless advocate of children's rights and has been instrumental in calling attention to the needs of children. *What are some of these needs?*
Courtesy of the Children's Defense Fund

Developmental psychologists and other researchers have examined the effects of many other government policies. They are seeking ways to help families living in poverty improve their well-being, and they have offered many suggestions for improving government policies (Cooper & Stewart, 2017; Duncan & others, 2012).

Review *Connect* Reflect

LG1 Identify five areas in which children's lives need to be improved, and explain the roles of resilience and social policy in children's development.

Review

- What are several aspects of children's development that need to be improved?
- What characterizes resilience in children's development? What is social policy, and how can it influence children's lives?

Connect

- How is the concept of resilience related to the story you read at the beginning of this chapter?

Reflect *Your Own Personal Journey of Life*

- Imagine what your development as a child would have been like in a culture that offered choices that were different from your own. How might your development have been different if your family had been significantly richer or poorer than it was as you were growing up?

Developmental Processes, Periods, and Issues

 LG2 Discuss the most important processes, periods, and issues in development.

| Biological, Cognitive, and Socioemotional Processes | Periods of Development | Cohort Effects | Issues in Development |

Each of us develops in certain ways like *all* other individuals, like *some* other individuals, and like *no* other individuals. Most of the time, our attention is directed to a person's uniqueness, but psychologists who study development are drawn to both our shared characteristics and those that make us unique. As humans, we all have traveled some common paths. Each of us—Leonardo da Vinci, Joan of Arc, George Washington, Martin Luther King, Jr., and you—walked at about the age of 1, engaged in fantasy play as a young child, and became more independent as a youth. What shapes this common path of human development, and what are its milestones?

BIOLOGICAL, COGNITIVE, AND SOCIOEMOTIONAL PROCESSES

The pattern of human development is created by the interplay of three key processes. They are biological, cognitive, and socioemotional in nature.

Biological Processes **Biological processes** produce changes in an individual's body. Genes inherited from parents, the development of the brain, height and weight gains, growth in motor skills, and hormonal changes during puberty all reflect the role of biological processes in development.

Cognitive Processes **Cognitive processes** lead to changes in an individual's thoughts, intelligence, and language. The tasks of watching a mobile swinging above a crib, putting together a two-word sentence, memorizing a poem, solving a math problem, and imagining what it would be like to be a movie star all involve cognitive processes.

biological processes Changes in an individual's body.

cognitive processes Changes in an individual's thinking, intelligence, and language skills.

Socioemotional Processes **Socioemotional processes** produce changes in relationships with other people, emotions, and personality. An infant's smile in response to her mother's touch, a toddler's attack on a playmate, a third-grader's development of assertiveness, and an adolescent's joy at the senior prom all reflect socioemotional development.

Connecting Biological, Cognitive, and Socioemotional Processes Biological, cognitive, and socioemotional processes are deeply intertwined (Diamond, 2013). Consider a baby smiling in response to a parent's touch. This response depends on biological processes (the physical nature of touch and responsiveness to it), cognitive processes (the ability to understand intentional acts of others), and socioemotional processes (smiling often reflects positive emotional feelings and helps connect us in positive ways with others). The connection across biological, cognitive, and socioemotional processes is most obvious in two rapidly emerging research fields:

- *developmental cognitive neuroscience,* which explores links between development, cognitive processes, and the brain (Johnson & de Haan, 2015)
- *developmental social neuroscience,* which examines connections between development, socioemotional processes, and the brain (Decety & Cowell, 2016)

Biological, cognitive, and socioemotional processes interact and can influence each other. For example, biological processes can influence cognitive processes and vice versa. Thus, although usually we will examine the processes of development (biological, cognitive, and socioemotional) separately rather than together, keep in mind that this discussion is referring to the development of an integrated individual with a mind and body that are interdependent (see Figure 4).

In many places throughout the chapters, we will call attention to connections between biological, cognitive, and socioemotional processes. A feature titled *Developmental Connection* appears multiple times in each chapter to highlight these as well as other content connections earlier or later in the text.

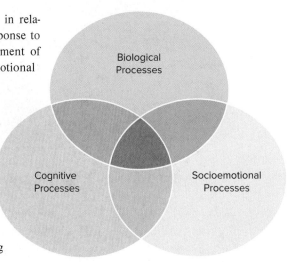

FIGURE **4**

CHANGES IN DEVELOPMENT ARE THE RESULT OF BIOLOGICAL, COGNITIVE, AND SOCIOEMOTIONAL PROCESSES. The processes interact as individuals develop.

developmental **connection**

Biological Processes

Can specific genes be linked to specific environmental experiences? Connect to "Biological Beginnings."

PERIODS OF DEVELOPMENT

For purposes of organization and understanding, a child's growth is commonly described in terms of developmental periods that correspond to specific age ranges. The most widely used classification of developmental periods includes the following sequence: the prenatal period, infancy, early childhood, middle and late childhood, and adolescence.

The **prenatal period** is the time from conception to birth, roughly a nine-month period. During this amazing time, a single cell grows into a fetus and then a baby, complete with a brain and a vast range of capabilities.

Infancy is the developmental period that extends from birth to about 18 to 24 months of age. Infancy is a time of extreme dependence on adults. Many psychological activities are just beginning—the abilities to speak, to coordinate sensations and physical actions, to think with symbols, and to imitate and learn from others.

Early childhood is the developmental period that extends from the end of infancy to about 5 or 6 years of age; sometimes this period is called the preschool years. During this time, young children learn to become more self-sufficient, they develop school readiness skills (following instructions, identifying letters), and they spend many hours in play and with peers. First grade typically marks the end of this period.

Middle and late childhood is the developmental period between about 6 and 11 years of age; sometimes this period is referred to as the elementary school years. Children master the fundamental skills of reading, writing, and arithmetic, and they are formally exposed to the larger world and its cultures. Achievement becomes a more central theme of the child's world, and self-control increases.

socioemotional processes Changes in an individual's interpersonal relationships, emotions, and personality.

prenatal period The time from conception to birth.

infancy The developmental period that extends from birth to about 18 to 24 months.

early childhood The developmental period that extends from the end of infancy to about 5 or 6 years of age, sometimes called the preschool years.

middle and late childhood The developmental period that extends from about 6 to 11 years of age, sometimes called the elementary school years.

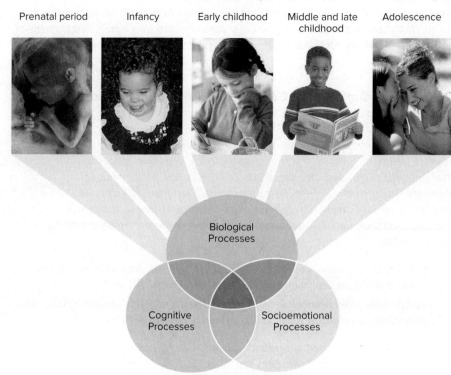

Periods of Development

Prenatal period | Infancy | Early childhood | Middle and late childhood | Adolescence

Biological Processes

Cognitive Processes

Socioemotional Processes

Processes of Development

FIGURE 5

PROCESSES AND PERIODS OF DEVELOPMENT. Development moves through the prenatal, infancy, early childhood, middle and late childhood, and adolescence periods. These periods of development are the result of interacting biological, cognitive, and socioemotional processes.

(*Left to right*): Steve Allen/Getty Images; Courtesy of Dr. John Santrock; Laurence Mouton/PhotoAlto/Getty Images; Ken Karp/McGraw-Hill Education; SW Productions/Brand X Pictures/Getty Images

Adolescence is the developmental period of transition from childhood to early adulthood, beginning at approximately 10 to 12 years of age and ending at about 18 to 19 years of age. Adolescence begins with rapid physical changes—dramatic gains in height and weight; changes in body shape; and the development of sexual characteristics such as enlargement of the breasts and widening of the hips, growth of pubic and facial hair, and deepening of the voice. The pursuit of independence and an identity are prominent features of this period of development, although this varies widely by culture. More and more time is spent outside the family. Thought becomes more abstract, idealistic, and logical.

Today, developmental psychologists do not believe that change ends with adolescence (Bornstein, 2018; Somerville & others, 2018). They describe development as a lifelong process. However, the purpose of this text is to describe the changes in development that take place from conception through adolescence. All of these periods of development are produced by the interplay of biological, cognitive, and socioemotional processes (see Figure 5).

COHORT EFFECTS

In addition to considering developmental periods that emerge and change with age, we also must consider when in time and history a group of people were born and grew up. A *cohort* is a group of people who are born at a similar point in history and share similar experiences as a result, such as growing up in the same city around the same time. These shared experiences can produce differences in development between cohorts (Halfon & Forrest, 2018). For example, adults who grew up during the Great Depression and World War II are likely to differ from their counterparts who grew up during the economically booming 1990s in their educational opportunities and economic status, in how they were raised, their attitudes and

adolescence The developmental period of transition from childhood to early adulthood, entered at approximately 10 to 12 years of age and ending at 18 or 19 years of age.

experiences related to gender, and their exposure to technology. In research on development, **cohort effects** are due to a person's time of birth, era, or generation but not to actual age.

Generations have been given labels by the popular culture. The most recent agreed-upon label is **millennials,** referring to the generation born after 1980—the first to come of age and enter emerging adulthood in the new millennium. Thus, today's children and many of their parents are millennials. Two characteristics of millennials stand out: (1) their ethnic diversity, and (2) their connection to technology (US Census Bureau, 2015).

As their ethnic diversity has increased over prior generations, many millennial adolescents and emerging adults are more tolerant and open-minded than their counterparts in previous generations (Frey, 2018).

Another major cohort change involving millennials is the dramatic increase in their use of media and technology (Medoff & Kaye, 2017). According to one analysis, the millennials were

> . . . history's first "always connected" generation. Steeped in digital technology and social media, they treat their multi-tasking hand-held gadgets almost like a body part—for better or worse. More than 8-in-10 say they sleep with a cell phone glowing by the bed, poised to disgorge texts, phone calls, e-mails, songs, news, videos, games, and wake-up jingles. But sometimes convenience yields to temptation. Nearly two-thirds admit to texting while driving (Pew Research Center, 2010, p. 1).

We will have much more to say about technology in childhood and adolescence in the "Culture and Diversity" chapter.

ISSUES IN DEVELOPMENT

Was Ted Kaczynski born a killer, or did his life turn him into one? Kaczynski himself thought that his childhood was the root of his troubles. He grew up as a genius in a boy's body and never fit in with other children. Did his early experiences determine his later life? Is your own journey through life marked out ahead of time, or can your experiences change your path? Are experiences that occur early in your journey more important than later ones? Is your journey like taking an elevator up a skyscraper with distinct stops along the way, or more like a boat ride down a river with smoother ebbs and flows? These questions point to three issues about the nature of development: the roles played by nature and nurture, continuity and discontinuity, and early and later experiences.

Nature and Nurture   The **nature-nurture issue** involves an old debate about whether development is primarily influenced by nature or by nurture. *Nature* refers to an organism's biological inheritance, *nurture* to its environmental experiences. Almost no one today argues that development can be explained by nature alone or by nurture alone, because we know they interact and work together in development. However, it is important to understand the history of the old nature-nurture positions. Some ("nature" proponents) claim that the most important influence on development is biological inheritance, and others ("nurture" proponents) claim that environmental experiences are the most important influence.

According to the nature proponents, just as a sunflower grows in an orderly way—unless it is defeated by an unfriendly environment—so does a person. The range of environments can be vast, but evolutionary and genetic foundations produce commonalities in growth and development (Buss, 2018). We walk before we talk, speak one word before two words, grow rapidly in infancy and less so in early childhood, and experience a rush of sexual hormones in puberty. Extreme environments—those that are psychologically barren or hostile—can stunt development, but nature proponents emphasize the influence of tendencies that are genetically wired into humans (Maxson, 2013).

By contrast, others have emphasized the importance of nurture, or environmental experiences, to development (Dweck, 2013). Experiences run the gamut from the individual's biological environment (nutrition, medical care, drugs, and physical accidents) to the social environment (family, peers, schools, community, media, and culture). For example, a child's diet can affect how tall the child grows and even how effectively the child can think and solve problems. Despite their genetic wiring, a child born and raised in a poor

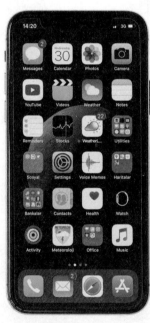

Zeynep Demir/Shutterstock

cohort effects Effects due to a person's time of birth, era, or generation but not to actual age.

millennials The generation born after 1980, the first to come of age and enter emerging adulthood in the new millennium.

nature-nurture issue Debate about whether development is primarily influenced by nature or nurture. The "nature" proponents claim biological inheritance is the most important influence on development; the "nurture" proponents claim that environmental experiences are the most influential factors.

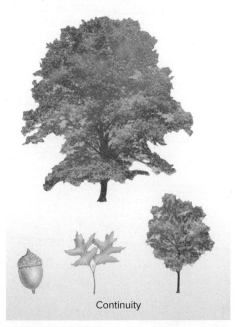

Continuity

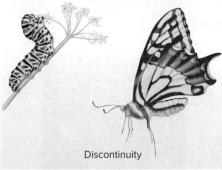

Discontinuity

FIGURE 6

CONTINUITY AND DISCONTINUITY IN DEVELOPMENT. Is human development more like that of a seedling gradually growing into a giant oak or more like that of a caterpillar suddenly becoming a butterfly?

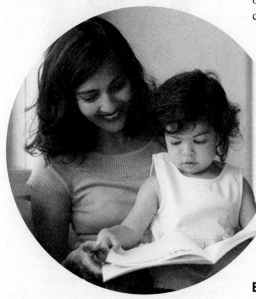

What is the nature of the early and later experience issue?
Photodisc/Stockbyte/Getty Images

village in Bangladesh and a child in the suburbs of Denver are likely to have different skills, different ways of thinking about the world, and different ways of relating to people. Today, we now understand that nature and nurture work together in explaining development.

Continuity and Discontinuity   Think about your own development for a moment. Did you become the person you are gradually, like the seedling that slowly, cumulatively grows into a giant oak? Or did you experience sudden, distinct changes, like the caterpillar that changes into a butterfly (see Figure 6)?

The **continuity-discontinuity issue** focuses on the extent to which development involves gradual, cumulative change (continuity) or distinct stages (discontinuity).

Consider continuity first. As the oak grows from seedling to giant oak, it becomes more oak—its development is continuous. Similarly, a child's first word, though seemingly an abrupt, discontinuous event, is actually the result of weeks and months of growth and practice. Puberty, another seemingly abrupt, discontinuous occurrence, is actually a gradual process occurring over several years.

Viewed in terms of discontinuity, each person is described as passing through a sequence of distinct stages. As the caterpillar changes to a butterfly, it does not become more caterpillar but a different kind of organism—its development is discontinuous. Similarly, at some point a child moves from not being able to think abstractly about the world to being able to do so. This change is a "qualitative," discontinuous change in development, not a "quantitative," continuous change.

Early and Later Experience   The **early-later experience issue** focuses on the degree to which early experiences (especially in infancy) or later experiences are the key determinants of the child's development. That is, if infants experience harmful circumstances, can those experiences be overcome by later, positive ones? Or are the early experiences so critical—possibly because they are the infant's first, essential experiences—that they cannot be overridden by a later, better environment? To those who emphasize early experiences, life is an unbroken trail on which a psychological quality can be traced back to its origin (Kagan, 2013). In contrast, to those who emphasize recent experiences, development is like a river, continually ebbing and flowing.

The early-later experience issue has a long history and continues to be hotly debated among developmental psychologists (Easterbrooks & others, 2013). The philosopher Plato was sure that infants who were rocked frequently became better athletes. Nineteenth-century New England ministers told parents in Sunday afternoon sermons that the way they handled their infants would determine their children's later character. Many developmentalists argue that unless infants and young children experience warm, nurturing care, their development will be compromised (Thompson, 2018).

In contrast, later-experience advocates argue that children readily change throughout development and that later sensitive caregiving is just as important as earlier sensitive caregiving. A number of developmentalists stress that too little attention has been given to later experiences in development (Schaie, 2012). They accept that early experiences are important contributors to development but assert that they are no more important than later experiences. Jerome Kagan (2013) points out that even children who show the qualities of an inhibited temperament, which is linked to heredity, have the capacity to change their behavior. In one classic study, almost one-third of a group of children who had an inhibited temperament at 2 years of age were not unusually shy or fearful when they were 4 years of age (Kagan & Snidman, 1991).

People in Western cultures, especially those influenced by Freudian theory (described later in this chapter), have tended to support the idea that early experiences are more important than later experiences (Fonagy & others, 2016). However, the majority of people in the world may not share this belief because their value systems and histories of psychology have not been heavily influenced by Freudian theory.

Evaluating the Developmental Issues   Most developmental psychologists recognize that it is unwise to take an extreme position on the issues of nature and nurture, continuity and discontinuity, and early and later experiences. Development is not all nature or all nurture, not all continuity or all discontinuity, and not all early or later experiences. Nature and nurture, continuity and discontinuity, and early and later experiences all play a part in development throughout the human life span. Along with this consensus, however, there is still spirited debate about how strongly development is influenced by each of these factors. Are there gender differences in certain skills because of inherited characteristics or because of society's expectations and because of how girls and boys are raised? Can enriched experiences during adolescence remove negative effects on development from poverty, neglect, and poor schooling during early childhood? The answers to these questions have a bearing on social policy decisions about children and adolescents, and consequently on each of our lives.

continuity-discontinuity issue Question about whether development involves gradual, cumulative change (continuity) or distinct stages (discontinuity).

early-later experience issue Controversy regarding the degree to which early experiences (especially during infancy) or later experiences are the key determinants of children's development.

Review *Connect* Reflect

 LG2 Discuss the most important processes, periods, and issues in development.

Review

- What are biological, cognitive, and socioemotional processes?
- What are the main periods of development?
- What are cohort effects?
- What are three important issues in development?

Connect

- Based on what you read earlier in this chapter, what do you think Ted Kaczynski would say about the early-later experience issue?

Reflect *Your Own Personal Journey of Life*

- Can you identify an early experience that you believe contributed in important ways to your development? Can you identify a recent or current (later) experience that you think had (or is having) a strong influence on your development?

The Science of Child Development

 LG3 Summarize why research is important in child development, the main theories of child development, and research methods, designs, and challenges.

| The Importance of Research | Theories of Child Development | Research Methods for Collecting Data | Research Designs | Challenges in Child Development Research |

Some people have difficulty thinking of child development as a science like physics, chemistry, and biology. Can a discipline that studies how parents nurture children, how peers interact, the ways in which children's thinking develops over time, and whether engaging in screen time hour after hour is linked with being overweight, be equated with scientific disciplines that study the molecular structure of a compound and how gravity works? Is child development really a science?

Science refines everyday thinking.

—Albert Einstein
German-born American physicist, 20th century

THE IMPORTANCE OF RESEARCH

The answer to the last question is "yes." Science is defined not by *what* it investigates, but by *how* it investigates. Whether you're studying photosynthesis, butterflies, Saturn's moons, or children's development, it is the way you study your topic that makes the approach scientific or not. How can we determine, for example, whether special care can repair the harm inflicted by child neglect or whether mentoring can improve children's achievement in school?

Scientific research provides the best answers to such questions. *Scientific research* is objective, systematic, and testable. It reduces the likelihood that information will be based on personal beliefs, opinions, and feelings (Stanovich, 2013). In conducting research, child

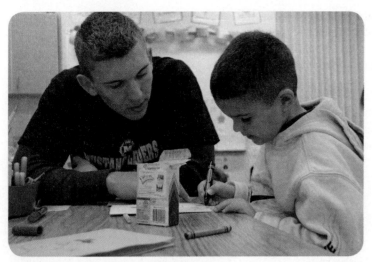

A high school senior mentors a kindergarten child as part of the Book Buddy mentoring program. *If a researcher wanted to study the effects of the mentoring program on children's academic achievement by following the scientific method, what steps would the researcher take in setting up the study?*
St. Petersburg Times/Zuma press inc/Alamy Stock Photo

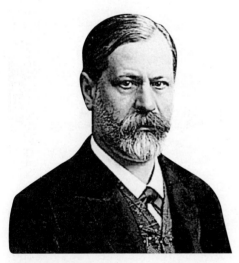

Sigmund Freud, the pioneering architect of psychoanalytic theory. *What are some characteristics of Freud's theory?*
Bettmann/Getty Images

FIGURE 7
FREUDIAN STAGES.

development researchers use the **scientific method**, a four-step process: (1) conceptualize a process or problem to be studied, (2) collect research information (data), (3) analyze data, and (4) draw conclusions.

THEORIES OF CHILD DEVELOPMENT

Theorizing is part of the scientific study of children's development. In the scientific method just described, theories often guide the conceptualization of a process or problem to be studied. A **theory** is an interrelated, coherent set of ideas that helps to explain and to make predictions. For example, a theory on mentoring might attempt to explain and predict why sustained support, guidance, and concrete experience make a difference in the lives of children from impoverished backgrounds. The theory might focus on children's opportunities to model the behavior and strategies of mentors, or it might focus on the effects of individual attention, which might otherwise be missing in the children's lives. A **hypothesis** is a specific, testable assumption or prediction. A hypothesis is often written as an *if-then* statement. In our example, a hypothesis might be: If children from impoverished backgrounds are given individual attention by mentors, then the children will spend more time studying and earn higher grades. Testing a hypothesis can inform researchers whether a theory is likely to be accurate.

Wide-ranging theories make understanding children's development a challenging undertaking. The current section outlines key aspects of five theoretical orientations to development: psychoanalytic, cognitive, behavioral and social cognitive, ethological, and ecological. Each contributes an important piece to the puzzle of understanding children's development. Although the theories disagree about certain aspects of development, many of their ideas are complementary rather than contradictory. Together they let us see the total landscape of children's development in all its richness.

Psychoanalytic Theories **Psychoanalytic theories** describe development as primarily unconscious (beyond awareness) and heavily colored by emotion. Psychoanalytic theorists emphasize that behavior is merely a surface characteristic and that a true understanding of development requires analyzing the symbolic meanings of behavior and the deep inner workings of the mind. Psychoanalytic theorists also stress that early experiences with parents extensively shape development. These characteristics are highlighted in the psychoanalytic theory of Sigmund Freud (1856–1939).

Freud's Theory As Freud listened to, probed, and analyzed his patients, he became convinced that their problems were the result of experiences early in life. He thought that as children grow up, their focus of pleasure and sexual impulses shifts from the mouth to the anus and eventually to the genitals. As a result, we go through five stages of psychosexual development: oral, anal, phallic, latency, and genital (see Figure 7). Our adult personality, Freud (1917) claimed, is determined by the way we resolve conflicts between sources of pleasure and the demands of reality at each stage.

Oral Stage	Anal Stage	Phallic Stage	Latency Stage	Genital Stage
Infant's pleasure centers on the mouth.	Child's pleasure focuses on the anus.	Child's pleasure focuses on the genitals.	Child represses sexual interest and develops social and intellectual skills.	A time of sexual reawakening; source of sexual pleasure becomes someone outside the family.
Birth to 1½ Years	**1½ to 3 Years**	**3 to 6 Years**	**6 Years to Puberty**	**Puberty Onward**

Freud's theory has been significantly revised by a number of psychoanalytic theorists. Many of today's psychoanalytic theorists maintain that Freud overemphasized sexual instincts; they place more emphasis on cultural experiences as determinants of an individual's development. Unconscious thought remains a central theme, but thought plays a greater role than Freud envisioned. Next, we will outline the ideas of an important revisionist of Freud's ideas—Erik Erikson.

Erikson's Psychosocial Theory   Erik Erikson (1902–1994) recognized Freud's contributions but believed that Freud misjudged some important dimensions of human development. For one thing, Erikson (1950, 1968) said we develop in psychosocial stages, rather than in psychosexual stages as Freud maintained. According to Freud, the primary motivation for human behavior is sexual in nature; according to Erikson, it is social and reflects a desire to affiliate with other people. According to Freud, our basic personality is shaped in the first five years of life; according to Erikson, developmental change occurs throughout the life span. Thus, in terms of the early-versus-later-experience issue described earlier in the chapter, Freud viewed early experience as far more important than later experiences, whereas Erikson emphasized the importance of both early and later experiences.

In **Erikson's theory,** eight stages of development unfold as we go through life (see Figure 8). At each stage, a unique developmental task confronts individuals with a crisis that must be resolved. According to Erikson, this crisis is not a catastrophe but a turning point marked by both increased vulnerability and enhanced potential. The more successfully an individual resolves the crises, the healthier development will be.

Trust versus mistrust is Erikson's first psychosocial stage, which is experienced in the first year of life. Trust in infancy sets the stage for a lifelong expectation that the world will be a good and pleasant place to live.

Autonomy versus shame and doubt is Erikson's second stage. This stage occurs in late infancy and toddlerhood (1 to 3 years). After gaining trust in their caregivers, infants begin to discover that their behavior is their own. They start to assert their sense of independence or autonomy. They realize their will. If infants and toddlers are restrained too much or punished too harshly, they are likely to develop a sense of shame and doubt.

Initiative versus guilt, Erikson's third stage of development, occurs during the preschool years. As preschool children encounter a widening social world, they face new challenges that require active, purposeful, responsible behavior. Feelings of guilt may arise, though, if the child is irresponsible and is made to feel too anxious.

Industry versus inferiority is Erikson's fourth developmental stage, occurring approximately in the elementary school years. Children now need to direct their energy toward mastering knowledge and intellectual skills. The negative outcome is that the child may develop a sense of inferiority—feeling incompetent and unproductive.

During adolescence, individuals confront the tasks of finding out who they are, what they are all about, and where they are going in life. This is Erikson's fifth developmental stage, *identity versus identity confusion*. If adolescents explore roles in a healthy manner and arrive at

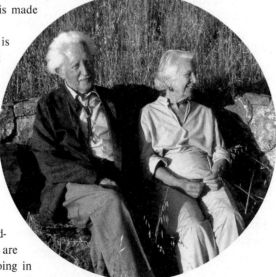

Erik Erikson with his wife, Joan, an artist. Erikson generated one of the most important developmental theories of the twentieth century. *Which stage of Erikson's theory are you in? Does Erikson's description of this stage characterize you?*

Jon Erikson/The Image Works

Erikson's Stages	Developmental Period
Integrity versus despair	Late adulthood (60s onward)
Generativity versus stagnation	Middle adulthood (40s, 50s)
Intimacy versus isolation	Early adulthood (20s, 30s)
Identity versus identity confusion	Adolescence (10 to 20 years)
Industry versus inferiority	Middle and late childhood (elementary school years, 6 years to puberty)
Initiative versus guilt	Early childhood (preschool years, 3 to 5 years)
Autonomy versus shame and doubt	Infancy (1 to 3 years)
Trust versus mistrust	Infancy (first year)

FIGURE 8

ERIKSON'S EIGHT LIFE-SPAN STAGES

scientific method An approach that can be used to obtain accurate information by carrying out four steps: (1) conceptualize the problem, (2) collect data, (3) draw conclusions, and (4) revise research conclusions and theory.

theory An interrelated, coherent set of ideas that helps to explain and make predictions.

hypotheses Specific assumptions and predictions that can be tested to determine their accuracy.

psychoanalytic theories Theories that describe development as primarily unconscious and heavily colored by emotion. Behavior is merely a surface characteristic, and the symbolic workings of the mind have to be analyzed to understand behavior. Early experiences with parents are emphasized.

Erikson's theory Description of eight stages of human development. Each stage consists of a unique developmental task that confronts individuals with a crisis that must be resolved.

caring *connections*

Strategies for Parenting, Educating, and Interacting with Children Based on Erikson's Theory

Parents, child care specialists, teachers, counselors, youth workers, and other adults can adopt positive strategies for interacting with children based on Erikson's theory. These strategies include the following:

1. ***Nurture infants and develop their trust, then encourage and monitor toddlers' autonomy.*** Because infants depend on others to meet their needs, it is critical for caregivers to consistently provide positive, attentive care for infants. Infants who experience consistently positive care feel safe and secure, sensing that people are reliable and loving, which leads them to develop trust in the world. Caregivers who neglect or abuse infants are likely to raise infants who develop a sense of mistrust in their world. After having developed a sense of trust in their world, children moving from infancy into the toddler years should be given the freedom to explore it. Toddlers whose caregivers are too restrictive or harsh are likely to develop shame and doubt, sensing that they can't adequately do things on their own. As toddlers gain more independence, caregivers need to monitor their exploration and curiosity because there are many things that can harm them, such as running into the street or touching a hot stove.

2. ***Encourage initiative in young children.*** Children should be given a great deal of freedom to explore their world. They should be allowed to choose some of the activities they engage in. If their requests for doing certain activities are reasonable, the requests should be honored. Children need to be provided exciting materials that will stimulate their imagination. Young children at this stage love to play. It not only benefits their socioemotional development but also serves as an important medium for their cognitive growth. Criticism should be kept to a minimum so that children will not develop high levels of guilt and anxiety. Young children are going to make lots of mistakes and have lots of spills. They need good models far more than harsh critics. Their activities and environment should be structured for success rather than failure by giving them developmentally appropriate tasks. For example, young children get frustrated when they have to sit for long periods of time and do academic paper-and-pencil tasks.

3. ***Promote industry in elementary school children.*** It was Erikson's hope that teachers could provide an atmosphere in which children would become passionate about learning. In Erikson's words, teachers should mildly but firmly coerce children into the adventure of finding out that they can learn to accomplish things that they themselves would never have thought they could do. In elementary school, children thirst to know. Most arrive at elementary school steeped in curiosity and fueled by a motivation to master tasks. In Erikson's view, it is important for teachers to nourish this motivation for mastery and curiosity. Teachers need to challenge students without overwhelming

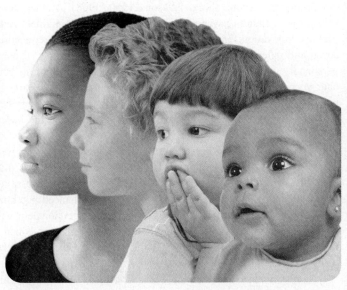

What are some applications of Erikson's theory for effective parenting?

(*Left to right*): Valeriebarry/iStock/Getty Images; Tomas Rodriguez/Corbis/Getty Images; Fuse/Corbis/Getty Images; Image Source/Getty Images

them; be firm in requiring students to be productive, but not be overly critical; and especially be tolerant of honest mistakes and make sure that every student has opportunities for many successes.

4. ***Stimulate identity exploration in adolescence.*** It is important to recognize that the adolescent's identity is multidimensional. Aspects include vocational goals; intellectual achievement; and interests in hobbies, sports, music, and other areas. Adolescents can be asked to write essays about such dimensions, exploring who they are and what they want to do with their lives. They should be encouraged to think independently and to freely express their views, which stimulates their self-exploration. Adolescents can also be encouraged to listen to debates on political and ideological issues, which stimulates them to examine different perspectives. Another good strategy is to encourage adolescents to talk with a school counselor about career options as well as other aspects of their identity. Teachers can invite people in different careers to come into the classroom and talk with their students about their work, regardless of students' grade levels.

In the strategies above, identify what Erikson called the "vulnerability" and the "potential" that adults need to take into account to help children accomplish the tasks of each developmental stage.

a positive path to follow in life, then they achieve a positive identity; if not, identity confusion reigns.

Intimacy versus isolation is Erikson's sixth developmental stage, which individuals experience during early adulthood. At this time, individuals face the developmental task of forming intimate relationships. If young adults form healthy friendships and an intimate relationship with another, intimacy will be achieved; if not, isolation will result.

Generativity versus stagnation, Erikson's seventh developmental stage, occurs during middle adulthood. By generativity Erikson means primarily a concern for helping the younger generation to develop and lead useful lives. The feeling of having done nothing to help the next generation is stagnation.

Integrity versus despair is Erikson's eighth and final stage of development, which individuals experience in late adulthood. During this stage, a person reflects on the past. If the person's life review reveals a life well spent, integrity will be achieved; if not, the retrospective glances likely will yield doubt or gloom—the despair Erikson described.

We will discuss Erikson's theory again in the chapters on socioemotional development. In *Caring Connections,* you can read about some effective strategies for improving the lives of children based on Erikson's view.

Evaluating Psychoanalytic Theories   Contributions of psychoanalytic theories include an emphasis on development, family relationships, and unconscious aspects of the mind. Criticisms include a lack of scientific support, too much emphasis on sexuality (Freud's theory), too much credit given to the unconscious mind, and an image of children that is too negative (Freud's theory).

Cognitive Theories   Whereas psychoanalytic theories stress the importance of the unconscious, cognitive theories emphasize conscious thoughts. Three important cognitive theories are Piaget's cognitive developmental theory, Vygotsky's sociocultural cognitive theory, and information-processing theory.

Piaget's Cognitive Developmental Theory   **Piaget's theory** states that children actively construct their understanding of the world and go through four stages of cognitive development. Two processes move us through the four stages of development in Piaget's theory: organization and adaptation. To make sense of our world, we *organize* our experiences. For example, we separate important ideas from less important ideas, and we connect one idea to another. In addition to organizing our observations and experiences, we *adapt,* adjusting to new environmental demands.

Piaget (1954) believed that we go through four stages in understanding the world (see Figure 9). Each stage is age-related and consists of a *different* way of understanding the world. Thus, according to Piaget, the child's cognition is *qualitatively* different in one stage compared with another.

The *sensorimotor stage,* which lasts from birth to about 2 years of age, is the first Piagetian stage. In this stage, infants construct an understanding of the world by coordinating sensory experiences (such as seeing and hearing) with physical, motoric actions— hence the term *sensorimotor.*

The *preoperational stage,* which lasts from approximately 2 to 7 years of age, is Piaget's second stage. In this stage, children begin to go beyond simply connecting sensory information with physical action by representing the world with words, images, and drawings. However, according to Piaget, preschool children still lack the ability to perform what he calls *operations,* which are internalized mental actions that allow children to do mentally what they previously could only do physically. For example, if you imagine putting two sticks together to see whether they would be as long as another stick, without actually moving the sticks, you are performing a concrete operation.

The *concrete operational stage,* which lasts from approximately 7 to 11 years of age, is the third Piagetian stage. In this stage, children can perform operations that involve objects, and they can reason logically as long as reasoning can be applied to specific or concrete examples. For instance, concrete operational thinkers cannot imagine the steps necessary to complete an algebraic equation, which is too abstract for thinking at this stage of development.

One's children's children's children.
Look back to us as we look to you; we are related by our imaginations. If we are able to touch, it is because we have imagined each other's existence, our dreams running back and forth along a cable from age to age.

—ROGER ROSENBLATT
American writer, 20th century

developmental **connection**

Cognitive Theory

The entire field of children's cognitive development began with Piaget, but a number of criticisms of his theory have been made. Connect to "Cognitive Developmental Approaches."

Piaget's theory Theory stating that children actively construct their understanding of the world and go through four stages of cognitive development: sensorimotor, preoperational, concrete operational, and formal operational.

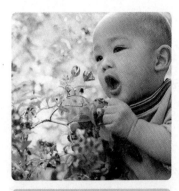

Sensorimotor Stage

The infant constructs an understanding of the world by coordinating sensory experiences with physical actions. An infant progresses from reflexive, instinctual action at birth to the beginning of symbolic thought toward the end of the stage.

Birth to 2 Years of Age

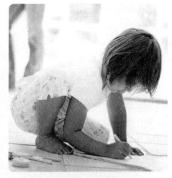

Preoperational Stage

The child begins to represent the world with words and images. These words and images reflect increased symbolic thinking and go beyond the connection of sensory information and physical action.

2 to 7 Years of Age

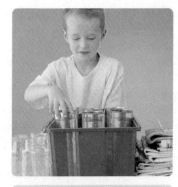

Concrete Operational Stage

The child can now reason logically about concrete events and classify objects into different sets.

7 to 11 Years of Age

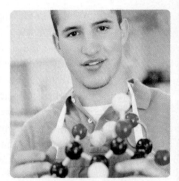

Formal Operational Stage

The adolescent reasons in more abstract, idealistic, and logical ways.

11 Years of Age Through Adulthood

FIGURE 9

PIAGET'S FOUR STAGES OF COGNITIVE DEVELOPMENT
(*Left to right*): Stockbyte/Getty Images; Jacobs Stock Photography/BananaStock/Getty Images; Fuse/image100/Corbis; Purestock/Getty Images

- - - - - - - - - - - ->

developmental **connection**

Education

Applications of Vygotsky's theory to children's education have been made in recent years. Connect to "Cognitive Developmental Approaches."

<- - - - - - - - - - - -

The *formal operational stage,* which appears between the ages of 11 and 15 and continues through adulthood, is Piaget's fourth and final stage. In this stage, individuals move beyond concrete experiences and think in abstract and more logical terms. As part of thinking more abstractly, adolescents develop images of ideal circumstances. They might think about what an ideal parent is like and compare their parents to this ideal standard. They begin to entertain possibilities for the future and are fascinated with what they can be. In solving problems, they become more systematic, developing hypotheses about why something is happening the way it is and then testing these hypotheses.

The preceding discussion is a brief introduction to Piaget's theory. It is provided here, along with other theories, to give you a broad understanding. In the chapter "Cognitive Developmental Approaches," we will return to Piaget and examine his theory in more depth.

Vygotsky's Sociocultural Cognitive Theory

Like Piaget, the Russian developmentalist Lev Vygotsky (1896–1934) argued that children actively construct their knowledge. However, Vygotsky (1962) gave social interaction and culture far more important roles in cognitive development than Piaget did. **Vygotsky's theory** is a sociocultural cognitive theory that emphasizes how culture and social interaction guide cognitive development.

Vygotsky portrayed the child's development as inseparable from social and cultural activities

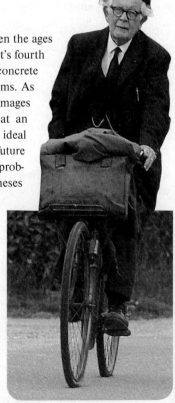

Jean Piaget, the famous Swiss developmental psychologist, changed the way we think about the development of children's minds. *What are some key ideas in Piaget's theory?*
Yves de Braine/Black Star/Stock Photo

Vygotsky's theory A sociocultural cognitive theory that emphasizes how culture and social interaction guide cognitive development.

(Veraksa & Sheridan, 2018). He argued that development of memory, attention, and reasoning involves learning to use the inventions of society, such as language, mathematical systems, and memory strategies. Thus, in one culture, children might learn to count with the help of a computer; in another, they might learn by using beads. According to Vygotsky, children's social interaction with more-skilled adults and peers is indispensable to their cognitive development. Through this interaction, they learn to use the tools that will help them adapt and be successful in their culture. For example, if you regularly help children learn how to read, you not only advance their reading skills but also communicate to them that reading is an important activity in their culture.

Vygotsky's theory has stimulated considerable interest in the view that knowledge is *situated* and *collaborative* (Gauvain, 2013). In this view, knowledge is not generated from within the individual but rather is constructed through interaction with other people and objects in the culture, such as books. This suggests that knowledge grows through interaction with others in cooperative activities.

Vygotsky's theory, like Piaget's, remained virtually unknown to American psychologists until the 1960s, but eventually both approaches became influential among educators as well as psychologists. We will further examine Vygotsky's theory in the chapter "Cognitive Developmental Approaches."

Information-Processing Theory Early computers may be the best candidates for the title of "creators" of information-processing theory. Although many factors stimulated the growth of this theory, none was more important than the computer. Psychologists began to wonder if the logical operations carried out by computers might tell us something about how the human mind works. They drew analogies between a computer's hardware and the brain and between computer software and cognition.

This line of thinking helped to generate **information-processing theory,** which emphasizes that individuals manipulate information, monitor it, and strategize about it. Unlike Piaget's theory but like Vygotsky's theory, information-processing theory does not describe development as happening in stages. Instead, according to this theory, individuals develop a gradually increasing capacity for processing information, which allows them to acquire increasingly complex knowledge and skills (Bjorklund & Causey, 2017).

Robert Siegler (2006, 2013), a leading expert on children's information processing, states that thinking is information processing. In other words, when individuals perceive, encode, represent, store, and retrieve information, they are thinking. Siegler emphasizes that an important aspect of development is learning good strategies for processing information. For example, becoming a better reader might involve learning to monitor the key themes of the material being read.

Evaluating the Cognitive Theories Contributions of cognitive theories include a positive view of development and an emphasis on the active construction of understanding. Criticisms include skepticism about the pureness of Piaget's stages and assertions that too little attention is paid to variations and differences between children.

Behavioral and Social Cognitive Theories At about the same time that Freud was interpreting patients' unconscious minds through their recollections of early childhood experiences, Ivan Pavlov and John B. Watson were conducting detailed observations of behavior in controlled laboratory settings. Their work provided the foundations of *behaviorism,* which holds that we can study scientifically only what can be directly observed and measured. Out of this tradition grew the belief that development is defined as observable behavior that can be learned through experience with the environment (Mazur, 2016). Do you recall the continuity-discontinuity issue discussed earlier in this chapter? The behavioral and social cognitive theories emphasize continuity and argue that development does not occur in stages. The three versions of the behavioral approach that we will explore are Pavlov's classical conditioning, Skinner's operant conditioning, and Bandura's social cognitive theory.

Pavlov's Classical Conditioning In the early 1900s, the Russian physiologist Ivan Pavlov (1927) knew that dogs salivate when they taste food. He became curious when he observed that dogs also salivate in response to various sights and sounds before

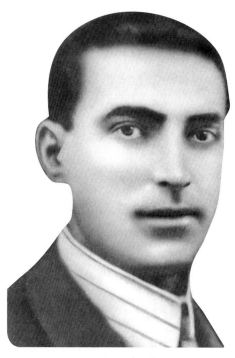

There is considerable interest today in Lev Vygotsky's sociocultural cognitive theory of child development. *What were Vygotsky's basic ideas about children's development?*
A.R. Lauria /Dr. Michael Cole, Laboratory of Human Cognition, University of California, San Diego

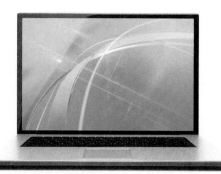

David Vernon/Getty Images

information-processing theory Emphasizes that individuals manipulate information, monitor it, and strategize about it. Central to this theory are the processes of memory and thinking.

eating their food. For example, when an individual paired the ringing of a bell with the food, the bell ringing subsequently elicited salivation from the dogs when it was presented by itself. With this experiment, Pavlov discovered the principle of *classical conditioning,* in which a neutral stimulus (in our example, hearing a bell ring) produces a response originally produced by another stimulus (in our example, tasting food).

In the early twentieth century, John Watson and Rosalie Rayner (1920) demonstrated that classical conditioning occurs in human beings. They showed an infant named Albert a white rat to see if he was afraid of it. He was not. As Albert played with the rat, a loud noise was made behind his head. As you might imagine, the noise caused little Albert to cry. After several pairings of the loud noise and the white rat, Albert began to cry at the sight of the rat even when the noise did not occur. Albert had been classically conditioned to fear the rat. Similarly, many of our fears may result from classical conditioning: fear of the dentist may be learned from a painful experience, fear of driving from being in an automobile accident, fear of heights from falling off a high chair when we were infants, and fear of dogs from being bitten.

Skinner's Operant Conditioning   Classical conditioning may explain how we develop many involuntary responses such as fears, but B. F. Skinner argued that a second type of conditioning accounts for the development of other types of behavior. According to Skinner (1938), through *operant conditioning* the consequences of a behavior produce changes in the future probability of the behavior. A behavior followed by a rewarding stimulus is more likely to recur, whereas a behavior followed by a punishing stimulus is less likely to recur. For example, when a person smiles at a child after the child has done something, the child is more likely to repeat that action than if the person gives the child a nasty look.

According to Skinner, such rewards and punishments shape development. For example, shy people learned to be shy as a result of experiences they had while growing up. It follows that modifications in an environment can help a shy person become more socially oriented. Also, for Skinner the key aspect of development is behavior, not thoughts and feelings. He emphasized that development consists of the pattern of behavioral changes that are brought about by rewards and punishments.

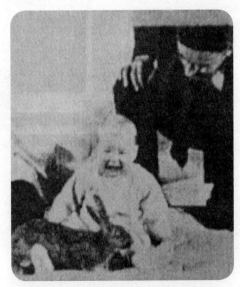

In 1920, Watson and Rosalie Rayner conditioned 11-month-old Albert to fear a white rat by pairing the rat with a loud noise. When little Albert was subsequently presented with other stimuli similar to the white rat, such as the rabbit shown here with little Albert, he was afraid of them, too. This illustrates the principle of stimulus generalization in classical conditioning.
Dr. Benjamin Harris

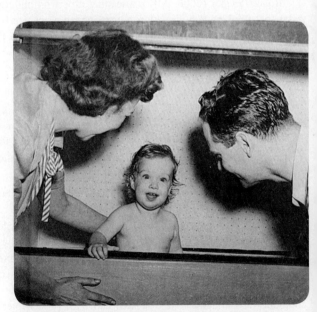

B. F. Skinner was a tinkerer who liked to make new gadgets. The younger of his two daughters, Deborah, spent much of her infancy in Skinner's enclosed Air-Crib, which he invented because he wanted to ensure her comfort while minimizing the need for heavy blankets and pajamas. The Air-Crib was temperature-controlled. Debbie, shown here as a child with her parents, is currently a successful artist, is married, and lives in London. *What do you think about Skinner's Air-Crib?*
AP Images

Bandura's Social Cognitive Theory   Some psychologists agree with the behaviorists' notion that development is learned and is influenced strongly by the environment. However, unlike Skinner, they argue that our thoughts—that is, cognition—is also important in understanding development. **Social cognitive theory** states that behavior, environment, and cognition are the key factors in development.

American psychologist Albert Bandura (1925-) is the leading architect of social cognitive theory. Bandura (2012, 2018) emphasizes that cognitive processes have important links with the environment and behavior. His early research focused heavily on *observational learning* (also called *imitation* or *modeling*), which is learning that occurs through observing what others do. For example, a young boy might observe his father yelling in anger and treating other people with hostility; with his peers, the young boy later acts very aggressively, showing the same characteristics his father displayed. A girl might adopt the dominant and sarcastic style of her teacher, saying to her younger brother, "You are so slow. How can you do this work so slowly?" Social cognitive theorists stress that people acquire a wide range of behaviors, thoughts, and feelings through observing others' behavior and that these observations powerfully influence children's development.

According to Bandura, what is *cognitive* about observational learning? He proposes that people cognitively represent the behavior of others and then sometimes adopt this behavior themselves. Bandura's (2018) most recent model of learning and development includes behavior, as well as the person/cognition and the environment. An individual's sense of being in control of his or her success is an example of a person/cognition factor; strategies are an example of a cognitive factor. As shown in Figure 10, behavior, person/cognition, and environmental factors operate interactively. Behavior can influence person factors and vice versa. Cognitive activities can influence the environment. The environment can change the person's cognition, and so on.

Evaluating the Behavioral and Social Cognitive Theories   Contributions of the behavioral and social cognitive theories include an emphasis on scientific research and environmental causes of behavior. Bandura's social cognitive theory emphasizes reciprocal links between the environment, behavior, and person/cognitive factors. Criticisms include too little emphasis on cognition in Skinner's theory, and giving inadequate attention to developmental changes and biological foundations.

Behavioral and social cognitive theories emphasize the importance of environmental experiences in human development. Next we turn our attention to a theory that underscores the importance of the biological foundations of development—ethological theory.

Ethological Theory   American developmental psychologists began to pay attention to the biological bases of development during the mid-twentieth century thanks to the work of European zoologists who pioneered the field of ethology. **Ethology** stresses that behavior is strongly influenced by biology, is tied to evolution, and is characterized by critical or sensitive periods. These are specific time frames during which, according to ethologists, the presence or absence of certain experiences has a long-lasting influence on individuals.

European zoologist Konrad Lorenz (1903-1989) helped bring ethology to prominence. In his best-known experiment, Lorenz (1965) studied the behavior of greylag geese, which will follow their mothers as soon as they hatch.

In a remarkable set of experiments, Lorenz separated the eggs laid by one goose into two groups. One group he returned to the goose to be hatched by her. The other group was hatched in an incubator. The goslings in the first group performed as predicted. They followed their mother as soon as they hatched. However, those in the second group, which saw Lorenz when they first hatched, followed him everywhere, as though he were their mother. Lorenz marked the goslings and then placed both groups under a box. Mother goose and "mother" Lorenz stood aside as the box was lifted. Each group of goslings went directly to its "mother." Lorenz called this *imprinting*—rapid, innate learning within a limited, critical period of time that involves attachment to the first moving object seen.

At first, ethology had little to say about the nature of social relationships across the *human* life span, and the theory stimulated few studies involving people. Ethologists' viewpoint that normal development requires that certain behaviors emerge during a *critical*

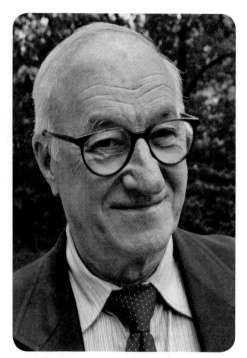

Albert Bandura has been one of the leading architects of social cognitive theory. *How does Bandura's theory differ from Skinner's?*
Courtesy of Dr. Albert Bandura

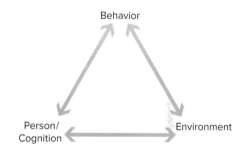

FIGURE **10**

BANDURA'S SOCIAL COGNITIVE MODEL. The arrows illustrate how relations between behavior, person/cognition, and environment reciprocally influence each other rather than being "unidirectional".

developmental **connection**

Theories

Bandura emphasizes that self-efficacy is a key person/cognition factor in children's achievement. Connect to "Schools and Achievement."

social cognitive theory The view of psychologists who emphasize behavior, environment, and cognition as the key factors in development.

ethology Stresses that behavior is strongly influenced by biology, is tied to evolution, and is characterized by critical or sensitive periods.

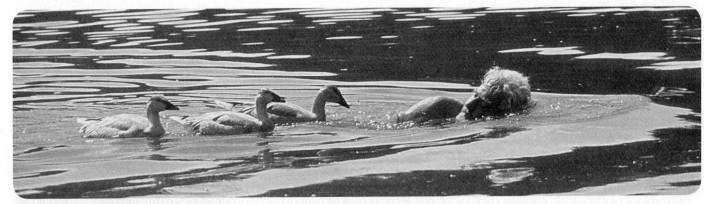

Konrad Lorenz, a pioneering student of animal behavior, is followed through the water by three imprinted greylag geese. *Describe Lorenz's experiment with the geese. Do you think his experiment would have the same results with human babies?* Explain.

Nina Leen//Time Life Pictures/Getty Images

┌ ─ ─ ─ ─ ─ ─ ─ ─ ─ ─►
developmental **connection**

Attachment

Human babies go through a series of phases in developing an attachment to a caregiver. Connect to "Emotional Development."

◄ ─ ─ ─ ─ ─ ─ ─ ─ ─ ─ ┘

period, a fixed time period very early in development, seemed to be overstated. However, John Bowlby's work (1989) illustrated an important application of ethology to human development. Bowlby argued that attachment to a caregiver during the first year of life has important consequences throughout the life span. Bowlby stated that if this attachment is positive and secure, the infant will likely develop positively in childhood and adulthood. If the attachment is negative and insecure, children's development will likely be less than optimal. Thus, the first year of life is a *sensitive period* for the development of social relationships. In the chapter, "Emotional Development," we will explore the concept of infant attachment in greater detail.

Contributions of ethological theory include a focus on the biological and evolutionary basis of development, and the use of careful observations in naturalistic settings. Critics assert that too much emphasis is placed on biological foundations and that the critical and sensitive period concepts might be too rigid.

Another theory that emphasizes the biological aspects of human development—evolutionary psychology—will be presented in the chapter "Biological Beginnings," along with views on the role of heredity in development.

Ecological Theory Whereas ethology stresses biological factors, ecological theory emphasizes environmental factors. One ecological theory that has important implications for understanding children's development was created by Urie Bronfenbrenner (1917–2005).

Bronfenbrenner's ecological theory (Bronfenbrenner, 1986; Hayes, O'Toole, & Halpenny, 2017) holds that development reflects the influence of several environmental systems. The theory identifies five environmental systems (see Figure 11):

- *Microsystem:* The setting in which the individual lives. These contexts include the person's family, peers, school, neighborhood, and work. It is within the microsystem that the most direct interactions with social agents take place—with parents, peers, and teachers, for example.

- *Mesosystem:* Relations between microsystems or connections between contexts. Examples are the relationships between family experiences and school experiences, school experiences and church experiences, and family experiences and peer experiences. For example, children whose parents have rejected them may have difficulty developing positive relationships with teachers.

- *Exosystem:* Links between a social setting in which the individual does not have an active role and the individual's immediate context. For example, a husband's or child's experience at home may be influenced by a mother's experiences at work. The mother might receive a promotion that requires more travel, which might increase conflict with the husband and change patterns of interaction with the child.

- *Macrosystem:* The culture in which individuals live. Remember from earlier in this chapter that *culture* refers to the behavior patterns, beliefs, and all other products of a group of people that are passed from generation to generation. Remember

Bronfenbrenner's ecological theory An environmental systems theory that focuses on five environmental systems: microsystem, mesosystem, exosystem, macrosystem, and chronosystem.

eclectic theoretical orientation An orientation that does not follow any one theoretical approach but instead selects the best aspects from each theory.

also that cross-cultural studies—comparisons of one culture with one or more other cultures—provide information about the generality of development (Mistry & Dutta, 2015).

- *Chronosystem:* The patterning of environmental events and transitions over the life course, as well as historical circumstances. For example, divorce is one transition. Researchers have found that the negative effects of divorce on children often peak in the first year after the divorce (Mahrer & others, 2018). By two years after the divorce, family interaction is less chaotic and more stable. As an example of historical circumstances, consider how career opportunities for women have increased during the last 40 years.

Bronfenbrenner has added biological influences to his theory and now describes it as a bioecological theory. Nonetheless, ecological, environmental contexts still predominate in Bronfenbrenner's theory (Hayes & others, 2017).

Contributions of ecological theory include a systematic examination of macro and micro dimensions of environmental systems, and attention to connections between environmental systems. A further contribution of Bronfenbrenner's theory is its emphasis on a range of social contexts beyond the family, such as neighborhood, religious organization, school, and workplace, as influential in children's development (Gauvain, 2013). Criticisms include giving inadequate attention to biological factors, as well as placing too little emphasis on cognitive factors.

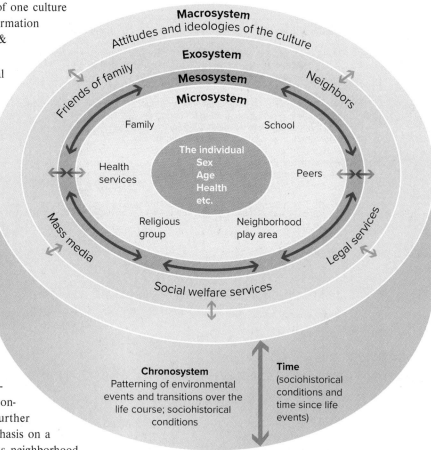

FIGURE 11

BRONFENBRENNER'S ECOLOGICAL THEORY OF DEVELOPMENT. Bronfenbrenner's ecological theory consists of five environmental systems: microsystem, mesosystem, exosystem, macrosystem, and chronosystem.

An Eclectic Theoretical Orientation No single theory described in this chapter can explain entirely the rich complexity of children's development, but each has contributed to our understanding of development. Psychoanalytic theory best explains the unconscious mind. Erikson's theory best describes the changes that occur in adult development. Piaget's, Vygotsky's, and the information-processing views provide the most complete description of cognitive development. The behavioral and social cognitive and ecological theories have been the most useful for identifying the environmental determinants of development. The ethological theories have highlighted biology's role and the importance of critical and sensitive periods in development.

In short, although theories are helpful guides, relying on a single theory to explain development is probably a mistake. This edition instead takes an **eclectic theoretical orientation,** which does not follow any one theoretical approach but rather selects from each theory whatever is considered its best features. With this orientation, you can view the study of development as it actually exists—with different theorists making different assumptions, stressing different research questions, and using different strategies to discover information. Figure 12 compares the main theoretical perspectives on important issues in children's development.

RESEARCH METHODS FOR COLLECTING DATA

If they follow an eclectic orientation, how do scholars and researchers determine that one feature of a theory is somehow better than another? The scientific method discussed earlier in this chapter provides the guide. Recall that the steps in the scientific method involve conceptualizing the problem, collecting data, drawing conclusions, and revising

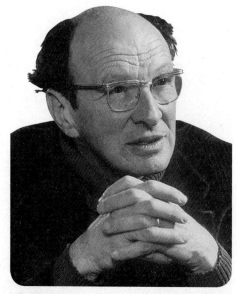

Urie Bronfenbrenner developed ecological theory, a perspective that is receiving increased attention. *What is the nature of ecological theory?*
Courtesy of Cornell University Photography

	Nature and nurture	Early and later experience	Continuity and discontinuity
Psychoanalytic	Freud's biological determinism interacting with early family experiences; Erikson's more balanced biological/cultural interaction perspective	Early experiences in the family very important influences	Emphasis on discontinuity between stages
Cognitive	Piaget's emphasis on interaction and adaptation; environment provides the setting for cognitive structures to develop. Vygotsky's theory involves the interaction of nature and nurture with strong emphasis on culture. The information-processing approach has not addressed this issue extensively; mainly emphasizes biological/environment interaction.	Childhood experiences important influences	Discontinuity between stages in Piaget's theory; no stages in Vygotsky's theory or the information-processing approach
Behavioral and Social Cognitive	Environment viewed as the main influence on development	Experiences important at all points in development	Continuity with no stages
Ethological	Strong biological view	Early experiences very important, which can contribute to change early in development; after early critical or sensitive period has passed, stability likely to occur	Discontinuity because of early critical or sensitive period; no stages
Ecological	Strong environmental view	Experiences involving the five environmental systems important at all points in development	No stages but little attention to the issue

FIGURE **12**

A COMPARISON OF THEORIES AND ISSUES IN CHILD DEVELOPMENT

laboratory A controlled setting from which many of the complex factors of the "real world" have been removed.

research conclusions and theories. Through scientific research, the features of theories can be tested and refined.

Whether we are interested in studying attachment in infants, the cognitive skills of children, or peer relations among adolescents, we can choose from several ways of collecting data. Here we outline the methods most often used, looking at the advantages and disadvantages of each.

Observation   Scientific observation requires an important set of skills (Gravetter & Forzano, 2019). Unless we are trained observers and practice our skills regularly, we might not know what to look for, we might not remember what we saw, we might not realize that what we are looking for is changing from one moment to the next, and we might not communicate our observations effectively.

For observations to be effective, they have to be systematic. We have to have some idea of what we are looking for. We have to know whom we are observing, when and where we will observe, how the observations will be made, and how they will be recorded.

Where should we make our observations? We have two choices: the laboratory and the everyday world. When we observe scientifically, we often need to control certain factors that determine behavior but are not the focus of our study (Rosnow & Rosenthal, 2013). For this reason, some research is conducted in a **laboratory,** a controlled setting from which many of the complex factors of the "real world" have been removed. For example, suppose you want to observe how children react when they see other people behave aggressively. If you observe children in their homes or schools, you have no control over how much aggression the children observe, what kind of aggression they see, which people they see acting aggressively, or how other people treat the children. In

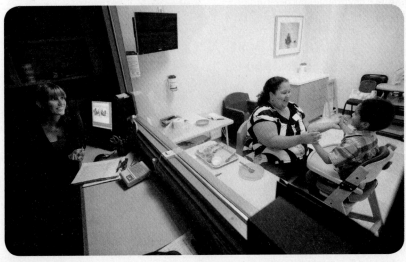

What are some important strategies in conducting observational research with children?
David Goldman/AP Images

contrast, if you observe the children in a laboratory, you can control these and other factors and therefore have more confidence about how to interpret your observations.

Laboratory research does have some drawbacks, however, including the following:

- It is almost impossible to conduct research without letting participants know they are being studied.
- The laboratory setting is unnatural and therefore can cause the participants to behave unnaturally.
- People who are willing to come to a university laboratory may not fairly represent groups from diverse cultural and socioeconomic backgrounds.
- People who are unfamiliar with university settings and with the idea of "helping science" may be intimidated by the laboratory setting.
- Some aspects of children's development are difficult, if not impossible, to examine in the laboratory.
- Laboratory studies of certain types of stress may even be unethical.

Naturalistic observation provides insights that we sometimes cannot achieve in the laboratory (Graziano & Raulin, 2013). **Naturalistic observation** means observing behavior in real-world settings, making no effort to manipulate or control the situation. Child development researchers conduct naturalistic observations in homes, child-care centers, schools, neighborhoods, malls, and other settings.

Naturalistic observation was used in one classic study that focused on conversations in a children's science museum (Crowley & others, 2001). Parents of boys were more than three times as likely as parents of girls to engage in explanatory talk while visiting exhibits at the science museum, suggesting a gender bias that encourages boys more than girls to be interested in science (see Figure 13). In another study, Mexican American parents who had completed high school used more explanations with their children when visiting a science museum than those who had not completed high school (Tenenbaum & others, 2002).

Survey and Interview Sometimes the best and quickest way to get information about people is to ask them for it. One technique is to interview them directly. A related method is the survey (sometimes referred to as a questionnaire), which is especially useful when information from many people is needed (Leedy & Ormrod, 2018). A standard set of questions is used to obtain people's self-reported attitudes or beliefs about a particular topic. In a good survey, the questions are clear and unbiased.

Surveys and interviews can be used to study a wide range of topics, from religious beliefs to sexual habits to attitudes about gun control to beliefs about how to improve schools. Surveys and interviews today are conducted in person, over the phone, and online through websites or social media.

One problem with surveys and interviews is the tendency for participants to answer questions in a way that they think is socially desirable rather than telling what they truly think or feel (Creswell, 2008). For example, on a survey or in an interview some individuals might say that they do not take drugs even though they do.

Standardized Test A **standardized test** has uniform procedures for administration and scoring. Many standardized tests allow a person's performance to be compared with the performance of other individuals to provide information about individual differences among people (Watson, 2012). One example is the Stanford-Binet intelligence test, which is described in the "Intelligence" chapter. Your score on the Stanford-Binet test shows how your performance compares with that of thousands of other people who have taken the test.

Standardized tests have three key weaknesses. First, they do not always predict behavior in non-test situations. Second, standardized tests are based on the belief that a person's behavior is consistent and stable, yet personality and intelligence—two primary targets of standardized testing—can vary with the situation. For example, individuals may perform poorly on a standardized intelligence test in an office setting but score much higher at home, where they are less anxious. This criticism is especially relevant for members of minority groups, some of whom have been inaccurately classified as intellectually disabled on the basis of their scores on intelligence tests. A third weakness of standardized tests

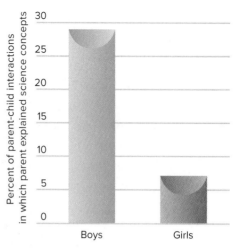

FIGURE **13**

PARENTS' EXPLANATIONS OF SCIENCE TO SONS AND DAUGHTERS AT A SCIENCE MUSEUM. In a classic naturalistic observation study at a children's science museum, parents were more than three times more likely to explain science to boys than to girls (Crowley & others, 2001). The gender difference occurred regardless of whether the father, the mother, or both parents were with the child, although the gender difference was greatest for fathers' science explanations to sons and daughters.

naturalistic observation Behavioral observation that takes place in real-world settings.

standardized test A test with uniform procedures for administration and scoring. Many standardized tests allow a person's performance to be compared with the performance of other individuals.

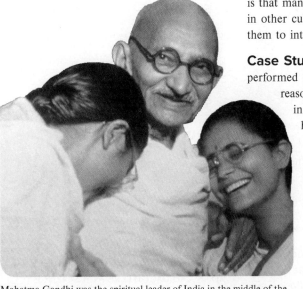

Mahatma Gandhi was the spiritual leader of India in the middle of the twentieth century. Erik Erikson conducted an extensive case study of his life to determine what contributed to his identity development. *What are some limitations of the case study approach?*

Bettmann/Getty Images

is that many psychological tests developed in Western cultures might not be appropriate in other cultures (Hall, 2018). The experiences of people in differing cultures may lead them to interpret and respond to questions differently.

Case Study   A **case study** is an in-depth look at a single individual. Case studies are performed mainly by mental health professionals when, for either practical or ethical reasons, the unique aspects of an individual's life cannot be duplicated and tested in other ways. A case study provides information about one person's fears, hopes, fantasies, traumatic experiences, upbringing, family relationships, health, or anything that helps the psychologist understand the person's mind and behavior. In later chapters, we discuss vivid case studies, such as that of Michael Rehbein, who had much of the left side of his brain removed at 7 years of age to end severe epileptic seizures.

Case studies provide dramatic, in-depth portrayals of people's lives, but remember that we must be cautious when generalizing from this information (McWhorter & Ellinger, 2018). The subject of a case study is unique, with a genetic makeup and personal history that no one else shares. In addition, psychologists who conduct case studies rarely check to see if other psychologists agree with their observations, so they may not be reliable.

Physiological Measures   Researchers are increasingly using physiological measures when they study children's development (Li & others, 2019). For example, as puberty unfolds, the blood levels of certain hormones increase. To determine the nature of these hormonal changes, researchers take blood samples from willing adolescents (Carmina & others, 2019).

Another physiological measure that is increasingly used to study children and adolescents is neuroimaging, especially *functional magnetic resonance imaging* (fMRI), in which electromagnetic waves are used to construct images of an individual's brain tissue and biochemical activity (White & Poldrack, 2018). Figure 14 compares the brain images of two adolescents—one a non-drinker and the other a heavy alcohol drinker—while engaged in a memory task. We will have much more to say about neuroimaging and other physiological measures in other chapters.

RESEARCH DESIGNS

Suppose you want to find out whether the children of permissive parents are more likely than other children to be rude and unruly. The data-collection method that researchers choose often depends on the goal of their research. The goal may be simply to describe a phenomenon, or it may be to describe relationships between phenomena, or to determine the causes or effects of a phenomenon.

case study An in-depth look at a single individual.

FIGURE **14**

BRAIN IMAGING OF 15-YEAR-OLD ADOLESCENTS. The two brain images indicate how alcohol can influence the functioning of an adolescent's brain. Notice the pink and red coloring (which indicates effective brain functioning involving memory) in the brain of the 15-year-old non-drinker while engaging in a memory task and the lack of those colors in the brain of the 15-year-old under the influence of alcohol.

(*left/right*): Dr. Susan F. Tapert, University of California, San Diego;

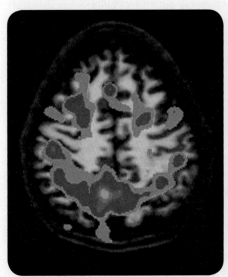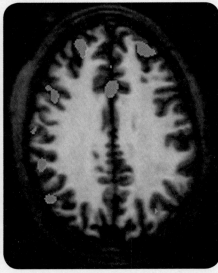

Perhaps you decide that you need to observe both permissive and strict parents with their children and compare them. How would you do that? In addition to choosing a method for collecting data, you would need to select a research design. There are three main types of research designs: descriptive, correlational, and experimental.

Descriptive Research All of the data-collection methods that we have discussed can be used in **descriptive research,** which aims to observe and record behavior. For example, a researcher might observe whether people behave altruistically or aggressively toward each other. By itself, descriptive research cannot prove what causes a specific behavior, but it can yield important information (Leedy & Ormrod, 2018).

Correlational Research In contrast with descriptive research, correlational research goes beyond describing phenomena and provides information that helps predict how people will behave. In **correlational research,** the goal is to describe the strength of the relationship between two or more events or characteristics. The more strongly the two events are correlated (or related or associated), the more effectively we can predict one event from the other (Leedy & Ormrod, 2018).

For example, to determine whether children of permissive parents have less self-control than other children, you would need to carefully record observations of parents' permissiveness and their children's self-control. The data could then be analyzed statistically to yield a numerical measure, called a **correlation coefficient,** a number based on a statistical analysis that is used to describe the degree of association between two variables. The correlation coefficient ranges from −1.00 to +1.00. A negative number means an inverse relation. For example, researchers often find a negative correlation between permissive parenting and children's self-control. By contrast, they often find a positive correlation between parental monitoring of children and children's self-control.

The higher the correlation coefficient (whether positive or negative), the stronger the association between the two variables. A correlation of 0 means that there is no association between the variables. A correlation of −.40 is stronger than a correlation of +.20 because we disregard whether the correlation is positive or negative in determining the strength of the correlation.

A caution is in order, however. Correlation does not equal causation (Graziano & Raulin, 2013). The correlational finding just mentioned does not mean that permissive parenting necessarily causes low self-control in children. It might mean that a child's lack of self-control caused the parents to simply give up trying to control the child. It might also mean that other factors, such as heredity or poverty, caused the correlation between permissive parenting and low self-control in children. Figure 15 illustrates these possible interpretations of correlational data.

Throughout the chapters you will read about numerous correlational research studies. Keep in mind how easy (and misleading) it can be to assume causality when two characteristics are merely correlated (Caldwell, 2013).

descriptive research Research that involves observing and recording behavior.

correlational research Research in which the goal is to describe the strength of the relationship between two or more events or characteristics.

correlation coefficient A number based on statistical analysis that is used to describe the degree of association between two variables.

Observed Correlation: As permissive parenting increases, children's self-control decreases.

Possible explanations for this observed correlation

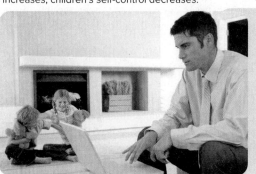

Permissive parenting   causes   Children's lack of self-control

Children's lack of self-control   causes   Permissive parenting

A third factor such as genetic tendencies or poverty   causes both   Permissive parenting and children's lack of self-control

An observed correlation between two events cannot be used to conclude that one event causes the second event. Other possibilities are that the second event causes the first event or that a third event causes the correlation between the first two events.

FIGURE **15**

POSSIBLE EXPLANATIONS OF THIS CORRELATION

JupiterImages/Getty Images

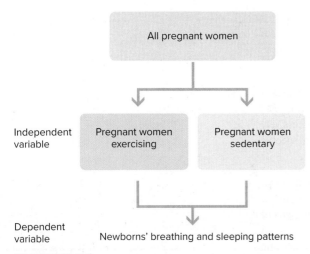

Independent variable

Pregnant women exercising | Pregnant women sedentary

Dependent variable

Newborns' breathing and sleeping patterns

FIGURE **16**

PRINCIPLES OF EXPERIMENTAL RESEARCH. Imagine that you conduct an experimental study of the effects of aerobic exercise by pregnant women on their newborns' breathing and sleeping patterns. You would randomly assign pregnant women to experimental and control groups. The experimental-group women would engage in aerobic exercise over a specified number of sessions and weeks. The control group would not. Then, when the infants are born, you would assess their breathing and sleeping patterns. If the breathing and sleeping patterns of newborns whose mothers were in the experimental group were more positive than those of the control group, you would conclude that aerobic exercise caused the positive effects.

experiment A carefully regulated procedure in which one or more of the factors believed to influence the behavior being studied are manipulated while all other factors are held constant.

cross-sectional approach A research strategy in which individuals of different ages are compared at the same point in time.

Experimental Research   To study causality, researchers turn to experimental research. An **experiment** is a carefully regulated procedure in which one or more factors believed to cause the behavior being studied are manipulated while all other factors are held constant. If the behavior under study changes when a factor is manipulated, we say that the manipulated factor has caused the behavior to change. In other words, the experiment has demonstrated cause and effect. The cause is the factor that was manipulated. The effect is the behavior that changed because of the manipulation. Descriptive and correlational research cannot establish cause and effect because it does not involve manipulating factors in a controlled way (Leedy & Ormrod, 2018).

Independent and Dependent Variables   Experiments include two types of changeable factors, or variables: independent and dependent. An independent variable is a manipulated, influential, experimental factor. It is a potential cause. The label *independent* is used because this variable can be manipulated independently of other factors to determine its effect. One experiment may include several independent variables.

A dependent variable is a factor that can change in an experiment, in response to changes in the independent variable. As researchers manipulate the independent variable, they measure the dependent variable for any resulting effect. See Figure 16 for an example. In the experiment described in Figure 16, the amount of exercise completed by the pregnant women is the independent variable, the factor being manipulated in the experiment. The infants' breathing and sleeping patterns are the dependent variable, the factor that changes as the result of your manipulation of the mothers' exercise.

Experimental and Control Groups   Experiments can involve one or more experimental groups and one or more control groups. An experimental group is a group whose experience is manipulated. A control group is a comparison group that is as much like the experimental group as possible and that is treated in every way like the experimental group except for the manipulated factor (independent variable). The manipulated condition can then be compared to the control group condition.

Random assignment is an important principle for deciding whether each participant will be placed in the experimental group or in the control group. Random assignment means that researchers assign participants to experimental and control groups by chance. It reduces the likelihood that the experiment's results will be due to any preexisting differences between groups (Gravetter & Forzano, 2019). In the example in Figure 16 of the effects of aerobic exercise by pregnant women on the breathing and sleeping patterns of their newborns, you would randomly assign half of the pregnant women to engage in aerobic exercise over a period of weeks (the experimental group) and the other half to not exercise over the same number of weeks (the control group).

Time Span of Research   Researchers in child development have a special concern with studies that focus on the relationship between age and some other variable. To do this, they study individuals of different ages and compare them, or they study the same individuals as they age over time.

Cross-Sectional Approach   The **cross-sectional approach** is a research strategy in which individuals of different ages are compared at one time. A typical cross-sectional study might include a group of 5-year-olds, 8-year-olds, and 11-year-olds. The groups can be compared with respect to a variety of dependent variables: intelligence, memory, peer relations, attachment to parents, hormonal changes, and so on. All of this can be accomplished in a short time. In some studies, data are collected in a single day. Even in large-scale cross-sectional studies with hundreds of participants, data collection does not usually take longer than several months to complete.

The main advantage of the cross-sectional study is that researchers don't have to wait for children to grow older. Despite its efficiency, the cross-sectional approach has its drawbacks. It gives no information about how individual children change or about the stability of their characteristics. It can obscure the increases and decreases of development—the hills and valleys of growth and development.

Longitudinal Approach   The **longitudinal approach** is a research strategy in which the same individuals are studied over time, usually several years or more. For example, if a study of the development of self-esteem were conducted longitudinally, the same children might be assessed three times—such as at 5, 8, and 11 years of age. Some longitudinal studies take place over time frames as short as one year or less.

Longitudinal studies provide a wealth of information about important issues such as stability and change in development and the influence of early experience on later development, but they are not without problems (Reznick, 2013). They are expensive and time-consuming. Also, the longer the study lasts, more participants drop out. For example, children's families may move, get sick, lose interest, and so forth. Those who remain in the study may be dissimilar to those who drop out, biasing the results. Those individuals who remain in a longitudinal study over a number of years may be more compulsive and conformity-oriented than average, for example, or they might lead more stable lives.

Earlier in the chapter we described *cohort effects,* which are effects due to a person's time of birth, era, or generation rather than to actual age. Cohort effects are important in research on children, adolescents, and their parents because they can powerfully affect the dependent measures in a study meant to be concerned with age (Halfon & Forrest, 2018). Cross-sectional studies can show how different cohorts develop, but they can confuse age and cohort changes. Longitudinal studies are effective in studying age changes but only within one cohort.

Theories are often linked with a particular research method or methods. Therefore, methods that researchers use are associated with their particular theoretical approaches. Figure 17 illustrates connections between research methods and theories.

So far we have discussed many aspects of scientific research in child development, but where can you read about this research firsthand? Read *Connecting Through Research* to find out.

longitudinal approach A research strategy in which the same individuals are studied over a period of time, usually several years.

Research Method	Theory
Observation	• All theories emphasize some form of observation. • Behavioral and social cognitive theories place the strongest emphasis on laboratory observation. • Ethological theory places the strongest emphasis on naturalistic observation.
Interview/survey	• Psychoanalytic and cognitive studies (Piaget, Vygotsky) often use interviews. • Behavioral, social cognitive, and ethological theories are the least likely to use surveys or interviews.
Standardized test	• None of the theories discussed emphasize the use of this method.
Correlational research	• All of the theories use this research method, although psychoanalytic theories are the least likely to use it.
Experimental research	• The behavioral and social cognitive theories and the information-processing theories are the most likely to use the experimental method. • Psychoanalytic theories are the least likely to use it.
Cross-sectional/longitudinal methods	• No theory described uses these methods more than any other.

FIGURE **17**
CONNECTIONS OF RESEARCH METHODS TO THEORIES

connecting through research

Where Is Child Development Research Published?

Regardless of whether you pursue a career in child development, psychology, or some related scientific field, you can benefit by learning about the journal process. As a student you might be required to look up original research in journals. As a parent, teacher, or nurse you might want to consult journals to obtain information that will help you understand and work more effectively with people. And as an inquiring person, you might look up information in journals after you have heard or read something that piqued your curiosity.

A journal publishes scholarly and academic information, usually in a specific domain such as physics, math, sociology, or our current interest, child development. Scholars in these fields publish most of their research in journals, which are the source of core information in virtually every academic discipline.

An increasing number of journals publish information about child development. Among the leading journals in child development are *Child Development, Developmental Psychology, Developmental Science, Development and Psychopathology, Pediatrics, Pediatric Nursing, Infant Behavior and Development, Journal of Research on Adolescence, Human Development, Social Development, Cognitive Development,* and many others. Also, a number of journals that do not focus solely on development include articles on various aspects of human development. These journals include *Journal of Educational Psychology, Sex Roles, Journal of Cross-Cultural Research, Journal of Marriage and the Family, Exceptional Children,* and *Journal of Consulting and Clinical Psychology.*

Every journal has a board of experts who evaluate articles submitted for publication. Each submitted paper is accepted or rejected on the basis of factors such as its contribution to the field, methodological excellence, and clarity of writing. Some of the most prestigious journals reject as many as 80 to 90 percent of the articles submitted.

Journal articles are usually written for other professionals in the specialized field of the journal's focus; therefore, they often contain technical language and terms specific to the discipline that are difficult for nonprofessionals to understand. They usually consist of the

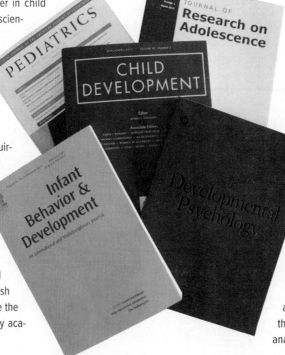

Research journals are the core of information in virtually every academic discipline. Those shown here are among the increasing number of research journals that publish information about child development. *What are the main parts of a research article that presents findings from original research?*
Mark Dierker/McGraw-Hill Education

following elements: abstract, introduction, method, results, discussion, and references. The *abstract* is a brief summary that appears at the beginning of the article. The abstract lets readers quickly determine whether the article is relevant to their interests. The *introduction* introduces the problem or issue that is being studied. It includes a concise review of research relevant to the topic, theoretical ties, and one or more hypotheses to be tested. The *method* section consists of a clear description of the subjects evaluated in the study, the measures used, and the procedures that were followed. The method section should be sufficiently clear and detailed so that reading it could allow another researcher to repeat or replicate the study. The *results* section reports the analysis of the data collected. In most cases, the results section includes statistical analyses that are difficult for nonprofessionals to understand. The *discussion* section describes the author's conclusions, inferences, and interpretation of what was found. Statements are usually made about whether the hypotheses presented in the introduction were supported, limitations of the study, and suggestions for future research. The last part of the journal article, called *references,* includes bibliographic information for each source cited in the article. The references section is often a good resource for finding other articles relevant to a topic that interests you.

Where do you find journals such as those we have described? Your college or university library likely has some of them, and some public libraries also carry journals. Online resources such as PsycINFO and Google Scholar, which can facilitate the search for journal articles, are available to students on many campuses.

The research published in the journals mentioned above shapes our lives. It not only informs the work of other child development researchers, but it also informs the practices of law and policy makers, physicians, educators, parents, and many others. In fact, much of what you will find that is new in this edition comes directly from research that can be found in the journals mentioned above.

CHALLENGES IN CHILD DEVELOPMENT RESEARCH

The scientific foundation of research in child development helps to minimize the effect of research bias and maximize the objectivity of the results. Still, subtle challenges remain for each researcher to resolve. One is to ensure that research is conducted in an ethical way; another is to recognize, and try to overcome, deeply buried personal biases.

Conducting Ethical Research   The explosion in technology has forced society to grapple with looming ethical questions that were unimaginable only a few decades ago. The same line of research that enables previously sterile couples to have children might someday let prospective parents "call up and order" the characteristics they prefer in their children or tip the balance of males and females in the world. For example, should embryos left over from procedures for increasing fertility be saved or discarded? Should people with inherited fatal diseases (such as Huntington's disease) be discouraged from having their own biological children?

Researchers also face ethical questions both new and old. They have a responsibility to anticipate the personal problems their research might cause and to at least inform the participants of the possible fallout. Safeguarding the rights of research participants is a challenge because the potential harm is not always obvious (Graziano & Raulin, 2013).

Ethics in research may affect you personally if you ever serve as a participant in a study. In that event, you need to know your rights as a participant and the responsibilities of researchers to assure that these rights are safeguarded. If you ever become a researcher in child development yourself, you will need an even deeper understanding of ethics. Even if you only carry out experimental projects in psychology courses, you must consider the rights of the participants in those projects.

Today, proposed research at colleges and universities must pass the scrutiny of a research ethics committee before the research can be initiated. In addition, the American Psychological Association (APA) has developed ethics guidelines for its members. The APA code of ethics instructs psychologists to protect their participants from mental and physical harm. The participants' best interests need to be kept foremost in the researcher's mind. APA's guidelines address four important issues: informed consent, confidentiality, debriefing, and deception.

- *Informed consent.* All participants must know what their participation will involve and what risks might develop. For example, participants in a study on dating should be told beforehand that a questionnaire might stimulate thoughts about issues in their relationship that they had not considered. Participants also should be informed that in some instances a discussion of the issues might improve their relationship, but in others it might worsen the relationship and even end it. Even after informed consent is given, participants have the right to withdraw from the study at any time and for any reason.

- *Confidentiality.* Researchers are responsible for keeping all of the data they gather on individuals completely confidential and, when possible, completely anonymous.

- *Debriefing.* After the study has been completed, participants should be informed of its purpose and the methods that were used. In most cases, the experimenter also can inform participants in a general manner beforehand about the purpose of the research without leading participants to behave in a way they think that the experimenter is expecting. When preliminary information about the study is likely to affect the results, participants can at least be debriefed after the study has been completed.

- *Deception.* This is an ethical issue that researchers debate extensively. In some circumstances, telling the participants beforehand what the research study is about substantially alters the participants' behavior and invalidates the researcher's data. In all cases of deception, however, the psychologist must ensure that the deception will not harm the participants and that the participants will be told the complete nature of the study (debriefed) as soon as possible after the study is completed.

Pam Reid, Educational and Developmental Psychologist

When she was a child, Pam Reid liked to play with chemistry sets. Reid majored in chemistry during college and wanted to become a doctor. However, when some of her friends signed up for a psychology class as an elective, she also decided to take the course. She was intrigued by learning about how people think, behave, and develop—so much so that she changed her major to psychology. Reid went on to obtain her Ph.D. in psychology (American Psychological Association, 2003, p. 16).

For many years Reid was a professor of education and psychology at the University of Michigan, where she also was a research scientist at the Institute for Research on Women and Gender, focusing on how children and adolescents develop social skills, with a special interest in the development of African American girls (Reid & Zalk, 2001). Reid then became provost and executive vice-president at Roosevelt University and served as President of the University of Saint Joseph from 2008 until she retired in 2015.

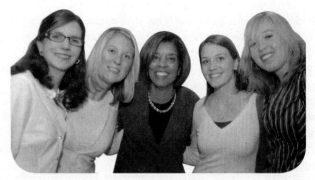

Pam Reid (*center*) with students at the University of Saint Joseph in Hartford, Connecticut, where she was the president of the university.
Courtesy of Dr. Pam Reid

For more information about what professors, researchers, and educational psychologists do, see the Careers in Child Development appendix.

Minimizing Bias   Studies of children's development are most useful when they are conducted without bias or prejudice toward any particular group of people. Of special concern is bias based on gender and bias based on culture or ethnicity.

Gender Bias   For most of its existence, our society has had a strong gender bias, a preconceived notion about the abilities of males and females that prevented individuals from pursuing their own interests and achieving their full potential (Garg & others, 2018). Gender bias also has had a less obvious effect within the field of child development. For example, it is not unusual for conclusions to be drawn about females' attitudes and behaviors from research conducted with males as the only participants.

Furthermore, when researchers find gender differences, their reports sometimes magnify those differences (Hyde & others, 2018). For example, a researcher might report that 74 percent of the boys in a study had high achievement expectations versus only 67 percent of the girls and go on to talk about the differences in some detail. In reality, this might be a rather small difference. It also might disappear if the study was repeated, or the study might have methodological problems that don't allow such strong interpretations.

Pam Reid is a leading researcher who studies gender and ethnic bias in development. To read about Pam's interests, see *Connecting with Careers.*

Cultural and Ethnic Bias   Research on children's development needs to include more children from diverse ethnic groups (Causadias & Umaña-Taylor, 2018). Historically, children from ethnic minority groups (African American, Latino, Asian American, and Native American) were excluded from most research in the United States and simply thought of as variations from the norm or average. If minority children were included in samples and their scores didn't fit the norm, the information was viewed as confounds or "noise" in data and discounted. Given the fact that children from diverse ethnic groups were excluded from research on child development for so long, we might reasonably conclude that children's real lives are perhaps more varied than research data have indicated in the past.

Researchers also have tended to overgeneralize about ethnic groups. **Ethnic gloss** is using an ethnic label such as *African American* or *Latino* in a superficial way that portrays an ethnic group as being more homogeneous than it really is (Trimble & Bhadra, 2013).

- - - - - - - - - ->

developmental **connection**

Culture and Ethnicity

What characterizes an adolescent's ethnic identity? Connect to "The Self and Identity."

<- - - - - - - - - - -

ethnic gloss Use of an ethnic label such as *African American* or *Latino* in a superficial way that portrays an ethnic group as being more homogeneous than it really is.

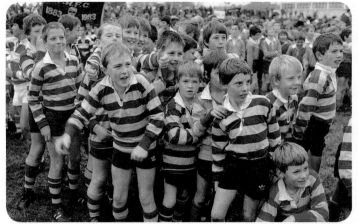 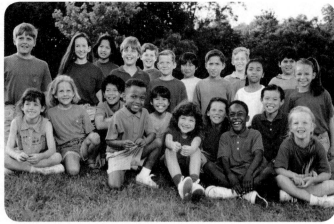

Look at these two photographs, one (*left*) of all non-Latino white boys, the other (*right*) of boys and girls from diverse ethnic backgrounds. Consider a topic in child development, such as independence seeking, cultural values, parenting education, or health care. *If you were conducting research on this topic, might the results of the study be different depending on whether the participants in your study were the children in the photo on the left or the photo on the right?*

(*left*): Kevin Fleming/Corbis Documentary/Getty Images; (*right*): C. Thatcher/Getty Images

For example, a researcher might describe a research sample like this: "The participants were 60 Latinos." A more complete description of the Latino group might be something like this: "The 60 Latino participants were Mexican Americans from low-income neighborhoods in the southwestern area of Los Angeles. Thirty-six were from homes in which Spanish is the dominant language spoken, 24 from homes in which English is the main language spoken. Thirty were born in the United States, 30 in Mexico. Twenty-eight described themselves as Mexican American, 14 as Mexican, 9 as American, 6 as Chicano, and 3 as Latino." Ethnic gloss can cause researchers to obtain samples of ethnic groups that are not representative of the group's diversity, which can lead to overgeneralization and stereotyping.

Research on ethnic minority children and their families has not been given adequate attention, especially in light of their significant rate of growth within the U.S. population (U.S. Census Bureau, 2017b). Until recently, ethnic minority families were combined in the category "minority," which masks important differences among ethnic groups as well as diversity within an ethnic group. At present and in the foreseeable future, the growth of minority families in the United States will be mainly due to the immigration of Latino and Asian families. Researchers need to take into account families' acculturation level and the generational status of both parents and adolescents (Gauvain, 2013). More attention needs to be given to biculturalism because many immigrant children and adolescents identify with two or more ethnic groups (Yip, 2018).

Review *Connect* Reflect

LG3 Summarize why research is important in child development, the main theories of child development, and research methods, designs, and challenges.

Review

- What is scientific research, what is it based on, and why is scientific research on child development important?
- What are the main theories of child development?
- What are the main research methods for collecting data about children's development?
- What types of research designs do child development researchers use?
- What are some research challenges in studying children's development?

Connect

- Which of the research methods for collecting data would be appropriate or inappropriate for studying Erikson's stage of trust versus mistrust? Why?

Reflect *Your Own Personal Journey of Life*

- Which of the theories of child development do you think best explains your own development? Why?

Introduction

Caring for Children

 LG1 Identify five areas in which children's lives need to be improved, and explain the roles of resilience and social policy in children's development.

Improving the Lives of Children

- Health and well-being is an important area in which children's lives can be improved. Today, many children in the United States and around the world need improved health care. We now recognize the importance of lifestyles and psychological states in promoting health and well-being. Parenting is an important influence on children's development. One-parent families, working parents, and child care are among the family issues that influence children's well-being. Education can also contribute to children's health and well-being. There is widespread concern that the education of children needs to be more effective, and there are many views in contemporary education about ways to improve schools.

Resilience, Social Policy, and Children's Development

- Some children triumph over adversity—they are resilient. Researchers have found that resilient children are likely to have a close relationship with a parent figure and to form bonds with caring people outside the family. Social policy is a government's course of action designed to promote the welfare of its citizens. The poor conditions of life for a significant percentage of U.S. children, and the lack of attention to prevention of these poor conditions, point to the need for revised social policies.

Developmental Processes, Periods, and Issues

LG2 Discuss the most important processes, periods, and issues in development.

Biological, Cognitive, and Socioemotional Processes

- Three key processes of development are biological, cognitive, and socioemotional. Biological processes (such as genes inherited from parents) involve changes in an individual's body. Cognitive processes (such as thinking) consist of changes in an individual's thought, intelligence, and language. Socioemotional processes (such as the advent of smiling) include changes in an individual's relationships with others, in emotions, and in personality.

Periods of Development

- Childhood's five main developmental periods are (1) prenatal, from conception to birth, (2) infancy, from birth to 18 to 24 months, (3) early childhood, from the end of infancy to about 5 or 6 years of age, (4) middle and late childhood, from about 6 to 11 years of age, and (5) adolescence, which begins at about 10 or 12 and ends at about 18 or 19 years of age.

Cohort Effects

- Cohort effects are due to a person's time of birth, era, or generation but not to actual age. Two characteristics of today's children and many of their parents—the generation labeled millennials—that stand out are their ethnic diversity and their connection to technology.

Issues in Development

- The nature-nurture issue focuses on the extent to which development is mainly influenced by nature (biological inheritance) or nurture (environmental experience). Some developmentalists describe development as continuous (gradual, cumulative change), while others describe it as discontinuous (a sequence of distinct stages). The early-later experience issue focuses on whether early experiences (especially in infancy) are more important in development than later experiences. Most developmentalists recognize that extreme positions on the nature-nurture, continuity-discontinuity, and early-later experience issues are not supported by research. Despite this consensus, they continue to debate the degree to which each issue influences children's development.

The Science of Child Development

LG3 Summarize why research is important in child development, the main theories of child development, and research methods, designs, and challenges.

The Importance of Research

- Scientific research is objective, systematic, and testable. Scientific research is based on the scientific method, which includes the following steps: (1) conceptualize the problem, (2) collect data, (3) draw conclusions, and (4) revise theory. Scientific research on child development reduces the likelihood that the information gathered is based on personal beliefs, opinions, and feelings.

Theories of Child Development

- Psychoanalytic theories describe development as primarily unconscious and as heavily colored by emotion. The two main psychoanalytic theories in developmental psychology are Freud's and Erikson's. Freud proposed that individuals go through five psychosexual stages—oral, anal, phallic, latency, and genital. Erikson's theory emphasizes eight psychosocial stages of development. The three main cognitive theories are Piaget's cognitive developmental theory, Vygotsky's sociocultural theory, and information-processing theory. Cognitive theories emphasize conscious thoughts. In Piaget's theory, children go through four cognitive stages: sensorimotor, preoperational, concrete operational, and formal operational. Vygotsky's sociocultural cognitive theory emphasizes how culture and social interaction guide cognitive development. The information-processing theory emphasizes that individuals manipulate information, monitor it, and strategize about it. Three versions of the behavioral and social cognitive theories are Pavlov's classical conditioning, Skinner's operant conditioning, and Bandura's social cognitive theory. Ethology stresses that behavior is strongly influenced by biology, is tied to evolution, and is characterized by critical or sensitive periods. Ecological theory is Bronfenbrenner's environmental systems view of development. It consists of five environmental systems: microsystem, mesosystem, exosystem, macrosystem, and chronosystem. An eclectic theoretical orientation does not follow any one theoretical approach but rather selects from each theory whatever is considered the best in it.

Research Methods for Collecting Data

- Research methods for collecting data about child development include observation (in a laboratory or a naturalistic setting), survey (questionnaire) or interview, standardized test, case study, and physiological measures.

Research Designs

- Descriptive research aims to observe and record behavior. In correlational research, the goal is to describe the strength of the relationship between two or more events or characteristics. Experimental research involves conducting an experiment that can determine cause and effect. An independent variable is the manipulated, influential, experimental factor. A dependent variable is a factor that can change in an experiment, in response to changes in the independent variable. Experiments can involve one or more experimental groups and control groups. In random assignment, researchers assign participants to experimental and control groups by chance. When researchers decide about the time span of their research, they can conduct cross-sectional or longitudinal studies.

Challenges in Child Development Research

- Researchers' ethical responsibilities include seeking participants' informed consent, ensuring their confidentiality, debriefing them about the purpose and potential personal consequences of participating, and avoiding unnecessary deception of participants. Researchers need to guard against gender, cultural, and ethnic bias in research. Every effort should be made to make research equitable for both females and males. Individuals from varied ethnic backgrounds need to be included as participants in child research, and overgeneralization about diverse members within a group must be avoided.

key **terms**

key **people**

appendix

Careers in Child Development

Each of us wants to find a rewarding career and enjoy the work we do. The field of child development offers an amazing breadth of career options that can provide extremely satisfying work.

If you decide to pursue a career in child development, what career options are available to you? There are many. College and university professors teach courses in areas of child development, education, family development, nursing, and medicine. Teachers impart knowledge, understanding, and skills to children and adolescents. Counselors, clinical psychologists, nurses, and physicians help parents and children of all ages to cope more effectively with their lives and well-being. Various professionals work with families to improve the quality of family functioning.

Although an advanced degree is not absolutely necessary in some areas of child development, you usually can expand your opportunities (and income) considerably by obtaining a graduate degree. Many careers in child development pay reasonably well. For example, psychologists earn well above the median salary in the United States. Also, by working in the field of child development you can guide people in improving their lives, understand yourself and others better, possibly advance the state of knowledge in the field, and have an enjoyable time while you are doing these things.

If you are considering a career in child development, would you prefer to work with infants, children, adolescents, parents or a combination of these? As you go through this term, try to spend some time with children of different ages. Observe their behavior. Talk with them about their lives. Think about whether you would like to work with children of this age in your life's work.

Another important way to explore careers is to talk with people who work in various jobs. For example, if you have some interest in becoming a school counselor, call a school, ask to speak with a counselor, and set up an appointment to discuss the counselor's career and work.

Something else that should benefit you is to work in one or more jobs related to your career interests while you are in college. Many colleges and universities have internships or work experiences for students who major in fields such as child development. In some instances, these jobs earn course credit or pay; in others, they are strictly on a volunteer basis. Take advantage of these opportunities. They can provide you with valuable experiences to help you decide whether this is the right career for you, and they can help you get into graduate school if you decide that you want to go.

In the upcoming sections, we will profile careers in four areas: education and research; clinical and counseling; medical, nursing, and physical development; and families and relationships. We have provided chapter references after some entries telling you where within the text you can find *Connecting with Careers,* the career profiles of people who hold some of these positions. These are not the only career options in child development, but they should provide you with an idea of the range of opportunities available and information about some of the main career avenues you might pursue. In profiling these careers, we will address the amount of education required, the type of training involved, and the nature of the work.

Education and Research

Numerous career opportunities in child development involve education or research. These positions range from college professor to child-care director to school psychologist.

College/University Professor

Courses in child development are taught in many programs and schools in colleges and universities, including psychology, education, nursing, child and family studies, social work, and medicine. The work that college professors do includes teaching courses at the undergraduate or graduate level (or both), conducting research in a specific area, advising students and/or directing their research, and serving on college or university committees. Some college instructors do not conduct research as part of their job but instead focus mainly on teaching. Research is most likely to be part of the job description at universities with master's and Ph.D. programs. A Ph.D. or master's degree almost always is required to teach in some area of child development in a college or university. Obtaining a doctoral degree usually takes four to six years of graduate work, and it is becoming common to do additional "postdoctoral" training to further build and refine skills. A master's degree requires approximately two years of graduate work. The training involves taking graduate courses, learning to conduct research, and attending and presenting papers at professional meetings. Many graduate students work as teaching or research assistants for professors in an apprenticeship relationship that helps them to become competent teachers and researchers.

If you are interested in becoming a college or university professor, you might want to make an appointment with your instructor in this class on child development to learn more about his or her profession and work. **Read a profile of a professor** in the chapter "Culture and Diversity."

Researcher

Some individuals in the field of child development work in research positions. In most instances, they have either a master's degree or Ph.D. in some area of child development. The researchers might work at a university, perhaps in a university professor's research program, in government at agencies such as the National Institutes of Health, or in private industry. Individuals who have full-time research positions in child development generate innovative research ideas, plan studies, carry out the research by collecting data, analyze the data, and then interpret it. Then they will usually attempt to publish the research in a scientific journal. A researcher often works in a collaborative manner with other researchers on a project and may present the research at scientific meetings. One researcher might spend much of his or her time in a laboratory while another researcher might work in the field, such as in schools, hospitals, and so on.

Elementary School Teacher

The work of an elementary or secondary school teacher involves teaching in one or more subject areas, preparing the curriculum, giving tests, assigning grades, monitoring students' progress, conducting parent-teacher conferences, and attending in-service workshops. Becoming an elementary or secondary school teacher requires a minimum of an undergraduate degree. The training involves taking a wide range of courses with a major or concentration in education as well as completing a supervised practice-teaching internship. **Read a profile of an elementary school teacher** in the chapter "Cognitive Developmental Approaches."

Exceptional Children (Special Education) Teacher

A teacher of exceptional children spends concentrated time with individual children who have a disability or are gifted. Among the students a teacher of exceptional children might work with are children with learning disabilities, ADHD (attention deficit hyperactivity disorder), intellectual disability, or a physical disability such as cerebral palsy. Some of this work will usually be done outside the student's regular classroom, and some of it will be carried out when the student is in the regular classroom. A teacher of exceptional children works closely with the student's regular classroom teacher and parents to create the best educational program for the student. Becoming a teacher of exceptional children requires a minimum of an undergraduate degree. The training consists of taking a wide range of courses in education and a concentration of courses in educating children with disabilities or children who are gifted. Teachers of exceptional children often continue their education after obtaining their undergraduate degree and attain a master's degree.

Early Childhood Educator

Early childhood educators work on college faculties and have a minimum of a master's degree in their field. In graduate school, they take courses in early childhood education and receive supervisory training in child-care or early childhood programs. Early childhood educators usually teach in community colleges that award an associate's degree in early childhood education.

Preschool/Kindergarten Teacher

Preschool teachers teach mainly 4-year-old children, and kindergarten teachers primarily teach 5-year-old children. They usually have an undergraduate degree in education, specializing in early childhood education. State certification to become a preschool or kindergarten teacher usually is required.

Family and Consumer Science Educator

Family and consumer science educators may specialize in early childhood education or instruct middle and high school students on topics such as nutrition, interpersonal relationships, human sexuality, parenting, and human development. Hundreds of colleges and universities throughout the United States offer two- and four-year degree programs in family and consumer science. These programs usually include an internship requirement. Additional education courses may be needed to obtain a teaching certificate. Some family and consumer educators go on to graduate school for further training, which provides a background for possible jobs in college teaching or research.

Educational Psychologist

An educational psychologist most often teaches in a college or university and conducts research in areas of educational psychology such as learning, motivation, classroom management, and assessment. Most educational psychologists have a doctorate in education, which takes four to six years of graduate work. They help to train students who will take various positions in education, including educational psychology, school psychology, and teaching.

School Psychologist

School psychologists focus on improving the psychological and intellectual well-being of elementary and secondary school students. They may work in a centralized office in a school district or in one or more schools. They give psychological tests, interview students and their parents, consult with teachers, and may provide counseling to students and their families.

School psychologists usually have a master's or doctoral degree in school psychology. In graduate school, they take courses in counseling, assessment, learning, and other areas of education and psychology.

Clinical and Counseling

A wide variety of clinical and counseling jobs are linked with child development. These range from child clinical psychologist to adolescent drug counselor.

Clinical Psychologist

Clinical psychologists seek to help people with psychological problems. They work in a variety of settings, including colleges and universities, clinics, medical schools, and private practice. Some clinical psychologists only conduct psychotherapy, others do psychological assessment and psychotherapy, and some also do research. Clinical psychologists may specialize in a particular age group, such as children (child clinical psychologist).

Clinical psychologists have either a Ph.D. (which involves clinical and research training) or a Psy.D. degree (which only involves clinical training). This graduate training usually takes five to seven years and includes courses in clinical psychology and a one-year supervised internship in an accredited setting toward the end of the training. In most cases, they must pass a test to become licensed in a state and to call themselves clinical psychologists. **Read a profile of a clinical child psychologist** in the chapter "Introduction."

Psychiatrist

Like clinical psychologists, psychiatrists might specialize in working with children (child psychiatry) or adolescents (adolescent psychiatry). Psychiatrists might work in medical schools in teaching and research roles, in a medical clinic, or in private practice. In addition to administering drugs to help improve the lives of people with psychological problems, psychiatrists also may conduct psychotherapy. Psychiatrists obtain a medical degree and then do a residency in psychiatry. Medical school takes approximately four years, and the psychiatry residency another three to four years. Unlike psychologists (who do not go to medical school), in most states psychiatrists can administer drugs to clients.

Counseling Psychologist

Counseling psychologists work in the same settings as clinical psychologists and may do psychotherapy, teach, or conduct research. In many instances, however, counseling psychologists do not work with individuals who have a severe mental disorder. A counseling psychologist might specialize in working with children, adolescents, and/or families.

Counseling psychologists go through much of the same training as clinical psychologists, although they are enrolled in a graduate program in counseling rather than clinical psychology. Counseling psychologists have either a master's

degree or a doctoral degree. They also must go through a licensing procedure. One type of master's degree in counseling leads to the designation of licensed professional counselor.

School Counselor

School counselors help to identify students' abilities and interests, guide students in developing academic plans, and explore career options with students. They may help students cope with adjustment problems. They may work with students individually, in small groups, or even in a classroom. They often consult with parents, teachers, and school administrators when trying to help students with their problems.

High school counselors advise students on choosing a major, satisfying admissions requirements for college, taking entrance exams, applying for financial aid, and pursuing appropriate vocational and technical training. Elementary school counselors are mainly involved in counseling students about social and personal problems. They may observe children in the classroom and at play as part of their work. School counselors usually have a master's degree in counseling.

Social Worker

Social workers often are involved in helping children and adults with social or economic problems. They may investigate, evaluate, and attempt to rectify reported cases of abuse, neglect, endangerment, or domestic disputes. They can intervene in families if necessary and provide counseling and referral services to children and families.

Social workers have a minimum of an undergraduate degree from a school of social work that includes coursework in various areas of sociology and psychology. Some social workers also have a master's or doctoral degree. They often work for publicly funded agencies at the city, state, or national level, although increasingly they work in the private sector in areas such as drug rehabilitation and family counseling.

In some cases, social workers specialize in a certain area, as is true of a medical social worker, who has a master's degree in social work (MSW). This involves graduate coursework and supervised clinical experiences in medical settings. A medical social worker might coordinate a variety of support services provided to people with severe or long-term disabilities. Family care social workers often work with families who need support services.

Drug Counselor

Drug counselors provide counseling to children and adults with drug abuse problems. They may work on an individual basis with a substance abuser or conduct group therapy sessions. They may work in private practice, with a state or federal government agency, with a company, or in a hospital setting. Some drug counselors specialize in working with adolescents or families. Most states provide a certification procedure for obtaining a license to practice drug counseling.

At a minimum, drug counselors go through an associate's or certificate program. Many have an undergraduate degree in substance-abuse counseling, and some have master's and doctoral degrees.

Medical, Nursing, and Physical Development

This third main area of careers in child development includes a wide range of careers in the medical and nursing areas, as well as jobs that focus on improving some aspect of the child's physical development.

Obstetrician/Gynecologist

An obstetrician/gynecologist prescribes prenatal and postnatal care and performs deliveries in maternity cases. The individual also treats diseases and injuries of the female reproductive system. Obstetricians may work in private practice, in a medical clinic, in a hospital, or in a medical school. Becoming an obstetrician/gynecologist requires a medical degree plus three to five years of residency in obstetrics/ gynecology.

Pediatrician

A pediatrician monitors infants' and children's health, works to prevent disease or injury, helps children attain optimal health, and treats children with health problems. Pediatricians may work in private practice, in a medical clinic, in a hospital, or in a medical school. As medical doctors, they can administer drugs to children and may counsel parents and children on ways to improve children's health. Many pediatricians on the faculties of medical schools also teach and conduct research on children's health and diseases. Pediatricians have attained a medical degree and completed a three-to five-year residency in pediatrics.

Neonatal Nurse

A neonatal nurse is involved in the delivery of care to newborn infants. The neonatal nurse may work to improve the health and well-being of infants born under normal circumstances or be involved in the delivery of care to premature and critically ill neonates.

A minimum of an undergraduate degree in nursing with a specialization in the newborn is required. This training involves coursework in nursing and the biological sciences, as well as supervisory clinical experiences.

Nurse-Midwife

A nurse-midwife formulates and provides comprehensive care to selected maternity patients, cares for the expectant mother as she prepares to give birth and guides her through the birth process, and cares for the postpartum patient. The nurse-midwife also may provide care to the newborn, counsel parents on the infant's development and parenting, and provide guidance about health practices. Becoming a nurse-midwife generally requires an undergraduate degree from a school of nursing. A nurse-midwife most often works in a hospital setting. **Read the profile of a perinatal nurse** in the chapter "Prenatal Development and Birth."

Pediatric Nurse

Pediatric nurses have a degree in nursing that takes from two to five years to complete. Some also may obtain a master's or doctoral degree in pediatric nursing. Pediatric nurses take courses in biological sciences, nursing care, and pediatrics, usually in a school of nursing. They also undergo supervised clinical experiences in medical settings. They monitor infants' and children's health, work to prevent disease or injury, and help children attain optimal health. They may work in hospitals, schools of nursing, or with pediatricians in private practice or at a medical clinic.

Audiologist

An audiologist has a minimum of an undergraduate degree in hearing science. This includes courses and supervisory training. Audiologists assess and identify the presence and severity of hearing loss as well as problems in balance. Some audiologists also go on to obtain a master's and/or doctoral degree. They may work in a medical clinic, with a physician in private practice, in a hospital, or in a medical school.

Speech Therapist

Speech therapists are health-care professionals who are trained to identify, assess, and treat speech and language problems. They may work with physicians, psychologists, social workers, and other health-care professionals as a team to help individuals with physical or psychological problems that include speech and language problems. Speech pathologists have a minimum of an undergraduate degree in speech and hearing science or communication disorders. They may work in private practice, in hospitals and medical schools, or in government agencies with individuals of any age. Some specialize in working with children or with a particular type of speech disorder. **Read a profile of a speech pathologist** in the chapter "Language Development."

Genetic Counselor

Genetic counselors work as members of a health care team, providing information and support to families who have members with birth defects or genetic disorders and to families who may be at risk for a variety of inherited conditions. They identify families at risk and provide supportive counseling. They serve as educators and resource people for other health care professionals and the public. Almost half work in university medical centers and another one-fourth work in private hospital settings.

Most genetic counselors enter the field after majoring in undergraduate school in such disciplines as biology, genetics, psychology, nursing, public health, and social work. They have specialized graduate degrees and experience in medical genetics and counseling. **Read a profile of a genetic counselor** in the chapter "Biological Beginnings."

Families and Relationships

A number of careers involve working with families and relationship problems. These range from being a child welfare worker to a marriage and family therapist.

Child Welfare Worker

A child welfare worker is employed by the child protective services unit of each state. The child welfare worker protects the child's rights, evaluates any maltreatment the child might experience, and may have the child removed from the home if necessary. A child social worker has a minimum of an undergraduate degree in social work.

Child Life Specialist

Child life specialists work with children and their families when the child needs to be hospitalized. They monitor the child patient's activities, seek to reduce the child's stress, help the child cope effectively, and assist the child in enjoying the hospital experience as much as possible. Child life specialists may provide parent education and develop individualized treatment plans based on an assessment of the child's development, temperament, medical plan, and available social supports.

Child life specialists have an undergraduate degree. As undergraduates, they take courses in child development and education and usually take additional courses in a child life program.

Marriage and Family Therapist

The work of marriage and family therapists is based on the principle that many individuals who have psychological problems benefit when psychotherapy is provided in the context of a marital or family relationship. Marriage and family therapists may provide marital therapy, couples therapy to individuals in a relationship who are not married, and family therapy to two or more members of a family.

Marriage and family therapists have a master's or doctoral degree. They go through a training program in graduate school similar to that of a clinical psychologist but with a focus on marital and family relationships. To practice marital and family therapy in most states, it is necessary to go through a licensing procedure.

These are only a handful of careers that require knowledge of developmental psychology. *Connecting with Careers* throughout this text highlight additional careers, including toy designer, infant assessment specialist, supervisor of gifted and talented education, English Language Learner (ELL) teacher, child-care director, health psychologist, and director of children's services. *What other careers can you think of that require knowledge of children's development?*

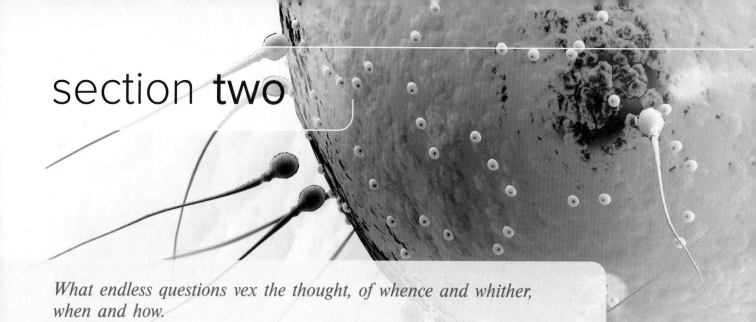

section two

What endless questions vex the thought, of whence and whither, when and how.

—SIR RICHARD BURTON
British explorer, 19th century

Biological Processes, Physical Development, and Perceptual Development

The rhythm and meaning of life involve beginnings, with questions raised about how, from so simple a beginning, complex forms develop, grow, and mature. What was this organism, what is this organism, and what will this organism be? In Section 2, you will read four chapters: "Biological Beginnings," "Prenatal Development and Birth," "Physical Development and Health," and "Motor, Sensory, and Perceptual Development."

chapter 2

BIOLOGICAL BEGINNINGS

chapter outline

1 The Evolutionary Perspective

Learning Goal 1 Discuss the evolutionary perspective on child development.

Natural Selection and Adaptive Behavior
Evolutionary Psychology

2 Genetic Foundations of Development

Learning Goal 2 Describe what genes are and how they influence children's development.

The Collaborative Gene
Genes and Chromosomes
Genetic Principles
Chromosomal and Gene-Linked Abnormalities

3 Reproductive Challenges and Choices

Learning Goal 3 Identify some important reproductive challenges and choices.

Prenatal Diagnostic Tests
Infertility and Reproductive Technology
Adoption

4 Heredity and Environment Interaction: Nature and Nurture

Learning Goal 4 Explain some of the ways that heredity and environment interact to produce individual differences in development.

Behavior Genetics
Heredity-Environment Correlations
Shared and Nonshared Environmental Experiences
The Epigenetic View and Gene × Environment (G × E) Interaction
Conclusions About Heredity-Environment Interaction

Image Source/Getty Images

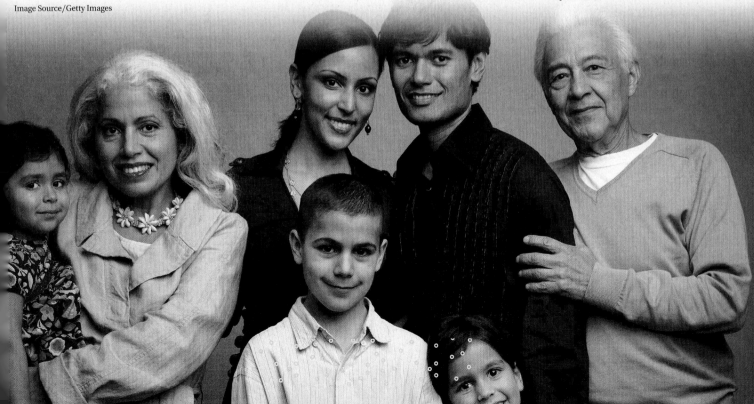

Jim Springer and Jim Lewis are identical twins. They were separated at 4 weeks of age and did not see each other again until they were 39 years old. Both worked as part-time deputy sheriffs, vacationed in Florida, drove Chevrolets, had dogs named Toy, and married and divorced women named Betty. One twin named his son James Allan, and the other named his son James Alan. Both liked math but not spelling, enjoyed carpentry and mechanical drawing, chewed their fingernails down to the nubs, had almost identical drinking and smoking habits, had hemorrhoids, put on 10 pounds at about the same point in development, first suffered headaches at the age of 18, and had similar sleep patterns.

Jim and Jim do have some differences. One wears his hair over his forehead; the other slicks it back and has sideburns. One expresses himself best orally; the other is more proficient in writing. But, for the most part, their profiles are remarkably similar.

Another pair of identical twins, Daphne and Barbara, are called the "giggle sisters" because, after being reunited, they were always making each other laugh. A thorough search of their adoptive families' histories revealed no gigglers. The giggle sisters ignored stress, avoided conflict and controversy whenever possible, and showed no interest in politics.

Jim and Jim and the giggle sisters were part of the Minnesota Study of Twins Reared Apart, directed by Thomas Bouchard and his colleagues. The study brings identical twins (identical genetically because they come from the same fertilized egg) and fraternal twins (who come from different fertilized eggs) from all over the world to Minneapolis to investigate their lives. There the twins complete personality and intelligence tests, and they provide detailed medical histories, including information about diet and smoking, exercise habits, chest X-rays, heart stress tests, and EEGs. The twins are asked more than 15,000 questions about their family and childhood, personal interests, vocational orientation, values, and aesthetic judgments (Bouchard & others, 1990).

When genetically identical twins who were separated as infants show such striking similarities in their tastes and habits and choices, can we conclude that their genes must have caused the development of those tastes and habits and choices? Other possible causes need to be considered. The twins shared not only the same genes but also some experiences. Some of the separated twins lived together for several months prior to their adoption; some of the twins had been reunited prior to testing (in some cases, many years earlier); adoption agencies often place twins in similar homes; and even strangers who spend several hours together and start comparing their lives are likely to come up with some coincidental similarities (Joseph, 2006). The Minnesota study of identical twins points to both the importance of the genetic basis of human development and the need for further research on genetic and environmental factors (Lykken, 2001).

preview

The examples of Jim and Jim and the giggle sisters stimulate us to think about our genetic heritage and the biological foundations of our existence. However, organisms are not like billiard balls, moved by simple external forces to predictable positions on life's table. Environmental experiences and biological foundations work together to make us who we are. Our coverage of life's biological beginnings focuses on evolution, genetic foundations, challenges and choices regarding reproduction, and the interaction of heredity and environment.

The Evolutionary Perspective Discuss the evolutionary perspective on child development.

> Natural Selection and Adaptive Behavior

> Evolutionary Psychology

In evolutionary time, humans are relative newcomers to Earth. As our earliest ancestors left the forest to feed on the savannahs and then to form hunting societies on the open plains, their minds and behaviors changed, and they eventually established humans as the dominant species on Earth. How did this evolution come about?

NATURAL SELECTION AND ADAPTIVE BEHAVIOR

Natural selection is the evolutionary process by which those individuals of a species that are best adapted are the ones that survive and reproduce. To understand what this means, let's return to the middle of the nineteenth century, when the British naturalist Charles Darwin was traveling around the world, observing many different species of animals in their natural surroundings. Darwin, who published his observations and thoughts in *On the Origin of Species* (1859), noted that most organisms reproduce at rates that would cause enormous increases in the population of most species and yet populations remain nearly constant. He reasoned that an intense, constant struggle for food, water, and resources must occur among the many young born each generation, because many of the young do not survive. Those that do survive and reproduce pass on their characteristics to the next generation. Darwin argued that these survivors are better *adapted* to their world than are the nonsurvivors (Simon, Dickey, & Reese, 2013). The best-adapted individuals survive to leave the most offspring. Over the course of many generations, organisms with the characteristics needed for survival make up an increasing percentage of the population. Over many, many generations, this could produce a gradual modification of the whole population (Brooker & others, 2014). If environmental conditions change, however, other characteristics might become favored by natural selection, moving the species in a different direction (Mader & Windelspecht, 2013).

All organisms must adapt to particular places, climates, food sources, and ways of life (Hoefnagels, 2013). An eagle's claws are a physical adaptation that facilitates predation. *Adaptive behavior* is behavior that promotes an organism's survival in the natural habitat. For example, attachment between a caregiver and a baby ensures the infant's closeness to a caregiver for feeding and protection from danger, thus increasing the infant's chances of survival.

EVOLUTIONARY PSYCHOLOGY

Although Darwin introduced the theory of evolution by natural selection in 1859, his ideas only recently have become a popular framework for explaining behavior. Psychology's newest approach, **evolutionary psychology,** emphasizes the importance of adaptation, reproduction, and "survival of the fittest" in shaping behavior. "Fit" in this sense refers to the ability to bear offspring that survive long enough to bear offspring of their own. In this view, natural selection favors behaviors that increase reproductive success—the ability to pass genes to the next generation (Cosmides, 2013; Durrant & Ellis, 2013).

> There are one hundred and ninety-three living species of monkeys and apes. One hundred and ninety-two of them are covered with hair. The exception is the naked ape, self-named Homo sapiens.
>
> **—DESMOND MORRIS**
> *British zoologist, 20th century*

evolutionary psychology Branch of psychology that emphasizes the importance of adaptation, reproduction, and "survival of the fittest" in shaping behavior.

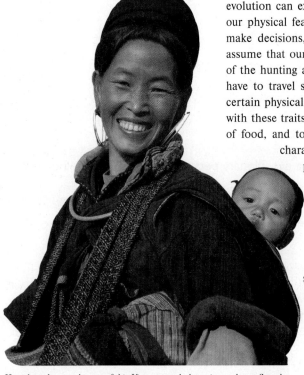

How does the attachment of this Vietnamese baby to its mother reflect the evolutionary process of adaptive behavior?

frans lemmens/age fotostock

David Buss (2015) has been especially influential in stimulating new interest in how evolution can explain human behavior. He reasons that just as evolution has contributed to our physical features such as body shape and height, it also pervasively influences how we make decisions, how aggressive we are, our fears, and our mating patterns. For example, assume that our ancestors were hunters and gatherers on the plains and that men did most of the hunting and women stayed close to home gathering seeds and plants for food. If you have to travel some distance from your home to find and slay a fleeing animal, you need certain physical traits along with the capacity for certain types of spatial thinking. Men born with these traits would be more likely than men without them to survive, to bring home lots of food, and to be considered attractive mates—and thus to reproduce and pass on these characteristics to their children. In other words, if these assumptions were correct, potentially these traits would provide a reproductive advantage for males. Over many generations, men with good spatial thinking skills might become more numerous in the population. Critics point out that this scenario might or might not have actually happened.

Anthropological research in current hunter-gatherer societies, such as the Hadza in Tanzania, suggests that mothers' and grandmothers' foraging supplies the large majority of families' caloric intake, as male hunters are successful on only 3.4 percent of hunting excursions (Hawkes, 2017). First-time mothers' foraging skills are correlated with infants' growth, but after the birth of a second infant, the correlation between mothers' foraging and infant growth disappears, and a correlation between grandmothers' foraging skills and infant growth emerges (Hawkes, 2017). These findings have several implications for understanding human evolution, including why humans are the only great apes in which women live long past reproductive age and why social orientation and cooperation are so central to our species (Hrdy, 2009).

Evolutionary Developmental Psychology   Recently, interest has grown in using the concepts of evolutionary psychology to understand human development (Belsky, 2013; Bjorklund, Hernandez Blasi, & Ellis, 2017; Narváez & others, 2013). Here we discuss some ideas proposed by evolutionary developmental psychologists (Bjorklund & Pellegrini, 2002).

An extended childhood period might have evolved because humans require time to develop a large brain and learn the complexity of human societies. Humans take longer to become reproductively mature than any other mammal (see Figure 1). During this extended childhood

FIGURE 1

THE BRAIN SIZES OF VARIOUS PRIMATES AND HUMANS IN RELATION TO THE LENGTH OF THE CHILDHOOD PERIOD. Compared with other primates, humans have both a larger brain and a longer childhood period. *What conclusions can you draw from the relation indicated by this graph?*

Tier Und Naturfotografie J und C Sohns/Getty Images

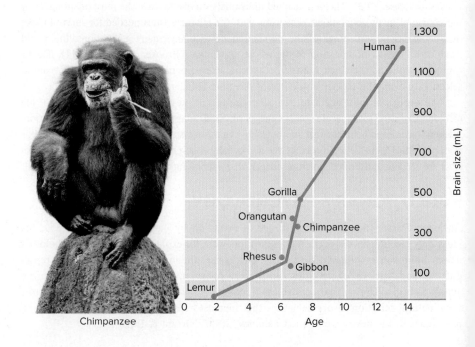

Chimpanzee

period, they develop a large brain and have the experiences needed to become competent adults in a complex society.

Many of our evolved psychological mechanisms are domain-specific—that is, the mechanisms apply only to a specific aspect of a person's psychological makeup. According to evolutionary psychology, the mind is not a general-purpose device that can be applied equally to a vast array of problems. Instead, as our ancestors dealt with certain recurring problems such as hunting and finding shelter, specialized modules evolved that process information related to those problems. For example, such specialized modules might include a module for physical knowledge for tracking animals, a module for mathematical knowledge for trading, and a module for language.

Evolved mechanisms are not always adaptive in contemporary society. Some behaviors that were adaptive for our prehistoric ancestors may not serve us well today. For example, the food-scarce environment of our ancestors likely led to humans' propensity to gorge when food is available and to crave high-caloric foods, a trait that might lead to an epidemic of obesity when food is plentiful.

Evaluating Evolutionary Psychology   Although the popular press gives a lot of attention to the ideas of evolutionary psychology, it remains just one theoretical approach among many. Like the theories described previously, it has limitations, weaknesses, and critics (Hyde & Else-Quest, 2013; Matlin, 2012). Albert Bandura (1998), whose social cognitive theory was described earlier, acknowledges the important influence of evolution on human adaptation. However, he rejects what he calls "one-sided evolutionism," which sees social behavior as strictly the product of evolved biology. An alternative is a bidirectional view, in which environmental and biological conditions influence each other. In this view, evolutionary pressures created changes in biological structures that allowed the use of tools, which enabled our ancestors to manipulate the environment, constructing new environmental conditions. In turn, environmental innovations produced new selection pressures that led to the evolution of specialized biological systems for consciousness, thought, and language.

In other words, evolution gave us biological potentialities, but it does not dictate behavior. People have used their biological capacities to produce diverse cultures—aggressive and peace-loving, egalitarian and autocratic. As American scientist Stephen Jay Gould (1981) concluded, in most domains of human functioning, biology allows a broad range of cultural possibilities.

The "big picture" idea of natural selection leading to the development of human traits and behaviors is difficult to refute or test because evolution is on a time scale that does not lend itself to empirical study. Thus, studying specific genes in humans and other species—and their links to traits and behaviors—may be the best approach for testing ideas coming out of the evolutionary psychology perspective.

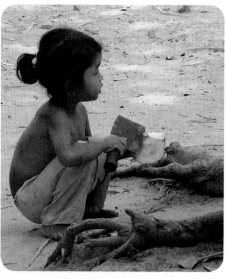

Children in all cultures are interested in the tools used by adults in their cultures. For example, this young child is using a machete near the Ankgor Temples in Cambodia. Children in this culture learn these skills at a very young age. *Might this child's behavior be evolutionary-based or be due to both biological and environmental conditions?*

Carol Adam/Moment Editorial/Getty Images

Review Connect Reflect

LG1 Discuss the evolutionary perspective on child development.

Review
- How can natural selection and adaptive behavior be defined?
- What is evolutionary psychology? What are some basic ideas about human development proposed by evolutionary psychologists? How might evolutionary influences have different effects at different points in the life span? How can evolutionary psychology be evaluated?

Connect
- Earlier, you learned about how different developmental processes interact. How was that principle reinforced by the information in this section?

Reflect *Your Own Personal Journey of Life*
- Which do you think is more persuasive in explaining your development: the views of evolutionary psychologists or those of their critics? Why?

Genetic Foundations of Development **LG2** Describe what genes are and how they influence children's development.

The Collaborative Gene | Genes and Chromosomes | Genetic Principles | Chromosomal and Gene-Linked Abnormalities

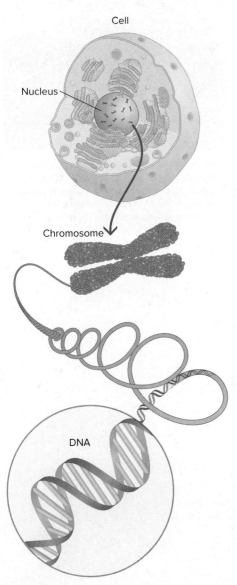

FIGURE 2

CELLS, CHROMOSOMES, DNA, AND GENES.
(*Top*) The body contains trillions of cells. Each cell contains a central structure, the nucleus. (*Middle*) Chromosomes are threadlike structures located in the nucleus of the cell. Chromosomes are composed of DNA. (*Bottom*) DNA has the structure of a spiral staircase. A gene is a segment of DNA.

chromosomes Threadlike structures that come in 23 pairs, with one member of each pair coming from each parent. Chromosomes contain the genetic substance DNA.

Genetic influences on behavior evolved over time and across many species. The many traits and characteristics that are genetically influenced have a long evolutionary history that is retained in our DNA. Our DNA is not just inherited from our parents; it includes what we inherited as a species from other species that were our ancestors.

How are characteristics that suit a species for survival transmitted from one generation to the next? Darwin did not know the answer to this question because genes and the principles of genetics had not yet been discovered. Each of us carries a human "genetic code" that we inherited from our parents. Because a fertilized egg carries this human code, a fertilized human egg cannot grow into an egret, eagle, or elephant.

THE COLLABORATIVE GENE

Each of us began life as a single cell weighing about one twenty-millionth of an ounce! This tiny piece of matter housed our entire genetic code—information that helps us grow from that single cell to a person made of trillions of cells, each containing a replica of the original code. That code is carried by our genes. What are genes and what do they do? For the answer, we need to look into our cells.

The nucleus of each human cell contains **chromosomes,** which are threadlike structures made up of deoxyribonucleic acid, or DNA. **DNA** is a complex molecule that has a double helix shape (like a spiral staircase) and contains genetic information. **Genes,** the units of hereditary information, are short segments of DNA, as you can see in Figure 2. They help cells to reproduce themselves and to assemble proteins. Proteins, in turn, are the building blocks of cells as well as the regulators that direct the body's processes (Belk & Maier, 2013; Tortora, Funke, & Case, 2013).

Each gene has its own location, its own designated place on a particular chromosome. Today, there is a great deal of enthusiasm about efforts to discover the specific locations of genes that are linked to certain functions and developmental outcomes (Oliver, 2017). An important step in this direction is the Human Genome Project's efforts to map the human genome—the complete set of developmental information for creating proteins that initiate the making of a human organism.

Among the major approaches to gene identification and discovery that are being used today are the genome-wide association method, linkage analysis, next-generation sequencing, and the 1,000 Genomes Project:

- Completion of the Human Genome Project has led to use of the *genome-wide association method* to identify genetic variations linked to a particular disorder, such as autism spectrum disorders, cancer, and cardiovascular disease (National Human Genome Research Institute, 2012). To conduct a genome-wide association study, researchers obtain DNA from individuals who have the disorder and from others who don't have it. Then each participant's complete set of DNA, or genome, is purified from the blood or cells and scanned on machines to determine markers of genetic variation. If the genetic variations occur more frequently in people who have the disorder, the variations point to the region in the human genome where the disorder-causing problem exists. Genome-wide association studies have been conducted for obesity (Dong & others, 2018), cardiovascular disease (Lieb & Vasan, 2018), and depression (Wray & others, 2018).

- *Linkage analysis,* in which the goal is to discover the location of a gene in relation to a marker gene (whose position is already known), is often used in the search for a disease gene (Li & others, 2017). Genes transmitted to offspring tend to be in close proximity to each other so that the gene involved in the disease is usually

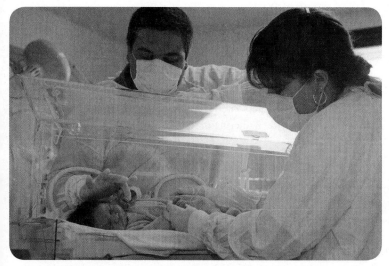
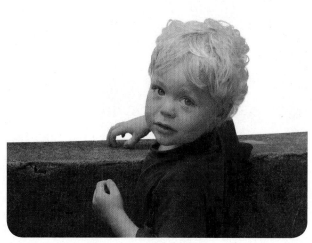

(*Left*) A positive result from the Human Genome Project. Shortly after Andrew Gobea was born, his cells were genetically altered to prevent his immune system from failing. (*Right*) A healthy Wilco Conradi, nearly 3 years old, suffered from the so-called "Bubble Boy" disease that attacked his immune system. He was isolated in a plastic enclosure for the first months of his life to protect him from fatal infections. Wilco was among the first to receive experimental gene therapy treatment which has given him a normal life.
(*Left*) Chris Martinez/AP Images; (*Right*) Peter Dejong/AP Images

located near the marker gene. Gene linkage studies are now being conducted on a wide variety of disorders and health conditions, including attention deficit hyperactivity disorder (Yuan & others, 2017), autism spectrum disorders (O'Roak & others, 2012), and depression (Wong & others, 2017).

- *Next-generation sequencing* is a term that is now used to describe the vast increase in genetic data generated at a much reduced cost and in a much shorter period of time. Next-generation sequencing has considerably increased knowledge about genetic influences on development in recent years (Goodwin, McPherson, & McCombie, 2016).

- The human genome varies between individuals in small but very important ways. To understand these variations will require examination of the whole genomes of many individuals. A current project that began in 2008, the 1,000 Genomes Project, is the most detailed study of human genetic variation to date, with the goal of determining the genomic sequences of at least 1,000 individuals from different ethnic groups around the world (Shibata & others, 2012). Compiling complete descriptions of the genetic variations of many people will make it possible for researchers to conduct studies of genetic variations in disease in a more detailed manner.

As scientists learn more about the human genome, estimates of the number of human genes have also changed. Current estimates are that humans have approximately 43,000 genes (Pertea & others, 2018). Previously, scientists had thought that humans had as many as 100,000 or more genes. They had also maintained that each gene programmed just one protein. In fact, humans have far more proteins than they have genes, so there cannot be a one-to-one correspondence between genes and proteins (Commoner, 2002). Each gene is not translated, in automaton-like fashion, into one and only one protein. A gene does not act independently but rather in combination with other genes and the environment (2018).

Rather than being a group of independent genes, the human genome consists of many genes that collaborate both with each other and with nongenetic factors inside and outside the body. The collaboration operates at many points (Lickliter & Witherington, 2017). For example, the cellular machinery mixes, matches, and links small pieces of DNA to reproduce the genes—and that machinery is influenced by what is going on around it (Moore, 2018).

Whether a gene is turned "on," working to assemble proteins, is also a matter of collaboration. The activity of genes (genetic expression) is affected by their environment (Lickliter & Witherington, 2017). For example, hormones that circulate in the blood make their way into the cell where they can turn genes "on" and "off." And the flow of hormones can be affected by environmental conditions such as light, day length, nutrition, and behavior. Numerous studies have shown that external events outside of the original cell and the

DNA A complex molecule that contains genetic information.

genes Units of hereditary information composed of DNA. Genes help cells to reproduce themselves and manufacture the proteins that maintain life.

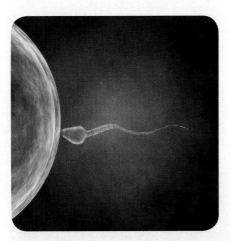

FIGURE 3

A SINGLE SPERM PENETRATING AN EGG AT THE POINT OF FERTILIZATION

3Dalia/Shutterstock

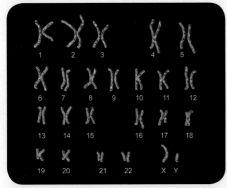

(a)

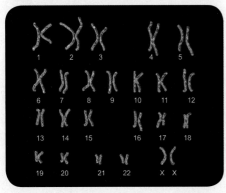

(b)

FIGURE 4

THE GENETIC DIFFERENCE BETWEEN MALES AND FEMALES. Set (*a*) shows the chromosome structure of a male, and set (*b*) shows the chromosome structure of a female. The last pair of 23 pairs of chromosomes is in the bottom right box of each set. Notice that the Y chromosome of the male is smaller than the X chromosome of the female. To obtain this kind of chromosomal picture, a cell is removed from a person's body, usually from the inside of the mouth. The chromosomes are stained by chemical treatment, magnified extensively, and then photographed.

Kateryna Kon/Shutterstock

person, as well as events inside the cell, can excite or inhibit gene expression (Gottlieb, Wahlsten, & Lickliter, 2006; Moore, 2018). Factors such as stress, radiation, and temperature can influence gene expression (Zhang & others, 2017). For example, an increase in the concentration of stress hormones such as cortisol produces an increase in DNA damage and slows the rate of repair if damage occurs (Hare & others, 2018). Exposure to radiation also changes the rate of DNA synthesis in cells (Kim & others, 2017).

In short, a single gene is rarely the source of a protein's genetic information, much less of an inherited trait (Lickliter & Witherington, 2017; Moore, 2018).

GENES AND CHROMOSOMES

Genes are not only collaborative, they are enduring. How do the genes manage to get passed from generation to generation and end up in all of the trillion cells in the body? Three processes explain the heart of the story: mitosis, meiosis, and fertilization.

Mitosis, Meiosis, and Fertilization   Every cell in your body, except the sperm and egg, has 46 chromosomes arranged in 23 pairs. These cells reproduce through a process called **mitosis.** During mitosis, the cell's nucleus—including the chromosomes—duplicates itself and the cell divides. Two new cells are formed, each containing the same DNA as the original cell, arranged in the same 23 pairs of chromosomes.

However, a different type of cell division—**meiosis**—forms eggs and sperm (which also are called *gametes*). During meiosis, a cell of the testes (in men) or ovaries (in women) duplicates its chromosomes but then divides twice, thus forming four cells, each of which has only half of the genetic material of the parent cell (Johnson, 2012). By the end of meiosis, each egg or sperm has 23 unpaired chromosomes.

During **fertilization,** an egg and a sperm fuse to create a single cell, called a **zygote** (see Figure 3). In the zygote, the 23 unpaired chromosomes from the egg and the 23 unpaired chromosomes from the sperm combine to form one set of 23 paired chromosomes—one chromosome of each pair from the mother's egg and the other from the father's sperm. In this manner, each parent contributes half of the offspring's genetic material.

Figure 4 shows 23 paired chromosomes of a male and a female. The members of each pair of chromosomes are both similar and different: Each chromosome in the pair contains varying forms of the same genes, at the same location on the chromosome. A gene that influences hair color, for example, is located on both members of one pair of chromosomes, in the same location on each. However, one of those chromosomes might carry a gene associated with blond hair; the other chromosome in the pair might carry a gene associated with brown hair.

Do you notice any obvious differences between the chromosomes of the male and the chromosomes of the female in Figure 4? The difference lies in the 23rd pair. Ordinarily, in females this pair consists of two chromosomes called X chromosomes; in males the 23rd pair consists of an X and a Y chromosome. The presence of a Y chromosome is one factor that makes a person male rather than female.

Sources of Variability   Combining the genes of two parents in their offspring increases genetic variability in the population, which is valuable for a species because it provides more characteristics for natural selection to operate on (Charlesworth & Charlesworth, 2017). In fact, the human genetic process creates several important sources of variability.

First, the chromosomes in the zygote are not exact copies of those in the mother's ovaries and the father's testes. During the formation of the sperm and egg in meiosis, the members of each pair of chromosomes are separated, but which chromosome in the pair goes to the gamete is a matter of chance. In addition, before the pairs separate, pieces of the two chromosomes in each pair are exchanged, creating a new combination of genes on each chromosome (Mader & Windelspecht, 2017). Thus, when chromosomes from the mother's egg and the father's sperm are brought together in the zygote, the result is a truly unique combination of genes.

If each zygote is unique, how do identical twins like those discussed in the opening of the chapter exist? *Identical twins* (also called monozygotic twins) develop from a single zygote that splits into two genetically identical replicas, each of which becomes a person. *Fraternal twins* (called dizygotic twins) develop when two eggs are each fertilized by a different sperm, creating two zygotes that are genetically no more similar than ordinary siblings.

Another source of variability comes from DNA (Starr & others, 2013). Chance events, a mistake by cellular machinery, or damage from an environmental agent such as radiation may produce a *mutated gene,* which is a permanently altered segment of DNA.

Even when their genes are identical, however, people vary. The difference between genotypes and phenotypes helps us to understand this source of variability. All of a person's genetic material makes up his or her **genotype.** However, not all of the genetic material is apparent in our observed and measurable characteristics. A **phenotype** consists of observable characteristics. Phenotypes include physical characteristics (such as height, weight, and hair color) and psychological characteristics (such as personality and intelligence).

For each genotype, a range of phenotypes can be expressed, providing another source of variability (Osório & others, 2017). An individual can inherit the genetic potential to grow very large, for example, but good nutrition, among other things, will be essential for achieving that potential.

GENETIC PRINCIPLES

What determines how a genotype is expressed to create a particular phenotype? Much is unknown about the answer to this question (Moore, 2013). However, a number of genetic principles have been discovered, among them those of dominant-recessive genes, sex-linked genes, genetic imprinting, and polygenically determined characteristics.

Dominant-Recessive Genes Principle   In some cases, one gene of a pair always exerts its effects; it is *dominant,* overriding the potential influence of the other gene, called the recessive gene. This is the *dominant-recessive genes principle.* A recessive gene exerts its influence only if the two genes of a pair are both recessive. If you inherit a recessive gene for a trait from each of your parents, you will show the trait. If you inherit a recessive gene from only one parent, you may never know you carry the gene. Brown hair, farsightedness, and dimples rule over blond hair, nearsightedness, and freckles in the world of dominant-recessive genes.

Can two brown-haired parents have a blond-haired child? Yes, they can. Suppose that each parent has a dominant gene for brown hair and a recessive gene for blond hair. Since dominant genes override recessive genes, the parents have brown hair, but both are carriers of blondness and pass on their recessive genes for blond hair. With no dominant gene to override them, the recessive genes can make the child's hair blond.

Sex-Linked Genes   Most mutated genes are recessive. When a mutated gene is carried on the X chromosome, the result is called *X-linked inheritance.* The implications for males may be very different from those for females (McClelland, Bowles, & Koopman, 2012). Remember that males have only one X chromosome. Thus, if there is an absent or altered, disease-relevant gene on the X chromosome, males have no "backup" copy to counter the harmful gene and therefore may develop an X-linked disease. However, females have a second X chromosome, which is likely to be unchanged. As a result, they are not likely to have the X-linked disease. Thus, most individuals who have X-linked diseases are males. Females who have one abnormal copy of the gene on the X chromosome are known as "carriers," and they usually do not show any signs of the X-linked disease. Hemophilia and fragile X syndrome, which we discuss later in the chapter, are examples of X-linked inherited diseases (Lykken & others, 2018).

Genetic Imprinting   *Genetic imprinting* occurs when genes have differing effects depending on whether they are inherited from the mother or the father (Nomura & others, 2017). A chemical process "silences" one member of the gene pair. For example, as a result of imprinting, only the maternally derived copy of a gene might be active, while the paternally derived copy of the same gene is silenced—or vice versa. Only a small percentage of human genes appears to undergo imprinting, but it is a normal and impor-

mitosis Cellular reproduction in which the cell's nucleus duplicates itself with two new cells being formed, each containing the same DNA as the parent cell, arranged in the same 23 pairs of chromosomes.

meiosis A specialized form of cell division that forms eggs and sperm (also known as gametes).

fertilization A stage in reproduction during which an egg and a sperm fuse to create a single cell, called a zygote.

zygote A single cell formed through fertilization.

genotype A person's genetic heritage; the actual genetic material present in each cell.

phenotype The way an individual's genotype is expressed in observed and measurable characteristics.

Name	Description	Treatment	Incidence
Down syndrome	An extra chromosome causes mild to severe intellectual disability and physical abnormalities.	Surgery, early intervention, infant stimulation, and special learning programs	1 in 1,900 births at age 20 1 in 300 births at age 35 1 in 30 births at age 45
Klinefelter syndrome (XXY)	An extra X chromosome causes physical abnormalities.	Hormone therapy can be effective	1 in 600 male births
Fragile X syndrome	An abnormality in the X chromosome can cause intellectual disability, learning disabilities, or short attention span.	Special education, speech and language therapy	More common in males than in females
Turner syndrome (XO)	A missing X chromosome in females can cause intellectual disability and sexual underdevelopment.	Hormone therapy in childhood and puberty	1 in 2,500 female births
XYY syndrome	An extra Y chromosome can cause above-average height.	No special treatment required	1 in 1,000 male births

FIGURE 5

SOME CHROMOSOMAL ABNORMALITIES. The treatments for these abnormalities do not necessarily erase the problem but may improve the individual's adaptive behavior and quality of life.

developmental **connection**

Conditions, Diseases, and Disorders

Intellectual disability can be classified in several ways. Connect to "Intelligence."

Down syndrome A chromosomally transmitted form of intellectual disability, caused by the presence of an extra copy of chromosome 21.

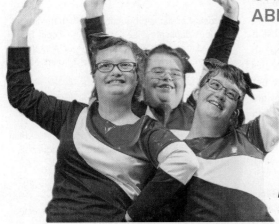

These athletes, who have Down syndrome, are on a cheerleading team for individuals with special needs. Notice the distinctive facial features characteristic of Down syndrome, such as a round face and a flattened skull. *What causes Down syndrome?*
kali9/E+/Getty Images

tant aspect of development. When imprinting goes awry, development is disturbed, as in the case of Beckwith-Wiedemann syndrome, a growth disorder, and Wilms tumor, a type of cancer (Nomura & others, 2017).

Polygenic Inheritance Genetic transmission is usually more complex than the simple examples we have examined thus far (Lewis, 2017). Few characteristics reflect the influence of only a single gene or pair of genes. Most are determined by the interaction of many different genes; they are said to be *polygenically determined*. Even simple characteristics such as height, for example, reflect the interaction of many genes, as well as the influence of the environment.

The term *gene-gene interaction* is used to describe studies that focus on the interdependence of two or more genes in influencing characteristics, behavior, diseases, and development (Ritchie & Van Steen, 2018). For example, studies have documented gene-gene interaction in children's immune system functioning (Törmänen & others, 2017), asthma (Su & others, 2012), cancer (Su & others, 2018), and cardiovascular disease (Luizon & others, 2018).

CHROMOSOMAL AND GENE-LINKED ABNORMALITIES

Abnormalities characterize the genetic process in some indviduals. Some of these abnormalities involve whole chromosomes that do not separate properly during meiosis. Other abnormalities are produced by harmful genes.

Chromosomal Abnormalities Sometimes a gamete is formed in which the male's sperm and/or the female's ovum do not have their normal set of 23 chromosomes. The most notable examples involve Down syndrome and abnormalities of the sex chromosomes (see Figure 5).

Down Syndrome An individual with **Down syndrome** has a round face, a flattened skull, an extra fold of skin over the eyelids, a protruding tongue, short limbs, and disabilities involving motor and intellectual development. The syndrome is caused by the presence of an extra copy of chromosome 21. It is not known why the extra chromosome is present, but the health of the male sperm or female ovum may be involved.

Down syndrome appears approximately once in every 700 live births. Women between the ages of 16 and 34 are less likely to give birth to a child with Down syndrome than are younger or older women. African American children are rarely born with Down syndrome.

Sex-Linked Chromosomal Abnormalities Recall that a newborn normally has either an X and a Y chromosome, or two X chromosomes. Human embryos must possess at least one X chromosome to be viable. The most common sex-linked chromosomal abnormalities involve the presence of an extra chromosome (either an X or Y) or the absence of one X chromosome in females.

Klinefelter syndrome is a chromosomal disorder in which males have an extra X chromosome, making them XXY instead of XY (Kanakis & Nieschlag, 2018). Males with this disorder have undeveloped testes, and they usually have enlarged breasts and become tall. Males with Klinefelter syndrome often have impairment in language, academic, attentional, and motor abilities (Van Rijn, de Sonneville, & Swaab, 2018). Klinefelter syndrome occurs approximately once in every 600 live male births.

Fragile X syndrome is a genetic disorder that results from an abnormality in the X chromosome, which becomes constricted and often breaks. The physical appearance of children with fragile X syndrome often appears normal, although these children typically have prominent ears, a long face, a high-arched palate, and soft skin. Mental deficiency often is an outcome, but it may take the form of intellectual disability, a learning disability, or a short attention span. Boys with fragile X syndrome are characterized by cognitive deficits in inhibition, memory, and planning (Hooper & others, 2018). This disorder occurs more frequently in males than in females, possibly because the second X chromosome in females negates the effects of the abnormal X chromosome (Hooper & others, 2018).

Turner syndrome is a chromosomal disorder in females in which either an X chromosome is missing, making the person XO instead of XX, or part of one X chromosome is deleted. Females with Turner syndrome are short in stature and have a webbed neck (Apperley & others, 2018). They might be infertile and have difficulty in mathematics, but their verbal ability often is quite good. Turner syndrome occurs in approximately 1 of every 2,500 live female births (Apperley & others, 2018).

XYY syndrome is a chromosomal disorder in which the male has an extra Y chromosome (Green, Flash, & Reiss, 2019). Early interest in this syndrome focused on the belief that the extra Y chromosome found in some males contributed to aggression and violence. However, researchers subsequently found that XYY males are no more likely to commit crimes than are XY males (Witkin & others, 1976).

Gene-Linked Abnormalities
Abnormalities can be produced not only by an abnormal number of chromosomes but also by harmful genes (Johnson, 2012). More than 7,000 such genetic disorders have been identified, although most of them are rare.

Phenylketonuria (PKU) is a genetic disorder in which the individual cannot properly metabolize phenylalanine, an amino acid. It results from a recessive gene and occurs about once in every 10,000 to 20,000 live births. Today, phenylketonuria is easily detected, and it is treated by a diet that prevents an excess accumulation of phenylalanine (Ahring & others, 2018). If phenylketonuria is left untreated, however, excess phenylalanine builds up in the child, producing intellectual disability and hyperactivity. Phenylketonuria accounts for approximately 1 percent of institutionalized individuals who are intellectually disabled, and it occurs primarily in non-Latino Whites.

The story of phenylketonuria has important implications for the nature-nurture issue. Although phenylketonuria is a genetic disorder (nature), how or whether a gene's influence in phenylketonuria is played out depends on environmental influences because the disorder can be treated (nurture) using an environmental manipulation. That is, the presence of a genetic defect *does not* inevitably lead to the development of the disorder *if* the individual develops in the right environment (one free of phenylalanine). This is one example of the important principle of heredity-environment interaction. Under one environmental condition (phenylalanine in the diet), intellectual disability results, but when other nutrients replace phenylalanine, intelligence develops in the normal range. The same

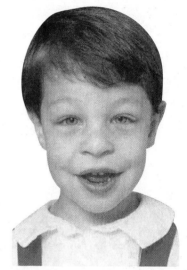

A boy with fragile X syndrome.
From R. Simensen and R. Curtis Rogers, "Fragile X Syndrome" in American Family Physician, 39(5): 186, May 1989 ©American Academy of Family Physicians

Klinefelter syndrome A chromosomal disorder in which males have an extra X chromosome, making them XXY instead of XY.

fragile X syndrome A genetic disorder involving an abnormality in the X chromosome, which becomes constricted and often breaks.

Turner syndrome A chromosomal disorder in females in which either an X chromosome is missing, making the person XO instead of XX, or the second X chromosome is partially deleted.

XYY syndrome A chromosomal disorder in which males have an extra Y chromosome.

phenylketonuria (PKU) A genetic disorder in which an individual cannot properly metabolize an amino acid. PKU is now easily detected but, if left untreated, results in intellectual disability and hyperactivity.

Name	Description	Treatment	Incidence
Cystic fibrosis	Glandular dysfunction that interferes with mucus production; breathing and digestion are hampered, resulting in a shortened life span.	Physical and oxygen therapy, synthetic enzymes, and antibiotics; most individuals live to middle age.	1 in 2,000 births
Diabetes	Body does not produce enough insulin, which causes abnormal metabolism of sugar.	Early onset can be fatal unless treated with insulin.	1 in 2,500 births
Hemophilia	Delayed blood clotting causes internal and external bleeding.	Blood transfusions/injections can reduce or prevent damage due to internal bleeding.	1 in 5,000 male births
Huntington disease	Central nervous system deteriorates, producing problems in muscle coordination and mental deterioration.	Does not usually appear until age 35 or older; death likely 10 to 20 years after symptoms appear.	1 in 20,000 births
Phenyketonuria (PKU)	Metabolic disorder that, left untreated, causes intellectual disability.	Special diet can result in average intelligence and normal life span.	1 in 10,000 to 1 in 20,000 births
Sickle-cell anemia	Blood disorder that limits the body's oxygen supply; it can cause joint swelling, as well as heart and kidney failure.	Penicillin, medication for pain, antibiotics, and blood transfusions.	1 in 400 African American children (lower among some but higher among other groups)
Spina bifida	Neural tube disorder that causes brain and spine abnormalities.	Corrective surgery at birth, orthopedic devices, and physical/medical therapy.	1 in 500 births
Tay-Sachs disease	Deceleration of mental and physical development caused by an accumulation of lipids in the nervous system.	Medication and special diet are used, but death is likely by 5 years of age.	1 in 30 American Jews is a carrier.

FIGURE 6

SOME GENE-LINKED ABNORMALITIES

genotype has different outcomes depending on the environment (in this case, the nutritional environment).

Sickle-cell anemia, which occurs most often in African Americans, is a genetic disorder that impairs the functioning of the body's red blood cells. Red blood cells carry oxygen to the body's other cells and are usually shaped like a disk. In sickle-cell anemia, a recessive gene causes the red blood cell to become a hook-shaped "sickle" that cannot carry oxygen properly and dies quickly. As a result, the body's cells do not receive adequate oxygen, causing anemia and early death (Pecker & Little, 2018). About 1 in 400 African American babies is affected by sickle-cell anemia. One in 10 African Americans is a carrier, as is 1 in 20 Latin Americans. The drug hydroxyurea has been used successfully to treat sickle cell anemia in children, adolescents, and adults (Phillips & others, 2018).

Other diseases that result from genetic abnormalities include cystic fibrosis, some forms of diabetes, hemophilia, spina bifida, and Tay-Sachs disease (Milunsky & Milunsky, 2016). Figure 6 provides further information about these diseases. Someday, scientists may identify why these and other genetic abnormalities occur and discover how to cure them.

Dealing with Genetic Abnormalities Every individual carries DNA variations that might predispose the person to serious physical disease or mental disorder. But not all individuals who carry a genetic disorder develop the disorder. Other genes or developmental events sometimes compensate for genetic abnormalities (Gottlieb, 2007; Lickliter, 2013). For example, recall the example of phenylketonuria from the previous section: Even though individuals might carry the genetic disorder associated with phenylketonuria, the phenotype does not develop when phenylalanine is replaced by other nutrients in their diet.

Thus, genes are not destiny, but genes that are missing, nonfunctional, or mutated can be associated with disorders (Wang & others, 2018). Identifying such genetic flaws could enable doctors to predict an individual's risks, recommend healthy practices, and prescribe the safest and most effective drugs (Chen & others, 2018). A decade or two from now, parents of a newborn baby may be able to leave the hospital with a full genome analysis of their offspring that identifies disease risks.

sickle-cell anemia A genetic disorder that affects the red blood cells and occurs most often in people of African descent.

Holly Ishmael, Genetic Counselor

Holly Ishmael is a genetic counselor at Children's Mercy Hospital in Kansas City. She obtained an undergraduate degree in psychology and a master's degree in genetic counseling from Sarah Lawrence College.

Genetic counselors like Ishmael work as members of a health care team, providing information and support to families with birth defects or genetic disorders. They identify families at risk by analyzing inheritance patterns, and they explore options with each family. Some genetic counselors, like Ishmael, become specialists in prenatal and pediatric genetics; others specialize in cancer genetics or psychiatric genetic disorders.

Ishmael says, "Genetic counseling is a perfect combination for people who want to do something science-oriented, but need human contact and don't want to spend all of their time in a lab or have their nose in a book" (Rizzo, 1999, p. 3).

Genetic counselors have specialized graduate degrees in the areas of medical genetics and counseling. They enter graduate school with undergraduate backgrounds from a variety of disciplines, including biology, genetics, psychology, public health, and social work. There are approximately 40 graduate genetic counseling programs in the United States. If you are interested in this profession, you can obtain

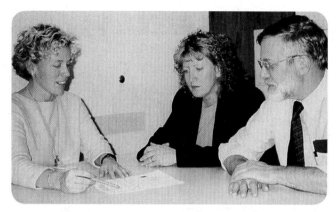

Holly Ishmael (*left*) in a genetic counseling session.
Courtesy of Holly Ishmael Welsh

further information from the National Society of Genetic Counselors at www.nsgc.org.

For more information about what genetic counselors do, see the Careers in Child Development appendix.

However, this knowledge might bring important costs as well as benefits. Who would have access to a person's genetic profile? An individual's ability to land and hold jobs or obtain insurance might be threatened if it is known that a person is considered at risk for some disease. For example, should an airline pilot or a neurosurgeon who is predisposed to develop a disorder that makes one's hands shake be required to leave that job early?

Genetic counselors, usually physicians or biologists who are well versed in the field of medical genetics, understand the kinds of problems just described, the odds of encountering them, and helpful strategies for offsetting some of their effects (Borle & others, 2018). Many individuals who receive genetic counseling find it difficult to quantify risk and tend to overestimate risk (Johansson & others, 2018). To read about the career and work of a genetic counselor, see the *Connecting with Careers* profile.

Review *Connect* Reflect

 Describe what genes are and how they influence children's development.

Review

- What are genes?
- How are genes passed on?
- What basic principles describe how genes interact?
- What are some chromosomal and gene-linked abnormalities?

Connect

- Explain how environment interacts with genes in gene-linked abnormalities.

Reflect *Your Own Personal Journey of Life*

- Would you want to be able to access a full genome analysis of yourself or your offspring? Why or why not?

Reproductive Challenges and Choices Identify some important reproductive challenges and choices.

Prenatal Diagnostic
Tests

Infertility and
Reproductive Technology

Adoption

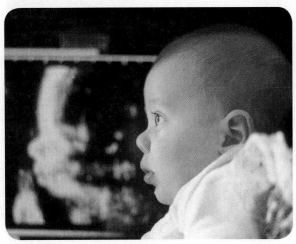

A 6-month-old infant poses with the ultrasound sonography record taken four months into the baby's prenatal development. *What is ultrasound sonography?*

Jacques Pavlovsky/Sygma/Corbis/Getty images

The facts and principles we have discussed regarding meiosis, genetics, and genetic abnormalities are a small part of the recent explosion of knowledge about human biology. This knowledge not only helps us understand human development but also opens up many new choices to prospective parents—choices that can also raise ethical questions.

PRENATAL DIAGNOSTIC TESTS

One choice open to prospective mothers is the extent to which they should undergo prenatal testing. A number of tests can indicate whether a fetus is developing normally; these include ultrasound sonography, fetal MRI, chorionic villus sampling, amniocentesis, maternal blood screening, and noninvasive prenatal diagnosis (NIPD). There has been a dramatic increase in research on the use of less invasive techniques, such as fetal MRI and NIPD, which pose lower risks to the fetus than more invasive techniques such as chorionic villus sampling and amniocentesis.

Ultrasound Sonography   An ultrasound test is often conducted seven weeks into a pregnancy and at various times later in pregnancy. *Ultrasound sonography* is a prenatal medical procedure in which high-frequency sound waves are directed into the pregnant woman's abdomen (Barišić & others, 2017). The echo from the sounds is transformed into a visual representation of the fetus's inner structures. This technique can detect many structural abnormalities in the fetus, including microencephaly, a form of intellectual disability involving an abnormally small brain; it can also determine the number of fetuses and give clues to the baby's sex (Barišić & others, 2017). This test poses virtually no risk to the woman or the fetus.

Fetal MRI   The development of brain-imaging techniques has led to increasing use of *fetal MRI* to diagnose fetal malformations (Manganaro & others, 2018) (see Figure 7). MRI, which stands for magnetic resonance imaging, uses a powerful magnet and radio images to generate detailed images of the body's organs and structure. Currently, ultrasound is still the first choice in fetal screening, but fetal MRI can provide more detailed images than ultrasound. In many instances, ultrasound will indicate a possible abnormality and then fetal MRI will be used to obtain a clearer, more detailed image (Manganaro & others, 2018). Among the fetal malformations that fetal MRI may be able to detect better than ultrasound sonography are certain abnormalities of the central nervous system, chest, gastrointestinal tract, genital/urinary system, and placenta (Robinson & Ederies, 2018).

Chorionic Villus Sampling   At some point between 10 and 14 weeks of pregnancy, chorionic villus sampling may be used to detect genetic defects and chromosomal abnormalities, such as the ones discussed in the previous section (Vink & Quinn, 2018). Diagnosis takes approximately 10 days. *Chorionic villus sampling (CVS)* is a prenatal medical procedure in which a small sample of the placenta (the vascular organ that links the fetus to the mother's uterus) is removed (Vink & Quinn, 2018). There is a small risk of limb deformity when CVS is used.

Amniocentesis   Between the 14th and 20th weeks of pregnancy, amniocentesis may be performed. *Amniocentesis* is a prenatal medical procedure in which a sample of amniotic fluid is withdrawn by syringe and tested for chromosomal or metabolic disorders

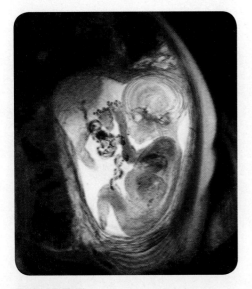

FIGURE **7**

A FETAL MRI, WHICH IS INCREASINGLY BEING USED IN PRENATAL DIAGNOSIS OF FETAL MALFORMATIONS

Du Cane Medical Imaging Ltd/Science Source

(Athanasiadis & others, 2011). The amniotic fluid is found within the amnion, a thin sac in which the embryo is suspended. Ultrasound sonography is often used during amniocentesis so that the syringe can be placed precisely. The later amniocentesis is performed, the better its diagnostic potential. The earlier it is performed, the more useful it is in deciding how to handle a pregnancy. It may take two weeks for enough cells to grow so that amniocentesis test results can be obtained. Amniocentesis brings a small risk of miscarriage—about 1 woman in every 200 to 300 miscarries after amniocentesis.

Both amniocentesis and chorionic villus sampling provide valuable information about the presence of birth defects, but they also raise difficult issues for parents about whether an abortion should be obtained if birth defects are present (Lotto, Smith, & Armstrong, 2018). Chorionic villus sampling allows a decision to be made sooner, at a time when abortion is safer and less traumatic. Although earlier reports indicated that chorionic villus sampling brings a slightly higher risk of pregnancy loss than amniocentesis, a subsequent U.S. study of more than 40,000 pregnancies found that loss rates for CVS decreased from 1998 to 2003 and that the risk of pregnancy loss was no greater for CVS than for amniocentesis (Caughey, Hopkins, & Norton, 2006).

Maternal Blood Screening During the 16th to 18th weeks of pregnancy, maternal blood screening may be performed. *Maternal blood screening* identifies pregnancies that have an elevated risk for birth defects such as spina bifida (a defect in the spinal cord) and Down syndrome (Ballard, 2011). The current blood test is called the *triple screen* because it measures three substances in the mother's blood. After an abnormal triple screen result, the next step is usually an ultrasound examination. If an ultrasound does not explain the abnormal triple screen results, amniocentesis is typically used.

Noninvasive Prenatal Diagnosis (NIPD) *Noninvasive prenatal diagnosis* (*NIPD*) is increasingly being explored as an alternative to procedures such as chorionic villus sampling and amniocentesis (Avent, 2012; Peterson & others, 2013). At this point, NIPD has mainly focused on brain-imaging techniques, the isolation and examination of fetal cells circulating in the mother's blood, and analysis of cell-free fetal DNA in maternal plasma (Byrou & others, 2018).

Researchers already have used NIPD to successfully test for genes inherited from a father that cause cystic fibrosis and Huntington's disease. They also are exploring the potential for using NIPD very early in fetal development to diagnose a baby's sex and detect Down syndrome (Palomaki & Kloza, 2018; Rita & others, 2018).

Fetal Sex Determination Chorionic villus sampling has often been used to determine the sex of the fetus at some point between 11 and 13 weeks of gestation. Recently, though, some noninvasive techniques have been able to detect the sex of the fetus at an earlier point (Mackie & others, 2017). A meta-analysis of studies confirmed that a baby's sex can be detected as early as 7 weeks into pregnancy (Devaney & others, 2011). Being able to detect an offspring's sex as well as the presence of various diseases and defects at such an early stage raises ethical concerns about couples' motivation to terminate a pregnancy (Gareth, 2017).

INFERTILITY AND REPRODUCTIVE TECHNOLOGY

Recent advances in biological knowledge have also opened up many choices for infertile people (Mahany & Smith, 2017). Approximately 10 to 15 percent of couples in the United States experience infertility, which is defined as the inability to conceive a child after 12 months of regular intercourse without contraception. The cause of infertility can rest with the woman or the man (Barbieri, 2019). The woman may not be ovulating (releasing

developmental **connection**

Biological Processes

Discover what the development of the fetus is like at the time chorionic villus sampling and amniocentesis can be used. Connect to "Prenatal Development and Birth."

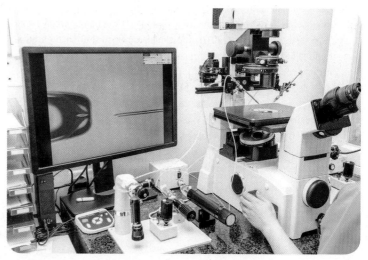

A technician using a micro-needle to inject human sperm into a human egg cell as part of an in vitro fertilization procedure. The injected sperm fertilizes the egg, and the resulting zygote is then grown in the laboratory until it reaches an early stage of embryonic development. Then it is implanted in the uterus.
Ideya/Shutterstock

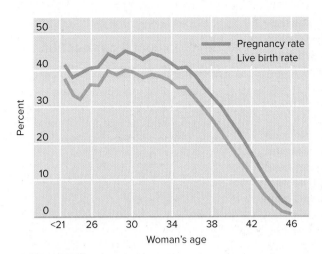

FIGURE 8

SUCCESS RATES OF IN VITRO FERTILIZATION VARY ACCORDING TO THE WOMAN'S AGE

From John Santrock, *Child Development*, 11/e, fig 2.9. Copyright © 2011 McGraw-Hill Companies. Reprinted by permission.

eggs to be fertilized), she may be producing abnormal ova, her fallopian tubes by which ova normally reach the womb may be blocked, or she may have a disease that prevents implantation of the embryo into the uterus. The man may produce too few sperm, the sperm may lack motility (the ability to move adequately), or he may have a blocked passageway (Kini & others, 2010).

In the United States, more than 2 million couples seek help for infertility every year. In some cases of infertility, surgery may correct the cause; in others, hormone-based drugs may improve the probability of having a child. Of the 2 million couples who seek help for infertility every year, about 40,000 try high-tech assisted reproduction. By far the most common technique used is *in vitro fertilization* (*IVF*), in which eggs and sperm are combined in a laboratory dish. If any eggs are successfully fertilized, one or more of the resulting fertilized eggs is transferred into the woman's uterus. A national study in the United States by the Centers for Disease Control and Prevention (2006) found the success rate for IVF depends on the mother's age (see Figure 8). Approximately 1.7% of births in the United States today result from IVF (Kawwass & Badell, 2018).

The creation of families by means of the new reproductive technologies raises important questions about the physical and psychological consequences for children (Wang & others, 2017). One result of fertility treatments is an increase in multiple births (Jones, 2007). Twenty-five to 30 percent of pregnancies achieved by fertility treatments—including in vitro fertilization—now result in multiple births. Twins born through IVF, compared with twins born through natural conception, are at slightly higher risk of low birth weight, prematurity, and adverse neonatal outcomes (Wang & others, 2018); therefore, additional prenatal care and attention following birth may be needed for twins born through assisted reproductive technology. To read about a study that addresses longer-term consequences of in vitro fertilization, see *Connecting Through Research*.

connecting through research

Do Children Conceived Through In Vitro Fertilization Show Significantly Different Developmental Outcomes in Childhood and Adolescence?

A longitudinal study sampled all singleton children and twins conceived through assisted reproductive technologies (ART) and born in Denmark in 1995 (Klausen & others, 2017). The sample included 858 children born through ART, each of whom was matched demographically to four spontaneously conceived children.

The children were assessed at ages 3, 7, 14, and 18 years to measure their rates of behavior problems (such as aggression and delinquency) and mental health problems (such as anxiety and depression). In a cumulative analysis of mental health disorders through age 18, no significant differences were found between the children born through ART and the spontaneously conceived children (see Figure 9).

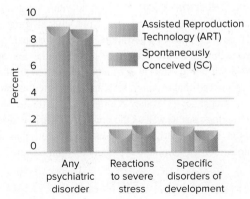

FIGURE 9

CUMULATIVE PREVALENCE OF PSYCHIATRIC DISORDERS AT AGE 18. No significant differences in any diagnostic categories were found between children who were born through assisted reproductive technologies and those who were spontaneously conceived. *Source:* Klausen, T., Hansen, K.J., Munk-Jørgensen, P., & Mohr-Jensen, C. (2017). Are assisted reproductive technologies associated with categorical or dimensional aspects of psychopathology in childhood, adolescence or early adulthood? Results from a Danish prospective nationwide cohort study. *European Child and Adolescent Psychiatry, 26,* 771–778. Retrieved from https://link.springer.com/article/10.1007/s00787-016-0937-z

The Increased Diversity of Adopted Children and Adoptive Parents

A number of changes have characterized adoptive children and adoptive parents in the last three to four decades (Zill, 2017). In the first half of the twentieth century, most U.S. adopted children were healthy, non-Latino White infants who were adopted at birth or soon after. However, in recent decades as contraception use increased, abortion became legal, and un-married mothers became increasingly likely to raise their children as single mothers or with the help of their own parents, fewer non-Latino White in-fants became available for adoption. Increasingly, U.S. couples adopted a much wider diversity of children—from other countries, from other ethnic groups, children with physical and/or mental problems, and children who had been neglected or abused. For example, between 1999 and 2011, the number of kindergarten adoptees being raised by a mother of a different ethnicity rose by 50 percent (Zill, 2017).

Changes also have characterized adoptive parents in the last three to four decades (Zill, 2017). In the first half of the twentieth century, most adoptive parents were married couples from non-Latino White middle or upper socioeconomic status backgrounds who did not have any type of disability. Although adoptive parents are still, on average, more likely to be White and from higher socioeconomic backgrounds than the general population, increased diversity has characterized adoptive parents in re-cent decades. Many adoption agencies today have no income require-ments for adoptive parents and now permit adoption by adults from a wide range of backgrounds, including single adults, gay and lesbian adults, and older adults. Further, many adoptions involve other family members (aunts/uncles/grandparents); currently, about 37 percent of U.S. domestic adoptions are made by relatives (Jones & Placek, 2017). And slightly more than 50 percent of U.S. adoptions occur through the foster care system; more than 100,000 children in the U.S. foster care system are waiting for someone to adopt them (U.S. Department of Health & Human Services, 2017).

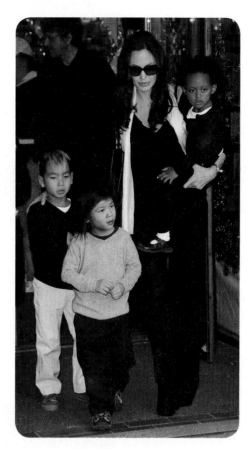

An increasing number of Hollywood celebrities are adopting children from developing countries. Actress Angelina Jolie (*above*) carries her adopted daughter Zahara with adopted sons Maddox and Pax walking beside them.
Jackson Lee/Tom Meinelt/Newscom

Many fertile adults adopt children, but many more adoptive parents are infertile. Based on what you read prior to this interlude, why might an infertile couple or individual decide to adopt rather than undergo repro-ductive technology procedures?

ADOPTION

Although surgery and fertility drugs can sometimes solve the infertility problem, another choice is to adopt a child (Sempowicz & others, 2018). Adoption is the social and legal process by which a parent-child relationship is established between persons unrelated at birth. As discussed in *Connecting with Diversity,* increased diversity has characterized the adoption of children in the United States in recent years.

How do adopted children fare after they are adopted? Children who are adopted very early in their lives are more likely to have positive outcomes than children adopted later in life, most likely because early adoption minimizes the amount of time children spend prior to adoption in adverse, traumatic situations that are often characterized by depriva-tion and other environmental risks (McCall & others, 2018). In a review of studies of children living in orphanages in the Russian Federation compared with children adopted within the Russian Federation or in the United States, children who were adopted before

caring *connections*

Parenting Adopted Children

Many of the keys to effectively parenting adopted children are no different from those for effectively parenting biological children: Be supportive and caring, be involved and monitor the child's behavior and whereabouts, be a good communicator, and help the child learn to develop self-control. However, parents of adopted children face some unique circumstances (Lee & others, 2018). They need to recognize the differences involved in adoptive family life, communicate about these differences, show respect for the birth family, and support the child's search for self and identity.

Following are some of the challenges parents face when their adopted children are at different points in development and some recommendations for how to face these challenges (Brodzinsky & Pinderhughes, 2002):

- **Infancy.** Researchers have found few differences in the attachment that adopted and non-adopted infants form with their parents. However, attachment can become problematic if parents have unresolved fertility issues or the child does not meet the parents' expectations. Counselors can help prospective adoptive parents develop realistic expectations.

- **Early childhood.** Because many children begin to ask where they came from when they are about 4 to 6 years old, this is a natural time to begin to talk in simple ways to children about their adoption status. Some parents (although not as many as in the past) decide not to tell their children about the adoption. This secrecy may create psychological risks for the child if he or she later finds out about the adoption. Adoptions today are more likely to be open adoptions rather than closed adoptions; in an open adoption the adoptive parents and adoptive children have information about the birth parents and the potential to have contact with the birth parents. Gay men and lesbian women who adopt have been found to maintain more contact with birth parents than do heterosexual couples who adopt (Brodzinsky & Goldberg, 2016).

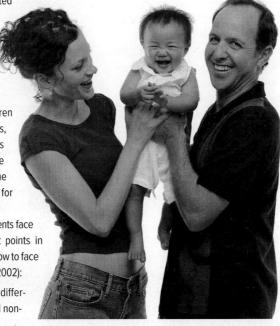

What are some strategies for parenting adopted children at different points in their development?
Photodisc/Getty Images

- **Middle and late childhood.** During the elementary school years, children begin to show more interest in their origins and may ask questions related to where they came from, what their birth parents looked like, and why their birth parents placed them for adoption. As they grow older, children may develop mixed feelings about being adopted and question their adoptive parents' explanations. It is important for adoptive parents to recognize that this ambivalence is normal. Also, problems may arise from the desire of adoptive parents to make life too perfect for the adoptive child and to present a perfect image of themselves to the child. The result too often is that adopted children feel that they cannot release any angry feelings or openly discuss problems.

- **Adolescence.** Adolescents are likely to develop more abstract and logical thinking processes, to focus their attention on their bodies, and to search for an identity. These characteristics provide the foundation for adopted adolescents to reflect on their adoption status in more complex ways, such as focusing on physical differences between themselves and their adoptive parents. As they explore their identity, adopted adolescents may have difficulty incorporating their adopted status into their identity in positive ways. It is important for adoptive parents to understand the complexity of the adopted adolescent's identity exploration and be patient with the adolescent's lengthy identity search.

According to the information presented in this box and in the text that precedes it, how can mental health professionals help adopting parents and adopted children?

the age of 18 months generally fared well (McCall & others, 2018). However, children adopted after the age of 18 months had higher levels of behavior problems and poorer cognitive function even years after the adoption. An intervention that focused on improving caregiver-child interactions in orphanages was found to improve orphans' physical, cognitive, and socioemotional outcomes (McCall & others, 2018).

Despite risks associated with early deprivation prior to adoption, the majority of adopted children and adolescents (including those adopted at older ages, transracially, and across national borders) adjust effectively, and their parents report considerable satisfaction with their decision to adopt (Castle & others, 2010). A research review of 88 studies also revealed no difference in the self-esteem of adopted and nonadopted children and adolescents, as well as no differences between transracial and same-race adoptees (Juffer & van IJzendoorn, 2007).

Also keep in mind that changes in adoption practice over the last several decades make it difficult to generalize about the average adopted child or average adoptive parent. To read more about adoption, see the *Caring Connections* interlude in which we discuss effective parenting strategies with adopted children.

Review *Connect* Reflect

LG3 Identify some important reproductive challenges and choices.

Review

- What are some common prenatal diagnostic tests?
- What are some techniques that help infertile people to have children?
- How does adoption affect children's development?

Connect

- Earlier, you learned about different methods for collecting data. How would you characterize the methods used in prenatal diagnostic testing?

Reflect *Your Own Personal Journey of Life*

- If you were an adult who could not have children, would you want to adopt a child? Why or why not?

Heredity and Environment Interaction: Nature and Nurture

LG4 Explain some of the ways that heredity and environment interact to produce individual differences in development.

- Behavior Genetics
- Heredity-Environment Correlations
- Shared and Nonshared Environmental Experiences
- The Epigenetic View and Gene × Environment (G × E) Interaction
- Conclusions about Heredity-Environment Interaction

Is it possible to untangle the influence of heredity from that of environment and discover the role of each in producing individual differences in development? When heredity and environment interact, how does heredity influence the environment, and vice versa?

BEHAVIOR GENETICS

Behavior genetics is the field that seeks to discover the influence of heredity and environment on individual differences in human traits and development (Kaplan, 2012; Maxson, 2013). Note that behavior genetics does not identify the extent to which genetics or the environment affects an individual's traits. Instead, behavior geneticists try to figure out what is responsible for the differences among people—that is, to what extent people vary because of differences in genes, environment, or a combination of these factors (Wang & others, 2012). To study the influence of heredity on behavior, behavior geneticists often use either twins or adoption situations (Kubarych & others, 2012).

In the most common **twin study,** the behavioral similarity of identical twins (who are genetically identical) is compared with the behavioral similarity of fraternal twins. Recall that although fraternal twins share the same womb, they are no more genetically alike than non-twin siblings. Thus, by comparing groups of identical and fraternal twins, behavior geneticists capitalize on the basic knowledge that identical twins are more similar

behavior genetics The field that seeks to discover the influence of heredity and environment on individual differences in human traits and development.

twin study A study in which the behavioral similarity of identical twins is compared with the behavioral similarity of fraternal twins.

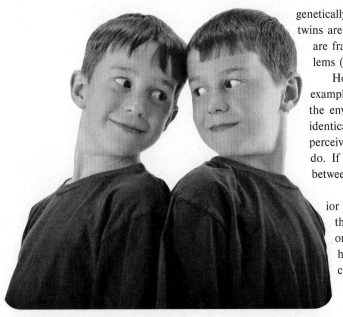

genetically than are fraternal twins (Li & others, 2018). For example, identical twins are more similar to one another on measures of conduct problems than are fraternal twins, suggesting the importance of heredity in conduct problems (Saunders & others, 2019).

However, several issues complicate interpretation of twin studies. For example, perhaps the environments of identical twins are more similar than the environments of fraternal twins. Adults might stress the similarities of identical twins more than those of fraternal twins, and identical twins might perceive themselves as a "set" and play together more than fraternal twins do. If so, the influence of the environment on the observed similarities between identical and fraternal twins might be very significant.

In an **adoption study,** investigators seek to discover whether the behavior and psychological characteristics of adopted children are more like those of their adoptive parents, who have provided a home environment, or more like those of their biological parents, who have contributed their heredity (Kendler & others, 2018). Another form of the adoption study compares adoptive and biological siblings.

HEREDITY-ENVIRONMENT CORRELATIONS

Twin studies compare identical twins with fraternal twins. Identical twins develop from a single fertilized egg that splits into two genetically identical organisms. Fraternal twins develop from separate eggs, making them genetically no more similar than nontwin siblings. *What is the nature of the twin study method?*
Compassionate Eye Foundation/Stockbyte/Getty Images

The difficulties that researchers encounter when they interpret the results of twin studies and adoption studies reflect the complexities of heredity-environment interaction. Some of these interactions are heredity-environment correlations, which means that individuals' genes may influence the types of environments to which they are exposed. In a sense, individuals "inherit" environments that may be related or linked to genetic "propensities." Behavior geneticist Sandra Scarr (1993) described three ways that heredity and environment are correlated (see Figure 10):

adoption study A study in which investigators seek to discover whether, in behavior and psychological characteristics, adopted children are more like their adoptive parents, who provided a home environment, or more like their biological parents, who contributed their heredity. Another form of the adoption study is one that compares adoptive and biological siblings.

passive genotype-environment correlations Correlations that exist when the natural parents, who are genetically related to the child, provide a rearing environment for the child.

evocative genotype-environment correlations Correlations that exist when the child's genetically influenced characteristics elicit certain types of environments.

- **Passive genotype-environment correlations** occur because biological parents, who are genetically related to the child, provide a rearing environment for the child. For example, the parents might have a genetic predisposition to be intelligent and read skillfully. Because they read well and enjoy reading, they provide their children with books to read. The likely outcome is that their children, given their own inherited predispositions from their parents and their book-filled environment, will become skilled readers.

- **Evocative genotype-environment correlations** occur because a child's genetically influenced characteristics elicit certain types of environments. For example, active, smiling children receive more social stimulation than passive, quiet

Heredity-Environment Correlation	Description	Examples
Passive	Children inherit genetic tendencies from their parents, and parents also provide an environment that matches their own genetic tendencies.	Musically inclined parents usually have musically inclined children and are likely to provide an environment rich in music for their children.
Evocative	The child's genetic tendencies elicit stimulation from the environment that supports a particular trait. Thus, genes evoke environmental support.	A happy, outgoing child elicits smiles and friendly responses from others.
Active (niche-picking)	Children actively seek out "niches" in their environment that reflect their own interests and talents and are thus in accord with their genotype.	Libraries, sports fields, and a store with musical instruments are examples of environmental niches children might seek out if they have intellectual interests in books, talent in sports, or musical talents, respectively.

FIGURE 10

EXPLORING HEREDITY-ENVIRONMENT CORRELATIONS

children do. Cooperative, attentive children evoke more pleasant and instructional responses from the adults around them than uncooperative, distractible children do.

- **Active (niche-picking) genotype-environment correlations** occur when children seek out environments that they find compatible and stimulating. Niche-picking refers to finding a setting that is suited to one's genetically influenced abilities. Children select from their surrounding environment some aspect that they respond to, learn about, or ignore. Their active selections of environments are related to their particular genotype. For example, outgoing children tend to seek out social contexts in which to interact with people, whereas shy children don't. Children who are musically inclined are likely to select musical environments in which they can successfully perform their skills. How these "tendencies" come about will be discussed shortly under the topic of the epigenetic view.

Scarr observes that the relative importance of the three genotype-environment correlations changes as children develop from infancy through adolescence. In infancy, much of the environment that children experience is provided by adults. Thus, passive genotype-environment correlations are more common in the lives of infants and young children than they are for older children and adolescents who can extend their experiences beyond the family's influence and create their environments to a greater degree.

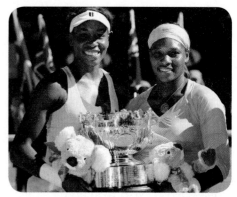

Tennis stars Venus and Serena Williams. *What might be some shared and nonshared environmental experiences they had while they were growing up that contributed to their tennis stardom?*
Greg Wood/AFP/Getty Images

SHARED AND NONSHARED ENVIRONMENTAL EXPERIENCES

Behavior geneticists have argued that to understand the environment's role in differences between people, we should distinguish between shared and nonshared environments. That is, we should consider experiences that children share in common with other children living in the same home, and experiences that are not shared (Salvy & others, 2017).

Shared environmental experiences are siblings' common experiences, such as their parents' personalities or intellectual orientation, the family's socioeconomic status, and the neighborhood in which they live. By contrast, **nonshared environmental experiences** are a child's unique experiences, both within the family and outside the family, that are not shared with a sibling. Even experiences occurring within the family can be part of the "nonshared environment." For example, parents often interact differently with each sibling, and siblings interact differently with parents. Siblings often have different peer groups, different friends, and different teachers at school, all of which contribute to nonshared environments.

Behavior geneticist Robert Plomin (2004) has found that shared environment accounts for little of the variation in children's personality or interests. In other words, even though two children live under the same roof with the same parents, their personalities are often very different. Further, Plomin argues that heredity influences the nonshared environments of siblings through the heredity-environment correlations we described earlier. For example, a child who has inherited a genetic tendency to be athletic is likely to spend more time in environments related to sports, and a child who has inherited a tendency to be musically inclined is more likely to spend time in environments related to music.

Longitudinal studies suggest that earlier in development, parenting or other environmental effects are stronger than these effects are later in development (Lansford & others, 2018). For example, maternal intelligence is related to higher-quality home environments, including books and other stimulating materials in the home as well as cognitively enriching outings such as trips to museums, for preschool-aged children. However, by the age of 8 or 9 and especially by adolescence, children's own intelligence becomes more predictive than their mothers' intelligence of the quality of their home environment (Hadd & Rodgers, 2017). More intelligent mothers are genetically more likely to have more intelligent children than are less intelligent mothers. Yet, even within a family, more intelligent children are likely to elicit more enriching experiences than are less intelligent siblings.

active (niche-picking) genotype-environment correlations Correlations that exist when children seek out environments they find compatible and stimulating.

shared environmental experiences Siblings' common environmental experiences, such as their parents' personalities and intellectual orientation, the family's socioeconomic status, and the neighborhood in which they live.

nonshared environmental experiences The child's own unique experiences, both within the family and outside the family, that are not shared by another sibling.

FIGURE 11
COMPARISON OF THE HEREDITY-ENVIRONMENT CORRELATION AND EPIGENETIC VIEWS

- - - - - - - - →

developmental **connection**

Biological Processes

A recent study revealed links between infant attachment, responsive parenting, and the short/long version of the 5-HTTLPR gene. Connect to "Emotional Development."

← - - - - - - -

epigenetic view Theory that development is the result of an ongoing, bidirectional interchange between heredity and environment.

gene × environment (G × E) interaction The interaction of a specific, measured variation in the DNA and a specific, measured aspect of the environment.

THE EPIGENETIC VIEW AND GENE × ENVIRONMENT (G × E) INTERACTION

Critics argue that the concept of heredity-environment correlation gives heredity too much of a one-sided influence in determining development because it does not consider the role of prior environmental influences in shaping the correlation itself (Gottlieb, 2007). However, earlier in this chapter we discussed how genes are collaborative, not determining an individual's traits in an independent manner but rather interacting with the environment.

The Epigenetic View   In line with the concept of a collaborative gene, Gilbert Gottlieb (2007) emphasizes the **epigenetic view,** which states that development is the result of an ongoing, bidirectional interchange between heredity and the environment. Figure 11 compares the heredity-environment correlation and epigenetic views of development.

Let's look at an example that reflects the epigenetic view. A baby inherits genes from both parents at conception. During prenatal development, toxins, nutrition, and stress can influence some genes to stop functioning while others become stronger or weaker. During infancy, environmental experiences such as toxins, nutrition, stress, learning, and encouragement continue to modify genetic activity and the activity of the nervous system that directly underlies behavior. Heredity and environment operate together—or collaborate—to produce a person's intelligence, temperament, height, weight, ability to pitch a baseball, ability to read, and so on (Gottlieb, 2007; Lickliter, 2013; Meaney, 2010; Moore, 2013).

Gene × Environment Interaction (G × E)   An increasing number of studies are exploring how the interaction between heredity and environment influences development, including interactions that involve specific DNA sequences (Zhou & others, 2018). The epigenetic mechanisms involve the actual molecular modification of the DNA strand as a result of environmental inputs in ways that alter genetic functioning (Feil & Fraga, 2012).

One study found that individuals who have a short version of a genotype labeled 5-HTTLPR (a gene involving the neurotransmitter serotonin) have an elevated risk of developing depression only if they *also* have stressful lives (Caspi & others, 2003). Thus, the specific gene did not directly cause depression to develop; rather, the gene interacted with a stressful environment in a way that allowed the researchers to predict whether individuals would develop depression. Recent studies also have found support for the interaction between the 5-HTTLPR gene and stress levels in predicting depression in adolescents and older adults (Saul & others, 2019).

Other research involving interaction between genes and environmental experience has focused on attachment, parenting, and supportive or adverse childrearing environments (Lovallo & others, 2017). For example, some genes are a risk factor for psychological disorders only if an individual has also experienced early adversity, such as physical or sexual abuse during childhood (Bulbena-Cabre, Nia, & Perez-Rodriguez, 2018). The type of research just described is referred to as **gene × environment (G × E) interaction**—the interaction of a specific, measured variation in DNA and a specific, measured aspect of the environment (Halldorsdottir & Binder, 2017).

Two main theories, each supported by empirical research, characterize G × E interactions. The first theory is known as the diathesis-stress or dual-risk model and characterizes G × E interactions in which a genetic risk factor leads to maladjustment only in the presence of a stressful or adverse environment (Zuckerman, 1999). Historically, this theory was the main way in which G × E interactions were understood. The second theory is known as the biological sensitivity to context model (Ellis & Boyce, 2008) or the differential susceptibility model (Belsky & Pluess, 2009). Both of these models characterize G × E interactions in which a genetic factor makes an individual more susceptible to both positive and negative environmental influences. Biological sensitivity to context has been illustrated by using an analogy of a dandelion, which can grow about the same in a wide range of environments, compared with an orchid, which thrives beautifully under the right environmental conditions but withers and dies in others (Ellis & Boyce, 2008).

CONCLUSIONS ABOUT HEREDITY-ENVIRONMENT INTERACTION

If an attractive, popular, intelligent girl is elected president of her senior class in high school, is her success due to heredity or to environment? Of course, the answer is both.

The relative contributions of heredity and environment are not additive. That is, we can't say that such-and-such a percentage of nature and such-and-such a percentage of experience make us who we are. Nor is it accurate to say that full genetic expression happens once, around conception or birth, after which we carry our genetic legacy into the world to see how far it takes us. Genes produce proteins throughout the life span, in many different environments. Or they don't produce these proteins, depending in part on how harsh or nourishing those environments are.

The emerging view is that complex behaviors are influenced by genes in a way that gives people a propensity for a particular developmental trajectory (Wertz & others, 2018). However, the actual development requires more: an environment. And that environment is complex, just like the mixture of genes we inherit (Gartstein & Skinner, 2018). Environmental influences range from the things we lump together under "nurture" (such as parenting, family dynamics, schooling, and neighborhood quality) to biological encounters (such as viruses, birth complications, and even biological events in cells).

Imagine for a moment that there is a cluster of genes somehow associated with youth violence (this example is hypothetical because we don't know of any such combination). The adolescent who carries this genetic mixture might experience a world of loving parents, regular nutritious meals, lots of books, and a series of masterful teachers. Or the adolescent's world might include parental neglect, a neighborhood in which gunshots and crime are everyday occurrences, and inadequate schooling. In which of these environments are the adolescent's genes likely to manufacture the biological underpinnings of criminality?

If heredity and environment interact to determine the course of development, is that all there is to answering the question of what causes development? Are children completely at the mercy of their genes and environment as they develop? Genetic heritage and environmental experiences are pervasive influences on development (Franke & Buitelaar, 2018). But children's development is not solely the outcome of their heredity and environment; children also can author a unique developmental path by changing their environment. As one psychologist concluded:

> In reality, we are both the creatures and creators of our worlds. We are . . . the products of our genes and environments. Nevertheless, . . . the stream of causation that shapes the future runs through our present choices . . . Mind matters . . . Our hopes, goals, and expectations influence our future. (Myers, 2010, p. 168)

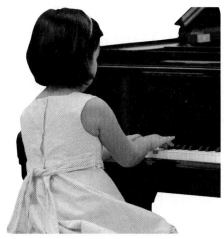

To what extent are this young girl's piano skills likely due to heredity, environment, or both? Explain.

Francisco Romero/E+/Getty Images

---

developmental **connection**

Nature and Nurture

The nature and nurture issue is one of the main issues in the study of children's development. Connect to "Introduction."

Review *Connect* Reflect

 LG4 Explain some of the ways that heredity and environment interact to produce individual differences in development.

Review

- What is behavior genetics?
- What are three types of heredity-environment correlations?
- What is meant by the concepts of shared and nonshared environmental experiences?
- What is the epigenetic view of development? What characterizes gene × environment (G × E) interaction?
- What conclusions can be reached about heredity-environment interaction?

Connect

- Of passive, evocative, and active genotype-environment correlations, which is the best explanation for the similarities discovered between the twins discussed in the story that opened this chapter?

Reflect *Your Own Personal Journey of Life*

- Imagine that someone tells you that he or she has analyzed your genetic background and environmental experiences and reached the conclusion that the environment you grew up in as a child definitely had little influence on your intelligence. What would you say about this analysis?

Biological Beginnings

The Evolutionary Perspective

Natural Selection and Adaptive Behavior

Evolutionary Psychology

 Discuss the evolutionary perspective on child development.

- Natural selection is the process by which those individuals of a species that are best adapted to the environment survive and reproduce. Darwin proposed that natural selection fuels evolution. In evolutionary theory, adaptive behavior is behavior that promotes the organism's survival in a natural habitat.

- Evolutionary psychology holds that adaptation, reproduction, and "survival of the fittest" are important in shaping behavior. Ideas proposed by evolutionary developmental psychology include the view that an extended childhood period is needed to develop a large brain and learn the complexity of human social communities. Like other theoretical approaches to development, evolutionary psychology has limitations. Bandura rejects "one-sided evolutionism" and argues for a bidirectional link between biology and environment. Biology allows for a broad range of cultural possibilities.

Genetic Foundations of Development

The Collaborative Gene

Genes and Chromosomes

Genetic Principles

Chromosomal and Gene-Linked Abnormalities

 Describe what genes are and how they influence children's development.

- Short segments of DNA constitute genes, the units of hereditary information that direct cells to reproduce and manufacture proteins. Genes act collaboratively, not independently.

- Genes are passed on to new cells when chromosomes are duplicated during the process of mitosis and meiosis, which are two ways in which new cells are formed. When an egg and a sperm unite in the fertilization process, the resulting zygote contains the genes from the chromosomes in the father's sperm and the mother's egg. Despite this transmission of genes from generation to generation, variability is created in several ways, including through the exchange of chromosomal segments during meiosis, through mutations, and through environmental influences.

- Genetic principles include those involving dominant-recessive genes, sex-linked genes, genetic imprinting, and polygenic inheritance.

- Chromosomal abnormalities produce Down syndrome, which is caused by the presence of an extra copy of chromosome 21. Other sex-linked chromosomal abnormalities include Klinefelter syndrome, fragile X syndrome, Turner syndrome, and XYY syndrome. Gene-linked abnormalities involve absent or harmful genes. Gene-linked disorders include phenylketonuria (PKU) and sickle-cell anemia. Genetic counseling offers couples information about their risk of having a child with inherited abnormalities.

Reproductive Challenges and Choices

Prenatal Diagnostic Tests

Infertility and Reproductive Technology

Adoption

 Identify some important reproductive challenges and choices.

- Ultrasound sonography, fetal MRI, chorionic villus sampling, amniocentesis, and maternal blood screening are used to determine whether a fetus is developing normally. Noninvasive prenatal diagnosis is increasingly being explored. Sex determination of the fetus is occurring much earlier than in the past.

- Approximately 10 to 15 percent of U.S. couples have infertility problems, some of which can be corrected through surgery or fertility drugs. An additional option is in vitro fertilization.

- The vast majority of adopted children adapt effectively. When adoption occurs very early in development, the outcomes for the child are improved. Because of the dramatic changes that occurred in adoption in recent decades, it is difficult to generalize about the average adopted child or average adoptive family.

Heredity and Environment Interaction: Nature and Nurture

 LG4 Explain some of the ways that heredity and environment interact to produce individual differences in development.

- Behavior Genetics

- Heredity-Environment Correlations

- Shared and Nonshared Environmental Experiences

- The Epigenetic View and Gene × Environment (G × E) Interaction

- Conclusions About Heredity-Environment Interaction

- Behavior genetics is the field concerned with the influence of heredity and environment on individual differences in human traits and development. Methods used by behavior geneticists include twin studies and adoption studies.

- In Scarr's view of heredity-environment correlations, heredity directs the types of environments that children experience. She describes three genotype-environment correlations: passive, evocative, and active (niche-picking). Scarr argues that the relative importance of these three genotype-environment correlations changes as children develop.

- Shared environmental experiences refer to siblings' common experiences, such as their parents' personalities and intellectual orientation, the family's socioeconomic status, and the neighborhood in which they live. Nonshared environmental experiences involve the child's unique experiences, both within a family and outside a family, that are not shared with a sibling. Many behavior geneticists argue that differences in the development of siblings are due to nonshared environmental experiences (and heredity) rather than shared environmental experiences.

- The epigenetic view emphasizes that development is the result of an ongoing, bidirectional interchange between heredity and environment. Gene × environment interaction involves the interaction of a specific, measured variation in the DNA and a specific, measured aspect of the environment. An increasing number of G × E studies are being conducted.

- Behaviors are influenced by genes in a way that gives people a propensity for a particular developmental trajectory. However, actual development also requires an environment, and that environment is complex. The interaction of heredity and environment is extensive. Much remains to be discovered about the specific ways that heredity and environment interact to influence development. Although heredity and environment are pervasive influences on development, humans can author a unique developmental path by changing their environment.

key terms

active (niche-picking) genotype-environment correlations 63
adoption study 62
behavior genetics 61
chromosomes 48
DNA 49
Down syndrome 52
epigenetic view 64

evocative genotype-environment correlations 62
evolutionary psychology 45
fertilization 51
fragile X syndrome 53
gene × environment (G × E) interaction 64
genes 49
genotype 51

Klinefelter syndrome 53
meiosis 51
mitosis 51
nonshared environmental experiences 63
passive genotype-environment correlations 62
phenotype 51
phenylketonuria (PKU) 53

shared environmental experiences 63
sickle-cell anemia 54
Turner syndrome 53
twin study 61
XYY syndrome 53
zygote 51

key people

Albert Bandura 47
Thomas Bouchard 44
David Buss 46

Charles Darwin 45
Gilbert Gottlieb 64
Stephen Jay Gould 47

Robert Plomin 63
Sandra Scarr 62

chapter 3

PRENATAL DEVELOPMENT AND BIRTH

chapter outline

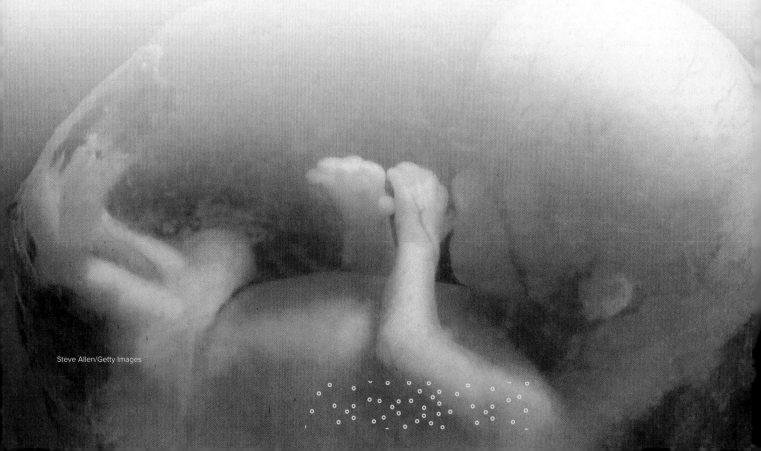

Steve Allen/Getty Images

D iana and Roger married when he was 38 and she was 34. Both worked full-time and were excited when Diana became pregnant. Two months later, Diana began to have some unusual pains and bleeding. Just two months into her pregnancy she had lost the baby. Diana thought deeply about possible reasons she had been unable to carry the baby to full term. At about the time she became pregnant, the federal government had begun to warn that eating certain types of fish with a high mercury content during pregnancy on a regular basis might cause a miscarriage. Now she eliminated these fish from her diet.

Six months later, Diana became pregnant again. She and Roger read about pregnancy and signed up for birth preparation classes. Each Friday night for eight weeks they practiced relaxation techniques during simulated contractions. They talked about what kind of parents they wanted to be and discussed how their lives would change after the baby was born. When they found out that their offspring was going to be a boy, they gave him a nickname: Mr. Littles.

This time, Diana's pregnancy went well and Alex was born. During the birth, however, Diana's heart rate dropped precipitously, and she was given a stimulant to raise it. Apparently the stimulant also increased Alex's heart rate and breathing to a dangerous point, and he was placed in a neonatal intensive care unit (NICU).

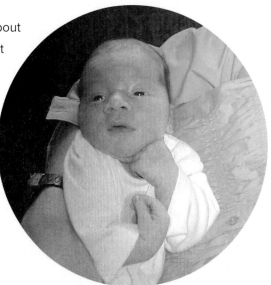

Alex, also known as "Mr. Littles."
Dr. John Santrock

Several times a day, Diana and Roger visited Alex in the NICU. A number of babies in the NICU who had a very low birth weight had been in intensive care for weeks, and some of these babies were not doing well. Fortunately, Alex was in better health. After several days in the NICU, his parents were permitted to take home a very healthy Alex.

preview

This chapter describes the truly remarkable developments from conception through birth. We will look at normal development as well as hazards to normal development (such as mercury, mentioned in the preceding story). We will outline the birth process and describe the tests used to assess the newborn. We will examine the physical, emotional, and psychological adjustments that a mother goes through during the time following birth—the postpartum period. And we will end the chapter by comparing theories on parent-infant bonding.

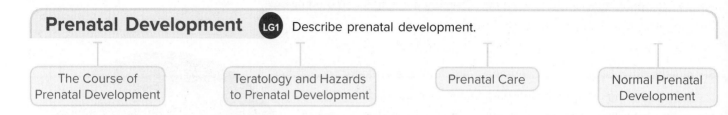

Prenatal Development (LG1) Describe prenatal development.

| The Course of Prenatal Development | Teratology and Hazards to Prenatal Development | Prenatal Care | Normal Prenatal Development |

The history of man for nine months preceding his birth would, probably, be far more interesting, and contain events of greater moment than all three score and ten years that follow it.

—SAMUEL TAYLOR COLERIDGE

English poet and essayist, 19th century

Imagine how Alex ("Mr. Littles") came to be. Out of thousands of eggs and millions of sperm, one egg and one sperm united to produce him. Had the union of sperm and egg come a day or even an hour earlier or later, he might have been very different—in his psychological and physical characteristics. *Conception* occurs when a single sperm cell from the male unites with an ovum (egg) in the female's fallopian tube in a process called fertilization. Over the next few months, the genetic code directs a series of changes in the fertilized egg, but many events and hazards will influence how that egg develops and becomes tiny Alex.

THE COURSE OF PRENATAL DEVELOPMENT

Typical prenatal development begins with fertilization and ends with birth, lasting between 266 and 280 days (from 38 to 40 weeks; around 9 months). It can be divided into three periods: germinal, embryonic, and fetal.

The Germinal Period   The **germinal period** is the period of prenatal development that takes place in the first two weeks after conception. It includes the creation of the fertilized egg, called a zygote, followed by cell division and attachment of the zygote to the uterine wall.

Rapid cell division by the zygote continues throughout the germinal period (recall that this cell division occurs through a process called *mitosis*). By approximately one week after conception, the differentiation of these cells—their specialization for different tasks—has already begun. At this stage, the group of cells, now called the **blastocyst,** consists of an inner mass of cells that will eventually develop into the embryo, and the **trophoblast,** an outer layer of cells that later provides nutrition and support for the embryo. *Implantation,* the attachment of the zygote to the uterine wall, takes place about 11 to 15 days after conception. Figure 1 illustrates some of the most significant developments during the germinal period.

The Embryonic Period   The **embryonic period** is the period of prenatal development that occurs from two to eight weeks after conception. During the embryonic period, the rate of cell differentiation intensifies, support systems for cells form, and organs appear.

This period begins as the blastocyst attaches to the uterine wall. The mass of cells is now called an *embryo,* and three layers of cells form. The embryo's *endoderm* is the inner layer of cells, which will develop into the digestive and respiratory systems. The *mesoderm* is the middle layer, which will become the circulatory system, bones, muscles, excretory system, and reproductive system. The *ectoderm* is the outermost layer, which

germinal period The period of prenatal development that takes place in the first two weeks after conception. It includes the creation of the zygote, continued cell division, and the attachment of the zygote to the uterine wall.

blastocyst The inner layer of cells that develops during the germinal period. These cells later develop into the embryo.

trophoblast The outer layer of cells that develops in the germinal period. These cells provide nutrition and support for the embryo.

embryonic period The period of prenatal development that occurs from two to eight weeks after conception. During the embryonic period, the rate of cell differentiation intensifies, support systems for the cells form, and organs appear.

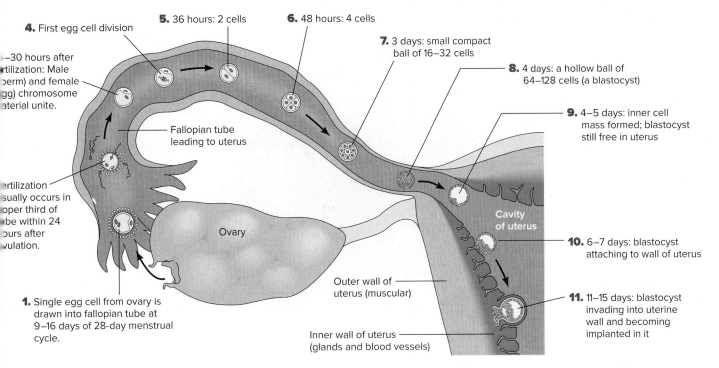

4. First egg cell division

5. 36 hours: 2 cells

6. 48 hours: 4 cells

7. 3 days: small compact ball of 16–32 cells

8. 4 days: a hollow ball of 64–128 cells (a blastocyst)

9. 4–5 days: inner cell mass formed; blastocyst still free in uterus

–30 hours after ...rtilization: Male ...erm) and female ...gg) chromosome ...aterial unite.

Fallopian tube leading to uterus

...rtilization ...sually occurs in ...pper third of ...ube within 24 ...ours after ...vulation.

Ovary

Cavity of uterus

10. 6–7 days: blastocyst attaching to wall of uterus

11. 11–15 days: blastocyst invading into uterine wall and becoming implanted in it

1. Single egg cell from ovary is drawn into fallopian tube at 9–16 days of 28-day menstrual cycle.

Outer wall of uterus (muscular)

Inner wall of uterus (glands and blood vessels)

FIGURE 1

SIGNIFICANT DEVELOPMENTS IN THE GERMINAL PERIOD. Just one week after conception, cells of the blastocyst have already begun specializing. The germination period ends when the blastocyst attaches to the uterine wall. *Which of the steps shown in the drawing occur in the laboratory when IVF is used?*

will become the nervous system and brain, sensory receptors (ears, nose, and eyes, for example), and skin parts (hair and nails, for example). Every body part eventually develops from these three layers. The endoderm primarily produces internal body parts, the mesoderm primarily produces parts that surround the internal areas, and the ectoderm primarily produces surface parts.

As the embryo's three layers form, life-support systems for the embryo develop rapidly. These life-support systems include the amnion, the umbilical cord (both of which develop from the fertilized egg, not the mother's body), and the placenta. The **amnion** is like a bag or an envelope and contains a clear fluid in which the developing embryo floats. The amniotic fluid provides an environment that is temperature and humidity controlled as well as shockproof. The **umbilical cord,** which contains two arteries and one vein, connects the baby to the placenta. The **placenta** consists of a disk-shaped group of tissues in which small blood vessels from the mother and the offspring intertwine but do not join.

Figure 2 illustrates the placenta, the umbilical cord, and the blood flow in the expectant mother and developing organism. Very small molecules—oxygen, water, salt, food from the mother's blood, as well as carbon dioxide and digestive wastes from the offspring's blood—pass back and forth between the mother and embryo or fetus (Kallol & others, 2018). Virtually any drug or chemical substance the pregnant woman ingests can cross the placenta to some degree, unless it is metabolized or altered during passage, or is too large (Kapur & Baber, 2017; Lye & others, 2018). A comprehensive review of the research revealed that cigarette smoke weakened and increased the oxidative stress of fetal membranes, from which the placenta develops (Lu & others, 2018). Large molecules that cannot pass through the placental wall include red blood cells and harmful substances, such as most bacteria, maternal wastes, and hormones. The complex mechanisms that control the movement of substances across the placental barrier are still not entirely understood (Saunders & others, 2018; Zhu & others, 2018).

By the time most women know they are pregnant, the major organs of the developing offspring have begun to form. **Organogenesis** is the name given to the process of organ

amnion Prenatal life-support system that is a bag or envelope containing a clear fluid in which the developing embryo floats.

umbilical cord A life-support system that contains two arteries and one vein and connects the baby to the placenta.

placenta A life-support system that consists of a disk-shaped group of tissues in which small blood vessels from the mother and offspring intertwine.

organogenesis Organ formation that takes place during the first two months of prenatal development.

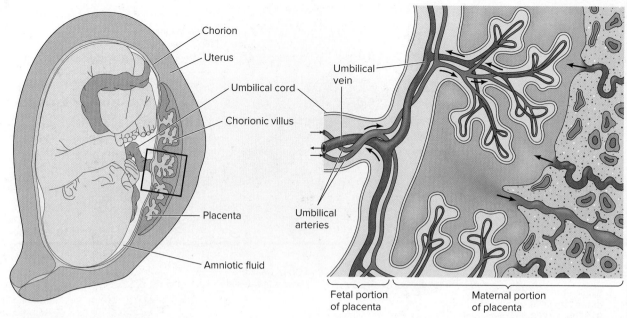

Chorion
Uterus
Umbilical cord
Chorionic villus
Umbilical vein
Placenta
Umbilical arteries
Amniotic fluid

Fetal portion of placenta   Maternal portion of placenta

FIGURE 2

THE PLACENTA AND THE UMBILICAL CORD. The area bound by the square in the illustration of the fetus and placenta is enlarged to show a segment of the placenta. Arrows indicate the direction of blood flow. Maternal blood flows through the uterine arteries to the spaces housing the placenta, and it returns through the uterine veins to the maternal circulation. Fetal blood flows through the umbilical arteries into the capillaries of the placenta and returns through the umbilical vein to the fetal circulation. The exchange of materials takes place across the layer separating the maternal and fetal blood supplies, so the bloods never come into contact. *What is known about how the placental barrier works and its importance?*

From John Santrock, Child Development, 13/e, fig 3.2. Copyright © 2011 McGraw-Hill Companies. Reprinted by permission.

formation during the first two months of prenatal development. While they are being formed, the organs are especially vulnerable to environmental changes (Sebastiani & others, 2018). In the third week after conception, the neural tube that eventually becomes the spinal cord forms. At about 21 days, eyes begin to appear, and at 24 days the cells for the heart begin to differentiate. During the fourth week, the urogenital system becomes apparent and arm and leg buds emerge. Four chambers of the heart take shape, and blood vessels appear. From the fifth to the eighth week, arms and legs differentiate further; at this time, the face starts to form but still is not very recognizable. The intestinal tract develops and the facial structures fuse. At eight weeks, the developing organism weighs about 1/30 ounce and is just over 1 inch long.

The Fetal Period   The **fetal period,** lasting about seven months, is the prenatal period between two months after conception and birth in typical pregnancies. Growth and development continue their dramatic course during this time.

Three months after conception, the fetus is about 3 inches long and weighs about 3 ounces. It has become active, moving its arms and legs, opening and closing its mouth, and moving its head. The face, forehead, eyelids, nose, and chin are distinguishable, as are the upper arms, lower arms, hands, and lower limbs. In most cases, the genitals can be identified as male or female. By the end of the fourth month of pregnancy, the fetus has grown to 6 inches in length and weighs 4 to 7 ounces. At this time, a growth spurt occurs in the body's lower parts. For the first time, the mother can feel arm and leg movements.

By the end of the fifth month, the fetus is about 12 inches long and weighs close to a pound. Structures of the skin have formed—toenails and fingernails, for example. The fetus is more active, showing a preference for a particular position in the womb. By the end of the sixth month, the fetus is about 14 inches long and has gained another half pound to a pound. The eyes and eyelids are completely formed, and a fine layer of hair covers the head. A grasping reflex is present and irregular breathing movements occur.

fetal period The period from two months after conception until birth, lasting about seven months in typical pregnancies.

As early as six months of pregnancy (about 24 to 25 weeks after conception), the fetus for the first time has a chance of surviving outside of the womb—that is, it is *viable.* Infants who are born early, or between 24 and 37 weeks of pregnancy, usually need help breathing because their lungs are not yet fully mature. By the end of the seventh month, the fetus is about 16 inches long and weighs about 3 pounds.

During the last two months of prenatal development, fatty tissues develop and various organ systems—heart and kidneys, for example—are functioning fully. During the eighth and ninth months, the fetus grows longer and gains substantial weight—about another 4 pounds. At birth, the average baby weighs 7½ pounds and is about 20 inches long. This average weight is remarkably consistent around the globe when the mother is healthy and has access to adequate prenatal care (Villar & others, 2014).

Figure 3 gives an overview of the main events during prenatal development. Notice that instead of describing development in terms of germinal, embryonic, and fetal periods, Figure 3

First trimester (first 3 months): Germinal and embryonic periods, and beginning of fetal period

Conception to 4 weeks
- Is less than ¹⁄₁₀ inch long
- Beginning development of spinal cord, nervous system, gastrointestinal system, heart, and lungs
- Amniotic sac envelops the preliminary tissues of entire body
- Is called a "zygote"

8 weeks
- Is just over 1 inch long
- Face is forming with rudimentary eyes, ears, mouth, and tooth buds
- Arms and legs are moving
- Brain is forming
- Fetal heartbeat is detectable with ultrasound
- Is called an "embryo"

12 weeks
- Is about 3 inches long and weighs about 1 ounce
- Can move arms, legs, fingers, and toes
- Fingerprints are present
- Can smile, frown, suck, and swallow
- Sex is distinguishable
- Can urinate
- Is called a "fetus"

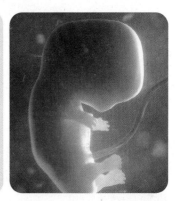

Second trimester (middle 3 months): Fetal period

16 weeks
- Is about 6 inches long and weighs about 4 to 7 ounces
- Heartbeat is strong
- Skin is thin, transparent
- Downy hair (lanugo) covers body
- Fingernails and toenails are forming
- Has coordinated movements; is able to roll over in amniotic fluid

20 weeks
- Is about 12 inches long and weighs close to 1 pound
- Heartbeat is audible with ordinary stethoscope
- Sucks thumb
- Hiccups
- Hair, eyelashes, eyebrows are present

24 weeks
- Is about 14 inches long and weighs 1 to 1½ pounds
- Skin is wrinkled and covered with protective coating (vernix caseosa)
- Eyes are open
- Waste matter is collected in bowel
- Has strong grip

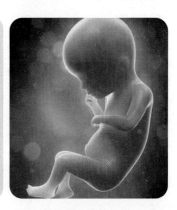

Third trimester (last 3 months): Fetal period

28 weeks
- Is about 16 inches long and weighs about 3 pounds
- Is adding body fat
- Is very active
- Rudimentary breathing movements are present

32 weeks
- Is 16½ to 18 inches long and weighs 4 to 5 pounds
- Has periods of sleep and wakefulness
- Responds to sounds
- May assume the birth position
- Bones of head are soft and flexible
- Iron is being stored in liver

36 to 38 weeks
- Is 19 to 20 inches long and weighs 6 to 7½ pounds
- Skin is less wrinkled
- Vernix caseosa is thick
- Lanugo is mostly gone
- Is less active
- Is gaining immunities from mother

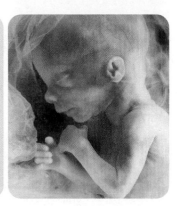

FIGURE 3

THE THREE TRIMESTERS OF PRENATAL DEVELOPMENT. Both the germinal and embryonic periods occur during the first trimester. The end of the first trimester as well as the second and third trimesters are part of the fetal period.

(*top*) unlim3d/123RF; (*middle*) SCIEPRO/Science Photo Library/Getty Images; (*bottom*) Steve Allen/Getty Images

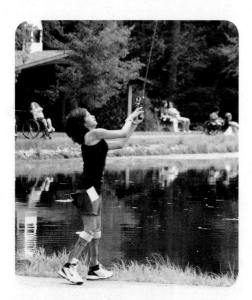

Yelyi Nordone of New York City, shown here as a 12-year-old casting her fishing rod line out into the pond during Camp Spifida in rural Pennsylvania. Camp Spifida is a week-long residential camp for children with spina bifida.

Bill Hughes/Bloomsburg Press Enterprise/AP Images

developmental **connection**

Brain Development

At birth, the brain's weight is approximately 25 percent of its adult weight. Connect to "Physical Development and Health."

neurons Nerve cells, which handle information processing at the cellular level in the brain.

teratogen From the Greek word *tera,* meaning "monster," this term refers to any agent that causes a birth defect. Teratology is the field of study that investigates the causes of birth defects.

divides prenatal development into equal periods of three months, called *trimesters.* Remember that the three trimesters are not the same as the three prenatal periods we have discussed. The germinal and embryonic periods occur in the first trimester. The fetal period begins toward the end of the first trimester and continues through the second and third trimesters. Viability (the possibility of surviving outside the womb) occurs at the very end of the second trimester.

The Brain   One of the most remarkable aspects of the prenatal period is the development of the brain (Arck & others, 2018). By the time babies are born, they have approximately 100 billion **neurons,** or nerve cells, which handle information processing at the cellular level in the brain. During prenatal development, neurons spend time moving to the right locations and are starting to become connected. The basic architecture of the human brain is assembled during the first two trimesters of prenatal development. In typical development, the third trimester of prenatal development and the first two years of postnatal life are characterized by connectivity and functioning of neurons (Moulson & Nelson, 2008).

As the human embryo develops inside its mother's womb, the nervous system begins forming as a long, hollow tube located on the embryo's back. This pear-shaped *neural tube,* which forms at about 18 to 24 days after conception, develops out of the ectoderm. The tube closes at the top and bottom at about 24 days after conception. Figure 4 shows that the nervous system still has a tubular appearance six weeks after conception.

Two birth defects related to a failure of the neural tube to close are anencephaly and spina bifida. The highest regions of the brain fail to develop when fetuses have *anencephaly* and the head end of the neural tube fails to close. Such infants die in the womb, during childbirth, or shortly after birth (Özel & others, 2018). Spina bifida results in varying degrees of paralysis of the lower limbs. Individuals with spina bifida usually need assistive devices such as crutches, braces, or wheelchairs. A strategy that can help to prevent neural tube defects is for women to take adequate amounts of the B vitamin folic acid, a topic we will discuss later in this chapter (Garrett & Bailey, 2018). And both maternal diabetes and obesity place the fetus at risk for developing neural tube defects (Huang, Chen, & Feng, 2017).

In a normal pregnancy, once the neural tube has closed, massive growth of new immature neurons begins to takes place at about the fifth prenatal week and continues throughout the remainder of the prenatal period. The generation of new neurons is called *neurogenesis* (Yang & others, 2014). At the peak of neurogenesis, it is estimated that as many as 200,000 neurons are being generated every minute.

At approximately 6 to 24 weeks after conception, *neuronal migration* occurs (Hadders-Algra, 2018). This involves cells moving outward from their point of origin to their appropriate locations and creating the different levels, structures, and regions of the brain. Once a cell has migrated to its target destination, it must mature and develop a more complex structure.

At about the 23rd prenatal week, connections between neurons begin to occur, a process that continues postnatally (Hadders-Algra, 2018). (We will have much more to say about the structure of neurons, their connectivity, and the development of the infant brain in the chapter "Physical Development and Health.")

TERATOLOGY AND HAZARDS TO PRENATAL DEVELOPMENT

For Alex, the baby discussed at the opening of this chapter, the course of prenatal development went smoothly. His mother's womb protected him as he developed. Despite this protection, the environment can affect the embryo or fetus in many well-documented ways.

General Principles   A **teratogen** is any agent that can potentially cause a birth defect or negatively alter cognitive and behavioral outcomes. (The word comes from the Greek word *tera,* meaning "monster.") So many teratogens exist that practically every fetus is exposed to at least some teratogens. For this reason, it is difficult to determine which teratogen causes which problem. In addition, it may take a long time for the effects of a teratogen to show up.

The field of study that investigates the causes of birth defects is called *teratology* (Teratology Society, 2017). Some exposures to teratogens do not cause physical birth defects but can alter the developing brain and influence cognitive and behavioral functioning, in which case the field of study is called *behavioral teratology*.

The dose, genetic susceptibility, and the time of exposure to a particular teratogen influence both the type of defect and the severity of the damage to an embryo or fetus:

- **Dose.** The greater the amount of exposure to a teratogen, such as a drug, the greater the effect.
- **Genetic susceptibility.** The type or severity of abnormalities caused by a teratogen is linked to the genes of both the pregnant woman and of her embryo or fetus (Gomes & others, 2018). For example, how a mother metabolizes a particular drug can influence the degree to which the drug effects are transmitted to the embryo or fetus. The extent to which an embryo or fetus is vulnerable to a teratogen may also depend on its genotype. Also, for unknown reasons, male fetuses are far more likely to be affected by teratogens than female fetuses (Hadley & Sheiner, 2017).
- **Time of exposure.** Teratogen exposure does more damage when it occurs at some points in development than at others. Damage during the germinal period may even prevent implantation. In general, the embryonic period is more vulnerable than the fetal period (Teratology Society, 2017).

Figure 5 summarizes additional information about the effects of time of exposure to a teratogen. The probability of a structural defect is greatest early in the embryonic period, when organs are being formed (Chudley, 2017). Each body structure has its own critical

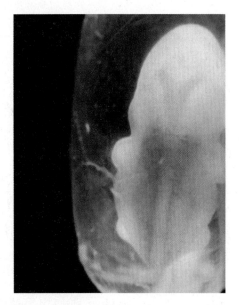

FIGURE **4**

EARLY FORMATION OF THE NERVOUS SYSTEM. The photograph shows the primitive, tubular appearance of the nervous system at six weeks in the human embryo.

Claude Edelmann/Science Source

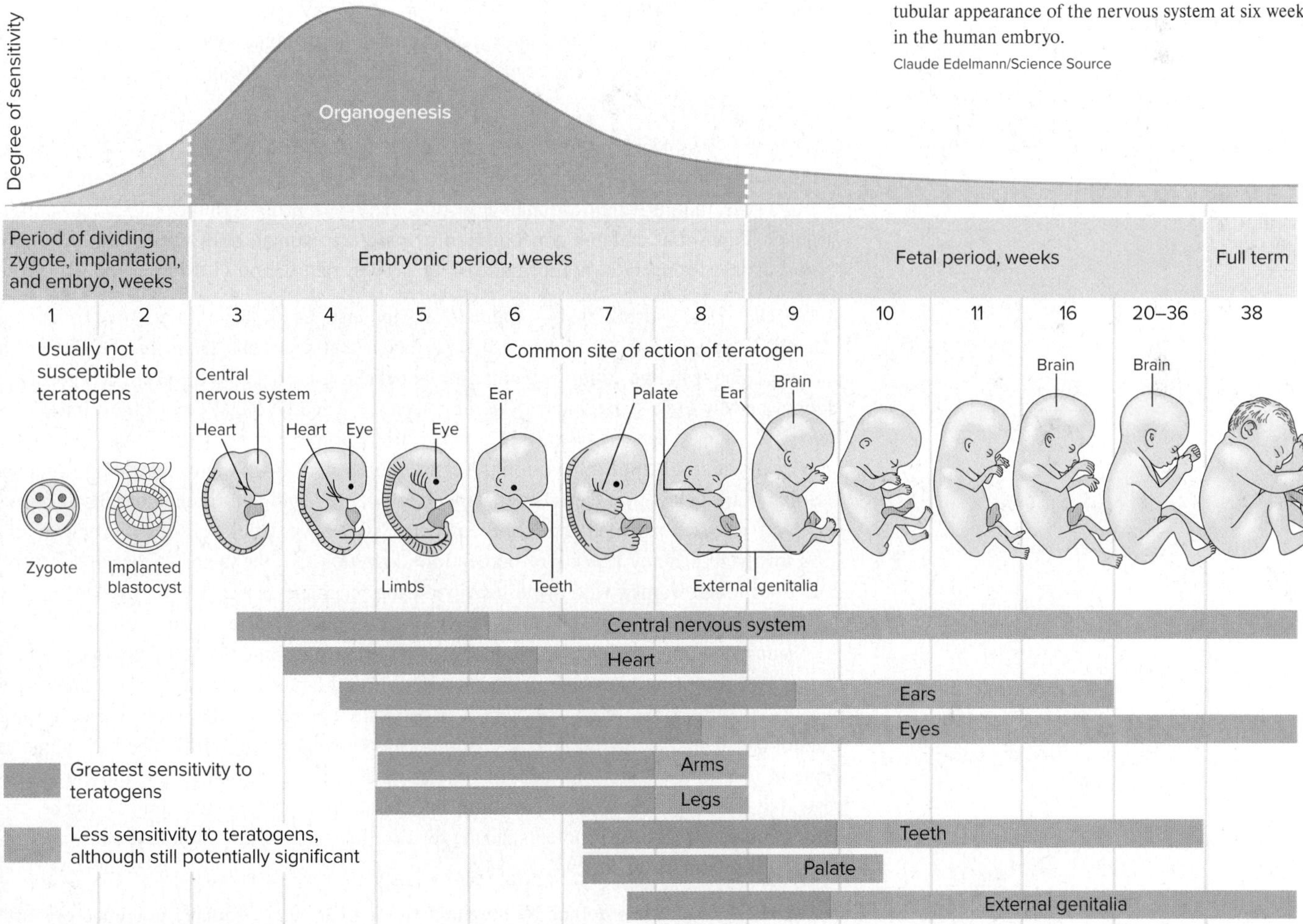

FIGURE **5**

TERATOGENS AND THE TIMING OF THEIR EFFECTS ON PRENATAL DEVELOPMENT. The danger of structural defects caused by teratogens is greatest early in embryonic development. The period of organogenesis (red color) lasts for about six weeks. Later effects of teratogens (blue-green color) mainly occur in the fetal period and instead of causing structural defects are more likely to stunt growth or cause problems with organ function.

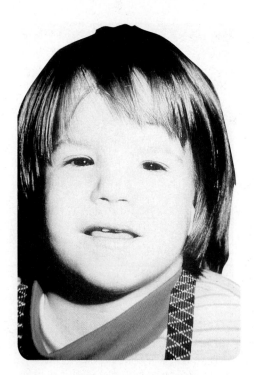

Fetal alcohol spectrum disorders (FASD) are characterized by a number of physical abnormalities and learning problems. Notice the wide-set eyes, flat cheekbones, and thin upper lip in this child with FASD.

Streissguth, AP, Landesman-Dwyer S, Martin, JC, & Smith, DW (1980). Teratogenic Effects of Alcohol in Humans and Laboratory Animals. Science, 209, 353–361.

period of formation. Recall that a critical period is a fixed time period very early in development during which certain experiences or events can have a long-lasting effect on development. The critical period for the nervous system (week 3) is earlier than for arms and legs (weeks 4 and 5).

After organogenesis is complete, teratogens are less likely to cause anatomical defects. Instead, exposure during the fetal period is more likely to stunt growth or to create problems in the way organs function. To examine some key teratogens and their effects, let's begin with drugs.

Prescription and Nonprescription Drugs   Many U.S. women are given prescriptions for drugs while they are pregnant—especially antibiotics, pain and fever reducers, and asthma medications. Prescription as well as nonprescription drugs, however, may have effects on the embryo or fetus that the women never imagine.

Prescription drugs that can function as teratogens include antibiotics, such as streptomycin and tetracycline; some antidepressants; certain hormones, such as progestin and synthetic estrogen; and Accutane (which often is prescribed for acne) (Campagne, 2018).

Nonprescription drugs that can be harmful include diet pills and high dosages of aspirin. However, recent research indicated that low doses of aspirin pose no harm for the fetus but that high doses can contribute to maternal and fetal bleeding (Roberge, Bujold, & Nicolaides, 2018).

Psychoactive Drugs   *Psychoactive drugs* are drugs that act on the nervous system to alter states of consciousness, modify perceptions, and change moods. Examples include caffeine, alcohol, and nicotine, as well as illicit drugs such as cocaine, methamphetamine, marijuana, and heroin.

Caffeine   People often consume caffeine when they drink coffee, tea, energy drinks, or colas, or when they eat chocolate. Although the U.S. Food and Drug Administration recommends that pregnant women consume it only sparingly or not at all, mounting evidence shows that caffeine consumption by pregnant women does not increase the risk of miscarriage, congenital malformations, or growth retardation (Leviton, 2018).

Alcohol   Heavy drinking by pregnant women can be devastating to their offspring (Zhang, Hashimoto, & Guizzetti, 2018). **Fetal alcohol spectrum disorders (FASD)** are a cluster of abnormalities and problems that appear in the offspring of mothers who drink alcohol heavily during pregnancy. The abnormalities include facial deformities and defective limbs, face, and heart (Brown & others, 2018). Some children with FASD have these body malformations, but others don't. Most children with FASD have learning problems, and many are below average in intelligence with some having an intellectual disability. A review of research revealed that children with FASD have deficiencies in the brain pathways involved in many aspects of perception, cognition, and behavior (Nguyen & others, 2017). Although women who drink heavily during pregnancy are at a higher risk of having a child with FASD, not all pregnant heavy drinkers have children with FASD.

What are some guidelines for alcohol use during pregnancy? Even drinking just one or two servings of beer or wine or one serving of hard liquor a few days a week may have negative effects on the fetus, although it is generally agreed that this level of alcohol use will not cause fetal alcohol spectrum disorders (Noor & Milligan, 2018). The U.S. Surgeon General recommends that no alcohol be consumed during pregnancy. And research suggests that it may not be wise to consume alcohol at the time of conception. Doing so can lead to increased risk for problems during fertilization and implantation that cause miscarriage (Kalisch-Smith & Moritz, 2018).

Nicotine   Cigarette smoking by pregnant women can also adversely influence prenatal development, birth, and postnatal development. Preterm births and low birth weights, fetal and neonatal deaths, and respiratory problems and sudden infant death syndrome (SIDS, also known as crib death) are all more common among the offspring of mothers who smoked during pregnancy (Dessì & others, 2018). Researchers also have found that maternal smoking during pregnancy is a risk factor for the development of attention deficit

fetal alcohol spectrum disorders (FASD) A cluster of abnormalities and problems that appear in the offspring of mothers who drink alcohol heavily during pregnancy.

hyperactivity disorder and closely related learning deficits in children (Abreu-Villaça & others, 2018). Researchers also have documented that environmental tobacco smoke is linked to an increased risk of low birth weight in offspring (Leonardo-Bee & others, 2008) and to diminished ovarian functioning in female offspring (Budani & Tiboni, 2017). Further, environmental tobacco smoke has been linked with alterations in gene functioning in the fetal cells of offspring (Dessì & others, 2018). Maternal smoking during pregnancy has even been linked to a modest increase in risk for childhood non-Hodgkin lymphoma (Antonopoulos & others, 2011).

Cocaine   Does cocaine use during pregnancy harm the developing embryo and fetus? Cocaine quickly crosses the placenta to reach the fetus. The most consistent finding is that cocaine exposure during prenatal development is associated with reduced birth weight, length, and head circumference (dos Santos & others, 2018). Also, although the results vary, prenatal cocaine exposure has been linked to lower arousal, less effective self-regulation, higher excitability, and poorer reflexes in neonates, impaired motor development, slower growth rate throughout childhood, higher blood pressure, impaired language development and information processing, attention deficits and impulsivity, learning disabilities, increased likelihood of needing special education supports in school, and increased rates of aggression and other conduct behavioral problems (Ackerman, Riggins, & Black, 2010; Buckingham-Howes & others, 2013; Viteri & others, 2015).

Some researchers argue that these findings should be interpreted cautiously. Why? Because other factors in the lives of pregnant women who use cocaine (such as poverty, malnutrition, and other substance abuse) often cannot be ruled out as possible contributors to the problems found in their children (Lowell & Mayes, 2019). For example, cocaine users are more likely than nonusers to smoke cigarettes, use marijuana, drink alcohol, and take amphetamines. Despite these cautions, the weight of research evidence just described indicates that children born to mothers who use cocaine are likely to have neurological and cognitive deficits. Cocaine use by pregnant women is never recommended.

Methamphetamine   Methamphetamine, like cocaine, is a stimulant, speeding up an individual's nervous system. Babies born to mothers who use methamphetamine, or "meth," during pregnancy are at risk for a number of problems, including high infant mortality, low birth weight, and developmental and behavioral problems (Kwiatkowski & others, 2018). A meta-analysis of studies revealed that prenatal meth exposure was associated with smaller head circumference, lower birth weight, and premature birth (Kalaitzopoulos & others, 2018). And another study of newborns found that prenatal exposure to meth was linked to smaller brain structures in a number of areas, especially in the thalamus and caudate areas in the center of the brain (Warton & others, 2018).

Marijuana   Recreational marijuana use is now legal or decriminalized in 23 states, even though it remains illegal in federal law. An increasing number of studies find that marijuana use by pregnant women has negative outcomes for offspring. For example, researchers have found that prenatal marijuana exposure was related to poorer functioning after birth, lower birth weight, premature birth, and higher likelihood of neonatal intensive care admission. However, most of these effects may be explained by other drugs that mothers were taking, since marijuana users often consume alcohol, tobacco, and other substances (Ryan, Ammerman, & O'Connor, 2018). Although interpreting its effects is complicated due to these "polydrug" effects, marijuana use is not recommended for pregnant women.

Heroin   It is well documented that infants whose mothers are addicted to heroin show several behavioral difficulties at birth. The difficulties include withdrawal symptoms, such as tremors, irritability, abnormal crying, disturbed sleep, and impaired motor control. Many still show behavioral problems at their first birthday, and attention deficits may appear later in development. The most common treatment for heroin addiction, methadone, is associated with very severe withdrawal symptoms in newborns as well as birth complications; these effects may be less severe for other heroin replacement drug therapies (Kelty & Hulse, 2017).

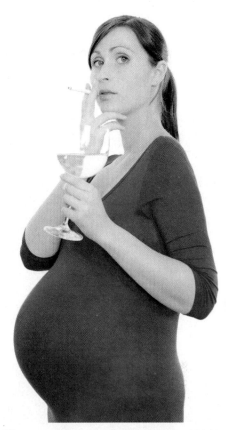

What are some links between expectant mothers' drinking and cigarette smoking and outcomes for their offspring?
Altafulla/Shutterstock

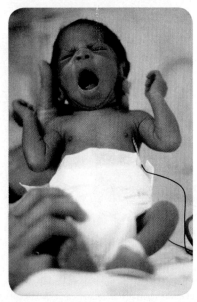

This baby was exposed to cocaine prenatally. *What are some of the possible effects on development of being exposed to cocaine prenatally?*
Chuck Nacke/Alamy Stock Photo

Incompatible Blood Types

Incompatible Blood Types Incompatibility between the mother's and father's blood types poses another risk to prenatal development. Blood types are created by differences in the surface structure of red blood cells. One type of difference in the surface of red blood cells creates the familiar blood groups—A, B, O, and AB. A second difference creates what is called Rh-positive and Rh-negative blood. If a surface marker, called the *Rh-factor,* is present in an individual's red blood cells, the person is said to be Rh-positive; if the Rh-marker is not present, the person is said to be Rh-negative. If a pregnant woman is Rh-negative and her partner is Rh-positive, the fetus may be Rh-positive. If the fetus' blood is Rh-positive and the mother's is Rh-negative, the mother's immune system may produce antibodies that will attack the fetus. This can result in any number of problems, including miscarriage or stillbirth, anemia, jaundice, heart defects, brain damage, or death soon after birth (Li & others, 2010).

Generally, the first Rh-positive baby of an Rh-negative mother is not at risk, but with each subsequent pregnancy the risk increases. A vaccine (RhoGAM) may be given to the mother within three days of the first child's birth to prevent her body from making antibodies that will attack any future Rh-positive fetuses in subsequent pregnancies. Also, babies affected by Rh incompatibility can be given blood transfusions before or immediately after birth (Na'Allah & Griebel, 2017).

Environmental Hazards Many aspects of our modern industrial world can endanger the embryo or fetus. Some specific hazards to the embryo or fetus include radiation, toxic wastes, and other chemical pollutants in neighborhoods as well as workplaces (Warembourg, Cordier, & Garlantézec, 2017).

X-ray radiation can affect the developing embryo or fetus, especially in the first several weeks after conception, when women do not yet know they are pregnant. Women and their physicians should weigh the risks against the benefits of an X-ray when an actual or potential pregnancy is involved (Rajaraman & others, 2011). However, a routine diagnostic X-ray of a body area other than the abdomen, with the woman's abdomen protected by a lead apron, is generally considered safe (Chansakul & Young, 2017).

Environmental pollutants and toxic wastes are also sources of danger to unborn children. Among the dangerous pollutants are carbon monoxide, mercury, and lead, as well as certain fertilizers and pesticides.

Maternal Diseases Maternal diseases and infections can produce defects in offspring by crossing the placental barrier, or they can cause damage during birth. Rubella (German measles) is one disease that can cause prenatal defects. Women who plan to have children should have a blood test before they become pregnant to determine whether they are immune to the disease (Bukasa & others, 2018).

Syphilis (a sexually transmitted infection) is more damaging later in prenatal development—four months or more after conception. Damage includes eye lesions, which can cause blindness, and skin lesions.

Another infection that has received widespread attention is genital herpes. Newborns contract this virus when they are delivered through the birth canal of a mother who has genital herpes (Contini & others, 2018). About one-third of babies delivered through an infected birth canal die; another one-fourth become brain damaged. If an active case of genital herpes is detected in a pregnant woman close to her delivery date, a cesarean section can be performed (in which the infant is delivered through an incision in the mother's abdomen) to keep the virus from infecting the newborn (Sénat & others, 2018).

AIDS is a sexually transmitted infection that is caused by the human immunodeficiency virus (HIV), which destroys the body's immune system. A mother can infect her offspring with HIV/AIDS in three ways: (1) during gestation across the placenta, (2) during delivery through contact with maternal blood or fluids, and (3) postpartum (after birth) through breast feeding. The transmission of AIDS through breast feeding is especially a problem in many developing countries (UNICEF, 2017). Babies born to HIV-infected mothers can be (1) infected and symptomatic (show HIV symptoms), (2) infected but asymptomatic (not show HIV symptoms), or (3) not infected at all. An infant who is infected and asymptomatic may still develop HIV symptoms until 15 months of age.

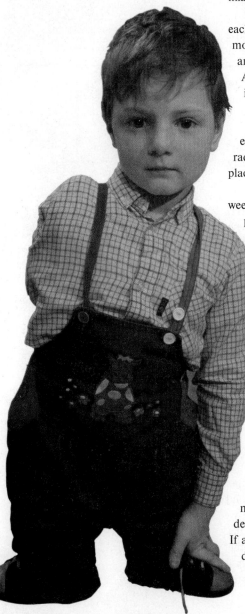

An explosion at the Chernobyl nuclear power plant in the Ukraine produced radioactive contamination that spread to surrounding areas. Thousands of infants were born with health problems and deformities as a result of the nuclear contamination, including this boy whose arm did not form. *Other than radioactive contamination, what are some other types of environmental hazards to prenatal development?*
Sergei Guneyev/The Life Images Collection/Getty Images

The more widespread disease of diabetes, characterized by high levels of sugar in the blood, also affects offspring (Desai, Beall, & Ross, 2013). Over the past three decades, there have been dramatic increases in the number of women giving birth who have diabetes (Freemark, 2018).

A research review indicated that newborns with physical defects are more likely to have diabetic mothers (Eriksson, 2009). Women who have gestational diabetes also may deliver very large infants (weighing 10 pounds or more), and these infants are at risk for diabetes themselves (Dugas & others, 2017).

Other Parental Factors   So far we have discussed a number of drugs, environmental hazards, maternal diseases, and incompatible blood types that can harm the embryo or fetus. Here we will explore other characteristics of the mother and father that can affect prenatal and child development, including nutrition, age, and emotional states and stress.

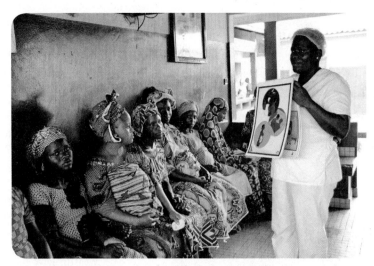

Because the fetus depends entirely on its mother for nutrition, it is important for the pregnant woman to have good nutritional habits. In Kenya, this government clinic provides pregnant women with information about how their diet can influence the health of their fetus and offspring. *What might the information about diet be like?*
Delphine Bousquet/AFP/Getty Images

Maternal Diet and Nutrition   A developing embryo or fetus depends completely on its mother for nutrition, which comes from the mother's blood. The nutritional status of the embryo or fetus is determined by the mother's total caloric intake and by her intake of proteins, vitamins, and minerals. Children born to malnourished mothers are more likely than other children to have malformations and other developmental problems.

Being overweight before and during pregnancy can also put the embryo or fetus at risk, and an increasing number of pregnant women in the United States are overweight (Desai, Beall, & Ross, 2013). Maternal obesity adversely affects pregnancy outcomes through elevated rates of hypertension, diabetes, respiratory complications, and infections in the mother. Management of obesity that includes weight loss and increased exercise prior to pregnancy is likely to benefit the mother and the baby (Mitanchez & Chavatte-Palmer, 2018).

One aspect of maternal nutrition that is important for normal prenatal development is consumption of folic acid, a B-complex vitamin (Garrett & Bailey, 2018). A classic study of more than 34,000 women indicated that taking folic acid either alone or as part of a multivitamin for at least one year prior to conceiving was linked with a 70 percent lower risk of delivering at 20 to 28 weeks and a 50 percent lower risk of delivering at 28 to 32 weeks (Bukowski & others, 2008). Another recent study revealed that young children of mothers who did not use folic acid or multivitamin supplements during pregnancy had more behavior problems (Virk & others, 2018). Also, as indicated earlier in the chapter, a lack of folic acid is related to neural tube defects in offspring, such as spina bifida (a defect in the spinal cord). The U.S. Department of Health and Human Services' Womenshealth.gov website (2018) recommends that pregnant women consume a minimum of 400 micrograms of folic acid per day (about twice the amount the average woman gets in one day). Orange juice and spinach are examples of foods rich in folic acid.

Eating fish is often recommended as part of a healthy diet, but pollution has made many types of fish a risky choice for pregnant women. Some fish contain high levels of mercury, which is released into the air both naturally and by industrial pollution (Kosik-Bogacka & others, 2018). When mercury falls into the water it can become toxic and accumulate in large fish, such as shark, swordfish, king mackerel, and some species of large tuna (American Pregnancy Association, 2018). Mercury is easily transferred across the placenta, and the embryo's developing brain and nervous system are highly sensitive to the metal. Researchers have found that prenatal mercury exposure is linked to adverse outcomes, including miscarriage, preterm birth, and lower intelligence, but these effects are reduced by public health knowledge about risk of mercury exposure during pregnancy (Murakami, Suzuki, & Yamaguchi, 2017).

developmental **connection**

Nutrition and Weight

What are some key factors that influence whether children become obese? Connect to "Physical Development and Heallth."

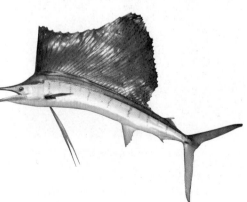

George Peters/Getty Images

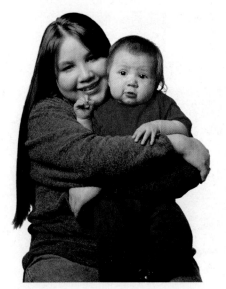

What are some of the risks for infants born to adolescent mothers?

Barbara Penoyar/Getty Images

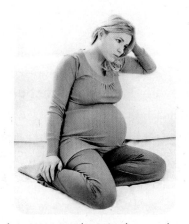

How do pregnant women's emotional states and stress affect prenatal development and birth?

Skynesher/E+/Getty Images

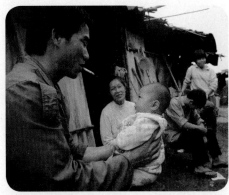

In a classic study in China, the longer fathers smoked, the greater the risk that their children would develop cancer (Ji & others, 1997). *What are some other paternal factors that can influence the development of the fetus and the child?*

David Butow/Corbis Historical/Getty Images

Maternal Age   When possible harmful effects on the fetus and infant are considered, two maternal ages are of special interest: adolescence and 35 years and older (Malizia, Hacker, & Penzias, 2009). The mortality rate of infants born to adolescent mothers is double that of infants born to mothers in their twenties. Adequate prenatal care decreases the probability that a child born to an adolescent girl will have physical problems. However, among women in all age groups adolescents are the least likely to obtain prenatal care from clinics and health services.

Maternal age is also linked to the risk that a child will have Down syndrome (Tamminga & others, 2018). As discussed previously, an individual with *Down syndrome* has distinctive facial characteristics, short limbs, and impaired motor and mental abilities. A baby with Down syndrome rarely is born to a mother 16 to 34 years of age. However, when the mother reaches 40 years of age, the probability is slightly over 1 in 100 that a baby born to her will have Down syndrome, and by age 50 it is almost 1 in 10. When mothers are 35 years and older, risks also increase for low birth weight, preterm delivery, and fetal death (Arya, Mulla, & Plavsic, 2018).

We still have much to learn about the role of the mother's age in pregnancy and childbirth. If women are physically active and are careful about their nutrition, their reproductive systems may remain healthier at older ages than was thought possible in the past.

Emotional States and Stress   When a pregnant woman experiences intense fears, anxieties, and other emotions or negative mood states, physiological changes occur that may affect her fetus (Breedlove & Fryzelka, 2011). A mother's stress may also influence the fetus indirectly by increasing the likelihood that the mother will engage in unhealthy behaviors such as taking drugs and receiving poor prenatal care.

High maternal anxiety and stress during pregnancy can have long-term consequences for the offspring (Fedock & Alvarez, 2018). A foundational research review indicated that pregnant women with high levels of stress are at increased risk for having a child with emotional or cognitive problems, attention deficit hyperactivity disorder (ADHD), and language delay (Taige & others, 2007). In the largest study of its kind, researchers examined more than 30,000 babies and found that across the nine months of pregnancy, their risk of being born preterm was highest when maternal exposure to stress occurred during the fifth and sixth months of pregnancy (Class & others, 2011). Maternal depression during pregnancy also has been linked to preterm birth and lower birth weight in some pregnancies (Dunkel Schetter, 2011).

Paternal Factors   So far, we have discussed how characteristics of the mother—such as drug use, disease, diet and nutrition, age, and emotional states—can influence prenatal development and the development of the child. This also is true for certain paternal risk factors. Men's exposure to lead, radiation, certain pesticides, and petrochemicals may cause abnormalities and genetic changes in sperm that lead to miscarriage or diseases such as childhood cancer (Soubry & others, 2014). The father's smoking during the mother's pregnancy also can cause problems for the offspring. In several studies conducted in multiple countries (for example, the United States and China), heavy paternal smoking was associated with the risk of early pregnancy loss (L. Wang & others, 2018). This negative outcome may be related to exposure to secondhand smoke. Paternal smoking around the time of the child's conception also has been linked to various cancers, physical deformities, and mental illnesses (Oldereid & others, 2018). And in another landmark study, children born to fathers who were 40 years of age or older had increased risk of developing autism because of an increase in random gene mutation in the older fathers (Kong & others, 2012).

PRENATAL CARE

Although prenatal care varies enormously, it usually involves a defined schedule of visits for medical care, which typically includes screening for manageable conditions and treatable diseases that can affect the baby or the mother. In addition to medical care, prenatal programs often include comprehensive educational, social, and nutritional services in most countries around the globe (Moller & others, 2017).

Exercise increasingly is recommended as part of a comprehensive prenatal care program (da Silva & others, 2017). Exercise during pregnancy helps prevent constipation, conditions the body, and is associated with a more positive mental state (Campolong & others, 2018; Vargas-Terrones & others, 2018). One experimental study found that pregnant women who completed a 3-month supervised aerobic exercise program showed improved health-related quality of life, including better physical functioning and reduced bodily pain, than their counterparts who did not participate in the program (Montoya Arizabaleta & others, 2010). A more recent experiment revealed that counseling to support increasing exercise and nutrition during pregnancy improved mothers' perception of their health (Engberg & others, 2018). However, it is important to remember not to overdo it. There is evidence from around the world that the incidence of exercise-related injuries is low, but pregnant women should always consult their healthcare professional before starting any exercise program (Evenson & others, 2014).

Does prenatal care matter? Information about pregnancy, labor, delivery, and caring for the newborn can be especially valuable for first-time mothers. A recent study revealed that pregnant women who have a broad network of social support have better mental health and functioning during and after the pregnancy (Hetherington & others, 2018).

Prenatal care is also very important for women in poverty and immigrant women because it links them with other social services (Hughson & others, 2018). An innovative program that is rapidly expanding in the United States is CenteringPregnancy (Kania-Richmond & others, 2017). This program is relationship-centered and provides complete prenatal care in a group setting. CenteringPregnancy replaces traditional 15-minute physician visits with 90-minute peer group support sessions and self-examination led by a physician or certified nurse-midwife. Groups of up to 10 women (and often their partners) meet regularly beginning at 12 to 16 weeks of pregnancy. The sessions emphasize empowering women to play an active role in experiencing a positive pregnancy. A recent study revealed that participants in CenteringPregnancy increased their prenatal visits, were more likely to breast feed, and their newborns were somewhat healthier (Grant & others, 2018).

Some prenatal programs for parents focus on home visitation (Michalopoulos & others, 2017). A classic series of program evaluations indicate that the most successful home visitation program is the Nurse Family Partnership created by David Olds and his colleagues (2004, 2007). The Nurse Family Partnership involves home visits by trained nurses beginning in the second or third trimester of prenatal development. The extensive program consists of approximately 50 home visits from the prenatal period through 2 years of age. The home visits focus on the mother's health, access to health care, parenting, and improvement of the mother's life by providing her with guidance in education, work, and relationships. Research revealed that the Nurse Family Partnership has numerous positive outcomes including fewer subsequent pregnancies, better work circumstances, and greater stability in relationship partners for the mother and improved academic success and social development for the child. Most recently, evidence for programs such as FamilyConnects suggests that many of these benefits can be generated with fewer visits (Dodge & others, 2014).

NORMAL PRENATAL DEVELOPMENT

Much of our discussion so far in this chapter has focused on what can go wrong with prenatal development. Prospective parents should take steps to avoid the vulnerabilities to fetal development that we have described. But it is important to keep in mind that most of the time prenatal development does not go awry and development occurs along the positive path that we described at the beginning of the chapter.

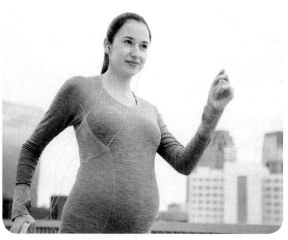

How might a woman's exercise in pregnancy benefit her health?
Jamie Grill/JGI/Getty Images

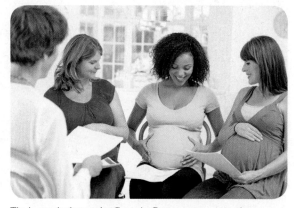

The increasingly popular CenteringPregnancy program alters routine prenatal care by bringing women out of exam rooms and into relationship-oriented groups.
MBI/Alamy Stock Photo

Review *Connect* Reflect

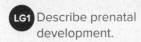

LG1 Describe prenatal development.

Review

- What is the course of prenatal development?
- What is teratology, and what are some of the main hazards to prenatal development?
- What are some good prenatal care strategies?
- Why is it important to take a positive approach to prenatal development?

Connect

- Earlier we discussed chromosomal and gene-linked abnormalities that can affect prenatal development. How are the symptoms of the related conditions or risks similar to or different from those caused by teratogens or other hazards?

Reflect *Your Own Personal Journey of Life*

- If you are a woman, imagine that you have just found out that you are pregnant. What health-enhancing strategies will you follow during the prenatal period? For men, imagine that you are the partner of a woman who has just found out she is pregnant. What will be your role in increasing the likelihood that the prenatal period will go smoothly?

Birth **LG2** Discuss the birth process.

The Birth Process	Assessing the Newborn	Preterm and Low Birth Weight Babies

There was a star danced, and under that I was born.

—WILLIAM SHAKESPEARE
English playwright, 17th century

Nature writes the basic script for how birth occurs, but parents make important choices about conditions surrounding birth. We look first at the sequence of physical steps that take place when a child is born.

THE BIRTH PROCESS

The birth process occurs in stages, takes place in different contexts, and in most cases involves one or more attendants.

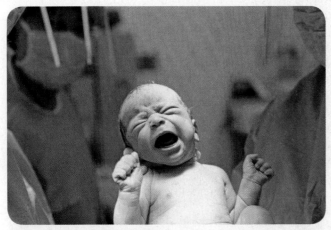

After the long journey of prenatal development, birth takes place. During birth the baby is on a threshold between two worlds. *What is the fetus/newborn transition like?*
ERproductions Ltd/Getty Images

afterbirth The third stage of birth, when the placenta, umbilical cord, and other membranes are detached and expelled.

Stages of Birth   The birth process occurs in three stages. The first stage is the longest of the three. Uterine contractions are 15 to 20 minutes apart at the beginning and last up to a minute each. These contractions cause the woman's cervix to stretch and open. As the first stage progresses, the contractions come closer together, appearing every two to five minutes. Their intensity increases. By the end of the first birth stage, contractions dilate the cervix to an opening of about 10 centimeters (4 inches), so that the baby can move from the uterus into the birth canal. For a woman having her first child, the first stage lasts an average of 6 to 12 hours; for subsequent children, this stage typically is much shorter.

The second birth stage begins when the baby's head starts to move through the cervix and the birth canal. It terminates when the baby emerges completely from the mother's body. With each contraction, the mother bears down hard to push the baby out of her body. By the time the baby's head is out of the mother's body, the contractions come almost every minute and last for about a minute each. This stage typically lasts approximately 45 minutes to an hour.

Afterbirth is the third stage, at which time the placenta, umbilical cord, and other membranes are detached and expelled. This final stage is the shortest of the three birth stages, lasting only minutes.

Childbirth Setting and Attendants   In the United States, the vast majority of births take place in hospitals, with about one percent taking place in the home (Martin & others, 2018). Home births are most common among non-Latino White women.

The people who help a mother during birth vary across cultures. In U.S. hospitals, it has become the norm for fathers or birth coaches to be with the mother throughout labor and delivery. In the East African Nigoni culture, by contrast, men are completely excluded from the childbirth process. When a woman is ready to give birth, female relatives move into the woman's hut and the husband leaves, taking his belongings (clothes, tools, weapons, and so on) with him. He is not permitted to return until after the baby is born. In some cultures, childbirth is an open, community affair. For example, in the Pukapukan culture in the Pacific Islands, women give birth in a shelter that is open for villagers to observe.

Midwives   Midwifery is practiced in most countries throughout the world. In Holland, more than 40 percent of babies are delivered by midwives rather than doctors. However, even though it is becoming more common in the United States, the most recent data available show that only 8 percent of women who delivered a baby were attended by a midwife (Weisband & others, 2018). Nearly all of the midwives who deliver babies in the United States are certified nurse-midwives. A recent research review concluded that for low-risk women, midwife-led care was characterized by a reduction in procedures during labor, greater satisfaction with care, and few adverse outcomes compared with physician-attended deliveries (Raipuria & others, 2018).

Doulas   In some countries, a doula attends a childbearing woman. Doula is a Greek word that means "a woman who helps." A **doula** is a caregiver who provides continuous physical, emotional, and educational support for the mother before, during, and after childbirth. Doulas remain with the parents throughout labor, assessing and responding to the mother's needs. Researchers have found positive effects when a doula is present at the birth of a child (McLeish & Redshaw, 2018).

In the United States, most doulas work as independent providers hired by the expectant parents. Doulas typically function as part of a "birthing team," serving as an adjunct to the midwife or the hospital's obstetric staff.

Methods of Childbirth   U.S. hospitals often allow the mother and her obstetrician a range of options regarding the method of delivery. Key choices involve the use of medication, whether to use any of a number of nonmedicated techniques to reduce pain, and when to have a cesarean delivery.

Medication   Three basic kinds of drugs that are used for labor are analgesia, anesthesia, and oxytocin/pitocin.

Analgesia is used to relieve pain. Analgesics include tranquilizers, barbiturates, and narcotics (such as Demerol).

Anesthesia is used in late first-stage labor and during delivery to block sensation in an area of the body or to block consciousness. Researchers are continuing to explore safer drug mixtures for use at lower doses to improve the effectiveness and safety of epidural anesthesia delivered directly to the spinal cord (Capogna & others, 2018).

Predicting how a drug will affect an individual woman and her fetus is difficult (Davidson & others, 2015). A particular drug might have only a minimal effect on one fetus yet have a much stronger effect on another. The drug's dosage also is a factor.

Natural and Prepared Childbirth   For a brief time not long ago, the idea of avoiding all medication during childbirth gained favor in the United States. Instead, many women chose to reduce the pain of childbirth through techniques known as

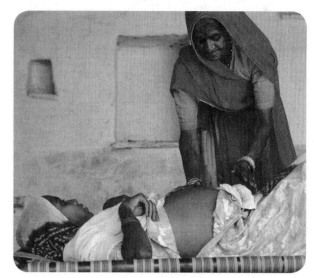

In India, a midwife checks on the size, position, and heartbeat of a fetus. Midwives deliver babies in many cultures around the world. *What are some cultural variations in prenatal care?*
Viviane Moos/Corbis Historical/Getty Images

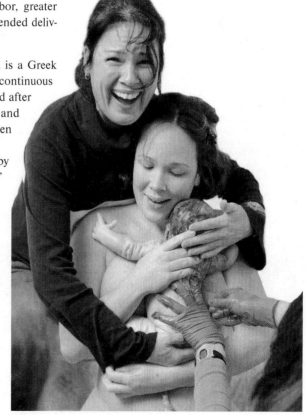

A doula assisting a birth. *What types of support do doulas provide?*
Brand X Pictures/Getty Images

doula A caregiver who provides continuous physical, emotional, and educational support for the mother before, during, and after childbirth.

connecting with careers

Linda Pugh, Perinatal Nurse

Perinatal nurses work with childbearing women to support health and well-being during the childbearing experience. Linda Pugh, Ph.D., R.N.C., is a perinatal nurse on the faculty at The University of North Carolina-Wilmington School of Nursing. She is certified as an inpatient obstetric nurse and specializes in the care of women during labor and delivery. She teaches undergraduate and graduate students, educates professional nurses, and conducts research. In addition, Pugh consults with hospitals and organizations about women's health issues and topics we discuss in this chapter.

Her research interests include nursing interventions with low-income breast-feeding women, discovering ways to prevent and ameliorate fatigue during childbearing, and using breathing exercises during labor.

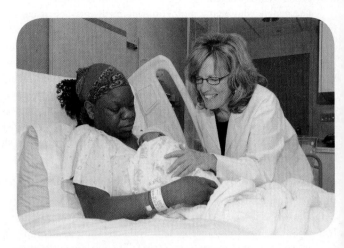

Linda Pugh (*right*) with a new mother and baby.
Courtesy Dr. Linda Pugh

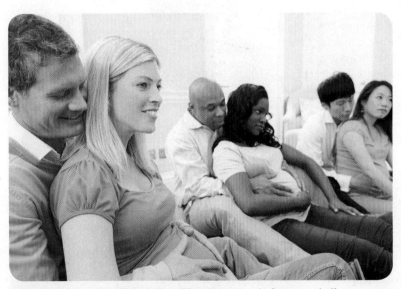

Expectant parents taking a Lamaze class. *What characterizes the Lamaze method?*
Monkey Business Images/Shutterstock

natural childbirth This method attempts to reduce the mother's pain by decreasing her fear through education about childbirth and relaxation techniques during delivery.

prepared childbirth Developed by French obstetrician Ferdinand Lamaze, this childbirth strategy is similar to natural childbirth but includes a special breathing technique to control pushing in the final stages of labor and a more detailed anatomy and physiology course.

breech position The baby's position in the uterus that causes the buttocks to be the first part to emerge from the vagina.

natural childbirth and prepared childbirth. Today, at least some medication is used in the typical childbirth, but elements of natural childbirth and prepared childbirth remain popular (Oates & Abraham, 2016).

Natural childbirth is the method that aims to reduce the mother's pain by decreasing her fear through education about childbirth and by teaching her and her partner to use breathing methods and relaxation techniques during delivery.

French obstetrician Ferdinand Lamaze developed a method similar to natural childbirth that is known as **prepared childbirth,** or the Lamaze method. It includes a special breathing technique to control pushing in the final stages of labor, as well as more detailed education about anatomy and physiology. The Lamaze method has become very popular in the United States. The pregnant woman's partner usually serves as a coach who attends childbirth classes with her and helps her with her breathing and relaxation during delivery.

In sum, proponents of current prepared childbirth methods conclude that when information and support are provided, women *know* how to give birth. To read about one nurse whose research focuses on fatigue during childbearing and breathing exercises during labor, see the *Connecting with Careers* profile on Linda Pugh. And to read about the increased variety of techniques now being used to reduce stress and control pain during labor, see *Caring Connections*.

Cesarean Delivery Normally, the baby's head comes through the vagina first. But if the baby is in a **breech position,** the baby's buttocks are the first part to emerge from the vagina. In 1 of every 25 deliveries, the baby's head is still in the uterus when the rest of the body is out. Breech births can cause respiratory problems. As a result, if the baby is in a breech position, a surgical procedure known as a cesarean section, or a cesarean

From Waterbirth to Music Therapy

The effort to reduce stress and control pain during labor has recently led to an increase in the use of some older and some newer nonmedicated techniques (Chaillet & others, 2014; Levett & others, 2016). These include waterbirth, massage, acupuncture, hypnosis, and music therapy.

Waterbirth

Waterbirth involves giving birth in a tub of warm water. Some women go through labor in the water and get out for delivery; others remain in the water for delivery. The rationale for waterbirth is that the baby has been in an amniotic sac for many months and that delivery in a similar environment is likely to be less stressful for the baby and the mother (Charles, 2018). Mothers get into the warm water when contractions become closer together and more intense. Getting into the water too soon can cause labor to slow or stop. Reviews of research have indicated mixed results for waterbirths. A recent study did find that waterbirth was linked with changes in labor and mothers' satisfaction with labor (Darsareh, Nourbakhsh, & Dabiri, 2018). Waterbirth has been practiced more often in European countries such as Switzerland and Sweden in recent decades than in the United States but is increasingly being included in U.S. birth plans.

Massage

Massage is increasingly used prior to and during delivery (Field & Hernandez-Reif, 2013). A recent experiment showed that massage during labor reduces pain and increases mothers' satisfaction (Erdogan, Yanikkerem, & Goker, 2017). Another now classic revealed that massage therapy reduced pain during labor and delivery and alleviated prenatal depression in both parents while improving their relationship (Field, Figueiredo, & others, 2008).

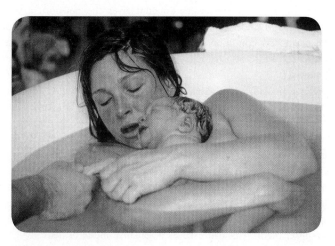

What characterizes the use of waterbirth in delivering a baby?
Eddie Lawrence/Science Source

Yoga

A research review concluded that practicing yoga during pregnancy was associated with a number of positive outcomes for mothers and a reduction in the incidence of low birth weight infants (Babbar, Parks-Savage, & Chauhan, 2012). Also, one experiment found that yoga and massage therapy sessions during pregnancy were associated with decreased levels of depression, anxiety, and back and leg pain (Field & others, 2012).

Acupuncture

Acupuncture, the insertion of very fine needles into specific locations in the body, is used as a standard procedure to reduce the pain of childbirth in China, although it only recently has begun to be used in the United States for this purpose. Recent research studies indicate that acupuncture can have positive effects on labor and delivery for a wide variety of women (Vixner, Schytt, & Mårtensson, 2017).

Hypnosis

Hypnosis, the induction of a psychological state of altered attention and awareness in which the individual is unusually responsive to suggestions, is also increasingly being used during childbirth. Some studies have indicated positive effects of hypnosis for reducing pain during childbirth (Eason & Parris, 2018).

Music Therapy

Music therapy during childbirth, which involves the use of music to reduce stress and manage pain, is becoming more prevalent (Kern & Tague, 2017). There is preliminary evidence that it may be effective for reducing labor pain and stress (Wan & Wen, 2018).

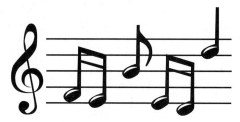

Megan Rhoades/McGraw-Hill Education

What are some reasons that childbirth methods such as these might be chosen along with or instead of the use of medication?

Score	0	1	2
Heart rate	Absent	Slow—less than 100 beats per minute	Fast—100–140 beats per minute
Respiratory effort	No breathing for more than one minute	Irregular and slow	Good breathing with normal crying
Muscle tone	Limp and flaccid	Weak, inactive, but some flexion of extremities	Strong, active motion
Body color	Blue and pale	Body pink, but extremities blue	Entire body pink
Reflex irritability	No response	Grimace	Coughing, sneezing and crying

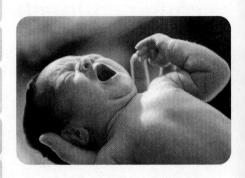

FIGURE 6

THE APGAR SCALE. A newborn's score on the Apgar Scale indicates whether the baby has urgent medical problems. *What are some trends in the Apgar scores of U.S. babies?*

Francisco Cruz/Purestock/SuperStock

delivery, is usually performed. In a **cesarean delivery,** the baby is removed from the mother's uterus through an incision made in her abdomen (Eden-Friedman & others, 2018).

The benefits and risks of cesarean sections continue to be debated (Belizán & others, 2018; Keag, Norman & Stock, 2018). Some critics believe that too many babies are delivered by cesarean section in the United States. More cesarean sections are performed in the United States than in any other country in the world. The most recent data show that 32 percent of babies in the United States are cesarean deliveries, and these numbers have increased dramatically over the past few decades (Martin & others, 2018).

ASSESSING THE NEWBORN

Almost immediately after birth, after the baby and its parents have been introduced, a newborn is taken to be weighed, cleaned up, and tested for signs of developmental problems that might require urgent attention (Ojodu & others, 2017). The **Apgar Scale** is widely used to assess the health of newborns at one and five minutes after birth. The Apgar Scale evaluates infants' heart rate, respiratory effort, muscle tone, body color, and reflex irritability. An obstetrician or a nurse does the evaluation and gives the newborn a score, or reading, of 0, 1, or 2 on each of these five health signs (see Figure 6). A total score of 7 to 10 indicates that the newborn's condition is good. A score of 5 indicates there may be developmental difficulties. A score of 3 or below signals an emergency and indicates that the baby might not survive.

The Apgar Scale is especially good at assessing the newborn's ability to cope with the stress of delivery and the new environment (Michalczyk, Torbé & Torbé, 2018). It also identifies high-risk infants who need resuscitation.

A recent study revealed that compared to children with a high Apgar score (9 to 10), the risk of developing attention deficit hyperactivity disorder (ADHD) in childhood was significantly higher for those with an Apgar score of 6 or less (Sucksdorff & others, 2018). For a more thorough assessment of the newborn, the Brazelton Neonatal Behavioral Assessment Scale or the Neonatal Intensive Care Unit Network Neurobehavioral Scale may be used.

The **Brazelton Neonatal Behavioral Assessment Scale (NBAS)** is typically performed within 24 to 36 hours after birth. It is also used as a sensitive index of neurological competence up to one month after birth for typical infants and as a measure in many studies of infant development (Lean, Smyser, & Rogers, 2017). The NBAS assesses the newborn's neurological development, reflexes, and reactions to people and objects. Sixteen reflexes, such as sneezing, blinking, and rooting, are assessed, along with reactions to animate stimuli (such as a face and voice) and inanimate stimuli (such as a rattle). (We will have more to say about reflexes when we discuss motor development in infancy.)

cesarean delivery Removal of the baby from the mother's uterus through an incision made in her abdomen.

Apgar Scale A widely used method to assess the health of newborns at one and five minutes after birth. The Apgar Scale evaluates infants' heart rate, respiratory effort, muscle tone, body color, and reflex irritability.

Brazelton Neonatal Behavioral Assessment Scale (NBAS) A measure that is used in the first month of life to assess the newborn's neurological development, reflexes, and reactions to people and objects.

A revised version of the NBAS, the **Neonatal Intensive Care Unit Network Neurobehavioral Scale (NNNS)** provides another assessment of the newborn's behavior, neurological and stress responses, and regulatory capacities (Provenzi & others, 2018). Whereas the NBAS was developed to assess normal, healthy, full-term infants, T. Berry Brazelton, along with Barry Lester and Edward Tronick, developed the NNNS to assess "at-risk" infants. The NNNS is especially useful for evaluating preterm infants (although it may not be appropriate for those of less than 30 weeks' gestational age) and substance-exposed infants. A very important NNNS assessment (at one month of age) of preterm infants who were exposed to substance abuse prenatally revealed that the NNNS predicted certain developmental outcomes, such as neurological difficulties, IQ, and reduced school readiness at 4.5 years of age (Liu & others, 2010).

PRETERM AND LOW BIRTH WEIGHT INFANTS

Conditions that pose threats for newborns have been given different labels. We will examine these conditions and discuss interventions that can improve outcomes of preterm infants.

Preterm and Small for Date Infants   Three related conditions pose threats to many newborns: low birth weight, preterm delivery, and being small for date. **Low birth weight infants** weigh less than 5½ pounds at birth. *Very low birth weight* newborns weigh under 3½ pounds, and *extremely low birth weight* newborns weigh under 2 pounds. **Preterm infants** are those born three weeks or more before the pregnancy has reached its full term—in other words, before the completion of 37 weeks of gestation (the time between fertilization and birth). **Small for date infants** (also called *small for gestational age infants*) are those whose birth weight is below normal when the length of the pregnancy is considered. They weigh less than 90 percent of all babies of the same gestational age. Small for date infants may be preterm or full term. Small for date infants have more birth complications, medical and developmental problems, and are at greater risk of dying soon after birth (Boghossian & others, 2018).

In 2016, 9.85 percent of U.S. infants were born preterm—a 30 percent increase since the 1980s but a decrease of nearly one percent since 2007 (Martin & others, 2018). The increase in preterm birth since the 1980s is likely due to several factors, including the increasing number of births to women 35 years and older, increasing rates of multiple births, increased management of maternal and fetal conditions (for example, inducing labor preterm if medical technology indicates it will increase the likelihood of survival), increased substance abuse (tobacco, alcohol), and increased stress (Goldenberg & Culhane, 2007). Ethnic variations characterize preterm birth (DeSisto & others, 2018). For example, the highest rate in 2016 was nearly 14 percent for African American infants (Martin & others, 2018).

Recently, there has been considerable interest in exploring the role that progestin might play in reducing preterm births. Research reviews indicate that progestin is most effective in reducing preterm births when it is administered to women with a history of a previous spontaneous birth at less than 37 weeks to women who have short cervixes, and to women pregnant with a singleton rather than twins (Choi, 2017; da Fonseca, Celik, & others, 2007; Norman & others, 2009).

The incidence of low birth weight varies considerably from country to country. To read about cross-cultural variations in low birth weight, see *Connecting with Diversity*.

Consequences of Preterm Birth and Low Birth Weight   Although most preterm and low birth weight infants are healthy, as a group they experience higher rates of illness and developmental problems than infants of normal birth weight. For preterm birth, the terms *extremely preterm* and *very preterm* are increasingly used. *Extremely preterm infants* are those born before the 28th week of pregnancy, and *very preterm infants* are those born before 33 weeks of gestational age. Figure 8 shows the results of a foundational Norwegian study indicating that the earlier preterm infants are born, the more likely they are to drop out of school (Swamy, Ostbye, & Skjaerven, 2008).

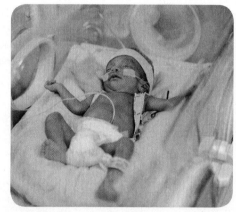

A "kilogram kid," weighing less than 2.3 pounds at birth. *What are some long-term outcomes for weighing so little at birth?*
Andresr/E+/Getty Images

Neonatal Intensive Care Unit Network Neurobehavioral Scale (NNNS) Based on the NBAS, the NNNS provides an assessment of the "at-risk" newborn's behavior, neurological and stress responses, and regulatory capacities.

low birth weight infant Infant that weighs less than 5½ pounds at birth.

preterm infants Those born before the completion of 37 weeks of gestation (the time between fertilization and birth).

small for date infants Also called small for gestational age infants, these infants have birth weights that are below normal when the length of pregnancy is considered. Small for date infants may be preterm or full term.

connecting with diversity

Cross-Cultural Variations in the Incidence and Causes of Low Birth Weight

In some countries, such as Pakistan and Uganda, where poverty is rampant and the health and nutrition of mothers are poor, the percentage of low birth weight babies reaches as high as 35 percent (see Figure 7). In the United States, there has been an increase in low birth weight infants in the last two decades. The U.S. low birth weight rate of 8.1 percent in 2016 is considerably higher than that of many other developed countries (Mahumud, Sultana, & Sarker, 2017; Organization for Economic Cooperation and Development, 2018). For example, only 4 percent of the infants born in Finland, Estonia, and Latvia are low birth weight, and only 5 percent of those born in New Zealand, Netherlands, and Israel are low birth weight.

In both developed and developing countries, adolescents who give birth when their bodies have not fully matured are at risk for having low birth weight babies. In the United States, the increase in the number of low birth weight infants has been attributed to drug use, poor nutrition, multiple births, reproductive technologies, and improved technology and pre-natal care that result in more high-risk babies surviving (Khatun & others, 2017). Nonetheless, poverty continues to be a major factor in preterm birth in the United States. Women living in poverty are more likely to be obese, have diabetes and hypertension, use cigarettes and illicit drugs, be depressed or anxious, and they are less likely to receive regular prenatal care (Congdon & others, 2016).

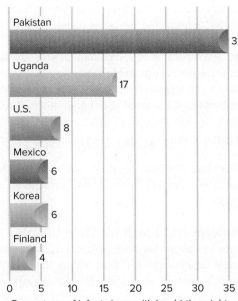

FIGURE 7
PERCENTAGE OF INFANTS BORN WITH LOW BIRTH WEIGHT IN SELECTED COUNTRIES

In the last sentence above, we learned that women living in poverty are less likely to receive regular prenatal care. What did you learn earlier in the chapter about the benefits of regular prenatal care? Aside from women living in poverty, which other demographic group is not likely to receive adequate prenatal care?

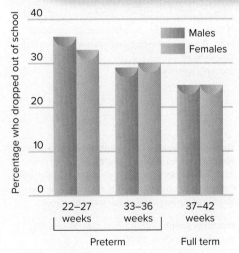

FIGURE 8
PERCENTAGE OF PRETERM AND FULL-TERM BIRTH INFANTS WHO DROPPED OUT OF SCHOOL

kangaroo care Treatment for preterm infants that involves skin-to-skin contact.

The number and severity of these problems increase when infants are born very early and as their birth weight decreases (Dilworth-Bart & others, 2018; FitzGerald & others, 2018). Survival rates for infants who are born very early and very small have risen in most countries, but with this improved survival rate have come increased rates of severe brain damage (as well as less severe developmental problems (Grisaru-Granovsky & others, 2018). Children born at low birth weights are more likely than their normal birth weight counterparts to develop a learning disability, attention deficit hyperactivity disorder, or breathing problem such as asthma (Johnson & Marlow, 2017). And a recent study found that very low birth weight was associated with childhood autism (Matheis, Matson & Burns, 2018). Low birth weight children also are overrepresented in special education programs.

Nurturing Low Birth Weight and Preterm Infants Two increasingly used interventions in the neonatal intensive care unit (NICU) are kangaroo care and massage therapy. **Kangaroo care** involves skin-to-skin contact in which the baby, wearing only a diaper, is held upright against the parent's bare chest, much as a baby kangaroo is carried inside its mother's pouch. Kangaroo care is typically practiced for two to three hours per day, skin-to-skin, over an extended time in early infancy; it is a strongly recommended intervention throughout the world (Chan & others, 2016).

Why use kangaroo care with preterm infants? Preterm infants often have difficulty coordinating their breathing and heart rate, and the close physical contact with the parent provided by kangaroo care can help to stabilize the preterm infant's heartbeat, temperature, and breathing (Kaffashi & others, 2013). Preterm infants who experience kangaroo care also gain more weight than their counterparts who are not given this care (Sharma, Murki & Pratap, 2016). This intervention also may have long-term positive effects on cognitive functioning into early adulthood (Ropars & others, 2018). Perhaps most importantly, a research review of clinical experiments concluded that kangaroo care decreased the risk of mortality in low birth weight infants (Conde-Agudelo & Diaz-Rossello, 2016).

Many adults will attest to the therapeutic effects of receiving a massage. In fact, many will pay a premium to receive one at a spa on a regular basis. But can massage play a role in improving developmental outcomes for preterm infants? To find out, see *Connecting Through Research*.

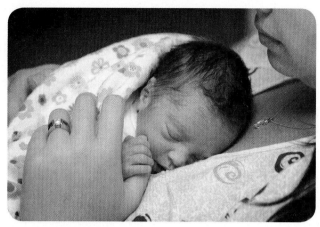

A new mother practicing kangaroo care. *What is kangaroo care?*
casenbina/iStockphoto.com

connecting through research

How Does Massage Therapy Affect the Mood and Behavior of Babies?

Throughout history and in many cultures, caregivers have massaged infants. In Africa and Asia, infants are routinely massaged by parents or other family members for several months after birth. In the United States, interest in using touch and massage to improve the growth, health, and well-being of infants has been stimulated by the foundational research and classic research studies of Tiffany Field (for a complete review of studies, see Field, 2016). Field is the director of the Touch Research Institute at the University of Miami School of Medicine.

In a typical experiment preterm infants in a neonatal intensive care unit (NICU) were randomly assigned to a massage therapy group or a control group. For five consecutive days, the preterm infants in the massage group were given three 15-minute moderate pressure massages. Behavioral observations of the following stress behaviors were made on the first and last days of the study: crying, grimacing, yawning, sneezing, jerky arm and leg movements, startles, and finger flaring. The various stress behaviors were summarized in a composite stress behavior index. As indicated in Figure 9, massage had a stress-reducing effect on the preterm infants, which is especially important because they encounter numerous stressors while they are hospitalized.

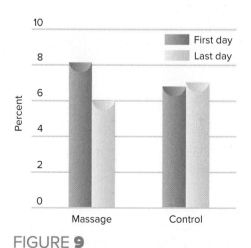

FIGURE 9

PRETERM INFANTS SHOW REDUCED STRESS BEHAVIORS AND ACTIVITY AFTER FIVE DAYS OF MASSAGE THERAPY (HERNANDEZ-REIF, DIEGO, & FIELD, 2007)

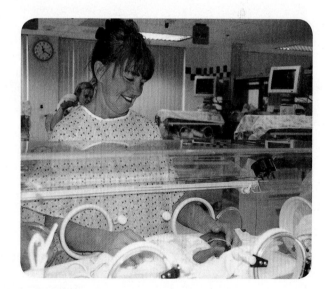

Tiffany Field massages a newborn infant. *What types of infants has massage therapy been shown to help?*
Courtesy of Dr. Tiffany Field

(continued)

(continued)

In the most comprehensive review of massage therapy with preterm infants, Field (2016) concluded that the most consistent findings involve two positive results: (1) increased weight gain and (2) discharge from the hospital several days earlier. One study revealed that the mechanisms responsible for increased weight gain as a result of massage therapy were stimulation of the vagus nerve (one of 12 cranial nerves leading to the brain) and in turn the release of insulin (a food absorption hormone) (Field, Diego, & Hernandez-Reif, 2010).

Infants are not the only ones who may benefit from massage therapy. In other studies, Field and her colleagues as well as other researchers have demonstrated the benefits of massage therapy with women in reducing labor pain, with children who have asthma, with autistic children's attentiveness, and with adolescents who have attention deficit hyperactivity disorder (as summarized in Field, 2016).

Review Connect Reflect

 LG2 Discuss the birth process.

Review

- What are the three main stages of birth? What are some different birth strategies? What is the transition from fetus to newborn like for the infant?
- What are three measures of neonatal health and responsiveness?
- What are the outcomes for children if they are born preterm or with a low birth weight?

Connect

- What correlations have been found between birth weight and country of birth, and what might the causes be?

Reflect *Your Own Personal Journey of Life*

- If you are a female who would like to have a baby, which birth strategy do you prefer? Why? If you are a male, how involved would you want to be in helping your partner through the birth of your baby? Explain.

The Postpartum Period

 LG3 Explain the changes that take place in the postpartum period.

Physical Adjustments

Emotional and Psychological Adjustments

Bonding

postpartum period The period after childbirth when the mother adjusts, both physically and psychologically, to the process of childbirth. This period lasts about six weeks or until her body has completed its adjustment and returned to a near prepregnant state.

The weeks after childbirth present challenges for many new parents and their offspring. This is the **postpartum period,** the period after childbirth or delivery that lasts for about six weeks or until the mother's body has completed its adjustment and has returned to a nearly prepregnant state. It is a time when the woman adjusts, both physically and psychologically, to the process of childbearing.

The postpartum period involves a great deal of adjustment and adaptation. The adjustments needed are physical, emotional, and psychological.

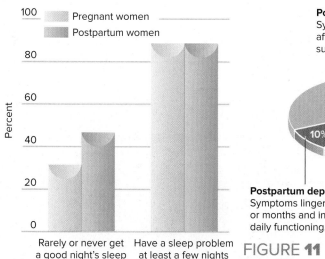

FIGURE **10**

SLEEP DEPRIVATION IN PREGNANT AND POSTPARTUM WOMEN

Source: Foundational 2007 Sleep in American poll, National Sleep Foundation

Postpartum blues
Symptoms appear 2 to 3 days after delivery and usually subside within 1 to 2 weeks.

Postpartum depression
Symptoms linger for weeks or months and interfere with daily functioning.

No symptoms

FIGURE **11**

POSTPARTUM BLUES AND POSTPARTUM DEPRESSION AMONG U.S. WOMEN. Some health professionals refer to the postpartum period as the "fourth trimester." Although the time span of the postpartum period does not necessarily cover three months, the term "fourth trimester" suggests continuity and the importance of the first several months after birth for the mother.

PHYSICAL ADJUSTMENTS

A woman's body makes numerous physical adjustments in the first days and weeks after childbirth (Mattson & Smith, 2015). She may have a great deal of energy or feel exhausted and let down. These changes are normal, but fatigue can undermine the new mother's sense of well-being and confidence in her ability to cope with a new baby and a new family life (Mathew, Phillips, & Sandanapitchai, 2018).

One often overlooked concern is the loss of sleep that the primary caregiver experiences in the postpartum period (Lillis & others, 2018). In many Western industrialized countries including the United States, a substantial percentage of women report poor sleep during pregnancy and in the postpartum period (Okun, 2015) (see Figure 10). The loss of sleep can contribute to stress, marital conflict, and impaired decision making (Meerlo, Sgoifo, & Suchecki, 2008).

After delivery, a mother's body undergoes sudden and dramatic changes in hormone production. When the placenta is delivered, estrogen and progesterone levels drop steeply and remain low until the ovaries start producing hormones again.

EMOTIONAL AND PSYCHOLOGICAL ADJUSTMENTS

Emotional fluctuations are common for mothers in the postpartum period. For some women, emotional fluctuations decrease within several weeks after the delivery, but other women experience longer-lasting mood swings.

As shown in Figure 11, about 70 percent of new mothers in the United States have what are called the postpartum blues. About two to three days after birth, they begin to feel depressed, anxious, and upset. These feelings may come and go for several months after the birth, often peaking about three to five days after birth. Even without treatment, these feelings usually go away after one or two weeks.

However, some women develop **postpartum depression,** which involves a major depressive episode that typically occurs about four weeks after delivery. Women with postpartum depression have such strong feelings of sadness, anxiety, or despair that for at least a

postpartum depression Characteristic of women who have such strong feelings of sadness, anxiety, or despair that they have trouble coping with daily tasks during the postpartum period.

Diane Sanford, Clinical Psychologist and Postpartum Expert

Diane Sanford has a doctorate in clinical psychology, and for many years she had a private practice that focused on marital and family relationships. But after she began collaborating with a psychiatrist whose clients included women with postpartum depression, Dr. Sanford, together with a women's health nurse, founded Women's Healthcare Partnership in St. Louis, Missouri, which specializes in women's adjustment during the postpartum period. Subsequently, they added a marriage and family relationships counselor and a social worker to their staff, and then later hired nurse educators, a dietician, and a fitness expert as consultants (Clay, 2001).

For more information about what clinical psychologists do, see the Careers in Child Development appendix.

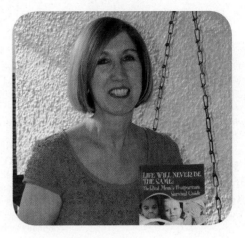

Diane Sanford holds a copy of her practical guidebook for new mothers who are coping with postpartum issues.
Courtesy of Dr. Diane Sanford

The postpartum period is a time of considerable adjustment and adaptation for both the mother and the father. Fathers can provide an important support system for mothers, especially in helping mothers care for young infants. *What kinds of tasks might the father of a newborn do to support the mother?*
Howard Grey/Getty Images

two-week period they have trouble coping with their daily tasks. Without treatment, postpartum depression may become worse and last for many months (Olin & others, 2017). Unfortunately, many women with postpartum depression don't seek help. For example, one study found that common barriers to seeking help included concern about stigma and a lack of encouragement from their partner (Silva, Canavarro & Fonseca, 2018). Estimates indicate that 10 to 14 percent of new mothers experience postpartum depression.

Several antidepressant drugs are effective in treating postpartum depression, although it is not yet clear whether these are safe to take while breast feeding (Brummelte & Galea, 2016). Psychotherapy, especially cognitive therapy, also is effective in treating postpartum depression for many women (Kleiman & Wenzel, 2017). And a recent experiment with new mothers showed that engaging in exercise may help in reducing postpartum depression, anxiety, stress, and fatigue (Yang & Chen, 2018).

Can a mother's postpartum depression affect the way she interacts with her infant? The most comprehensive review of the research literature concluded that the interaction difficulties of depressed mothers and their infants occur across cultures and socioeconomic status groups, and encompass less sensitivity of the mothers and less responsiveness on the part of their infants (Field, 2010). Several caregiving activities also are compromised, including feeding (especially breast feeding), sleep routines, and safety practices. To read about one individual who specializes in helping women adjust during the postpartum period, see *Connecting with Careers.*

Fathers also undergo considerable adjustment during the postpartum period, even when they work away from home all day. When the mother experiences postpartum depression, many fathers also develop depressed feelings (O'Brien & others, 2017). Sometimes fathers feel that the baby comes first and gets all of the mother's attention; some feel that they have been replaced by the baby.

The father's support and caring can play a role in whether the mother develops postpartum depression. A recent study in Taiwan revealed that higher support by fathers was related to lower rates of postpartum depression in women, especially among women who were not working outside the home (Lin & others, 2017).

BONDING

A special component of the parent-infant relationship is **bonding,** the formation of a connection, especially a physical bond between parents and the newborn in the period shortly after birth. Sometimes hospitals seem determined to deter bonding. Drugs given to the mother to make her delivery less painful can make the mother drowsy, interfering with her ability to respond to and stimulate the newborn. Mothers and newborns are often separated shortly after delivery, and preterm infants are isolated from their mothers even more than full-term infants.

Do these practices do any harm? Some physicians believe that during the period shortly after birth, direct skin-to-skin contact between the parents and newborn is necessary to form an emotional attachment as a foundation for optimal development in the years to come. Is there evidence that close contact between mothers and infants in the first several days after birth is critical for optimal development later in life? Although some research supports this bonding hypothesis (Kennell, 2006), a body of research, including several classic studies, challenges the significance of the first few days of life as a critical period (Bakeman & Brown, 1980; Rode & others, 1981). Indeed, the extreme form of the bonding hypothesis—that the newborn must have close contact with the mother in the first few days of life to develop optimally—simply is not true.

Nonetheless, the weakness of the bonding hypothesis should not be used as an excuse to keep motivated mothers from interacting with their newborns. Such contact brings pleasure to many mothers. In some mother-infant pairs—including preterm infants, adolescent mothers, and mothers from disadvantaged circumstances—early close contact may establish a climate for improved interaction after the mother and infant leave the hospital.

Most hospitals offer a *rooming-in* arrangement, in which the baby remains in the mother's room most of the time during its hospital stay. However, if parents choose not to use this rooming-in arrangement, the weight of the research suggests that this decision will not harm the infant (Theo & Drake, 2017).

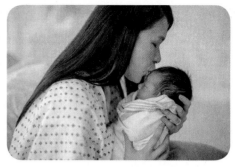

A mother bonds with her infant moments after it is born. *How critical is bonding for the development of social competence later in childhood?*
FatCamera/Getty Images

bonding The formation of a close connection, especially a physical bond, between parents and their newborn in the period shortly after birth.

developmental **connection**

Theories

Lorenz demonstrated the importance of bonding in greylag geese, but the first few days of life are unlikely to be a critical period for bonding in human infants. Connect to "Introduction."

Review Connect Reflect

 LG3 Explain the changes that take place in the postpartum period.

Review

- What does the postpartum period involve? What physical adjustments does the woman's body make during this period?
- What emotional and psychological adjustments characterize the postpartum period?
- Is bonding critical for optimal development?

Connect

- How can exercise help pregnant women before delivery and women with postpartum depression after giving birth?

Reflect *Your Own Personal Journey of Life*

- If you are a female who plans to have children, what can you do to adjust effectively in the postpartum period? If you are the partner of a new mother, what can you do to help during the postpartum period?

Prenatal Development and Birth

Prenatal Development

LG1 Describe prenatal development.

The Course of Prenatal Development

- Prenatal development is divided into three periods: germinal (conception until 10 to 14 days later), which ends when the zygote (fertilized egg) attaches to the uterine wall; embryonic (two to eight weeks after conception), during which the embryo differentiates into three layers, life-support systems develop, and organ systems form (organogenesis); and fetal (from two months after conception until about nine months, or when the infant is born), a time when organ systems have matured to the point at which life can be sustained outside of the womb. Neurogenesis is the formation of new neurons. The nervous system begins with the formation of a neural tube at 18 to 24 days after conception, and by the time babies are born they have approximately 100 billion neurons, or nerve cells. Proliferation and migration are two processes that characterize brain development in the prenatal period. The basic architecture of the brain is formed in the first two trimesters of prenatal development.

Teratology and Hazards to Prenatal Development

- Teratology is the field that investigates the causes of congenital (birth) defects. Any agent that causes birth defects is called a teratogen. The dose, genetic susceptibility, and time of exposure influence the severity of the damage to an unborn child and the type of defect that occurs. Prescription drugs that can be harmful include antibiotics, some antidepressants, certain hormones, and Accutane. Nonprescription drugs that can be harmful include diet pills and aspirin. Legal psychoactive drugs that are potentially harmful to prenatal development include caffeine, alcohol, and nicotine. Fetal alcohol spectrum disorders are a cluster of abnormalities that appear in offspring of mothers who drink heavily during pregnancy. Even when pregnant women drink moderately (one to two drinks a few days a week), negative effects on their offspring have been found. Cigarette smoking by pregnant women has serious adverse effects on prenatal and child development (such as low birth weight). Illegal psychoactive drugs that are potentially harmful to offspring include methamphetamine, marijuana, cocaine, and heroin. Incompatibility of the mother's and the father's blood types can also be harmful to the fetus. Environmental hazards include radiation, environmental pollutants, and toxic wastes. Syphilis, rubella (German measles), genital herpes, and AIDS are infectious diseases that can harm the fetus. Other parental factors include maternal diet and nutrition, age, emotional states and stress, and paternal factors. A developing fetus depends entirely on its mother for nutrition. Maternal age can negatively affect the offspring's development if the mother is an adolescent or over 35. High stress in the mother is linked with less than optimal prenatal and birth outcomes. Paternal factors that can adversely affect prenatal development include exposure to lead, radiation, certain pesticides, and petrochemicals.

Prenatal Care

- Prenatal care varies extensively but usually involves medical care services with a defined schedule of visits.

Normal Prenatal Development

- It is important to remember that, although things can and do go wrong during pregnancy, most of the time pregnancy and prenatal development go well.

Birth

LG2 Discuss the birth process.

The Birth Process

- Childbirth occurs in three stages. The first stage, which lasts about 6 to 12 hours for a woman having her first child, is the longest stage. The cervix dilates to about 10 centimeters (4 inches) at the end of the first stage. The second stage begins when the baby's head starts to move through the cervix and ends with the baby's complete emergence. The third stage involves the delivery of the placenta after birth. Childbirth strategies involve the childbirth setting and attendants. In many countries, a doula attends a childbearing woman. Methods of delivery include medicated, natural or prepared, and cesarean. Being born involves considerable stress for the baby, but the baby is well prepared and adapted to handle the stress.

- For many years, the Apgar Scale has been used to assess the health of newborn babies. The Brazelton Neonatal Behavioral Assessment Scale (NBAS) examines the newborn's neurological development, reflexes, and reactions to people. More recently, the Neonatal Intensive Care Unit Network Neurobehavioral Scale (NNNS) was created to assess at-risk infants.

- Low birth weight infants weigh less than 5½ pounds, and they may be preterm (born before the completion of 37 weeks of gestation) or small for date (also called small for gestational age), which refers to infants whose birth weight is below normal when the length of pregnancy is considered. Small for date infants may be preterm or full term. Although most low birth weight and preterm infants are normal and healthy, as a group they experience more illness and developmental problems than infants of normal birth weight. Kangaroo care and massage therapy have been shown to benefit preterm infants.

The Postpartum Period

LG3 Explain the changes that take place in the postpartum period.

- The postpartum period is the period after childbirth or delivery. The period lasts for about six weeks or until the woman's body has completed its adjustment. Physical adjustments in the postpartum period include fatigue, involution (the process by which the uterus returns to its prepregnant size five or six weeks after birth), and hormonal changes.

- Emotional fluctuations on the part of the mother are common in this period, and they can vary greatly from one mother to the next. Postpartum depression characterizes women who have such strong feelings of sadness, anxiety, or despair that they have trouble coping with daily tasks in the postpartum period. Postpartum depression occurs in about 10 to 14 percent of new mothers. The father also goes through a postpartum adjustment.

- Bonding is the formation of a close connection, especially a physical bond, between parents and the newborn shortly after birth. Early bonding has not been found to be critical in the development of a competent infant.

key **terms**

afterbirth 82
amnion 71
Apgar Scale 86
blastocyst 70
bonding 93
Brazelton Neonatal Behavioral
   Assessment Scale (NBAS) 86
breech position 84

cesarean delivery 86
doula 83
embryonic period 70
fetal alcohol spectrum disorders
   (FASD) 76
fetal period 72
germinal period 70
kangaroo care 88

low birth weight infants 87
natural childbirth 84
Neonatal Intensive Care Unit
   Network Neurobehavioral
   Scale (NNNS) 87
neurons 74
organogenesis 71
placenta 71

postpartum depression 91
postpartum period 90
prepared childbirth 84
preterm infants 87
small for date infants 87
teratogen 74
trophoblast 70
umbilical cord 71

key **people**

T. Berry Brazelton 87

Tiffany Field 89

Ferdinand Lamaze 84

David Olds 81

chapter 4

PHYSICAL DEVELOPMENT AND HEALTH

chapter **outline**

1 Body Growth and Change

Learning Goal 1 Discuss developmental changes in the body.

Patterns of Growth
Infancy and Childhood
Adolescence

2 The Brain

Learning Goal 2 Describe how the brain changes.

The Neuroconstructivist View
Brain Physiology
Infancy
Childhood
Adolescence

3 Sleep

Learning Goal 3 Summarize how sleep patterns change as children and adolescents develop.

Infancy
Childhood
Adolescence

4 Health

Learning Goal 4 Characterize children's health.

Illness and Injuries Among Children
Nutrition and Eating Behavior
Exercise

Christopher Futcher/Getty Images

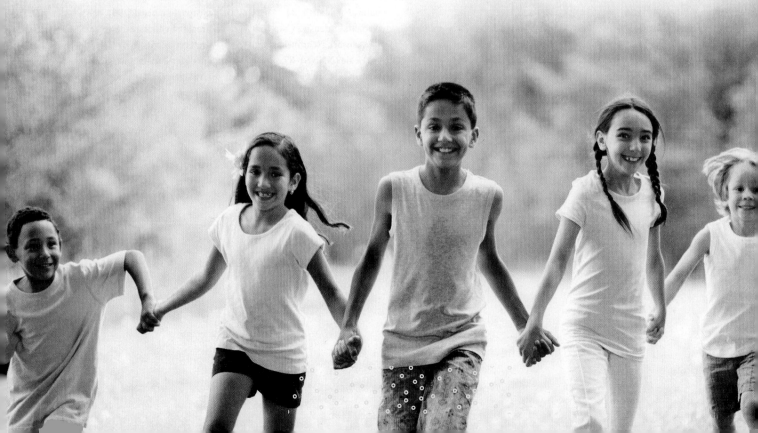

Angie, an elementary-school-aged girl, provided the following comments about losing weight:

When I was eight years old, I weighed 125 pounds. My clothes were the size that large teenage girls wear. I hated my body and my classmates teased me all the time. I was so overweight and out of shape that when I took a P.E. class my face would get red and I had trouble breathing. I was jealous of the kids who played sports and weren't overweight like I was.

I'm nine years old now and I've lost 30 pounds. I'm much happier and proud of myself. How did I lose the weight? My mom said she had finally decided enough was enough. She took me to a pediatrician who specializes in helping children lose weight and keep it off. The pediatrician counseled my mom about my eating and exercise habits, then had us join a group that he had created for overweight children and their parents. My mom and I go to the group once a week and we've now been participating in the program for six months. I no longer eat fast food meals and my mom is cooking more healthy meals. Now that I've lost weight, exercise is not as hard for me and I don't get teased by the kids at school. My mom's pretty happy too because she's lost 15 pounds herself since we've been in the counseling program.

Not all overweight children are as successful as Angie at reducing their weight. Indeed, being overweight in childhood has become a major national concern in the United States (Centers for Disease Control and Prevention, 2018). Later in the chapter, we will explore the causes and consequences of being overweight in childhood.

preview

Think about how much you changed physically as you grew up. You came into this life as a small being but grew very rapidly in infancy, more slowly in childhood, and once again more rapidly during puberty. In this chapter, we will explore changes in body growth, the brain, and sleep. We also will examine aspects of children's health.

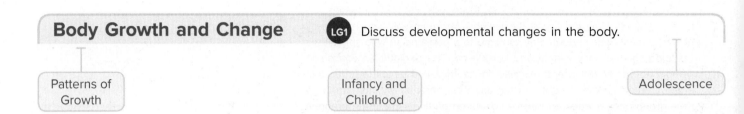

Body Growth and Change

LG1 Discuss developmental changes in the body.

Patterns of Growth

Infancy and Childhood

Adolescence

In the journey of childhood, we go through many bodily changes. Let's begin by studying some basic patterns of growth and then turn to the bodily changes that occur from infancy through adolescence.

PATTERNS OF GROWTH

During prenatal development and early infancy, the head constitutes an extraordinarily large portion of the total body (see Figure 1). Gradually, the body's proportions change. Why? Growth is not random. Instead, it generally follows two patterns: the cephalocaudal pattern and the proximodistal pattern.

The **cephalocaudal pattern** is the sequence in which the fastest growth always occurs at the top—the head. Physical growth in size, weight, and feature differentiation gradually works its way down from the top to the bottom—for example, from neck to shoulders, to middle trunk, and so on. This same pattern occurs in the head area; the top parts of the head—the eyes and brain—grow faster than the lower parts, such as the jaw.

cephalocaudal pattern The sequence in which the fastest growth occurs at the top of the body—the head—with physical growth in size, weight, and feature differentiation gradually working from top to bottom.

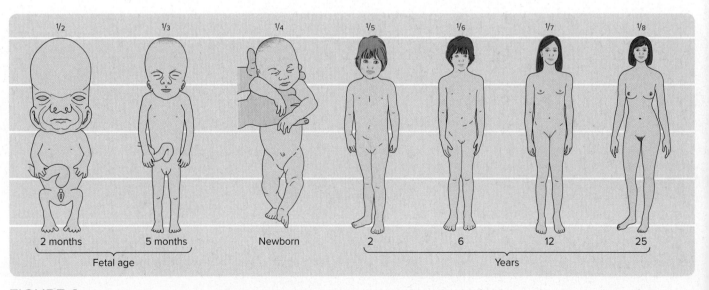

FIGURE 1

CHANGES IN PROPORTIONS OF THE HUMAN BODY DURING GROWTH. As individuals develop from infancy through adulthood, one of the most noticeable physical changes is that the head becomes smaller in relation to the rest of the body. The fractions listed refer to head size as a proportion of total body length at different ages.

Sensory and motor development also generally proceed according to the cephalocaudal principle. For example, infants see objects before they can control their torso, and they can use their hands long before they can crawl or walk. However, infants reach for toys with their feet prior to using their hands (Adolph & Franchak, 2017). On average, infants first touch toys with their feet when they are 12 weeks old and with their hands when they are 16 weeks old. (We will have much more to say about sensory and motor development in the "Motor, Sensory, and Perceptual Development" chapter.)

The **proximodistal pattern** is the growth sequence that starts at the center of the body and moves toward the extremities. For example, muscle control of the trunk and arms matures before control of the hands and fingers. Further, infants use their whole hand as a unit before they can control several fingers.

INFANCY AND CHILDHOOD

Height and weight increase rapidly in infancy (Lampl, 2008). Growth takes a slower course during the childhood years.

Infancy   The average North American newborn is 20 inches long and weighs 7½ pounds. Ninety-five percent of full-term newborns are 18 to 22 inches long and weigh between 5½ and 10 pounds.

In the first several days of life, most newborns lose 5 to 7 percent of their body weight. Once infants adjust to sucking, swallowing, and digesting, they grow rapidly, gaining an average of 5 to 6 ounces per week during the first month. They have doubled their birth weight by the age of 4 months and have nearly tripled it by their first birthday. Infants grow about one inch per month during the first year, reaching approximately 1½ times their birth length by their first birthday.

In the second year of life, infants' rate of growth slows considerably (Burns & others, 2013). By 2 years of age, infants weigh approximately 26 to 32 pounds, having gained a quarter to half a pound per month during the second year; at age 2 they have reached about one-fifth of their adult weight. The average 2-year-old is 32 to 35 inches tall, which is nearly one-half of adult height.

Early Childhood   As the preschool child grows older, the percentage of increase in height and weight decreases with each additional year (McMahon & Stryjewski, 2011). Girls are only slightly smaller and lighter than boys during these years. Both boys and girls slim down as the trunks of their bodies lengthen. Although their heads are still somewhat large for their bodies, by the end of the preschool years most children have lost their top-heavy look. Body fat declines slowly but steadily during the preschool years. Girls have more fatty tissue than boys; boys have more muscle tissue.

Growth patterns vary individually (Florin & Ludwig, 2011). Much of the variation is due to heredity, but environmental experiences also are involved. The height and weight of children around the world largely reflect nutrition, with around 3 million children dying each year and millions more experiencing stunted growth because of undernutrition (UNICEF, 2018). Also, urban, middle-socioeconomic-status, and firstborn children are taller than rural, lower-socioeconomic-status, and later-born children. Children whose mothers smoked during pregnancy are half an inch shorter than children whose mothers did not smoke during pregnancy. In the United States, African American children are taller than White children.

Why are some children unusually short? The culprits are congenital factors (genetic or prenatal problems), growth hormone deficiency, a physical problem that develops in childhood, or an emotional difficulty (Wit, Kiess, & Mullis, 2011). When congenital growth problems are the cause of unusual shortness, often the child can be treated with hormones (Collett-Solberg, 2011). Usually this treatment is directed at the pituitary, the body's master gland, located at the base of the brain. This gland secretes growth-related hormones. Physical problems during childhood that can stunt growth include malnutrition and chronic infections. However, if the problems are properly treated, normal growth usually is attained.

developmental **connection**

Dynamic Systems Theory

Sensory and motor development are coupled in many aspects of children's acquisition of skills. Connect to "Motor, Sensory, and Perceptual Development."

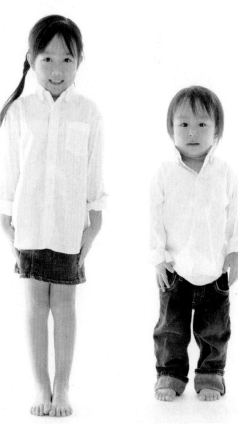

The bodies of 5-year-olds and 2-year-olds have different proportions. Notice how the 5-year-old not only is taller and weighs more, but also has a longer trunk and legs than the 2-year-old. *What might be some other physical differences between 2- and 5-year-olds?*
Michael Hitoshi/Getty Images

proximodistal pattern The sequence in which growth starts at the center of the body and moves toward the extremities.

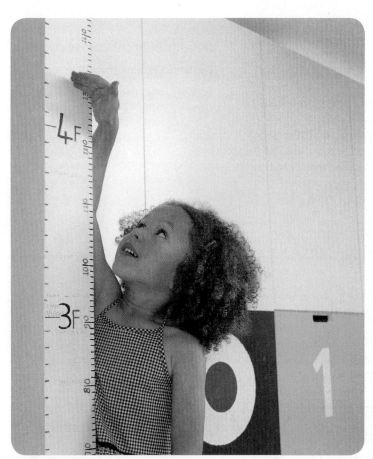

What characterizes physical growth during middle and late childhood?
Chris Windsor/Digital Vision/Getty Images

Middle and Late Childhood The period of middle and late childhood—from about 6 to 11 years of age—involves slow, consistent growth. This is a period of calm before the rapid growth spurt of adolescence.

During the elementary school years, children grow an average of 2 to 3 inches a year. At the age of 8 the average girl and the average boy are 4 feet 2 inches tall. During the middle and late childhood years, children gain about 5 to 7 pounds a year. The average 8-year-old girl and the average 8-year-old boy weigh 56 pounds (National Center for Health Statistics, 2017). The weight increase is due mainly to increases in the size of the skeletal and muscular systems, as well as the size of some body organs. Muscle mass and strength gradually increase as "baby fat" decreases in middle and late childhood.

The loose movements of early childhood give way to improved muscle tone in middle and late childhood. Children also double their strength capacity during these years. The increase in muscular strength is due to heredity and to exercise. Because they have more muscle cells, boys tend to be stronger than girls.

Changes in proportions are among the most pronounced physical changes in middle and late childhood. Head circumference, waist circumference, and leg length decrease in relation to body height (Burns & others, 2013). A less noticeable physical change is that bones continue to harden during middle and late childhood; still, they yield to pressure and pull more than mature bones.

ADOLESCENCE

After slowing through childhood, growth surges during puberty. **Puberty** is a period of rapid physical maturation involving hormonal and bodily changes that occur primarily in early adolescence. The features and proportions of the body change as the individual becomes capable of reproducing. We will begin our exploration of puberty by describing its determinants and then examine important physical changes and psychological accompaniments of puberty.

Determinants of Puberty Puberty is not the same as adolescence. For virtually everyone, puberty has ended long before adolescence is over. Puberty is often thought of as the most important marker for the beginning of adolescence.

There are wide variations in the onset and progression of puberty (Vijayakumar & others, 2018). On average, girls usually go through puberty between the ages of 10 and 14. For boys, puberty usually occurs between the ages of 12 and 16.

In fact, over the years the timing of puberty has changed. Imagine a 3-year-old girl with fully developed breasts or a boy just slightly older with a deep male voice. That is what toddlers would be like by the year 2250 if the age at which puberty arrives were to continue decreasing as it did for much of the twentieth century. For example, in Norway, **menarche**—a girl's first menstruation—now occurs at just over 13 years of age, compared with 17 years of age in the 1840s (Petersen, 1979). In the United States, where children mature up to a year earlier than in European countries, the average age of menarche dropped an average of two to four months per decade for much of the twentieth century, to about 12½ years today. Some researchers have found evidence that the age of puberty is still dropping for American girls; others suggest that the evidence is inconclusive or that the decline in age is slowing down (Herman-Giddens, 2007). One study found that puberty is continuing to occur earlier for boys, although critics say the study sample is skewed toward including more early maturing boys because parents likely brought their sons to see the participating physicians because of health concerns (Herman-Giddens & others, 2012). The earlier onset of puberty is likely the result of improved health and nutrition (Herman-Giddens, 2007; Herman-Giddens & others, 2012).

puberty A period of rapid physical maturation involving hormonal and bodily changes that take place primarily in early adolescence.

menarche A girl's first menstruation.

The normal range for the onset and progression of puberty is wide enough that, given two boys of the same chronological age, one might complete the pubertal sequence before the other one has begun it. For girls, the age range of menarche is even wider. It is considered within a normal range when it occurs between the ages of 9 and 15.

Precocious puberty is the term used to describe the very early onset and rapid progression of puberty. Precocious puberty is usually diagnosed when pubertal onset occurs before 8 years of age in girls and before 9 years of age in boys (Sultan & others, 2017). Precocious puberty occurs approximately 10 times more often in girls than in boys. When precocious puberty takes place, it often is managed through endocrinology interventions to try to stop pubertal change temporarily (Sultan & others, 2017). This treatment is recommended because children who experience precocious puberty are ultimately likely to have short stature, early sexual capability, and the potential for engaging in age-inappropriate behavior (Blakemore, Berenbaum, & Liben, 2009).

Heredity and Environmental Influences   Puberty is not an environmental accident. It does not take place at 2 or 3 years of age, and it does not occur in the twenties. Programmed into the genes of every human being is a timing for the emergence of puberty. Recently, scientists have begun to conduct molecular genetic studies in an attempt to identify specific genes that are linked to the onset and progression of puberty (Dvornyk & Waqar-ul-Haq, 2012).

Environmental factors, such as family influences and stress, can also influence the onset and duration of puberty (Joos & others, 2018). Experiences that are linked to earlier pubertal onset include adoption, father absence, low socioeconomic status, family conflict, maternal harshness, child maltreatment, and early substance use (Savage & others, 2018). In many cases, puberty comes months earlier in these situations, and this earlier onset of puberty is likely explained by high rates of conflict and stress in these social contexts. One study revealed that maternal harshness in early childhood was linked to early maturation as well as sexual risk taking in adolescence (Belsky & others, 2010). Another study found that early onset of menarche was associated with severe child sexual abuse (Noll & others, 2017).

Hormones   Behind the first whisker in boys and the widening of hips in girls is a flood of hormones. **Hormones** are powerful chemical substances secreted by the endocrine glands and carried through the body by the bloodstream. In the case of puberty, the secretion of key hormones is controlled by the interaction of the hypothalamus, the pituitary gland, and the gonads (sex glands). The *hypothalamus* is a structure in the brain best known for monitoring eating, drinking, and sex. The *pituitary gland* is an important endocrine gland that controls growth and regulates other glands. The *gonads* are the sex glands—the testes in males, the ovaries in females.

The key hormonal changes involve two classes of hormones that have significantly different concentrations in males and females (Susman & Dorn, 2013). **Androgens** are the main class of male sex hormones. **Estrogens** are the main class of female sex hormones.

Testosterone is an androgen that is a key hormone in the development of puberty in boys (Colvin & Abdullatif, 2012). As the testosterone level rises during puberty, external genitals enlarge, height increases, and the voice changes. **Estradiol** is an estrogen that plays an important role in female pubertal development. As the estradiol level rises, breast development, uterine development, and skeletal changes occur. In one study, testosterone levels increased eighteenfold in boys but only twofold in girls across puberty; estradiol levels increased eightfold in girls but only twofold in boys across puberty (Nottleman & others, 1987) (see Figure 2).

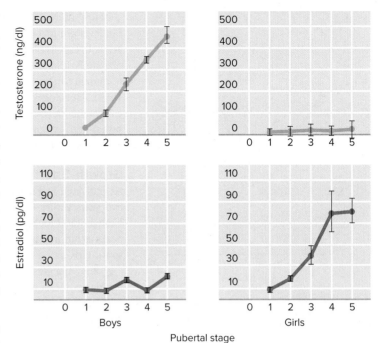

FIGURE **2**

HORMONE LEVELS BY SEX AND PUBERTAL STAGE FOR TESTOSTERONE AND ESTRADIOL. The five stages range from the early beginning of puberty (stage 1) to the most advanced stage of puberty (stage 5). Notice the significant increase in testosterone in boys and the significant increase in estradiol in girls.

precocious puberty Very early onset and rapid progression of puberty.

hormones Powerful chemical substances secreted by the endocrine glands and carried through the body by the bloodstream.

androgens The main class of male sex hormones.

estrogens The main class of female sex hormones.

testosterone An androgen that is a key hormone in boys' pubertal development.

estradiol An estrogen that is a key hormone in girls' pubertal development.

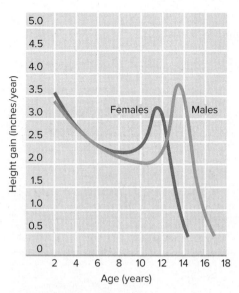

FIGURE 3

PUBERTAL GROWTH SPURT. On average, the peak of the growth spurt that characterizes pubertal change occurs two years earlier for girls (11½) than for boys (13½).

Source: J. M. Tanner et al., "Standards from Birth to Maturity for Height, Weight, Height Velocity: British Children in 1965" in *Archives of Diseases in Childhood*, 41(219), pp. 454–471, 1966.

Are there links between concentrations of hormones and adolescent behavior? Findings are inconsistent (Welker & others, 2019). In any event, hormonal factors alone are not responsible for adolescent behavior (Yeager, Dahl, & Dweck, 2018). For example, one study found that social factors accounted for two to four times as much variance as hormonal factors in young adolescent girls' depression and anger (Brooks-Gunn & Warren, 1989). Hormones do not act independently; hormonal activity is influenced by many environmental factors, including parent-adolescent relationships. Stress, eating patterns, sexual activity, and depression can also activate or suppress various aspects of the hormone system (Susman & Dorn, 2013).

Growth Spurt Puberty ushers in the most rapid increases in growth since infancy. As indicated in Figure 3, the growth spurt associated with puberty occurs approximately two years earlier for girls than for boys. The mean beginning of the growth spurt in the United States today is 9 years of age for girls and 11 years of age for boys. Pubertal change peaks at an average of 11.5 years for girls and 13.5 years for boys. During their growth spurt, girls increase in height about 3.5 inches per year, boys about 4 inches.

Boys and girls who are shorter or taller than their peers before adolescence are likely to remain so during adolescence. At the beginning of adolescence, girls tend to be as tall as or taller than boys their age, but by the end of the middle school years most boys have caught up, or, in many cases, even surpassed girls in height. And although height in elementary school is a good predictor of height later in adolescence, as much as 30 percent of the height of individuals in late adolescence is unexplained by height in the elementary school years.

Sexual Maturation Think back to the onset of your puberty. Of the striking changes that were taking place in your body, what was the first change that occurred? Researchers have found that male pubertal characteristics develop in this order: increase in penis and testicle size, appearance of straight pubic hair, minor voice change, first ejaculation (which usually occurs through masturbation or a wet dream), appearance of curly pubic hair, onset of maximum body growth, growth of hair in armpits, more detectable voice changes, and growth of facial hair. Three of the most noticeable areas of sexual maturation in boys are penis elongation, testes development, and growth of facial hair. The normal range and average age of development in boys and girls for these sexual characteristics, along with height spurt, is shown in Figure 4.

What is the order of appearance of physical changes in females? First, on average the breasts enlarge and then pubic hair appears. These are two of the most noticeable aspects of female pubertal development. A longitudinal study revealed that on average, girls' breast development preceded their pubic hair development by about 2 months (Susman & others, 2010). Later, hair appears in the armpits. As these changes occur, the female grows in height, and her hips become wider than her shoulders. Her first menstruation (menarche) occurs rather late in the pubertal cycle; it is considered normal if it occurs between the ages of 9 and 15. Initially, her menstrual cycles may be highly irregular. For the first several years, she might not ovulate during every menstrual cycle. Some girls do not become fertile until two years after their periods begin. Pubertal females do not experience voice changes comparable to those in pubertal males. By the end of puberty, the female's breasts have become more fully rounded.

Psychological Dimensions of Puberty A host of psychological changes accompany an adolescent's pubertal development. Two of the most pronounced psychological changes involve body image and early and late maturation.

Body Image One psychological aspect of physical change in puberty is certain: Adolescents are preoccupied with their bodies and develop images of what their bodies are like (Zsakai & others, 2017). Preoccupation with body image is strong throughout adolescence, but it is especially acute during early adolescence, a time when adolescents are more dissatisfied with their bodies than in late adolescence. Nonetheless, when the entirety of adolescence was considered, not just puberty, a study found that both boys' and girls' body images became more positive as they moved from the beginning to the end of adolescence (Holsen, Carlson Jones, & Skogbrott Birkeland, 2012).

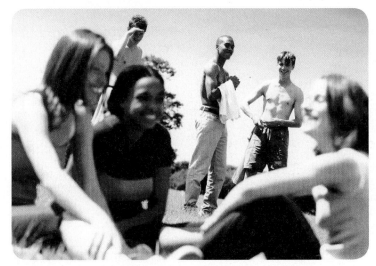

What gender differences characterize adolescents' body image? What might explain the differences?
Corbis/VCG/Getty Images

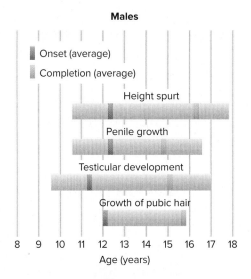

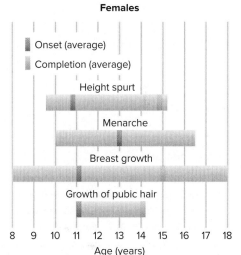

FIGURE 4
NORMAL RANGE AND AVERAGE DEVELOPMENT OF SEXUAL CHARACTERISTICS IN MALES AND FEMALES

Gender differences characterize adolescents' perceptions of their bodies. In general, girls are less happy with their bodies and have more negative body images than boys throughout puberty (Benowitz-Fredericks & others, 2012). As pubertal change proceeds, girls often become more dissatisfied with their bodies, probably because their body fat increases. In contrast, boys become more satisfied as they move through puberty, probably because their muscle mass increases.

Although we have described gender differences in the body images of adolescents, emphasizing that girls tend to have more negative body images than boys, keep in mind that there is considerable variation, with many adolescent girls having positive body images and many adolescent boys having negative body images. Different trajectories of body images have been tracked over time for individuals' perceptions of their own appearance, weight, and attributions related to their bodies (Nelson & others, 2018). Differences in body image trajectories are related to gender, identity, and psychological functioning.

Early and Late Maturation   Did you enter puberty early, late, or on time? When adolescents mature earlier or later than their peers, they often perceive themselves differently and their maturational timing is linked to their socioemotional development and whether they develop problems (Negriff, Susman, & Trickett, 2011). In the Berkeley Longitudinal Study conducted some years ago, early-maturing boys perceived themselves more positively and had more successful peer relations than did late-maturing boys (Jones, 1965). The findings for early-maturing girls were similar but not as strong as for boys. When the late-maturing boys were in their thirties, however, they had developed a more positive identity than the early-maturing boys had (Peskin, 1967). Perhaps the late-maturing boys had more time to explore life's options, or perhaps the early-maturing boys continued to focus on their physical status instead of paying attention to career development and achievement.

An increasing number of researchers have found that early maturation increases girls' vulnerability to a number of problems (Pomerantz & others, 2017). Early-maturing girls are more likely to smoke, drink, be depressed, have an eating disorder, engage in delinquency, struggle for earlier independence from their parents, and have older friends; and their bodies are likely to elicit responses from males that lead to earlier dating and earlier sexual experiences (Chen, Rothman, & Jaffee, 2017). And early-maturing girls are more likely to drop out of high school and to cohabit and marry earlier (Cavanagh, 2009). Apparently as a result of their social and cognitive immaturity, combined with early physical development, early-maturing girls are easily lured into problem behaviors, not recognizing the possible long-term effects of these on their development.

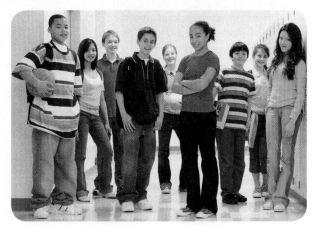

How does early and late maturation influence adolescent development?
Fuse/Getty Images

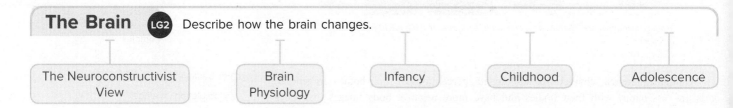

The Brain **LG2** Describe how the brain changes.

The Neuroconstructivist View | Brain Physiology | Infancy | Childhood | Adolescence

---

developmental connection

Nature and Nurture

In the epigenetic view, development is an ongoing, bidirectional interchange between heredity and the environment. Connect to "Biological Beginnings."

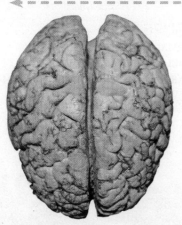

FIGURE 5

THE HUMAN BRAIN'S HEMISPHERES. The two halves (hemispheres) of the human brain are clearly seen in this photograph.

IgorZD/Shutterstock

neuroconstructivist view Theory of brain development emphasizing the following points: (a) biological processes and environmental conditions influence the brain's development, (b) the brain has plasticity and is context dependent, and (c) the development of the brain and the child's cognitive development are closely linked.

In every physical change we have described so far, the brain is involved in some way. Structures of the brain help to regulate not only behavior but also metabolism, the release of hormones, and other aspects of the body's physiology.

We have described the amazing growth of the brain from conception to birth. In this section, we initially will explore the neuroconstructivist view, describe basic structures and function of the brain, and then examine developmental changes in the brain from infancy through adolescence.

THE NEUROCONSTRUCTIVIST VIEW

Until recently, little was known for certain about how the brain changes as children develop. Not long ago, scientists thought that our genes determined how our brains were "wired" and that the cells in the brain responsible for processing information just maturationally unfolded with little or no input from environmental experiences. Whatever brain your heredity dealt you, you were essentially stuck with it. This view, however, turned out to be wrong. Instead, the brain has plasticity, and its development depends on context (Diamond, 2013; Nelson, 2012).

In the increasingly popular **neuroconstructivist view,** (a) biological processes (genes, for example) and environmental conditions (enriched or impoverished, for example) influence the brain's development, (b) the brain has plasticity and is context dependent, and (c) development of the brain is closely linked with the child's cognitive development. These factors constrain or advance the child's construction of cognitive skills (Diamond, 2013). The neuroconstructivist view emphasizes the importance of considering interactions between experience and gene expression in the brain's development, much in the same way the epigenetic view proposes (see the chapter, "Biological Beginnings").

BRAIN PHYSIOLOGY

The brain includes a number of major structures. The key components of these structures are *neurons,* the nerve cells that handle information processing.

Structure and Function Looked at from above, the brain has two halves, or hemispheres (see Figure 5). The top portion of the brain, farthest from the spinal cord,

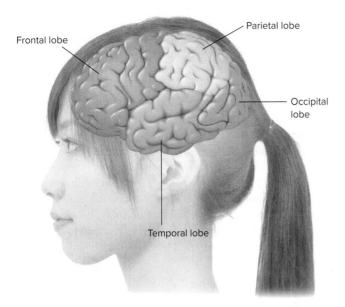

Frontal lobe

Parietal lobe

Occipital lobe

Temporal lobe

FIGURE 6

THE BRAIN'S FOUR LOBES. Shown here are the locations of the brain's four lobes: frontal, occipital, temporal, and parietal.

(photo) Takayuki/Shutterstock

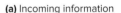

developmental **connection**

Intelligence

Are some regions of the brain linked with children's intelligence more than others? Connect to "Intelligence."

is known as the forebrain. Its outer layer of cells, the cerebral cortex, covers it like a cap. The cerebral cortex is responsible for about 80 percent of the brain's volume and is critically important in perception, thinking, language, and other functions.

Each hemisphere of the cortex has four major areas, called lobes (see Figure 6). Although the lobes usually work together, each has a somewhat different primary function:

- *Frontal lobes* are involved in voluntary movement, thinking, personality, and intentionality or purpose.
- *Occipital lobes* function in vision.
- *Temporal lobes* facilitate hearing, language processing, and memory.
- *Parietal lobes* help to register spatial location, direct attention, and maintain motor control.

Deeper in the brain, beneath the cortex, lie other key structures. These include the hypothalamus and the pituitary gland as well as the *amygdala,* which plays an important role in emotions, and the *hippocampus,* which is especially active in memory and emotion.

Neurons   How do neurons work? As we indicated, these nerve cells process information. Figure 7 shows some important parts of the neuron, including the *axon* and *dendrites.* Basically, an axon sends electrical signals away from the central part of the neuron. At the end of the axon are terminal buttons, which release chemicals called *neurotransmitters* into *synapses,* which are tiny gaps between neurons' fibers. Chemical interactions in synapses connect axons and dendrites, allowing information to pass from neuron to neuron (Schreiner & others, 2017). Think of the synapse as a river that blocks a road. A grocery truck arrives at one bank of the river, crosses by ferry, and continues its journey to market. Similarly, a message in the brain is "ferried" across the synapse by a neurotransmitter, which pours out information contained in chemicals when it reaches the other side of the river.

Most axons are covered by a myelin sheath, which is a layer of fat cells. The sheath helps impulses travel faster along the axon, increasing the speed with which information travels from neuron to neuron (Buttermore, Thaxton, & Bhat, 2013). The myelin sheath developed as the brain evolved. As brain size increased, it became necessary for information to travel faster over longer distances in the nervous system. We can compare the myelin sheath's development to the evolution of freeways as cities grew. A freeway is a shielded road, and it keeps fast-moving, long-distance traffic from getting snarled by slow local traffic.

Which neurons get which information? Clusters of neurons known as *neural circuits* work together to handle particular types of information (Dehaene-Lambertz, 2017). The brain is organized in many neural circuits (Gilmore, Knickmeyer, & Gao, 2018). For example, one neural circuit is important in attention and working memory (the type of memory that holds

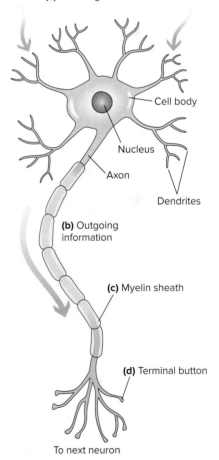

(a) Incoming information

Cell body

Nucleus

Axon

Dendrites

(b) Outgoing information

(c) Myelin sheath

(d) Terminal button

To next neuron

FIGURE 7

THE NEURON. (*a*) The dendrites receive information from other neurons, muscles, or glands. (*b*) Axons transmit information away from the cell body. (*c*) A myelin sheath covers most axons and speeds information transmission. (*d*) As the axon ends, it branches out into terminal buttons.

information for a brief time and serves as a "mental workbench" as we perform a task) (Standage & Pare, 2018). This neural circuit uses the neurotransmitter dopamine and lies in the prefrontal cortex and midbrain areas of the brain (D'Ardenne & others, 2012).

To some extent, the type of information handled by neurons depends on whether they are in the left or right hemisphere of the cortex (Yang, Marslen-Wilson, & Bozic, 2017). Speech and grammar, for example, depend on activity in the left hemisphere in most people; humor and the use of metaphors depend on activity in the right hemisphere (McGettigan & others, 2017). This specialization of function in one hemisphere of the cerebral cortex or the other is called **lateralization.** However, most neuroscientists agree that complex functions such as reading or performing music involve both hemispheres (Rao & Vaid, 2017). Labeling people as "left-brained" because they are logical thinkers and "right-brained" because they are creative thinkers does not correspond to the way the brain's hemispheres work. Complex thinking in normal people is the outcome of communication between both hemispheres of the brain (Tzourio-Mazoyer & others, 2017). For example, a meta-analysis revealed no hemispheric specialization in creative thinking (Mihov, Denzler, & Forster, 2010).

INFANCY

Brain development occurs extensively during the prenatal period. The brain's development is also substantial during infancy and later on (Hodel, 2018).

Because the brain is still developing so rapidly in infancy, the infant's head should be protected from falls or other injuries and the baby should never be shaken. *Shaken baby syndrome,* which includes brain swelling and hemorrhaging, affects hundreds of babies in the United States each year (Swaiman & others, 2012). One analysis found that fathers were the most frequent perpetrators of shaken baby syndrome, followed by child care providers and by a boyfriend of the victim's mother (National Center on Shaken Baby Syndrome, 2011).

Studying the brain's development in infancy is not as easy as it might seem. Even the latest brain-imaging technologies cannot make out fine details in adult brains and cannot be used with babies (Nelson, 2012). Positron-emission tomography (PET) scans pose a radiation risk to babies, and infants wriggle too much to allow technicians to capture accurate images using magnetic resonance imaging (MRI). However, researchers have been successful in using the electroencephalogram (EEG), a measure of the brain's electrical activity, to learn about the brain's development in infancy (Anderson & Perone, 2018) (see Figure 8).

As an infant walks, talks, runs, shakes a rattle, smiles, and frowns, changes in its brain are occurring. Consider that the infant began life as a single cell and nine months later

developmental **connection**

Gender

How large are gender differences in the brain? Connect to "Gender."

developmental **connection**

Brain Development

How does the brain change from conception to birth? Connect to "Prenatal Development and Birth."

lateralization Specialization of function in one hemisphere of the cerebral cortex or the other.

FIGURE 8

MEASURING THE ACTIVITY OF AN INFANT'S BRAIN. By attaching up to 128 electrodes to a baby's scalp to measure the brain's activity, Charles Nelson (2003, 2012) has found that even newborns produce distinctive brain waves that reveal they can distinguish their mother's voice from another woman's, even while they are asleep. *Why is it so difficult to measure infants' brain activity?*

Owen Humphreys/PA Images/Getty Images

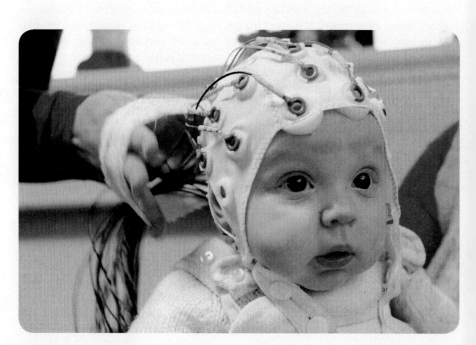

was born with a brain and nervous system that contained approximately 100 billion nerve cells, or neurons. What determines how those neurons are connected to communicate with each other?

Early Experience and the Brain Children who grow up in a deprived environment may also have depressed brain activity (Zeanah, Fox, & Nelson, 2012). As shown in Figure 9, a child who grew up in the unresponsive and unstimulating environment of a Romanian orphanage showed considerably depressed brain activity compared with a child who grew up in a normal environment.

Are the effects of deprived environments irreversible? There is reason to think the answer is no (Bryck & Fisher, 2012; Sharma, Classen, & Cohen, 2013). The brain demonstrates both flexibility and resilience. Consider 14-year-old Michael Rehbein. At age 7, he began to experience uncontrollable seizures—as many as 400 a day. Doctors said the only solution was to remove the left hemisphere of his brain where the seizures were occurring. Recovery was slow, but his right hemisphere began to reorganize and take over functions that normally occur in the brain's left hemisphere, including speech (see Figure 10). A study that compared children and young adults who had brain damage in the left hemisphere (where language functions are generally controlled) to children and young adults without brain damage found that in more than 80 percent of the individuals with damage to the left hemisphere of their brain, the right hemisphere dominated the language functions usually controlled by the left side of the brain (Chilosi & others, 2019).

Neuroscientists believe that what wires the brain—or rewires it, in the case of Michael Rehbein—is repeated experience. Each time a baby tries to touch an attractive object or gazes intently at a face, tiny bursts of electricity shoot through the brain, knitting together neurons into circuits. The results are some of the behavioral milestones we discuss in this chapter.

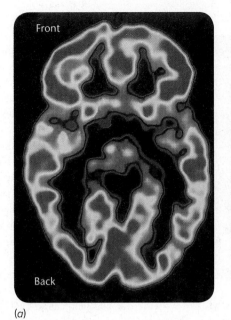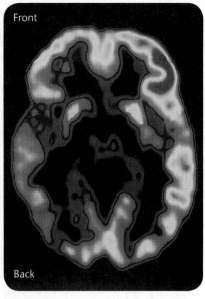

(a)　　　　　　　　　(b)

FIGURE 9

EARLY DEPRIVATION AND BRAIN ACTIVITY.
These two photographs are PET (positron emission tomography) scans (which use radioactive tracers to image and analyze blood flow and metabolic activity in the body's organs) of the brains of (*a*) a normal child and (*b*) an institutionalized Romanian orphan who experienced substantial deprivation since birth. In PET scans, the highest to lowest brain activity is reflected in the colors of red, yellow, green, blue, and black, respectively. As can be seen, red and yellow show up to a much greater degree in the PET scan of the normal child than the deprived Romanian orphan.

(a-b) Courtesy of Dr. Harry T. Chugani, Children's Hospital of Michigan

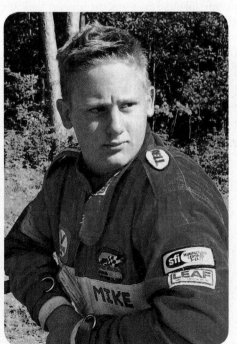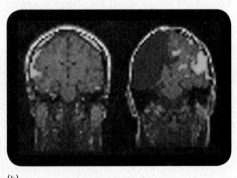

(b)

FIGURE 10

PLASTICITY IN THE BRAIN'S HEMISPHERES.
(*a*) Michael Rehbein at 14 years of age. (*b*) Michael's right hemisphere (*right*) has reorganized to take over the language functions normally carried out by corresponding areas in the left hemisphere of an intact brain (*left*). However, the right hemisphere is not as efficient as the left, and more areas of the brain are recruited to process speech.

(a-b) Courtesy Crystal Rehbein

(a)

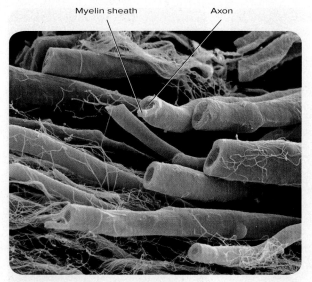

Myelin sheath   Axon

FIGURE 11

MYELINATED NERVE FIBER. The myelin sheath, shown in brown, encases the axon (white). This image was produced by an electron microscope that magnified the nerve fiber 12,000 times. *What role does myelination play in the brain's development?*

Science Photo Library/Getty Images

myelination The process of encasing axons with a myelin sheath that increases the speed of processing information.

FIGURE 12

THE DEVELOPMENT OF DENDRITIC SPREADING. Note the increase in connectedness between neurons over the course of the first two years of life.

The Postnatal Development of the Human Cerebral Cortex, Volumes I–VIII by Jesse LeRoy Conel, Cambridge, Mass.: Harvard University Press, Copyright © 1939, 1941, 1947, 1951, 1955, 1959, 1963, 1967 by the President and Fellows of Harvard College. Copyright © renewed 1967, 1969, 1975, 1979, 1983, 1987, 1991.

In sum, the infant's brain is waiting for experiences to determine how connections are made (Meltzoff, Saby, & Marshall, 2019). Before birth, it appears that genes mainly direct basic wiring patterns. Neurons grow and travel to distant places awaiting further instructions (Nelson, 2012). After birth, the inflowing stream of sights, sounds, smells, touches, language, and eye contact help shape the brain's neural connections (Diamond, 2013; Lamb, 2013a, b; Narváez & others, 2013).

Changing Neurons   At birth, the newborn's brain is about 25 percent of its adult weight. By the second birthday, the brain is about 75 percent of its adult weight. Two key developments during these first two years involve the myelin sheath (the layer of fat cells that speeds up the electrical impulse along the axon) and connections between dendrites.

Myelination, the process of encasing axons with a myelin sheath, begins prenatally and continues after birth (see Figure 11). The myelin sheath insulates axons and helps electrical signals travel faster down the axon (Hodel, 2018). As we indicated earlier, myelination increases the speed at which information is processed. It also is involved in providing energy to neurons and in communication (Micu & others, 2018). Myelination for visual pathways occurs rapidly after birth and is completed during the first six months. Auditory myelination is not completed until 4 or 5 years of age. Some aspects of myelination continue even into adolescence. Indeed, the most extensive changes in myelination in the frontal lobes occur during adolescence (Giedd, 2012).

Dramatic increases in dendrites and synapses (the tiny gaps between neurons across which neurotransmitters carry information) also characterize the development of the brain in the first two years of life (see Figure 12). Nearly twice as many of these connections are made as will ever be used (Huttenlocher & others, 1991; Huttenlocher & Dabholkar, 1997). The connections that are used become strengthened and survive; the unused ones are replaced by other pathways or disappear. That is, connections are "pruned" (Lieberman & others, 2019). Figure 13 vividly illustrates the growth and later pruning of synapses in the visual, auditory, and prefrontal cortex areas of the brain (Huttenlocher & Dabholkar, 1997).

As shown in Figure 13, "blooming and pruning" vary considerably by brain region in humans. For example, the peak synaptic overproduction in the area concerned with vision occurs about the fourth postnatal month, followed by a gradual pruning until the middle to end of the preschool years (Huttenlocher & Dabholkar, 1997). In areas of the brain involved in hearing and language, a similar, though somewhat later, course is detected. However, in the prefrontal cortex (the area of the brain where higher-level thinking and self-regulation occur), the peak of overproduction occurs at just after 3 years of age. Both heredity and environment are thought to influence synaptic overproduction and subsequent pruning.

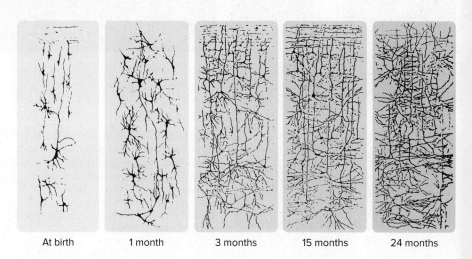

At birth   1 month   3 months   15 months   24 months

Changing Structures At birth, the hemispheres already have started to specialize: Newborns show greater electrical activity in the left hemisphere than in the right hemisphere when they are making or listening to speech sounds (Imada & others, 2007).

In general, some areas of the brain, such as the primary motor areas, develop earlier than others, such as the primary sensory areas. The frontal lobes are immature in the newborn. However, as neurons in the frontal lobes become myelinated and interconnected during the first year of life, infants develop an ability to regulate their physiological states, such as sleep, and gain more control over their reflexes. Cognitive skills that require deliberate thinking do not emerge until later in the first year (Bell & Cuevas, 2013).

CHILDHOOD

The brain and other parts of the nervous system continue developing through childhood and adolescence. These changes enable children to plan their actions, to attend to stimuli more effectively, and to make considerable strides in language development (Diamond, 2013).

During early childhood, the brain and head grow more rapidly than any other part of the body. Figure 14 shows how the growth curve for the head and brain advances more rapidly than the growth curve for height and weight. Some of the brain's increase in size is due to myelination and some is due to an increase in the number and size of dendrites. Some developmentalists conclude that myelination is important in the maturation of a number of abilities in children (Fair & Schlaggar, 2008). For example, myelination in the areas of the brain related to hand-eye coordination is not complete until about 4 years of age. More advanced myelination is related to more advanced verbal and nonverbal cognitive abilities and has been described as a mechanism through which breast feeding promotes cognitive development, as breast feeding results in better myelination than does formula feeding (Deoni & others, 2018). Myelination in the areas of the brain related to focusing attention is not complete until middle or late childhood.

The brain in early childhood is not growing as rapidly as it did in infancy. However, the anatomical changes in the child's brain between the ages of 3 and 15 are dramatic. By repeatedly obtaining brain scans of the same children for up to four years, scientists have found that children's brains experience rapid, distinct bursts of growth (Gogtay & Thompson, 2010). The amount of brain material in some areas can nearly double in as little as one year, followed by a drastic loss of tissue as unneeded cells are purged and the brain continues to reorganize itself. The overall size of the brain does not increase dramatically from 3 to 15. What does dramatically change are local patterns within the brain (Gogtay & Thompson, 2010). From 3 to 6 years of age, the most rapid growth occurs in the frontal lobe areas involved in planning and organizing new actions and in maintaining attention to tasks (Diamond, 2013). From age 6 through puberty, the most dramatic growth takes place in the temporal and parietal lobes, especially in areas that play major roles in language and spatial relations.

Developmental neuroscientist Mark Johnson and his colleagues (2009) proposed that the prefrontal cortex likely orchestrates the functions of many other brain regions during development. As part of this neural leadership and organizational role, the prefrontal cortex may provide an advantage to neural connections and networks that include

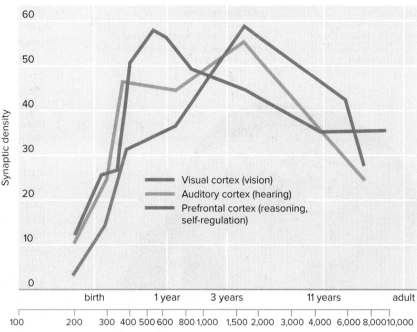

FIGURE 13

SYNAPTIC DENSITY IN THE HUMAN BRAIN FROM INFANCY TO ADULTHOOD. The graph shows the dramatic increase and then pruning in synaptic density for three regions of the brain: visual cortex, auditory cortex, and prefrontal cortex. Synaptic density is believed to be an important indication of the extent of connectivity between neurons.

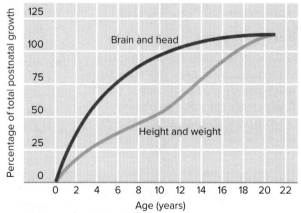

FIGURE 14

GROWTH CURVES FOR THE HEAD AND BRAIN AND FOR HEIGHT AND WEIGHT. The more rapid growth of the brain and head can easily be seen. Height and weight advance more gradually over the first two decades of life.

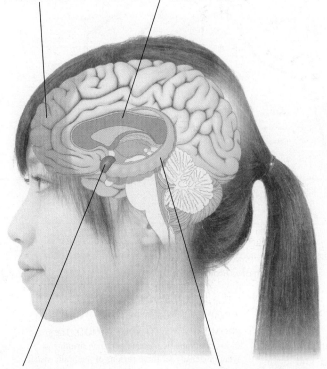

Prefrontal cortex
This "judgment" region reins in intense emotions but doesn't finish developing until at least emerging adulthood.

Corpus callosum
These nerve fibers connect the brain's two hemispheres; they thicken in adolescence to process information more effectively.

Amygdala
Limbic system structure especially involved in emotion.

Limbic system
A lower, subcortical system in the brain that is the seat of emotions and experience of rewards. This system is almost completely developed in early adolescence.

FIGURE 15

CHANGES IN THE ADOLESCENT BRAIN

(photo) Takayauki/Shutterstock

---

developmental **connection**

Brain Development

How might developmental changes in the adolescent's brain be linked to adolescents' decision-making skills? Connect to "Information Processing."

---

corpus callosum Brain area where fibers connect the brain's left and right hemispheres.

prefrontal cortex The highest level of the frontal lobes that is involved in reasoning, decision making, and self-control.

amygdala The seat of emotions in the brain.

the prefrontal cortex. In the view of these researchers, the prefrontal cortex likely coordinates the best neural connections for solving a problem.

Links between the changing brain and children's cognitive development involve activation of brain areas, with some areas increasing in activation while others decrease. One shift in activation that occurs as children develop in middle and late childhood is from diffuse, larger areas to more focal, smaller areas (Durston & others, 2006). This shift is characterized by synaptic pruning in which areas of the brain not being used lose synaptic connections and those being used show an increase in connections. Researchers have found less diffusion and more focal activation in the prefrontal cortex (the highest level of the frontal lobes) from 7 to 30 years of age (Durston & others, 2006). The activation change was accompanied by increased efficiency in cognitive performance, especially in *cognitive control,* which involves flexible and effective control in a number of areas. These areas include controlling attention, reducing interfering thoughts, inhibiting motor actions, and being flexible in switching between competing choices (Friedman & Miyake, 2017).

ADOLESCENCE

Along with the rest of the body, the brain is changing during adolescence (Blakemore & Mills, 2014; Giedd & others, 2012). As advances in technology take place, significant strides will also likely be made in charting developmental changes in the adolescent brain. What do we know now?

Earlier we indicated that connections between neurons become "pruned" as children and adolescents develop. The pruning means that the connections that are used strengthen and survive, while the unused ones are replaced by other pathways or disappear. As a result of this pruning, by the end of adolescence individuals have "fewer, more selective, more effective neuronal connections than they did as children" (Kuhn, 2009, p. 153). And this pruning indicates that the activities adolescents choose to engage in and not to engage in influence which neural connections will be strengthened and which will disappear.

Using fMRI brain scans, scientists have discovered that adolescents' brains undergo significant structural changes (Foulkes & Blakemore, 2018). The **corpus callosum,** where fibers connect the brain's left and right hemispheres, thickens in adolescence; this improves adolescents' ability to process information. We just described advances in the development of the **prefrontal cortex**—the highest level of the frontal lobes involved in reasoning, decision making, and self-control. The prefrontal cortex doesn't finish maturing until the emerging adult years (approximately 18 to 25 years of age) or later, but the **amygdala**—the seat of emotions such as anger—matures earlier than the prefrontal cortex (Romeo, 2017). Figure 15 shows the locations of the corpus callosum, prefrontal cortex, and amygdala. Larger amygdala volumes, as well as different patterns of connectivity with other brain regions, are associated with more aggressive behavior during adolescence (Saxbe & others, 2018).

Many of the changes in the adolescent brain that have been described involve the rapidly emerging field of *developmental social neuroscience,* which involves connections between development, the brain, and socioemotional processes (Blakemore & Mills, 2014; Salley, Miller, & Bell, 2013). For example, consider leading researcher Charles Nelson's (2003) view that although adolescents are capable of very strong emotions, their prefrontal cortex hasn't developed to the point at which they can control these passions. It is as if their brain doesn't have the brakes to slow down their emotions. Or consider this interpretation of the development of emotion and cognition in adolescents: "early activation of strong 'turbo-charged' feelings with a relatively un-skilled set of 'driving skills' or cognitive abilities to modulate strong emotions and motivations" (Dahl, 2004, p. 18).

Of course, a major issue in adolescent brain development is which comes first: biological changes in the brain or experiences that stimulate these changes (Lerner, Boyd, & Du, 2009). Consider a study in which the prefrontal cortex thickened and more brain connections formed when adolescents resisted peer pressure (Paus & others, 2007). A recent study found that Mexican American adolescents' adjustment was predicted by both biological and psychosocial factors (Qu & others, 2018). Namely, smaller hippocampal volume and parental cultural socialization both independently predicted better academic achievement. In addition, smaller nucleus accumbens volume and less affiliation with deviant peers both independently predicted less substance use.

Scientists have yet to determine whether the brain changes come first or whether they result from experiences with peers, parents, and others. Once again, we encounter the nature/nurture issue that is so prominent in examining development (Giedd & others, 2012).

developmental **connection**

Brain Development

Developmental social neuroscience is a recently emerging field that focuses on connections between development, socioemotional factors, and neuroscience. Connect to "Introduction."

Review Connect Reflect

 LG2 Describe how the brain changes.

Review

- What are some key features of the neuroconstructivist view?
- What is the nature of brain physiology?
- How does the brain change in infancy?
- What characterizes the development of the brain in childhood?
- How does the brain change in adolescence, and how might this change be linked to adolescents' behavior?

Connect

- Both infancy and adolescence are times of significant change in the brain. Compare and contrast these changes.

Reflect *Your Own Personal Journey of Life*

- A parent tells you that his or her child is "left-brained" and that this aspect of the brain explains why the child does well in school. Is the parent likely to be providing an accurate explanation or probably off-base? Explain.

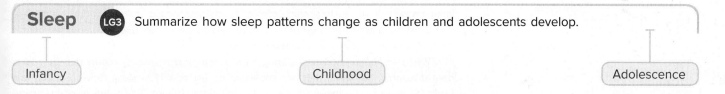

Sleep **LG3** Summarize how sleep patterns change as children and adolescents develop.

| Infancy | Childhood | Adolescence |

Sleep restores, replenishes, and rebuilds our brains and bodies. Some neuroscientists believe that sleep gives neurons that have been used while we are awake a chance to shut down and repair themselves (National Institute of Neurological Disorders and Stroke, 2018). How do sleeping patterns change during the childhood years?

INFANCY

When we were infants, sleep consumed more of our time than it does now. Newborns sleep 16 to 17 hours a day, although some sleep more and others less—the range is from a low of about 10 hours to a high of about 21 hours per day. A research review concluded that infants 0 to 2 years of age slept an average of 12.8 hours out of the 24, within a range of 9.7 to 15.9 hours (Galland & others, 2012). By 6 months of age the majority of infants sleep through the night, awakening their parents only once or twice a week (Weinraub & others, 2012).

Although total sleep remains somewhat consistent for young infants, their sleep during the day does not always follow a rhythmic pattern. An infant might change from

Sleep that knits up the ravelled sleave of care . . . Balm of hurt minds, nature's second course. Chief nourisher in life's feast.

—**WILLIAM SHAKESPEARE**
English playwright, 17th century

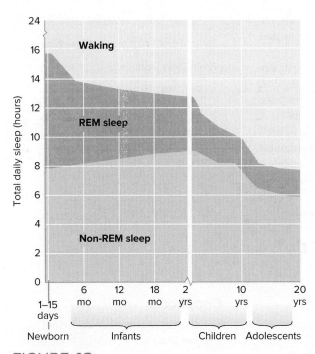

FIGURE 16

DEVELOPMENTAL CHANGES IN REM AND NON-REM SLEEP

sleeping several long bouts of 7 or 8 hours to three or four shorter sessions only several hours in duration. By about 1 month of age, most infants have begun to sleep longer at night. By 6 months of age, they usually have moved closer to adult-like sleep patterns, spending their longest span of sleep at night and their longest span of waking during the day (Sadeh, 2008).

The most common infant sleep-related problem reported by parents is nighttime waking (The Hospital for Sick Children & others, 2010). Surveys indicate that 20 to 30 percent of infants have difficulty going to sleep at night and staying asleep (Sadeh, 2008). Less disrupted infant sleep is predicted by mothers' emotional availability at bedtime as well as less household chaos, suggesting that better-regulated infant sleep is promoted by feelings of safety and security (Whitesell & others, 2018). Infant sleep problems have been related to a range of family difficulties, including marital conflict, and are reduced by sensitive caregiving from both mothers and fathers (El-Sheikh & Kelly, 2017). Infant sleep problems can also be a source of marital discord, as mothers and fathers who disagree about how to respond to infants' nighttime wakings perceive themselves as having lower-quality co-parenting relationships (Reader, Teti, & Cleveland, 2017). Maternal depression during pregnancy, early introduction of solid foods, infant TV viewing, and child care attendance are related to shorter duration of sleep during early childhood (Plancoulaine & others, 2018). Also, nighttime wakings at 1 year of age predict lower sleep efficiency at 4 years of age (Tikotzky & Shaashua, 2012).

REM Sleep   In REM sleep, the eyes flutter beneath closed lids; in non-REM sleep, this type of eye movement does not occur and sleep is quieter. Figure 16 shows developmental changes in the average number of total hours spent in REM and non-REM sleep. By the time they reach adulthood, individuals spend about one-fifth of their night in REM sleep, and REM sleep usually appears about one hour after non-REM sleep. However, about half of an infant's sleep is REM sleep, and infants often begin their sleep cycle with REM sleep rather than non-REM sleep (Sadeh, 2008). A much greater amount of time is taken up by REM sleep in infancy than at any other point in the life span. By the time infants reach 3 months of age, the percentage of time they spend in REM sleep falls to about 40 percent, and REM sleep no longer begins their sleep cycle.

Why do infants spend so much time in REM sleep? Researchers are not certain. The large amount of REM sleep may provide infants with added self-stimulation, since they spend less time awake than do older children. REM sleep also might promote the brain's development in infancy (Dereymaeker & others, 2017).

When adults are awakened during REM sleep, they frequently report that they have been dreaming, but when they are awakened during non-REM sleep they are much less likely to report having been dreaming (Cartwright & others, 2006). Since infants spend more time than adults in REM sleep, can we conclude that they dream a lot? We don't know whether infants dream or not, because they don't have any way of reporting dreams.

Shared Sleeping   Some child experts stress that there are benefits to shared sleeping (as when an infant sleeps in the same bed with its mother). They state that it can promote breast feeding, lets the mother respond more quickly to the baby's cries, and allows her to detect breathing pauses in the baby that might be dangerous (Mileva-Seitz & others, 2017). Sharing a bed with a mother is common practice in many countries, such as Guatemala and China, whereas in others, such as the United States and Great Britain, most newborns sleep in a crib, either in the same room as the parents or in a separate room.

Shared sleeping remains a controversial issue, with some experts recommending it and others arguing against it, although recently the recommendation trend has been to avoid infant-parent bed sharing, especially until the infant is at least six months of age (Mileva-Seitz & others, 2017). The American Academy of Pediatrics (Moon & Task Force on Sudden Infant Death Syndrome, 2016) recommends against shared sleeping. AAP members argue that in some instances bed sharing might lead to sudden infant death syndrome (SIDS), as could be the case if a sleeping mother rolls over on her baby. Bed sharing is linked with a greater incidence of SIDS, especially when parents smoke (Byard, 2018). And a study of 2-month-old infants revealed that they had more sleep problems such as disordered breathing when they shared the bed with parents (Kelmanson, 2010).

SIDS **Sudden infant death syndrome (SIDS)** is a condition that occurs when infants stop breathing, usually during the night, and die suddenly without an apparent cause. SIDS remains the highest cause of infant death in the United States, with nearly 3,000 infant deaths attributed to it annually (Montagna & Chokroverty, 2011). Risk of SIDS is highest at 2 to 4 months of age (National Institute of Child Health and Human Development, 2013).

Since 1992, The American Academy of Pediatrics (AAP) has recommended that infants be placed to sleep on their backs to reduce the risk of SIDS, and the frequency of prone (on the stomach) sleeping among U.S. infants has dropped dramatically (Moon & Task Force on Sudden Infant Death Syndrome, 2016). Researchers have found that SIDS does indeed decrease when infants sleep on their backs rather than their stomachs or sides (Darrah & Bartlett, 2013). Among the reasons given for prone sleeping being a high-risk factor for SIDS are that it reduces an infant's cardiac output and the amount of blood pumped from the left ventricle of the heart on each beat (Wu & others, 2017).

In addition to sleeping in a prone position, researchers have found that the following are risk factors for SIDS:

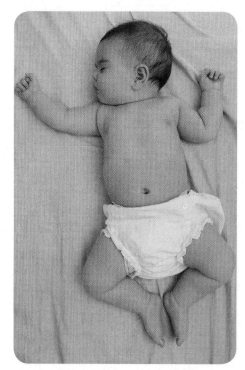

Is this a good sleep position for infants? Why or why not?
Maria Teijeiro/Cultura/Getty Images

- SIDS occurs more often in infants with abnormal brain stem functioning involving the neurotransmitter serotonin (Haynes & others, 2017).
- Heart arrhythmias linked to rare genetic variants are estimated to occur in as many as 15 percent of SIDS cases, and other genetic risks have been estimated to occur in up to 35 percent of SIDS cases (Baruteau & others, 2017; Neubauer & others, 2017).
- Six percent of infants with sleep apnea, a temporary cessation of breathing in which the airway is completely blocked, usually for 10 seconds or longer, die of SIDS (Ednick & others, 2010; McNamara & Sullivan, 2000).
- Low birth weight infants are 5 to 10 times more likely to die of SIDS than are their normal-weight counterparts (Horne & others, 2002).
- Infants whose siblings have died of SIDS are five to six times as likely to die of it (Corwin, 2018).
- African American and Eskimo infants are four to six times as likely as all others to die of SIDS (Ige & Shelton, 2004; Kitsantas & Gaffney, 2010).
- SIDS is more common in lower socioeconomic groups (Mitchell & others, 2000).
- Breast feeding for at least two months is linked to a lower incidence of SIDS, with greater protection against SIDS provided by breast feeding of longer duration (Thompson & others, 2017).
- Infants whose mothers smoked during pregnancy are two to three times more likely to die of SIDS than are infants whose mothers did not smoke during pregnancy (England & others, 2017).
- SIDS is more common when infants and parents share the same bed (Senter & others, 2010).
- SIDS is more common if infants sleep in soft bedding (Moon & Fu, 2012).

CHILDHOOD

A good night's sleep is an important aspect of a child's development (El-Sheikh & Kelly, 2017). The American Academy of Sleep Medicine recommends that young children get 11 to 14 hours of sleep each night and that first- to fifth-graders get 9 to 12 hours of sleep each night (Paruthi & others, 2016). Most young children sleep through the night and have one daytime nap. Not only is the amount of sleep children get important, but so is uninterrupted sleep (Verschuren, Gorter, & Pritchard-Wiart, 2017). However, it sometimes is difficult to get young children to go to sleep as they drag out their bedtime routine.

sudden infant death syndrome (SIDS) A condition that occurs when an infant stops breathing, usually during the night, and suddenly dies without an apparent cause.

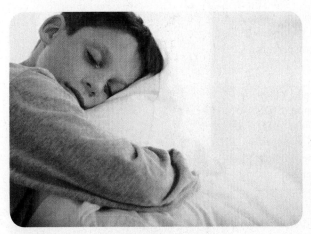

What characterizes children's sleep?
Sigrid Olsson/PhotoAlto

To improve sleep, Mona El-Sheikh and other sleep experts recommend ensuring that children have a bedroom that is cool, dark, and comfortable; consistent bed times and wake times; and positive family relationships (El-Sheikh & Kelly, 2017). Also, helping the child slow down before bedtime often contributes to less resistance in going to bed. Reading the child a story, playing quietly with the child in the bath, and letting the child sit on the caregiver's lap while listening to music are quieting activities.

Children can experience a number of sleep problems (Foley & Weinraub, 2017). One estimate indicates that more than 40 percent of children experience a sleep problem at some point in their development (Boyle & Cropley, 2004). The following research studies indicate links between children's sleep problems and negative developmental outcomes:

- Shorter sleep duration at age 12 predicted a greater likelihood of heavy alcohol use and marijuana use later in adolescence (Miller, Janssen, & Jackson, 2017).
- Sleep problems in early childhood predict subsequent problems with emotional regulation and attention, which in turn predict future sleep problems in a cycle that perpetuates over time (Williams & others, 2017).
- A review of research studies concluded that inadequate sleep during childhood is related to impairments in brain structures and functions (Dutil & others, 2018).
- Emotional security in parent-child and marital relationships is predictive of children's better sleep quality (El-Sheikh & Kelly, 2017).

ADOLESCENCE

There has recently been a surge of interest in adolescent sleep patterns (Tsai & others, 2018). This interest focuses on the belief that many adolescents are not getting enough sleep, that there are physiological underpinnings to the desire of adolescents, especially older ones, to stay up later at night and sleep longer in the morning, and that these findings have implications for understanding the times of day when adolescents learn most effectively in school (Agostini & others, 2017). For example, a national survey found that 8 percent of middle school students and 14 percent of high school students are late for school or miss school because they oversleep (National Sleep Foundation, 2006). Also in this survey, 6 percent of middle school students and 28 percent of high school students fall asleep in U.S. schools on any given day. Studies have confirmed that adolescents in other countries also are not getting adequate sleep (Leger & others, 2012; Short & others, 2012). For example, Asian adolescents have later bedtimes and get less sleep than U.S. adolescents (Gradisar, Gardner, & Dohnt, 2011).

Getting too little sleep in adolescence is linked to a number of problems, including risk-taking behaviors and substance use (Short & Weber, 2018), sleep disturbances in emerging and early adulthood (Fatima & others, 2017), and less effective attention (Beebe, Rose, & Amin, 2010). In one longitudinal study, Mexican American adolescents completed nightly sleep diaries for two weeks at the age of 15 and then again about a year later. The amount of sleep associated with the best mental health (in terms of less anxiety and depression and fewer behavior problems) was about one hour more than the amount of sleep associated with having the highest grades, suggesting complex trade-offs in different aspects of adjustment related to sleep (Fuligni & others, 2018).

Mary Carskadon (2011; Crowley & others, 2018) has conducted a number of research studies on adolescent sleep patterns. She has found that adolescents sleep an average of 9 hours and 25 minutes when given the opportunity to sleep as long as they like. Most adolescents get considerably less sleep than this, especially during the week. This creates a sleep debt, which adolescents often try to make up on the weekend. Carskadon also found that older adolescents are often more sleepy during the day than are younger adolescents and concluded that this was not because of factors such as academic work and social pressures. Rather, her research suggests that adolescents' biological clocks undergo a hormonal phase shift as they get older. This pushes the time of wakefulness to an hour later than when they were young adolescents. Carskadon found that this shift was caused by a delay in the nightly presence of the hormone *melatonin,* which is produced by the brain's pineal gland in preparing the body for sleep. Melatonin is secreted at about 9:30 p.m. in younger adolescents but is produced approximately an hour later in older adolescents, which delays the onset of sleep.

Carskadon determined that early school starting times can result in grogginess and lack of attention in class and poor performance on tests. Based on this research, some schools are now starting later (Gariépy & others, 2017). The American Academy of Sleep Medicine issued a position statement recommending that school boards and educational institutions implement start times no earlier than 8:30 a.m. in middle and high schools (Watson & others, 2017). Adolescents who attend schools with later start times get more sleep and have better school performance, better physical and mental health, and engage in less risky behavior, such as unsafe driving.

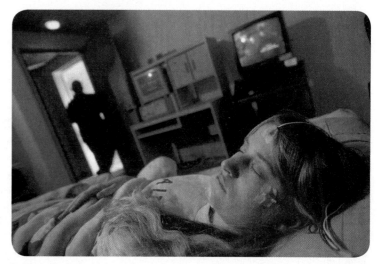

In Mary Carskadon's sleep laboratory at Brown University, an adolescent girl's brain activity is being monitored. Carskadon (2005) says that in the morning, sleep-deprived adolescents' "brains are telling them it's nighttime . . . and the rest of the world is saying it's time to go to school" (p. 19).
Courtesy of Jim LoScalzo

Review Connect Reflect

LG3 Summarize how sleep patterns change as children and adolescents develop.

Review

- How can sleep be characterized in infancy?
- What changes occur in sleep during childhood?
- How does adolescence affect sleep?

Connect

- In this section, you learned that exposure to cigarette smoke can affect an infant's risk for SIDS. What have you learned about cigarette smoke's effect on fetal development?

Reflect *Your Own Personal Journey of Life*

- Did your sleep patterns start to change when you became an adolescent? Have they changed since you went through puberty? If so, how?

Health **LG4** Characterize children's health.

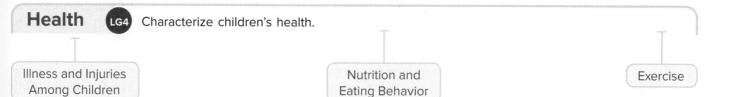

Illness and Injuries Among Children

Nutrition and Eating Behavior

Exercise

What are the major threats to children's health today? We will look first at the major illnesses and injuries experienced by children and adolescents before turning to less obvious threats to healthy development: poor nutrition and eating habits, and lack of exercise. The formation of healthy habits in childhood, such as eating fruits and vegetables and engaging in regular exercise, not only has immediate benefits but also contributes to the delay or prevention of premature disability and mortality in adulthood from heart disease, stroke, diabetes, and cancer. And adolescence is a critical juncture in the adoption of many health-enhancing behaviors, such as regular exercise, and health-compromising behaviors, such as smoking (Dunne & others, 2017).

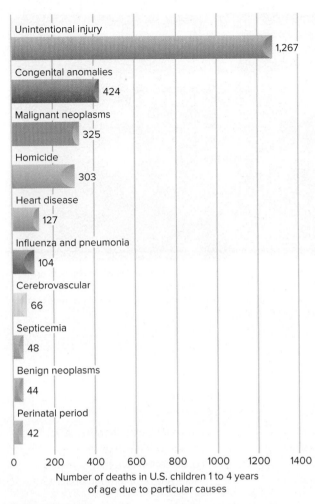

FIGURE **17**

MAIN CAUSES OF DEATH IN CHILDREN 1 THROUGH 4 YEARS OF AGE. These figures show the 10 leading causes of death for children 1 to 4 years of age in 2017 (National Vital Statistics Reports, 2017).

ILLNESS AND INJURIES AMONG CHILDREN

In this section, we first examine broad patterns in the causes of illness and death among children and adolescents. Then we turn to the difficulties faced by poor children in the United States and around the world.

Early Childhood Young children's active and exploratory nature, coupled with being unaware of danger in many instances, often puts them in situations in which they are at risk for injuries. Most of the cuts, bumps, and bruises sustained by young children are minor, but some accidental injuries can produce serious impairment or even death. In the United States, unintentional injuries (such as in motor vehicle accidents) are the leading cause of death in young children, followed by congenital anomalies and cancer (Centers for Disease Control and Prevention, 2016) (see Figure 17). In addition to motor vehicle accidents, other accidental deaths in children involve drowning, falls, burns, and poisoning (McDonald & others, 2018).

An increasing number of studies reach the conclusion that children are at risk for health problems when they live in homes in which a parent smokes (Been & others, 2013; Hwang & others, 2012). Children exposed to tobacco smoke in the home are more likely to develop wheezing symptoms and asthma than children in nonsmoking homes (Yi & others, 2012). Parental smoking is a risk factor for higher blood pressure in children (Cabral & others, 2017). Exposure to secondhand smoke is also related to young children's sleep problems (Plancoulaine & others, 2018).

An estimated 4 million U.S. households include children who are exposed to high levels of lead (Centers for Disease Control and Prevention, 2018). Half a million American children between 1 and 5 years of age have blood lead levels that exceed the threshold at which intervention is recommended. The negative effects of high lead levels in children's blood include lower intelligence, lower achievement, attention deficit hyperactivity disorder, and elevated blood pressure (Hauptman, Bruccoleri, & Woolf, 2017). Children in poverty face a higher risk for lead poisoning than children living in higher socioeconomic conditions (Muller, Sampson, & Winter, 2018).

Middle and Late Childhood For the most part, middle and late childhood is a time of excellent health (Centers for Disease Control and Prevention, 2018). Disease and death are less prevalent in this period than in early childhood and adolescence.

The most common cause of severe injury and death in middle and late childhood is motor vehicle accidents, either as a pedestrian or as a passenger (Centers for Disease Control and Prevention, 2018). Using safety-belt restraints is important in reducing the severity of motor vehicle injuries.

Most accidents occur in or near the child's home or school. The most effective strategy for preventing injury is to educate the child about the hazards of risk taking and improper use of equipment (Centers for Disease Control and Prevention, 2018). Appropriate safety helmets, protective eye and mouth shields, and protective padding are recommended for children who engage in active sports.

Cancer Children not only are vulnerable to injuries but also may develop life-threatening diseases. Cancer is the leading cause of disease-related deaths during childhood, with approximately 10,600 new cases of childhood cancer diagnosed each year in the United States (National Cancer Institute, 2018).

Childhood cancers have a different profile from adult cancers. Cancers in adults attack mainly the lungs, colon, breast, prostate, and pancreas. In children, cancers mainly attack the white blood cells (leukemia), brain, bone, lymphatic system, muscles, kidneys, and nervous system. Researchers are intensely searching for possible genetic links to childhood cancers (Karlsson & others, 2018).

The most common cancer in children is leukemia, a cancer of the tissues that make blood cells (Kelly & others, 2013). In leukemia, the bone marrow makes an abundance of white blood cells that don't function properly. They crowd out normal cells, making the child susceptible to bruising and infection.

Because of advancements in cancer treatment, children with cancer are surviving longer (Loeffen & others, 2017). Approximately 80 percent of children with acute lymphoblastic leukemia are cured with current chemotherapy treatment (Wayne, 2011). Death rates from childhood cancer have declined by 57 percent in the last four decades (National Cancer Institute, 2018).

Cardiovascular Disease   Cardiovascular disease is uncommon in children. Nonetheless, environmental experiences and behavior in the childhood years can sow the seeds for cardiovascular disease in adulthood. Many elementary-school-aged children already possess one or more of the risk factors for cardiovascular disease, such as hypertension and obesity (Malatesta-Muncher & Mitsnefes, 2012; Peters & others, 2012). Hypertension and high blood pressure during childhood are under-recognized and under-diagnosed (Dionne, 2017). Nevertheless, treating these conditions is important not only to promote children's health but also to prevent health problems stemming from early hypertension and high blood pressure that otherwise will likely continue and worsen during adulthood (Baker-Smith & others, 2018).

Health, Illness, and Poverty Among the World's Children   An estimated 7 percent of U.S. children receive no health care, and the vast majority of these children live in poverty. One approach to children's health aims to treat not only medical problems of the individual child but also the conditions of the entire family. In fact, some programs seek to identify children who are at risk for problems and then try to alter the risk factors in an effort to prevent illness and disease.

Poverty in the United States is dwarfed by poverty in developing countries around the world. Each year UNICEF produces a report entitled *The State of the World's Children.* In recent years, the following factors that are especially influenced by poverty are linked

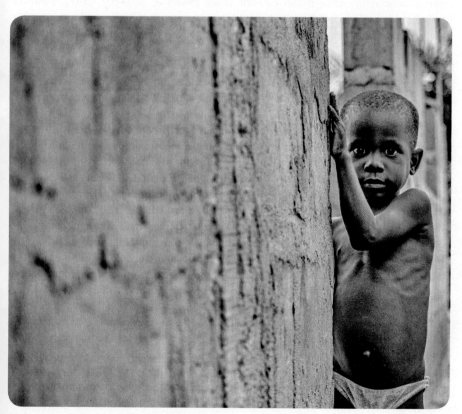

What are some of the main causes of death in young children around the world?
Bojstudios/Shutterstock

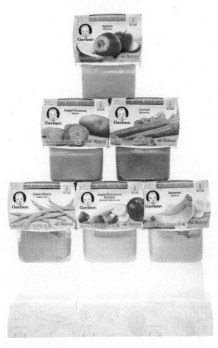

Keith Homan/Shutterstock

to the under-5 mortality rate: the nutritional health and health knowledge of mothers, levels of immunization, dehydration, availability of maternal and child health services, income and food availability in the family, availability of clean water and safe sanitation, and the overall safety of the child's environment.

Devastating effects on the health of young children occur in countries where poverty rates are high (UNICEF, 2017). The poor are the majority in nearly one of every five nations in the world (UNICEF, 2017). They often experience hunger, malnutrition, illness, inadequate access to health care, unsafe water, and a lack of protection from harm (Ahmed & others, 2017).

Worldwide, HIV/AIDS is a serious problem faced by millions of children whose parents have died of the virus, transmitted it to their children, or both (UNICEF, 2018). About 2.3 million children globally are estimated to be living with HIV, and over 15 million children have lost one or both parents to AIDS.

Many of the deaths of young children around the world can be prevented by a reduction in poverty and improvements in nutrition, sanitation, education, and health services (Riumallo-Herl & others, 2018).

NUTRITION AND EATING BEHAVIOR

Poverty influences health in part through its effects on nutrition. However, it is not just children living in low-income families who have health-related nutrition problems; across the spectrum of income levels, recent decades have seen a dramatic increase in the percent of U.S. children who are overweight.

Infancy From birth to 1 year of age, human infants nearly triple their weight and increase their length by 50 percent. What do they need to sustain this growth?

Nutritional Needs and Eating Behavior Individual differences among infants in terms of their nutrient reserves, body composition, growth rates, and activity patterns make it difficult to define actual nutrient needs (Miles & Siega-Riz, 2017). However, because parents need guidelines, nutritionists recommend that infants consume approximately 50 calories per day for each pound they weigh—more than twice an adult's requirement per pound.

A national study of Americans indicated that by 6 months, 37 percent of infants were already consuming snacks and that by the age of 12 months, 25 percent of daily energy intake was from snacks (Deming & others, 2017). Infants are consuming more junk food and fewer fruits and vegetables than recommended by nutrition experts. For example, 25 percent of 6- to 11-month-olds and 20 percent of 12- to 23-month-olds consumed no vegetables over the course of the study period in a national sample of Americans (Miles & Siega-Riz, 2017).

Such poor dietary patterns early in development can result in more infants being overweight (Thorisdottir, Gunnarsdottir, & Thorisdottir, 2013). The Centers for Disease Control and Prevention (2018) defines overweight as having a body mass index (BMI) between the 85th and 95th percentile and defines obesity as having a BMI at or above the 95th percentile for children of the same age and sex. BMI is computed by dividing an individual's weight in kilograms by the square of his or her height in meters.

One analysis revealed that in 1980, 3.4 percent of U.S. babies less than 6 months old were overweight, a percentage that increased to 5.9 percent in 2001 (Kim & others, 2006). As shown in Figure 18, as younger infants become older infants, an even greater percentage are overweight. Also in this study, in addition to the 5.9 percent of infants less than 6 months old who were overweight in 2001, another 11 percent were categorized as at risk for being overweight.

In addition to consuming too many French fries, sweetened drinks, and desserts, are there other factors that might explain this increase in overweight U.S. infants? A mother's weight gain during pregnancy and a mother's own

FIGURE **18**

PERCENTAGE OF OVERWEIGHT U.S. INFANTS IN 1980–1981 AND 2000–2001. *Note:* Infants above the 95th percentile for their age and gender on a weight-for-height index were categorized as overweight.

high weight before pregnancy may be factors (Rios-Castillo & others, 2013). One important factor seems to be whether an infant is breast-fed or bottle-fed. Breast-fed infants have lower rates of weight gain than bottle-fed infants by school age, and it is estimated that breast feeding reduces the risk of obesity by approximately 20 percent (Li & others, 2007).

Breast Versus Bottle Feeding   For the first four to six months of life, human milk or an alternative formula is the baby's source of nutrients and energy. A large body of scientific research demonstrates that breast feeding provides better nutrition and a number of other benefits for infants compared with formula feeding (Hakala & others, 2017). Since the 1970s, breast feeding by U.S. mothers has soared. The World Health Organization (2018) recommends exclusive breast feeding in the first six months followed by continued breast feeding as complementary foods are introduced, and further breast feeding for one year or longer as mutually desired by the mother and infant. Figure 19 shows current rates of breast feeding for infants born in the United States.

What are some of the benefits of breast feeding? The following conclusions are based on the current status of research:

Evaluation of Outcomes for Child

- *Gastrointestinal infections.* Breast-fed infants have fewer gastrointestinal infections (Stuebe & others, 2017).

- *Lower respiratory tract infections.* Breast-fed infants have fewer infections of the lower respiratory tract (Prameela, 2011).

- *Allergies.* A research review by the American Academy of Pediatrics indicated that there is no evidence that breast feeding reduces the risk of allergies in children (Greer & others, 2008). The research review also concluded that modest evidence exists for feeding hypoallergenic formulas to susceptible babies if they are not solely breast-fed.

- *Asthma.* The research review by the American Academy of Pediatrics concluded that exclusive breast feeding for three months protects against wheezing in babies, but whether it prevents asthma in older children is unclear (Greer & others, 2008).

- *Otitis media.* Breast-fed infants are less likely to develop this middle ear infection (Stuebe & others, 2017).

- *Atopic dermatitis.* Breast-fed babies are less likely to have this chronic inflammation of the skin (Vaughn & others, 2017).

- *Overweight and obesity.* Research indicates that breast-fed infants are less likely to become overweight or obese in childhood, adolescence, and adulthood (Uwaezuoke, Eneh, & Ndu, 2017).

- *Diabetes.* Breast-fed infants are less likely to develop type 1 diabetes in childhood (Ping & Hagopian, 2006) and type 2 diabetes in adulthood (Villegas & others, 2008).

- *SIDS.* Breast-fed infants are less likely to experience SIDS (Zotter & Pichler, 2012).

In large-scale research reviews, no conclusive evidence for the benefits of breast feeding was found for children's cognitive development and cardiovascular health (Agency for Healthcare Research and Quality, 2007; Ip & others, 2009).

Evaluation of Outcomes for Mother

- *Breast cancer.* Consistent evidence indicates a lower incidence of breast cancer in women who breast feed their infants (Unar-Munguía & others, 2017).

- *Ovarian cancer.* Evidence also reveals a reduction in ovarian cancer in women who breast feed their infants (Danial & others, 2018).

- *Type 2 diabetes.* Some evidence suggests a small reduction in type 2 diabetes in women who breast feed their infants (Ip & others, 2009; Stuebe & Schwartz, 2010).

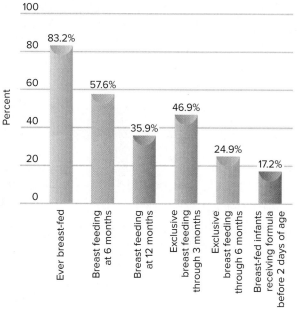

FIGURE **19**

BREAST FEEDING RATES FOR INFANTS BORN IN THE UNITED STATES IN 2015. Statistics are based on data released in 2018 by the Centers for Disease Control and Prevention.
Source: https://www.cdc.gov/breastfeeding/data/reportcard.htm

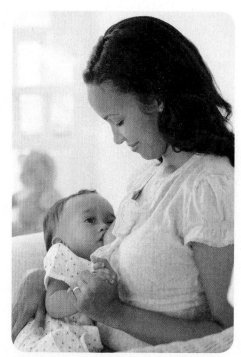

Human milk or an alternative formula is a baby's source of nutrients for the first four to six months. The growing consensus is that breast feeding is better for the baby's health, although controversy still swirls about the issue of breast feeding versus bottle feeding. *Why is breast feeding strongly recommended by pediatricians?*
Blend Images/Getty Images

In large-scale research reviews, no conclusive evidence could be found for maternal benefits of breast feeding with regard to return to prepregnancy weight, protection from osteoporosis, and reduced rates of postpartum depression (Agency for Healthcare Research and Quality, 2007; Ip & others, 2009). However, women who breast feed their infants have a lower risk of cardiovascular disease and a lower incidence of metabolic syndrome (a disorder characterized by obesity, hypertension, and insulin resistance) in midlife (Nguyen, Jin, & Ding, 2017).

Many health professionals have argued that breast feeding facilitates the development of an attachment bond between the mother and infant (Gibbs, Forste, & Lybbert, 2018). However, a research review found that the positive role of breast feeding on the mother-infant relationship is not supported by research (Jansen, de Weerth, & Riksen-Walraven, 2008). The review concluded that recommending breast feeding should not be based on its role in improving the mother-infant relationship but rather on its positive effects on infant and maternal health.

The World Health Organization (2018) strongly endorses breast feeding throughout the first year of life. Are there circumstances when mothers should not breast feed? Yes, a mother should not breast feed (1) when she is infected with HIV or some other infectious disease that can be transmitted through her milk, (2) if she has active tuberculosis, or (3) if she is taking any drug that may not be safe for the infant (Goga & others, 2012).

Some women cannot breast feed their infants because of physical difficulties; others feel guilty if they terminate breast feeding early. Mothers may also worry that they are depriving their infants of important emotional and psychological benefits if they bottle feed rather than breast feed.

A further issue in interpreting the benefits of breast feeding was underscored in large-scale research reviews (Agency for Healthcare Research and Quality, 2007; Ip & others, 2009). While highlighting a number of breast feeding benefits for children and mothers, the report issued a caution about breast feeding research: None of the findings imply causality. Breast versus bottle feeding studies are correlational rather than experimental, and women who breast feed are wealthier, older, more educated, and likely more health-conscious than their bottle-feeding counterparts, which could explain why breast-fed children are healthier.

Malnutrition in Infancy   Early weaning of infants from breast milk to inadequate sources of nutrients, such as unsuitable and unsanitary cow's milk formula, can cause protein deficiency and malnutrition in infants (World Health Organization, 2018). Something that looks like milk but is not, usually a form of tapioca or rice, is also often substituted for breast milk. In many of the world's developing countries, mothers used to breast feed their infants for at least two years. To become more modern, they stopped breast feeding much earlier and replaced it with bottle feeding. Comparisons of breast-fed and bottle-fed infants in countries such as Afghanistan, Haiti, Ghana, and Chile document that the mortality rate of bottle-fed infants is as much as five times that of breast-fed infants (Grant, 1997). However, in the *Connecting with Diversity* interlude, you can read about a recent concern regarding breast feeding.

Two life-threatening conditions that can result from malnutrition are marasmus and kwashiorkor. **Marasmus** is caused by a severe protein-calorie deficiency and results in a wasting away of body tissues in the infant's first year. The infant becomes grossly underweight and his or her muscles atrophy. **Kwashiorkor,** caused by severe protein deficiency, usually appears between 1 and 3 years of age. Children with kwashiorkor sometimes appear to be well fed even though they are not because the disease can cause the child's abdomen and feet to swell with water. Kwashiorkor causes a child's vital organs to collect the nutrients that are present and deprive other parts of the body of them. The child's hair becomes thin, brittle, and colorless, and the child's behavior often becomes listless.

Even if it is not fatal, severe and lengthy malnutrition is detrimental to physical, cognitive, and socioemotional development (Schiff, 2013). A study of Indian children documented the negative influence of chronic malnutrition on children's cognitive development. Children who had a history of malnutrition had more problems with executive functioning (cognitive processes to control behavior) than their counterparts who were not malnourished (Selvam & others, 2018).

developmental **connection**

Research Methods

How does a correlational study differ from an experimental study? Connect to "Introduction."

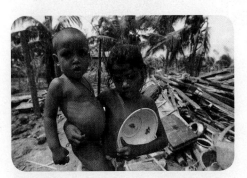

This *Bangladeshi* child has kwashiorkor. Notice the telltale sign of kwashiorkor—a greatly expanded abdomen. *What are some other characteristics of kwashiorkor?*
Peter Charlesworth/LightRocket/Getty Images

marasmus Severe malnutrition caused by an insufficient protein-calorie intake, resulting in a shrunken, elderly appearance.

kwashiorkor Severe malnutrition caused by a protein-deficient diet, causing the feet and abdomen to swell with water.

connecting with diversity

The Stories of Latonya and Ramona: Breast and Bottle Feeding in Africa

Latonya is a newborn baby in Ghana. During her first days of life, she has been kept apart from her mother and bottle-fed. Manufacturers of infant formula provide free or subsidized milk powder to the hospital where she was born. Her mother has been persuaded to bottle feed rather than breast feed Latonya. When her mother bottle feeds Latonya, she overdilutes the milk formula with unclean water. Latonya's feeding bottles have not been sterilized. Latonya becomes very sick, and she dies before her first birthday.

Ramona was born in Nigeria, where her family takes part in a "baby-friendly" program. In this program, babies are not separated from their mothers when they are born, and the mothers are encouraged to breast feed them. The mothers are told of the perils that bottle feeding can bring because of unsafe water and unsterilized bottles. They also are informed about the advantages of breast milk, which include its nutritious and hygienic qualities, its ability to immunize babies against common illnesses, and its role in reducing the mother's risk of breast and ovarian cancer. Ramona's mother is breast feeding her. At 1 year of age, Ramona is very healthy.

For many years, maternity units in hospitals favored bottle feeding and did not give mothers adequate information about the benefits of breast feeding. In recent years, the World Health Organization and UNICEF have tried to reverse the trend toward bottle feeding of infants in many impoverished countries. They instituted the "baby-friendly" program in many countries. They also persuaded the International Association of Infant Formula Manufacturers to stop marketing their baby formulas to hospitals in countries where the governments support the baby-friendly initiatives (Grant, 1997). For the hospitals themselves, costs actually were reduced as infant formula, feeding bottles, and separate nurseries became unnecessary. For example, baby-friendly Jose Fabella Memorial Hospital in the Philippines reported saving 8 percent of its annual budget.

The advantages of breast feeding in impoverished countries are substantial. However, these advantages must be balanced against the risk of passing HIV to babies through breast milk if the mothers have the virus; the majority of mothers don't know that they are infected (Fox & others, 2018). In some areas of Africa, more than 30 percent of mothers have the human immunodeficiency virus (HIV).

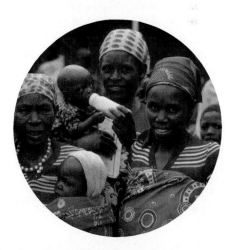

(Top) An HIV-infected mother breast feeding her baby in Nairobi, Africa. (Bottom) A Rwandan mother bottle feeding her baby. What are some concerns about breast versus bottle feeding in impoverished African countries?
(Top): Wendy Stone/Corbis Documentary/Getty Images; *(Bottom)*: Dave Bartruff/Corbis Documentary/Getty Images

In what ways does education play a role in the health decisions discussed in this interlude?

Improving the Nutrition of Infants and Young Children Living in Low-Income Families

Poor nutrition is a special concern in the lives of infants from low-income families. To address this problem in the United States, the WIC (Women, Infants, and Children) program provides federal grants to states for healthy supplemental foods, health care referrals, and nutrition education for women from low-income families beginning in pregnancy, and to infants and young children up to 5 years of age who are at nutritional risk (Ng & others, 2018). WIC serves approximately 7,500,000 participants in the United States.

Positive influences on infants' and young children's nutrition and health have been found for participants in WIC (Koleilat & others, 2017). One study revealed that a WIC program that introduced peer counseling services for pregnant women increased breast feeding initiation by 27 percent (Olson & others, 2010a, b). Another study found that entry during the first trimester of pregnancy to the WIC program in Rhode Island reduced maternal cigarette smoking (Brodsky, Viner-Brown, & Handler, 2009). And a multiple-year literacy intervention with Spanish-speaking families in the WIC program in Los Angeles increased literacy resources and activities at home, which in turn led to a higher level of school readiness in children (Whaley & others, 2011).

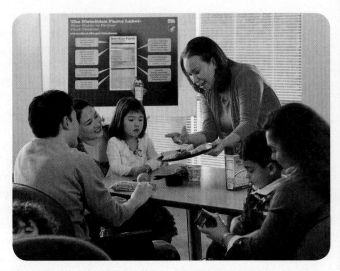

Participants in the WIC program. *What characterizes the WIC program?*
Source: USDA Food and Nutrition Service, Supplemental Nutrition Assistance Program

Why would the WIC program provide lactation counseling as part of its services?

Several studies in different countries have examined the effects of nutritional supplements by randomly assigning children to experimental conditions that involve nutritional supplements or control groups that do not. In Guatemala, for example, children whose mothers received nutritional supplements during pregnancy and up to 6 months postpartum and who themselves received nutritional supplements from 6 to 24 months of age were less likely to be stunted (low height for age) than were children who received no supplements (Olney & others, 2018). The benefits of nutritional supplements extend beyond physical growth and include enhanced cognitive and psychosocial development. In a review of 67 interventions in 20 low- and middle-income countries, nutritional supplements were found to enhance children's cognitive development; in addition to benefits of administering nutritional supplements to children, providing nutritional supplements to mothers during the first trimester of pregnancy was found to boost their children's cognitive development (Ip & others, 2017). To read further about improving infants' and young children's nutrition, as well as other aspects of their lives, see *Caring Connections*.

Adequate early nutrition is an important aspect of healthy development (Hurley & others, 2013; Schiff, 2013). In addition to sound nutrition, children need a nurturing, supportive environment (Johnson & others, 2018). Caregivers who are not sensitive to developmental changes in infants' nutritional needs, neglectful caregivers, and conditions of poverty can contribute to the development of eating problems in infants (Galloway & others, 2018). Low maternal sensitivity is a risk factor for children's obesity, particularly when children are more genetically susceptible to environmental influences (Levitan & others, 2017).

One individual who has stood out as an advocate of caring for children is T. Berry Brazelton, who is featured in the *Connecting with Careers* profile.

T. Berry Brazelton, Pediatrician

T. Berry Brazelton is America's best-known pediatrician as a result of his numerous books, television appearances, and newspaper and magazine articles about parenting and children's health. He takes a family-centered approach to child development issues and communicates with parents in easy-to-understand ways.

Dr. Brazelton founded the Child Development Unit at Boston Children's Hospital and created the Brazelton Neonatal Behavioral Assessment Scale, a widely used measure of the newborn's health and well-being. He also has conducted a number of research studies on infants and children and has been president of the Society for Research in Child Development, a leading research organization.

For more information about what pediatricians do, see the Careers in Child Development appendix.

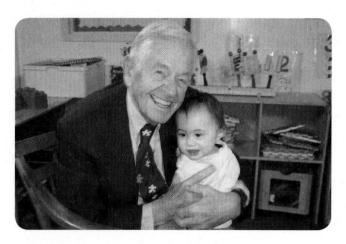

T. Berry Brazelton, pediatrician, with a young child.
Courtesy Brazelton Touchpoints Center

Childhood   Poor nutrition in childhood can lead to a number of problems and occurs more frequently in low-income than in higher-income families. A special concern is the increasing epidemic of overweight children.

Eating Behavior and Parental Feeding Styles   For most children in the United States, insufficient food is not the key problem. Instead, unhealthy eating habits and being overweight threaten their present and future health. A study of 2- and 3-year-olds found that French fries and other fried potatoes were the vegetable they were most likely to consume (Fox, Levitt, & Nelson, 2010).

Children's eating behavior is strongly influenced by their caregivers' behavior (Campbell & others, 2018). Children's eating behavior improves when caregivers eat with children on a predictable schedule, model eating healthy food, make mealtimes pleasant occasions, and engage in certain feeding styles. Distractions from television, family arguments, and competing activities should be minimized so children can focus on eating. A sensitive/responsive caregiver feeding style is recommended, in which the caregiver is nurturant, provides clear information about what is expected, and responds appropriately to children's cues (Campbell & others, 2018). Forceful and restrictive caregiver behaviors are not recommended. For example, a restrictive feeding style is linked to children being overweight (Johnson & others, 2018).

Overweight Children   Being overweight has become a serious health problem in early childhood (Centers for Disease Control and Prevention, 2018). A national study revealed that 45 percent of children's meals exceed recommendations for saturated and trans fat, which can raise cholesterol levels and increase the risk of heart disease (Center for Science in the Public Interest, 2008). This study also found that one-third of children's daily caloric intake comes from restaurants, twice the percentage consumed away from home in the 1980s. Further, 93 percent of almost 1,500 possible choices at 13 major fast food chains exceeded 430 calories—one-third of what the National Institute of Medicine recommends that 4- to 8-year-old children consume in a day. Nearly all of the children's meal options offered at KFC, Taco Bell, Sonic, Jack in the Box, and Chick-fil-A were too high in calories.

The percentages of young children who are overweight or at risk of becoming overweight in the United States have increased dramatically in recent decades, and these percentages are likely to grow unless changes occur in children's lifestyles (Ward & others, 2017).

In the United States, obesity is more prevalent in Hispanic (26 percent) and non-Hispanic African American (22 percent) children than in non-Hispanic White (14 percent) or Asian American (11 percent) children (Centers for Disease Control and Prevention, 2018).

It is not just in the United States that children are becoming more overweight. Childhood obesity is one of the most pressing public health challenges of the 21st century, according to the World Health Organization (2018), with an estimated 41 million children under the age of 5 years currently classified as obese and the proportion of obese children worldwide increasing at an alarming rate.

The risk that overweight young children will continue to be overweight when they are older was documented in a study in which 80 percent of the children who were at risk for being overweight at age 3 were also at risk for being overweight or were overweight at age 12 (Nader & others, 2006). Another study revealed that preschool children who were overweight were at significant risk for being overweight/obese at age 12 (Shankaran & others, 2011).

Being overweight in childhood also is linked to being overweight in adulthood. One study revealed that girls who were overweight in childhood were 11 to 30 times more likely to be obese in adulthood than girls who were not overweight in childhood (Thompson & others, 2007).

The increase in overweight children in recent decades is cause for great concern because being overweight raises the risk for many medical and psychological problems (Anspaugh & Ezell, 2013). Diabetes, hypertension (high blood pressure), and elevated blood cholesterol levels are common in children who are overweight (Pulgaron, 2013; Riley & Bluhm, 2012). Once considered rare in childhood, hypertension has become increasingly common in overweight children (Lytle, 2012). Social and psychological consequences of being overweight in childhood include low self-esteem, depression, and some exclusion of obese children from peer groups (Lin & others, 2018). In one study, obese children were found to spend less time with friends after school, to communicate less with friends through social media, to be bullied, and to be less likely to perceive their best friend as a confidant (Kjelgaard & others, 2017). In a nationally representative sample of American children, being overweight was related to a number of later negative physical and psychological outcomes, effects that were partly accounted for by overweight children's greater likelihood of being bullied (Lee, Jeong, & Roh, 2018).

Both heredity and environment influence whether children will become overweight. Genetic analysis indicates that heredity is an important factor in children becoming overweight (Loos & Janssens, 2017). Overweight parents tend to have overweight children, even if they are not living in the same household (Schiff, 2013). One study found that the greatest risk factor for being overweight at 9 years of age was having a parent who was overweight (Agras & others, 2004). Having two overweight/obese parents significantly increases the likelihood of a child being overweight/obese (Xu & others, 2011).

Environmental factors that influence whether children become overweight or not include the greater availability of food (especially food high in fat content), energy-saving devices, declining physical activity, parents' eating habits and monitoring of children's eating habits, the context in which a child eats, and heavy screen time (watching TV, playing video games, texting, and so on) (Potter & others, 2018). A behavior modification study of overweight and obese children made watching TV contingent on their engagement in exercise (Goldfield, 2011). The intervention markedly increased their exercise and reduced their TV viewing time.

Parents play an important role in preventing children from becoming overweight (Wilson & others, 2017). Intervention programs that emphasize getting parents to engage in healthier lifestyles themselves, as well as feeding their children healthier food and getting them to exercise more, can produce weight reduction in overweight and obese children (Campbell-Voytal & others, 2017). For example, in a 3-month intervention that compared weight loss of children randomly assigned to different intervention conditions, children lost the most weight if they participated jointly with their parents in the intervention, and these

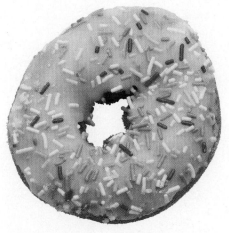

Jules Frazier/Getty Images

Faize Mustafa-Infante, Pediatrician

Dr. Faize Mustafa-Infante grew up in Colombia, South America. She initially taught elementary school students in Colombia and then obtained her medical degree with a specialty in pediatrics. Once she finished her medical training, she moved to San Bernardino, California, working as a health educator with a focus on preventing and treating child obesity in low-income communities. Dr. Mustafa-Infante currently works at Mission Pediatrics in Riverside, California, where she mainly treats infants. She continues her effort to prevent obesity in children and also serves as a volunteer for Ayacucho Mission, a nonprofit organization that provides culturally sensitive medical care for people living in poverty in Ayacucho, Peru. In regard to her cultural background, Dr. Mustafa-Infante describes herself as a Latino doctor with a middle-eastern name that reflects her strong family commitments to both heritages. Dr. Mustafa-Infante says that hard work and education have been the keys to her success and personal satisfaction.

positive effects were sustained up to 2 years following the intervention (Yackobovitch-Gavan & others, 2018). Some intervention programs with overweight children are conducted through schools and often focus on teaching children and parents about developing a healthy diet, exercising more, and reducing screen time (Ward & others, 2017). A promising strategy is to provide students with healthier foods to eat at school. Several states now have laws that require healthier foods to be sold in vending machines at schools. In one intervention, reducing soft drink consumption at schools was linked with a subsequent reduction in the number of 7- to 11-year-old children who were overweight (James & others, 2004).

In sum, healthy eating and an active rather than sedentary lifestyle play important roles in children's development (Kotte, Winkler, & Takken, 2013; Wang & others, 2013). Pediatricians can influence the health of children by providing advice to parents about ways to improve their children's eating habits and activity levels. To read about the work of one pediatrician, see the *Connecting with Careers* profile of Dr. Faize Mustafa-Infante.

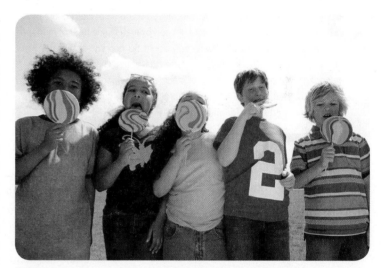

What are some concerns about overweight children?
Image Source/Getty Images

EXERCISE

Exercise can make significant contributions not only to children's physical development but also to their cognitive development and mental health (Petruzzello & others, 2018). In this section we will explore developmental aspects of children's exercise and the roles of parents, schools, and screen-based activity.

Early Childhood   Routine physical activity should be a daily occurrence for young children. Guidelines recommend that preschool children engage in two hours of physical activity per day, divided into one hour of structured activity and at least one hour of unstructured free play (Society of Health and Physical Educators, 2018). The child's life should be centered around activities, not meals.

Following are descriptions of research studies that examine young children's exercise and activities:

- Observations of 3- to 5-year-old children during outdoor play at preschools revealed that the preschool children were mainly sedentary even when participating in outdoor play (Brown & others, 2009). In this study, throughout the day the preschoolers were sedentary 89 percent of the time, engaged in light activity 8 percent of the time, and participated in moderate to vigorous physical activity only 3 percent of the time.

Are Preschool Children Getting Enough Physical Activity?

One study examined the activity level of 281 3- to 5-year-olds in nine preschools (Pate & others, 2004). Each child wore an accelerometer (a small activity monitor) for four to five hours a day. Height and weight assessments of the children were made to calculate each child's body mass index (BMI).

Activity guidelines recommend that preschool children engage in two hours of physical activity per day, divided into one hour of structured activity and one hour of unstructured free play (Society of Health and Physical Educators, 2018). In this study, the young children participated in an average of 7.7 minutes per hour of moderate to vigorous activity, usually in a block of time when they were outside. Over the course of eight hours of a preschool day, these children would get approximately one hour of moderate and vigorous physical activity, only about 50 percent of the amount recommended. The researchers concluded that young children are unlikely to engage in another hour per day of moderate and vigorous physical activity outside their eight hours spent in preschool and thus are not getting adequate opportunities for physical activity.

Gender and age differences characterized the preschool children's physical activity. Boys were more likely to engage in moderate or vigorous physical activity than girls. Children who were 4 or 5 years old were more likely to be sedentary than 3-year-old children.

The young children's physical activity also varied according to the particular preschool they attended. The extent to which they participated in moderate and vigorous physical activity ranged from 4.4 to 10.2 minutes per hour across the nine preschools. Thus, the policies and practices of particular preschools influence the extent to which children engage in physical activity. The researchers concluded that young children need more vigorous play and organized activities. Unfortunately, there is a trend toward reducing time for physical activity, especially eliminating recess, in U.S. elementary schools that is trickling down to kindergarten and preschool programs. This decrease is part of a larger trend that involves narrowing early childhood programs to focus on academic learning and moving away from more comprehensive programs that focus on the whole child (Hyson, Copple, & Jones, 2006).

- Preschool children's physical activity is enhanced by participating in sports and play together, but less than 1 percent of time that mothers and young children spend together is in moderate to vigorous physical activity (Dlugonski, DuBose, & Rider, 2017).
- Preschool children are more physically active if they spend time outdoors and live in a safe neighborhood (Schmutz & others, 2017).
- A research review concluded that more screen time (watching TV, using a computer) at 4 to 6 years of age was linked to a lower activity level and being overweight from preschool through adolescence (te Velde & others, 2012).

To find out how much activity most preschool students are currently getting, see *Connecting Through Research.*

Middle and Late Childhood   A large number of studies document the importance of exercise in children's physical development (Han & others, 2017). Vigorous physical

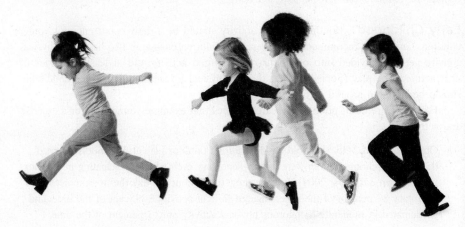

What are some positive outcomes when young children exercise regularly?
RubberBall Productions/Getty Images

activity has benefits for children above and beyond the benefits of moderate physical activity (Owens, Galloway, & Gutin, 2017). A higher level of physical activity is linked to a lower level of metabolic disease (Nyström & others, 2017). Interventions have found that even brief interruptions in sedentary behavior (with 3 minutes of moderate-intensity walking every 30 minutes across 3 hours) improve glucose metabolism and are a promising strategy for reducing metabolic risk in overweight and obese children (Broadney & others, 2018).

A research review concluded that aerobic exercise also increasingly is linked to children's cognitive skills (Best, 2010). Researchers have found that aerobic exercise benefits children's attention, memory, effortful and goal-directed thinking and behavior, and creativity (Fair & others, 2017).

Adolescence   Gender and ethnic differences in exercise participation rates are noteworthy, and they reflect the trend of decreasing exercise from early through late adolescence. One study revealed that 40 percent of female and 57 percent of male adolescents met U.S. guidelines for physical activity (Butcher & others, 2008). A national study also found that adolescent boys were much more likely to engage in 60 minutes or more of vigorous exercise per day than were girls (Eaton & others, 2012). Also, as indicated in Figure 20, in the National Youth Risk Survey, non-Latino White boys exercised the most, African American girls the least (Eaton & others, 2012).

Exercise is linked to a number of positive outcomes in adolescence, including weight regulation as well as lower levels of blood pressure and type 2 diabetes (Goldfield & others, 2012; So & others, 2013). Consider also these studies that found positive effects of exercise on a range of adolescent outcomes:

- Adolescents who engaged in higher levels of exercise had lower levels of alcohol, cigarette, and marijuana use (Teery-McElrath, O'Malley, & Johnston, 2012).

- A daily morning running program for three weeks improved the sleep quality, mood, and concentration of adolescents (Kalak & others, 2012).

- Engaging in a 12-week exercise intervention lowered the depression of adolescents who were depressed and not regular exercisers (Dopp & others, 2012).

- Participating in regular exercise is associated with better cognition, including memory, creativity, and perception (Misuraca, Miceli, & Teuscher, 2017).

Parents, Peers, Schools, and the Media   Parents play important roles in children's and adolescents' exercise habits and physical activity (Lindsay & others, 2018). Growing up with parents who regularly exercise provides positive models of exercise for children and adolescents.

Peers also can play an important role in children's and adolescents' physical activity (Mollborn & Lawrence, 2018). Peer/friend support of exercise, better friendship quality and acceptance, and not having experienced peer victimization all have been linked to adolescents' physical activity.

Some of the blame for inactivity also falls on the nation's schools, many of which fail to provide daily physical education classes (Fung & others, 2012). A national survey revealed that only about 50 percent of U.S. ninth- through twelfth-graders participated in physical education classes on one or more days in an average school week and only 31.5 percent did so five days per week (Eaton & others, 2012).

Screen-based activity (watching television or using computers, tablets, or cell phones for long hours) is linked to lower levels of physical fitness in children and adolescents (Potter & others, 2018). Children and adolescents who engage in the most daily screen-based activity (TV/video/video games in one study) are less likely to exercise daily (Sisson & others, 2010). Children and adolescents who engage in low physical activity and high screen-based activity are almost twice as likely to be overweight as their more active, less sedentary counterparts (Sisson & others, 2010).

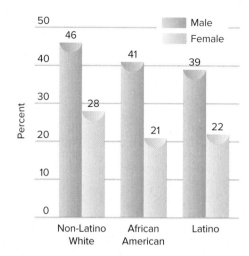

FIGURE 20

EXERCISE RATES OF U.S. HIGH SCHOOL STUDENTS IN 2011: GENDER AND ETHNICITY.
Note: Data are for high school students who were physically active doing any kind of physical activity that increased their heart rate and made them breathe hard some of the time for a total of at least 60 minutes a day on five or more of the seven days preceding the survey. (Source: After Eaton & others, 2012, Table 91).

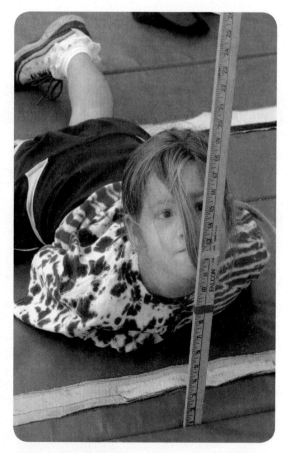

In 2007, Texas became the first state to test students' physical fitness. The student shown here is performing the trunk lift. Other assessments include aerobic exercise, muscle strength, and body fat. Assessments will be done annually.
St Petersburg Times/ZUMAPRESS/Newscom

A research review concluded that screen-based activity is linked to a number of adolescent health problems (Costigan & others, 2013). In this review, screen-based sedentary behavior was associated with being overweight, sleep problems, lower levels of physical activity/ fitness and well-being, and a higher level of depression.

Here are some ways to get children and adolescents to exercise more:

- Improve physical fitness classes in schools.
- Offer more physical activity programs run by volunteers at school facilities.
- Have children plan community and school exercise activities that interest them.
- Encourage families to focus on physical activity, and challenge parents to exercise more.

Review Connect Reflect

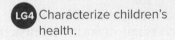 Characterize children's health.

Review

- What are the key health problems facing children?
- What are some important aspects of children's nutrition and eating behavior?
- What role does exercise play in children's development?

Connect

- Nutrition was discussed earlier in the chapter as well. What did you learn about nutrition's effect on growth?

Reflect *Your Own Personal Journey of Life*

- What were your eating habits like as a child? In what ways are they similar to or different from your current eating habits? Do you think your early eating habits predicted whether you would have weight problems in adulthood?

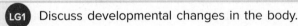

reach your **learning goals**

Physical Development and Health

Body Growth and Change

LG1 Discuss developmental changes in the body.

Patterns of Growth

- Human growth follows cephalocaudal and proximodistal patterns. In a cephalocaudal pattern, the fastest growth occurs at the top—the head. Physical growth in size, weight, and feature differentiation occurs gradually and moves from the top to the bottom. In a proximodistal pattern, growth begins at the center of the body and then moves toward the extremities.

Infancy and Childhood

- Height and weight increase rapidly in infancy and then take a slower course during childhood. The average North American newborn is 20 inches long and weighs 7½ pounds. Infants grow about 1 inch per month during their first year. In early childhood, girls are only slightly smaller and lighter than boys. Growth is slow and consistent in middle and late childhood, and head circumference, waist circumference, and leg length decrease in relation to body height.

Adolescence

- Puberty is a rapid maturation involving hormonal and body changes that occur primarily in early adolescence. Puberty began to occur at younger ages during the twentieth century. There are wide individual variations in the age at which puberty begins. Heredity plays an important role in determining the onset of puberty. Key hormones involved in puberty are testosterone and estradiol. Rising testosterone levels in boys cause voice changes, enlargement of external genitals, and increased height. In girls, increased levels of estradiol influence breast and uterine development and skeletal change. Key physical changes of puberty include a growth spurt as well as sexual maturation. The growth spurt occurs an average of two years earlier for girls than for boys. Adolescents are preoccupied with their bodies and develop images of their bodies. Adolescent girls have more negative body images than adolescent boys. Early maturation favors boys during adolescence, but in adulthood late-maturing boys have a more successful identity. Early-maturing girls are vulnerable to a number of problems including eating disorders, smoking, and depression.

The Brain

LG2 Describe how the brain changes.

The Neuroconstructivist View

- The old view was that genes determined how a child's brain is wired and that environmental experiences play little or no role in the brain's development. However, in the neuroconstructivist view, (a) biological processes and environmental conditions influence the brain's development, (b) the brain has plasticity and is context dependent, and (c) the development of the brain and the child's cognitive development are closely linked.

Brain Physiology

- Each hemisphere of the brain's cerebral cortex has four lobes (frontal, occipital, temporal, and parietal) with somewhat different primary functions. Neurons are nerve cells in the brain that process information. Communication between neurons occurs through the release of neurotransmitters at gaps called synapses. Communication is speeded by the myelin sheath that covers most axons. Clusters of neurons, known as neural circuits, work together to handle particular types of information. Specialization of functioning occurs in the brain's hemispheres, as in speech and grammar, but for the most part both hemispheres are involved in most complex functions, such as reading or performing music.

Infancy

- Researchers have found that experience influences the brain's development. Early experiences are very important in brain development, and growing up in deprived environments can harm the brain. Myelination continues throughout the childhood years and even into adolescence for some brain areas such as the frontal lobes. Dramatic increases in dendritic and synaptic connections occur in infancy. These connections are overproduced and later pruned.

Childhood

- During early childhood, the brain and head grow more rapidly than any other part of the body. Rapid, distinct bursts of growth occur in different areas of the brain between 3 and 15 years of age. One shift in brain activation in middle and late childhood is from diffuse, larger areas to more focal, smaller areas, especially in cognitive control.

Adolescence

- In adolescence, the corpus callosum thickens, and this improves information processing. Also, the amygdala, which is involved in emotions such as anger, develops earlier than the prefrontal cortex, which functions in reasoning and self-regulation. This gap in development may help to explain the increase in risk-taking behavior that characterizes adolescence.

Sleep

LG3 Summarize how sleep patterns change as children and adolescents develop.

Infancy

- The typical newborn sleeps 16 to 17 hours a day. REM sleep occurs more in infancy than in childhood and adulthood. Sleeping arrangements vary across cultures, and there is controversy about infants sharing a bed with parents while sleeping. SIDS is a special concern in early infancy.

Childhood

- Most young children sleep through the night and have one daytime nap. It is recommended that preschool children sleep 11 to 14 hours each night and 5- to 12-year-old children 9 to 12 hours each night. Sleep problems in childhood are linked to negative outcomes in other areas of children's development.

Adolescence

- Many adolescents stay up later than when they were children and are getting less sleep than they need. Research suggests that as adolescents get older, the hormone melatonin is released later at night, shifting the adolescent's biological clock. Inadequate sleep is linked to an unhealthy diet, low exercise level, depression, and ineffective stress management.

Health

 Characterize children's health.

Illness and Injuries Among Children

- Motor vehicle accidents are the number one cause of death in childhood. Parental smoking is a major danger for young children. For the most part, middle and late childhood is a time of excellent health. Caregivers play an important role in preventing childhood injuries. Two diseases of special concern in childhood are cancer and cardiovascular disease. A special concern also is the health of children living in poverty in the United States and abroad. Improvements are needed in sanitation, nutrition, education, and health services in addition to a reduction in poverty. In low-income countries, there has been a dramatic increase in the number of children who have died from HIV/AIDS that was transmitted to them by their parents.

Nutrition and Eating Behavior

- The importance of adequate energy intake consumed in a loving and supportive environment during infancy cannot be overstated. Breast feeding is recommended over bottle feeding. Marasmus and kwashiorkor are diseases caused by severe malnutrition. Concerns about nutrition in childhood focus especially on unhealthy food choices and overweight/obese children. The percentage of overweight/obese children has increased dramatically in recent decades. Being overweight increases a child's risk of developing many medical and psychological problems. Parents play an important role in helping children avoid weight problems.

Exercise

- Most children and adolescents are not getting nearly enough exercise. Boys and girls become less active as they reach and progress through adolescence. Parents, schools, and screen-based activity play important roles in whether children and adolescents are physically fit or unfit.

key terms

amygdala 110
androgens 101
cephalocaudal pattern 98
corpus callosum 110
estradiol 101

estrogens 101
hormones 101
kwashiorkor 120
lateralization 106
marasmus 120

menarche 100
myelination 108
neuroconstructivist view 104
precocious puberty 101
prefrontal cortex 110

proximodistal pattern 99
puberty 100
sudden infant death syndrome (SIDS) 113
testosterone 101

key people

Mary Carskadon 114

Mona El-Sheikh 114

Mark Johnson 109

Charles Nelson 110

chapter 5

MOTOR, SENSORY, AND PERCEPTUAL DEVELOPMENT

chapter outline

1 Motor Development

Learning Goal 1 Describe how motor skills develop.

The Dynamic Systems View
Reflexes
Gross Motor Skills
Fine Motor Skills

2 Sensory and Perceptual Development

Learning Goal 2 Outline the course of sensory and perceptual development.

What Are Sensation and Perception?
The Ecological View
Visual Perception
Other Senses
Intermodal Perception
Nature, Nurture, and Perceptual Development

3 Perceptual-Motor Coupling

Learning Goal 3 Discuss perceptual-motor coupling.

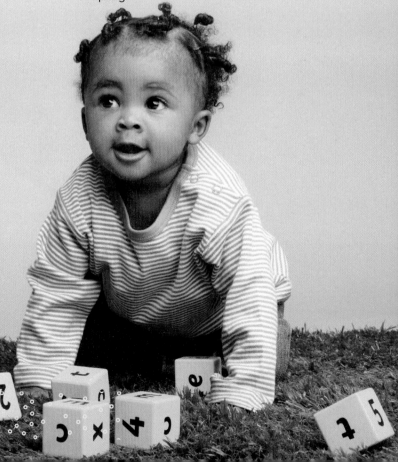

Image Source/Getty Images

In 1950, the newly born Steveland Morris was placed in an incubator in which he was given too much oxygen. The result was permanent blindness. In 1962, as 12-year-old singer and musician Stevie Wonder, he began a career that has included such hits as "My Cherie Amour" and "Signed, Sealed, Delivered." In the twenty-first century, his music is still perceived by some as "wondrous."

At age 12, Andrea Bocelli lost his sight in a soccer mishap. Today, in his sixties and after a brief career as a lawyer, Andrea has taken the music world by storm with his magnificent, classically trained voice.

Although Bocelli's and Stevie Wonder's accomplishments are great, imagine how very difficult it must have been for them as children to do many of the things we take for granted in sighted children. Yet children who lose one channel of sensation—such as vision—often compensate for the loss by enhancing their sensory skills in another area, such as hearing or touch. For example, researchers have found that blind individuals are more accurate at locating a sound source and have greater sensitivity to touch than sighted individuals do (Lewald, 2012; Proulx & others, 2013). In one study, blind children were more skillful than blindfolded sighted children at using hearing to detect walls (Ashmead & others, 1998). In this study, acoustic information was most useful when the blind children were within one meter of a wall—at which point, sound pressure increases.

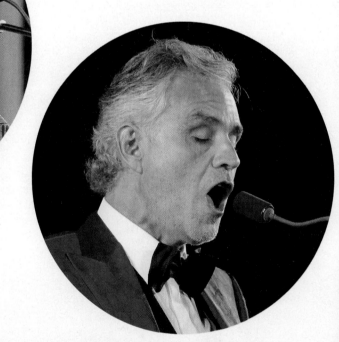

Two "sensations": Stevie Wonder (*left*) and Andrea Bocelli (*right*). *How have they adapted to life without sight?*

preview

Think about what is required for children to find their way around their environment, to play sports, or to create art. These activities require both active perception and precisely timed motor actions. Neither innate, automatic movements nor simple sensations are enough to let children do the things they do every day. How do children develop perceptual and motor abilities? In this chapter, we will focus first on the development of motor skills, then on sensory and perceptual development, and finally on the coupling of perceptual-motor skills.

A baby is the most complicated object made by unskilled labor.

—ANONYMOUS

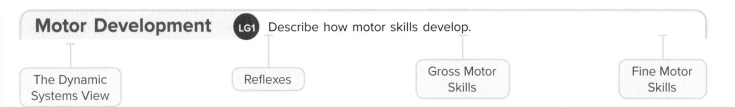

Motor Development **LG1** Describe how motor skills develop.

| The Dynamic Systems View | Reflexes | Gross Motor Skills | Fine Motor Skills |

Most adults are capable of coordinated, purposeful actions requiring considerable skill, including driving a car, playing golf, and typing accurately on a keyboard. Some adults have extraordinary motor skills, such as those involved in winning an Olympic pole vault competition, performing heart surgery, painting a masterpiece, or in the case of Stevie Wonder, being extraordinarily talented at playing the piano. Look all you want at a newborn infant, and you will observe nothing even remotely approaching these skilled actions. How, then, do the motor behaviors of adults develop?

THE DYNAMIC SYSTEMS VIEW

Arnold Gesell (1934a, b) thought his painstaking observations had revealed how people develop their motor skills. He had discovered that infants and children develop rolling over, sitting, standing, and other motor skills in a fixed order and within specific time frames. These observations, said Gesell, show that motor development comes about through the unfolding of a genetic plan, or *maturation.*

Later studies, however, have demonstrated that the sequence of developmental milestones is not as fixed as Gesell indicated and not due as much to heredity as Gesell argued (Lee & others, 2018). In the last two decades, the study of motor development experienced a renaissance as psychologists developed new insights about *how* motor skills develop (Thelen & Smith, 2006). One increasingly influential theory is dynamic systems theory, proposed by Esther Thelen (1941–2004).

According to **dynamic systems theory,** infants assemble motor skills for perceiving and acting. Notice that perception and action are coupled. To develop motor skills, infants must perceive something in the environment that motivates them to act and then use their perceptions to fine-tune their movements. Motor skills represent solutions to the infant's goals (Dineva & Schöner, 2018).

How is a motor skill developed, according to this theory? When infants are motivated to do something, they might create a new motor behavior. The new behavior is the result of many converging factors: the development of the nervous system, the body's physical properties and its possibilities for movement, the goal the child is motivated to reach, and the environmental support for the skill. For example, babies learn to walk only when maturation of the nervous system allows them to control certain leg muscles, when their legs have grown enough to support their weight, and when they want to move.

Mastering a motor skill requires the infant's active efforts to coordinate several components of the skill. Infants explore and select possible solutions to the demands of a new task; they assemble adaptive patterns by modifying their current movement patterns. The first step occurs when the infant is motivated by a new challenge—such as the desire to cross a room—and gets into the "ballpark" of the task demands by taking a couple of stumbling steps. Then the infant "tunes" these movements to make them smoother and more effective.

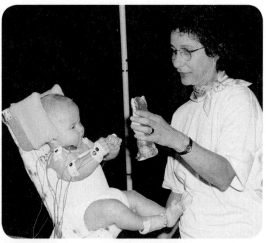

Esther Thelen (1941-2004) is shown conducting an experiment to discover how infants learn to control their arms to reach and grasp for objects. A computer was used to monitor the infant's arm movements and to track muscle patterns. Thelen's research was conducted from a dynamic systems perspective. *What is the nature of this perspective?*
Courtesy of Esther Thelen

dynamic systems theory A theory, proposed by Esther Thelen, that seeks to explain how motor behaviors are assembled for perceiving and acting.

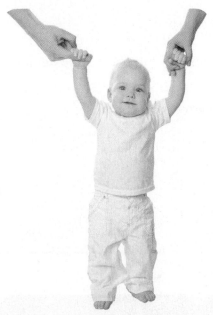

How might dynamic systems theory explain the development of learning to walk?
Vitalinka/Shutterstock

---

developmental connection

Nature and Nurture

The epigenetic view states that development is an ongoing, bidirectional interchange between heredity and environment. Connect to "Biological Beginnings."

---

reflexes   Built-in automatic reactions to stimuli.

rooting reflex   A newborn's built-in reaction that occurs when the infant's cheek is stroked or the side of the mouth is touched. In response, the infant turns its head toward the side that was touched, in an apparent effort to find something to suck.

sucking reflex   A newborn's built-in reaction of automatically sucking an object placed in its mouth. The sucking reflex enables the infant to get nourishment before it has associated a nipple with food.

Moro reflex   A newborn's startle response that occurs in reaction to a sudden, intense noise or movement. When startled, the newborn arches its back, throws its head back, and flings out its arms and legs. Then the newborn rapidly closes its arms and legs to the center of the body.

grasping reflex   A newborn's built-in reaction that occurs when something touches the infant's palms. The infant responds by grasping tightly.

The tuning is achieved through repeated cycles of action and perception of the consequences of that action. According to the dynamic systems view, even culturally "universal" milestones, such as crawling, reaching, and walking, are learned through this process of adaptation: infants modulate their movement patterns to fit a new task by exploring and selecting possible configurations (Adolph & Berger, 2013). Motor development does appear to be similar across nations and cultures. For example, this was confirmed in a large study in Argentina, India, South Africa, and Turkey (Ertem & others, 2018).

To see how dynamic systems theory explains motor behavior, imagine that you offer a new toy to a baby named Gabriel (Thelen & others, 1993). There is no exact program that can tell Gabriel ahead of time how to move his arm and hand and fingers to grasp the toy. Gabriel must adapt to his goal—grasping the toy—and the context. From his sitting position, he must make split-second adjustments to extend his arm, holding his body steady so that his arm and torso don't plow into the toy. Muscles in his arm and shoulder contract and stretch in a host of combinations, exerting a variety of forces. He improvises a way to reach out with one arm and wrap his fingers around the toy.

Thus, according to dynamic systems theory, motor development is not a passive process in which genes dictate the unfolding of a sequence of skills over time. Rather, the infant actively puts together a skill to achieve a goal within the constraints set by the infant's body and environment. Nature and nurture, the infant and the environment, work together as part of an ever-developing system.

As we examine the course of motor development, we will describe how dynamic systems theory applies to some specific skills. First, though, let's see how the story of motor development begins with reflexes.

REFLEXES

The newborn is not completely helpless. Among other things, it has some basic reflexes. For example, the newborn automatically holds its breath and contracts its throat to keep water out. **Reflexes** are built-in reactions to stimuli; they govern the newborn's movements, which are automatic and beyond the newborn's control. Reflexes are genetically carried survival mechanisms. They allow infants to respond adaptively to their environment before they have had an opportunity to learn. An overview of reflexes, some discussed below, is given in Figure 1.

The rooting and sucking reflexes are important examples. Both have survival value for newborn humans and other mammals, who must find a mother's breast to obtain nourishment. The **rooting reflex** occurs when the infant's cheek is stroked or the side of the mouth is touched. In response, the infant turns its head toward the side that was touched in an apparent effort to find something to suck. The **sucking reflex** occurs when newborns automatically suck an object placed in their mouth. This reflex enables newborns to get nourishment before they have associated a nipple with food; sucking also serves as a self-soothing mechanism.

Another example is the **Moro reflex,** which occurs in response to a sudden, intense noise or movement. When startled, the newborn arches its back, throws back its head, and flings out its arms and legs. Then the newborn rapidly closes its arms and legs. The Moro reflex is believed to be a way of grabbing for support while falling; it would have had survival value for our primate ancestors.

Some reflexes—coughing, sneezing, blinking, shivering, and yawning, for example—persist throughout life. They are as important for the adult as they are for the infant. Other reflexes, though, disappear several months following birth, as the infant's brain matures and it develops voluntary control over many behaviors (Gieysztor, Choińska, & Paprocka-Borowicz, 2018). The rooting and Moro reflexes, for example, tend to disappear when the infant is 3 to 4 months old.

The movements of some reflexes eventually become incorporated into more complex, voluntary actions. One important example is the **grasping reflex,** which occurs when something touches the infant's palms. The infant responds by grasping tightly. By the end of the third month, the grasping reflex diminishes, and the infant shows a more voluntary grasp. As its motor development becomes smoother, the infant will grasp objects, carefully manipulate them, and explore their qualities.

Reflex	Stimulation	Infant's Response	Developmental Pattern
Blinking	Flash of light, puff of air	Closes both eyes	Permanent
Babinski	Sole of foot stroked	Fans out toes, twists foot in	Disappears after 9 months to 1 year
Grasping	Palms touched	Grasps tightly	Weakens after 3 months, disappears after 1 year
Moro (startle)	Sudden stimulation, such as hearing loud noise or being dropped	Startles, arches back, throws head back, flings out arms and legs and then rapidly closes them to center of body	Disappears after 3 to 4 months
Rooting	Cheek stroked or side of mouth touched	Turns head, opens mouth, begins sucking	Disappears after 3 to 4 months
Stepping	Infant held above surface and feet lowered to touch surface	Moves feet as if to walk	Disappears after 3 to 4 months
Sucking	Object touching mouth	Sucks automatically	Disappears after 3 to 4 months
Swimming	Infant put face down in water	Makes coordinated swimming movements	Disappears after 6 to 7 months
Tonic neck	Infant placed on back	Forms fists with both hands and usually turns head to the right (sometimes called the "fencer's pose" because the infant looks like it is assuming a fencer's position)	Disappears after 2 months

FIGURE 1

INFANT REFLEXES. This chart describes some of the infant's reflexes.

Although reflexes are automatic and inborn, differences in reflexive behavior are soon apparent. For example, the sucking capabilities of newborns vary among babies. Some newborns are efficient at forcefully sucking and obtaining milk; others are not as efficient and get tired before they are full. Most infants take several weeks to establish a sucking style that is coordinated with the way the mother is holding the infant, the way milk is coming out of the bottle or breast, and the infant's temperament. This transition reflects actual changes in the nervous system and the brain (Muscatelli & Bouret, 2018). Cross-cultural brain science research shows that there are corresponding changes in the new mother's brain, to better coordinate and respond to the infant's needs (Bornstein & others, 2017).

The old view of reflexes is that they were exclusively genetic, built-in mechanisms that govern the infant's movements. The new perspective on infant reflexes is that they are not automatic or completely beyond the infant's control. For example, infants can control such movements as alternating their legs to make a mobile jiggle or change their sucking rate to listen to a recording (Adolph & Berger, 2013).

In a classic and important study, pediatrician T. Berry Brazelton (1956) observed how infants' sucking changed as they grew older. Over 85 percent of the infants engaged in considerable sucking behavior unrelated to feeding. They sucked their fingers, their fists, and pacifiers. By the age of 1 year, most had stopped the sucking behavior, but as many as 40 percent of children continued to suck their thumbs after starting school (Kessen, Haith, & Salapatek, 1970).

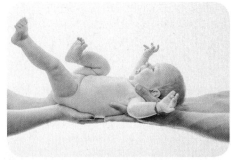

Moro reflex

The Moro reflex usually disappears around the age of 3 months.

Volodymyr Tverdokhlib/Shutterstock

GROSS MOTOR SKILLS

Ask any parents about their baby, and sooner or later you are likely to hear about motor milestones, such as "Cassandra just learned to crawl," "Jesse is finally sitting alone," or "Angela took her first step last week." Parents proudly announce such milestones as their children transform themselves from babies unable to lift their heads to toddlers who grab things off the grocery store shelf, chase a cat, and participate actively in the family's social

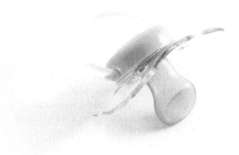

Laurence Mouton/PhotoAlto/Getty Images

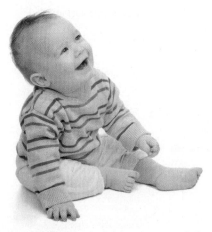

What are some developmental changes in posture during infancy?

Serhiy Kobyakov/Shutterstock

gross motor skills Motor skills that involve large-muscle activities, such as moving one's arms and walking.

life. These milestones are examples of **gross motor skills,** which are skills that involve large-muscle activities, such as moving one's arms and walking.

The Development of Posture   How do gross motor skills develop? As a foundation, these skills require postural control (Hadders-Algra, 2018). For example, to track moving objects, you must be able to control your head in order to stabilize your gaze; before you can walk, you must be able to balance on one leg. Posture is more than just holding still and straight. Posture is a dynamic process that is linked with sensory information in the skin, joints, and muscles, which tell us where we are in space; in vestibular organs in the inner ear that regulate balance and equilibrium; and in vision and hearing.

Newborn infants cannot voluntarily control their posture. Within a few weeks, though, they can hold their heads erect, and soon they can lift their heads while prone. By 2 months of age, babies can sit while supported on a lap or an infant seat, but they cannot sit independently until they are 6 or 7 months of age. Standing also develops gradually during the first year of life. By about 8 to 9 months of age, infants usually learn to pull themselves up and hold on to a chair, and they often can stand alone by about 10 to 12 months of age. Though there is general consistency across places and cultures in this developmental progression, there are important cultural differences in caregivers' understanding and beliefs about development that can influence how parents stimulate and support gross motor skills in infancy (van Schaik, Oudgenoeg-Paz, & Atun-Einy, 2018).

Learning to Walk   Locomotion and postural control are closely linked, especially in walking upright (Adolph & Hoch, 2018). To walk upright, the baby must be able both to balance on one leg as the other is swung forward and to shift the weight from one leg to the other.

Even young infants can make the alternating leg movements that are needed for walking. The neural pathways that control leg alternation are in place from a very early age, even at birth or before. Indeed, researchers have found that alternating leg movements occur during the fetal period and at birth (van Merendonk & others, 2017).

When infants learn to walk, they typically take small steps because of their limited balance control and strength. However, one study revealed that infants occasionally take a few large steps that even exceed their leg length, and these large steps indicate increased balance and strength (Hallemans & others, 2018).

In learning to locomote, infants learn what kinds of places and surfaces are safe for locomotion. In a classic series of studies, Karen Adolph (1997) investigated how experienced and inexperienced crawling infants and walking infants go down steep slopes (see Figure 2). Newly crawling infants, who averaged about 8½ months in age, rather indiscriminately went down the steep slopes, often falling in the process (with their mothers next to the slope to catch them). After weeks of practice, the crawling babies became more adept

FIGURE **2**

THE ROLE OF EXPERIENCE IN CRAWLING AND WALKING INFANTS' JUDGMENTS OF WHETHER TO GO DOWN A SLOPE. Karen Adolph (1997) found that locomotor *experience* rather than *age* was the primary predictor of adaptive responding on slopes of varying steepness. Newly crawling and walking infants could not judge the safety of the various slopes. With experience, they learned to avoid slopes where they would fall. When expert crawlers began to walk, they again made mistakes and fell, even though they had judged the same slope accurately when crawling. Adolph referred to this as the *specificity of learning* because it does not transfer across crawling and walking.

Dr. Karen Adolph, New York University

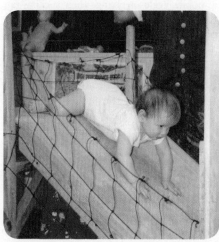

Newly crawling infant

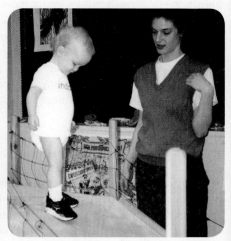

Experienced walker

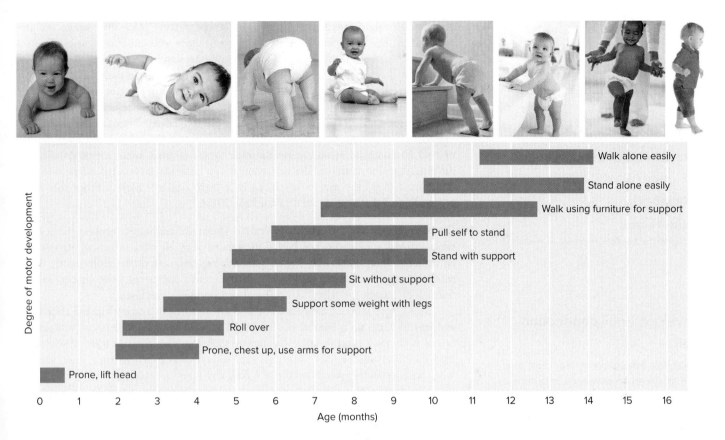

FIGURE **3**

MILESTONES IN GROSS MOTOR DEVELOPMENT

(Left to right): Barbara Penoyar/Getty Images; Evan Kafka/Iconica/Getty Images; Image Source/Alamy Stock Photo; Victoria Blackie/Getty Images; Cohen/Ostrow/Digital Vision/Getty Images; Fotosearch/Getty Images; Tom Grill/Corbis; amaviael/123RF

at judging which slopes were too steep to crawl down and which ones they could navigate safely. New walkers also could not judge the safety of the slopes, but experienced walkers accurately matched their skills with the steepness of the slopes. They rarely fell downhill, either refusing to go down the steep slopes or going down backward in a cautious manner. Experienced walkers perceptually assessed the situation—looking, swaying, touching, and thinking before they moved down the slope. With experience, both the crawlers and the walkers learned to avoid the risky slopes where they would fall, integrating perceptual information with the development of a new motor behavior. In a follow-up study, Adolph and her colleagues (2012) observed 12- to 19-month-olds during free play. Locomotor experience was extensive, with the infants averaging 2,368 steps and 17 falls per hour.

An important conclusion from Adolph's classic (1997) study involves the *specificity of learning*—the idea that infants who have experience with one mode of locomotion (crawling, for example) don't seem to appreciate the dangers inherent in another mode of locomotion—risky walkways when they are making the transition to walking. Also in Adolph's research, we again see the importance of perceptual-motor coupling in the development of motor skills.

Practice is especially important in learning to walk. However, practice does not involve exact repetition. Infants and toddlers accumulate an immense number of experiences with balance and locomotion. From the perspective of Adolph and her colleagues (2003, p. 495):

> Thousands of daily walking steps, each step slightly different from the last because of variations in the terrain and the continually varying bio-mechanical constraints on the body, may help infants to identify the relevant combination of strength and balance required to improve their walking skills.

The First Year: Motor Development Milestones and Variations   Figure 3 summarizes important accomplishments in gross motor skills during the first year, culminating in the ability to walk easily. The timing of these milestones, especially the later ones, may vary among children by several months, and experiences can accelerate or delay the onset of these milestones (Hadders-Algra, 2018). For example, a classic study found

- - - - - - - - →

developmental connection

Exercise

Children's engagement in aerobic exercise in linked to advances in a number of aspects of cognitive development. Connect to "Physical Development and Health."

←- - - - - - -

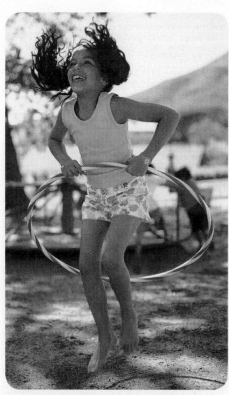

What are some developmental changes in children's motor development that occur in early, middle, and late childhood?

Charlie Edwards/Getty Images

that, when pediatricians began recommending that parents place their babies on their backs when they sleep, fewer babies crawled, and those who did crawled later (Davis & others, 1998). Also, some infants do not follow the standard sequence of motor milestones. For example, many infants never crawl on their belly or on their hands and knees, and this is more common in some cultures than in others. Furthermore, these non-crawling infants may discover a different form of locomotion before walking, such as rolling, or they might never locomote until they get upright (Adolph, Hoch, & Cole, 2018).

The latest compelling evidence, utilizing frequent text messaging to survey mothers of 3- to 12-month-old infants, shows the wide variety of gross motor accomplishments in the first year. Furthermore, the environment (for example, how often infants are held, transported in a baby carrier, or placed in a "baby walker") plays a major role in the progression of these motor skills (Franchak, 2018).

Development in the Second Year   The motor accomplishments of the first year bring increasing independence during the second year, allowing infants to explore their environment more extensively and to initiate interaction with others more readily. Motor activity during the second year is vital to the child's competent development, and few restrictions, except for safety, should be placed on their adventures.

By 13 to 18 months, toddlers can pull a toy attached to a string and use their hands and legs to climb up a number of steps. By 18 to 24 months, toddlers can walk quickly or run stiffly for a short distance, balance on their feet in a squatting position while playing with objects on the floor, walk backward without losing their balance, stand and kick a ball without falling, stand and throw a ball, and jump in place.

Can parents give their babies a head start on becoming physically fit and skilled through structured exercise classes? Most infancy experts recommend against structured exercise classes for babies. But there are other ways of guiding infants' motor development. Caregivers in some cultures handle babies vigorously, and this might advance motor development, as we discuss in *Connecting with Diversity*.

Childhood   Our exploration of motor development in childhood begins with a focus on developmental changes in gross motor skills, and then we examine the role of sports in children's development.

Developmental Changes   Unlike a 2-year-old, the older preschool child no longer has to make an effort to stay upright and to move around. As children move their legs with more confidence and carry themselves more purposefully, moving around in the environment becomes more automatic.

At 3 years of age, children enjoy simple movements, such as hopping, jumping, and running back and forth, just for the sheer delight of performing these activities. They take considerable pride in showing how they can run across a room and jump all of 6 inches. The run-and-jump will win no Olympic gold medals, but for the 3-year-old the activity is a source of pride.

At 4 years of age, children are still enjoying the same kind of activities, but they have become more adventurous. They scramble over low jungle gyms as they display their athletic prowess. Although they have been able to climb stairs with one foot on each step for some time, they are just beginning to be able to come down the same way.

At 5 years of age, children are even more adventuresome than they were at 4. It is not unusual for self-assured 5-year-olds to perform hair-raising stunts on practically any climbing object. They run hard and enjoy races with each other and their parents.

During middle and late childhood, children's motor development becomes much smoother and more coordinated than it was in early childhood. For example, only one child in a thousand can hit a tennis ball over the net at the age of 3, yet by the age of 10 or 11 most children can learn to play the sport. Running, climbing, skipping rope, swimming, bicycle riding, and skating are just a few of the many physical skills elementary school children can master. And, when mastered, these physical skills are a source of great pleasure and a sense of accomplishment. Several research studies of children and adolescents have revealed that those who are more physically fit have a better mastery of motor skills (Weedon & others, 2018). In gross motor skills involving large-muscle activity,

Cultural Variations in Guiding Infants' Motor Development

Mothers in developing countries tend to stimulate their infants' motor skills more than mothers in industrialized countries. For instance, in many African, Indian, and Caribbean cultures, mothers massage and stretch their infants during daily baths and at other times (Adolph, Karasik, & Tamis-LeMonda, 2010). And in sub-Saharan Africa, traditional practices in many villages involve mothers and siblings engaging babies in exercises, such as frequent exercise for trunk and pelvic muscles (Super & Harkness, 2010).

Do these cultural variations make a difference in the development of motor skills? When caregivers provide babies with physical guidance by physically handling them in special ways (such as stroking, massaging, or stretching) or by giving them opportunities for exercise, the infants often reach motor milestones earlier than infants whose caregivers have not provided these activities (Adolph, Karasik, & Tamis-LeMonda, 2010). These differences in practices also are reflected in parents' different expectations for motor development.

Many forms of restricted movement—such as Chinese sandbags, orphanage restrictions, and failure of caregivers to encourage movement in Budapest—have been found to produce substantial delays in motor development (Adolph, Hoch, & Cole, 2018). In some rural Chinese provinces, babies are placed in a bag of fine sand, which acts as a diaper and is changed once a day. The baby is left alone, face up, and is visited only when being fed by the mother. Some studies of swaddling show slight delays in motor development, but other studies show no delays. Cultures that do swaddle infants usually do

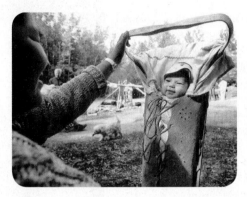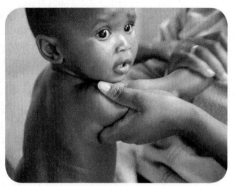

(*Left*) In the Algonquin culture in Quebec, Canada, babies are strapped to a cradle board for much of their infancy. (*Right*) In Jamaica, mothers massage and stretch their infants' arms and legs. *To what extent do cultural variations in the activity infants engage in influence the time at which they reach motor milestones?*

(*Left*): Michael Greenlar/The Image Works; (*right*): Pippa Hetherington/Earthstock/Newscom

so early in the infant's development when the infant is not mobile; when the infant becomes more mobile, swaddling decreases.

Nonetheless, even when infants' motor activity is restricted, many infants still reach the milestones of motor development at a normal age. For example, Algonquin infants in Quebec, Canada, spend much of their first year strapped to a cradle board. Despite their inactivity, these infants still sit up, crawl, and walk within an age range similar to that of infants in cultures where they have had much greater opportunity for activity.

To help babies with their motor development, is stroking, massaging, or stretching their arms and legs a better or worse strategy than engaging them in a structured exercise class?

---

boys usually outperform girls on average, although there is a wide range of skills within both genders that overlaps.

As children move through the elementary school years, they gain greater control over their bodies and can sit and pay attention for longer periods of time. However, elementary school children are far from being physically mature, and they need to be active. Elementary school children become more fatigued by long periods of sitting than by running, jumping, or bicycling (Walton-Fisette & Wuest, 2018). Physical action is essential for these children to refine their developing skills, such as batting a ball, skipping rope, or balancing on a beam. Children benefit from exercise breaks several times during the school day. For example, cross-cultural research on school-age children in Greece, Italy, and Norway revealed national differences in fine and gross motor skills that were influenced in part by cultural differences in physical activities and attitudes about exercise (Haga & others, 2018). In sum, children should be engaged in active, rather than passive, activities, because of many benefits to not only motor development and physical health but also cognitive functioning and overall well-being (Hillman, Erickson, & Hatfield, 2017).

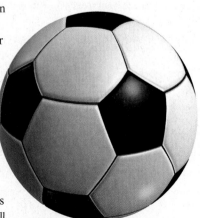

Ryan McVay/Getty Images

caring *connections*

Parents, Coaches, and Children's Sports

Most sports psychologists stress that it is important for parents to show an interest in their children's sports participation. Most children want their parents to watch them perform in sports. Many children whose parents do not come to watch them play in sporting events feel that their parents do not adequately support them. However, some children become extremely nervous when their parents watch them perform, or they get embarrassed when their parents cheer too loudly or make a fuss. If children request that their parents not watch them perform, parents should respect their children's wishes.

Parents should compliment their children for their sports performance, and if they don't become overinvolved, they can help their children build their physical skills and help them emotionally—discussing with them how to deal with a difficult coach, how to cope with a tough loss, and how to put in perspective a poorly played game. The following are some guidelines based on the Women's Sports Foundation's (2009) and the Families in Sport Lab's (Dorsch & others, 2014) suggestions, that can benefit both parents and coaches of all children in sports:

The Dos

- Make sports fun; the more children enjoy sports, the more they will want to play.
- Remember that it is okay for children to make mistakes; it means they are trying.
- Allow children to ask questions about the sport and discuss the sport in a calm, supportive manner.
- Show respect for the child's sports participation.
- Be positive and acknowledge that the child is making a good effort.
- Be a positive role model for the child in sports.

The Don'ts

- Yell or scream at the child.
- Condemn the child for poor play or continue to bring up failures long after they happen.
- Point out the child's errors in front of others.
- Expect the child to learn something immediately.
- Expect the child to become a pro.
- Ridicule or make fun of the child.

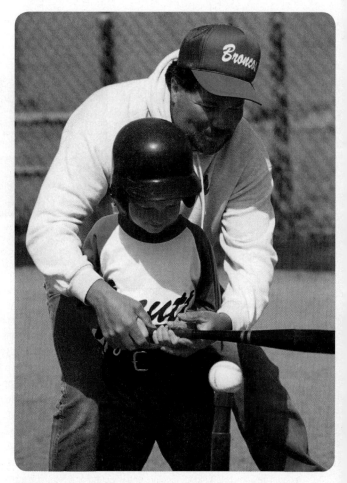

What are some guidelines that can benefit parents and coaches of children in sports?
SW Productions/Photodisc/Getty Images

- Compare the child to siblings or to more talented children.
- Make sports all work and no fun.

What are some of the potentially positive and negative aspects of children's participation in sports?

Sports   Organized sports are one way of encouraging children to be active and to develop their motor skills. Schools and community agencies offer programs for children that involve baseball, soccer, football, basketball, swimming, gymnastics, and other sports. For children who participate in them, these programs may play a central role in their lives.

Participation in sports can have both positive and negative consequences for children (Foss & others, 2018). Participation can provide exercise and self-esteem, opportunities to learn how to compete and be persistent, and a setting for developing peer relations and friendships (Van Boekel & others, 2016). Further, participating in sports reduces the likelihood that children will become obese (Lee, Pope, & Gao, 2018). One study of Australian children and teens revealed that youth who participated in organized sports activities were far more physically active and less likely to be overweight than their nonparticipating counterparts (Telford & others, 2016). However, sports also can bring pressure to achieve and win, physical injuries and burnout, and stressful expectations for success as an athlete (Foss & others, 2018; Pelka & Kellmann, 2017). The *Caring Connections* interlude examines the roles of parents and coaches in children's sports.

FINE MOTOR SKILLS

Whereas gross motor skills involve large-muscle activity, **fine motor skills** involve finely tuned movements. Grasping a toy, using a spoon, buttoning a shirt, or doing anything that requires finger dexterity demonstrates fine motor skills.

fine motor skills Motor skills that involve more finely tuned movements, such as finger dexterity.

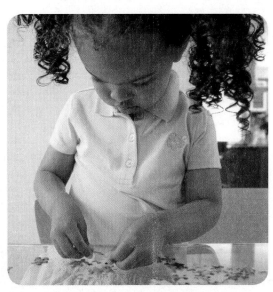

A young girl using a pincer grip to pick up puzzle pieces.
Newstockimages/SuperStock

Infancy Infants have hardly any control over fine motor skills at birth, but they do have many components of what will become finely coordinated arm, hand, and finger movements. The onset of reaching and grasping marks a significant achievement in infants' ability to interact with their surroundings. During the first two years of life, infants refine how they reach and grasp (Gonzalez & Sacrey, 2018). Initially, infants reach by moving their shoulders and elbows crudely, swinging toward an object. Later, when infants reach for an object they move their wrists, rotate their hands, and coordinate thumb and forefinger movements. Infants do not have to see their own hands in order to reach for an object or person. "Proprioceptive" cues from muscles, tendons, and joints, not sight of the limb, guide reaching by 4 months of age (Corbetta & others, 2018).

Infants refine their ability to grasp objects by developing two types of grasps. Initially, infants grip with the whole hand, which is called the *palmer grasp*. Later, toward the end of the first year, infants also grasp small objects with their thumb and forefinger, which is called the *pincer grip*. Their grasping system is very flexible. They vary their grip on an object depending on its size, shape, and texture, as well as the size of their own hands relative to the object's size. Infants grip small objects with their thumb and forefinger (and sometimes their middle finger too), whereas they grip large objects with all of the fingers of one hand or both hands.

Perceptual-motor coupling is necessary for the infant to coordinate grasping. Which perceptual system the infant is most likely to use to coordinate grasping varies with age. Four-month-old infants rely greatly on touch to determine how they will grip an object; 8-month-olds are more likely to use vision as a guide (Thomas, Karl & Whishaw, 2015). This developmental change is efficient because vision lets infants "preshape" their hands as they reach for an object.

Experience plays a role in reaching and grasping. In one clever experiment, 3-month-old infants participated in play sessions wearing "sticky mittens . . . mittens with palms that stuck to the edges of toys and allowed the infants to pick up the toys" (Needham, Barrett, & Peterman, 2002, p. 279) (see Figure 4). Infants who used the mittens grasped and manipulated objects earlier in their development than a control group of infants who did not get to use the mittens. The experienced infants looked at the objects longer, swatted at them more during visual contact, and were more likely to mouth the objects. In subsequent research using the mittens, 5-month-old infants whose parents trained them to use the sticky mittens for 10 minutes a day over a two-week period showed advances in their reaching behavior compared with infants who did not have this experience (Libertus & Needham, 2011).

Thus, just as infants need to exercise their gross motor skills, they also need to exercise their fine motor skills. Infants delight in picking up small objects after they begin using a pincer grip. Many develop the pincer grip and begin to crawl at about the same time, and infants at this time pick up virtually everything in sight, especially on the floor, and put the objects in

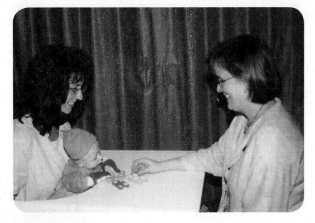

FIGURE 4

INFANTS' USE OF "STICKY MITTENS" TO EXPLORE OBJECTS. Amy Needham and her colleagues (2002) found that "sticky mittens" enhanced young infants' object exploration skills.
Courtesy of Dr. Amy Needham

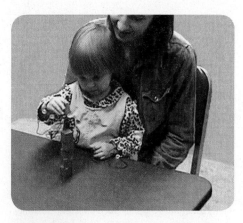

FIGURE 5

TOWER-BUILDING TODDLERS. This 18-month-old is building a block tower in the study by Chen & Others, 2011. Note the "kinematic" sensors on the toddler's wrists for obtaining data on speed, location, and timing of movement.

Courtesy Rachel Keen

their mouth. Thus, parents need to be vigilant in regularly monitoring what objects are within the infant's reach (Morrongiello & Cox, 2016).

Around 18 to 24 months of age, toddlers show mounting fine motor coordination. For example, they begin to build towers with blocks (see Figure 5). Initially, they can only balance two- to three-block towers, but soon the tower increases to four, five, and even more blocks. To build a tower, toddlers must engage in the cognitive activity of planning, in this case a plan that involves a number of sequential movements in picking up and stacking blocks in a precise way (Keen, 2011). Also, they need to have developed the motor skill to release blocks smoothly so the tower won't topple. In one study, substantial individual differences in the tower building skills of 18- to 21-month-olds was observed (Chen & others, 2010). Interestingly, toddlers who built higher towers at this age continued to be more advanced in tower building at 3 years of age.

Childhood As children get older, their fine motor skills continue to improve. At 3 years of age, children have had the ability to pick up the tiniest objects between their thumb and forefinger for some time, but they are still somewhat clumsy at it. Many 3-year-olds can build surprisingly high block towers, each block placed with intense concentration but often not in a completely straight line. When 3-year-olds play with a form board or a simple puzzle, they are rough in placing the pieces. When they try to position a piece in a hole, they often try to force the piece or pat it vigorously.

By 4 years of age, children's fine motor coordination is much more precise. Sometimes 4-year-old children have trouble building high towers with blocks because, in their desire to place each of the blocks perfectly, they upset those already stacked. By age 5, children's fine motor coordination has improved further. Hand, arm, and fingers all move together under better command of the eye. Mere towers no longer interest the 5-year-old, who now wants to build a house or skyscraper. The child's imagination drives their building activities.

Increased myelination of the central nervous system is reflected in the improvement of fine motor skills during middle and late childhood. Recall that myelination involves the covering of the axon with a myelin sheath, a process that increases the speed of information transfer from neuron to neuron. By middle childhood, children can use their hands as sophisticated tools. Six-year-olds can hammer, paste, tie shoes, and fasten clothes. By 7 years of age, children's hands have become steadier. At this age, children prefer a pencil to a crayon for printing, and reversal of letters is less common. Printing becomes smaller. At 8 to 10 years of age, children can use their hands independently with more ease and precision; children can now write rather than print words. Letter size becomes smaller and more even. At 10 to 12 years of age, children begin to show manipulative skills similar to the abilities of adults. The complex, intricate, and rapid movements needed to produce fine-quality crafts or to play a difficult piece on a musical instrument can be mastered. Girls usually outperform boys in fine motor skills on average, although there is a wide range within both genders.

Review Connect Reflect

 Describe how motor skills develop.

Review

- What is the dynamic systems view of motor development?
- What are some reflexes of infants?
- How do gross motor skills develop?
- How do fine motor skills develop?

Connect

- In this section, you learned how infants explore their environment as they develop gross and fine motor skills. How does this experience affect infants' neural connections?

Reflect *Your Own Personal Journey of Life*

- If and when you become a parent, how would you evaluate the benefits and drawbacks of allowing your 7-year-old to play for a soccer team in a competitive league in your town or city?

Sensory and Perceptual Development   **LG2** Outline the course of sensory and perceptual development.

What Are Sensation and Perception?	The Ecological View	Visual Perception	Other Senses	Intermodal Perception	Nature, Nurture, and Perceptual Development

How do sensations and perceptions develop? Can a newborn see? If so, what can it perceive? What about the other senses—hearing, smell, taste, and touch? What are they like in the newborn, and how do they develop? Can an infant put together information from two modalities, such as sight and sound? What is the role of gene-environment interplay in perceptual development? These are among the intriguing questions that we will explore in this section.

WHAT ARE SENSATION AND PERCEPTION?

How does a newborn know that her mother's skin is soft rather than rough? How does a 5-year-old know what color his hair is? Infants and children "know" these things as a result of information that comes through the senses. Without vision, hearing, touch, taste, and smell, we would be isolated from the world; we would live in dark silence, a tasteless, colorless, feelingless void.

Sensation occurs when information interacts with sensory *receptors*—the eyes, ears, tongue, nostrils, and skin. The sensation of hearing occurs when waves of pulsating air are collected by the outer ear and transmitted through the bones of the inner ear to the auditory nerve. The sensation of vision occurs as rays of light contact the eyes, become focused on the retina, and are transmitted by the optic nerve to the visual centers of the brain.

Perception is the interpretation of what is sensed. The air waves that contact the ears might be interpreted as noise or as musical sounds, for example. The physical energy of light being transmitted to the retina of the eye might be interpreted as a particular color, pattern, or shape, depending on how it is perceived.

THE ECOLOGICAL VIEW

Much of the research on perceptual development in infancy has been guided by the ecological view of Eleanor and James J. Gibson (E. Gibson, 1989; J. Gibson, 2014). They argue that we do not have to take bits and pieces of data from sensations and build up representations of the world in our minds. Instead, our perceptual system can select from the rich information that the environment itself provides.

According to the Gibsons' **ecological view,** we directly perceive information that exists in the world around us. The view is called *ecological* "because it connects perceptual capabilities to information available in the world of the perceiver" (Kellman & Arterberry, 2006, p. 112). Thus, perception brings us into contact with the environment so that we can interact with and adapt to it. Perception is designed for action. Perception gives people such information as when to duck, when to turn their bodies to get through a narrow passageway, and when to put their hands up to catch something.

In the Gibsons' view, objects have **affordances,** which are opportunities for interaction offered by objects that fit within our capabilities to perform activities. A pot may afford you something to cook with, and it may afford a toddler something to bang. Adults typically know when a chair is appropriate for sitting, when a surface is safe for walking, or when an object is within reach. We directly and accurately perceive these affordances by sensing information from the environment—the light or sound reflecting from the surfaces of the world—and from our own bodies through muscle receptors, joint receptors, and skin receptors; this information, in turn, informs the motor actions we make (Plumert, 2018).

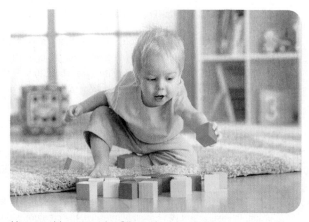

How would you use the Gibsons' ecological theory of perception and the concept of affordance to explain the role that perception is playing in this baby's activity?
Oksana Kuzmina/Shutterstock

sensation Reaction that occurs when information contacts sensory receptors—the eyes, ears, tongue, nostrils, and skin.

perception The interpretation of sensation.

ecological view The view, proposed by the Gibsons, that people directly perceive information in the world around them. Perception brings people in contact with the environment so that they can interact with and adapt to it.

affordances Opportunities for interaction offered by objects that are necessary to perform activities.

A helpful example of affordances was described earlier in the section on motor development. Infants who were just learning to crawl or just learning to walk were less cautious when confronted with a steep slope than experienced crawlers or walkers were (Adolph, 1997). The more experienced crawlers and walkers perceived that a slope *affords* the possibility for not only faster locomotion but also for falling. Again, infants coupled perception and action to make a decision about what to do in their environment. Through perceptual development, children become more efficient at discovering and using affordances.

In Karen Adolph's research, slopes, gaps, apertures, and dropoffs, coupled with experimental manipulation of infants' body properties (slippery shoes or floors, for example), are used to examine infants' success in connecting their motor decisions to actual affordances for action. Using such observational measures as checklist diaries, telephone diaries, step-counters, and video tracking, she and her colleagues (Adolph & Franchak, 2017; Adolph & Hoch, 2018) collected information about infants' everyday locomotor experiences. They have discovered that the extent of infants' experiences help explain developmental changes beyond their body dimensions and chronological age.

Studying the infant's perception has not been an easy task. For instance, if newborns have limited communication abilities and are unable to tell us what they are seeing, hearing, smelling, and so on, how can we study their perception? *Connecting Through Research* describes some of the ingenious ways researchers study infants' perception.

visual preference method A method developed by Fantz to determine whether infants can distinguish one stimulus from another by measuring the length of time they attend to different stimuli.

habituation Decreased responsiveness to a stimulus after repeated presentations of the stimulus.

dishabituation The recovery of a habituated response after a change in stimulation.

connecting through research

How Can We Study Newborns' Perception?

The creature has poor motor coordination and can move itself only with great difficulty. Although it cries when uncomfortable, it uses few other vocalizations. In fact, it sleeps most of the time, about 16 to 17 hours a day. You are curious about this creature and want to know more about what it can do. You think to yourself, "I wonder if it can see. How could I find out?"

You obviously have a communication problem with the creature. You must devise a way that will allow the creature to "tell" you that it can see. While examining the creature one day, you make an interesting discovery. When you move an object horizontally in front of the creature, its eyes follow the object's movement.

The creature's head movement suggests that it has at least some vision. In case you haven't already guessed, the creature you have been reading about is the human infant, and the role you played is that of a researcher interested in devising techniques to learn about the infant's visual perception. Across many decades, scientists have developed research methods and tools sophisticated enough to examine the subtle abilities of infants and to interpret their complex actions. The following discussion describes several of these techniques.

Visual Preference Method

Robert Fantz (1963) was a pioneer in the study of infants' perception. Fantz made an important discovery that advanced the ability of researchers to investigate infants' visual perception: Infants look at different things for different lengths of time. Fantz placed infants in a "looking chamber," which had two visual displays on the ceiling above the infant's head. An experimenter viewed the infant's eyes by looking through a peephole.

If the infant was fixating on one of the displays, the experimenter could see the display's reflection in the infant's eyes. This allowed the experimenter to determine how long the infant looked at each display. Fantz (1963) found that infants only 2 days old look longer at patterned stimuli, such as faces and concentric circles, than at patternless red, white, or yellow discs. Infants 2 to 3 weeks old preferred to look at patterns—a face, a piece of printed matter, or a bull's-eye—longer than at patternless red, yellow, or white discs (see Figure 6). Fantz's research method—studying whether infants can distinguish one stimulus from another by measuring the length of time they attend to different stimuli—is referred to as the **visual preference method.**

Habituation and Dishabituation

Another way that researchers have studied infants' perception is to repeatedly present a stimulus (such as a sight or a sound). If the infant decreases the time spent looking at the stimulus after several presentations, this indicates that the infant is no longer interested in it. If the researcher now presents a new stimulus, the infant's looking behavior will recover, indicating that the infant could discriminate between the old and new stimuli (Colombo, Brez, & Curtindale, 2013).

Habituation is the name given to decreased responsiveness to a stimulus after repeated presentations of the stimulus. **Dishabituation** is the recovery of a habituated response after a change in stimulation. Newborn infants can habituate to repeated sights, sounds, smells, or touches (Addabbo & others, 2018). Among the measures researchers use in habituation studies are sucking behavior (sucking stops when the young

connecting through research

(continued)

FIGURE 6

FANTZ'S EXPERIMENT ON INFANTS' VISUAL PERCEPTION. (*a*) Infants 2 to 3 weeks old preferred to look at some stimuli more than others. In Fantz's experiment, infants preferred to look at patterns rather than at color or brightness. For example, they looked longer at a face, a piece of printed matter, or a bull's-eye than at patternless red, yellow, or white discs. (*b*) Fantz used a "looking chamber" to study infants' perception of stimuli.

(b) David Linton, Courtesy of the Linton Family

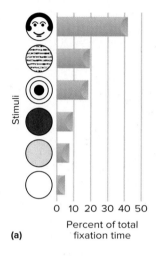

(a)

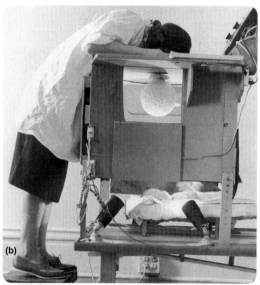

(b)

infant attends to a new object), heart and breathing rates, and the length of time the infant looks at an object. Figure 7 shows the results of one illustrative study of habituation and dishabituation with newborns (Slater, Morison, & Somers, 1988).

High-Amplitude Sucking

To assess an infant's attention to sound, researchers often use a method called *high-amplitude sucking*. In this method, infants are given a nonnutritive nipple to suck (like those used on bottles or pacifiers), and the

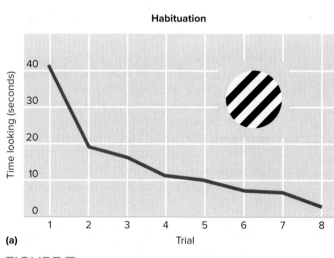

(a)

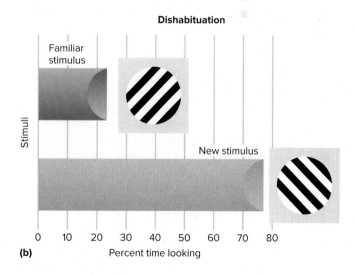

(b)

FIGURE 7

HABITUATION AND DISHABITUATION. In the first part of one study, 7-hour-old newborns were shown the stimulus in (*a*). As indicated, the newborns looked at it an average of 41 seconds when it was first presented to them (Slater, Morison, & Somers, 1988). Over seven more presentations of the stimulus, they looked at it less and less. In the second part of the study, infants were presented with both the familiar stimulus to which they had just become habituated (*a*) and a new stimulus (shown in *b*, which was rotated 90 degrees). The newborns looked at the new stimulus three times as much as the familiar stimulus.

(continued)

(continued)

nipple is connected to a sound-generating system. The researcher computes a baseline high-amplitude sucking rate in a one-minute silent period (that is, the frequency or number of times the infant sucks the nipple). Following the baseline, presentation of a sound is made contingent on the rate of sucking. The sound is interesting, so initially the babies suck frequently so that the same sound occurs often. Gradually, they lose interest in hearing the same sound so they begin to suck less often. Then the researcher changes the sound that is being presented. If the babies again increase their rate of sucking, the interpretation is that they have discriminated the sound change and are sucking more because they want to hear the interesting new sound (Pelaez & Monlux, 2017).

The Orienting Response

A technique that can be used to determine whether an infant can see or hear is the *orienting response*, which involves turning one's head toward a sight or sound. Also, a startle response can be used as an indicator of an infant's reaction to a noise (Shultz, Klin, & Jones, 2018).

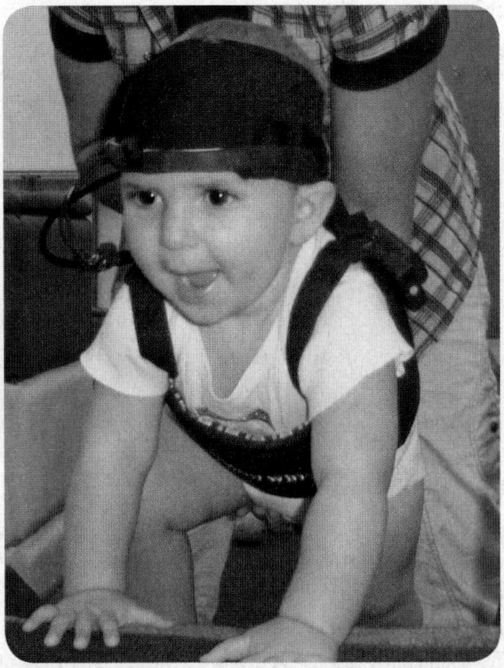

Equipment

Technology can facilitate the use of most methods for investigating the infant's perceptual abilities. Video equipment allows researchers to investigate elusive behaviors. High-speed computers make it possible to perform complex data analysis in minutes to seconds. Other equipment records respiration, heart rate, body movement, visual fixation, and sucking behavior, which provide clues to what the infant is sensing and perceiving. For example, some researchers use equipment that detects whether a change in infants' respiration follows a change in the pitch of a sound. If so, it suggests that the infants heard the pitch change.

FIGURE 8

AN INFANT WEARING EYE-TRACKING HEADGEAR. Using the ultralight, wireless, head-mounted eye-tracking equipment shown here, researchers can record where infants are looking while they freely locomote. (Source: Courtesy of Dr. Karen Adolph's laboratory, New York University.)

Eye Tracking

One very important technical advance in measuring infant perception is the development of sophisticated eye-tracking equipment (Franchak & others, 2011; Slone & others, 2018). Figure 8 shows an infant wearing an eye-tracking headgear in a study on visually guided movement and social interaction.

One of the main reasons that infant perception researchers are so enthusiastic about sophisticated eye-tracking equipment is that "looking time" is among the most important measures of infant perceptual and cognitive development, but this behavior is difficult to assess (Oakes, 2017). The new eye-tracking equipment allows for much greater precision than human observation in assessing various aspects of infant looking and gaze. Among the areas of infant perception in which eye-tracking equipment is being used are memory, joint attention, and face processing (Falck-Ytter & others, 2012). Further, eye-tracking equipment is improving our understanding of infants at risk for atypical developmental outcomes, including preterm infants and infants at risk for developing autism (Wagner & others, 2018).

An illustrative study using eye-tracking technology shed light on the effectiveness of TV programs and videos that claim to educate infants (Kirkorian, Anderson, & Keen, 2012). In this study, 1-year-olds, 4-year-olds, and adults watched *Sesame Street* and the eye-tracking equipment recorded precisely what they looked at on the screen. The 1-year-olds were far less likely to consistently look at the same part of the screen than their older counterparts, suggesting that the 1-year-olds showed little understanding of the *Sesame Street* video but instead were attracted to what was visually salient and not by the meaningful content.

VISUAL PERCEPTION

What do newborns see? How does visual perception develop across infancy and childhood?

Infancy　Some important changes in visual perception with age can be traced to differences in how the eye itself functions over time. For example, changes in eye function influence how clearly we can see an object, whether we can differentiate its colors, at what distance, and in what light.

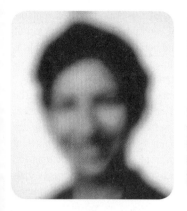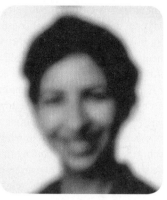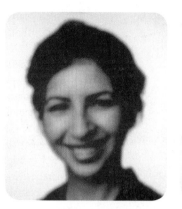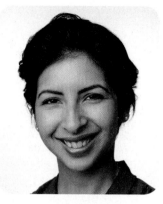

Visual Acuity   Psychologist William James (1890/1950) called the newborn's perceptual world a "blooming, buzzing confusion." More than a century later, we can safely say that he was wrong (Maurer & Lewis, 2018). Even the newborn perceives a world with some order. That world, however, is far different from the one perceived by the toddler or the adult.

Just how well can infants see? At birth, the nerves and muscles and lens of the eye are still developing. As a result, newborns cannot see small things that are far away. The newborn's vision is estimated to be 20/240 on the well-known Snellen chart used for eye examinations, which means that a newborn can see at 20 feet only as much as an adult with normal vision can see at 240 feet. In other words, an object 20 feet away is only as clear to the newborn as it would be if it were 240 feet away from an adult with normal vision (20/20). By 6 months of age, though, on *average* vision is 20/40 (Aslin & Lathrop, 2008). Although this may seem like an initial disadvantage for newborns, this progression of visual acuity is a typical and important part of visual sensory and perceptual development (Vogelsang & others, 2018).

Face Perception   Infants show an interest in human faces soon after birth (Sugden & Marquis, 2017). Figure 9 shows a computer estimation of what a picture of a face looks like to an infant at different ages from a distance of about 6 inches. Infants spend more time looking at their mother's face than a stranger's face as early as 12 hours after being born. By 4 months of age, infants match voices to faces, distinguish between male and female faces, and discriminate between faces of their own racial and ethnic group compared with those of other groups (Lee, Quinn, & Pascalis, 2017; Otsuka, 2017).

As infants develop, they change the way they gather information from the visual world, including human faces. A study that illustrates this progression recorded eye movements of 3-, 6-, and 9-month-old infants as they viewed clips from an animated film—*A Charlie Brown Christmas* (Frank, Vul, & Johnson, 2009). From 3 to 9 months of age, infants gradually began focusing their attention more on the faces of the characters in the animated film and less on salient background stimuli.

Pattern Perception   As we discussed in the *Connecting Through Research* interlude, young infants can perceive certain patterns. With the help of his "looking chamber," Robert Fantz (1963) revealed that even 2- to 3-week-old infants prefer to look at patterned displays rather than nonpatterned displays. For example, they prefer to look at a normal human face rather than one with scrambled features, and they prefer to look at a bull's-eye target or black-and-white stripes rather than a plain circle.

Color Vision   The infant's color vision also improves over time. By 8 weeks, and possibly as early as 4 weeks, infants can discriminate between some colors. By 4 months of age, they have color preferences that mirror those of adults in some cases, preferring saturated colors such as royal blue over pale blue, for example (Bornstein, 2015). One study of 4- to 5-month-olds found that they looked longest at reddish hues and shortest at greenish hues (Franklin & others, 2010). In part, these changes in vision reflect maturation. Experience, however, is also necessary for color vision to develop normally (Sugita, 2004).

Perceptual Constancy   Some perceptual accomplishments are especially intriguing because they indicate that the infant's perception goes beyond the information provided by the senses (Arterberry & Kellman, 2016; Johnson, 2013). This is the case in *perceptual constancy*,

FIGURE 9

VISUAL ACUITY DURING THE FIRST MONTHS OF LIFE. The four photographs represent a computer estimation of what a picture of a face looks like to a 1-month-old, 2-month-old, 3-month-old, and 1-year-old (which approximates the visual acuity of an adult).

Kevin Peterson/Photodisc/Getty Images

developmental **connection**

Research Methods

The still-face paradigm has been used to study face-to-face interaction between infants and caregivers. Connect to "Emotional Development."

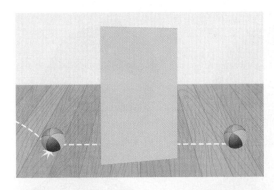

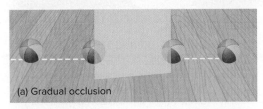

(a) Gradual occlusion

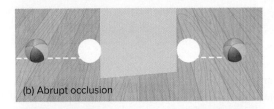

(b) Abrupt occlusion

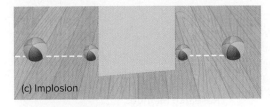

(c) Implosion

FIGURE 10

INFANTS' PREDICTIVE TRACKING OF A BRIEFLY OCCLUDED MOVING BALL. The top drawing shows a visual scene that infants experienced. At the beginning of each event, a multicolored ball bounded up and down with an accompanying bouncing sound, and then rolled across the floor until it disappeared behind the partition. The bottom drawing shows the three stimulus events the 5- to 9-month-old infants experienced: occlusion, disappearance, and implosion. (*a*) *Gradual Occlusion:* The ball gradually disappears behind the right side of the occluding partition located in the center of the display. (*b*) *Abrupt Occlusion:* The ball abruptly disappears when it reaches the location of the white circle and then abruptly reappears 2 seconds later at the location of the second white circle on the other side of the occluding partition. (*c*) *Implosion:* The rolling ball quickly decreases in size as it approaches the occluding partition and rapidly increases in size as it reappears on the other side of the occluding partition.

size constancy Recognition that an object remains the same even though the retinal image of the object changes.

shape constancy Recognition that an object remains the same even though its orientation to the viewer changes.

in which sensory stimulation is changing but perception of the physical world remains constant. If infants did not develop perceptual constancy, each time they saw an object at a different distance or in a different orientation, they would perceive it as a different object. Thus, the development of perceptual constancy allows infants to perceive their world as stable. Two types of perceptual constancy are size constancy and shape constancy.

Size constancy is the recognition that an object remains the same even though the retinal image of the object changes as you move toward or away from the object (Chen, Sperandio & Goodale, 2018). The farther away from us an object is, the smaller is its image on our eyes. Thus, the size of an object on the retina is not sufficient to tell us its actual size. For example, you perceive a bicycle standing right in front of you as smaller than the car parked across the street, even though the bicycle casts a larger image on your eyes than the car does. When you move away from the bicycle, you do not perceive it to be shrinking even though its image on your retinas shrinks; you perceive its size as constant.

But what about babies? Do they have size constancy? Researchers have long known that babies as young as 3 months of age show size constancy (Bower, 1966). However, at 3 months of age, this ability is not full-blown. It continues to develop across early and middle childhood (Johnson & Hannon, 2015).

Shape constancy is the recognition that an object remains the same shape even though its orientation to us changes. Look around the room you are in right now. You likely see objects of varying shapes, such as tables and chairs. If you get up and walk around the room, you will see these objects from different sides and angles. Even though your retinal image of the objects changes as you walk and look, you will still perceive the objects as the same shape.

Do babies have shape constancy? As with size constancy, researchers have found that babies as young as 3 months of age have shape constancy (Bower, 1966). Three-month-old infants, however, do not have shape constancy for *irregularly* shaped objects with distinct features, edges, and shadowing (Woods & Schuler, 2014).

Perception of Occluded Objects　Look around the place where you are now. You likely see that some objects are partly occluded by other objects that are in front of them—possibly a desk behind a chair, some books behind a computer, or a car parked behind a tree. Do infants perceive an object as complete when it is occluded by an object in front of it?

In the first two months of postnatal development, infants don't perceive occluded objects as complete, instead only perceiving what is visible (Johnson, 2013). Beginning at about 2 months of age, infants develop the ability to perceive that occluded objects are whole. How does perceptual completion develop? In Scott Johnson's research (2004, 2013, 2019), learning, experience, and self-directed exploration via eye movements play key roles in the development of perceptual completion in young infants.

Many objects that are occluded appear and disappear behind closer objects, as when you are walking down the street and see cars appear and disappear behind buildings as they move or you move. Can infants predictively track briefly occluded moving objects? They develop the ability to track briefly occluded moving objects at about 3 to 5 months of age (Bremner & others, 2016). One illustrative study explored 5- to 9-month-old infants' ability to track moving objects that disappeared gradually behind an occluded partition, disappeared abruptly, or imploded (shrank quickly in size) (Bertenthal, Longo, & Kenny, 2007) (see Figure 10). In this study, the infants were more likely to accurately predict the path of the moving object when it disappeared gradually than when it disappeared abruptly or imploded.

Depth Perception　Might infants be able to perceive depth? To investigate this question, in a classic experiment Eleanor Gibson and Richard Walk (1960) constructed in their laboratory a miniature cliff with a dropoff covered by glass. They placed infants on the edge of this visual cliff and had their mothers coax them to crawl onto the glass (see Figure 11). Most infants would not crawl out on the glass, choosing instead to remain on the shallow side, an indication that they could perceive depth, according to Gibson and Walk. However, critics point out that the visual cliff likely is a better test of social referencing and fear of heights than depth perception.

The 6- to 12-month-old infants in the visual cliff experiment had extensive visual experience. Do younger infants without this experience behave the same way? Since younger infants do not crawl, this question is difficult to answer. Early on, the evidence showed that 2- to 4-month-old infants show differences in heart rate when they are placed directly on the deep side instead of on the shallow side (Campos, Langer, & Krowitz, 1970). However, these differences might mean that young infants respond to differences in some visual characteristics of the deep and shallow cliffs, with no actual knowledge of depth (Adolph & Kretch, 2012). Although researchers do not know exactly how early in life infants can perceive depth, we do know that infants develop the ability to use "binocular" cues to discern depth by about 3 to 4 months of age.

Childhood Perceptual development continues in early childhood (Johnson & Hannon, 2015; Vida & Maurer, 2012). Children become increasingly efficient at detecting the boundaries between colors (such as red and orange) at 3 to 4 years of age. When they are about 4 or 5 years old, most children's eye muscles are developed enough for them to move their eyes efficiently across a series of letters. Many toddlers are farsighted, unable to see close up as well as they can see far away (Mutti & others, 2018). By the time they enter kindergarten, though, most children can focus their eyes and sustain their attention effectively on close-up objects.

After infancy, children's visual expectations about the physical world continue to develop (Keen, 2011). In another illustrative study, 2- to 4½-year-old children were given a task in which the goal was to find a toy ball that had been dropped through an opaque tube (Hood, 1995). As shown in Figure 12, if the ball is dropped into the opaque tube, it will land in the box that is farthest away. However, in this task, most of the 2-year-olds, and even some of the 4-year-olds, persisted in searching in the box immediately beneath the dropping point. For them, gravity ruled, and they had failed to perceive the end location of the curved tube.

In a subsequent study, 3-year-olds were presented with a task that was similar to the one shown in Figure 12 (Palmquist, Keen, & Jaswal, 2018). In the group that was told to imagine the ball rolling through the tube, the young children were more accurate in predicting where the ball would land. In another study, 3-year-olds improved their performance on the ball-dropping task when they were instructed to follow the tube with their eyes to the bottom (Bascandziev & Harris, 2011). Thus, in these two studies, 3-year-olds were able to overcome the gravity bias and their impulsive tendencies when they were given verbal instructions from a knowledgeable adult.

How do children learn to deal with situations like that in Figure 12, and how do they come to understand other laws of the physical world? These questions are addressed by research on children's cognitive development, which we will discuss in the chapters on "Cognitive Developmental Approaches" and "Information Processing."

OTHER SENSES

Other sensory systems besides vision also develop during infancy. We will explore development in hearing, touch and pain, smell, and taste.

Hearing During the last two months of pregnancy, as the fetus nestles in its mother's womb, it can hear sounds such as music and the mother's voice (Moon, 2017). In a classic study, two psychologists wanted to find out if a fetus that heard Dr. Seuss' classic story *The Cat in the Hat* while still in the mother's womb would prefer hearing the story after birth (DeCasper & Spence, 1986). During the last months of pregnancy, 16 women read *The Cat in the Hat* to their fetuses. Then shortly after they were born, the mothers read either *The Cat in the Hat* or a story with a different rhyme and pace, *The King, the Mice and the Cheese* (which was not read to them during prenatal development). The infants sucked on a nipple in a

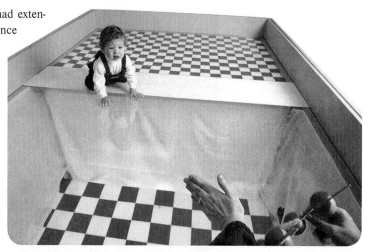

FIGURE 11

EXAMINING INFANTS' DEPTH PERCEPTION ON THE VISUAL CLIFF.
Eleanor Gibson and Richard Walk (1960) found that most infants would not crawl out on the glass, which, according to Gibson and Walk, indicated that they had depth perception. However, critics point out that the visual cliff is a better indication of the infant's social referencing and fear of heights than the infant's perception of depth.
Mark Richard/PhotoEdit

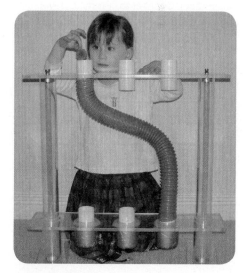

FIGURE 12

VISUAL EXPECTATIONS ABOUT THE PHYSICAL WORLD. When young children see a ball dropped into the tube, many of them will search for it immediately below the dropping point. *How might verbal instructions from a knowledgeable adult help younger children overcome a gravity bias?*
Courtesy of Dr. Bruce Hood, University of Bristol

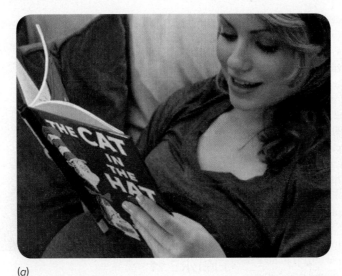
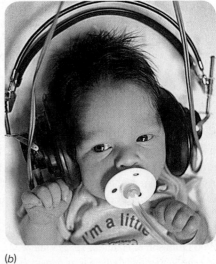

(a)   (b)

FIGURE 13

HEARING IN THE WOMB. (*a*) Pregnant mothers read *The Cat in the Hat* to their fetuses during the last few months of pregnancy. (*b*) When they were born, the babies preferred listening to a recording of their mothers reading *The Cat in the Hat*—as evidenced by the way they sucked on a nipple—rather than another story, *The King, the Mice and the Cheese.*

(a) Jill Braaten/McGraw-Hill Education; (b) Courtesy of Dr. Melanie J. Spence

developmental **connection**

Biological Processes

Prenatal development is divided into three periods: germinal (first 2 weeks after conception), embryonic (2 to 8 weeks after conception), and fetal (begins at 2 months after conception and lasts for 7 months on average). Connect to "Prenatal Development and Birth."

different way when the mothers read the two stories, suggesting that the infants recognized the pattern and tone of *The Cat in the Hat* (see Figure 13). This study illustrates not only that a fetus can hear but also that it has a remarkable ability to learn even before birth. Contemporary brain-imaging research inspired by this classic study has demonstrated that the fetal brain is sensing and processing auditory signals in a sophisticated way (Draganova & others, 2018).

The fetus can also recognize the mother's and the father's voice, but they prefer the mother's voice (Lee & Kisilevsky, 2014). Thirty-nine third-trimester fetuses near the end of the pregnancy were exposed to a tape recording of their mother and their father reading a passage. The sounds of the tape were delivered through a loudspeaker held just above the mother's abdomen. Fetal heart rate increased more in response to the mother's voice than the father's voice, and postnatally the newborns showed a preference for the mother's voice by turning their head toward the sound of the mother's voice but not the father's voice.

What kind of changes in hearing take place during infancy? They involve perception of a sound's loudness, pitch, and localization:

- *Loudness.* Immediately after birth, infants cannot hear soft sounds quite as well as adults can; a stimulus must be louder to be heard by a newborn than by an adult. For example, an adult can hear a whisper from about 4 to 5 feet away, but a newborn requires that sounds be closer to a normal conversational level to be heard at that distance. This can make it challenging for medical professionals to accurately evaluate potential hearing impairment in newborns (Kanji, Khoza-Shangase, & Moroe, 2018).

- *Pitch.* Infants are also less sensitive to the pitch of a sound than adults are. *Pitch* is the perception of the frequency of a sound. A soprano voice sounds high-pitched, a bass voice low-pitched. Infants are less sensitive to low-pitched sounds and are more likely to hear high-pitched sounds, yet from early in infancy they can demonstrate that they hear the difference (Pietraszewski & others, 2017). One study revealed that by 7 months of age, infants can process simultaneous pitches when they hear voices but they are more likely to encode the higher-pitched voice (Marie & Trainor, 2012). By 2 years of age, infants have considerably improved their ability to distinguish between sounds with different pitches.

- *Localization.* Even newborns can determine the general location from which a sound is coming, but by 7 months of age, they are more proficient at *localizing* sounds or detecting their origins. Their ability to localize sounds continues to improve during infancy and toddlerhood (Kezuka, Amano, & Reddy, 2017).

Cochlear implants—small, electronic devices that directly stimulate the auditory nerve—are done routinely for children who are born deaf, even as early as 12 months of age. Many of the hearing-impaired children who have early cochlear implant surgery show good progress in learning speech and in understanding others' speech, although traditional hearing aids also can be effective (Percy-Smith & others, 2018). The most effective outcomes are likely found for children who also are exposed to frequent, supportive spoken and sign language at home (Lavelli & others, 2018).

Otitis media is a middle-ear infection that can impair hearing temporarily. If it continues too long, it can interfere with language development and socialization (Schilder & others, 2017). As many as one-third of all U.S. children have three or more episodes between birth and age 3. In some cases, the infection can develop into a more chronic condition in which the middle ear becomes filled with fluid, and this can seriously impair hearing. Treatments for otitis media include antibiotics and placement of a tube in the inner ear to drain fluid (Klopp-Dutote & others, 2018; Simon & others, 2018).

Touch and Pain Do newborns respond to touch? Can they feel pain?

Newborns do respond to touch. A touch to the cheek produces a turning of the head; a touch to the lips produces sucking movements. These are aspects of the "rooting" reflex.

Newborns can also feel pain (Gunnar & Quevado, 2007). There are customary medical procedures, such as pricking the heel for blood testing or inserting needles and tubes for newborns requiring intensive care to survive and heal after a difficult or premature birth. Research examining the behavior, physiology, and even brain activity of newborns undergoing these procedures shows that they experience pain (Bellieni & others, 2018; Verriotis & others, 2018).

In the past, doctors performed operations on newborns without anesthesia. This practice was accepted because of the dangers of anesthesia and because of the supposition that newborns did not feel pain. Over the past few decades, major advances have been made so that anesthesia and pain relievers can be effectively used with newborns (Steward, 2015).

Smell Newborns can differentiate odors (Schaal, 2017). The expressions on their faces seem to indicate that they like the way pleasant odors such as vanilla and strawberry smell but do not like the way unpleasant odors like rotten eggs and fish smell. In one classic study, 6-day-old infants who were breast fed showed a clear preference for smelling their mother's breast pad rather than a clean breast pad (MacFarlane, 1975) (see Figure 14). However, when they were 2 days old, they did not show this preference, indicating that they require several days of experience to recognize this odor. Since then, many studies have shown the importance of early experience with odors in the development of olfactory perception (Schaal, 2017).

Taste Sensitivity to taste is present even before birth. Human newborns learn tastes prenatally through the amniotic fluid and in breast milk after birth (Podzimek & others, 2018). In another classic study, even at only 2 hours of age, babies made different facial expressions when they tasted sweet, sour, and bitter solutions (Rosenstein & Oster, 1988) (see Figure 15). During their first several months of life infants begin to prefer salty tastes, which is adaptive given the important role of salt in the diet (Liem, 2017).

INTERMODAL PERCEPTION

Imagine yourself playing basketball or tennis. You are experiencing many visual inputs: the ball coming and going, other players moving around, and so on. However, you are experiencing many auditory inputs as well: the sound of the ball bouncing or being hit, the grunts and groans of the players, and so on. There is a good correspondence between much of the visual and auditory information: When you see the ball bounce, you hear a bouncing sound; when a player stretches to hit a ball, you hear a groan. When you look at

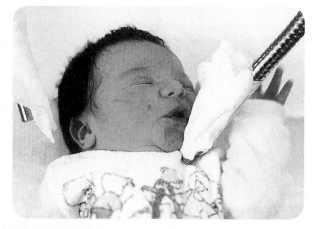

FIGURE 14

NEWBORNS' PREFERENCE FOR THE SMELL OF THEIR MOTHER'S BREAST PAD. In the classic experiment by MacFarlane (1975), 6-day-old infants preferred to smell their mother's breast pad rather than a clean one that had never been used, but 2-day-old infants did not show this preference, indicating that this odor preference requires several days of experience to develop.
Jean Guichard

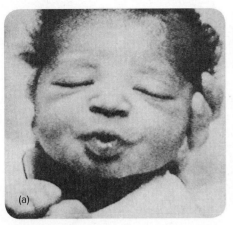
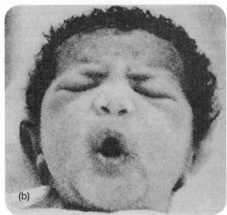
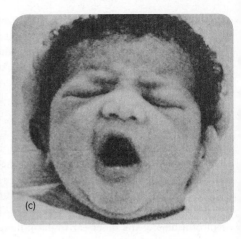

FIGURE 15

NEWBORNS' FACIAL RESPONSES TO BASIC TASTES. Facial expression elicited by (*a*) a sweet solution, (*b*) a sour solution, and (*c*) a bitter solution.

Rosenstein, D & Oster, H (1988) Differential facial responses to four basic tastes in newborns. Child Development, 59, p.1561

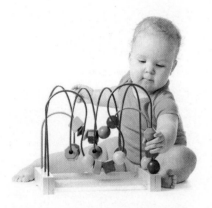

What is intermodal perception? Which two senses is this infant using to integrate information about the blocks?

Oksana Kuzmina/Shutterstock

intermodal perception The ability to relate and integrate information about two or more sensory modalities, such as vision and hearing.

and listen to what is going on, you do not experience just the sounds or just the sights separately—you put all these things together. You experience a single episode. This is **intermodal perception,** which involves integrating information from two or more sensory modalities, such as vision and hearing. Most perception is intermodal (Bahrick, Todd, & Soska, 2018).

Early, exploratory forms of intermodal perception exist even in newborns. For example, newborns turn their eyes and their head toward the sound of a voice or rattle when the sound is maintained for several seconds, but this orienting behavior is reflexive and it is only with rapid brain development over the first few months of life that this orienting behavior becomes controlled (Small, Ishida, & Stapells, 2017). In another classic study, infants as young as 3 months old looked more at their mother when they also heard her voice and longer at their father when they also heard his voice (Spelke & Owsley, 1979). Thus, even young infants can coordinate visual-auditory information involving people. These early forms of intermodal perception become sharpened with experience and development over the first year of life (Hannon, Schachner, & Nave-Blodgett, 2017). For instance, in the first six months, infants have difficulty connecting sensory input from different modes, but in the second half of the first year they show an increased ability to make this connection mentally.

The important ability to connect information about vision with information about touch also is evident early in infancy. Coordination of vision and touch has been demonstrated in 2- to 3-month-olds and develops rapidly across the first year (Bremner & Spence, 2017).

In sum, babies are born into the world with some abilities to perceive relations among sensory modalities, but their intermodal abilities improve considerably through experience. As with all aspects of development, in perceptual development, biological factors and experience interact and work together.

NATURE, NURTURE, AND PERCEPTUAL DEVELOPMENT

Now that we have discussed many aspects of perceptual development, let's explore one of developmental psychology's key issues as it relates to perceptual development: the nature-nurture issue. Historically, there has been a long-standing interest in how strongly infants' perception is influenced by nature, nurture, and their interaction (Aslin, 2009; Johnson, 2013). In the field of perceptual development, nature proponents were referred to as *nativists* and those who emphasized learning and experience were called *empiricists.*

In the strict nativist view, the ability to perceive the world in a competent, organized way is inborn or innate. At the beginning of our discussion of perceptual development, we examined the ecological view of the Gibsons because it has played such a pivotal role in guiding research in perceptual development. The Gibsons' ecological view leans toward a nativist explanation of perceptual development because it holds that perception is direct and evolved over time to allow the detection of size and shape constancy, a three-dimensional world, intermodal perception, and so on early in infancy. However, the Gibsons' view is not entirely nativist because they emphasized that distinct features in perception were detected at different ages. Further, the Gibsons argued that a key question in infant perception is what information is available in the environment and how infants learn to generate, differentiate, and discriminate the information—certainly not a nativist view.

This view is quite different from Piaget's constructivist view, which reflects an empiricist approach to explaining perceptual development. According to Piaget, much of perceptual development in infancy must await the development of a sequence of cognitive stages for infants to construct more complex perceptual tasks as they learn from experience with the world. Thus, in Piaget's view, the ability to perceive size and shape constancy, a three-dimensional world, intermodal perception, and so on develops later in infancy than the Gibsons envision.

Today, it is clear that an extreme empiricist position on perceptual development is unwarranted. As described in this chapter, much of early perception develops from innate foundations and the basic foundation of many perceptual abilities can be detected in newborns, whereas other abilities unfold gradually as infants develop. However, as infants develop, environmental experiences refine or modify many perceptual functions and may be the driving force behind still others (Amso & Johnson, 2010).

The longitudinal research of Daphne Maurer and her colleagues (Maurer, 2017; Maurer & Lewis, 2018) has focused on infants born with cataracts—a thickening of the lens of the eye that causes vision to become cloudy, opaque, and distorted, severely restricting infants' ability to experience their visual world. As they studied infants whose cataracts were removed at different points in development, they discovered that those whose cataracts were removed and new lenses placed in their eyes in the first several months after birth subsequently showed a normal pattern of visual development. However, the longer the delay in removing the cataracts, the more their visual development was impaired. In their research, Maurer and her colleagues (Hadad, Maurer, & Lewis, 2017) have found that experiencing patterned visual input early in infancy is important for holistic and detailed perception of patterns and contours after infancy. Their research program illustrates how deprivation and experience influence visual development, particularly during an early sensitive period in which visual input is necessary for normal visual development.

To summarize, the accumulation of experience with and knowledge about their perceptual world contributes to infants' ability to form coherent perceptions of people and things. A full portrait of perceptual development includes the interacting influence of nature, nurture, and a developing sensitivity to information in the environment.

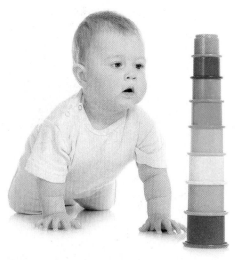
What roles do nature and nurture play in the infant's perceptual development?
Boris Ryaposov/Shutterstock

developmental **connection**

Cognitive Development

Piaget's theory states that children construct their understanding of the world and go through four stages of cognitive development. Connect to "Introduction."

Review Connect Reflect

LG2 Outline the course of sensory and perceptual development.

Review

- What are sensation and perception?
- What is the ecological view of perception? What are some research methods used to study infant perception?
- How does vision develop?
- How do the senses other than vision develop?
- What is intermodal perception, and how does it develop?
- What roles do nature and nurture play in perceptual development?

Connect

- One of the topics we discussed in this section was vision. What did you learn about development, vision loss, and the other senses in the story that opened the chapter?

Reflect *Your Own Personal Journey of Life*

- Imagine that you are the parent of a 1-year-old infant. What would you do to effectively stimulate the sensory development of your very young child?

Perceptual-Motor Coupling **LG3** Discuss perceptual-motor coupling.

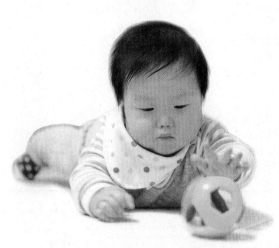

How are perception and action coupled in infants' development?

Kevin Liu/Getty Images

As we come to the end of this chapter, we return to the important theme of perceptual-motor coupling. The distinction between perceiving and doing has been a time-honored tradition in psychology. However, a number of experts on perceptual and motor development have questioned for some time whether this distinction makes sense. Instead, they view perception and action as being coupled (Adolph & Berger, 2013; Keen, 2011; Thelen & Smith, 2006). The main thrust of research in Esther Thelen's dynamic systems approach is to explore how people assemble motor behaviors for perceiving and acting. The main theme of the ecological approach of Eleanor and James J. Gibson is to discover how perception guides action. Action can guide perception, and perception can guide action. Only by moving one's eyes, head, hands, and arms and by moving from one location to another can an individual fully experience his or her environment and learn how to adapt to it.

Babies, for example, continually coordinate their movements with perceptual information to learn how to maintain balance, reach for objects in space, and move across various surfaces and terrains. They are motivated to move by what they perceive. For example, consider the sight of an attractive toy across the room. In this situation, infants must perceive the current state of their bodies and learn how to use their limbs to reach the toy. Although their movements at first are awkward and uncoordinated, babies soon learn to select patterns that are appropriate for reaching their goals.

Equally important is the other part of the perception-action coupling. That is, action influences and educates perception. For example, watching an object while exploring it with their hands helps infants to discriminate its texture, size, and hardness. Locomoting in the environment teaches babies about how objects and people look from different perspectives, or whether surfaces will support their weight.

How do infants develop new perceptual-motor couplings? Recall from our discussion earlier in this chapter that in the traditional view of Gesell, infants' perceptual-motor development is prescribed by a genetic plan to follow a fixed sequence of stages in development. The genetic determination view has been replaced by the dynamic systems view that infants learn new perceptual-motor couplings by assembling skills for perceiving and acting. New perceptual-motor coupling is not passively accomplished; rather, the infant actively develops a skill to achieve a goal within the limits set by the infant's body and the environment.

Thus, children perceive in order to move and move in order to perceive. Perceptual and motor development do not occur in isolation from each other but instead are coupled.

Review Connect Reflect

LG3 Discuss perceptual-motor coupling.

Review

- How are perception and motor actions coupled in development?

Connect

- In this section, you learned that perceptual and motor development do not occur in isolation from each other but instead are coupled. How is this distinction similar to the distinction psychologists make when speaking of nature and nurture when describing development?

Reflect *Your Own Personal Journey of Life*

- Think about your development as a child. Describe two examples, not given in the text, in which your perception guided your action. Then describe two examples, not given in the text, in which your action guided your perception.

Motor, Sensory, and Perceptual Development

Motor Development

LG1 Describe how motor skills develop.

The Dynamic Systems View

- Thelen's dynamic systems theory describes the development of motor skills as the assembling of behaviors for perceiving and acting. Perception and action are coupled. According to this theory, the development of motor skills depends on the development of the nervous system, the body's physical properties and its movement possibilities, the goal the child is motivated to reach, and environmental support for the skill. In the dynamic systems view, motor development is far more complex than the result of a genetic blueprint; the infant or child actively puts together a skill in order to achieve a goal within constraints set by the body and the environment.

Reflexes

- Reflexes—built-in reactions to stimuli—govern the newborn's movements. They include the sucking, rooting, and Moro reflexes, all of which typically disappear after three to four months. Some reflexes, such as blinking and yawning, persist throughout life; components of other reflexes are incorporated into voluntary actions.

Gross Motor Skills

- Gross motor skills involve large-muscle activities. Key skills developed during infancy include control of posture and walking. Gross motor skills improve dramatically during the childhood years. On average, boys usually outperform girls in gross motor skills involving large-muscle activity.

Fine Motor Skills

- Fine motor skills involve finely tuned movements. The onset of reaching and grasping marks a significant accomplishment. Fine motor skills continue to develop through the childhood years and by 4 years of age are much more precise. Children can use their hands as tools by middle childhood, and at 10 to 12 years of age start to show manipulative fine motor skills similar to those of adults.

Sensory and Perceptual Development

LG2 Outline the course of sensory and perceptual development.

What Are Sensation and Perception?

The Ecological View

- Sensation occurs when information interacts with sensory receptors. Perception is the interpretation of sensation.

- The Gibsons' ecological view states that people directly perceive information that exists in the world. Perception brings people in contact with the environment so that they can interact with and adapt to it. Affordances are opportunities for interaction offered by objects that are necessary to perform activities. Researchers have developed a number of methods to assess infants' perception, including the visual preference method (which Fantz used to determine young infants' interest in looking at patterned over nonpatterned displays), habituation and dishabituation, high-amplitude sucking, and tracking.

Visual Perception

- The infant's visual acuity increases dramatically in the first year of life. Infants show an interest in human faces soon after birth, and young infants systematically scan faces. Possibly by 4 weeks of age, infants can discriminate some colors. By 3 months of age, infants show size and shape constancy. At approximately 2 months of age, infants develop the ability to perceive that occluded objects are complete. Infants as young as 6 months of age have depth perception. After infancy, children's visual expectations continue to develop, and further color differentiation occurs from 3 to 4 years of age. A number of children experience vision problems.

- The fetus can hear several weeks prior to birth. Developmental changes in the perception of loudness, pitch, and localization of sound occur during infancy. Newborns can respond to touch and feel pain. Newborns can differentiate between odors, and sensitivity to taste may be present before birth.

- Intermodal perception is the ability to relate and integrate information from two or more sensory modalities. Crude, exploratory forms of intermodal perception are present in newborns and become sharpened over the first year of life.

- With regard to the study of perception, nature advocates were referred to as nativists and nurture proponents were called empiricists. A full contemporary account of perceptual development includes the intersecting roles of nature, nurture, and increasing sensitivity to information.

Perceptual-Motor Coupling

 Discuss perceptual-motor coupling.

- Perception and action are coupled—individuals perceive in order to move and move in order to perceive. New perceptual-motor couplings do not occur as the result of genetic predetermination but rather because the infant actively assembles skills for perceiving and acting.

key **terms**

affordances 143
dishabituation 144
dynamic systems
    theory 133
ecological view 143

fine motor skills 141
grasping reflex 134
gross motor skills 136
habituation 144
intermodal perception 152

Moro reflex 134
perception 143
reflexes 134
rooting reflex 134
sensation 143

shape constancy 148
size constancy 148
sucking reflex 134
visual preference
    method 144

key **people**

Karen Adolph 136
T. Berry Brazelton 135
Robert Fantz 144

Eleanor and James J. Gibson 143
William James 147
Scott Johnson 148

Daphne Maurer 153
Esther Thelen 133
Richard Walk 148

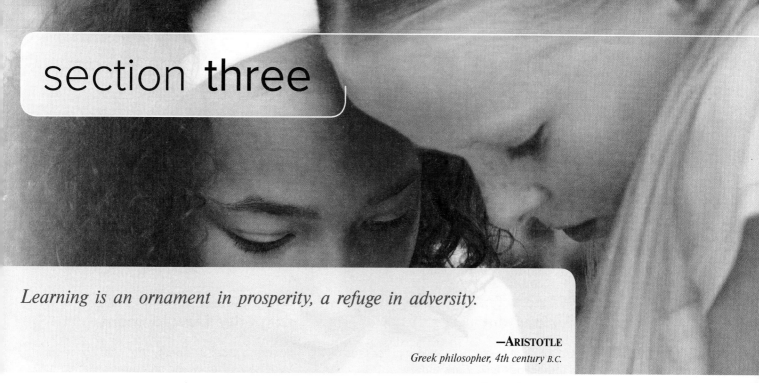

Learning is an ornament in prosperity, a refuge in adversity.

—ARISTOTLE
Greek philosopher, 4th century B.C.

Beau Lark/Glow Images

Cognition and Language

Children thirst to know and understand. In their effort to know and understand, they construct their own ideas about the world around them. They are remarkable for their curiosity and their intelligence. In Section 3, you will read four chapters: "Cognitive Developmental Approaches," "Information Processing," "Intelligence," and "Language Development."

chapter 6

COGNITIVE DEVELOPMENTAL APPROACHES

chapter outline

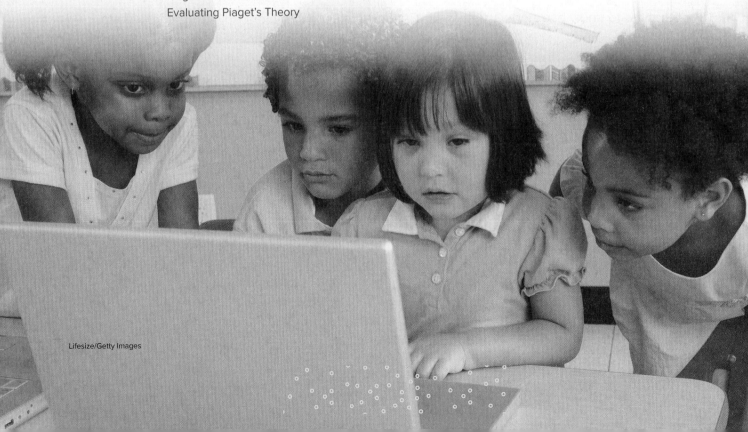

Lifesize/Getty Images

Jean Piaget, the famous Swiss psychologist, was a meticulous observer of his three children—Laurent, Lucienne, and Jacqueline. His books on cognitive development are filled with these observations. Here are a few of Piaget's observations of his children in infancy (Piaget, 1952):

- At 21 days of age, "Laurent found his thumb after three attempts: prolonged sucking begins each time. But, once he has been placed on his back, he does not know how to coordinate the movement of the arms with that of the mouth and his hands draw back even when his lips are seeking them" (p. 27).
- During the third month, thumb sucking becomes less important to Laurent because of new visual and auditory interests. But, when he cries, his thumb goes to the rescue.
- Toward the end of Lucienne's fourth month, while she is lying in her crib, Piaget hangs a doll above her feet. Lucienne thrusts her feet at the doll and makes it move. "Afterward, she looks at her motionless foot for a second, then recommences. There is no visual control of her foot, for the movements are the same when Lucienne only looks at the doll or when I place the doll over her head. On the other hand, the tactile control of the foot is apparent: after the first shakes, Lucienne makes slow foot movements as though to grasp and explore" (p. 159).
- At 11 months, "Jacqueline is seated and shakes a little bell. She then pauses abruptly in order to delicately place the bell in front of her right foot; then she kicks hard. Unable to recapture it, she grasps a ball which she then places at the same spot in order to give it another kick" (p. 225).
- At 1 year, 2 months, "Jacqueline holds in her hands an object which is new to her: a round, flat box which she turns all over, shakes, (and) rubs against the bassinet. . . . She lets it go and tries to pick it up. But she only succeeds in touching it with her index finger, without grasping it. She nevertheless makes an attempt and presses on the edge. The box then tilts up and falls again" (p. 273). Jacqueline shows an interest in this result and studies the fallen box.

For Piaget, these observations reflect important changes in the infant's cognitive development. Later in the chapter, you will learn that Piaget argued that infants go through six substages of development and that the behaviors you have just read about characterize those substages.

preview

Cognitive developmental approaches place a special emphasis on how children actively construct their thinking. They also focus heavily on how thinking changes from one point in development to another. In this chapter, we will highlight the cognitive developmental approaches of Jean Piaget and Lev Vygotsky.

Piaget's Theory of Cognitive Development

LG1 Discuss the key processes and four stages in Piaget's theory.

| Processes of Development | Sensorimotor Stage | Preoperational Stage | Concrete Operational Stage | Formal Operational Stage |

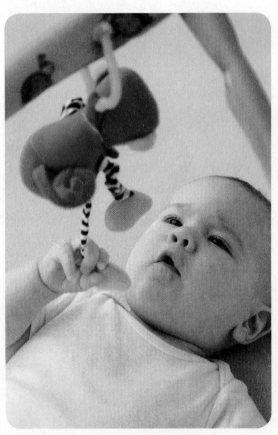

In Piaget's view, what is a scheme? What schemes might this young infant be displaying?
Maya Kovacheva Photography/Getty Images

schemes In Piaget's theory, actions or mental representations that organize knowledge.

assimilation Piagetian concept of the incorporation of new information into existing knowledge.

accommodation Piagetian concept of adjusting schemes to fit new information and experiences.

Poet Nora Perry asked, "Who knows the thoughts of a child?" As much as anyone, Piaget knew. Through careful observations of his own three children—Laurent, Lucienne, and Jacqueline—and observations and interviews with other children, Piaget changed perceptions of the way children think about the world.

Piaget's theory is a general, unifying story of how biology and experience sculpt cognitive development. Piaget thought that, just as our physical bodies have structures that enable us to adapt to the world, we build mental structures that help us adapt to the world. *Adaptation* involves adjusting to new environmental demands. Piaget stressed that children actively construct their own cognitive worlds; information is not just poured into their minds from the environment. He sought to discover how children at different points in their development think about the world and how systematic changes in their thinking occur.

PROCESSES OF DEVELOPMENT

What processes do children use as they construct their knowledge of the world? Piaget stressed that the following processes are especially important in this regard: schemes, assimilation, accommodation, organization, and equilibration.

Schemes Piaget (1954) said that as the child seeks to construct an understanding of the world, the developing brain creates **schemes.** These are actions or mental representations that organize knowledge. In Piaget's theory, behavioral schemes (physical activities) characterize infancy, and mental schemes (cognitive activities) develop in childhood (Waite-Stupiansky, 2017). A baby's schemes are structured by simple actions that can be performed on objects, such as sucking, looking, and grasping. Older children have schemes that include strategies and plans for solving problems. For example, a 5-year-old might have a scheme that involves the strategy of classifying objects by size, shape, or color. By the time we have reached adulthood, we have constructed an enormous number of diverse schemes, ranging from driving a car to balancing a budget to achieving fairness.

Assimilation and Accommodation To explain how children use and adapt their schemes, Piaget proposed two concepts: assimilation and accommodation. Recall that **assimilation** occurs when children incorporate new information into their existing schemes. **Accommodation** occurs when children adjust their schemes to fit new information and experiences.

Think about a toddler who has learned the word *car* to identify the family's car. The toddler might call all moving vehicles on roads "cars," including motorcycles and trucks;

the child has assimilated these objects into his or her existing scheme. But the child soon learns that motorcycles and trucks are not cars and then fine-tunes the category to exclude motorcycles and trucks, accommodating the scheme.

Assimilation and accommodation operate even in very young infants. Newborns reflexively suck everything that touches their lips; they assimilate all sorts of objects into their sucking scheme. By sucking different objects, they learn about their taste, texture, shape, and so on. After several months of experience, though, they construct their understanding of the world differently. Some objects, such as fingers and the mother's breast, can be sucked, and others, such as fuzzy blankets, should not be sucked. In other words, babies accommodate their sucking scheme.

Organization To make sense out of their world, said Piaget, children cognitively organize their experiences. **Organization** in Piaget's theory is the grouping of isolated behaviors and thoughts into a higher-order system. Continual refinement of this organization is an inherent part of development. A boy who has only a vague idea about how to use a hammer may also have a vague idea about how to use other tools. After learning how to use each one, he relates these uses, grouping items into categories and organizing his knowledge.

Equilibration and Stages of Development **Equilibration** is a mechanism that Piaget proposed to explain how children shift from one stage of thought to the next. The shift occurs as children experience cognitive conflict, or disequilibrium, in trying to understand the world. Eventually, they resolve the conflict and reach a balance, or equilibrium, of thought. Piaget argued that there is considerable movement between states of cognitive equilibrium and disequilibrium as assimilation and accommodation work in concert to produce cognitive change. For example, if a child believes that the amount of a liquid changes simply because the liquid is poured into a container with a different shape—for instance, from a container that is short and wide into a container that is tall and narrow—she might be puzzled by such issues as where the "extra" liquid came from and whether there is actually more liquid to drink. The child will eventually resolve these puzzles as her thought becomes more advanced. In the everyday world, the child is constantly faced with such counterexamples and inconsistencies.

Assimilation and accommodation always take the child to a higher ground. For Piaget, the motivation for change is an internal search for equilibrium. As old schemes are adjusted and new schemes are developed, the child organizes and reorganizes the old and new schemes. Eventually, the organization is fundamentally different from the old organization; it is a new way of thinking, a new stage. The result of these processes, according to Piaget, is that individuals go through four stages of development. A different way of understanding the world makes one stage more advanced than another. Cognition is *qualitatively* different in one stage compared with another. In other words, the way children reason at one stage is different from the way they reason at another stage.

Each of Piaget's stages is age-related and consists of distinct ways of thinking. Piaget identified four stages of cognitive development: sensorimotor, preoperational, concrete operational, and formal operational (see Figure 1).

SENSORIMOTOR STAGE

The **sensorimotor stage** lasts from birth to about 2 years of age. In this stage, infants construct an understanding of the world by coordinating sensory experiences (such as seeing and hearing) with physical, motoric actions—hence the term "sensorimotor." At the beginning of this stage, newborns have little more than reflexive patterns with which to work. At the end of the sensorimotor stage, 2-year-olds can produce complex sensorimotor patterns and use primitive symbols. We first will summarize Piaget's descriptions of how infants develop. Later we will consider criticisms of his views.

Substages Piaget divided the sensorimotor stage into six substages: (1) simple reflexes; (2) first habits and primary circular reactions; (3) secondary circular reactions;

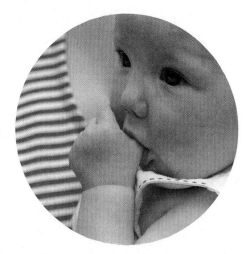

How might assimilation and accommodation be involved in infants' sucking?
Brand X Pictures/Stockbyte/Getty Images

We are born capable of learning.

—Jean-Jacques Rousseau
Swiss-born French philosopher, 18th century

organization Piaget's concept of grouping isolated behaviors into a higher-order, more smoothly functioning cognitive system; the grouping or arranging of items into categories.

equilibration A mechanism that Piaget proposed to explain how children shift from one stage of thought to the next. The shift occurs as children experience cognitive conflict, or disequilibrium, in trying to understand the world. Eventually, they resolve the conflict and reach a balance, or equilibrium, of thought.

sensorimotor stage The first of Piaget's stages, which lasts from birth to about 2 years of age, when infants construct an understanding of the world by coordinating sensory experiences (such as seeing and hearing) with motoric actions.

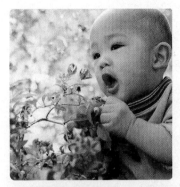
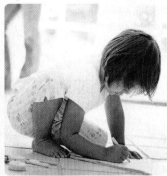
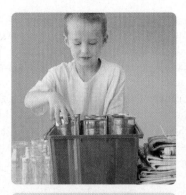
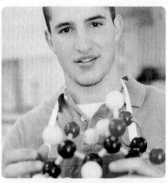

Sensorimotor Stage	**Preoperational Stage**	**Concrete Operational Stage**	**Formal Operational Stage**
The infant constructs an understanding of the world by coordinating sensory experiences with physical actions. An infant progresses from reflexive, instinctual action at birth to the beginning of symbolic thought toward the end of the stage.	The child begins to represent the world with words and images. These words and images reflect increased symbolic thinking and go beyond the connection of sensory information and physical action.	The child can now reason logically about concrete events and classify objects into different sets.	The adolescent reasons in more abstract, idealistic, and logical ways.
Birth to 2 Years of Age	**2 to 7 Years of Age**	**7 to 11 Years of Age**	**11 Years of Age Through Adulthood**

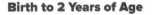

FIGURE 1

PIAGET'S FOUR STAGES OF COGNITIVE DEVELOPMENT

(a) Stockbyte/Getty Images; (b) Jacobs Stock Photography/BananaStock/Getty Images; (c) Fuse/image100/Corbis; (d) Purestock/Getty Images

(4) coordination of secondary circular reactions; (5) tertiary circular reactions, novelty, and curiosity; and (6) internalization of schemes (see Figure 2).

- *Simple reflexes,* the first sensorimotor substage, corresponds to the first month after birth. In this substage, sensation and action are coordinated primarily through reflexive behaviors, such as the rooting and sucking reflexes. Soon the infant produces behaviors that resemble reflexes in the absence of the usual stimulus for the reflex. For example, a newborn will suck a nipple or bottle only when it is placed directly in the baby's mouth or touched to the lips. But soon the infant might suck when a bottle or nipple is only nearby. The infant is initiating action and is actively structuring experiences in the first month of life.

- *First habits and primary circular reactions* is the second sensorimotor substage, which develops between 1 and 4 months of age. In this substage, the infant coordinates sensation and two types of schemes: habits and primary circular reactions. A *habit* is a scheme based on a reflex that has become completely separated from its eliciting stimulus. For example, infants in substage 1 suck when bottles are put to their lips or when they see a bottle. Infants in substage 2 might suck even when no bottle is present. A *circular reaction* is a repetitive action. A *primary circular reaction* is a scheme based on the attempt to reproduce an event that initially occurred by chance. For example, suppose an infant accidentally sucks his fingers when they are placed near his mouth. Later, he searches for his fingers to suck them again, but the fingers do not cooperate because the infant cannot coordinate visual and manual actions.

  Habits and circular reactions are stereotyped—that is, the infant repeats them the same way each time. During this substage, the infant's own body remains the infant's center of attention. There is no outward pull by environmental events.

- *Secondary circular reactions* is the third sensorimotor substage, which develops between 4 and 8 months of age. In this substage, the infant becomes more object-oriented,

Substage	Age	Description	Example
1 Simple reflexes	Birth to 1 month	Coordination of sensation and action through reflexive behaviors.	Rooting, sucking, and grasping reflexes; newborns suck reflexively when their lips are touched.
2 First habits and primary circular reactions	1 to 4 months	Coordination of sensation and two types of schemes: habits (reflex) and primary circular reactions (reproduction of an event that initially occurred by chance). Main focus is still on the infant's body.	Repeating a body sensation first experienced by chance (sucking thumb, for example); then infants might accommodate actions by sucking their thumb differently from how they suck on a nipple.
3 Secondary circular reactions	4 to 8 months	Infants become more object-oriented, moving beyond self-preoccupation; repeat actions that bring interesting or pleasurable results.	An infant coos to make a person stay near; as the person starts to leave, the infant coos again.
4 Coordination of secondary circular reactions	8 to 12 months	Coordination of vision and touch—hand-eye coordination; coordination of schemes and intentionality.	Infant manipulates a stick in order to bring an attractive toy within reach.
5 Tertiary circular reactions, novelty, and curiosity	12 to 18 months	Infants become intrigued by the many properties of objects and by the many things they can make happen to objects; they experiment with new behavior.	A block can be made to fall, spin, hit another object, and slide across the ground.
6 Internalization of schemes	18 to 24 months	Infants develop the ability to use primitive symbols and form enduring mental representations.	An infant who has never thrown a temper tantrum before sees a playmate throw a tantrum; the infant retains a memory of the event, then throws one himself the next day.

FIGURE 2
PIAGET'S SIX SUBSTAGES OF SENSORIMOTOR DEVELOPMENT

moving beyond preoccupation with the self. By chance, an infant might shake a rattle. The infant repeats this action for the sake of its fascination. The infant also imitates some simple actions, such as the baby talk or burbling of adults, and some physical gestures. However, the baby imitates only actions that he or she is already able to produce. Although directed toward objects in the world, the infant's schemes are not intentional or goal-directed.

- *Coordination of secondary circular reactions* is Piaget's fourth sensorimotor substage, which develops between 8 and 12 months of age. To progress into this substage, the infant must coordinate vision and touch, hand and eye. Actions become more outwardly directed. Significant changes during this substage involve the coordination of schemes and intentionality. Infants readily combine and recombine previously learned schemes in a coordinated way. They might look at an object and grasp it simultaneously, or they might visually inspect a toy, such as a rattle, and finger it simultaneously, exploring it tactilely. Actions are even more outwardly directed than before. Related to this coordination is the second achievement—the presence of intentionality. For example, infants might manipulate a stick in order to bring a desired toy within reach, or they might knock over one block to reach for another one and play with it.

- *Tertiary circular reactions, novelty, and curiosity* is Piaget's fifth sensorimotor substage, which develops between 12 and 18 months of age. In this substage, infants become intrigued by the many properties of objects and by the many things that they can make happen to objects. A block can be made to fall, spin, hit another object, and slide across the ground. *Tertiary circular reactions* are schemes in which the infant purposely explores new possibilities with objects, continually doing new things to them and exploring the results. Piaget says that this stage marks the starting point for human curiosity and interest in novelty.

- *Internalization of schemes* is Piaget's sixth and final sensorimotor substage, which develops between 18 and 24 months of age. In this substage, the infant develops the ability to use primitive symbols. For Piaget, a *symbol* is an internalized sensory image or word that represents an event. Primitive symbols permit the infant to think about concrete events without directly acting them out or perceiving them. Moreover, symbols allow the infant to manipulate and transform the represented events in simple ways. In a favorite Piagetian example, Piaget's young daughter saw a matchbox being opened and closed. Later, she mimicked the event by opening and closing her mouth. This was an obvious expression of her image of the event.

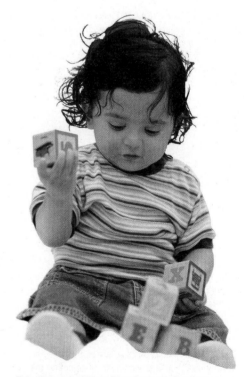

This 17-month-old is in Piaget's stage of tertiary circular reactions. *What might the infant do that suggests he is in this stage?*
Tom Grill/Getty Images

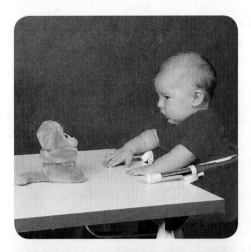

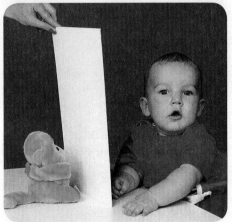

FIGURE 3

OBJECT PERMANENCE. Piaget argued that object permanence is one of infancy's landmark cognitive accomplishments. For this 5-month-old boy, "out of sight" is literally out of mind. The infant looks at the toy monkey (*top*), but when his view of the toy is blocked (*bottom*), he does not search for it. Several months later, he will search for the hidden toy monkey, reflecting the presence of object permanence.

Doug Goodman/Science Source

object permanence The Piagetian term for one of an infant's most important accomplishments: understanding that objects and events continue to exist even when they cannot directly be seen, heard, or touched.

A-not-B error Also called A$\overline{\text{B}}$ error, this occurs when infants make the mistake of selecting the familiar hiding place (A) to locate an object, rather than looking in the new hiding place (B), as they progress into substage 4 in Piaget's sensorimotor stage.

Object Permanence   Imagine how chaotic and unpredictable your life would be if you could not distinguish between yourself and your world. This is what the life of a newborn must be like, according to Piaget. There is no differentiation between the self and world; objects have no separate, permanent existence.

By the end of the sensorimotor period, children understand that objects are both separate from the self and permanent. **Object permanence** is the understanding that objects and events continue to exist even when they cannot be seen, heard, or touched. Acquiring the sense of object permanence is one of the infant's most important accomplishments. According to Piaget, infants develop object permanence in a series of substages that correspond to the six substages of sensorimotor development.

How can anyone know whether an infant has developed a sense of object permanence? The principal way that object permanence is studied is by watching an infant's reaction when an interesting object disappears (see Figure 3). If infants search for the object, it is assumed that they believe it continues to exist.

Object permanence is just one of the basic concepts about the physical world developed by babies. To Piaget, children—even infants—are much like little scientists, examining the world to see how it works. But how can adult scientists determine what these "baby scientists" are finding out about the world and at what age they're finding it out? To answer this question, read the *Connecting Through Research* interlude that follows.

Evaluating Piaget's Sensorimotor Stage   Piaget opened up a new way of looking at infants with his view that their main task is to coordinate their sensory impressions with their motor activity. However, the infant's cognitive world is not as neatly packaged as Piaget portrayed it, and some of Piaget's explanations for the cause of cognitive changes in development are debated. In the past several decades, sophisticated experimental techniques have been devised to study infants, and there have been a large number of research studies on infant development. Much of the new research suggests that Piaget's view of sensorimotor development needs to be modified (Anderson, Hespos, & Rips, 2018; Krist & others, 2018; Meltzoff & Marshall, 2018).

The A-not-B Error   One modification concerns Piaget's claim that certain processes are crucial in transitions from one stage to the next. The data do not always support his explanations. For example, in Piaget's theory, an important feature in the progression into substage 4, *coordination of secondary circular reactions,* is an infant's inclination to search for a hidden object in a familiar location rather than to look for the object in a new location. For example, if a toy is hidden twice, initially at location A and subsequently at location B, 8- to 12-month-old infants search correctly at location A initially. But when the toy is subsequently hidden at location B, they make the mistake of continuing to search for it at location A. **A-not-B error** (also called A$\overline{\text{B}}$ error) is the term used to describe this common mistake. Older infants are less likely to make the A-not-B error because their concept of object permanence is more complete.

Researchers have found, however, that a variety of parameters affect whether infants make A-not-B errors. For example, when only the hands and arms rather than the full body of an experimenter are visible, 9-month-old infants are less likely to make A-not-B errors, suggesting that part of the error is due to infants' imitation of body movements (Boyer, Harding, & Bertenthal, 2017). Likewise, A-not-B errors are sensitive to the delay between hiding the object at B and the infant's attempt to find it (Buss, Ross-Sheehy, & Reynolds, 2018). Thus, the A-not-B error might be due to a failure in memory. Another explanation is that infants tend to repeat a previous motor behavior (MacNeill & others, 2018).

Perceptual Development and Expectations   One of the major strengths of Piaget's theory is that it formed a set of hypotheses for the developmental course of cognition and perception that could be tested in future research. Since Piaget's time, infants' perceptual abilities and cognition have been found to be more advanced at earlier ages than theorized by Piaget (Barrouillet, 2015).

How Do Researchers Determine Infants' Understanding of Object Permanence and Causality?

Two accomplishments of infants that Piaget examined were the development of object permanence and the child's understanding of causality. Let's examine two research studies that address these topics.

In both studies, Renée Baillargeon and her colleagues used a research method that involves violation of expectations. In this method, infants see an event happen as it normally would. Then the event is changed in a way that violates what the infant expects to see. When infants look longer at the event that violates their expectations, it indicates they are surprised by it.

In one study focused on object permanence, researchers showed infants a toy car that moved down an inclined track, disappeared behind a screen, and then reemerged at the other end, still on the track (Baillargeon & DeVoe, 1991). After this sequence was repeated several times, something different occurred: A toy mouse was placed behind the tracks but was hidden by the screen while the car rolled by. This was the "possible" event. Then the researchers created an "impossible event": The toy mouse was placed on the tracks but was secretly removed after the screen was lowered so that the car seemed to go through the mouse. In this study, infants as young as 3½ months of age looked longer at the impossible event than at the possible event, indicating that they were surprised by it. Their surprise suggested that not only did they remember that the toy mouse still existed (object permanence), but they also recalled its location.

Another study focused on infants' understanding of causality (Kotovsky & Baillargeon, 1994). In this research, a cylinder rolls down a ramp and hits a toy bug at the bottom of the ramp. By 5½ and 6½ months of age, after infants have seen how far the bug will be pushed by a medium-sized cylinder, their reactions indicate that they understand that the bug will roll farther if it is hit by a large cylinder than if it is hit by a small cylinder. Thus, by the middle of the first year of life infants understand that the size of a moving object determines how far it will move a stationary object that it collides with.

In Baillargeon's (2008; Baillargeon & others, 2012) view, infants have a pre-adapted, innate bias called the principle of persistence that explains their assumption that objects don't change their properties—including how solid they are, their location, their color, and their form—unless some external factor (a person who moves the object, for example) obviously intervenes. Shortly, we will revisit the extent to which nature and nurture are at work in the changes that take place in the infant's cognitive development.

The research findings discussed in this interlude and other research indicate that infants develop object permanence and causal reasoning much earlier than Piaget proposed (Baillargeon, 2014; Baillargeon & others, 2012). Indeed, as you will see in the next section, a major theme of infant cognitive development today is that infants are more cognitively competent than Piaget envisioned.

Research also suggests that infants develop the ability to understand how the world works at a very early age (Baillargeon & DeJong, 2017). In experiments designed to test infants' expectations of how physical objects and people will behave, infants are often placed before a puppet stage and shown a series of actions that would either be expected or unexpected depending on one's understanding of how the world works. How long infants look at each series of actions is used as a measure of surprise, because babies look longer at surprising than at expected events. Infants look longer in experiments that violate their expectations about the physical or social world than in experiments in which objects and people behave as infants expect them to. For example, by as early as 5 months of age, infants understand differences between how solid substances and liquid substances will behave and even have expectations about how potentially trickier granular substances, such as sand, will behave (Hespos & others, 2016). Likewise, from early in life, infants have expectations about how other people will behave. In a study in which infants were shown videos of a stranger either comforting or ignoring a crying infant, even 4-month-old infants were more surprised by the video in which the stranger ignored rather than comforted the infant (Jin & others, 2018).

One criticism of studies that use how long infants look at different types of events as a measure of their understanding of how the world works is that looking time might be a better measure of perceptual expectations than knowledge. Thus, researchers advocate using different types of methodologies to study infant cognition rather than relying on any single approach. New neuroimaging techniques and measures of psychophysiology offer options for assessing infants' cognitive development (Ellis & Turk-Browne, 2018). For example, infants' visual attention is related to changes in heart rate (Reynolds & Richards, 2017).

Within the first year of life, infants have learned how objects behave in relation to other objects and in relation to laws of the physical world, such as gravity. Infants also have learned that people generally behave in goal-directed ways toward objects (Corbetta

& Fagard, 2017). As infants develop, their experiences and actions on objects help them to understand physical laws, and their experiences with people help them to understand the social world (Ullman & others, 2018).

Nature and Nurture   Both nature and nurture play important roles in infant development. The **core knowledge approach** states that infants are born with domain-specific innate knowledge systems. Among these domain-specific knowledge systems are those involving space, number sense, object permanence, and language (which we will discuss later in this chapter). Strongly influenced by evolution, the core knowledge domains are theorized to be prewired to allow infants to make sense of their world. After all, how could infants possibly grasp the complex world in which they live if they didn't come into the world equipped with core sets of knowledge? In this approach, the innate core knowledge domains form a foundation on which more mature cognitive functioning and learning develop. Proponents of the core knowledge approach argue that Piaget greatly underestimated the cognitive abilities of infants, especially young infants (Jin & Baillargeon, 2017).

An intriguing domain of core knowledge that has been investigated in young infants is whether they have a sense of number. Using the violations of expectations method discussed in the *Connecting Through Research* interlude, Karen Wynn (1992) conducted an early experiment on infants' sense of number. Five-month-old infants were shown one or two Mickey Mouse dolls on a puppet stage. Then the experimenter hid the doll(s) behind a screen and visibly removed or added one. Next, when the screen was lifted, the infants looked longer when they saw the incorrect number of dolls. Other researchers also have found that infants can distinguish between different numbers of objects, actions, and sounds (Odic, 2018; Smith & others, 2017).

Not everyone agrees that young infants have early math skills. One criticism is that infants in the number experiments are merely responding to changes in the display that violated their expectations.

In criticizing the core knowledge approach, British developmental psychologist Mark Johnston (2008) says that infants already have accumulated hundreds, and in some cases even thousands, of hours of experience in grasping what the world is about, which gives considerable room for the environment's role in the development of infant cognition. According to Johnston (2008), infants likely come into the world with "soft biases to perceive and attend to different aspects of the environment, and to learn about the world in particular ways." Although debate about the cause and course of infant cognitive development continues, most developmentalists today agree that Piaget underestimated the early cognitive accomplishments of infants and that both nature and nurture are involved in infants' cognitive development (Baillargeon, 2014).

Conclusions   In sum, many researchers conclude that Piaget wasn't specific enough about how infants learn about their world and that infants, especially young infants, are more competent than Piaget thought. As researchers have examined the specific ways that infants learn, the field of infant cognition has become very specialized. Many researchers are at work on different questions, with no general theory emerging that can connect all of the different findings. Their theories often are local theories, focused on specific research questions, rather than grand theories like Piaget's. If there is a unifying theme, it is that investigators in infant development seek to understand more precisely how developmental changes in cognition take place. As they seek to identify more precisely the contributions of nature and nurture to infant development, researchers face the difficult task of determining whether the course of acquiring information, which is very rapid in some domains, is better accounted for by an innate set of biases (that is, core knowledge) or by the extensive input of environmental experiences to which the infant is exposed (Aslin, 2012). Recall that exploring connections between brain, cognition, and development involves the field of *developmental cognitive neuroscience* (Steinbeis & others, 2017).

PREOPERATIONAL STAGE

The cognitive world of the preschool child is creative, free, and fanciful. The imaginations of preschool children work overtime, and their mental grasp of the world improves. Piaget described the preschool child's cognition as *preoperational*. What did he mean?

developmental **connection**

Theories

Eleanor Gibson was a pioneer in crafting the ecological perception view of development. Connect to "Motor, Sensory, and Perceptual Development."

developmental **connection**

Nature and Nurture

Development is influenced by both nature (biological inheritance) and nurture (environmental experiences). Connect to "Introduction" and "Biological Beginnings."

core knowledge approach States that infants are born with domain-specific innate knowledge systems, such as those involving space, number sense, object permanence, and language.

operations Internalized actions that allow children to do mentally what before they had done only physically. Operations also are reversible mental actions.

Because Piaget called this stage preoperational, it might sound unimportant. Not so. Preoperational thought is anything but a convenient waiting period for the next stage, concrete operational thought. However, the label *preoperational* emphasizes that the child does not yet perform **operations,** which are internalized actions that allow children to do mentally what they could formerly do only physically. Operations are reversible mental actions. Mentally adding and subtracting numbers are examples of operations. *Preoperational thought* is the beginning of the ability to reconstruct in thought what has been established in behavior.

The **preoperational stage,** which lasts from approximately 2 to 7 years of age, is the second Piagetian stage. In this stage, children begin to represent the world with words, images, and drawings. Symbolic thought goes beyond simple connections of sensory information and physical action. Stable concepts are formed, mental reasoning emerges, egocentrism is present, and magical beliefs are constructed. Preoperational thought can be divided into substages: the symbolic function substage and the intuitive thought substage.

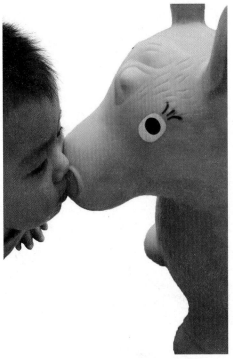

What revisions in Piaget's theory of sensorimotor development do contemporary researchers conclude need to be made? How do nature and nurture affect infant cognitive development?
Baobao ou/Getty Images

The Symbolic Function Substage The **symbolic function substage** is the first substage of preoperational thought, occurring roughly between the ages of 2 and 4. In this substage, the young child gains the ability to mentally represent an object that is not present. This ability vastly expands the child's mental world; how early symbolic representation abilities develop is related to children's exposure to symbols in everyday life, such as exposure to video and print materials and drawing with parents (Salsa & Gariboldi, 2018). Young children use scribble designs to represent people, houses, cars, clouds, and so on; they begin to use language and engage in pretend play. However, although young children make distinct progress during this substage, their thought still has several important limitations, two of which are egocentrism and animism.

Egocentrism is the inability to distinguish between one's own perspective and someone else's perspective. The following telephone conversation between 4-year-old Mary, who is at home, and her father, who is at work, typifies Mary's egocentric thought:

Father: Mary, is Mommy there?

Mary: (Silently nods)

Father: Mary, may I speak to Mommy?

Mary: (Nods again silently)

Mary's response is egocentric in that she fails to consider her father's perspective before replying. A nonegocentric thinker would have responded verbally.

Piaget and Barbel Inhelder (1969) initially studied young children's egocentrism by devising the three-mountains task (see Figure 4). The child walks around the model of the mountains and becomes familiar with what the mountains look like from different perspectives,

preoperational stage The second Piagetian developmental stage, which lasts from about 2 to 7 years of age, when children begin to represent the world with words, images, and drawings.

symbolic function substage The first substage of preoperational thought, occurring roughly between the ages of 2 and 4. In this substage, the young child gains the ability to represent mentally an object that is not present.

egocentrism An important feature of preoperational thought: the inability to distinguish between one's own and someone else's perspective.

Model of Mountains

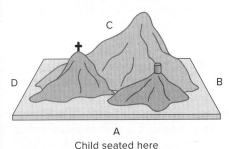

A
Child seated here

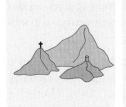
Photo 1
(View from A)

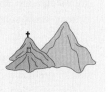
Photo 2
(View from B)

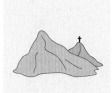
Photo 3
(View from C)

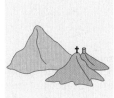
Photo 4
(View from D)

FIGURE 4

THE THREE-MOUNTAINS TASK. The mountain model on the far left shows the child's perspective from view A, where he or she is sitting. The four squares represent photos showing the mountains from four different viewpoints of the model—A, B, C, and D. The experimenter asks the child to identify the photo in which the mountains look as they would from position B. To identify the photo correctly, the child has to take the perspective of a person sitting at spot B. Invariably, a child who thinks in a preoperational way cannot perform this task. When asked what a view of the mountains looks like from position B, the child selects Photo 1, taken from location A (the child's own view at the time) instead of Photo 2, the correct view.

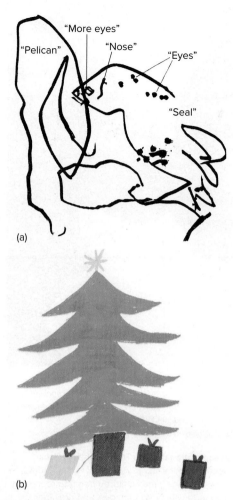

FIGURE 5

THE SYMBOLIC DRAWINGS OF YOUNG CHILDREN. (*a*) A 3½-year-old's symbolic drawing. Halfway into this drawing, the 3½-year-old artist said it was "a pelican kissing a seal." (*b*) This 11-year-old's drawing is neater and more realistic but also less inventive.

animism A facet of preoperational thought: the belief that inanimate objects have lifelike qualities and are capable of action.

intuitive thought substage The second substage of preoperational thought, occurring between approximately 4 and 7 years of age, when children begin to use primitive reasoning.

centration Focusing attention on one characteristic to the exclusion of all others.

conservation The realization that altering an object's or substance's appearance does not change its basic properties.

and she can see that there are different objects on the mountains. The child is then seated on one side of the table on which the mountains are placed. The experimenter moves a doll to different locations around the table, at each location asking the child to select from a series of photos the one photo that most accurately reflects the view the doll is seeing. Children in the preoperational stage often pick their own view rather than the doll's view. Preschool children frequently show perspective skills on some tasks but not others.

Animism, another limitation of preoperational thought, is the belief that inanimate objects have lifelike qualities and are capable of action (Poulin-Dubois, 2018). A young child might show animism by saying, "That tree pushed the leaf off, and it fell down" or "The sidewalk made me mad; it made me fall down." A young child who uses animism fails to distinguish the appropriate occasions for using human and nonhuman perspectives.

Possibly because young children are not very concerned about reality, their drawings are fanciful and inventive. Suns are blue, skies are yellow, and cars float on clouds in their symbolic, imaginative world. One 3½-year-old looked at a scribble he had just drawn and described it as a pelican kissing a seal (see Figure 5a). The symbolism is simple but strong, like abstractions found in some modern art. Twentieth-century Spanish artist Pablo Picasso commented, "I used to draw like Raphael but it has taken me a lifetime to draw like young children." In the elementary school years, a child's drawings become more realistic, neat, and precise (see Figure 5b). Improvements in fine motor control and working memory contribute to increased realism with age in children's drawings (Morra & Panesi, 2017).

The Intuitive Thought Substage The **intuitive thought substage** is the second substage of preoperational thought, occurring between approximately 4 and 7 years of age. In this substage, children begin to use primitive reasoning and want to know the answers to all sorts of questions. Consider 4-year-old Tommy, who is at the beginning of the intuitive thought substage. Although he is starting to develop his own ideas about the world he lives in, his ideas are still simple, and he is not very good at thinking things out. He has difficulty understanding events that he knows are taking place but which he cannot see. His fantasized thoughts bear little resemblance to reality. He cannot yet answer the question "What if?" in any reliable way. For example, he has only a vague idea of what would happen if a car were to hit him. He also has difficulty negotiating traffic because he cannot do the mental calculations necessary to estimate whether an approaching car will hit him when he crosses the road.

By the age of 5, children have just about exhausted the adults around them with "why" questions. The child's questions signal the emergence of interest in reasoning and in figuring out why things are the way they are. By the time children enter preschool, they ask an average of 76 questions per hour seeking information and, by the age of 5, their questions are well-formulated to elicit information children need to learn new concepts (Kurkul & Corriveau, 2018). Some of the questions children ask require simple, one-word answers such as naming an unfamiliar object, but "how" and "why" questions require more complex explanations.

Piaget called this substage *intuitive* because young children seem so sure about their knowledge and understanding yet are unaware of how they know what they know. That is, they know something but know it without the use of rational thinking.

Centration and the Limitations of Preoperational Thought One limitation of preoperational thought is **centration,** a centering of attention on one characteristic to the exclusion of all others. Centration is most clearly evidenced in young children's lack of **conservation,** the awareness that altering an object's or a substance's appearance does not change its basic properties. For example, to adults, it is obvious that a certain amount of liquid stays the same, regardless of a container's shape. But this is not at all obvious to young children. Instead, they are struck by the height of the liquid in the container; they focus on that characteristic to the exclusion of others.

The situation that Piaget devised to study conservation is his most famous task. In the conservation task, a child is presented with two identical beakers, each filled to the same level with liquid (see Figure 6). The child is asked if these beakers have the same amount of liquid, and she usually says "yes." Then the liquid from one beaker is poured

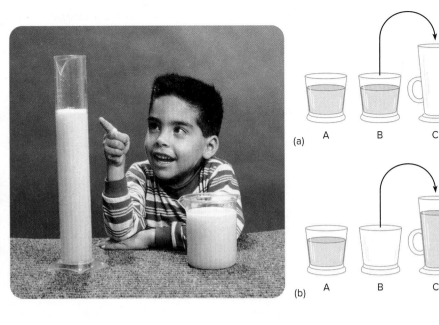

FIGURE **6**

PIAGET'S CONSERVATION TASK. The beaker test is a well-known Piagetian task to determine whether a child can think operationally—that is, whether he or she can mentally reverse actions and show conservation of the substance. (*a*) Two identical beakers are presented to the child. Next, the experimenter pours the liquid from B into C, which is taller and thinner than A or B. (*b*) The child is asked if these beakers (A and C) have the same amount of liquid. The preoperational child says "no." When asked to point to the beaker that has more liquid, the preoperational child points to the tall, thin beaker.

Tony Freeman/PhotoEdit

into a third beaker, which is taller and thinner than the first two. The child is then asked if the amount of liquid in the tall, thin beaker is equal to that which remains in one of the original beakers. Children who are less than 7 or 8 years old usually say "no" and justify their answers in terms of the differing height or width of the beakers. Older children usually answer "yes" and justify their answers appropriately ("If you poured the water back, the amount would still be the same").

In Piaget's theory, failing the conservation-of-liquid task is a sign that children are at the preoperational stage of cognitive development. The preoperational child fails to show conservation not only of liquid but also of number, matter, length, volume, and area. Figure 7 portrays several of these dimensions of conservation.

Children often vary in their performance on different conservation tasks. Thus, a child might be able to conserve volume but not number. Researchers have discovered links between children's performance on Piagetian tasks and the brain's development, particularly the prefrontal cortex (Bolton & Hattie, 2017). For example, a fMRI brain imaging study of conservation of number revealed that advances in a network in the parietal and frontal lobes were linked to 9- and 10-year-olds' conservation success when compared to non-conserving 5- and 6-year-olds (Houde & others, 2011).

Some developmentalists do not believe Piaget was entirely correct in his estimate of when children's conservation skills emerge. For example, early research by Rochel Gelman (1969) showed that when the child's attention to relevant aspects of the conservation task is improved, the child is more likely to conserve. Gelman has also demonstrated that attentional training on one dimension, such as number, improves the preschool child's performance on another dimension, such as mass. Thus, Gelman suggests that conservation appears earlier than Piaget thought and that attention is especially important in explaining conservation.

CONCRETE OPERATIONAL STAGE

The **concrete operational stage,** which lasts approximately from 7 to 11 years of age, is the third Piagetian stage. In this stage, logical reasoning replaces intuitive reasoning as long as the reasoning can be applied to specific or concrete examples. For instance, concrete operational thinkers cannot imagine the steps necessary to complete an algebraic equation, which is too abstract for thinking at this stage of development. Children at this stage can perform *concrete operations,* which are reversible mental actions on real, concrete objects.

Conservation   The conservation tasks demonstrate a child's ability to perform concrete operations. In the test of reversibility of thought involving conservation of matter (shown in Figure 7), a child is presented with two identical balls of clay. An experimenter rolls one ball

concrete operational stage Piaget's third stage, which lasts from approximately 7 to 11 years of age, when children can perform concrete operations, and logical reasoning replaces intuitive reasoning as long as the reasoning can be applied to specific or concrete examples.

Type of Conservation	Initial Presentation	Manipulation	Preoperational Child's Answer
Number	Two identical rows of objects are shown to the child, who agrees they have the same number.	One row is lengthened and the child is asked whether one row now has more objects.	Yes, the longer row.
Matter	Two identical balls of clay are shown to the child. The child agrees that they are equal.	The experimenter changes the shape of one of the balls and asks the child whether they still contain equal amounts of clay.	No, the longer one has more.
Length	Two sticks are aligned in front of the child. The child agrees that they are the same length.	The experimenter moves one stick to the right, then asks the child if they are equal in length.	No, the one on the top is longer.

FIGURE 7

SOME DIMENSIONS OF CONSERVATION: NUMBER, MATTER, AND LENGTH. *What characteristics of preoperational thought do children demonstrate when they fail these conservation tasks?*

horizontal décalage Piaget's concept that similar abilities do not appear at the same time within a stage of development.

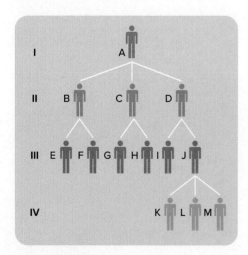

FIGURE 8

CLASSIFICATION: AN IMPORTANT ABILITY IN CONCRETE OPERATIONAL THOUGHT. A family tree of four generations (*I to IV*): The preoperational child has trouble classifying the members of the four generations; the concrete operational child can classify the members vertically, horizontally, and obliquely (up and down and across). For example, the concrete operational child understands that a family member can be a son, a brother, and a father, all at the same time.

into a long, thin shape; the other remains in its original ball shape. The child is then asked if there is more clay in the ball or in the long, thin piece of clay. By the time children reach the age of 7 or 8, most answer that the amount of clay is the same. To answer this problem correctly, children have to imagine the clay ball rolling back into a ball after it has been changed into a long, thin shape; they need to mentally reverse the action on the ball.

Concrete operations allow children to coordinate several characteristics rather than focus on a single property of an object. In the clay example, a preoperational child is likely to focus on height or width, while a concrete operational child coordinates information about both dimensions. Conservation involves recognizing that the length, number, mass, quantity, area, weight, and volume of objects and substances are not changed by transformations that merely alter their appearance.

Children do not conserve all quantities or conserve on all tasks simultaneously. The order of their mastery is number, length, liquid quantity, mass, weight, and volume. **Horizontal décalage** is Piaget's concept that similar abilities do not appear at the same time within a stage of development. During the concrete operational stage, conservation of number usually appears first and conservation of volume last. Also, an 8-year-old child may know that a long stick of clay can be rolled back into a ball but not understand that the ball and the stick weigh the same. At about 9 years of age, the child recognizes that they weigh the same, and eventually, at about 11 to 12 years of age, the child understands that the clay's volume is unchanged by rearranging it. Children initially master tasks in which the dimensions are more salient and visible, only later mastering those not as visually apparent, such as volume.

Classification Many of the concrete operations identified by Piaget involve the ways children reason about the properties of objects. One important skill that characterizes children in the concrete operational stage is the ability to classify things and to consider their relationships. Specifically, concrete operational children can understand (1) the interrelationships among sets and subsets, (2) seriation, and (3) transitivity.

The ability of the concrete operational child to divide things into sets and subsets and understand their relationships is illustrated by a family tree of four generations (Furth & Wachs, 1975) (see Figure 8). This family tree suggests that the grandfather (A) has three children (B, C, and D), each of whom has two children (E through J), and that one of these children (J) has three children (K, L, and M). The concrete operational child understands that person J can, at the same time, be father, brother, and grandson. A child who comprehends this classification system can move up and down a level (vertically), across a level (horizontally), and up and down and across (obliquely) within the system.

Seriation is the ordering of stimuli along a quantitative dimension (such as length). To see if children can serialize, a teacher might haphazardly place eight sticks of varying lengths on a table. The teacher then asks the children to order the sticks by length. Many young children put the sticks into two or three small groups of "big" sticks or "little" sticks, rather than a correct ordering of all eight sticks. Or they line up the tops of the sticks but ignore the bottoms. The concrete operational thinker simultaneously understands that each stick must be longer than the one that precedes it and shorter than the one that follows it.

Transitivity involves the ability to reason about and logically combine relationships. If a relation holds between a first object and a second object, and also holds between the second object and a third object, then it also holds between the first and third objects. For example, consider three sticks (A, B, and C) of differing lengths. A is the longest, B is intermediate in length, and C is the shortest. Does the child understand that if A is longer than B, and B is longer than C, then A is longer than C? In Piaget's theory, concrete operational thinkers do; preoperational thinkers do not.

seriation The concrete operation that involves ordering stimuli along a quantitative dimension (such as length).

transitivity Principle that says if a relation holds between a first object and a second object, and holds between the second object and a third object, then it holds between the first object and the third object. Piaget argued that an understanding of transitivity is characteristic of concrete operational thought.

FORMAL OPERATIONAL STAGE

So far we have studied the first three of Piaget's stages of cognitive development: sensorimotor, preoperational, and concrete operational. What are the characteristics of the fourth stage?

The **formal operational stage,** which appears between 11 and 15 years of age, is the fourth and final Piagetian stage. In this stage, individuals move beyond concrete experiences and think in abstract and more logical ways. As part of thinking more abstractly, adolescents develop images of ideal circumstances. They might think about what an ideal parent is like and compare their parents to their ideal standards. They begin to entertain possibilities for the future and are fascinated with what they might become. In solving problems, formal operational thinkers are more systematic and use logical reasoning.

Abstract, Idealistic, and Logical Thinking The abstract quality of the adolescent's thought at the formal operational level is evident in the adolescent's verbal problem-solving ability. The concrete operational thinker needs to see the concrete elements A, B, and C to be able to make the logical inference that if $A = B$ and $B = C$, then $A = C$. The formal operational thinker can solve this problem merely through verbal presentation.

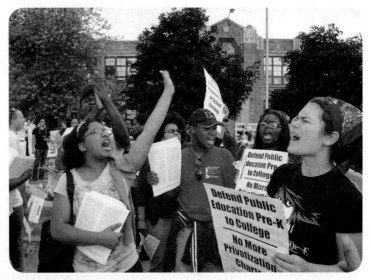

Might adolescents' ability to reason hypothetically and to evaluate what is ideal versus what is real lead them to engage in demonstrations, such as this protest of school privatization? What other causes might be attractive to adolescents' newfound cognitive abilities of hypothetical-deductive reasoning and idealistic thinking?
Jim West/Alamy Stock Photo

Another indication of the abstract quality of adolescents' thought is their increased tendency to think about thought itself. One adolescent commented, "I began thinking about why I was thinking about what I was. Then I began thinking about why I was thinking about what I was thinking about what I was." If this sounds abstract, it is, and it characterizes the adolescent's enhanced focus on thought and its abstract qualities.

Accompanying the abstract thought of adolescence is thought full of idealism and possibilities. While children frequently think in concrete ways, or in terms of what is real and limited, adolescents begin to engage in extended speculation about ideal characteristics— qualities they desire in themselves and in others. Such thoughts often lead adolescents to compare themselves with others in regard to ideal standards. And the thoughts of adolescents are often fantasy flights into future possibilities. It is not unusual for the adolescent to become impatient with these newfound ideal standards and to become perplexed over which of many ideal standards to adopt.

As adolescents are learning to think more abstractly and idealistically, they are also learning to think more logically. Children are likely to solve problems in a trial-and-error fashion. Adolescents begin to think more as a scientist thinks, devising plans to solve problems and systematically testing solutions. They use **hypothetical-deductive reasoning,** which means that they develop hypotheses, or best guesses, and systematically deduce, or conclude, which is the best path to follow in solving the problem.

formal operational stage Piaget's fourth and final stage, which occurs between the ages of 11 and 15, when individuals move beyond concrete experiences and think in more abstract and logical ways.

hypothetical-deductive reasoning Piaget's formal operational concept that adolescents have the cognitive ability to develop hypotheses about ways to solve problems and can systematically deduce which is the best path to follow in solving the problem.

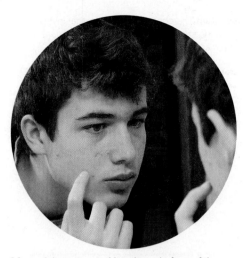

Many adolescents spend long hours in front of the mirror, checking their appearance. *How might this behavior be related to changes in adolescent cognitive and physical development?*
Syldavia/iStock/Getty Images

adolescent egocentrism The heightened self-consciousness of adolescents, which is reflected in adolescents' beliefs that others are as interested in them as they are in themselves, and in adolescents' sense of personal uniqueness and invulnerability.

imaginary audience The aspect of adolescent egocentrism that involves attention-getting behavior motivated by a desire to be noticed, visible, and "onstage."

personal fable The part of adolescent egocentrism that involves an adolescent's sense of uniqueness and invincibility.

Assimilation (incorporating new information into existing knowledge) dominates the initial development of formal operational thought, and these thinkers perceive the world subjectively and idealistically. Later in adolescence, as intellectual balance is restored, these individuals accommodate to the cognitive upheaval that has occurred (they adjust to the new information).

Some of Piaget's ideas on formal operational thought are being challenged (Blakemore & Mills, 2014). There is much more individual variation in formal operational thought than Piaget envisioned. Only about one in three young adolescents is a formal operational thinker. Many American adults never become formal operational thinkers, and neither do many adults in other cultures.

Adolescent Egocentrism   In addition to thinking more logically, abstractly, and idealistically—characteristics of Piaget's formal operational thought stage—in what other ways do adolescents change cognitively? David Elkind (1978) described how adolescent egocentrism governs the way that adolescents think about social matters. **Adolescent egocentrism** is the heightened self-consciousness of adolescents, which is reflected in their belief that others are as interested in them as they are themselves, and in their sense of personal uniqueness and invincibility. Elkind argued that adolescent egocentrism can be dissected into two types of social thinking—imaginary audience and personal fable.

The **imaginary audience** refers to the aspect of adolescent egocentrism that involves feeling one is the center of everyone's attention and sensing that one is on stage. An adolescent boy might think that others are as aware of a few hairs that are out of place as he is. An adolescent girl walks into her classroom and thinks that all eyes are riveted on her complexion. Adolescents especially sense that they are "on stage" in early adolescence, believing they are the main actors and all others are the audience.

According to Elkind, the **personal fable** is the part of adolescent egocentrism that involves an adolescent's sense of personal uniqueness and invincibility. Adolescents' sense of personal uniqueness makes them feel that no one can understand how they really feel. For example, an adolescent girl thinks that her mother cannot possibly sense the hurt she feels because her boyfriend has broken up with her. As part of their effort to retain a sense of personal uniqueness, adolescents might craft stories about themselves that are filled with fantasy, immersing themselves in a world that is far removed from reality. Personal fables frequently show up in adolescent diaries.

Research studies, however, suggest that, rather than perceiving themselves to be invulnerable, many adolescents portray themselves as vulnerable (Reyna, 2018). For example, 12- to 18-year-olds greatly overestimate their chance of dying in the next year and prior to age 20 (de Bruin & Fischhoff, 2017).

Some researchers have questioned the view that invulnerability is a unitary concept and argued rather that it consists of two dimensions (Kim, Park, & Kang, 2018; Potard & others, 2018):

- *Danger invulnerability,* which involves adolescents' sense of indestructibility and tendency to take on physical risks (driving recklessly at high speeds, for example)
- *Psychological invulnerability,* which captures an adolescent's felt invulnerability related to personal or psychological distress (getting one's feelings hurt, for example)

Adolescents who score low on perceptions of risks (or high on perceptions of danger invulnerability) are more likely to engage in a given behavior than are adolescents who perceive the behavior as more risky. For example, misuse of opioids is higher among adolescents who do not perceive opioid use as risky (Voepel-Lewis & others, 2018). Adolescents who face traumatic experiences that disrupt their sense of psychological invulnerability are more at risk of developing depression, anxiety, and other mental health problems (Chen & others, 2017). In terms of psychological invulnerability, adolescents often benefit from the normal developmental challenges of exploring identity options, making new friends, asking someone to go out on a date, and learning a new skill. All of these important adolescent tasks involve risk and failure as an option, but if successful result in enhanced self-image.

Other researchers argue that the separation-individuation process—which involves adolescents separating from their parents and developing independence and identity—is responsible for the findings just discussed, rather than cognitive developmental changes (Lapsley & Woodbury, 2015). With respect to personal fables, they argue that invulnerability and personal uniqueness are forms of adolescent narcissism.

Review Connect Reflect

 LG1 Discuss the key processes and four stages in Piaget's theory.

Review

- What are the key processes in Piaget's theory of cognitive development?
- What are the main characteristics of the sensorimotor stage? What revisions of Piaget's sensorimotor stage have been proposed?
- What are the main characteristics of the preoperational stage?
- What are the main characteristics of the concrete operational stage?
- What are the main characteristics of the formal operational stage? How has Piaget's formal operational stage been criticized?

Connect

- How does Piaget's sensorimotor stage relate to what you learned about perceptual-motor coupling?

Reflect *Your Own Personal Journey of Life*

- Do you consider yourself to be a formal operational thinker? Do you still sometimes feel like a concrete operational thinker? Give examples.

Applying and Evaluating Piaget's Theory **LG2** Apply Piaget's theory to education and evaluate his theory.

Piaget and Education

Evaluating Piaget's Theory

What are some applications of Piaget's theory to education? What are the main contributions and criticisms of Piaget's theory?

PIAGET AND EDUCATION

Piaget was not an educator, but he provided a sound conceptual framework for viewing learning and education. Following are some ideas in Piaget's theory that can be applied to teaching children (Waite-Stupiansky, 2017):

1. *Take a constructivist approach.* Piaget emphasized that children learn best when they are active and seek solutions for themselves. Piaget opposed teaching methods that treat children as passive receptacles. The educational implication of Piaget's view is that, in all subjects, students learn best by making discoveries, reflecting on them, and discussing them, rather than by blindly imitating the teacher or doing things by rote.

2. *Facilitate rather than direct learning.* Effective teachers design situations that allow students to learn by doing. These situations promote students' thinking and discovery. Teachers listen, watch, and question students, to help them gain better understanding.

3. *Consider the child's knowledge and level of thinking.* Students do not come to class with empty minds. They have concepts of space, time, quantity, and causality. These ideas differ from the ideas of adults. Teachers need to interpret what a student is saying and respond in a way that is not too far from the student's level. Also, Piaget suggested that it is important to examine children's mistakes in thinking, not just what they get correct, to help guide them to a higher level of understanding.

4. *Promote the student's intellectual health.* When Piaget came to lecture in the United States, he was asked, "What can I do to get my child to a higher cognitive stage sooner?" He was asked this question so often here compared with other countries

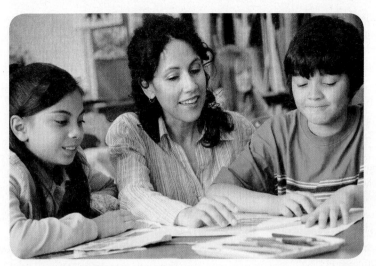

What are some educational strategies that can be derived from Piaget's theory?
Fuse/Getty Images

that he called it the American question. For Piaget, children's learning should occur naturally. Children should not be pushed and pressured into achieving too much too early in their development, before they are maturationally ready. Some parents spend long hours every day holding up large flash cards with words on them to improve their baby's vocabulary. In the Piagetian view, this is not the best way for infants to learn. It places too much emphasis on speeding up intellectual development, involves passive learning, and will not lead to positive outcomes.

5. *Turn the classroom into a setting of exploration and discovery.* What do actual classrooms look like when the teachers adopt Piaget's views? Montessori methods build on Piaget's work (Povell, 2017). The teachers emphasize students' own exploration and discovery. The classrooms are less structured than what we think of as a typical classroom. Workbooks and predetermined assignments are not used. Rather, the teachers observe the students' interests and natural participation in activities to determine what the course of learning will be. For example, a math lesson might be constructed around counting the day's lunch money or dividing supplies among students. Games are often used in the classroom to stimulate mathematical thinking.

EVALUATING PIAGET'S THEORY

What were Piaget's main contributions? Has his theory withstood the test of time?

Contributions   Piaget was a giant in the field of developmental psychology, the founder of the present field of children's cognitive development. Psychologists owe him for a long list of masterful concepts of enduring power and fascination: assimilation, accommodation, object permanence, egocentrism, conservation, and others (Bjorklund, 2018). Psychologists also owe him for the current vision of children as active, constructive thinkers. And they are indebted to him for creating a theory that generated a huge volume of research on children's cognitive development.

Piaget also was a genius when it came to observing children. His careful observations demonstrated inventive ways to discover how children act on and adapt to their world. Piaget showed us some important things to look for in cognitive development, such as the shift from preoperational to concrete operational thinking. He also showed us how children need to make their experiences fit their schemes (cognitive frameworks) yet simultaneously adapt their schemes to experience. Piaget also revealed how cognitive change is likely to occur if the context is structured to allow gradual movement to the next higher level. Concepts do not emerge suddenly, full-blown, but instead develop through a series of partial accomplishments that lead to increasingly comprehensive understanding (Baillargeon & DeJong, 2017).

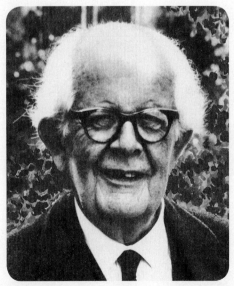

Jean Piaget, the main architect of the field of cognitive development.
Bettmann/Getty Images

Criticisms   Piaget's theory has not gone unchallenged. Questions are raised about estimates of children's competence at different developmental levels, stages, the training of children to reason at higher levels, and culture and education.

Estimates of Children's Competence   Some cognitive abilities emerge earlier than Piaget thought (Baillargeon, 2014; Bauer, 2013). For example, as previously noted, some aspects of object permanence emerge earlier than he proposed. Even 2-year-olds are nonegocentric in some contexts. When they realize that another person will not see an object, they investigate whether the person is blindfolded or looking in a different direction. Some understanding of the conservation of number has been demonstrated as early as age 3, although Piaget did not think it emerged until 7. Young children are not as uniformly "pre" this and "pre" that (precausal, preoperational) as Piaget thought.

Cognitive abilities also can emerge later than Piaget thought. Many adolescents still think in concrete operational ways or are just beginning to master formal operations. Even many adults are not formal operational thinkers. For example, college students are better at solving formal operations problems in their majors than in unfamiliar subject areas (Bjorklund & Causey, 2018). In sum, recent theoretical revisions highlight more cognitive competencies of infants and young children and more cognitive shortcomings of adolescents and adults.

Stages   Piaget conceived of stages as unitary structures of thought. Thus, his theory assumes developmental synchrony—that is, various aspects of a stage should emerge at the same time. However, some concrete operational concepts do not appear in synchrony. For example, children do not learn to conserve at the same time that they learn to cross-classify. Thus, most contemporary developmentalists agree that children's cognitive development is not as stage-like as Piaget thought (Bjorklund & Causey, 2017).

Effects of Training   Some children who are at one cognitive stage (such as preoperational) can be trained to reason at a higher cognitive stage (such as concrete operational). This poses a problem for Piaget's theory. He argued that such training is only superficial and ineffective, unless the child is at a maturational transition point between the stages. Contemporary interventions that target spatial visualization skills, for example, capitalize on the potential of training to improve children's performance in early math skills, such as symbolic number comparisons (Hawes & others, 2017).

Culture and Education   Culture and education exert stronger influences on children's development than Piaget reasoned (Sternberg, 2018). For example, the age at which children acquire conservation skills is related to how much practice their culture provides in these skills. However, great caution is needed in taking a procedure, such as a standard Piagetian task, and applying it in a new cultural context in which the materials and even the manner of an adult questioning a child about a problem to which the adult already knows the answer may be quite unusual, leading children to respond in ways that do not reflect knowledge they hold in situations that are closer to their lived experiences (Rogoff, Dahl, & Callanan, 2018).

The Neo-Piagetian Approach   **Neo-Piagetians** argue that Piaget got some things right but that his theory needs considerable revision. They give more emphasis to how children use attention, memory, and strategies to process information (Morra & Panesi, 2017). They especially believe that a more accurate portrayal of children's thinking requires attention to children's strategies, the speed at which children process information, the particular task involved, and the division of problems into smaller, more precise steps (Demetriou & others, 2018).

neo-Piagetians Developmentalists who have elaborated on Piaget's theory, believing that children's cognitive development is more specific in many respects than Piaget thought and giving more emphasis to how children use memory, attention, and strategies to process information.

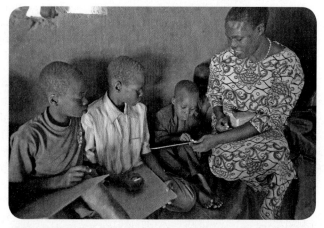

An outstanding teacher and education in the logic of science and mathematics are important cultural experiences that promote the development of operational thought. *Might Piaget have underestimated the roles of culture and schooling in children's cognitive development?*
Majority World/Universal Images Group Editorial/Getty Images

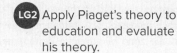

Review *Connect* Reflect

LG2 Apply Piaget's theory to education and evaluate his theory.

Review

- How can Piaget's theory be applied to educating children?
- What are some key contributions and criticisms of Piaget's theory?

Connect

- In this section, you learned that culture exerts a strong influence on cognitive development. What have you learned about the influence of different cultural practices on infants' motor skills?

Reflect *Your Own Personal Journey of Life*

- How might thinking in formal operational ways rather than concrete operational ways help you to develop better study skills?

Vygotsky's Theory of Cognitive Development Identify the main concepts in Vygotsky's theory and compare it with Piaget's theory.

| The Zone of Proximal Development | Scaffolding | Language and Thought | Teaching Strategies | Evaluating Vygotsky's Theory |

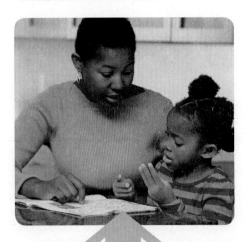

Upper limit

Level of additional responsibility child can accept with assistance of an able instructor

Zone of proximal development (ZPD)

Lower limit

Level of problem solving reached on these tasks by child working alone

FIGURE 9

VYGOTSKY'S ZONE OF PROXIMAL DEVELOPMENT. Vygotsky's zone of proximal development has a lower limit and an upper limit. Tasks in the ZPD are too difficult for the child to perform alone. They require assistance from an adult or a more-skilled child. As children experience the verbal instruction or demonstration, they organize the information in their existing mental structures so that they can eventually perform the skill or task alone.
Ariel Skelley/Blend Images LLC

zone of proximal development (ZPD) Vygotsky's term for tasks that are too difficult for children to master alone but can be mastered with assistance from adults or more-skilled children.

scaffolding In cognitive development, Vygotsky used this term to describe the practice of changing the level of support provided over the course of a teaching session, with the more-skilled person adjusting guidance to fit the child's current performance level.

Piaget's theory is a major developmental theory. Another developmental theory that focuses on children's cognition is Vygotsky's theory. Like Piaget, Lev Vygotsky (1962) emphasized that children actively construct their knowledge and understanding. In Piaget's theory, children develop ways of thinking and understanding by their actions and interactions with the physical world. In Vygotsky's theory, children are more often described as social creatures than in Piaget's theory. They develop their ways of thinking and understanding primarily through social interaction (Bodrova & Leong, 2017). Their cognitive development depends on the tools provided by society, and their minds are shaped by the cultural context in which they live (Legare, Sobel, & Callanan, 2017).

Previously, we briefly described Vygotsky's theory. Here we take a closer look at his ideas about how children learn and his view of the role of language in cognitive development.

THE ZONE OF PROXIMAL DEVELOPMENT

Vygotsky's belief in the importance of social influences, especially instruction, on children's cognitive development is reflected in his concept of the zone of proximal development. **Zone of proximal development (ZPD)** is Vygotsky's term for the range of tasks that are too difficult for the child to master alone but that can be learned with guidance and assistance of adults or more-skilled children. Thus, the lower limit of the ZPD is the level of skill reached by the child working independently. The upper limit is the level of additional responsibility the child can accept with the assistance of an able instructor (see Figure 9). The ZPD captures the child's cognitive skills that are in the process of maturing and can be accomplished only with the assistance of a more-skilled person (Rowe, 2018). Vygotsky (1962) called these the "buds" or "flowers" of development, to distinguish them from the "fruits" of development, which the child already can accomplish independently.

Vygotsky's concept of the zone of proximal development—that children learn by interacting with more experienced adults and peers, who help them think beyond the "zone" in which they would be able to perform without assistance—has been applied primarily to academic learning. Barbara Rogoff (Rogoff, 2016; Rogoff & others, 2017) argues that many of Vygotsky's ideas, including the zone of proximal development, are important in understanding children's development beyond the classroom in everyday interactions with adults and peers. To read further about Rogoff's ideas, see *Connecting with Diversity*.

SCAFFOLDING

Closely linked to the idea of the ZPD is the concept of scaffolding. **Scaffolding** means changing the level of support. Over the course of a teaching session, a more-skilled person (a teacher or advanced peer) adjusts the amount of guidance to fit the child's current performance (Wright, 2018). When the student is learning a new task, the skilled person may use direct instruction. As the student's competence increases, less guidance is given.

Dialogue is an important tool of scaffolding in the zone of proximal development (Muhonen & others, 2018). Vygotsky viewed children as having rich but unsystematic, disorganized, and spontaneous concepts. In a dialogue, these concepts meet with the skilled helper's more systematic, logical, and rational concepts. As a result, the child's concepts become more systematic, logical, and rational. For example, a dialogue might take place between a teacher and a child when the teacher uses scaffolding to help a child understand a concept like "transportation."

Guided Participation and Cultural Contexts

According to Rogoff, children serve a sort of apprenticeship in thinking through *guided participation* in social and cultural activities. Guided participation may occur, for example, when adults and children share activities.

Parents can broaden or limit children's opportunities through their decisions about how much and when to expose children to books, television, and child care. They may give children opportunities to learn about cultural traditions and practices through their routines and play. For example, in the Zambian culture of Chewa, children play numerous games, such as "hide-and-seek, guessing games, complex sand drawing games, imaginative games representing local work and family routines, skill games like jacks and a rule game requiring considerable strategic planning and numerical calculations, and constructing models of wire or clay" (Rogoff, 2003, p. 297). In addition, through observational learning, or as Rogoff calls it, learning by "osmosis," children adopt values, skills, and mannerisms by simply watching and listening to peers and adults.

Guided participation is widely used around the world, but cultures may differ in the goals of development—what content is to be learned—and the means for providing guided participation (Rogoff, Dahl, & Callanan, 2018). Around the world, caregivers and children arrange children's activities and revise children's responsibilities as they gain skill and knowledge. With guidance, children participate in cultural activities that socialize them into skilled activities. For example, Mayan mothers in Guatemala help their daughters learn to weave through guided participation. Throughout the world, learning occurs, not just by studying or by attending classes, but also through interaction with knowledgeable people.

Two contrasting approaches characterize cultural variations in children's attention and learning (Coppens & others, 2018): (1) Participation of children in a wide variety of family and community activities, which

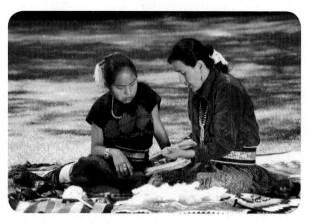

A Native American woman teaches her daughter how to weave. *What are some other ways that children learn through guided participation?*
Coral Coolahan/Getty Images

characterizes many Indigenous-heritage communities in North and South America; and (2) Separation of children from the variety of family and community activities and creating activities for them in specialized settings, such as school, which is prevalent in middle-SES European-heritage communities. In the United States, children's out-of-school time provides limited opportunities to learn by observing and participating in a variety of valued family and community activities. According to research on guided participation, including children in meaningful family and community activities would help them to better understand valued work and other activities in their culture.

How does Rogoff's concept of guided participation relate to Vygotsky's concept of the zone of proximal development?

LANGUAGE AND THOUGHT

The use of dialogue as a tool for scaffolding is only one example of the important role of language in a child's development. According to Vygotsky, children use speech not only for social communication, but also to help them solve tasks. Vygotsky (1962) further concluded that young children use language to plan, guide, and monitor their behavior. This use of language for self-regulation is called *private speech.* Piaget viewed private speech as egocentric and immature, but Vygotsky saw it as an important tool of thought during the early childhood years (Sawyer, 2017).

Vygotsky said that language and thought initially develop independently of each other and then merge. He emphasized that all mental functions have external, or social, origins. Children must use language to communicate with others before they can focus inward on their own thoughts. Children also must communicate externally and use language for a long period of time before they can make the transition from external

developmental **connection**

Parenting

Scaffolding also is an effective strategy for parents to adopt in interacting with their infants. Connect to "Families, Lifestyles, and Parenting."

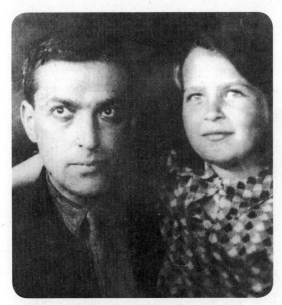

Lev Vygotsky (1896–1934), shown here with his daughter, believed that children's cognitive development is advanced through social interaction with skilled individuals embedded in a sociocultural backdrop.
Courtesy of James V. Wertsch, Washington University

developmental **connection**

Language

In thinking about links between language and cognition, we might ask: (1) Is language necessary for cognition? and (2) Is cognition necessary for language? Connect to "Language Development."

to internal speech. This transition period occurs between 3 and 7 years of age and involves talking to oneself. After a while, the self-talk becomes second nature to children, and they can act without verbalizing. When this occurs, children have internalized their egocentric speech in the form of *inner speech,* which becomes their thoughts.

Vygotsky reasoned that children who use a lot of private speech are more socially competent than those who don't. He argued that private speech represents an early transition in becoming more socially communicative. For Vygotsky, when young children talk to themselves, they are using language to govern their behavior and guide themselves. For example, a child working on a puzzle might say to herself, "Which pieces should I put together first? I'll try those green ones first. Now I need some blue ones. No, that blue one doesn't fit there. I'll try it over here."

Piaget stressed that self-talk is egocentric and reflects immaturity. However, researchers have found support for Vygotsky's view that private speech plays a positive role in children's development (Day & others, 2018). Preschoolers who use private speech are better able to regulate their behaviors and internalize new information (Day & Smith, 2019). Preschoolers who use positive private speech are more motivated to master challenging tasks (Sawyer, 2017).

TEACHING STRATEGIES

Vygotsky's theory has been embraced by many teachers and has been successfully applied to education (Bodrova & Leong, 2017). Here are some ways Vygotsky's theory can be incorporated in classrooms:

1. *Assess the child's ZPD.* Like Piaget, Vygotsky did not think that formal, standardized tests are the best way to assess children's learning. Rather, Vygotsky argued that assessment should focus on determining the child's zone of proximal development. The skilled helper presents the child with tasks of varying difficulty to determine the best level at which to begin instruction. Today, standardized test results often are reported using a ZPD for reading or math instruction, such as by providing a reading level range to guide teachers and students in choosing books that are at a reading level that is neither too difficult nor too easy for the child (Poehner, Davin, & Lantolf, 2017).

2. *Use the child's ZPD in teaching.* Teaching should begin toward the zone's upper limit, so that the child can reach the goal with help and move to a higher level of skill and knowledge. Offer just enough assistance. You might ask, "What can I do to help you?" Or simply observe the child's intentions and attempts and provide support when needed. When the child hesitates, offer encouragement. And encourage the child to practice the skill. You may watch and appreciate the child's practice or offer support when the child forgets what to do.

3. *Use more-skilled peers as teachers.* Remember that it is not just adults who are important in helping children learn. Children also benefit from the support and guidance of more-skilled children (Kirova & Jamison, 2018).

4. *Monitor and encourage children's use of private speech.* Be aware of the developmental change from externally talking to oneself when solving a problem during the preschool years to privately talking to oneself in the early elementary school years. In the elementary school years, encourage children to internalize and self-regulate their talk to themselves.

5. *Place instruction in a meaningful context.* Educators today are moving away from abstract presentations of material, instead providing students with opportunities to experience learning in real-world settings. For example, instead of just memorizing math formulas, students work on math problems with real-world implications.

How can Vygotsky's ideas be applied to educating children?
IT Stock Free/Alamy Stock Photo

Donene Polson, Elementary School Teacher

Donene Polson teaches at Washington Elementary School in Salt Lake City, Utah. Washington is an innovative school that emphasizes the importance of people learning together as part of a community of learners. Children as well as adults plan learning activities. Throughout the school day, children work in small groups.

Polson says that she loves working in a school in which students, teachers, and parents work together as a community to help children learn. Before the school year begins, Polson meets with parents at the family's home to prepare for the upcoming year, get acquainted, and establish schedules to determine when parents can contribute to classroom instruction.

At monthly parent-teacher meetings, Polson and the parents plan the curriculum and discuss how children's learning is progressing. They brainstorm about resources in the community that can be used effectively to promote children's learning.

For more information about what elementary school teachers do, see the Careers in Child Development appendix.

6. *Transform the classroom with Vygotskian ideas.* What does a Vygotskian classroom look like? Flipped classrooms, in which student-centered learning activities, such as team problem-solving, are prioritized over teacher-centered delivery of information, represent one approach based on Vygotsky's theory (Lo, Hew, & Chen, 2017). Flipped classrooms can benefit students' learning by providing time for in-class practice, enabling students to receive immediate feedback from teachers and peers, and helping students take more responsibility for their own learning.

To read about the work of a teacher who applies Vygotsky's theory to her teaching, see the *Connecting with Careers* profile. The *Caring Connections* interlude further explores the implications of Vygotsky's theory for children's education.

EVALUATING VYGOTSKY'S THEORY

Even though their theories were proposed at about the same time, most of the world learned about Vygotsky's theory later than they learned about Piaget's theory, so Vygotsky's theory has not yet been evaluated as thoroughly. Vygotsky's view of the importance of sociocultural influences on children's development fits with the current belief that it is important to evaluate the contextual factors in learning (Gauvain, 2018).

We already have mentioned several distinctions between Vygotsky's and Piaget's theories, such as Vygotsky's emphasis on the importance of inner speech in development and Piaget's view that such speech is immature. Although both theories are constructivist, Vygotsky's is a **social constructivist approach,** which emphasizes the social contexts of learning and the construction of knowledge through social interaction (van Hover & Hicks, 2017).

In moving from Piaget to Vygotsky, the conceptual shift is from the individual to collaboration, social interaction, and sociocultural activity (Bodrova & Leong, 2017). The end point of cognitive development for Piaget is formal operational thought. For Vygotsky, the endpoint can differ, depending on which skills are considered to be the most important in a particular culture. For Piaget, children construct knowledge by transforming, organizing, and reorganizing previous knowledge. For Vygotsky, children construct knowledge through social interaction (Bodrova & Leong, 2017). The implication of Piaget's theory for teaching is that children need support to explore their world and discover knowledge. The main implication of Vygotsky's theory for teaching is that students need many opportunities to learn with their teachers and more-skilled

developmental connection

Education and Achievement

Whether to adopt a direct instruction or constructivist approach is a major issue in educating children. Connect to "Schools, Achievement, and Work."

social constructivist approach An emphasis on the social contexts of learning and the construction of knowledge through social interaction. Vygotsky's theory reflects this approach.

caring *connections*

Tools of the Mind

Tools of the Mind is an early childhood education curriculum that emphasizes children's development of self-regulation and the cognitive foundations of literacy (Diamond, 2013). The curriculum was created by Elena Bodrova and Deborah Leong (2007) and has been implemented in more than 200 classrooms. Most of the children in the Tools of the Mind programs are at risk because of their living circumstances, which in many instances involve poverty and other difficult conditions such as being homeless and having parents with drug problems.

Tools of the Mind is grounded in Vygotsky's (1962) theory, with special attention given to cultural tools and developing self-regulation, the zone of proximal development, scaffolding, private speech, shared activity, and play as important activity. In a Tools of the Mind classroom, dramatic play has a central role. Teachers guide children in creating themes that are based on the children's interests, such as treasure hunt, store, hospital, and restaurant. Teachers also incorporate field trips, visitor presentations, videos, and books in the development of children's play. They help children develop a play plan, which increases the maturity of their play. Play plans describe what the children expect to do during the play period, including the imaginary context, roles, and props to be used. The play plans increase the quality of their play and self-regulation.

Scaffolding writing is another important theme in the Tools of the Mind classroom. Teachers guide children in planning their own message by drawing a line to stand for each word the child says. Children then repeat the message, pointing to each line as they say the word. Next, the child writes on the lines, trying to represent each word with some letters or symbols. Figure 10 shows how the scaffolding writing process improved a 5-year-old child's writing over the course of two months.

Research assessments of children's writing in Tools of the Mind classrooms revealed that they have more advanced writing skills than children in other early childhood programs (Bodrova & Leong, 2007) (see Figure 10). For example, they write more complex messages, use more words, spell more accurately, show better letter recognition, and have a better understanding of the concept of a sentence.

In a study of 759 students in 29 schools, kindergarten children in schools that were randomly assigned to use the Tools of the Mind curriculum showed greater improvements in executive functioning, reasoning, attention control, and performance in math, reading, and vocabulary over the course of the school year and into first grade than did students in control schools that did not use the Tools of the Mind curriculum (Blair & Raver, 2014). The effects of using the Tools of the Mind curriculum were especially pronounced for students in schools with high levels of poverty.

Earlier in this section of the chapter, we outlined strategies for incorporating Vygotsky's theory into teaching. Revisit that list and explain how the Tools of the Mind curriculum uses those strategies.

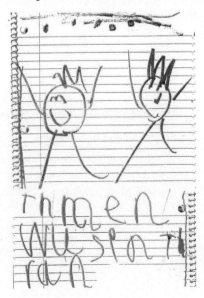 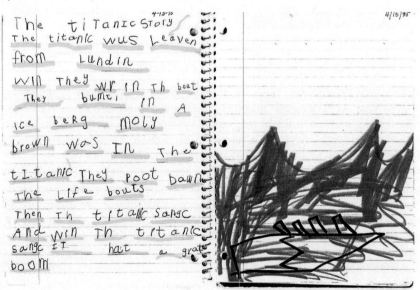

(a) Five-year-old Aaron's independent journal writing prior to the scaffolded writing technique.

(b) Aaron's journal two months after using the scaffolded writing technique.

FIGURE **10**

WRITING PROGRESS OF A 5-YEAR-OLD BOY OVER TWO MONTHS USING THE SCAFFOLDING WRITING PROCESS IN TOOLS OF THE MIND
Bodrova, Elena and Leong, Deborah J. "Tools of the Mind: A Case Study of Implementing the Vygotskian Approach in American Early Childhood and Primary Classrooms," Geneva, Switzerland: International Bureau of Education, 2001, 36-38.

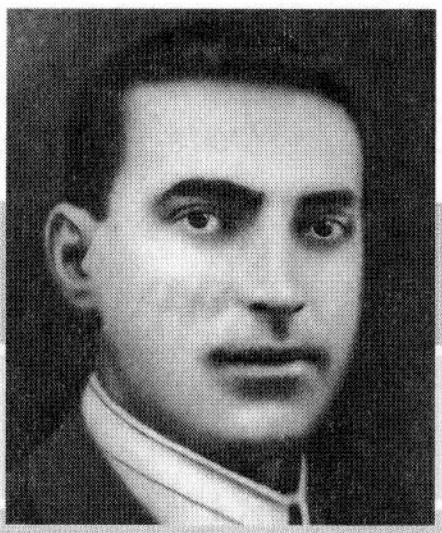

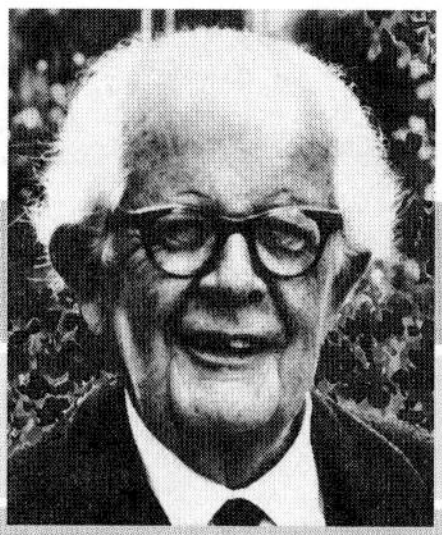

	Vygotsky		Piaget	
Sociocultural Context	Strong emphasis		Little emphasis	
Constructivism	Social constructivist		Cognitive constructivist	
Stages	No general stages of development proposed		Strong emphasis on stages (sensorimotor, preoperational, concrete operational, and formal operational)	
Key Processes	Zone of proximal development, language, dialogue, tools of the culture		Schema, assimilation, accommodation, operations, conservation, classification	
Role of Language	A major role; language plays a powerful role in shaping thought		Language has a minimal role; cognition primarily directs language	
View on Education	Education plays a central role, helping children learn the tools of the culture		Education merely refines the child's cognitive skills that have already emerged	
Teaching Implications	Teacher is a facilitator and guide, not a director; establish many opportunities for children to learn with the teacher and more-skilled peers		Also views teacher as a facilitator and guide, not a director; provide support for children to explore their world and discover knowledge	

FIGURE 11

COMPARISON OF VYGOTSKY'S AND PIAGET'S THEORIES

(Vygotsky) A.R. Lauria/(Piaget) Dr. Michael Cole, Laboratory of Human Cognition, University of California, San Diego; Bettmann/Getty Images

peers. In both Piaget's and Vygotsky's theories, teachers serve as facilitators and guides, rather than as directors and molders of learning. Figure 11 compares Vygotsky's and Piaget's theories.

Criticisms of Vygotsky's theory also have surfaced (Daniels, 2017). Some critics point out that Vygotsky was not specific enough about age-related changes. Another criticism asserts that Vygotsky did not adequately describe how changes in socioemotional capabilities contribute to cognitive development. Yet another criticism is that he overemphasized the role of language in thinking. Also, his emphasis on collaboration and guidance has potential pitfalls. Might facilitators be too helpful in some cases, as when a parent becomes overbearing and controlling? Further, some children might become lazy and expect help when they might have learned more by doing something on their own.

Review Connect Reflect

LG3 Identify the main concepts in Vygotsky's theory and compare it with Piaget's theory.

Review

- What is the zone of proximal development?
- What is scaffolding?
- How did Vygotsky view language and thought?
- How can Vygotsky's theory be applied to education?
- What are some similarities and differences between Vygotsky's and Piaget's theories?
- What are some criticisms of Vygotsky's theory?

Connect

- Compare the strategies that were laid out in the section for using Piaget's theories in teaching to those for applying Vygotsky's theories in teaching. What are the similarities? Differences?

Reflect *Your Own Personal Journey of Life*

- Which theory—Piaget's or Vygotsky's—do you think is more effective in explaining your own cognitive development as a child?

Cognitive Developmental Approaches

Piaget's Theory of Cognitive Development (LG1) Discuss the key processes and four stages in Piaget's theory.

Processes of Development

- According to Piaget's theory, children construct their own cognitive worlds, building mental structures to adapt to their world. Schemes are actions or mental representations that organize knowledge. Behavioral schemes (physical activities) characterize infancy, and mental schemes (cognitive activities) develop in childhood. Adaptation involves assimilation and accommodation. Assimilation occurs when children incorporate new information into their existing schemes. Accommodation refers to children's adjustment of their schemes to fit new information and experiences. Through organization, children group isolated behaviors into a higher-order, more smoothly functioning cognitive system. Equilibration is a mechanism Piaget proposed to explain how children shift from one cognitive stage to the next. As children experience cognitive conflict in trying to understand the world, they seek equilibrium. The result is equilibration, which brings the child to a new stage of thought. According to Piaget, there are four qualitatively different stages of thought: sensorimotor, preoperational, concrete operational, and formal operational.

Sensorimotor Stage

- In sensorimotor thought, the first of Piaget's four stages, the infant organizes and coordinates sensory experiences (such as seeing and hearing) with physical movements. This stage lasts from birth to about 2 years of age and is nonsymbolic throughout, according to Piaget. Sensorimotor thought has six substages: simple reflexes; first habits and primary circular reactions; secondary circular reactions; coordination of secondary circular reactions; tertiary circular reactions, novelty, and curiosity; and internalization of schemes. One key aspect of this stage is object permanence, the ability to understand that objects continue to exist even though the infant is no longer observing them. Another aspect involves infants' understanding of cause and effect. In the past two decades, revisions of Piaget's view have been proposed based on research. For example, researchers have found that a stable and differentiated perceptual world is established earlier than Piaget envisioned. However, controversy surrounds the question of when object permanence emerges. Most developmentalists conclude that nature and nurture are both important in infant cognitive development.

Preoperational Stage

- Preoperational thought is the beginning of the ability to reconstruct at the level of thought what has been established in behavior. It involves a transition from a primitive to a more sophisticated use of symbols. In preoperational thought, the child does not yet think in an operational way. The symbolic function substage occurs roughly from 2 to 4 years of age and is characterized by symbolic thought, egocentrism, and animism. The intuitive thought substage stretches from about 4 to 7 years of age. It is called intuitive because children seem sure about their knowledge yet are unaware of how they know what they know. The preoperational child lacks conservation and asks a barrage of questions.

Concrete Operational Stage

- Concrete operational thought occurs roughly from 7 to 11 years of age. During this stage, children can perform concrete operations, think logically about concrete objects, classify things, and reason about relationships among classes of things. Concrete thought is not as abstract as formal operational thought.

Formal Operational Stage

- Formal operational thought appears between 11 and 15 years of age. Formal operational thought is more abstract, idealistic, and logical than concrete operational thought. Piaget maintains that adolescents become capable of engaging in hypothetical-deductive reasoning. But Piaget did not give adequate attention to individual variation in adolescent thinking. Many young adolescents do not think in hypothetical-deductive ways but rather are consolidating their concrete operational thinking. In addition, according to Elkind, adolescents develop a special kind of egocentrism that involves an imaginary audience and a personal fable about being unique and invulnerable. However, recent research questions the accuracy of the invulnerability aspect of the personal fable.

Applying and Evaluating Piaget's Theory Apply Piaget's theory to education and evaluate his theory.

Piaget and Education

- Piaget was not an educator, but his constructivist views have been applied to teaching. These applications include an emphasis on facilitating rather than directing learning, considering the child's level of knowledge, using ongoing assessment, promoting the student's intellectual health, and turning the classroom into a setting for exploration and discovery.

Evaluating Piaget's Theory

- We owe to Piaget the field of cognitive development. He was a genius at observing children, and he gave us a number of masterful concepts such as assimilation, accommodation, object permanence, and egocentrism. Critics question his estimates of competence at different developmental levels, his stage concept, and other ideas. Neo-Piagetians, who emphasize the importance of information processing, stress that children's cognition is more specific than Piaget thought.

Vygotsky's Theory of Cognitive Development Identify the main concepts in Vygotsky's theory and compare it with Piaget's theory.

The Zone of Proximal Development

- Zone of proximal development (ZPD) is Vygotsky's term for the range of tasks that are too difficult for children to master alone but can be learned with the guidance and assistance of adults or more-skilled peers.

Scaffolding

- Scaffolding is a teaching technique in which a more-skilled person adjusts the level of guidance to fit the child's current performance level. Dialogue is an important aspect of scaffolding.

Language and Thought

- Vygotsky stressed that language plays a key role in cognition. Language and thought initially develop independently, but then children internalize their egocentric speech in the form of inner speech, which becomes their thoughts. This transition to inner speech occurs between 3 and 7 years of age.

Teaching Strategies

- Applications of Vygotsky's ideas to education include using the child's ZPD and scaffolding, using more-skilled peers as teachers, monitoring and encouraging children's use of private speech, and accurately assessing the ZPD. These practices can transform the classroom and establish a meaningful context for instruction.

Evaluating Vygotsky's Theory

- Like Piaget, Vygotsky emphasized that children actively construct their understanding of the world. Unlike Piaget, he did not propose stages of cognitive development, and he emphasized that children construct knowledge through social interaction. According to Vygotsky's theory, children depend on tools provided by the culture, which determines which skills they will develop. Vygotsky's view contrasts with Piaget's view that young children's private speech is immature and egocentric. Critics of Vygotsky's theory assert that it lacks specificity about age-related changes and overemphasizes the role of language in thinking.

key terms

accommodation 160
adolescent egocentrism 172
animism 168
A-not-B error 164
assimilation 160
centration 168
concrete operational stage 169
conservation 168

core knowledge approach 166
egocentrism 167
equilibration 161
formal operational stage 171
horizontal décalage 170
hypothetical-deductive reasoning 171
imaginary audience 172

intuitive thought substage 168
neo-Piagetians 175
object permanence 164
operations 166
organization 161
personal fable 172
preoperational stage 167
scaffolding 176

schemes 160
sensorimotor stage 160
seriation 171
social constructivist approach 179
symbolic function substage 167
transitivity 171
zone of proximal development (ZPD) 176

key people

Renée Baillargeon 165
David Elkind 172
Rochel Gelman 169

Barbel Inhelder 167
Jean Piaget 159
Lev Vygotsky 176

Karen Wynn 166

chapter 7

INFORMATION PROCESSING

chapter outline

Hero Images Inc/Corbis

Laura Bickford is a master teacher who chairs the English Department at La Quinta High School in California. She spoke about how she encourages her students to think:

I believe the call to teach is a call to teach students how to think. In encouraging critical thinking, literature itself does a good bit of work for us but we still have to be guides. We have to ask good questions. We have to show students the value in asking their own questions, in having discussions and conversations. In addition to reading and discussing literature, the best way to move students to think critically is to have them write. We write all the time in a variety of modes: journals, formal essays, letters, factual reports, news articles, speeches, or other formal oral presentations. We have to show students where they merely scratch the surface in their thinking and writing. I call these moments "hits and runs." When I see this "hit and run" effort, I draw a window on the paper. I tell them it is a "window of opportunity" to go deeper, elaborate, and clarify. Many students don't do this kind of thinking until they are prodded to do so.

I also ask them to keep reading logs so they can observe their own thinking as it happens. In addition, I ask students to comment on their own learning by way of grading themselves. This year a student gave me one of the most insightful lines about her growth as a reader I have ever seen from a student. She wrote, "I no longer think in a monotone when I'm reading." I don't know if she grasps the magnitude of that thought or how it came to be that she made that change. It is magic when students see themselves growing like this.

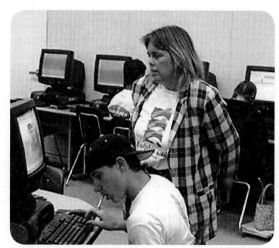

Laura Bickford (standing), working with students who are writing papers.
Courtesy of Laura Johnson Bickford

preview

What do children notice in the environment? What do they remember? And how do they think about it? These questions illustrate the information-processing approach. Using this approach, researchers usually do not describe children as being in one stage of cognitive development or another. But they do describe and analyze how information processing, attention, memory, thinking, and metacognition change over time.

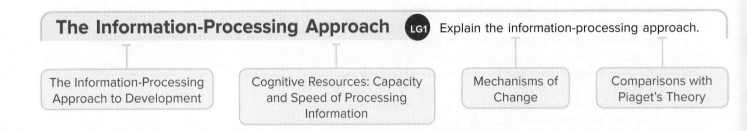

The Information-Processing Approach LG1 Explain the information-processing approach.

- The Information-Processing Approach to Development
- Cognitive Resources: Capacity and Speed of Processing Information
- Mechanisms of Change
- Comparisons with Piaget's Theory

What are some of the basic ideas in the information-processing approach? How is it similar to and different from the cognitive developmental approaches we described previously?

THE INFORMATION-PROCESSING APPROACH TO DEVELOPMENT

The information-processing approach shares a basic characteristic with the theories of cognitive development that were discussed previously. Like those theories, the information-processing approach rejected the behavioral perspective that dominated psychology during the first half of the twentieth century. As we discussed earlier, the behaviorists argued that to explain behavior it is important to examine associations between stimuli and behavior. In contrast, the theories of Piaget and Vygotsky and the information-processing approach focus on how children think.

The **information-processing approach** analyzes how children manipulate information, monitor it, and create strategies for handling it (Siegler, 2013, 2016). A computer metaphor can illustrate how the information-processing approach can be applied to development. A computer's information processing is *limited* by its hardware and software. The hardware limitations include the amount of data the computer can process—its capacity—and its speed. The software limits the kind of data that can be used as input and the ways that data can be manipulated; text editing programs will not handle music, for example. Similarly, children's information processing may be limited by capacity and speed as well as by their ability to manipulate information—in other words, their ability to apply appropriate strategies to acquire and use knowledge. In the information-processing approach, children's cognitive development results from their ability to overcome processing limitations by increasingly executing basic operations, expanding information-processing capacity, and acquiring new knowledge and strategies.

COGNITIVE RESOURCES: CAPACITY AND SPEED OF PROCESSING INFORMATION

Developmental changes in information processing are likely to be influenced by increases in both capacity and speed of processing. These two characteristics are often referred to as *cognitive resources* because they have an important influence on memory and problem solving.

> The mind is an enchanting thing.
>
> —MARIANNE MOORE
> *American poet, 20th century*

information-processing approach An approach that focuses on the ways children process information about their world—how they manipulate information, monitor it, and create strategies to deal with it.

Both biology and experience contribute to growth in cognitive resources (Bjorklund & Causey, 2017; Kuhn, 2013). Think about how much faster you can process information in your native language than in a second language. Developmental changes in the brain provide a biological foundation for increased cognitive resources (Battista & others, 2018). Important biological changes occur both in brain structures, such as changes in the frontal lobes, and at the level of neurons, such as the blooming and pruning of connections between neurons. Also, myelination (the process in which the axon is covered with a myelin sheath) increases the speed of electrical impulses in the brain. Myelination and changes in connectivity continue throughout childhood and adolescence (Oyefiade & others, 2018).

Most information-processing psychologists argue that an increase in capacity also improves processing of information (Camos & Barrouillet, 2018; Kuhn, 2013). For example, as children's information-processing capacity increases, they likely can hold in mind several dimensions of a topic or problem simultaneously, whereas younger children are more prone to attend to only one dimension.

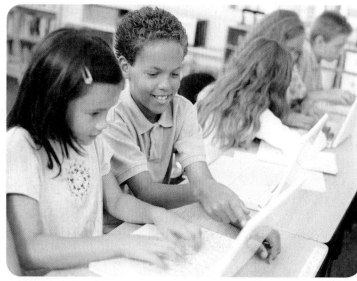

How does speed of processing information change during the childhood and adolescent years?
Bananastock/age fotostock

What is the role of processing *speed*? Children's speed in processing information is linked with their competence in thinking (Bjorklund & Causey, 2017). For example, the speed at which children can articulate a series of words affects how many words they can remember. This is because how quickly children can process information often influences what they can do with that information (Robinson-Riegler & Robinson-Riegler, 2016). For instance, a number of studies, spanning English and other European and Middle Eastern languages, have shown that faster processing speed is linked with faster and more reliable reading skills in childhood and adolescence (Tibi & Kirby, 2018). However, the downside of slower processing speed can be offset by creating effective strategies for processing information, in reading and many other domains of cognitive skills.

Researchers have devised a number of ways to assess processing speed. For example, it can be assessed through a *reaction-time task* in which individuals are asked to push a button or keyboard key as soon as they see a stimulus such as a light. Or individuals might be asked to match letters or match numbers with symbols on a computer screen. Another method involves having the person name a series of stimuli (for example, numbers, letters, colors) as quickly and accurately as possible.

There is abundant evidence that the speed with which such tasks are completed improves dramatically across the childhood years (Kuhn, 2013). For example, a 2.5-year longitudinal study of 8- to 13-year-olds revealed that processing speed increased with age, and furthermore, that the developmental change in processing speed predicted an increase in working memory capacity and complex abstract reasoning skills (Kail, Lervåg, & Hulme, 2016).

MECHANISMS OF CHANGE

Robert Siegler (2013, 2016) argues that mechanisms of change are especially important in the advances children make in cognitive development. According to Siegler, three mechanisms work together to create changes in children's cognitive skills: encoding, automaticity, and strategy construction.

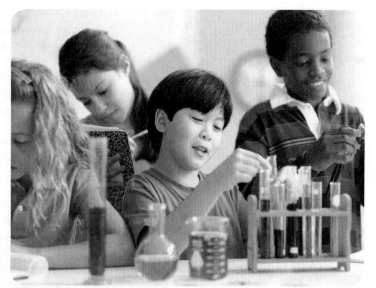

What are some important mechanisms of change in the development of children's information processing?
American Images, Inc/Digital Vision/Getty Images

encoding The mechanism by which information gets into memory.

Encoding is how information gets into memory. Changes in children's cognitive skills depend on increased skill at encoding relevant information and ignoring irrelevant information. For example, to a 4-year-old, an *s* in cursive writing is a shape very different from an *s* that is printed. But a 10-year-old has learned to encode the relevant fact that both are the letter *s* and to ignore the irrelevant differences in their shape.

automaticity The ability to process information with little or no effort.

Automaticity refers to the processing of information with little or no effort. Practice allows children to encode increasing amounts of information automatically. For example, once children have learned to read well, they do not think about each letter in a word as a letter; instead, they encode whole words. Once a task is automatic, it does not require conscious effort. As a result, as information processing becomes more automatic, we can complete tasks more quickly and handle more than one task at a time. If you did not encode words automatically but instead read this page by focusing your attention on each letter in each word, imagine how long it would take you to read it.

strategy construction Creation of new procedures for processing information.

metacognition Cognition about cognition, or "knowing about knowing."

Strategy construction is the creation of new procedures for processing information. For example, children's reading comprehension improves when they develop the strategy of stopping periodically to think about what they have read so far (Dimmitt & McCormick, 2012).

In addition, Siegler (2013, 2016) argues that children's information processing is characterized by *self-modification.* That is, children learn to use what they have learned in previous circumstances to adapt their responses to a new situation. Part of this self-modification draws on **metacognition,** which means knowing about knowing (Flavell, 2004; McCormick, Dimmitt, & Sullivan, 2013). One example of metacognition is what children know about the best ways to remember what they have read. Do they know that they will remember what they have read better if they can relate it to their own lives in some way? Thus, in Siegler's application of the information-processing approach to development, children play an active role in their cognitive development. More broadly, interventions aimed at helping children use metacognition strategies to "think about thinking" as they learn new things have been shown to be effective; and these interventions are particularly effective for children from lower-socioeconomic-status households (de Boer & others, 2018).

developmental **connection**

Cognitive Theory

Piaget theorized that cognitive development occurs in four stages: sensorimotor, preoperational, concrete operational, and formal operational. Connect to "Cognitive Developmental Approaches."

developmental **connection**

Theories

In Skinner's behavioral view, it is external rewards and punishment that determine behavior, not thoughts. Connect to "Introduction."

COMPARISONS WITH PIAGET'S THEORY

How does the information-processing approach compare with Piaget's theory? According to Piaget, children actively construct their knowledge and understanding of the world. Their thinking develops in distinct stages. At each stage, children develop qualitatively different types of mental structures (or schemes) that allow them to think about the world in new ways.

Like Piaget's theory, some versions of the information-processing approach are constructivist; they see children as directing their own cognitive development. And like Piaget, information-processing psychologists identify cognitive capabilities and limitations at various points in development (Siegler, 2016). They describe ways in which individuals do and do not understand important concepts at different points in life and try to explain how more advanced understanding grows out of a less advanced version as we acquire the capacity to understand how thinking "works" (Demetriou & others, 2018). They emphasize the impact that existing understanding has on the ability to acquire a new understanding of something.

Unlike Piaget, however, the information-processing approach does not see development as occurring abruptly in distinct stages with a brief transition period from one stage to the next. Instead, individuals gradually develop the capacity to process information, which allows them to acquire increasingly complex knowledge and skills (Kuhn, 2013). Compared with Piaget's theory, the information-processing approach also focuses on more precise analysis of change and on the contributions made by ongoing cognitive activity—such as encoding and strategies—to that change.

Review Connect Reflect

 LG1 Explain the information-processing approach.

Review

- What is the information-processing approach to development?
- How do capacity and processing speed change developmentally?
- What are three important mechanisms of change involved in information processing?
- How can the information-processing approach be compared to Piaget's theory?

Connect

- In this section, we learned that changes in the brain are linked to advances in information processing. What did you learn earlier about changes in brain structure and the cognitive abilities of infants, children, and adolescents?

Reflect *Your Own Personal Journey of Life*

- In terms of your ability to learn, think about your early childhood, elementary, and middle school years. Describe a task on which you were faster in processing information in elementary school than in preschool. Then describe a task on which you were faster in processing information in middle school than in elementary school.

Attention **LG2** Define attention and outline its developmental changes.

What Is Attention?   Infancy   Childhood   Adolescence

The world holds a lot of information to perceive. Right now, you are perceiving the letters and words that make up this sentence. Now look around you and pick out something else to look at. After that, curl up the toes on your right foot. In each of these circumstances, you engaged in the process of paying attention. What is attention, and what effect does it have on processing information? How does attention change with age?

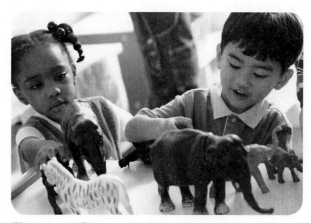

What are some different ways that children allocate their attention?
Photodisc Collection/EyeWire/Getty Images

WHAT IS ATTENTION?

Attention is the focusing of mental resources. Attention improves cognitive processing for many tasks, from grabbing a toy to hitting a baseball or adding numbers. But like adults, children can pay attention to only a limited amount of information. One study that examined 7- and 8-month-old infants' visual attention to sequences of events found that the amount of information had to be "just right"; the infants tended to look away from events that were too simple or complex, preferring instead to look at those of intermediate complexity (Kidd, Piantadosi, & Aslin, 2012).

Children allocate their attention in different ways (Colombo, Brez, & Curtindale, 2013; Rueda, 2018). Psychologists have labeled some of these types, including selective attention, divided attention, sustained attention, and executive attention.

- **Selective attention** is focusing on a specific aspect of experience that is relevant while ignoring others that are irrelevant (Isbell & others, 2017). Focusing on one voice among many in a crowded room or a noisy restaurant is an example of selective attention. Earlier, when you switched your attention to the toes on your right foot, you were engaging in selective attention.

attention Concentrating and focusing mental resources.

selective attention Focusing on a specific aspect of experience that is relevant while ignoring others that are irrelevant.

divided attention Concentrating on more than one activity at the same time.

sustained attention Maintaining attention to a selected stimulus for a prolonged period of time. Sustained attention is also called *focused attention* and *vigilance*.

executive attention Involves planning actions, allocating attention to goals, detecting and compensating for errors, and monitoring progress on tasks while sometimes dealing with novel or difficult circumstances.

developmental **connection**

Brain Development

Orienting attention to an object or event involves the parietal lobes in the cerebral cortex. Connect to "Physical Development and Health."

developmental **connection**

Research Methods

Among the measures researchers use in habituation studies are sucking behavior, heart and respiration rates, and how long an infant looks at an object. Connect to "Motor, Sensory, and Perceptual Development."

- **Divided attention** involves concentrating on more than one activity at the same time. If you are listening to music or a television program while you are reading this, you are engaging in divided attention.
- **Sustained attention** is maintaining attention to a selected stimulus for a prolonged period of time. Sustained attention is also sometimes called *focused attention* and *vigilance.* An example is when you stay focused for 30 minutes on a series of math problems for an assignment, without stopping or becoming distracted.
- **Executive attention** is broader and involves planning actions, attending to goals, detecting and compensating for errors, and monitoring progress on tasks, while sometimes dealing with novel or difficult circumstances. For example, you are using executive attention when you are playing a complex multi-player game in which you have to keep in mind various rules, must apply several strategies, and have to quickly adjust your plans and strategies in response to another player's actions.

INFANCY

How effectively can infants attend to something? Even newborns can visually detect a contour and fixate on it. Older infants scan patterns more thoroughly. By 4 months, infants can selectively attend to an object.

Orienting/Investigative Process Attention in the first year of life is dominated by an *orienting/investigative process* (Colombo, Brez, & Curtindale, 2013). This process involves directing attention to potentially important locations in the environment (that is, *where*) and recognizing objects and their features (such as color and form) (that is, *what*). From 3 to 9 months of age, infants rapidly change to deploy their attention more flexibly and quickly (Xie, Mallin, & Richards, 2018).

Another important type of attention is *sustained attention,* also referred to as *focused attention* (Lewis & others, 2017). New stimuli typically cause an orienting response followed by sustained attention. Sustained attention allows infants to learn about and remember characteristics of a stimulus as it becomes familiar. Infants as young as 3 months of age can engage in 5 to 10 seconds of sustained attention. The length of sustained attention increases through the second year (Reynolds & Romano, 2016).

Habituation and Dishabituation Closely linked with attention are the processes of habituation and dishabituation (Kavsek, 2013). Recall that if a stimulus—a sight or sound—is presented to infants several times in a row, they usually pay less attention to it each time. This suggests they are bored with it. This is the process of *habituation*—decreased responsiveness to a stimulus after repeated presentations of the stimulus. *Dishabituation* is the recovery of a habituated response after the stimulus changes to something new.

Infants' attention is so strongly affected by novelty that when an object becomes familiar, attention becomes shorter, making infants vulnerable to distraction. Researchers study habituation to determine the extent to which infants can see, hear, smell, taste, and experience touch (Colombo, Brez, & Curtindale, 2013).

Parents can use knowledge of habituation and dishabituation to improve interaction with their infant. If parents keep repeating the same words or actions, the infant will stop responding. It is important for parents to do novel things and to repeat them often until the infant stops responding. Sensitive parents can tell when the infant shows interest and know that many repetitions of the stimulus may be necessary for the infant to process the information. The parents stop or change their behavior when the infant redirects attention, and the parent notices this as part of a pattern of sensitive and responsive caregiving (Deák & others, 2018).

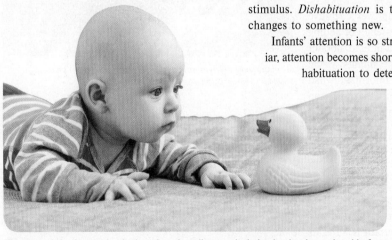

This young infant's attention is riveted on the yellow toy duck that has just been placed in front of him. The young infant's attention to the toy duck will be strongly regulated by the processes of habituation and dishabituation. *What characterizes these processes?*
Sporrer/Rupp/Getty Images

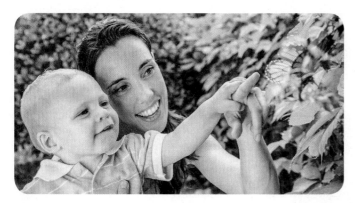

FIGURE 1

GAZE FOLLOWING IN INFANCY. Researcher Rechele Brooks and colleague Andrew Meltzoff (2005) found that infants begin to engage in a behavior called "gaze following" at 10 to 11 months of age. *Why might gaze following be an important accomplishment for an infant?*
XiXinXing/age fotostock

Joint Attention Another aspect of attention that is important to infant development is **joint attention,** in which individuals focus together on the same object or event. Joint attention requires (1) an ability to track another's behavior, such as following someone else's gaze; (2) one person directing another's attention; and (3) reciprocal interaction. Early in infancy, joint attention usually involves a caregiver pointing or using words to direct an infant's attention (Mundy, 2018). In many cultures, emerging forms of joint attention occur at about 7 to 8 months, but it is not until toward the end of the first year that joint attention skills are frequently observed (Kinard & Watson, 2015). In an illustrative study (Brooks & Meltzoff, 2005), at 10 to 11 months of age infants first began engaging in "gaze following," which involves looking where another person has just looked (see Figure 1). By their first birthday, infants have begun to use vocalizations and gestures to direct adults to objects that capture their interest (Cochet & Byrne, 2016).

Joint attention plays important roles in many aspects of infant development and considerably increases infants' ability to learn from other people (Carpenter, 2011). Nowhere is this more apparent than in observations of interchanges between caregivers and infants as infants are learning language (Salo, Rowe, & Reeb-Sutherland, 2018). When caregivers and infants frequently engage in joint attention, infants say their first word earlier and develop a larger vocabulary. These differences are related to subsequent language and non-language cognitive skills in the toddler years (Miller & Marcovitch, 2015). An illustrative study revealed that the extent to which 9-month-old infants engaged in joint attention was linked to their long-term memory (a one-week delay), possibly because joint attention enhances the relevance of attended items (Kopp & Lindenberger, 2012). Another study of 12- to 14-month-old infants found that a region of the temporal cortex was activated when they engaged in interaction and joint attention with another person (Hakuno & others, 2018). Later in the chapter in our discussion of language, we further discuss joint attention as an early predictor of language development in older infants and toddlers.

Joint attention skills in infancy and beyond also are associated with the development of self-regulation later in childhood. For example, one detailed observational study revealed that mother and school-age children's joint attention was linked to self-regulation and other scaffolded learning skills; and, these mother and child attentive behaviors were dynamic and co-coordinated during play (Leith, Yuill, & Pike, 2018).

CHILDHOOD

The child's ability to pay attention improves significantly during the preschool years, as seen in children's behavior as well as measures of brain activity and functioning (Rueda, 2018). A toddler typically wanders around, shifts attention from one activity to another, and seems to spend little time focused on any one object or event.

joint attention Individuals focusing on the same object or event; requires the ability to track another's behavior, one person directing another's attention, and reciprocal interaction.

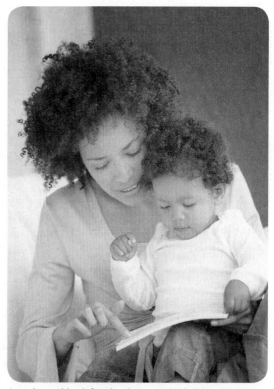

A mother and her infant daughter engaging in joint attention. *What about this photograph tells you that joint attention is occurring? Why is joint attention an important aspect of infant development?*
Tom Merton/OJO Images/Getty Images

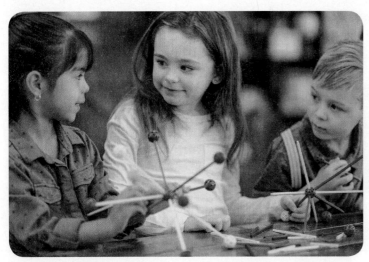

What are some advances in children's attention as they go through early childhood and middle and late childhood?
FatCamera/E+/Getty Images

In contrast, a preschool child might watch television for a half-hour at a time. In one classic study in which 99 families were observed in their homes for 4,672 hours, visual attention to television dramatically increased during the preschool years (Anderson & others, 1985). However, contemporary evidence shows that spending more time on screens in early childhood may be associated with poorer attention regulation (Anderson & Subrahmanyam, 2017).

Young children especially make advances in two aspects of attention—executive attention and sustained attention. Mary Rothbart and Maria Gartstein (2008, p. 332) described why advances in executive and sustained attention are so important in early childhood:

> The development of the . . . executive attention system supports the rapid increases in effortful control in the toddler and preschool years. Increases in attention are due, in part, to advances in comprehension and language development. As children are better able to understand their environment, this increased appreciation of their surroundings helps them to sustain attention for longer periods of time.

In certain aspects of daily activity and curricula in preschool and kindergarten, children participate in exercises designed to improve their attention (Posner & Rothbart, 2007). For example, in one eye-contact exercise, the teacher sits in the center of a circle of children, and each child is required to catch the teacher's eye before being permitted to leave the group. In other exercises created to improve attention, teachers have children participate in stop-go activities during which they have to listen for a specific signal, such as a drumbeat or an exact number of rhythmic beats, before stopping the activity. Other examples include games like "red light/green light" and "Simon Says"—activities that help children practice attending to relevant information and disregarding irrelevant information. Contemporary approaches utilize digital media (for example, computerized tasks and games) to exercise and "train" attention (Posner, Rothbart, & Tang, 2015). There are many such games and tools available now commercially. These and other types of cognitive skills training methods—for young children as well as teens and adults—tend to be effective for training the specific skill; but for the most part the training does not appear to have general effects beyond the specific skill that is being practiced (Kassai & others, 2019).

Control over attention continues to show shows important changes during middle and late childhood (Cragg, 2016; Jiang & others, 2018). For preschoolers, external stimuli are likely to determine the target of attention; in other words, what is salient, or obvious, grabs the preschooler's attention. For example, suppose a flashy, attractive interactive toy presents the directions for solving a problem. Preschool children are likely to pay attention to the toy and ignore the directions, because they are influenced strongly by the salient features of the toy's sounds and visual features and actions. After the age of 6 or 7, children start to pay more attention to features relevant to performing a task or solving a problem, such as the directions. Thus, instead of being drawn to the most striking stimuli in their environment, school-age children can direct their attention to more important and relevant information. This change reflects a shift to *cognitive control* of attention, so that children are less impulsive and more reflective. Recall that the increase in cognitive control during the elementary school years is linked to changes in the brain, especially more focal activation in the prefrontal cortex (Rueda, 2018).

Preschool children's ability to control and sustain their attention is related to school readiness and academic success. For example, a now classic longitudinal study of more than 1,000 children revealed that their ability to sustain their attention at 54 months of age was linked to their school readiness, measured as scholastic and language skills (NICHD Early Child Care Research Network, 2005). And in a follow-up study, those children whose parents and teachers rated them as having fewer attention problems at 54 months of age had stronger social skills in peer relations in the first and third grades (NICHD Early Child Care Research Network, 2009).

developmental **connection**

Brain Development

One shift in activation of some areas of the brain more than others in middle and late childhood is from diffuse, large areas to more focused, smaller areas, which especially involves more focal activation in the prefrontal cortex. Connect to "Physical Development and Health."

ADOLESCENCE

Adolescents typically have better attentional skills than children do, although there are wide individual differences in how effectively adolescents and children deploy their attention. Sustained and executive attention are very important aspects of adolescent cognitive development. As adolescents are required to engage in larger, increasingly complex tasks that take longer to complete, their ability to sustain attention is critical for succeeding on the tasks. An increase in executive attention supports the increase in effortful control required to effectively engage in these complex academic tasks (Kim-Spoon & others, 2019).

One trend involving divided attention is adolescents' multitasking, which in some cases involves dividing attention not just between two activities, but even among three or more (Mills & others, 2015). A major influence on the increase in multitasking is availability of multiple electronic media. Many adolescents have a range of electronic media at their disposal. It is not unusual for adolescents to simultaneously divide their attention among working on homework, engaging in text messaging, surfing the Web, and listening to music—all on their phones. And a 2015 national survey revealed that just over one-third of adolescents wrote and/or read text messages while driving (Li & others, 2018).

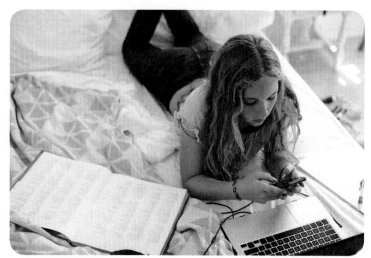

Is multitasking beneficial or distracting for adolescents?
Monkey Business Images/Shutterstock

Is multitasking beneficial or distracting? Multitasking expands the information adolescents attend to and forces the brain to share processing resources, which can distract the adolescent's attention from what might be most important at the moment (Toh & others, 2019). And, if the key task is at all complex and challenging, such as trying to figure out how to solve a homework problem, multitasking considerably reduces attention to the key task; overall, youth who more frequently engage in multitasking have poorer academic and cognitive performance (May & Elder, 2018).

Controlling attention is a key aspect of learning and thinking in adolescence and emerging adulthood (Bjorklund & Causey, 2017). Distractions that can interfere with attention in adolescence and emerging adulthood come from the external environment. Examples include other students talking while the student is trying to listen to a lecture, or when someone uses Facebook on their laptop during a lecture and looks at messages and friends' photos. Other intrusive distractions can come from competing thoughts in the individual's mind. Self-oriented thoughts, such as worrying, self-doubt, and intense emotions, may especially interfere with focusing attention on thinking tasks and can also affect mental health (Blake, Trinder, & Allen, 2018).

Review Connect Reflect

LG2 Define attention and outline its developmental changes.

Review

- What is attention? What are four ways in which children can allocate attention?
- How does attention develop in infancy?
- How does attention develop in childhood?
- What are some characteristics of attention in adolescence?

Connect

- In this section, you learned about joint attention. How might a child's ability to engage in joint attention be important in the successful implementation of a zone of proximal development teaching strategy?

Reflect *Your Own Personal Journey of Life*

- Imagine that you are an elementary school teacher. Devise some strategies to help children pay attention in class.

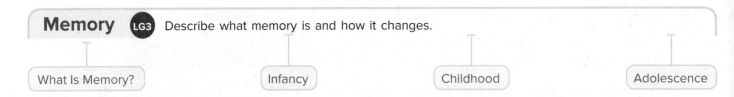
Twentieth-century American playwright Tennessee Williams once commented that life is all memory except for that one present moment that goes by so quickly that you can hardly catch it going. But just what do we do when we remember something, and how does our ability to remember develop?

WHAT IS MEMORY?

memory Retention of information over time.

Memory is the retention of information over time. Without memory you would not be able to connect what happened to you yesterday with what is going on in your life today. Human memory is truly remarkable when you consider how much information we put into our memories and how much we must retrieve to perform all of life's activities.

Processes and Types of Memory   Researchers study how information is initially placed or encoded into memory, how it is retained or stored after being encoded, and how it is found or retrieved for a certain purpose later (see Figure 2). Encoding, storage, and retrieval are the basic processes required for memory. Failures can occur in any of these processes. Some part of an event might not be encoded, the mental representation of the event might not be stored, or even if the memory exists, you might not be able to retrieve it.

short-term memory Limited-capacity memory system in which information is usually retained for up to 30 seconds if there is no rehearsal of the information. Using rehearsal, individuals can keep the information in short-term memory longer.

long-term memory A relatively permanent and long-lasting type of memory.

Examining the storage process led psychologists to classify memories based on their permanence. **Short-term memory** is a memory system with a limited capacity in which information is usually retained for 15 to 30 seconds unless strategies are used to retain it longer. **Long-term memory** is a relatively permanent, long-lasting type of memory. People are usually referring to long-term memory when they talk about "memory." When you remember the type of games you enjoyed playing as a child or the details of your first love, you are drawing on your long-term memory. But when you remember a word you just read a few seconds ago, you are using short-term memory.

When psychologists first analyzed short-term memory, they described it as if it were a passive storage room with shelves to store information until it is moved to long-term memory. But we do many other things with the information stored in short-term memory. For example, the words in this sentence are part of your short-term memory, and you are manipulating them to form a meaningful whole as you read them.

working memory A mental "workbench" where individuals actively use memory to manipulate and assemble information when making decisions, solving problems, and comprehending written and spoken language.

The concept of working memory is used to describe how we manipulate the information in short-term memory. **Working memory** is a kind of mental "workbench" where individuals actively use memory to manipulate and assemble information when they make decisions, solve problems, and comprehend written and spoken language (Baddeley, 2018). Many psychologists prefer the term *working memory* over *short-term memory* to describe how memory works.

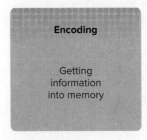
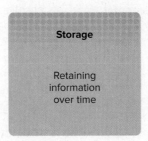
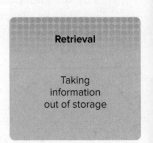

Encoding

Getting information into memory

Storage

Retaining information over time

Retrieval

Taking information out of storage

FIGURE 2

PROCESSING INFORMATION IN MEMORY. As you read about the many aspects of memory in this chapter, think about the organization of memory in terms of these three main activities.

Figure 3 shows Alan Baddeley's model of working memory. Notice that it includes two short-term "storage compartments"—one for speech and one for visual and spatial information—as well as a central executive. It is the job of the central executive to monitor and control the system—determining what information is stored, relating information from long-term memory to the information in short-term storage, and moving information into long-term memory.

Working memory is linked to many aspects of children's development (Camos & Barrouillet, 2018). For example, children who have better working memory have better reading comprehension, math skills, and problem-solving skills than their counterparts with less effective working memory (Gray & others, 2017; Kroesbergen, van 't Noordende, & Kolkman, 2014).

The following four recent studies illustrate the importance of working memory in children's cognitive development:

- Working memory and executive function predicted emergent literacy skills in young children in ethnically diverse low-income families (Chang & Gu, 2018).
- Working memory capacity among fourth-grade English speakers predicted rate of learning Chinese Mandarin vocabulary as part of their foreign language education (Wei, 2015).
- A computerized working memory intervention with 9- to 11-year-old children improved their reading performance (Loosli & others, 2012).
- Assessment of working memory in kindergarten was a key process in predicting reading and math academic achievement, as well as cognitive flexibility, at the end of the first grade (Vandenbroucke, Verschueren, & Baeyens, 2017).

Constructing Memories   Memory is not like a smartphone or computer memory; we don't store and retrieve bits of data in computer-like fashion. Instead, children and adults construct and reconstruct their memories (Camos & others, 2018; De Brigard & Parikh, 2018).

Schema Theory   According to **schema theory,** people mold memories to fit information that already exists in their minds. This process is guided by **schemas,** which are mental frameworks that organize concepts and information. Suppose a basketball fan and a visitor from a country where basketball isn't played are eating at a restaurant and overhear a conversation about last night's game. Because the visitor doesn't have a schema for information about basketball, he or she is more likely than the fan to mishear what is said. Perhaps the visitor will interpret the conversation in terms of a schema for another sport, constructing a false memory of the conversation.

Schemas influence the way we encode, interpret, and retrieve information. We reconstruct the past rather than take an exact recording of it, and the mind can distort an event as it encodes and stores impressions of it. Often when we retrieve information, we fill in the gaps with fragmented information.

Fuzzy Trace Theory   Another variation of how individuals reconstruct their memories has been proposed by Charles Brainerd and Valerie Reyna (Holliday, Brainerd, & Reyna, 2011). **Fuzzy trace theory** states that when individuals encode information, they create two types of memory representations: (1) a *verbatim memory trace,* which consists of precise details; and (2) a *fuzzy trace,* or *gist,* which is the central idea of the information. For example, consider a child who is presented with information about a pet store that has 10 birds, 6 cats, 8 dogs, and 7 rabbits. Then the child is asked two types of questions: (1) verbatim questions, such as "How many cats are in the pet store, 6 or 8?" and (2) gist questions, such as "Are there more cats or more dogs in the pet

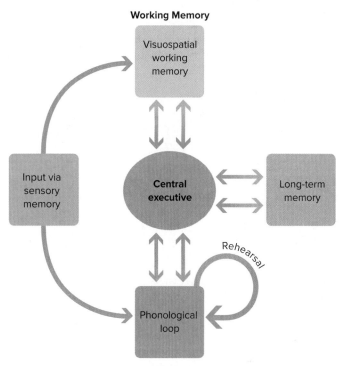

Working Memory

FIGURE 3

WORKING MEMORY. In Baddeley's classic working memory model, working memory is like a mental workbench where a great deal of information processing is carried out. Working memory consists of three main components: the phonological loop and visuospatial working memory serve as assistants, helping the central executive do its work. Input from sensory memory goes to the phonological loop, where information about speech is stored and rehearsal takes place, and visuospatial working memory, where visual and spatial information, including imagery, are stored. Working memory is a limited-capacity system, and information is stored there for only a brief time. Working memory interacts with long-term memory, using information from long-term memory in its work and transmitting information to long-term memory for longer storage. Most recently, Baddeley added an "episodic buffer" component, to help explain how information about the timing and location of memories gets stored and used.

schema theory States that when people reconstruct information, they fit it into information that already exists in their minds.

schemas Mental frameworks that organize concepts and information.

developmental **connection**

Gender

Gender schema theory emphasizes children's gender schemas that organize the world in terms of male and female. Connect to "Gender."

fuzzy trace theory States that memory is best understood by considering two types of memory representations: (1) verbatim memory trace; and (2) fuzzy trace, or gist. According to this theory, older children's better memory is attributed to the fuzzy traces created by extracting the gist of information.

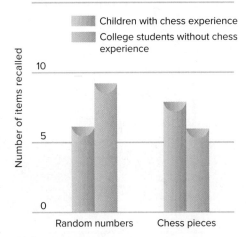

FIGURE 4

MEMORY FOR NUMBERS AND CHESS PIECES. Notice that when 10- and 11-year-old children and college students were asked to remember a string of random numbers that had been presented to them, the college students fared better. However, the 10- and 11-year-olds who had experience playing chess ("experts") had better memory for the location of chess pieces on a chess board than college students with no chess experience ("novices") (Chi, 1978).

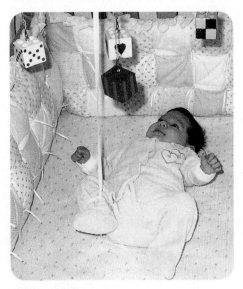

FIGURE 5

THE TECHNIQUE USED IN ROVEE-COLLIER'S INVESTIGATION OF INFANT MEMORY. In Rovee-Collier's experiment, infants as young as 2½ months of age retained information from the experience of being conditioned. *What did infants recall in Rovee-Collier's experiment?*

Courtesy of Dr. Carolyn Rovee-Collier

store?" Preschool children tend to remember verbatim information more than gist information, but elementary-school-aged children and adults are more likely to remember gist information (Kiraly & others, 2017). The increased use of gist by elementary-school-aged children accounts for their improved memory compared to preschoolers because fuzzy traces are less likely to be forgotten than verbatim traces (Reyna & Rivers, 2008).

Content Knowledge and Expertise Our ability to remember new information about something depends on what we already know about it (Gobet, 2018). Much of the research on the role of knowledge in memory has compared experts and novices (Ericsson & others, 2018). *Experts* have acquired extensive knowledge about a particular content area; this knowledge influences what they notice and how they organize, represent, and interpret information. This in turn affects their ability to remember, reason, and solve problems. When individuals have expertise about a particular subject, their memory also tends to be good regarding material related to that subject.

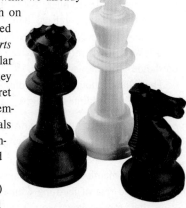

Tetra Images/Alamy Stock Photo

For example, one illustrative study (see Figure 4) found that 10- and 11-year-olds who were experienced chess players ("experts") were able to remember more information about chess pieces than college students who were not chess players ("novices") (Chi, 1978). In contrast, when the college students were presented with "non-chess" stimuli, they were able to remember them better than the children were. Even though the children were much younger than the college students, the children's expertise in chess gave them superior memories, but only in chess.

There are developmental changes in expertise that help to explain improvements in memory with age. Older children usually have more expertise about many subjects than younger children do, which can contribute to their better memory for the subject. However, it is important to consider that expertise is gained in a broader context of family, school and neighborhood, and culture. In their investigation of memory, researchers generally have not examined the roles that sociocultural factors might play. In *Connecting with Diversity*, we will explore culture's role in children's memory.

INFANCY

In the past, popular child-rearing expert Penelope Leach (2010) told parents that 6- to 8-month-old babies cannot hold in their mind a picture of their mother or father. Child development researchers, however, have revealed that infants as young as 3 months of age show early stages of memory development (Howe, Courage, & Rooksby, 2009).

First Memories Carolyn Rovee-Collier (Rovee-Collier & Barr, 2010) conducted research demonstrating that infants can remember perceptual-motor information. In a characteristic experiment, a baby was placed in a crib underneath an elaborate mobile and one end of a ribbon would be tied to the baby's ankle and the other end to the mobile. The baby would kick and make the mobile move (see Figure 5). Weeks later, the baby would be returned to the crib, but its foot would not be tied to the mobile. The baby would kick, apparently trying to make the mobile move. However, if the look of the mobile was changed even slightly, the baby usually would not kick. If the mobile was then restored to being exactly as it was when the baby's ankle was originally tied to it, the baby would begin kicking again. According to Rovee-Collier, even by 2½ months the baby's memory is incredibly detailed.

How well can infants remember? Some researchers such as Rovee-Collier have concluded that infants as young as 2 to 6 months of age can remember some experiences

connecting with diversity

Culture and Children's Memory

A culture sensitizes its members to certain objects, events, and strategies, which in turn can influence the nature of memory (Bauer & Fivush, 2013; Wagoner, 2017). In schema theory, a child's background, which is encoded in schemas, is revealed in the way the child reconstructs a story. This effect of cultural background on memory is called the *cultural-specificity hypothesis*. It states that cultural experiences determine what is relevant in a person's life and thus what the person is likely to remember. For example, imagine a child living on a remote island in the Pacific Ocean whose parents make their livelihood by fishing. The child's memory about how weather conditions affect fishing is likely to be highly developed. By contrast, a Pacific Islander child might struggle to encode and recall the details of a job involving work on large farms, or cutting lumber on forested mountains.

Cultures may vary in the strategies that children use to remember information, and these cultural variations are due in part to schooling (Packer & Cole, 2016). Children who have experienced schooling are more likely to cluster items together in broader categories, which helps them to remember the items. Schooling also provides children with specialized information-processing tasks, such as committing large amounts of information to memory in a short time frame and using logical reasoning, that may generate specialized strategies. However, there is no evidence that schooling increases memory capacity per se; rather, it influences the strategies for remembering (Packer & Cole, 2016).

Scripts are schemas for an event. In one older but illustrative study, adolescents in the United States and Mexico remembered according to script-based knowledge (Harris, Schoen, & Hensley, 1992). In line with common practices in their respective cultures, adolescents in the United States remembered information about a dating script better when no chaperone was present on a date, whereas adolescents in Mexico remembered the information better when a chaperone was present.

American children, especially American girls, describe autobiographical narratives

that are longer, more detailed, more specific, and more 'personal' (both in terms of mention of self, and mention of internal states), than

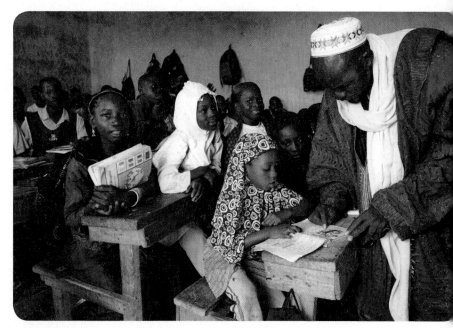

Students in class at a school in Mali, Africa. *How might their schooling influence their memory?*
Pascal Deloche/Corbis Documentary/Getty Images

narratives by children from China and Korea. The pattern is consistent with expectations derived from the finding that in their conversations about past events, American mothers and their children are more elaborative and more focused on autonomous themes . . . and that Korean mothers and their children have less frequent and less detailed conversations about the past. . . . (Bauer, 2006, p. 411)

Family narratives and stories pass down memories from one generation to the next, and these family memories may be particularly salient in cultures in which individuals are highly "interdependent" with each other (Reese & others, 2017).

How might guided participation, which is used in many different cultures, support the influence of culture on memory?

---

through 1½ to 2 years of age (Rovee-Collier & Barr, 2010). However, the infants in Rovee-Collier's experiments are displaying only implicit memory (Jabès & Nelson, 2015; Mandler, 2012). **Implicit memory** refers to memory without conscious recollection—for example, procedural long-term memories of routine activities that are performed automatically after being practiced and repeated, such as riding a bicycle. In contrast, **explicit memory** refers to the conscious memory of facts and experiences.

implicit memory Memory without conscious recollection; memory of routine activities that are performed automatically.

explicit memory Conscious memory of facts and experiences.

Age Group	Length of Delay
6-month-olds	24 hours
9-month-olds	1 month
10–11-month-olds	3 months
13–14-month-olds	4–6 months
20-month-olds	12 months

FIGURE 6

AGE-RELATED CHANGES IN THE LENGTH OF TIME OVER WHICH MEMORY OCCURS.

Source: Bauer, P. (2009). Learning and memory: Like a horse and carriage. In A. Needham & A. Woodward (Eds.), Learning and the infant mind . New York: Oxford University Press.

When people think about long-term memory, they are usually referring to explicit memory. Most researchers find that babies do not show explicit memory until the second half of the first year (Bauer & Fivush, 2013). Then, explicit memory improves substantially during the second year of life. In an illustrative longitudinal study, infants were assessed several times during their second year (Bauer & others, 2000). Older infants showed more accurate memory and required fewer reminders to demonstrate their memory than younger infants did. Figure 6 summarizes how long infants of different ages can remember information (from Bauer, 2009). Six-month-olds can remember information for 24 hours, but by 20 months of age infants can remember information they encountered 12 months earlier.

What changes in the brain are linked to infants' memory development? From about 6 to 12 months of age, the maturation of the hippocampus and the surrounding cerebral cortex, especially the frontal lobes, makes the emergence of explicit memory possible (Bauer & Fivush, 2013; Jabès & Nelson, 2015) (see Figure 7). Explicit memory continues to improve in the second year and beyond, as these brain structures further mature and connections between them increase. Less is known about the areas of the brain involved in implicit memory in infancy.

Infantile Amnesia Let's examine another aspect of long-term memory. Do you remember your third birthday party? Probably not. Most adults can remember little, if anything, from the first three years of their life (Riggins & others, 2016). This is called *infantile,* or *childhood, amnesia.* The few reported adult memories of life at age 2 or 3 are at best somewhat unclear and inaccurate (Howe, Courage, & Rooksby, 2009). Even elementary school children do not remember much about their early childhood years.

What is the cause of infantile amnesia? One reason older children and adults have difficulty recalling events from their infant and early child years is that during these early years the prefrontal lobes of the brain are immature; this area of the brain, along with its network of connections with the hippocampus, is believed to play an important role in long-term memories (Jabès & Nelson, 2015; Riggins & others, 2016).

In sum, most of young infants' conscious memories appear to be fragile and short-lived, although their implicit memory of perceptual-motor actions can be substantial. By the end of the second year, long-term memory is more substantial and reliable.

CHILDHOOD

Children's memory improves considerably after infancy (Bauer & Fivush, 2013; Bjorklund & Causey, 2017). Sometimes the long-term memories of preschoolers seem erratic, but young children can remember a great deal of information if they are given appropriate cues and prompts.

One reason children remember less than adults is that they are far less expert in most areas, but their growing knowledge is one likely source of their memory improvement. For example, a child's ability to recount what she has seen on a trip to a farm depends greatly on what she already knows about farms, such as what kinds of animals are commonly found there, how to feed and look after animals, and so on. If a child knows little about farms, she will have a much more difficult time recounting what she saw there.

Fuzzy trace theory suggests another way in which memory develops during childhood. Recall from our earlier discussion that young children tend to encode, store, and retrieve verbatim traces, whereas elementary-school-aged children begin to use gist more. The increased use of gist likely produces more enduring memory traces of information. Other sources of improvement in children's memory include changes in memory span and their use of strategies.

Memory Span Unlike long-term memory, short-term memory has a very limited capacity. One method of assessing that capacity is the *memory-span task.* You simply hear

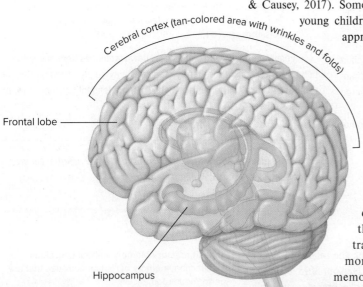

Cerebral cortex (tan-colored area with wrinkles and folds)

Frontal lobe

Hippocampus

FIGURE 7

KEY BRAIN STRUCTURES INVOLVED IN EXPLICIT MEMORY DEVELOPMENT IN INFANCY

a short list of stimuli—such as digits—presented at a rapid pace (one per second, for example). Then you are asked to repeat the digits.

Research with the memory-span task suggests that short-term memory increases during childhood. For example, in one classic study, memory span increased from about two digits in 2-year-old children to about five digits in 7-year-old children. Between 7 and 12 years of age, memory span increased by only one and a half digits (Dempster, 1981) (see Figure 8). Keep in mind, though, that individuals have different memory spans.

Why does memory span increase with age? Speed of processing information is important, especially the speed with which memory items can be identified. For example, an important early study tested children on their speed at repeating words presented orally (Case, Kurland, & Goldberg, 1982). Speed of repetition was a powerful predictor of memory span. Indeed, when the speed of repetition was controlled, the 6-year-olds' memory spans were equal to those of young adults. Rehearsal of information is also important; older children rehearse the digits more than younger children do.

Strategies Learning to use effective strategies is a key aspect of improving memory and other related cognitive capacities (Dawson & Guare, 2018). Rehearsal is just one of the strategies that can sometimes aid memory, although rehearsal is a better strategy for short-term memory than long-term memory. Following are some strategies that benefit children's long-term retention of information.

Organization If children logically organize information when they encode it, their memory benefits. Consider this demonstration: Recall the 12 months of the year as quickly as you can. How long did it take you? What was the order of your recall? You probably answered something like "a few seconds" and "in chronological order." Now try to remember the months of the year in alphabetical order. Did you make any errors? How long did it take you? It should be obvious that your memory for the months of the year is organized in a particular way.

By middle or late childhood, organizing is a strategy that older children (and adults) typically use, and it helps them to remember information. In contrast, younger preschool children usually don't use strategies like organization (Schneider & Ornstein, 2015).

Elaboration Another important strategy is elaboration, which involves engaging in more extensive processing of information. When individuals engage in elaboration, their memory benefits. Thinking of examples is a good way to elaborate information. For example, self-reference is an effective way to elaborate information. Thinking about personal associations with information makes the information more meaningful and helps children to remember it.

The use of elaboration changes developmentally and enhancing its use influences memory and attention skills in childhood (Jonkman, Hurks, & Schleepen, 2016; Schneider, 2015). Adolescents are more likely than children to use elaboration spontaneously. Elementary-school-aged children can be taught to use elaboration strategies on a learning task, but they will be less likely than adolescents to use the strategies on other learning tasks in the future. Nonetheless, verbal elaboration can be an effective strategy even for young elementary-school-aged children.

Imagery Creating mental images is another strategy for improving memory. However, using imagery to remember verbal information works better for older children than for younger children. Still, using mental imagery can help young schoolchildren to remember pictures (Schneider, 2015).

Teaching Strategies So far we have described several important strategies adults can adopt when guiding children to remember information more effectively over the long term. These strategies include guiding children to organize information, elaborate the information, and develop images of the information. Another good strategy is to encourage children to understand the material that needs to be remembered rather than rotely

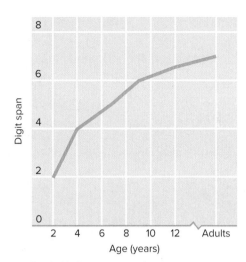

FIGURE 8

DEVELOPMENTAL CHANGES IN MEMORY SPAN. In a classic study, memory span increased by about three digits from 2 years of age to 7 years of age (Dempster, 1981). By 12 years of age, memory span had increased on average another one and a half digits.

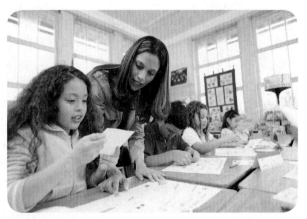

What are some good teaching strategies for guiding children's long-term memory?
Stretch Photography/Blend Images/Getty Images

memorizing it. Two other strategies adults can use to guide children's retention of memory have been proposed:

- Repeat with variation on the instructional information, and link early and often. These are memory development research expert Patricia Bauer's (2009) recommendations to improve children's consolidation and reconsolidation of the information they are learning. Variations on a lesson theme increase the number of associations in memory storage, and linking expands the network of associations in memory storage; both strategies expand the routes for retrieving information from storage.
- Embed memory-relevant language when instructing children. Teachers vary considerably in how much they use memory-relevant language that encourages students to remember information. In research that involved extensive observations of a number of first-grade teachers in the classroom, Peter Ornstein & his colleagues (Ornstein & others, 2010) found that in the time segments observed, the teachers rarely used strategy suggestions or metacognitive (thinking about thinking) questions. In this research, when lower-achieving students were placed in classrooms in which teachers frequently embedded memory-relevant information in their teaching, student achievement increased.

Reconstructive Memory and Children as Eyewitnesses Children's memories, like those of adults, are constructive and reconstructive. Children have schemas for all sorts of information, and these schemas affect how they encode, store, and retrieve memories. If a teacher tells her class a story about two men and two women who were involved in a train crash in France, students won't remember every detail of the story and will reconstruct the story, putting their own individual stamp on it. One student might reconstruct the story by saying the characters died in a plane crash, another might describe three men and three women, another might say the crash was in Germany, and so on.

Reconstruction and distortion are nowhere more apparent than in clashing testimony given by eyewitnesses at trials. A special concern is susceptibility to suggestion and how this can alter memory (Otgaar & others, 2018). Consider a study of individuals who had visited Disneyland (Loftus, 2003). Four groups of participants read ads and answered questionnaires about a trip to Disneyland. One group saw an ad that mentioned no cartoon characters; the second read the same ad and saw a 4-foot-tall cardboard figure of Bugs Bunny; the third read a fake ad for Disneyland with Bugs Bunny on it; and the fourth saw the same fake ad along with cardboard Bugs. Participants were asked whether they had ever met Bugs Bunny at Disneyland. Less than 10 percent of those in the first two groups reported having met Bugs Bunny at Disneyland, but approximately 30 to 40 percent of the third and fourth groups remembered meeting Bugs there. People were persuaded they had met Bugs Bunny at Disneyland, even though Bugs is a Warner Brothers character who would never appear at a Disney theme park.

The following conclusions about children as eyewitnesses indicate that a number of factors can influence the accuracy of a young child's memory:

- *There are age differences in children's susceptibility to suggestion.* Preschoolers are the most suggestible age group in comparison with older children and adults (Ceci, Hritz, & Royer, 2016). For example, preschool children are more susceptible to believing misleading or incorrect information given after an event. Despite these age differences, there is still concern about the reaction of older children when they are subjected to suggestive interviews (La Rooy, Brown, & Lamb, 2013).
- *There are individual differences in susceptibility.* Some preschoolers as well as older children are highly resistant to interviewers' suggestions, whereas others immediately succumb to the slightest suggestion (Klemfuss & Olaguez, 2018).
- *Interviewing techniques can produce substantial distortions in children's reports about highly salient events.* Children are suggestible not just about peripheral details but

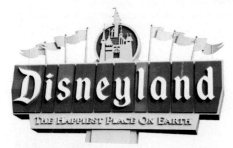

Pictures Colour Library/Alamy Stock Photo

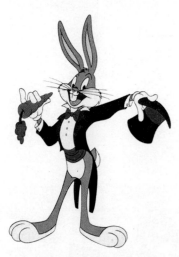

United Archives/age fotostock

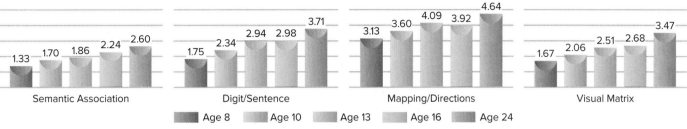

Verbal tasks

Semantic Association: 1.33, 1.70, 1.86, 2.24, 2.60

Digit/Sentence: 1.75, 2.34, 2.94, 2.98, 3.71

Visuospatial tasks

Mapping/Directions: 3.13, 3.60, 4.09, 3.92, 4.64

Visual Matrix: 1.67, 2.06, 2.51, 2.68, 3.47

■ Age 8   ■ Age 10   ■ Age 13   ■ Age 16   ■ Age 24

FIGURE 9

DEVELOPMENTAL CHANGES IN WORKING MEMORY. *Note:* The scores shown here are the means for each age group, and the age also represents a mean age. Higher scores reflect superior working memory performance (Swanson, 1999).

also about the central aspects of an event. When children do accurately recall information about an event, the interviewer often has a neutral tone, there is limited use of misleading questions, and there is an absence of any motivation for the child to make a false report (Malloy & others, 2012; Turoy-Smith & Powell, 2017).

In sum, whether a young child's eyewitness testimony is accurate may depend on a number of factors such as the type, number, and intensity of the suggestive techniques the child has experienced.

ADOLESCENCE

There has been relatively little research on memory changes in adolescence, compared with the research in childhood. As you saw in Figure 8, memory span (which is a measure of short-term memory) increases during adolescence. There also is evidence that working memory increases during adolescence. In one extensive cross-sectional study, the performances of individuals from 6 to 57 years of age were examined on both verbal and visuospatial working memory tasks (Swanson, 1999). As shown in Figure 9, working memory increased substantially from 8 through 24 years of age no matter what the task. Another study using brain imaging found that these improvements during adolescence and young adulthood were due to shifts in neural functioning in specific brain regions (Simmonds, Hallquist, & Luna, 2017). Thus, the adolescent years are likely to be an important developmental period for improvement in working memory. Note that working memory continues to improve through the transition to adulthood and beyond.

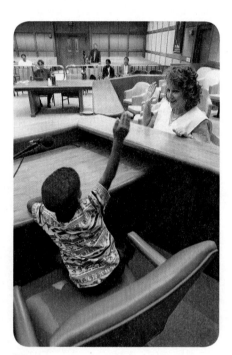

What are some issues involved in whether young children should be allowed to testify in court?
Buddy Norris/KRT/Newscom

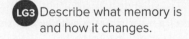

Review *Connect* Reflect

LG3 Describe what memory is and how it changes.

Review

- What is memory? What are some important processes and types of memory?
- How does memory develop in infancy?
- How does memory change in childhood?
- How does memory change in adolescence?

Connect

- In this section, we learned about *schemas* as they relate to memory.

How is this concept similar to or different from the concept of *schemes*, as related to Piaget's theory of development?

Reflect *Your Own Personal Journey of Life*

- What is your earliest memory? Why do you think you can remember this particular situation?

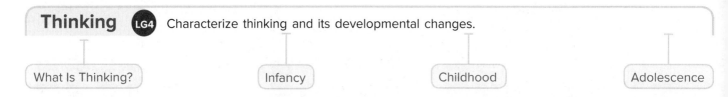

Thinking LG4 Characterize thinking and its developmental changes.

What Is Thinking?   Infancy   Childhood   Adolescence

Attention and memory are often steps toward another level of information processing—thinking. What is thinking? How does it change developmentally? What is children's scientific thinking like, and how do they solve problems? Let's explore these questions.

WHAT IS THINKING?

thinking Transforming and manipulating information in memory. Individuals think in order to reason, reflect, evaluate ideas, solve problems, and make decisions.

concepts Cognitive groupings of similar objects, events, people, or ideas.

Thinking involves manipulating and transforming information in memory; it is the job of the central executive in Baddeley's model of working memory shown in Figure 3. We think in order to reason, reflect, evaluate ideas, solve problems, and make decisions. Let's explore how thinking changes developmentally, beginning with infancy.

INFANCY

Interest in thinking during infancy has especially focused on concept formation and categorization (Gelman, 2013; Rakison & Lawson, 2013). **Concepts** are cognitive groupings of similar objects, events, people, or ideas. Without concepts, you would see each object and event as unique; you would not be able to make any generalizations.

Do infants have concepts? Yes, they do, although we do not know just how early concept formation begins (Ferguson & Waxman, 2017).

Using habituation experiments, some researchers have found that infants as young as 3 to 4 months of age can group together objects with similar appearances, such as animals (Quinn, 2016). This research capitalizes on the knowledge that infants are more likely to look at a novel object than a familiar object.

Jean Mandler (2012) argues that these early categorizations are best described as *perceptual categorization*. That is, the categorizations are based on similar perceptual features of objects, such as size, color, and movement, as well as parts of objects, such as legs for animals. Mandler concludes that it is not until about 7 to 9 months of age that infants form *conceptual* categories rather than just making perceptual discriminations between different categories. In one illustrative study of 9- to 11-month-olds, infants classified birds as animals and airplanes as vehicles even though the objects were perceptually similar—airplanes and birds with their wings spread (Mandler & McDonough, 1993) (see Figure 10).

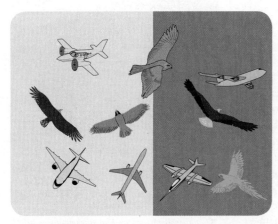

FIGURE 10

CATEGORIZATION IN 9- TO 11-MONTH-OLDS. These are the type of stimuli used in the study that indicated 9- to 11-month-old infants categorized birds as animals and airplanes as vehicles even though the objects were perceptually similar (Mandler & McDonough, 1993).

Further advances in categorization occur in the second year of life (Poulin-Dubois & Pauen, 2017). Early concepts in infancy are very broad, such as "food" or "animal." As cognitive development proceeds in the second year, these categories become more distinct and precise, such as "fruit" then "apple," or "flying animal" then "bird." Also in the second year, infants often categorize objects on the basis of their shape—a strategy that they move beyond later in early childhood (Ware, 2017).

Learning to put things into the correct categories—what makes something one kind of thing rather than another kind of thing, such as what makes a bird a bird, or a fish a fish—is an important aspect of learning. As infant development researcher Alison Gopnik (2010, p. 159) once pointed out, "If you can sort the world into the right categories—put things in the right boxes—then you've got a big advance on understanding the world."

Do some very young children develop an intense, passionate interest in a particular category of objects or activities? They do, and this emerges strongly from late infancy into early childhood. One study found clear gender difference in preferences, with an intense interest in particular objects or categories as well as repeated procedures stronger for boys than girls, and preference for creative and socially interactive interests more evident in girls than in boys (Neitzel, Alexander, & Johnson, 2019). When Alex, a grandson of one

Infants are creating concepts and organizing their world into conceptual domains that will form the backbone of their thought throughout life.

—JEAN MANDLER

Contemporary psychologist, University of California–San Diego

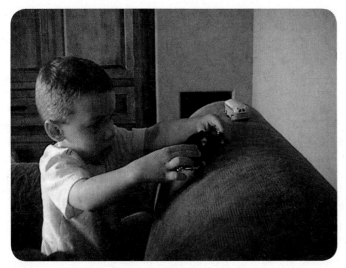

Two-year-old Alex shows his intense, passionate interest in the category of vehicles while playing with a London taxi and a funky Malta bus.

Dr. John Santrock

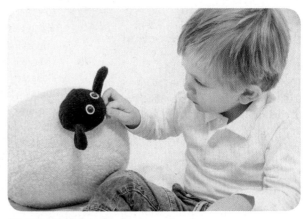

FIGURE **11**

STUDYING EXECUTIVE FUNCTION IN YOUNG CHILDREN.
Researcher Stephanie Carlson has conducted a number of research studies on young children's executive function. In one study, young children were read either *Planet Opposite*—a fantasy book in which everything is turned upside down—or *Fun Town*—a reality-oriented fiction book (Carlson & White, 2013). After being read one of the books, the young children completed the Less Is More Task, in which they were shown two trays of candy—one with 5 pieces, the other with 2—and told that the tray they pick will be given to the stuffed animal seated at the table. This task is difficult for 3-year-olds who tend to pick up the tray that they themselves want (and so ending up losing the tray to the stuffed animal). Sixty percent of the 3-year-olds who heard the *Planet Opposite* story selected the smaller number of candies (hence keeping the five pieces of candy), compared with only 20 percent of their counterparts who heard the more straightforward story. The results indicated that learning about a topsy-turvy imaginary world likely helped the young children become more flexible in their thinking.

vwPix/Shutterstock

of the authors, was 18 to 24 months old, he already had developed an intense, passionate interest in the category of vehicles. For example, at this age, he categorized vehicles into such subcategories as cars, trucks, earth-moving equipment, and buses. In addition to common classifications of cars into police cars, jeeps, taxis, and such, and trucks into fire trucks, dump trucks, and the like, his categorical knowledge of earth-moving equipment included bulldozers and excavators, and he categorized buses into school buses, London buses, and funky Malta buses (retro buses on the island of Malta). Later, at 2 to 3 years of age, Alex developed an intense, passionate interest in categorizing dinosaurs.

In sum, the infant's advances in processing information—through attention, memory, imitation, and concept formation—is much richer, more gradual and less stage-like, and occurs earlier than was envisioned by earlier theorists, such as Piaget (Bauer, 2009; Bjorklund & Causey, 2017; Mandler, 2012; Quinn, 2016).

CHILDHOOD

To explore thinking in childhood, we will examine four important types of thinking: executive function, critical thinking, scientific thinking, and problem solving.

Executive Function Recently, increasing research attention has focused on the development of children's **executive function,** an umbrella-like concept that encompasses a number of higher-level cognitive processes linked to the development of the brain's prefrontal cortex. Executive function involves managing one's thoughts to engage in goal-directed behavior and to exercise self-control (Carlson, Zelazo, & Faja, 2013; Miller & Marcovitch, 2015). Earlier in this chapter, we described the recent interest in *executive attention,* which comes under the umbrella of executive function.

In early childhood, executive function especially involves developmental advances in cognitive inhibition (such as inhibiting a strong tendency that is incorrect), cognitive flexibility (such as shifting attention to another item or topic), goal-setting (such as sharing a toy or mastering a skill like catching a ball), and delay of gratification (the ability to forego an immediate pleasure or reward for a more desirable one later) (McDermott & Fox, 2018). During early childhood, the relatively stimulus-driven toddler is transformed into a child capable of flexible, goal-directed problem solving that characterizes executive function (Zelazo, 2015). Figure 11 describes a research study on young children's executive function (Carlson & White, 2013).

executive function An umbrella-like concept that consists of a number of higher-level cognitive processes linked to the development of the brain's prefrontal cortex. Executive function involves managing one's thoughts to engage in goal-directed behavior and to exercise self-control.

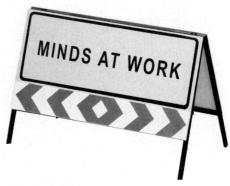

Anthony Harvie/Getty Images

developmental **connection**

The Brain

The prefrontal cortex is the location in the brain where much of executive function occurs. Connect to "Physical Development and Health."

Researchers have discovered that advances in executive function in the preschool years are linked with school readiness (Ursache, Blair, & Raver, 2012). Parents and teachers play important roles in the development of executive function. Ann Masten and her colleagues (Masten, 2013; Masten & others, 2015) have found that executive function and parenting skills are linked to homeless children's success in school. Masten believes that executive function and good parenting skills are related. In her words, "When we see kids with good executive function, we often see adults around them that are good self-regulators. . . . Parents model, they support, and they scaffold these skills" (Masten, 2012, p. 11). Mounting evidence supports this view (Deater-Deckard & Sturge-Apple, 2017).

How might executive function change during the middle and late childhood years and affect success in school? The following dimensions of executive function are particularly important for 4- to 11-year-old children's cognitive development and school success (Diamond & Lee, 2011; Kassai & others, 2019):

- *Self-control/inhibition.* Children need to develop self-control that will allow them to concentrate and persist on learning tasks, to inhibit their tendencies to repeat incorrect responses, and to resist the impulse to do something now that they would regret later.

- *Working memory.* Children need an effective working memory to process the masses of information they will encounter as they go through school and beyond.

- *Flexibility.* Children need to be flexible in their thinking to consider different strategies and perspectives.

Some researchers have found that executive function and related aspects of self-regulation may be an even better predictor of school readiness than general IQ (Duckworth & others, 2019). A number of diverse activities have been found to increase children's executive function, such as computerized training that uses games to improve working memory (CogMed, 2013), aerobic exercise (Chu & others, 2017), mindfulness (the Tools of the Mind program, for example) (Blair & Raver, 2014), and some types of school curricula, such as the Montessori curriculum (Diamond, 2013; Lillard, 2016).

Further, the largest and longest-running longitudinal study of an important dimension of executive function—inhibitory control—found that 3- to 11-year-old children who had better inhibitory control (they were able to wait their turn, not easily distracted, more persistent, and less impulsive) were more likely to still be in school, less likely to engage in risk-taking behavior, and less likely to be taking drugs in adolescence (Moffitt & others, 2011). In addition, thirty years after they were initially assessed, the children with better inhibitory control had better physical and mental health (they were less likely to be overweight, for example), had better earnings in their career, were more law-abiding, and were happier.

Some critics argue that not much benefit is derived from placing various cognitive processes under the broader concept of executive function. Although we have described a number of components of executive function here—working memory, cognitive inhibition, cognitive flexibility, and so on—a consensus has not been reached on what the components are, how they are connected, and how they develop. In addition, it has been a challenge to show that training specific executive function skills leads to broader improvements in cognition and academic skills (Kassai & others, 2019). Further research will provide a clearer picture of executive function and how it develops (Friedman & Miyake, 2017).

critical thinking Thinking reflectively and productively, and evaluating the evidence.

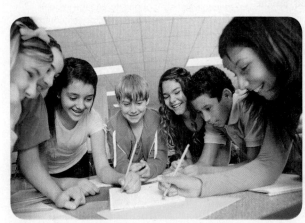

What are some good strategies for guiding students to think critically?
Steve Debenport/Getty Images

Critical Thinking Executive function also involves the ability to think critically in effective ways. There is considerable interest among psychologists and educators in **critical thinking** that involves thinking reflectively and productively, and evaluating evidence. If you think critically, you will do the following things:

- Ask not only what happened but how and why.

- Examine supposed "facts" to determine whether there is evidence to support them.

- Argue in a reasoned way rather than through emotions.
- Recognize that there is sometimes more than one good answer or explanation.
- Compare various answers and judge which is the best answer.
- Evaluate what other people say rather than immediately accepting it as the truth.
- Ask questions and speculate beyond what is known to create new ideas and new information.

Too few schools teach students to think critically. Schools push students to give a single correct answer rather than encouraging them to come up with new ideas and rethink conclusions. Too often teachers ask students to recite, define, describe, state, and list rather than to analyze, infer, connect, synthesize, criticize, create, evaluate, think, and rethink. As a result, many schools graduate students who think superficially, staying on the surface of problems rather than becoming deeply engaged in meaningful thinking.

However, this deficiency in education can be addressed through teaching methods that emphasize critical thinking and creativity (Grigg & Lewis, 2019). One way to encourage students to think critically is to present them with controversial topics or both sides of an issue to discuss (Litman & Greenleaf, 2018). Debates can motivate students to delve more deeply into a topic and examine issues, especially if teachers refrain from stating their own views so that students feel free to explore multiple perspectives.

Mindfulness—being alert, mentally present, and cognitively flexible while going through life's everyday activities and tasks—is an important aspect of thinking critically (Farrar & Tapper, 2018; Langer, 2005). Mindful children and adults maintain an active awareness of the circumstances in their life and are motivated to find the best solutions to tasks. Mindful individuals create new ideas, are open to new information, and can operate from more than one perspective. By contrast, mindless individuals are entrapped in old ideas, engage in automatic behavior, and operate from a single perspective.

Mindfulness is an important mental process that children can engage in to improve a number of cognitive and socioemotional skills, such as executive function, focused attention, emotion regulation, and empathy (Roeser & Zelazo, 2012). Mindfulness training can be implemented in schools by using age-appropriate activities that increase children's reflection on moment-to-moment experiences to improve self-regulation (Carsley, Khoury, & Heath, 2018; Sheinman & others, 2018). In addition to mindfulness, techniques such as yoga, meditation, and tai chi have been proposed as candidates for improving children's cognitive and socioemotional development. To read about one developmental psychologist who used her training in cognitive development to pursue a career in an applied area, see the *Connecting with Careers* profile.

mindfulness Being alert, mentally present, and cognitively flexible while going through life's everyday activities and tasks.

developmental **connection**

Exercise

Recent research indicates that more physically fit children have better thinking skills, including those involving executive function, than less physically fit children. Connect to "Physical Development and Health."

Scientific Thinking Some aspects of thinking are specific to a particular domain, such as mathematics, science, or reading. We will explore reading in the chapter on "Language Development." Here we will examine scientific thinking by children.

Like scientists, children ask fundamental questions about reality and seek answers to questions that seem trivial or unanswerable to other people (such as "Why is the sky blue?"). Do children generate hypotheses, perform experiments, and reach conclusions about their data in ways resembling those of scientists?

Scientific reasoning often is aimed at identifying causal relations. Like scientists, children place a great deal of emphasis on causal mechanisms. Their understanding of how events are caused weighs more heavily in their reasoning than even such strong influences as whether the cause happened immediately before the effect.

There also are important differences between the reasoning of children and the reasoning of scientists (Kuhn, 2013). Children are more influenced by coincidence than by an overall pattern. Often, children maintain their old theories regardless of the evidence (Lehrer & Schauble, 2015).

Children might go through mental gymnastics trying to reconcile seemingly contradictory new information with their existing beliefs. Children also have difficulty designing experiments that can distinguish among alternative causes. Instead, they tend to bias the experiments in favor of whatever hypothesis they began with. Sometimes they see the results as supporting their original hypothesis even when the results directly contradict it.

Helen Hadani, Developmental Psychologist, Toy Designer, and Research Practitioner

Helen Hadani obtained a Ph.D. from Stanford University in developmental psychology, but she now spends her days talking with computer engineers, designing "smart" toys for children, and connecting these technologies to children's learning at the Center for Childhood Creativity in California. Smart toys are designed to improve children's problem-solving and symbolic thinking skills.

When she was a graduate student, Hadani worked part-time for Hasbro toys, testing its children's software on preschoolers. Her first job after graduate school was with Zowie Entertainment, which was subsequently bought by LEGO. According to Hadani, "Even in a toy's most primitive stage of development, . . . you see children's creativity in responding to challenges, their satisfaction when a problem is solved or simply their delight when they are having fun" (Schlegel, 2000, p. 50). In addition to conducting experiments and focus groups at different stages of a toy's development, she also assesses the age appropriateness of learning materials.

For more information about what researchers do, see the Careers in Child Development appendix.

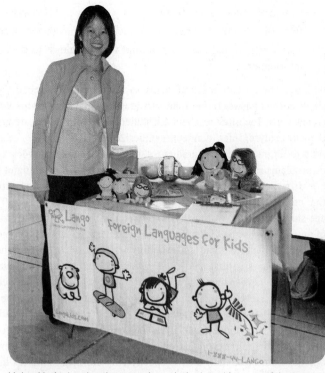

Helen Hadani, a developmental psychologist, with some of the toys she designed for her work on teaching foreign languages to children.
Courtesy of Helen Hadani

Thus, although there are important similarities between children and scientists, in their basic curiosity and in the kinds of questions they ask, there are also important differences in the degree to which they can separate theory from evidence and in their ability to design conclusive experiments (Lehrer & Schauble, 2015).

Too often, the skills scientists use, such as careful observation, graphing, self-regulatory thinking, and knowing when and how to apply one's knowledge to solve problems, are not routinely taught in schools (Zembal-Saul, McNeill, & Hershberger, 2013). Children hold many concepts that are incompatible with science and reality. Good teachers perceive and understand a child's underlying scientific concepts, then use the concepts as a scaffold for learning. Effective science teaching helps children distinguish between fruitful errors and misconceptions, and detect plainly wrong ideas that need to be replaced with more accurate conceptions (Harlen & Qualter, 2018). It is important for teachers to initially scaffold students' science learning, extensively monitor their progress, and ensure that they are learning science content because these practices are most essential to scientific reasoning and critical thinking (Novak & Treagust, 2018). Thus, in pursuing science investigations, students need to learn inquiry skills and science content simultaneously (Lehrer & Schauble, 2015).

Solving Problems   Children face many problems, both in school and out of school. *Problem solving* involves finding an appropriate way to attain a goal. Let's examine two ways children solve problems—by applying rules and by using analogies—and then consider some ways to help children learn effective strategies for solving problems.

Using Rules to Solve Problems   As noted earlier, during early childhood the relatively stimulus-driven toddler is transformed into a child capable of flexible, goal-directed problem solving. One element in this change is children's developing ability to form representations of reality.

For example, because they struggle with the concept that there are multiple perspectives, 3- to 4-year-olds cannot understand that a single stimulus can be redescribed in a different, incompatible way (Perner & Leahy, 2016). Consider a problem in which children must sort stimuli using the rule of *color* (Doebel & Zelazo, 2015). In the course of the color sorting, a child may describe a red rabbit as a *red one* to solve the problem. However, in a subsequent task, the child may need to discover a rule that describes the rabbit as just a *rabbit* to solve the problem. If 3- to 4-year-olds fail to understand that it is possible to provide multiple descriptions of the same stimulus, they persist in describing the stimulus as a red rabbit; this is sometimes called representational inflexibility. Researchers have found that it is at about 4 years of age that children acquire the concept of perspectives so that they can appreciate that a single thing can be described in different ways.

With age, children also learn better rules to apply to problems (Li & others, 2017). Figure 12 provides an example; it shows the balance scale problem that has been used to examine children's use of rules in solving problems. The scale includes a fulcrum and an arm that can rotate around it. The arm can tip left or right or remain level, depending on how weights (metal disks with holes in the center) are arranged on the pegs in each side of the fulcrum. The child's task is to look at the configuration of weights on the pegs in each problem and then predict whether the left side will go down, the right side will go down, or the arm will balance.

Robert Siegler hypothesized that children would use one of the four rules listed in Figure 12. He reasoned that presenting problems on which different rules would generate different outcomes would allow assessment of each child's rules. Through a child's pattern of correct answers and errors on a set of such problems, that child's underlying rule could be inferred. The findings from this and many other studies that followed have informed our understanding of how children develop their use of rules for problem solving (Lemaire, 2017).

What were the results? Almost all 5-year-olds used Rule I, in which the child considers only the weight on the scales. Almost all 9-year-olds used either Rule II, which takes both weight and distance into account, or Rule III, which calls for guessing if the weight and distance dimensions would give conflicting information. Both 13-year-olds and 17-year-olds generally used Rule III.

In other words, the older children performed better at solving the problems because they used a better rule. But even 5-year-old children can be trained to use Rule III if they are taught to pay attention to differences in distance. As children learn more about what is relevant to a problem and learn to encode the relevant information, they are better at using rules in problem solving.

Interestingly, despite the 17-year-olds' having studied balance scales in their physics course, almost none of them used the only rule that generated consistently correct answers, Rule IV. Discussions with their teachers revealed why: The balance scale the students had

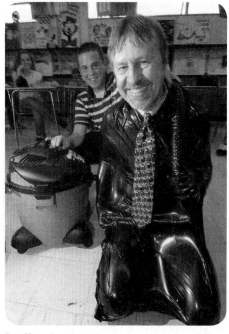

Pete Karpyk, who taught chemistry in Weirton, West Virginia, would use an extensive array of activities that bring science to life for students. He received the Presidential Award for Excellence in Mathematics and Science Teaching in 2015–the highest recognition of teaching skill in the United States. Here he has shrink-wrapped himself to demonstrate the effects of air pressure. He has some students give chemistry demonstrations at elementary schools and has discovered that in some cases students who don't do well on tests excel when they teach children. He also adapted his teaching based on feedback from former students and incorporated questions from their college chemistry tests as bonus questions on the tests he would give his high school students. (Source: Wong Briggs, 2005. p. 6D).
Dale Sparks

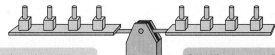

Rule I. If the weight is the same on both sides, predict that the scale will balance. If the weight differs, predict that the side with more weight will go down.

Balance scale apparatus

Rule II. If the weight is greater on one side, say that that side will go down. If the weights on the two sides are equal, choose the side on which the weight is farther from the fulcrum.

Rule III. Act as in Rule II, except that if one side has more weight and the weight on the other side is farther from the fulcrum, then guess.

Rule IV. Proceed as in Rule III, unless one side has more weight and the other more distance. In that case, calculate torques by multiplying weight times distance on each side. Then predict that the side with the greater torque will go down.

FIGURE 12

THE TYPE OF BALANCE SCALE USED BY SIEGLER (1976). Weights could be placed on pegs on each side of the fulcrum; the torque (the weight on each side times the distance of that weight from the fulcrum) determined which side would go down.

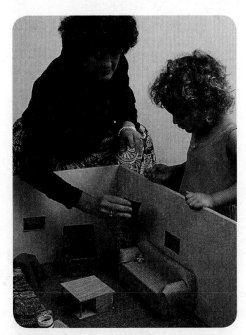

Judy DeLoache has conducted research that focuses on young children's developing cognitive abilities. She has demonstrated that children's symbolic representation between 2½ and 3 years of age enables them to find a toy in a real room that is a much bigger version of the scale model.

Courtesy of Judy DeLoache

studied was a pan balance, on which small pans could be hung from various locations along the arm, rather than an arm balance, with pegs extending upward. Retesting the high school students showed that most could consistently solve the problems when the familiar pan balance was used. This example illustrates a set of lessons that frequently emerge from studies of problem solving—learning is often quite narrow, generalization beyond one's existing knowledge is difficult, and even analogies that seem straightforward are often missed.

Using Analogies to Solve Problems   An *analogy* involves correspondence in some respects between things that are dissimilar. Even very young children can draw reasonable analogies under some circumstances and use them to solve problems (Whitaker & others, 2018; Yuan, Uttal, & Gentner, 2017). Under other circumstances, even college students fail to draw seemingly obvious analogies (as in the high school students' difficulty in extrapolating from the familiar pan balance to the unfamiliar arm balance).

In one effort to discover developmental changes in young children's analogical problem solving, in an illustrative study Judy DeLoache (2011) created a situation in which 2½- and 3-year-olds were shown a small toy hidden within a scale model of a room. The child was then asked to find the toy in a real room that was a bigger version of the scale model. If the toy was hidden under the armchair in the scale model, it was also hidden under the armchair in the real room. Substantial development occurred in just six months between 2½ and 3 years of age on this task. Thirty-month-old children rarely could solve the problem, but most 36-month-old children could.

Why was the task so difficult for the 2½-year-olds? Their problem was not an inability to understand that a symbol can represent another situation. Shown line drawings or photographs of the larger room, 2½-year-olds had no difficulty finding the object. Instead, the difficulty seemed to come from the toddlers' simultaneously viewing the scale model as a symbol of the larger room and as an object in itself. When children were allowed to play with the scale model before using it as a symbol, their performance actually got worse, presumably because playing with it made them think of it more as an object in itself. Conversely, when the scale model was placed in a glass case, where the children could not handle it at all, more children used it successfully to find the object hidden in the larger room. Thus, young children can use a variety of tools to draw analogies, but they easily can forget that an object is being used as a symbol of something else and instead treat it as an object in its own right (Yuan, Uttal, & Gentner, 2017).

Using Strategies to Solve Problems   Good thinkers routinely use strategies and effective planning to solve problems (Bjorklund & Causey, 2017). One study revealed that children's selection of effective strategies in solving math and memory problems improves from the third grade to the seventh grade (Geurten, Meulemans, & Lemaire, 2018).

Children often use more than one strategy when problem solving. Most children benefit from generating a variety of alternative strategies and experimenting with different approaches to a problem, discovering what works well, when, and where. This is especially true for children from the middle elementary school grades on, although some cognitive psychologists stress that even young children should be encouraged to practice varying strategies (Siegler, 2013, 2016). To read further about guiding children to learn effective strategies, see the *Caring Connections* interlude.

ADOLESCENCE

By adolescence, considerable variation in cognitive functioning is present across individuals. This variability supports the argument that adolescents are producers of their own development, perhaps to a greater extent than are children.

A very important cognitive change in adolescence is improvement in *executive function,* which we discussed earlier in this chapter. Our coverage of executive function in adolescence focuses on monitoring and managing cognitive resources, critical thinking, and decision making.

The error of youth is to believe that intelligence is a substitute for experience, while the error of age is to believe that experience is a substitute for intelligence.

—LYMAN BRYSON

American author, 20th century

Helping Children Learn Strategies

Michael Pressley's [1951–2006] view about academic success has been very influential (Pressley, 2007; Pressley & Hilden, 2006). Accordingly, the key to education is helping students learn a rich repertoire of strategies for solving problems. Pressley argued that when children are given instruction about effective strategies, they often can apply strategies that they had not used on their own. Pressley emphasized that children benefit when the teacher (1) models the appropriate strategy, (2) verbalizes the steps in the strategy, and (3) guides the children to practice the strategy and supports their practice with feedback. "Practice" means that children use the strategy over and over until they perform it automatically. To execute strategies effectively, they need to have the strategies in long-term memory, and extensive practice makes this possible.

Just having children learn a new strategy is usually not enough for them to continue to use it and to transfer the strategy to new situations. Children need to be motivated to learn and to use the strategies. For effective maintenance and transfer, children should be encouraged to monitor the effectiveness of the new strategy by comparing their performance on tests and other assessments.

Let's examine an example of effective strategy instruction. Good readers extract the main ideas from text and summarize them. In contrast, novice readers (for example, most children) usually don't store the main ideas of what they read. One classic intervention based on what we know about the summarizing strategies of good readers consisted of instructing children to (1) skim over trivial information, (2) ignore redundant information, (3) replace less inclusive terms with more inclusive ones, (4) use a more inclusive action term to combine a series of events, (5) choose a topic sentence, and (6) create a topic sentence if none is given (Brown & Day, 1983). Instructing elementary school students to use these summarizing strategies improves their reading performance, and similar effects are observed in other subjects and among older children and teenagers (Santi & Reed, 2015).

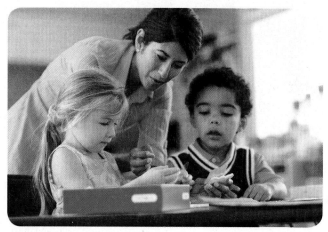

What are some effective ways that teachers can help students learn to develop a rich repertoire of strategies for solving problems?
John Lund/Marc Romanelli/Blend Images/Getty Images

Pressley and his colleagues (Pressley & Hilden, 2006; Pressley & others, 2007) spent considerable time observing the use of strategy instruction by teachers and strategy use by students in elementary and secondary school classrooms. They concluded that teachers' use of strategy instruction is far less complete and intense than what is needed for students to learn how to use strategies effectively. Pressley's colleagues continue to argue that education needs to be restructured so that students are provided with more opportunities to become competent strategic learners.

How do the research findings of Peter Ornstein and his colleagues (2010) regarding teachers' use of strategy suggestions or metacognitive questions in the classroom (mentioned earlier in this chapter) compare with the findings of Pressley and his colleagues about teaching strategies?

Monitoring and Managing Cognitive Resources   Executive function strengthens not only in childhood but also during adolescence (Crone, Peters, & Steinbeis, 2017; Kuhn, 2009). This executive function

> assumes a role of monitoring and managing the deployment of cognitive resources as a function of task demands. As a result, cognitive development and learning itself become more effective. . . . Emergence and strengthening of this executive (functioning) is arguably the single most important and consequential intellectual development to occur in the second decade of life (Kuhn & Franklin, 2006, p. 987).

Critical Thinking   Adolescence is an important transitional period in the development of critical thinking (Sanders, 2013). Among the cognitive changes that allow improvement in critical thinking during this period are the following:

- Increased speed, automaticity, and capacity of information processing, which free cognitive resources for other purposes
- Greater breadth of content knowledge in a variety of domains

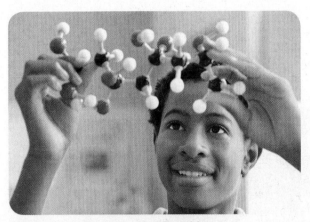

What are some cognitive changes that allow adolescents to think more critically than children?
Fuse/Getty Images

- Increased ability to construct new combinations of knowledge
- A greater range and more spontaneous use of strategies and procedures for obtaining and applying knowledge, such as planning, considering the alternatives, and cognitive monitoring

Adolescence is an important period in the development of critical-thinking skills. However, if a solid basis of fundamental literacy and math skills was not developed during childhood, critical-thinking skills are unlikely to develop adequately in adolescence, although some youth can "catch up" to their peers over development (Geary, Nicholas, & Sun, 2017; Huang, Moon, & Boren, 2014).

Decision Making   Adolescence is a time of increased decision making—which friends to choose, which person to date, whether to have sex, buy a car, go to college, and so on (Hartley & Somerville, 2015; Steinberg & others, 2018). How competent are adolescents at making decisions? Overall, the research shows that, older adolescents are more competent than younger adolescents, who in turn are more competent than children. Compared with children, young adolescents are more likely to generate different options, examine a situation from a variety of perspectives, anticipate the consequences of decisions, and consider the credibility of sources.

However, older adolescents' (as well as adults') decision-making skills are far from perfect, and having the capacity to make competent decisions does not guarantee they will be made in everyday life, where breadth of experience often comes into play (Kuhn, 2009). As an example, driver-training courses improve adolescents' cognitive and motor skills to levels equal to, or sometimes superior to, those of adults. However, driver training has not been effective in reducing adolescents' high rate of traffic accidents. Still, graduated driver licensing (GDR) does reduce crash and fatality rates for adolescent drivers (Alderman & Johnston, 2018). GDR components include a learner's holding period, practice-driving certification, night-driving restriction, and passenger restriction. GDR is now commonly used throughout North America, Europe, and Australia, as well as certain countries on other continents.

Most people make better decisions when they are calm rather than emotionally aroused, which often is especially true for adolescents. Recall that adolescents have a tendency to be emotionally intense, in part due to hormonal changes due to puberty (Hoyt & others, 2015). Thus, the same adolescent who makes a wise decision when calm may make an unwise decision when emotionally aroused. In the heat of the moment, then, adolescents' emotions may especially overwhelm their decision-making ability.

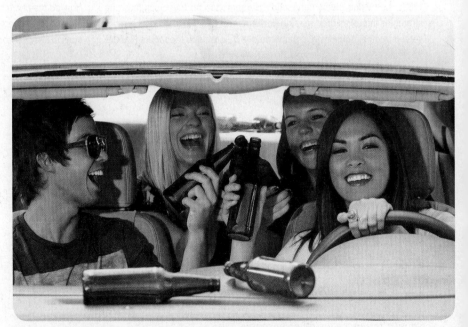

How do emotions and social contexts influence adolescents' decision making?
Jodi Jacobson/Getty Images

The social context plays a key role in adolescent decision making (Silva, Chein, & Steinberg, 2016). For example, adolescents' willingness to make risky decisions is more likely to occur in contexts where alcohol, drugs, and other temptations are readily available (Reyna, 2018). Research reveals that the presence of peers in risk-taking situations increases the likelihood that adolescents will make risky decisions. In one study of risk taking involving a simulated driving task, the presence of peers increased an adolescent's decision to engage in risky driving by 50 percent but had no effect on adults (Gardner & Steinberg, 2005). The presence of peers may activate the brain's reward system, especially its dopamine pathways (Hartley & Somerville, 2015).

It also is important to consider how the stress level of situations and individual differences in risk taking can influence adolescents' decisions. Few research studies have examined how trait-like tendencies might influence the types of decisions adolescents make when faced with stressful and risky situations. Several studies have found that adolescents take more risks in stressful than in non-stressful situations (Jamieson & Mendes, 2016; Johnson, Dariotis, & Wang, 2012). However, the effects of stress likely depend on each adolescent's general tendency toward sensation seeking and risk taking.

Adolescents need more opportunities to practice and discuss realistic decision making. Many real-world decisions on matters such as sex, drugs, and dangerous driving occur in an atmosphere of stress that includes time constraints and emotional involvement. One strategy for improving adolescent decision making in such circumstances is to provide more opportunities for them to engage in role playing and group problem solving. Another strategy is for parents to involve adolescents in appropriate decision-making activities.

To better understand adolescent decision making, Valerie Reyna and her colleagues (Reyna, 2018; Reyna & Brainerd, 2011; Reyna & Rivers, 2008) have proposed the **dual-process model,** which states that decision making is influenced by two cognitive systems—one analytical and one experiential—that compete with each other. The dual-process model emphasizes that it is the experiential system—monitoring and managing actual experiences—that benefits adolescents' decision making, not the analytical system. In this view, adolescents don't benefit from engaging in reflective, detailed, higher-level cognitive analysis about a decision, especially in high-risk, real-world contexts. In such contexts, adolescents just need to know that there are some circumstances that are so dangerous that they need to be avoided at all costs.

In the experiential system, in risky situations, it is important for an adolescent to quickly get the *gist,* or meaning, of what is happening and perceive that the situation is a dangerous context. This can cue personal values that will protect the adolescent from making a risky decision. Further, adolescents who have higher impulse control are less likely to show risky behavior compared with more impulsive peers. However, some experts on adolescent cognition argue that in many cases adolescents benefit from both analytical and experiential systems, arising in part from continuing improvements in executive function (Kuhn, 2009).

dual-process model States that decision making is influenced by two systems, one analytical and one experiential, that compete with each other. In this model, it is the experiential system—monitoring and managing actual experiences—that benefits adolescent decision making.

Review Connect Reflect

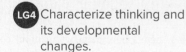 Characterize thinking and its developmental changes.

Review

- What is thinking?
- How does thinking develop in infancy?
- What characterizes children's development of executive function, critical thinking, scientific thinking, and problem solving?
- What are some important aspects of thinking in adolescence?

Connect

- In this section, you learned about a study that found a difference between boys' and girls' interests in particular categories of objects or activities. Why do researchers need to be cautious about making conclusions regarding gender-linked aspects of their findings?

Reflect *Your Own Personal Journey of Life*

- How good was your decision making in adolescence? What factors do you think contributed to whether you made good decisions during adolescence?

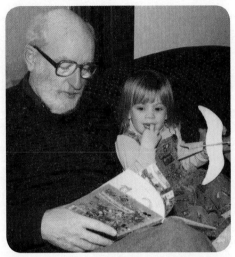

Cognitive developmentalist John Flavell is a pioneer in providing insights about children's thinking. Among his many contributions are establishing the field of metacognition and conducting numerous studies in this area, including metamemory and theory of mind studies.
Courtesy of Dr. John Flavell

metamemory Knowledge about memory.

theory of mind Awareness of one's own mental processes and the mental processes of others.

As discussed earlier in this chapter, *metacognition* is cognition about cognition, or "knowing about knowing" (de Boer & others, 2018; Flavell, 2004). It is partly a function of the central executive in Baddeley's model (see Figure 3).

WHAT IS METACOGNITION?

Metacognition can take many forms. It includes thinking about and knowing when and where to use particular strategies for learning or for solving problems. Conceptualization of metacognition includes several dimensions of executive function, such as planning (deciding on how much time to focus on the task, for example), evaluation (monitoring progress toward task completion, for example), and self-regulation (modifying strategies as work on the task progresses, for example) (Dimmitt & McCormick, 2012).

Metacognition helps children to perform many cognitive tasks more effectively (McCormick, Dimmitt, & Sullivan, 2013). In one illustrative experimental study, students were taught metacognitive skills to help them solve math problems (Cardelle-Elawar, 1992). In each of 30 daily lessons involving math story problems, a teacher guided low-achieving students to recognize when they did not know the meaning of a word, did not have all of the information necessary to solve a problem, did not know how to subdivide the problem into specific steps, or did not know how to carry out a computation. After the 30 daily lessons, the students who were given this metacognitive training had better math achievement and attitudes toward math. Since then, there have been many studies examining the effects of metacognitive skill training, and these have shown many of these skills to be effective (de Boer & others, 2018).

Metacognition can take many forms. It includes knowledge about when and where to use particular strategies for learning or for solving problems. **Metamemory** (Schneider, 2015), individuals' knowledge about memory, is an especially important form of metacognition. Metamemory includes general knowledge about memory, such as knowing that recognition tests (such as multiple-choice questions) are easier than recall tests (such as essay questions). It also encompasses knowledge about one's own memory, such as knowing whether you have studied enough for an upcoming test.

THE CHILD'S THEORY OF MIND

Even young children are curious about the nature of the human mind (Gelman, 2013; Low & others, 2016). They have a **theory of mind,** which refers to awareness of one's own mental processes and the mental processes of others. Studies of theory of mind investigate how children acquire the skills to notice, think about, explain, and understand the feelings and thoughts of others.

Developmental Changes Although whether infants have a theory of mind continues to be heavily investigated and debated (Burge, 2018; Fizke & others, 2017; Slaughter, 2015), the consensus is that some changes occur quite early in development, as we see next. From 18 months to 3 years of age, children begin to understand three mental states:

- *Perceptions.* By 2 years of age, children recognize that another person will see what's in front of her own eyes instead of what's in front of the child's eyes and by 3 years of age, they realize that looking leads to knowing what's inside a container.
- *Emotions.* The child can distinguish between positive (for example, happy) and negative (for example, sad) emotions. A child might say, "Tommy feels bad."

- *Desires.* All humans have some sort of desires. But when do children begin to recognize that someone else's desires may differ from their own? Toddlers recognize that if people want something, they will try to get it. For instance, a child might say, "I want my mommy."

Two- to 3-year-olds understand the way that desires are related to actions and to simple emotions. For example, they understand that people will search for what they want and that if they obtain it, they are likely to feel happy, but if they don't get it they will keep searching for it and are likely to feel sad or angry (Wu, Muentener, & Schulz, 2017). Children also refer to desires earlier and more frequently than they refer to cognitive states such as thinking and knowing (Bartsch & Wellman, 1995).

One of the landmark developments in understanding others' desires is recognizing that someone else may have different desires from one's own (Wellman, 2011). In one illustrative example, 18-month-olds understood that their own food preferences might not match the preferences of others—they would give an adult the food to which she says "Yummy!" even if the food was something that the infants detested (Repacholi & Gopnik, 1997). As they get older, young children can recognize and verbalize that they themselves do not like something but another person might (Rostad & Pexman, 2015).

Between the ages of 3 and 5, children come to understand that the mind can represent objects and events accurately or inaccurately (Low & others, 2016). The realization that people can have *false beliefs*—beliefs that are not true—develops in a majority of children by the time they are 5 years old (see Figure 13). This awareness is often described as a pivotal milestone in understanding the mind—recognizing that beliefs are not just mapped directly into the mind from the surrounding world, but also that different people can have different, and sometimes incorrect, beliefs (Tomasello, 2018). In a classic false-belief task, young children are shown a Band-Aids box and asked what is inside. To the children's surprise, the box actually contains pencils. When asked what a child who had never seen the box would think was inside, 3-year-olds typically respond, "Pencils." However, the 4- and 5-year-olds, grinning at the anticipation of the false beliefs of other children who had not seen what is inside the box, are more likely to say "Band-Aids."

In a similar task, children are told a story about Sally and Anne: Sally places a toy in a basket and then leaves the room (see Figure 14). In her absence, Anne takes the toy from the basket and places it in a box. Children are asked where Sally will look for the toy when she returns. The major finding is that 3-year-olds tend to fail false-belief tasks, saying that Sally will look in the box (even though Sally could not know that the toy has been moved to this new location). Four-year-olds and older children tend to pass the task, correctly saying that Sally will have a "false belief"— she will think the object is in the basket, even though that belief is now false. The conclusion from these studies is that children younger than 4 years old do not understand that it is possible to have a false belief.

It is only beyond the preschool years—at approximately 5 to 7 years of age—that children have a deepening appreciation of the mind itself rather than just an understanding of mental states (Wellman, 2011). For example, they begin to recognize that people's behaviors do not necessarily reflect their thoughts and feelings. Not until middle and late childhood do children see the mind as an active constructor of knowledge or a processing center and move from understanding that beliefs can be false to realizing that the same event can be open to multiple interpretations (Brandone & Klimek, 2018; Magid & others, 2018). For example, in one study, children saw an ambiguous line drawing (for example, a drawing that could be seen as either a duck or a rabbit); one puppet told the child she believed the drawing was a duck while another puppet

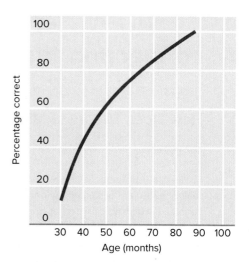

FIGURE **13**

DEVELOPMENTAL CHANGES IN FALSE-BELIEF PERFORMANCE. False-belief recognition dramatically increases from 2½ years of age through the middle of the elementary school years. In a summary of the results of many studies, 2½-year-olds gave incorrect responses about 80 percent of the time (Wellman, Cross, & Watson, 2001). At 3 years, 8 months, they were correct about 50 percent of the time, and after that, gave increasingly correct responses.

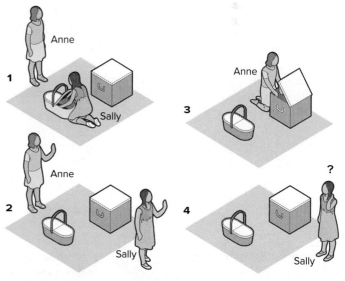

FIGURE **14**

THE SALLY AND ANNE FALSE-BELIEF TASK. In the false-belief task, the skit above in which Sally has a basket and Anne has a box is shown to children. Sally places a toy in her basket and then leaves. While Sally is gone and can't watch, Anne removes the toy from Sally's basket and places it in her box. Sally then comes back and the children are asked where they think Sally will look for her toy. Children are said to "pass" the false-belief task if they understand that Sally looks in her basket first before realizing the toy isn't there.

How Does Theory of Mind Differ in Children with Autism?

Approximately 1 in 59 children is estimated to have some sort of autism spectrum disorder (National Autism Association, 2019). Autism can usually be diagnosed by the age of 3 years, and sometimes earlier. Children with autism show a number of behaviors different from typically developing children their age, including deficits in social interaction and communication as well as repetitive behaviors or interests. They often show indifference toward others, in many instances preferring to be alone and showing more interest in objects than people. It now is accepted that autism is linked to genetic and brain abnormalities (Tremblay & Jiang, 2019). Children and adults with autism have difficulty in social interactions. These deficits are generally greater than deficits in children the same mental age with intellectual disability (Greenberg & others, 2018). Researchers have found that children with autism have difficulty in developing a theory of mind, especially in understanding others' beliefs and emotions (Fletcher-Watson & Happé, 2019). Although children with autism tend to do poorly when reasoning on false-belief tasks, they can perform much better on reasoning tasks requiring an understanding of physical causality. Individuals with autism might have

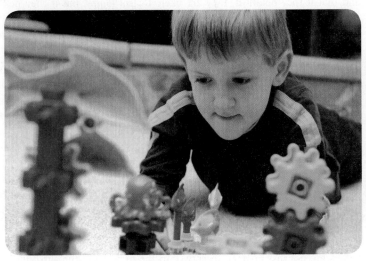

A young boy with autism. *What are some characteristics of children who are autistic? What are some deficits in their theory of mind?*
Robin Nelson/PhotoEdit

difficulty in understanding others' beliefs and emotions not solely because of theory of mind deficits but also due to other aspects of cognition such as problems in focusing attention, eye gaze, face recognition, memory, language impairment, or some general intellectual impairment (Boucher, 2017).

In relation to theory of mind, however, it is important to consider the effects of individual variations in the abilities of children with autism. Children with autism are not a homogeneous group, and some have less severe social and communication problems than others. Thus, it is not surprising that children who have less severe forms of autism do better than those who have more severe forms of the disorder on some theory of mind tasks (Jones & others, 2018). A further important consideration in

thinking about autism and theory of mind is that children with autism might have difficulty in understanding others' beliefs and emotions not solely due to theory of mind deficits but to other aspects of cognition such as problems in focusing attention or some general intellectual impairment. For instance, weaknesses in executive function may be related to the problems experienced by those with autism in performing theory of mind tasks. Other theories have pointed out that typically developing individuals process information by extracting the big picture, whereas those with autism process information in a very detailed, almost obsessive way. It may be that in autism, a number of different but related deficits lead to social cognitive deficits (Moseley & Pulvermueller, 2018; Rajendran & Mitchell, 2007).

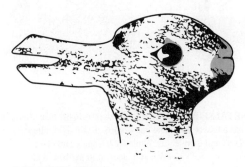

FIGURE **15**

AMBIGUOUS LINE DRAWING

told the child he believed the drawing was a rabbit (see Figure 15). Before the age of 7, children said that there was one right answer, and it was not okay for both puppets to have different opinions.

While most research on children's theory of mind focuses on children around or before their preschool years, at 7 years of age and beyond there are important developments in the ability to understand the beliefs and thoughts of others. Although understanding that people may have different interpretations is important, it is also necessary to recognize that some interpretations and beliefs may still be evaluated on the basis of the merits of arguments and evidence (Osterhaus, Koerber, & Sodian, 2017). In late childhood and early adolescence, children can understand that people can have mixed and ambivalent feelings and that people's thoughts, feelings, and decisions can be consistent or inconsistent in different situations (Lagattuta, Elrod, & Kramer, 2016).

Individual Differences   As in other developmental research, there are individual differences in the ages when children reach certain milestones in their theory of mind. For example, children who talk with their parents about desires and feelings frequently as 2-year-olds show better performance on theory of mind tasks (Ruffman & others, 2018), as do children who frequently engage in pretend play (Giménez-Dasí, Pons, & Bender, 2016).

Executive function, which describes several functions (such as inhibition and planning) that are important for flexible, future-oriented behavior, also may be connected to theory of mind development (Wade & others, 2018). For example, in one executive function task, children are asked to say the word "night" when they see a picture of a sun, and the word "day" when they see a picture of a moon and stars. Children who perform better at executive function tasks seem also to have a better understanding of theory of mind.

Another individual difference in understanding the mind involves autism (Fletcher-Watson & Happé, 2019). To learn how theory of mind differs in children with autism, see *Connecting Through Research.*

METACOGNITION IN CHILDHOOD

By 5 or 6 years of age, children usually know that familiar items are easier to learn than unfamiliar ones, that short lists are easier to remember than long ones, that recognition is easier than recall, and that forgetting becomes more likely over time (Lyon & Flavell, 1993). However, in other ways young children's metamemory is limited. They don't understand that related items are easier to remember than unrelated ones or that remembering the gist of a story is easier than remembering information verbatim (Kreutzer & Flavell, 1975). By fifth grade, students understand that gist recall is easier than verbatim recall.

Preschool children also have an inflated opinion of their memory abilities. For example, in one classic study, a majority of preschool children predicted that they would be able to recall all 10 items on a list of 10 items. When tested, none of the young children managed this feat (Flavell, Friedrichs, & Hoyt, 1970). As they move through the elementary school years, children give more realistic evaluations of their memory skills.

Preschool children also have little appreciation for the importance of cues to memory, such as "It helps when you can think of an example of it." By 7 or 8 years of age, children better appreciate the importance of cueing for memory. In general, children's understanding of their memory abilities and their skill in evaluating their performance on memory tasks is relatively poor at the beginning of the elementary school years but improves considerably by 11 to 12 years of age (Bjorklund & Causey, 2017).

METACOGNITION IN ADOLESCENCE

Important changes in metacognition take place during adolescence (Kuhn, 2009). Compared with when they were children, adolescents have an increased capacity to monitor and manage cognitive resources to effectively meet the demands of a learning task. This increased metacognitive ability results in cognitive functioning and learning becoming more effective.

Two studies illustrate this pattern. The first revealed that from 12 to 14 years of age, young adolescents increasingly used metacognitive skills and used them more effectively in math and history classes (van der Stel & Veenman, 2010). For example, 14-year-olds monitored their own text comprehension more frequently and did so more effectively than their younger counterparts. The other study documented the importance of metacognitive skills, such as planning, strategies, and monitoring, in college students' ability to think critically (Magno, 2010).

An important aspect of cognitive functioning and learning is determining how much attention will be allocated to an available resource. Evidence is accumulating that adolescents have a better understanding of how to effectively

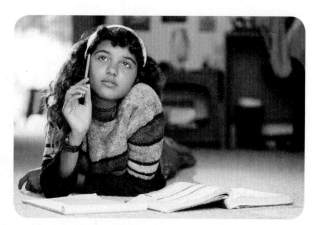

How does metacognition change in childhood and adolescence?
Thinkstock/Comstock Images/Getty Images

deploy their attention to different aspects of a task than children do. Further, adolescents have a better meta-level understanding of strategies—that is, knowing the best strategy to use and when to use it in performing a learning task.

Keep in mind, though, that there is considerable individual variation in adolescents' metacognition. Indeed, some experts argue that individual variation in metacognition becomes much more pronounced in adolescence than in childhood (Kuhn, 2009). Thus, some adolescents are quite good at using metacognition to improve their learning, while others are far less so.

Review Connect Reflect

LG5 Define metacognition and summarize its developmental changes.

Review

- What is metacognition?
- What is theory of mind? How does children's theory of mind change developmentally?
- How does metacognition change during childhood?

Connect

- Compare the classic false-belief task study you learned about in this section with what you learned earlier about A-not-B error studies. What is similar and what is different about these studies and what they are assessing?

Reflect *Your Own Personal Journey of Life*

- Do you remember your teachers ever instructing you in ways to improve your use of metacognition—that is, your "knowing about knowing" and "thinking about thinking," when you were in elementary and secondary school? To help you to think further about this question, connect the discussion of metacognition that you just read with the discussion of strategies earlier in the chapter.

Information Processing

The Information-Processing Approach Explain the information-processing approach.

> The Information-
> Processing Approach to
> Development

- The information-processing approach analyzes how individuals manipulate information, monitor it, and create strategies for handling it. Attention, memory, and thinking are involved in effective information processing. The computer has served as a model for how humans process information. In the information-processing approach, children's cognitive development results from their ability to overcome processing limitations by increasingly executing basic operations, expanding information-processing capacity, and acquiring new knowledge and strategies.

> Cognitive Resources:
> Capacity and Speed of
> Processing Information

- Capacity and speed of processing information, often referred to as cognitive resources, increase across childhood and adolescence. Changes in the brain serve as biological foundations for developmental changes in cognitive resources. In terms of capacity, the increase is reflected in older children being able to hold in mind several dimensions of a topic simultaneously. A reaction-time task has often been used to assess speed of processing. Processing speed continues to improve in early adolescence.

> Mechanisms of Change

- According to Siegler, three important mechanisms of change are encoding (how information gets into memory), automaticity (ability to process information with little or no effort), and strategy construction (creation of new procedures for processing information). Children's information processing is characterized by self-modification, and an important aspect of this self-modification involves metacognition—that is, knowing about knowing.

> Comparisons with
> Piaget's Theory

- Unlike Piaget's theory, the information-processing approach does not portray development as occurring in distinct stages. Instead, this approach holds that individuals develop a gradually increasing capacity for processing information, which allows them to develop increasingly complex knowledge and skills. Like Piaget's theory, some versions of the information-processing approach are constructivist—they see children directing their own cognitive development.

Attention Define attention and outline its developmental changes.

> What Is Attention?

- Attention is the focusing of mental resources. Four ways that children can allocate their attention are selective attention (focusing on a specific aspect of experience that is relevant while ignoring others that are irrelevant); divided attention (concentrating on more than one activity at the same time); sustained attention (maintaining attention to a selected stimulus for a prolonged period of time, also referred to as focused attention and vigilance); and executive attention (planning actions, allocating attention to goals, detecting errors and compensating for them, monitoring progress on tasks, and dealing with novel or difficult tasks).

> Infancy

- Even newborns can fixate on a contour, but as infants get older they can scan a pattern more thoroughly. Attention in the first year of life is dominated by the orienting/investigative process. Attention in infancy is often studied through habituation and dishabituation. Habituation can provide a measure of an infant's maturity and well-being. Joint attention increases an infant's ability to learn from others.

> Childhood

- Salient stimuli tend to capture the attention of the preschooler. After 6 or 7 years of age, there is a shift to more cognitive control of attention. Young children especially make advances in executive and sustained attention. Selective attention also improves through childhood. Children's attentional skills are increasingly being found to predict later cognitive competencies, such as school readiness.

Adolescence

- Adolescents typically have better attentional skills than children do, although there are wide individual differences in how effectively adolescents deploy their attention. Sustained attention and executive attention are especially important as adolescents are required to work on increasingly complex tasks that take longer to complete. Multitasking is an example of divided attention, and it can harm adolescents' attention when they are engaging in a challenging task.

Memory

LG3 Describe what memory is and how it changes.

What Is Memory?

- Memory is the retention of information over time. Psychologists study the processes of memory: how information is initially placed or encoded into memory, how it is retained or stored, and how it is found or retrieved for a certain purpose later. Short-term memory involves retaining information for up to 30 seconds, assuming there is no rehearsal of the information. Long-term memory is a relatively permanent and unlimited type of memory. Working memory is a kind of "mental workbench" where individuals manipulate and assemble information when they make decisions, solve problems, and comprehend written and spoken language. Many contemporary psychologists prefer the term *working memory* over *short-term memory*. Working memory is linked to children's reading comprehension and problem solving. People construct and reconstruct their memories. Schema theory states that people mold memories to fit the information that already exists in their minds. Fuzzy trace theory states that memory is best understood by considering two types of memory representation: (1) verbatim memory trace, and (2) fuzzy trace, or gist. According to this theory, older children's better memory is attributed to the fuzzy traces created by extracting the gist of information. Children's ability to remember new information about a subject depends on what they already know about it. The contribution of content knowledge is especially relevant in the memory of experts. Experts have a number of characteristics that can explain why they solve problems better than novices do.

Infancy

- Infants as young as 2 to 3 months of age display implicit memory, which is memory without conscious recollection, as in memory of perceptual-motor skills. However, many experts stress that explicit memory, which is the conscious memory of facts and experiences, does not emerge until the second half of the first year of life. Older children and adults remember little if anything from the first three years of their lives.

Childhood

- Young children can remember a great deal of information if they are given appropriate cues and prompts. One method of assessing short-term memory is with a memory-span task, on which there are substantial developmental changes through the childhood years. Children's memory improves in the elementary school years as they begin to use gist more, acquire more content knowledge and expertise, develop large memory spans, and use more effective strategies. Organization, elaboration, and imagery are important memory strategies. Current research focuses on how accurate children's long-term memories are and the implications of this accuracy for children as eyewitnesses.

Adolescence

- Short-term memory, as assessed in memory span, increases during adolescence. Working memory also increases in adolescence.

Thinking

LG4 Characterize thinking and its developmental changes.

What Is Thinking?

- Thinking involves manipulating and transforming information in memory. We can think about the past, reality, and fantasy. Thinking helps us reason, reflect, evaluate, solve problems, and make decisions.

Infancy

- Studies of thinking in infancy focus on concept formation and categorization. Concepts refer to cognitive groupings of similar objects, events, people, or ideas. Infants form concepts early in their development, with perceptual categorization appearing as early as 3 months of age. Mandler argues that it is not until about 7 to 9 months of age that infants form conceptual categories. Infants' first concepts are broad. Over the first two years of life, these broad concepts gradually become more differentiated.

- Advances in executive function, an umbrella-like concept that consists of a number of higher-level cognitive processes linked to the development of the prefrontal cortex, occur in childhood. Executive function involves managing one's thoughts to engage in goal-directed behavior and to exercise self-control. Critical thinking involves thinking reflectively and productively, and evaluating the evidence. Mindfulness is an important aspect of critical thinking. A lack of emphasis on critical thinking in schools is a special concern. Children and scientists think alike in some ways but not in others. Problem solving relies on the use of strategies, rules, and analogies. Even young children can use analogies to solve problems in some circumstances.

- Key changes in information processing during adolescence especially focus on executive function. These changes include monitoring and managing cognitive resources, engaging in critical thinking, and making decisions. It is increasingly thought that executive function strengthens during adolescence. Adolescence is an important transitional period in critical thinking because of cognitive changes such as increased speed, automaticity, and capacity of information processing; more breadth of content knowledge; increased ability to construct new combinations of knowledge; and increased use of spontaneous strategies.

Metacognition

LG5 Define metacognition and summarize its developmental changes.

- Metacognition is cognition about cognition, or knowing about knowing.

- Theory of mind refers to a child's awareness of his or her own mental processes and the mental processes of others. Young children are curious about the human mind, and this has been studied under the topic of theory of mind. A number of developmental changes characterize children's theory of mind. For example, by 5 years of age most children realize that people can have false beliefs—beliefs that are untrue. Individual variations also are involved in theory of mind. For example, autistic children have difficulty in developing a theory of mind.

- Metamemory improves in middle and late childhood. As children progress through the elementary school years, they make more realistic judgments about their memory skills and increasingly understand the importance of memory cues.

- Adolescents have an increased capacity to monitor and manage resources to effectively meet the demands of a learning task, although there is considerable individual variation in metacognition during adolescence.

key **terms**

attention 189
automaticity 188
concepts 202
critical thinking 204
divided attention 190
dual-process model 211
encoding 188
executive attention 190

executive function 203
explicit memory 197
fuzzy trace theory 195
implicit memory 197
information-processing
    approach 186
joint attention 191
long-term memory 194

memory 194
metacognition 188
metamemory 212
mindfulness 205
schemas 195
schema theory 195
selective attention 189

short-term memory 194
strategy construction 188
sustained attention 189
theory of mind 212
thinking 202
working memory 194

key **people**

Alan Baddeley 195
Charles Brainerd 195
Rechele Brooks 191
Stephanie Carlson 203

Judy DeLoache 208
Maria Gartstein 192
Jean Mandler 202
Andrew Meltzoff 191

Michael Pressley 209
Valerie Reyna 195
Mary Rothbart 192
Carolyn Rovee-Collier 196

Robert Siegler 207

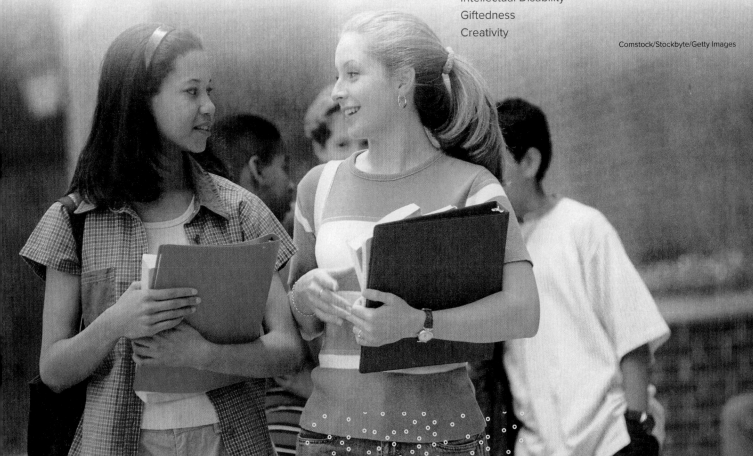

chapter 8

INTELLIGENCE

chapter outline

Comstock/Stockbyte/Getty Images

Take a moment to think about your favorite teachers over the years. What have you liked best about them? How did they foster your learning? Often, students connect best with teachers who tailor their teaching styles to meet students' diverse needs rather than relying on a one-size-fits-all approach.

The most effective teachers recognize that students demonstrate intelligence in different ways, and they provide students with opportunities to learn in ways that build on their abilities. For example, some students may learn well from lectures and reading. Others may learn better by getting more actively involved in the process. Effective teachers use innovative methods to target different kinds of intelligence. Instead of having children passively absorb science texts, for example, one third-grade teacher helps her students learn about science by having them go outside to observe plants and animals and record their findings. Instead of simply reading a play, another teacher has his students create costumes and enact the play to get them physically and socially engaged with one another. In these ways, children who may not shine in traditional academic pursuits have opportunities to achieve through other abilities such as interpersonal or physical competence. Recognizing that students learn in different ways and have diverse profiles of abilities, schools increasingly build socioemotional content into the curriculum and require physical education. These schools not only build on different skills that children already possess but take a holistic approach to education. The goal is to foster a wide range of abilities in addition to traditional cognitive aspects of learning, such as reading and math.

preview

The teaching strategies just described build on various theories of intelligence that we will explore in this chapter. We will examine the concept of intelligence and its assessment, trace the development of intelligence from infancy through adolescence, and look at the extremes of intelligence and creativity.

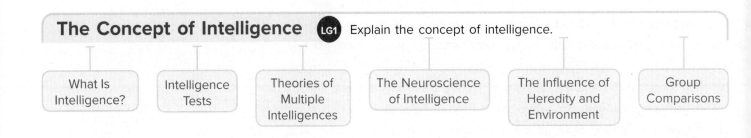

The Concept of Intelligence LG1 Explain the concept of intelligence.

| What Is Intelligence? | Intelligence Tests | Theories of Multiple Intelligences | The Neuroscience of Intelligence | The Influence of Heredity and Environment | Group Comparisons |

Intelligence is one of our most prized attributes. However, even the most intelligent people do not agree on how to define it and how to measure it.

WHAT IS INTELLIGENCE?

> As many people, as many minds, each in his own way.
>
> —TERENCE
> *Roman playwright, 2nd century B.C.*

What does the term *intelligence* mean to psychologists? Some experts describe intelligence as the ability to solve problems. Others describe it as the capacity to adapt and learn from experience. Still others argue that intelligence includes characteristics such as creativity and interpersonal skills.

The problem with intelligence is that, unlike height, weight, and age, intelligence cannot be directly measured. We can evaluate intelligence only *indirectly* by studying and comparing the intelligent acts that people perform.

The primary components of intelligence are similar to the cognitive processes of memory and thinking. The differences in how these cognitive processes are described, and how we will discuss intelligence, lie in the concepts of individual differences and assessment (Bjorklund & Causey, 2018). *Individual differences* are the stable, consistent ways in which people differ from one another. Individual differences in intelligence generally have been measured by intelligence tests designed to tell us whether a person can reason better than others who have taken the test.

We will use as our definition of **intelligence** the ability to solve problems and to adapt and learn from experiences. But even this broad definition doesn't satisfy everyone. As you will see shortly, Howard Gardner proposes that musical skills should be considered part of intelligence. Also, a definition of intelligence based on a theory such as Vygotsky's, would have to include the ability to use the tools of the culture with help from more-skilled individuals. Because intelligence is such an abstract, broad concept, it is not surprising that there are different ways to define it.

INTELLIGENCE TESTS

The two main intelligence tests that are administered to children on an individual basis today are the Stanford-Binet test and the Wechsler scales. As you will see next, an early version of the Binet was the first intelligence test to be devised.

The Binet Tests In 1904, the French Ministry of Education asked psychologist Alfred Binet to devise a method of identifying children who were unable to learn in school. School officials wanted to reduce crowding by placing in special schools students who

---

- - - - - - - - - - - - - - →

developmental connection

Information Processing

The information-processing approach emphasizes how children manipulate, monitor, and create strategies for handling information. Connect to "Information Processing."

← - - - - - - - - - - - - -

intelligence The ability to solve problems and to adapt to and learn from experiences.

would not benefit from regular classroom teaching. Binet and his student Theophile Simon developed an intelligence test to meet this request. The test is called the 1905 Scale. It consisted of 30 questions, ranging from the ability to touch one's ear to the abilities to draw designs from memory and define abstract concepts.

Binet developed the concept of **mental age (MA),** an individual's level of mental development relative to others. In 1912, William Stern created the concept of **intelligence quotient (IQ),** which refers to a person's mental age divided by chronological age (CA), multiplied by 100. That is, IQ = MA/CA × 100.

If mental age is the same as chronological age, then the person's IQ is 100. If mental age is above chronological age, then IQ is more than 100. For example, a 6-year-old with a mental age of 8 would have an IQ of 133. If mental age is below chronological age, then IQ is less than 100. For example, a 6-year-old with a mental age of 5 would have an IQ of 83.

The Binet test has been revised many times to incorporate advances in the understanding of intelligence and intelligence testing (Wasserman, 2018). These revisions are called the *Stanford-Binet tests* (because the revisions were made at Stanford University). By administering the test to large numbers of people of different ages from different backgrounds, researchers have found that scores on a Stanford-Binet test approximate a normal distribution (see Figure 1). A **normal distribution** is symmetrical, with a majority of the scores falling in the middle of the possible range of scores and far fewer scores appearing toward the extremes of the range.

The current Stanford-Binet test is administered individually to people aged 2 through adult. It includes a variety of items, some of which require verbal responses, others nonverbal responses. For example, items that reflect a typical 6-year-old's level of performance on the test include the verbal ability to define at least six words, such as *orange* and *envelope,* as well as the nonverbal ability to trace a path through a maze. Items that reflect an average adult's level of performance include defining such words as *disproportionate* and *regard,* explaining a proverb, and comparing idleness and laziness.

The fifth edition of the Stanford-Binet was published in 2003. The current version of the Stanford-Binet includes both verbal and nonverbal subscales that assess knowledge, quantitative reasoning, visual-spatial processing, working memory, and fluid reasoning. A general composite score is still obtained to reflect overall intelligence. The Stanford-Binet continues to be one of the most widely used tests to assess intelligence (Twomey & others, 2018).

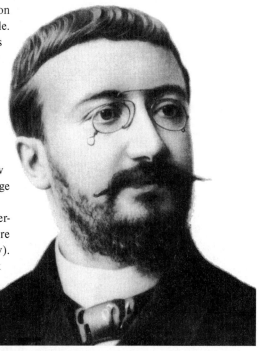

Alfred Binet constructed the first intelligence test after being asked to create a measure to determine which children could benefit from instruction in France's schools and which could not.
Universal History Archive/Getty Images

mental age (MA) An individual's level of mental development relative to others.

intelligence quotient (IQ) An individual's mental age divided by chronological age and multiplied by 100; devised in 1912 by William Stern.

normal distribution A symmetrical distribution with a majority of the cases falling in the middle of the possible range of scores and few scores appearing toward the extremes of the range.

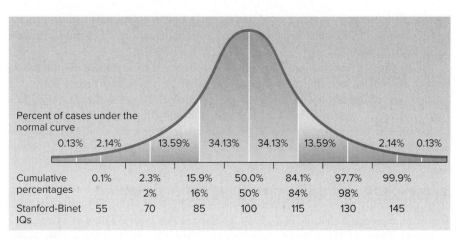

FIGURE 1

THE NORMAL CURVE AND STANFORD-BINET IQ SCORES. The distribution of IQ scores approximates a normal curve. Most of the population falls in the middle range of scores. Notice that extremely high and extremely low scores are very rare. Slightly more than two-thirds of the scores fall between 84 and 116. Only about 1 in 50 individuals has an IQ above 132, and only about 1 in 50 individuals has an IQ below 68.

Verbal Subscales

Similarities

A child must think logically and abstractly to answer a number of questions about how things might be similar.

Example: "In what way are a lion and a tiger alike?"

Comprehension

This subscale is designed to measure an individual's judgment and common sense.

Example: "What is the advantage of keeping money in a bank?"

Nonverbal Subscales

Block Design

A child must assemble a set of multicolored blocks to match designs that the examiner shows.
Visual-motor coordination, perceptual organization, and the ability to visualize spatially are assessed.

Example: "Use the four blocks on the left to make the pattern on the right."

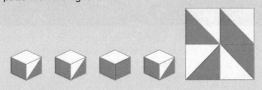

FIGURE 2

SAMPLE SUBSCALES OF THE WECHSLER INTELLIGENCE SCALE FOR CHILDREN–FIFTH EDITION (WISC-V).
The Wechsler includes 11 subscales—6 verbal and 5 nonverbal. Three of the subscales are shown here.
Source: Wechsler Intelligence Scale for Children®, Fifth Edition (WISC-V), Upper Saddle River, NJ: Pearson Education, Inc., 2014.

The Wechsler Scales   Another set of tests widely used to assess intelligence is called the *Wechsler scales,* developed by psychologist David Wechsler. They include the Wechsler Preschool and Primary Scale of Intelligence–Fourth Edition (WPPSI-IV) to test children from 2 years 6 months to 7 years 3 months of age; the Wechsler Intelligence Scale for Children–Fifth Edition (WISC-V) for children and adolescents 6 to 16 years of age; and the Wechsler Adult Intelligence Scale–Fourth Edition (WAIS-IV).

The Wechsler scales not only provide an overall IQ score and scores on a number of subtests but also yield several composite indexes (for example, the Verbal Comprehension Index, the Working Memory Index, and the Processing Speed Index). The subtest and composite scores allow the examiner to quickly identify the areas in which the child is strong or weak. Three of the Wechsler subscales are shown in Figure 2.

Intelligence tests such as the Stanford-Binet and Wechsler are given on an individual basis. A psychologist approaches an individual assessment of intelligence as a structured interaction between the examiner and the child. This provides the psychologist with an opportunity to sample the child's behavior. During the testing, the examiner observes the ease with which rapport is established, the child's enthusiasm and interest, whether anxiety interferes with the child's performance, and the child's degree of tolerance for frustration.

The Use and Misuse of Intelligence Tests   Intelligence tests have real-world applications as predictors of longevity, school success, and work success (Demetriou & Spanoudis, 2018). Researchers have found that lower intelligence in childhood is linked to illness, chronic disease, and how long people will live (Dobson & others, 2017). Also, scores on tests of general intelligence are substantially correlated with school grades and achievement test performance, both at the time of the test and years later (Yu & others, 2017). Intelligence tests also are moderately correlated with work performance and are sometimes used in hiring decisions (Ones, Viswesvaran, & Dilchert, 2017).

Despite the links between IQ and academic achievement and occupational success, it is important to keep in mind that many other factors contribute to success in school and work. These include the motivation to succeed, physical and mental health, social skills, and grit (Steinmayr, Weidinger, & Wigfield, 2018).

The single number provided by many IQ tests can easily lead to false expectations about an individual. Sweeping generalizations are too often made on the basis of an IQ score. If IQ scores are misused, they have the potential to lead to self-fulfilling processes if teachers and others provide more learning opportunities to students with a high IQ, and IQ is then further bolstered by enhanced learning opportunities (Murdock-Perriera & Sedlacek, 2018).

To be effective, information about a child's performance on an intelligence test should be used in conjunction with other information about the child (McCluskey, 2017). For example, an intelligence test alone should not determine whether a child is placed in a special education or gifted class. The child's developmental history, medical background, performance in school, social competencies, and family experiences should be taken into account, too.

THEORIES OF MULTIPLE INTELLIGENCES

Is it more appropriate to think of a child's intelligence as a general ability or as a number of specific abilities? Psychologists have thought about this question since early in the twentieth century and continue to debate the issue.

Sternberg's Triarchic Theory   According to Robert J. Sternberg's (2018b) **triarchic theory of intelligence,** intelligence comes in three forms: analytical, creative, and practical. *Analytical intelligence* involves the ability to analyze, judge, evaluate, compare,

triarchic theory of intelligence Sternberg's theory that intelligence comes in three forms: analytical, creative, and practical.

and contrast. *Creative intelligence* consists of the ability to create, design, invent, originate, and imagine. *Practical intelligence* focuses on the ability to use, apply, implement, and put into practice.

Sternberg (2018a) says that students with different triarchic patterns look different in school. Students with high analytical ability tend to be favored in conventional schools. They often do well in classes in which the teacher lectures and gives objective tests. These students typically get good grades, do well on traditional IQ tests and the SAT, and later gain admission to competitive colleges.

Students high in creative intelligence often are not in the top rung of their class. Creatively intelligent students might not conform to teachers' expectations about how assignments should be done. They give unique answers, for which they might get reprimanded or marked down.

Like students high in creative intelligence, students who are practically intelligent often do not relate well to the demands of school. However, these students frequently do well outside the classroom's walls. Their social skills and common sense may allow them to become successful managers or entrepreneurs, despite undistinguished school records.

Sternberg (2018b) argues that wisdom is linked to both practical and academic intelligence. In his view, academic intelligence is a necessary but in many cases insufficient requirement for wisdom. Practical knowledge about the realities of life also is needed for wisdom. For Sternberg, balance between self-interest, the interests of others, and contexts produces a common good. Thus, wise individuals don't just look out for themselves—they also need to consider others' needs and perspectives, as well as the particular context involved. Sternberg assesses wisdom by presenting problems that require solutions highlighting various intrapersonal, interpersonal, and contextual interests. He also emphasizes that such aspects of wisdom should be taught in schools (Sternberg, 2018b).

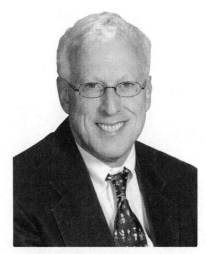

Robert J. Sternberg, who developed the triarchic theory of intelligence.
Courtesy of Dr. Robert Sternberg

Gardner's Eight Frames of Mind   Howard Gardner (1983; Chen & Gardner, 2018) says there are many specific types of intelligence, or frames of mind. They are described here along with examples of the occupations in which they are regarded as strengths (Campbell, Campbell, & Dickinson, 2004):

- *Verbal skills:* The ability to think in words and to use language to express meaning.
  Occupations: Authors, journalists, speakers.
- *Mathematical skills:* The ability to carry out mathematical operations.
  Occupations: Scientists, engineers, accountants.
- *Spatial skills:* The ability to think three-dimensionally.
  Occupations: Architects, artists, sailors.
- *Bodily-kinesthetic skills:* The ability to manipulate objects and be physically adept.
  Occupations: Surgeons, craftspeople, dancers, athletes.
- *Musical skills:* A sensitivity to pitch, melody, rhythm, and tone.
  Occupations: Composers, musicians, and music therapists.
- *Intrapersonal skills:* The ability to understand oneself and effectively direct one's life.
  Occupations: Theologians, psychologists.
- *Interpersonal skills:* The ability to understand and effectively interact with others.
  Occupations: Teachers, mental health professionals.
- *Naturalist skills:* The ability to observe patterns in nature and understand natural and human-made systems.
  Occupations: Farmers, botanists, ecologists, landscapers.

Entity vs. Incremental Theories of Intelligence   Rather than representing a theory developed by scientific researchers (as Sternberg's and Gardner's theories are), implicit theories of intelligence describe what laypeople believe to be the causes of intelligence. Individuals who hold *entity* theories believe that intelligence is primarily something people are born with that does not change much over time. By contrast,

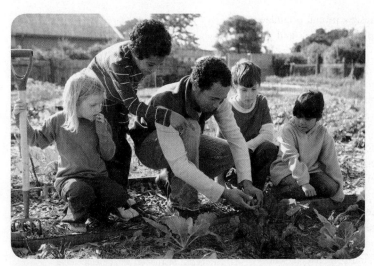

Children learn not only in classrooms but also by engaging in meaningful activities of everyday life.

Alistair Berg/Getty Images

emotional intelligence The ability to perceive and express emotion accurately and adaptively, to understand emotion and emotional knowledge, to use feelings to facilitate thought, and to manage emotions in oneself and others.

individuals who hold *incremental* theories of intelligence believe that intelligence can grow over time and be improved through hard work. Students who hold incremental theories of intelligence are more motivated to work hard in school, and parents and teachers who hold incremental theories of intelligence are more likely to praise effort rather than ability and to convey to students that improvement is possible with hard work (Gunderson & others, 2017).

Emotional Intelligence Both Gardner's and Sternberg's theories include one or more categories related to the ability to understand oneself and others and to get along in the world. In Gardner's theory, the categories are called interpersonal intelligence and intrapersonal intelligence; in Sternberg's theory, practical intelligence. Other theorists who emphasize interpersonal, intrapersonal, and practical aspects of intelligence focus on what is called *emotional intelligence,* which was popularized by Daniel Goleman (1995) in his book *Emotional Intelligence.*

The concept of emotional intelligence was initially developed by Peter Salovey and John Mayer (1990). They conceptualize **emotional intelligence** as the ability to perceive and express emotion accurately and adaptively (such as taking the perspective of others), to understand emotion and emotional knowledge (such as understanding the roles that emotions play in friendship and other relationships), to use feelings to facilitate thought (such as being in a positive mood, which is linked to creative thinking), and to manage emotions in oneself and others (such as being able to control one's anger).

There continues to be considerable interest in the concept of emotional intelligence (Chen & Chen, 2018; Karle & others, 2018). For example, interventions to improve emotional intelligence that focus on teaching children how to regulate emotions more effectively have been found to reduce not only anger and other negative emotions but also to reduce physical and verbal aggression (Castillo-Gualda & others, 2018). Furthermore, for adolescents who have been cyberbullied, higher emotional intelligence plays a protective role in reducing negative outcomes such as suicidal ideation and low self-esteem that are otherwise associated with being bullied (Extremera & others, 2018).

Critics argue that emotional intelligence broadens the concept of intelligence too far to be useful and has not been adequately assessed and researched (Keefer, Parker, & Saklofske, 2018). They also argue that emotional intelligence is a combination of emotional self-regulation and the ability to read or predict the emotional responses of others, rather than intelligence per se. Challenges arise in coding certain responses as correct or not in emotional domains (Fiori & Vesely-Maillefer, 2018).

Do People Have One or Many Intelligences? In comparing Sternberg's, Gardner's, and Salovey/Mayer's views of intelligence, notice that Sternberg's view is unique in emphasizing creative intelligence and that Gardner's includes a number of types of intelligence that are not addressed by the other views. These theories of multiple intelligence have much to offer. They have stimulated us to think more broadly about what makes up people's intelligence and competence (Sternberg, 2018b), and they have motivated educators to develop programs that instruct students in different domains.

Theories of multiple intelligences have critics who conclude that the research base to support these theories has not yet been developed (Jensen, 2008). In particular, some argue that Gardner's classification seems arbitrary. For example, if musical skills represent a type of intelligence, why don't we also refer to chess intelligence, prizefighter intelligence, and so on?

A number of psychologists still support the concept of *g* (general intelligence) (Hill & others, 2018). They point out that people who excel at one type of intellectual task are

What characterizes emotional intelligence?

Walter Hodges/Jetta Productions/Getty Images

likely to excel at other intellectual tasks (Zaboski, Kranzler, & Gage, 2018). Thus, individuals who do well at memorizing lists of digits are also likely to be good at solving verbal problems and spatial layout problems. This general intelligence includes abstract reasoning or thinking, the capacity to acquire knowledge, and problem-solving ability (Schneider & McGrew, 2018).

Advocates of the concept of general intelligence point to its success in predicting school and job performance (Demetriou & Spanoudis, 2018). For example, scores on tests of general intelligence are substantially correlated with school grades and achievement test performance, both at the time of the test and years later (Yu & others, 2017). And intelligence tests are moderately correlated with job performance (Ones, Viswesvaran, & Dilchert, 2017). Individuals with higher scores on tests designed to measure general intelligence tend to get higher-paying, more prestigious jobs (Ones, Viswesvaran, & Dilchert, 2017). However, many factors in addition to intelligence, such as motivation, contribute to success in the workplace (Van Iddekinge & others, 2018).

Some experts who argue for the existence of general intelligence conclude that individuals also have specific intellectual abilities (Zaboski, Kranzler, & Gage, 2018). In sum, controversy still characterizes whether it is more accurate to conceptualize intelligence as a general ability, specific abilities, or both (Flanagan & McDonough, 2018).

developmental **connection**

Brain Development

The frontal lobes continue to develop through the adolescent and emerging adult years. Connect to "Physical Development and Health."

THE NEUROSCIENCE OF INTELLIGENCE

In the current era of extensive research on the brain, interest in the neuroscience underpinnings of intelligence has increased (Haier, 2017). Among the questions asked about the brain's role in intelligence are the following: Is having a big brain linked to higher intelligence? Is intelligence located in certain brain regions? Is intelligence related to how fast the brain processes information?

Early consensus was that the frontal lobes are the likely location of intelligence. However, researchers now agree that intelligence is distributed more widely across brain regions and depends on connectivity and coordination among different areas of the brain (Avena-Koenigsberger, Misic, & Sporns, 2017) (see Figure 3). Albert Einstein's total brain size was average, but a region of his brain's parietal lobe that is very active in processing math and spatial information was 15 percent larger than average (Witelson, Kigar, & Harvey, 1999). Rather than looking for intelligence in any specific part of the brain, more recent studies using newer technology have been able to examine brain functioning, not just size. Brain-imaging studies have found, for example, that children 6 to 18 years of age with higher verbal intelligence have structural brain differences from children with lower verbal intelligence, not just in localized regions of the brain but in patterns of connectivity among different brain regions, suggesting that more intelligent children are able to process information more efficiently across different brain regions (Khundrakpam & others, 2017).

Examining the neuroscience of intelligence has also led to study of the role that processing speed might play in intelligence (DiTrapani & others, 2016). Recent work in neuroscience suggests that as much as 80 percent of the variance in general intelligence can be explained by the speed with which individuals process information, which leads to more efficient communication among brain regions responsible for attention, working memory, and long-term storage (Schubert, Hagemann, & Frischkorn, 2017).

As the technology to study the brain's functioning continues to advance in coming decades, we are likely to see more specific conclusions about the brain's role in intelligence (Haier, 2017). As this research proceeds, keep in mind that both heredity and environment contribute to links between the brain and intelligence.

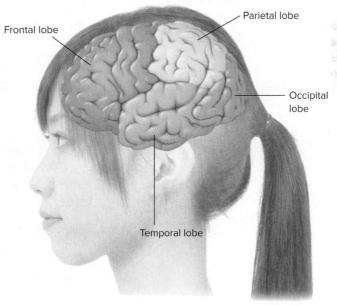

Frontal lobe

Parietal lobe

Occipital lobe

Temporal lobe

FIGURE **3**

INTELLIGENCE AND THE BRAIN. Researchers have found that a higher level of intelligence is linked to a distributed neural network in the frontal and parietal lobes. To a lesser extent than the frontal/parietal network, the temporal and occipital lobes, as well as the cerebellum, also have been found to have links to intelligence. The current consensus is that intelligence is likely to be distributed across brain regions rather than being localized in a specific region such as the frontal lobes.
Photo: Takayuki/Shutterstock

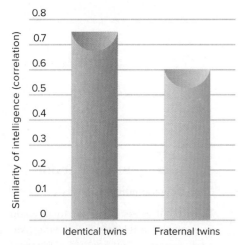

FIGURE 4

CORRELATION BETWEEN INTELLIGENCE TEST SCORES AND TWIN STATUS. The graph represents a summary of research findings that have compared the intelligence test scores of identical and fraternal twins. An approximate .15 difference has been found, with a higher correlation for identical twins (.75) and a lower correlation for fraternal twins (.60).

heritability The fraction of the variance in a population that is attributed to genetics.

THE INFLUENCE OF HEREDITY AND ENVIRONMENT

We have seen that intelligence is a slippery concept with competing definitions, tests, and theories. It is not surprising, therefore, that attempts to understand the concept of intelligence are filled with controversy. Researchers agree that both heredity and environment influence intelligence. Genetic and environmental influences interact so that genetic proclivities are malleable in different environments, and environments are able to influence genes (Sauce & Matzel, 2018).

Genetic Influences To what degree do our genes make us smart? A research review found that the difference in the average correlations for identical and fraternal twins was not very high—only .15 (Grigorenko, 2000) (see Figure 4).

Have scientists been able to pinpoint specific genes that are linked to intelligence? Using genome-wide association studies, a method that looks at individuals' entire genome in relation to observed traits, researchers have identified polygenic scores that integrate thousands of genetic sequences that contribute to intelligence (Plomin & von Stumm, 2018).

Adoption studies are also used in attempts to analyze the relative importance of heredity and environment in intelligence (Haier, 2017). In most *adoption studies,* researchers determine whether the behavior of adopted children is more like that of their biological parents or their adoptive parents. In two studies, the educational levels attained by biological parents were better predictors of children's IQ scores than were the IQs of the children's adoptive parents (Petrill & Deater-Deckard, 2004; Scarr & Weinberg, 1983). But studies of adoption also document the influence of environments. A research analysis by Richard Nisbett and his colleagues (2012) revealed a 12 to 18 point increase in IQ when children were adopted from low-income families into middle- and upper-income families.

How strong is the effect of heredity on intelligence? The concept of heritability attempts to tease apart the effects of heredity and environment in a population. **Heritability** is the fraction of the variance within a population that is attributed to genetics. The heritability index is computed using correlational techniques. Thus, the highest degree of heritabilty is 1.00, and correlations of .70 and above suggest a strong genetic influence. Genome-wide association studies that look at individuals' entire genetic profile have identified gene sequences that account for 20 to 50 percent of the heritability of intelligence (Plomin & von Stumm, 2018).

A key point to keep in mind about heritability is that it refers to a specific group (population), *not* to individuals. Researchers use the concept of heritability to try to describe why people differ. Heritability says nothing about why a single individual has a certain intelligence. Nor does heritability say anything about differences *between* groups.

Most research on heredity and environment does not include environments that differ radically. Thus, it is not surprising that many genetic studies show environment to be a fairly weak influence on intelligence.

The heritability index has a number of flaws (Sandoval-Motta & others, 2017). It is only as good as the data that are entered into its analysis and the interpretations made from it. The data are virtually all from traditional IQ tests, which some experts believe are not always the best indicator of intelligence (Sternberg, 2018b). Also, the heritability index assumes that we can treat genetic and environmental influences as factors that can be separated, with each part contributing a distinct amount of influence. Genes and the environment always work together: Genes always exist in an environment, and the environment shapes the activity of genes.

Environmental Influences The environment also plays an important role in intelligence (Haier, 2017). This means that improving children's environments can raise their intelligence (McLeod & others, 2018). One argument for the importance of environment in intelligence involves the increasing scores on IQ tests around the world. Scores on these tests have been increasing so rapidly that a high percentage of people regarded as having average intelligence in the early 1900s would be considered below

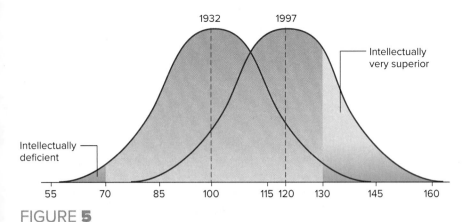

1932   1997

Intellectually
very superior

Intellectually
deficient

55   70   85   100   115 120   130   145   160

FIGURE 5

THE INCREASE IN IQ SCORES FROM 1932 TO 1997. As measured by the Stanford-Binet intelligence test, American children seem to be getting smarter. Scores of a group tested in 1932 fell along a bell-shaped curve with half below 100 and half above. Studies show that if children took that same test today, half would score above 120 on the 1932 scale. Very few of them would score in the "intellectually deficient" range on the left side, and about one-fourth would rank in the "very superior" range.

average in intelligence today (Flynn, 2018) (see Figure 5). If a representative sample of today's children took the Stanford-Binet test used in 1932, about one-fourth would be defined as very superior, a label usually accorded to less than 3 percent of the population. Because the increase has taken place in a relatively short period of time, it can't be due to heredity (Bratsberg & Rogeberg, 2018). Rather, it might result from environmental factors such as increased exposure to information and education. Factors such as prenatal and postnatal nutrition also are related to intelligence (Freitas-Vilela & others, 2018) and have been proposed as explanations for historical changes in intelligence test scores (Bratsberg & Rogeberg, 2018). The worldwide increase in intelligence test scores over a short time frame is called the *Flynn effect* after the researcher who discovered it, James Flynn (2018).

Studies of schooling also reveal effects on intelligence. In a meta-analysis of 42 data sets including over 600,000 participants, each additional year of formal education was found to raise IQ scores by 1 to 5 points, even taking into account the fact that people of higher intelligence tend to stay in school longer (Ritchie & Tucker-Drob, 2018). The biggest effects occur when large groups of children are deprived of formal education for an extended period, resulting in lower intelligence. For example, an increase in IQ of 8 to 13 points in children ages 6 to 9 years between 2004 and 2016 in Khartoum, Sudan, could be attributed to the absence of compulsory schooling in the earlier cohorts of children (Dutton & others, 2018).

Researchers, educators, and policy makers are interested in manipulating the early environment of children who are at risk for impoverished intelligence (Dunst, 2017). The emphasis is on prevention rather than remediation. Many low-income parents have difficulty providing an intellectually stimulating environment for their children. Programs that educate parents to be more sensitive caregivers and better teachers, as well as support services such as quality child-care programs, can enhance a child's intellectual development (McLeod & others, 2018).

What can we learn from research on the influence of early intervention on intelligence? To find out, see *Connecting Through Research.*

Revisiting the Nature and Nurture Issue

In sum, there is a consensus among psychologists that both heredity and environment influence intelligence (Sauce & Matzel, 2018). As in other areas of development, genetic factors interact with factors in the environment to influence intelligence.

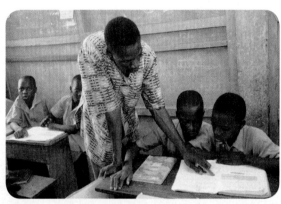

Students in an elementary school in South Africa. *How might schooling influence the development of children's intelligence?*
Owen Franken/Corbis Documentary/Getty Images

The highest-risk children often benefit the most cognitively when they experience early interventions.

—CRAIG RAMEY
Contemporary psychologist, Virginia Tech

developmental **connection**

Nature and Nurture

The epigenetic view emphasizes that development is an ongoing, bidirectional interchange between heredity and environment. Connect to "Biological Beginnings."

The Abecedarian Project

In the Abecedarian Intervention program at the University of North Carolina at Chapel Hill, conducted by Craig Ramey and his colleagues (Ramey, 2018), 111 young children from low-income, poorly educated families were randomly assigned to either an intervention group, which received full-time, year-round child care along with medical and social work services, or a control group, which received medical and social benefits but no child care. The child-care program included game-like learning activities aimed at improving language, motor, social, and cognitive skills.

The success of the program in improving IQ was evident by the time the children were 3 years of age. At that age, the experimental group showed normal IQs averaging 101, a 17-point advantage over the control group. Recent follow-up results suggest that the effects are long-lasting. More than a decade later at age 15, children from the intervention group maintained an IQ advantage of 5 points over the control-group children (97.7 to 92.6) (Ramey, 2018). They also did better on standardized tests of reading and math and were less likely to be held back a year in school. Also, the greatest IQ gains were made by the children whose mothers had especially low IQs—below 70. At age 15, these children showed a 10-point IQ advantage over a group of children whose mothers' IQs were below 70 but who had not experienced the child-care intervention. By age 30, the children who had experienced the early intervention were almost four times more likely to have graduated from college, were more likely to be employed full-time, and were less likely to receive extensive welfare support (Ramey, 2018). A benefit-cost ratio of 7.3 to 1 suggests a large financial return on this investment in early childhood (Ramey, 2018).

The results of the Abecedarian Intervention program are not unprecedented. A review of the research on early interventions reached the following conclusions (Brooks-Gunn, 2003):

- High-quality center-based interventions are associated with increases in children's intelligence and school achievement.
- Early interventions are most successful with poor children and children whose parents have little education.
- The positive benefits continue through adolescence but are stronger in early childhood and at the beginning of elementary school.
- The programs that are continued into middle and late childhood have the best long-term results.

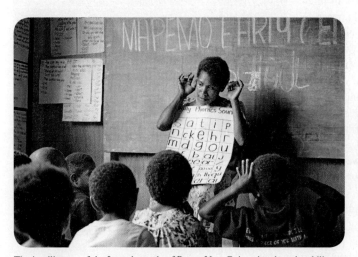

The intelligence of the Iatmul people of Papua New Guinea involves the ability to remember the names of many clans.
Robertharding/Alamy Stock Photo

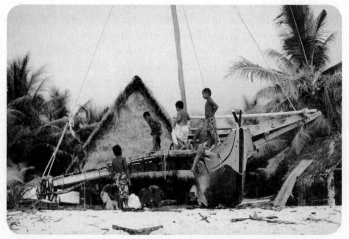

On the 680 Caroline Islands in the Pacific Ocean east of the Philippines, the intelligence of their inhabitants includes the ability to navigate by the stars. *Why might it be difficult to create a culture-fair intelligence test for the Iatmul children, Caroline Islands children, and U.S. children?*
Anders Ryman/Corbis NX/Getty Images

GROUP COMPARISONS

For decades, many controversies surrounding intelligence tests have grown from the tendency to compare one group with another.

Why Is It So Hard to Create Culture-Fair Tests?

Why is it so hard to create culture-fair tests? Most tests tend to reflect what the dominant culture thinks is important (Sternberg, 2018b). If tests have time limits, that will bias the test against groups that are not concerned with time. If languages differ, the same words might have different meanings for different language groups. Even pictures can produce bias because some cultures have less experience with drawings and photographs. Within the same culture, different groups could have different attitudes, values, and motivation, and this could affect their performance on intelligence tests (Barnett & others, 2011). Items that ask why buildings should be made of brick are biased against children with little or no experience with brick houses. Questions about railroads, furnaces, seasons of the year, distances between cities, and so on can be biased against groups who have less experience than others with these contexts. Because of such difficulties in creating culture-fair tests, Robert Sternberg (Sternberg, 2018b) concludes that there are no culture-fair tests, but only culture-reduced tests.

Cross-Cultural Comparisons Cultural groups, and individuals within cultures, vary in the way they describe what it means to be intelligent (Sternberg, 2017). People in Western cultures tend to view intelligence in terms of reasoning and thinking skills, but individuals can demonstrate intellectual skills in different ways. For example, children in an Inuit community in Canada performed poorly in traditional classrooms but were able to navigate for long distances between villages in the Arctic during winter with no visible landmarks (Sternberg, 2017). Likewise, Kenyan children who performed poorly in school were able to administer hundreds of herbal treatments for illnesses, suggesting that intelligence encompasses a broader array of intellectual abilities than those captured in traditional tests (Sternberg, 2017).

Cultural Bias in Testing Many of the early intelligence tests were culturally biased, favoring people who were from urban rather than rural environments, of middle socioeconomic status rather than lower socioeconomic status, and White rather than African American ethnicity, leading to a deficit perspective on the intelligence and abilities of individuals from groups that were not those creating the tests (Rogoff & others, 2017). For example, one question on an early test asked what you should do if you find a 3-year-old child in the street. The correct answer was "call the police." But children from inner-city families who perceive the police as adversaries are unlikely to choose this answer. Also, members of minority groups who do not speak English or who speak nonstandard English are at a disadvantage in trying to understand questions framed in standard English (Romstad & Xiong, 2017).

culture-fair tests Intelligence tests that aim to avoid cultural bias.

Psychologists have developed **culture-fair tests,** which are intelligence tests that aim to avoid cultural bias. Two types of culture-fair tests have been developed. The first includes questions that are familiar to people from all socioeconomic and ethnic backgrounds. For example, a child might be asked how a bird and a dog are different, on the assumption that virtually all children are familiar with birds and dogs. The second type of culture-fair test contains no verbal questions. To read further about culture-fair tests, see the *Connecting with Diversity* interlude.

Ethnic and Gender Comparisons Sometimes intelligence tests are used to compare one demographic group with another. In any group comparison, it is important to keep in mind that average scores of groups are being compared and that the overlap in the distribution of scores is generally extensive. Group averages sometimes favor one group over

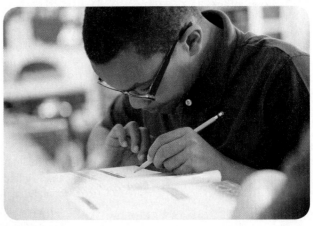

How might stereotype threat be involved in ethnic minority students' performance on standardized tests?
Pradeep Edussuriya/McGraw-Hill Education

stereotype threat Anxiety that one's behavior might confirm a stereotype about one's group.

another, such as when males outperform females on tests of math abilities or when European Americans outperform African Americans on intelligence tests.

One potential influence on intelligence test performance is **stereotype threat,** the anxiety that one's behavior might confirm a negative stereotype about one's group (Wasserberg, 2017). For example, when African Americans take an intelligence test, they may experience anxiety about confirming the old stereotype that African Americans are "intellectually inferior." Some studies have confirmed the existence of stereotype threat (Van Loo & Boucher, 2017). For example, African American students do more poorly on standardized tests if they perceive that they are being evaluated. If they think the test doesn't count, they perform as well as White students (Aronson, 2002). However, stereotype threat explains less of the variance in African American students' test performance than do other factors, such as schools' racial climate, cultural competence training initiatives for teachers, and faculty diversity (Whaley, 2018).

Review Connect Reflect

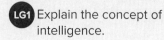 Explain the concept of intelligence.

Review

- What is intelligence?
- What are the main individual tests of intelligence?
- What theories of multiple intelligences have been developed? Do people have one intelligence or many intelligences?
- What are some links between the brain and intelligence?
- What evidence indicates that heredity influences IQ scores? What evidence indicates that environment influences IQ scores?
- What is known about the intelligence of people from different cultures and ethnic groups?

Connect

- In this section you learned that different cultures have different concepts of intelligence. Earlier you learned about culture's effect on motor development. What do these findings have in common?

Reflect *Your Own Personal Journey of Life*

- An assessment product is being sold to parents for testing their child's IQ. Several parents tell you that they purchased the product and assessed their children's IQs. Why might you be skeptical about giving your children an IQ test and interpreting the results yourself?

The Development of Intelligence Discuss the development of intelligence.

Tests of Infant Intelligence

Stability and Change in Intelligence Through Adolescence

How can the intelligence of infants be assessed? Is intelligence stable through childhood? These are some of the questions we will explore as we examine the development of intelligence.

TESTS OF INFANT INTELLIGENCE

The infant-testing movement grew out of the tradition of IQ testing. However, tests that assess infants are necessarily less verbal than IQ tests for older children. Tests for infants contain far more items related to perceptual-motor development. They also include measures of social interaction. To read about the work of one infant assessment specialist, see *Connecting with Careers.*

The most important early contributor to the testing of infants was Arnold Gesell (1934). He developed a measure that helped sort out typically developing from atypically

Toosje Thyssen Van Beveren, Infant Assessment Specialist

Toosje Thyssen Van Beveren has a master's degree in child clinical psychology and a Ph.D. in human development. Van Beveren has been involved in a 12-week program called New Connections, which is a comprehensive intervention for young children who were affected by substance abuse prenatally and for their caregivers.

In the New Connections program, Van Beveren assesses infants' developmental status and progress. She might refer the infants to a speech, physical, or occupational therapist and monitor the infants' services and progress. Van Beveren trains the program staff and encourages them to use the exercises she recommends. She also discusses the child's problems with the primary caregivers, suggests activities, and assists them in enrolling infants in appropriate programs.

During her graduate work at the University of Texas at Dallas, Van Beveren was author John Santrock's teaching assistant in his undergraduate course on life-span development for four years. As a teaching assistant, she attended classes, graded exams, counseled students, and occasionally gave lectures. Each semester, Van Beveren returns to give a lecture on prenatal development and infancy. She also teaches a number of courses

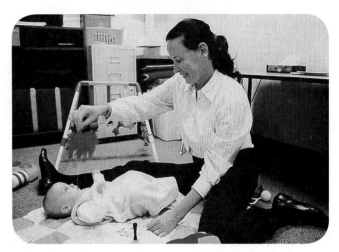

Toosje Thyssen Van Beveren conducts an infant assessment.
Dr. John Santrock

in the psychology department at UT–Dallas, including the course "Child Development." In Van Beveren's words, "My days are busy and full. The work is often challenging. There are some disappointments, but mostly the work is enormously gratifying."

---

developing babies. This was especially useful to adoption agencies, which had large numbers of babies awaiting placement. Gesell's examination was used widely for many years and still is frequently employed by pediatricians to distinguish between typically developing and atypically developing infants. The current version of the Gesell test has four categories of behavior: motor, language, adaptive, and personal-social. The **developmental quotient (DQ)** combines subscores in these categories to provide an overall score.

The widely used **Bayley Scales of Infant Development** were developed by Nancy Bayley (1969) to assess infant behavior and predict later development. The current version, Bayley-III, has five scales: cognitive, language, motor, socioemotional, and adaptive (Bayley, 2006). The first three scales are administered directly to the infant; the latter two are questionnaires given to the caregiver. The Bayley-III also is more appropriate for use in clinical settings than the two previous editions (Lennon & others, 2008).

How should a 6-month-old perform on the Bayley cognitive scale? The 6-month-old infant should be able to vocalize pleasure and displeasure, persistently search for objects that are just out of immediate reach, and approach a mirror that is placed in front of the infant by the examiner. By 12 months of age, the infant should be able to inhibit behavior when commanded to do so, imitate words the examiner says (such as *Mama*), and respond to simple requests (such as "Take a drink").

Several studies have found that measures of intelligence in infancy are correlated with measures of intelligence later in childhood. For example, the efficiency of infants' play (which was measured by dividing the amount of time an infant played with a novel toy by the number of the toy's functions the infant discovered) predicted larger vocabulary and higher IQ scores by age 3 (Muentener, Herrig, & Schulz, 2018). Measures of implicit memory at age 9 months are related to measures of implicit memory at age 3 years (Vöhringer & others, 2018).

developmental quotient (DQ) An overall developmental score that combines subscores on motor, language, adaptive, and personal-social domains in the Gesell assessment of infants.

Bayley Scales of Infant Development Initially created by Nancy Bayley, these scales are widely used in assessing infant development. The current version has five scales: cognitive, language, motor, socioemotional, and adaptive.

developmental connection

Information Processing

Habituation and dishabituation are important aspects of attention in infancy. Connect to "Information Processing."

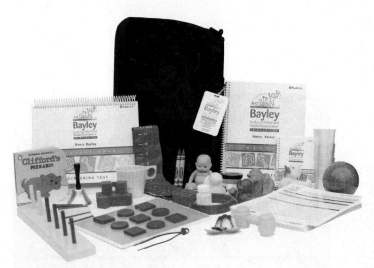

Items used in the Bayley Scales of Infant Development.
Amy Kiley Photography

It is important, however, not to go too far and think that connections between cognitive development in early infancy and later cognitive development are so strong that no discontinuity takes place. Some important changes in cognitive development occur after infancy.

STABILITY AND CHANGE IN INTELLIGENCE THROUGH ADOLESCENCE

IQ measured at ages 1 and 2 years is correlated about .90 with IQ in preschool, .69 with IQ in childhood, and .57 with IQ in adolescence, with stronger correlations in IQ measured at developmentally closer time points (Yu & others, 2018). Developmentally close assessments of IQ are likely to be more highly correlated than assessments conducted at greater time intervals, in part because the tests themselves are more similar (for example, a test of infant IQ is more similar to a test of preschool IQ than a test of adolescent IQ). Life experiences, such as starting school, may contribute to or disrupt the stabilization of IQ over time.

What has been said so far about the stability of intelligence has been based on measures of groups of individuals. The stability of intelligence also can be evaluated through studies of individuals. Robert McCall and his associates (McCall, Appelbaum, & Hogarty, 1973) studied 140 children between the ages of 2½ and 17. They found that the average range of IQ scores was more than 28 points. The scores of one out of three children changed by as much as 40 points.

What can we conclude about stability and changes in intelligence during childhood? Intelligence test scores can fluctuate dramatically across the childhood years, indicating that intelligence is not as stable as the original intelligence theorists envisioned. Children are adaptive beings. They have the capacity for intellectual change, but they do not become entirely new intelligent beings. In a sense, children's intelligence changes but remains connected with early points in development.

Review Connect Reflect

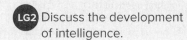 Discuss the development of intelligence.

Review

- How is intelligence assessed during infancy?
- How much does intelligence change through childhood and adolescence?

Connect

- In this section, you learned about research on the development of intelligence. Identify which research methods and designs were used in these research studies and describe their pros and cons relative to their subject matter.

Reflect *Your Own Personal Journey of Life*

- As a parent, would you want to have your infant's intelligence tested? Why or why not?

The Extremes of Intelligence and Creativity

 Describe the characteristics of intellectual disability, giftedness, and creativity.

Intellectual Disabilty

Giftedness

Creativity

Intellectual disability and intellectual giftedness are the extremes of intelligence. Often intelligence tests are used to identify exceptional individuals. After discussing intellectual disability and giftedness, we'll explore how creativity differs from intelligence.

INTELLECTUAL DISABILITY

The most distinctive feature of intellectual disability (formerly called mental retardation) is inadequate intellectual functioning. Long before formal tests were developed to assess intelligence, individuals with an intellectual disability were identified by a lack of age-appropriate skills in learning and caring for themselves. Once intelligence tests were developed, they were used to identify the degree of intellectual disability. But of two individuals with an intellectual disability who have the same low IQ, one might be married, employed, and involved in the community and the other might require constant supervision in an institution. Such differences in social competence led psychologists to include deficits in adaptive behavior in their definition of intellectual disability.

Intellectual disability is a condition of limited mental ability in which the individual (1) has a low IQ, usually below 70 on a traditional intelligence test; (2) has difficulty adapting to everyday life; and (3) first exhibits these characteristics by age 18 (Hodapp, 2016). The age limit is included in the definition of intellectual disability because, for example, we don't usually think of a college student who suffers massive brain damage in a car accident, resulting in an IQ of 60, as having an "intellectual disability." The low IQ and low adaptiveness should be evident in childhood, not after normal functioning is interrupted by damage of some form. About 5 million Americans fit this definition of intellectual disability.

There are several ways to define degrees of intellectual disability (Hodapp, 2016). Most school systems use the classifications shown in Figure 6, in which IQ scores categorize intellectual disability as mild, moderate, severe, or profound.

Note that a large majority of individuals diagnosed with an intellectual disability fit into the mild category. However, these categories are not perfect predictors of functioning. A different classification system is based on the degree of support required for a person with an intellectual disability to function at the highest level. These categories of support are intermittent (supports given as needed), limited (supports are intense over time), extensive (supports needed are regular, typically occurring every day), and pervasive (supports are constant, intense, and are needed in all settings).

Some cases of intellectual disability have an organic cause. *Organic intellectual disability* describes a genetic disorder or a lower level of intellectual functioning caused by brain damage. Down syndrome is one form of organic intellectual disability, and it occurs when an extra chromosome is present. Other causes of organic intellectual disability include fragile X syndrome (an abnormality in the X chromosome); prenatal malformation; metabolic disorders; and diseases that affect the brain. Most people who suffer from organic intellectual disability have IQs between 0 and 50.

When no evidence of organic brain damage can be found, cases are labeled *cultural-familial intellectual disability*. Individuals with this type of disability have IQs between 55 and 70. Psychologists suspect that this type of disability often results from growing up in a below-average intellectual environment. Children with this type of disability can be identified in schools, where they often fail, need tangible rewards (candy rather than praise), and are highly sensitive to what others expect of them. However, as adults, these individuals are usually able to function in society without notice perhaps because adult settings don't tax their cognitive skills as heavily. It may also be that they increase their intelligence as they move toward adulthood.

GIFTEDNESS

There have always been people whose abilities and accomplishments have surpassed others'—the whiz kid in class, the star athlete, the natural musician. People who are **gifted** have above-average intelligence (an IQ of 130 or higher) and/or superior talent for something. When it comes to programs for the gifted, most school systems select children who have intellectual superiority and academic aptitude, whereas children who are talented in the visual and performing arts (arts, drama, dance), who are skilled athletes, or who possess other special aptitudes tend to be overlooked (Gubbels & others, 2016). Estimates vary but indicate that approximately 3 to 5 percent of U.S. students are gifted

Type of Intellectual Disability	IQ Range	Percentage
Mild	55–70	89
Moderate	40–54	6
Severe	25–39	4
Profound	Below 25	1

FIGURE 6

CLASSIFICATION OF INTELLECTUAL DISABILITY BASED ON IQ

intellectual disability A condition of limited mental ability in which the individual (1) has a low IQ, usually below 70 on a traditional intelligence test; (2) has difficulty adapting to everyday life; and (3) has an onset of these characteristics by age 18.

gifted Possession of above-average intelligence (an IQ of 130 or higher) and/or superior talent for something.

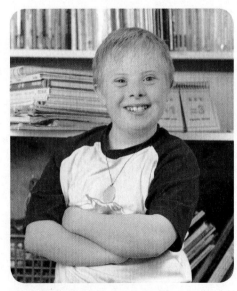

This young boy has Down syndrome. *What causes a child to develop Down syndrome? In what major classification of intellectual disability does the condition fall?*
George Doyle/Stockbyte/Getty Images

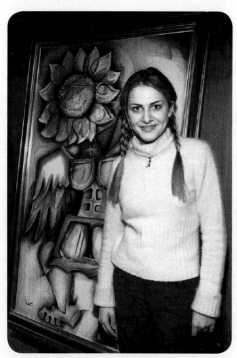

At 2 years of age, art prodigy Alexandra Nechita (shown here as a teenager) colored in coloring books for hours and also took up pen and ink drawing. She had no interest in dolls or friends. By age 5 she was using watercolors. Once she started school, she would start painting as soon as she got home. At the age of 8, she saw the first public exhibit of her work. In succeeding years, working quickly and impulsively on canvases as large as 5 feet by 9 feet, she has completed hundreds of paintings, some of which sell for close to $100,000 apiece. As an adult, she continues to paint—relentlessly and passionately. It is, she says, what she loves to do. *What are some characteristics of children who are gifted?*
Koichi Kamoshida/Hulton Archive/Getty Images

(National Association for Gifted Children, 2015). This percentage is likely conservative because it focuses more on children who are gifted intellectually and academically, often failing to include those who are gifted in creative thinking as well as the visual and performing arts (Ford, 2012).

What are the characteristics of children who are gifted? Despite speculation that giftedness is linked with having a mental disorder, no connection between giftedness and mental disorder has been found. Similarly, the idea that gifted children are maladjusted is a myth, as Lewis Terman (1925) found when he conducted an extensive study of 1,500 children whose Stanford-Binet IQs averaged 150. The children in Terman's study were socially well adjusted, and many went on to become successful doctors, lawyers, professors, and scientists. Studies support the conclusion that gifted people tend to be more mature than others, have fewer emotional problems than average, and grow up in a positive family climate (Worrell & others, 2019).

Noncognitive contributors to giftedness have received increasing attention in recent years (Reis & Renzulli, 2011). Creativity, motivation, optimism, and physical and mental energy are examples of noncognitive factors that can influence whether children display giftedness.

Three key criteria characterize gifted children, whether in art, music, or academic domains (Winner & Drake, 2018):

1. *Precocity.* Gifted children are precocious. They begin to master an area earlier than their peers. Learning in their domain is more effortless for them than for ordinary children. In most instances, these gifted children are precocious because they have an inborn high ability in a particular domain or domains.

2. *Marching to their own drummer.* Gifted children learn in a qualitatively different way from ordinary children. One way that they march to a different drummer is that they need minimal help, or scaffolding, from adults to learn. In many instances, they resist any kind of explicit instruction. They often make discoveries on their own and solve problems in unique ways.

3. *A passion to master.* Gifted children are driven to understand the domain in which they have high ability. They display an intense, obsessive interest and an ability to focus. They motivate themselves and do not need to be "pushed" by their parents.

Nature and Nurture Giftedness, like other aspects of development, is a product of both heredity and environment. Individuals who are gifted often demonstrate special abilities from an early age, even before they receive formal training (Comeau & others, 2018). This suggests the importance of innate ability in giftedness. However, researchers have also found that individuals with world-class status in the arts, mathematics, science, and sports all report strong family support and years of training and practice (Ericsson & others, 2018). Deliberate practice is an important characteristic of individuals who become experts in a particular domain. For example, in one study, the best musicians engaged in twice as much deliberate practice over their lives as did the least successful ones (Ericsson, Krampe, & Tesch-Romer, 1993).

Developmental Changes and Domain-Specific Giftedness Can we predict from infancy who will be gifted as children, adolescents, and adults? John Colombo and his colleagues (2004, 2009) have found that measures of infant attention and habituation are not good predictors of high cognitive ability later in development. However, they have discovered a link between assessment with the Home Observation for Measure of the Environment at 18 months of age and high cognitive ability in the preschool years. The best predictor at 18 months of high cognitive ability in the preschool years was the provision of materials and a variety of experiences in the home. These findings illustrate the importance of the cognitive environment provided by parents in the development of children's giftedness.

Individuals who are highly gifted are typically not gifted in many domains, and research on giftedness is increasingly focused on domain-specific developmental trajectories (Chang & Lane, 2018). During the childhood years, the domains in which individuals

connecting with careers

Sterling Jones, Supervisor of Gifted and Talented Education

Sterling Jones is program supervisor for gifted and talented children in the Detroit Public School System. Jones has been working for more than three decades with children who are gifted. He believes that students' mastery of skills mainly depends on the amount of time devoted to instruction and the length of time allowed for learning. Thus, he believes that many basic strategies for challenging children who are gifted to develop their skills can be applied to a wider range of students than once believed. He has rewritten several pamphlets for use by teachers and parents, including *How to Help Your Child Succeed* and *Gifted and Talented Education for* Everyone.

Jones holds undergraduate and graduate degrees from Wayne State University, and he taught English for a number of years before becoming involved in the program for gifted children. He also has written materials on African Americans, such as *Voices from the Black Experience,* that are used in the Detroit schools.

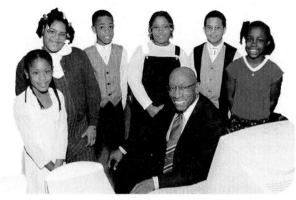

Sterling Jones with some of the children in the gifted program in the Detroit Public School System.

Courtesy of Helen Dove-Jones

For more information about what teachers of exceptional children (special education) do, see the Careers in Child Development appendix.

are gifted usually emerge. Thus, at some point in the childhood years, the child who will become a gifted artist or the child who will become a gifted mathematician begins to show expertise in that domain. Regarding domain-specific giftedness, software genius Bill Gates (1998), the founder of Microsoft and one of the world's richest persons, commented that when you are good at something you may have to resist the urge to think that you will be good at everything. Gates says that because he has been so successful at software development, people expect him to be brilliant about other domains in which he is far from being a genius.

Identifying an individual's domain-specific talent and providing the individual with individually appropriate and optional educational opportunities needs to be accomplished by adolescence at the latest (Lo & Porath, 2017). During adolescence, individuals who are talented become less reliant on parental support and increasingly pursue their own interests.

Some children who are gifted become gifted adults, but many gifted children do not become gifted and highly creative adults. In Terman's research on children with superior IQs, the children typically became experts in a well-established domain, such as medicine, law, or business. However, they did not become major creators (Winner, 2000). That is, they did not create a new domain or revolutionize an old domain.

Education of Children Who Are Gifted

A number of experts argue that the education of children who are gifted in the United States requires a significant overhaul (Ecker-Lyster & Niileksela, 2017). Gifted children who are insufficiently challenged can become disruptive, skip classes, and lose interest in achieving. Sometimes these children just disappear into the woodwork, becoming passive and apathetic toward school. It is extremely important for teachers to challenge children who are gifted to reach high expectations.

Too often, children who are gifted are socially isolated and underchallenged in the classroom (Winner & Drake, 2018). It is not unusual for them to be ostracized and labeled

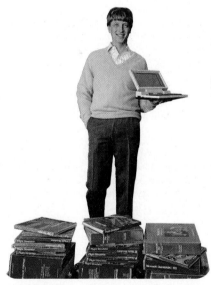

A young Bill Gates, founder of Microsoft and one of the world's richest persons. Like many highly gifted students, Gates was not especially fond of school. He hacked a computer security system when he was 13 and as a high school student, he was allowed to take some college math classes. He dropped out of Harvard University and began developing a plan for what was to become Microsoft Corporation. *What are some ways that schools can enrich the education of such highly talented students as Gates to make it a more challenging, interesting, and meaningful experience?*
Joe McNally/Hulton Archive/Getty Images

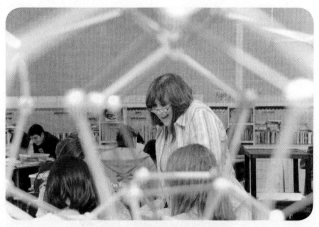

Margaret (Peg) Cagle with some of the gifted seventh- and eighth-grade math students she teaches at Lawrence Middle School in Chatsworth, California. Cagle especially advocates challenging students who are gifted to take intellectual risks. To encourage collaboration, she often has students work together in groups of four, and frequently tutors students during lunch hour. As 13-year-old Madeline Lewis commented, "If you don't get it one way, she'll explain it another and talk to you about it and show you until you do get it." Cagle says it is important to be passionate about teaching math and to open up a world for students that shows them how beautiful learning math can be (Wong Briggs, 2007, p. 6D).
Scott Buschman

creativity The ability to think in novel and unusual ways and come up with unique solutions to problems.

divergent thinking Thinking that produces many answers to the same question; characteristic of creativity.

convergent thinking Thinking that produces one correct answer; characteristic of the kind of thinking required on conventional intelligence tests.

brainstorming A technique in which children are encouraged to come up with creative ideas in a group, play off one another's ideas, and say practically whatever comes to mind.

"nerds" or "geeks." A child who is truly gifted often is the only child in the classroom who does not have the opportunity to learn with students of like ability. Many eminent adults report that school was a negative experience for them, that they were bored and sometimes knew more than their teachers (Bloom, 1985). Raising standards can benefit all children, but when some children are still underchallenged, one option is to allow them to attend advanced classes in their domain of exceptional ability (Worrell & others, 2019). For example, some especially precocious middle school students should be allowed to take college classes in their area of expertise. Bill Gates, founder of Microsoft, took college math classes and hacked a computer security system at 13; Yo-Yo Ma, famous cellist, graduated from high school at 15 and attended Juilliard School of Music in New York City.

A final concern is that African American, Latino, and Native American children are underrepresented in gifted programs (Worrell & others, 2019). Much of the underrepresentation involves the lower test scores for these children compared with non-Latino White and Asian American children, which may be due to test bias and fewer opportunities to develop language skills such as vocabulary and comprehension (Owens & others, 2018).

A number of individuals work in various capacities in school systems with children who are gifted. To read about the work of Sterling Jones, specialist in gifted and talented education, see *Connecting with Careers*.

CREATIVITY

We brought up the term "creative" on several occasions in our discussion of intelligence and giftedness. What does it mean to be creative? **Creativity** is the ability to think about something in novel and unusual ways and come up with unique solutions to problems.

Intelligence and creativity are not the same thing (Sternberg 2018a). Most creative people are quite intelligent, but the reverse is not necessarily true. Many highly intelligent people (as measured by high scores on conventional tests of intelligence) are not very creative (Sternberg, 2018a). Many highly intelligent people produce large numbers of products that are not necessarily novel.

Why don't IQ scores predict creativity? Creativity requires divergent thinking (Cortes & others, 2019). **Divergent thinking** produces many answers to the same question. In contrast, conventional intelligence tests require **convergent thinking.** For example, a typical question on a conventional intelligence test is, "How many quarters will you get in return for 60 dimes?" There is only one correct answer to this question. In contrast, a question such as "What image comes to mind when you hear the phrase 'sitting alone in a dark room'?" has many possible answers; it calls for divergent thinking.

Just as in being gifted, children show creativity in some domains more than others (Huang & others, 2017). For example, a child who shows creativity in mathematics might not be as creative in art.

A special concern is that children's creative thinking appears to be declining. A study of approximately 300,000 U.S. children and adults found that creativity scores rose until 1990, but since then have been steadily declining (Kim, 2010). Among the likely causes of the creativity decline are the number of hours U.S. children spend watching TV and playing video games instead of engaging in creative activities, as well as the lack of emphasis on creative thinking skills in schools (Gregorson, Kaufman, & Snyder, 2013; Kaufman & Sternberg, 2012, 2013). Some countries, though, are placing increasing emphasis on creative thinking in schools. For example, creative thinking historically was discouraged in Chinese schools. However, Chinese educators are now encouraging teachers to spend more classroom time on creative activities (Plucker, 2010). To read about some strategies for helping children become more creative, see *Caring Connections*.

Guiding Children's Creativity

An important goal of teachers is to help children become more creative (Bereczki & Kárpáti, 2018). What are the best strategies for accomplishing this goal? We examine some of these strategies next.

Encourage Creative Thinking on a Group and Individual Basis

Brainstorming is a technique in which children are encouraged to come up with creative ideas in a group, play off each other's ideas, and say practically whatever comes to mind that seems relevant to a particular issue. Participants are usually told to hold off from criticizing others' ideas at least until the end of the brainstorming session.

Provide Environments That Stimulate Creativity

Some environments nourish creativity, while others inhibit it. Parents and teachers who encourage creativity often rely on children's natural curiosity (Moore, Tank, & English, 2018). They provide exercises and activities that stimulate children to find insightful solutions to problems, rather than ask a lot of questions that require rote answers (Jónsdóttir, 2017). Teachers also encourage creativity by taking students on field trips to locations where creativity is valued, such as science, discovery, and children's museums that offer rich opportunities to stimulate creativity.

Don't Overcontrol Students

Telling children exactly how to do things might leave them feeling that originality is a mistake and exploration is a waste of time. If, instead of dictating which activities they should engage in, you let children select activities that match their interests and you support their inclinations, you will be less likely to inhibit their natural curiosity (Bereczki & Kárpáti, 2018). When parents and teachers hover over students all of the time, they make students feel that they are constantly being watched while they are working. When children are under constant surveillance, their creative risk taking and adventurous spirit diminish. Children's creativity also is diminished when adults have grandiose expectations for children's performance and expect perfection from them.

Encourage Internal Motivation

Excessive use of prizes, such as gold stars, money, or toys, can stifle creativity by undermining the intrinsic pleasure students derive from creative activities (Malik & Butt, 2017). Creative children's motivation is the satisfaction generated by the work itself. Competition for prizes and formal evaluations often undermine intrinsic motivation and creativity. However, this should not rule out material rewards altogether.

Guide Children to Help Them Think in Flexible Ways

Creative thinkers approach problems in many different ways, rather than getting locked into rigid patterns of thought. Give children opportunities to exercise this flexibility in their thinking.

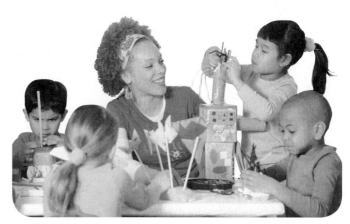

What are some good strategies teachers can use to guide children in thinking more creatively?
Ariel Skelley/Blend Images LLC

Build Children's Confidence

To expand children's creativity, encourage them to believe in their own ability to create something innovative and worthwhile. Building children's confidence in their creative skills aligns with Bandura's (2018) concept of *self-efficacy,* the belief that one can master a situation and produce positive outcomes.

Guide Children to Be Persistent and Delay Gratification

Most highly successful creative products take years to develop. Most creative individuals work on ideas and projects for months and years without being rewarded for their efforts (Sternberg, 2018a). Children don't become experts at sports, music, or art overnight. It usually takes many years of working at something to become an expert at it; the same is true for a creative thinker who produces a unique, worthwhile product.

Encourage Children to Take Intellectual Risks

Creative individuals take intellectual risks and seek to discover or invent something never before discovered or invented (Sternberg, 2018a). They risk spending a lot of time on an idea or project that may not work. Failure can be useful in the creative process (Hannigan, 2018). Creative people often see failure as an opportunity to learn. They might go down 20 dead-end streets before they come up with an innovative idea.

Which of the strategies described above specifically encourages divergent thinking?

Review Connect Reflect

LG3 Describe the characteristics of intellectual disability, giftedness, and creativity.

Review

- What is intellectual disability, and what are its causes?
- What makes individuals gifted?
- What makes individuals creative?

Connect

- In this section you learned how intellectual disability is assessed and classified. What have you learned about the prevalence of Down syndrome in the population and the factors that might cause an infant to be born with Down syndrome?

Reflect *Your Own Personal Journey of Life*

- If you were an elementary school teacher, what would you do to encourage students' creativity?

Intelligence

The Concept of Intelligence

LG1 Explain the concept of intelligence.

What Is Intelligence?

Intelligence Tests

Theories of Multiple Intelligences

- Intelligence consists of the ability to solve problems and to adapt and learn from experiences. A key aspect of intelligence focuses on its individual variations. Traditionally, intelligence has been measured by tests designed to compare people's performance on cognitive tasks.

- Alfred Binet developed the first intelligence test and created the concept of mental age. William Stern developed the concept of IQ for use with the Binet test. Revisions of the Binet test are called the Stanford-Binet. The test scores on the Stanford-Binet approximate a normal distribution. The Wechsler scales, created by David Wechsler, are the other main intelligence assessment tool. These tests provide an overall IQ, scores on a number of subtests, and several composite indexes. When used by a judicious examiner, tests can be valuable tools for determining individual differences in intelligence. Test scores should be only one type of information used to evaluate an individual. IQ scores can produce unfortunate stereotypes and false expectations.

- Sternberg's triarchic theory states that there are three main types of intelligence: analytical, creative, and practical. Sternberg created the Sternberg Triarchic Abilities Test to assess these three types of intelligence and has described applications of triarchic theory to children's education. Gardner maintains that there are eight types of intelligence, or frames of mind: verbal skills, mathematical skills, spatial skills, bodily-kinesthetic skills, musical skills, interpersonal skills, intrapersonal skills, and naturalist skills. Emotional intelligence is the ability to perceive and express emotion accurately and adaptively, to understand emotion and emotional knowledge, to use feelings to facilitate thought, and to manage emotions in oneself and others. The multiple-intelligences approaches have broadened the definition of intelligence and motivated educators to develop programs that instruct students in different domains. Critics maintain that Gardner's multiple-intelligence classification seems arbitrary. Critics also say that there is insufficient research to support the concept of multiple intelligences.

The Neuroscience of Intelligence

The Influence of Heredity and Environment

- Interest in discovering links between the brain and intelligence has been stimulated by advances in brain imaging. Neuroimaging studies have found that intelligence is not localized in a specific area of the brain but rather depends on patterns of connectivity among different brain regions that enable people to process information quickly and efficiently.

- Genetic similarity might explain why identical twins show stronger correlations on intelligence tests than fraternal twins do. Some studies indicate that the IQs of adopted children are more similar to the IQs of their biological parents than to those of their adoptive parents. Many studies show that intelligence has a reasonably strong heritability component, but environmental influences also are important. Intelligence test scores have risen considerably around the world in recent decades—this trend is called the Flynn effect—and this supports the role of environment in intelligence. Researchers have found that being deprived of formal education lowers IQ scores. Ramey's research revealed the positive effects of educational child care on intelligence.

Group Comparisons

- Cultures vary in the way they define intelligence. Early intelligence tests favored White, middle-socioeconomic-status, urban individuals. Tests may be biased against certain groups that are not familiar with a standard form of English, with the content tested, or with the testing situation. Tests are likely to reflect the values and experience of the dominant culture.

The Development of Intelligence Discuss the development of intelligence.

Tests of Infant Intelligence

- A test developed by Gesell was an important early contributor to the developmental testing of infants. Tests designed to assess infant intelligence include the widely used Bayley scales. Infant information-processing tasks that involve attention—especially habituation and dishabituation—are related to scores on standardized tests of intelligence in childhood.

Stability and Change in Intelligence Through Adolescence

- Intelligence is not as stable across childhood and adolescence as the original theorists believed. Many children's scores on intelligence tests fluctuate considerably.

The Extremes of Intelligence and Creativity Describe the characteristics of intellectual disability, giftedness, and creativity.

Intellectual Disability

- Intellectual disability is a condition of limited mental ability in which the individual (1) has a low IQ, usually below 70; (2) has difficulty adapting to everyday life; and (3) has an onset of these characteristics by age 18. Most affected individuals have an IQ in the 55 to 70 range (mild intellectual disability). Intellectual disability can have an organic cause (called organic intellectual disability) or be social and cultural in origin (called cultural-familial intellectual disability).

Giftedness

- Individuals who are gifted have above-average intelligence (an IQ of 130 or higher) and/or superior talent for something. Three characteristics of gifted children are precocity, marching to their own drummer, and a passion to master their domain. Giftedness is a consequence of both heredity and environment. Developmental changes characterize giftedness, and increasingly the domain-specific aspect of giftedness is emphasized. Concerns exist about the education of children who are gifted.

Creativity

- Creativity is the ability to think about something in novel and unusual ways and come up with unique solutions to problems. Although most creative people are intelligent, individuals with high IQs are not necessarily creative. Creative people tend to be divergent thinkers; traditional intelligence tests measure convergent thinking. Parents and teachers can use a number of strategies to increase children's creative thinking.

key **terms**

Bayley Scales of Infant Development 233
brainstorming 238
convergent thinking 238
creativity 238

culture-fair tests 231
developmental quotient (DQ) 233
divergent thinking 238
emotional intelligence 226
gifted 235

heritability 228
intellectual disability 235
intelligence 222
intelligence quotient (IQ) 223
mental age (MA) 223

normal distribution 223
stereotype threat 232
triarchic theory of intelligence 224

key **people**

Nancy Bayley 233
Alfred Binet 222
John Colombo 236
James Flynn 229

Arnold Gesell 232
Daniel Goleman 226
John Mayer 226
Robert McCall 234

Craig Ramey 230
Peter Salovey 226
Theophile Simon 223
Robert J. Sternberg 223

Lewis Terman 236
David Wechsler 224

chapter 9

LANGUAGE DEVELOPMENT

chapter outline

1 What Is Language?

Learning Goal 1 Define language and describe its rule systems.

Defining Language
Language's Rule Systems

2 How Language Develops

Learning Goal 2 Describe how language develops.

Infancy
Early Childhood
Middle and Late Childhood
Adolescence

3 Biological and Environmental Influences

Learning Goal 3 Discuss the biological and environmental contributions to language development.

Biological Influences
Environmental Influences
An Interactionist View of Language

4 Language and Cognition

Learning Goal 4 Evaluate how language and cognition are linked.

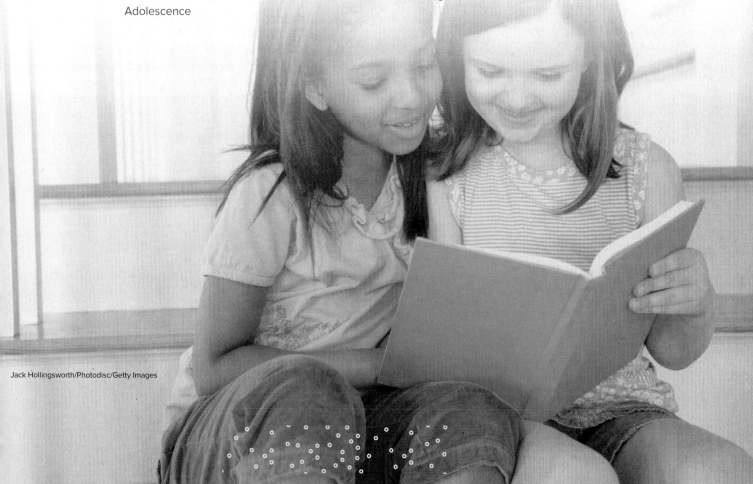

Jack Hollingsworth/Photodisc/Getty Images

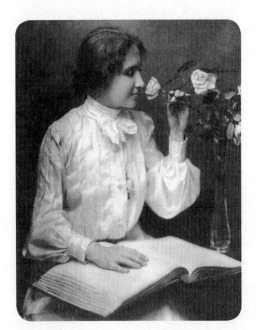

Helen Keller.
Whitman Studio/Library of Congress, Prints and Photographs Division, LC-USZ61-326

A stunning portrayal of a child isolated from the mainstream of language is the case of Helen Keller (1880–1968). At 18 months of age, Helen was an intelligent toddler in the process of learning to say her first words. Then she developed an illness that left her both deaf and blind, suffering the double affliction of sudden darkness and silence. For the next five years, she lived in a world she learned to fear because she could not see or hear.

Even with her fears, Helen spontaneously invented a number of gestures to reflect her wants and needs. For example, when she wanted ice cream, she turned toward the freezer and shivered. When she wanted bread and butter, she imitated the motions of cutting and spreading. But this homemade language system severely limited her ability to communicate with the surrounding community, which did not understand her idiosyncratic gestures.

Alexander Graham Bell, the famous inventor of the telephone, suggested to her parents that they hire a tutor named Anne Sullivan to help Helen overcome her fears. By using sign language, Anne was able to teach Helen to communicate. Anne realized that language learning needs to occur naturally, so she did not force Helen to memorize words out of context as in the drill methods that were in vogue at the time. Sullivan's success depended not only on the child's natural ability to organize language according to form and meaning but also on introducing language in the context of communicating about objects, events, and feelings about others. Helen Keller eventually graduated from Radcliffe with honors, became a very successful educator, and crafted books about her life and experiences. She had this to say about language:

> Whatever the process, the result is wonderful. Gradually from naming an object we advance step by step until we have traversed the vast distance between our first stammered syllable and the sweep of thought in a line of Shakespeare.

preview

In this chapter, we will tell the remarkable story of language and how it develops. The questions we will explore include these: What is language? What is the developmental course of language? What does biology contribute to language? How does experience influence language? How are language and cognition linked?

What Is Language? Define language and describe its rule systems.

```
Defining          Language's
Language          Rule Systems
```

In 1799, a nude boy was observed running through the woods in France. The boy was captured when he was 11 years old. He was called the Wild Boy of Aveyron and was believed to have lived in the woods alone for six years (Lane, 1976). When found, he made no effort to communicate. He never learned to communicate effectively. Sadly, a modern-day wild child named Genie was discovered in Los Angeles in 1970. Despite intensive intervention, Genie acquired only a limited form of spoken language. Both cases—the Wild Boy of Aveyron and Genie—raise questions about the biological and environmental determinants of language—topics that we will examine later in the chapter. First, though, we need to define language.

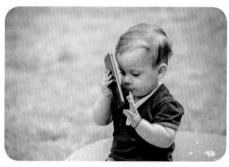

Language allows us to communicate with others. *What are some important characteristics of language?*
LiandStudio/Shutterstock

DEFINING LANGUAGE

Language is a form of communication—whether spoken, written, or signed—that is based on a system of symbols. Language consists of the words used by a community and the rules for varying and combining them.

Think how important language is in our everyday lives. It is difficult to imagine what Helen Keller's life would have been like if she had never learned language. We need language to communicate with others—to speak, listen, read, and write. Our language enables us to describe past events in detail and to plan for the future. Language lets us pass down information from one generation to the next and create a rich cultural heritage.

All human languages have some common characteristics (Berko Gleason & Ratner, 2017). These include infinite generativity and organizational rules. **Infinite generativity** is the ability to produce an endless number of meaningful sentences using a finite set of words and rules. When we say "rules," we mean that language is orderly and that rules describe the way language works. Let's further explore what these rules involve.

LANGUAGE'S RULE SYSTEMS

When nineteenth-century American writer Ralph Waldo Emerson said, "The world was built in order and the atoms march in tune," he must have had language in mind. Language is highly ordered and organized (Berko Gleason & Ratner, 2017). The organization involves five systems of rules: phonology, morphology, syntax, semantics, and pragmatics.

Phonology   Every language is made up of basic sounds. **Phonology** is the sound system of a language, including the sounds that are used and how they may be combined (Kuhl, 2017). For example, English has the sounds *sp*, *ba*, and *ar*, but the sound sequences *zx* and *qp* do not occur. A *phoneme* is the basic unit of sound in a language; it is the smallest unit of sound that affects meaning. A good example of a phoneme in English is /k/, the sound represented by the letter *k* in the word *ski* and the letter *c* in the word *cat*. The /k/ sound is slightly different in these two words, and in some languages such as

> Words not only affect us temporarily; they change us, they socialize us, and they unsocialize us.
>
> —**David Riesman**
> *American social scientist, 20th century*

language A form of communication, whether spoken, written, or signed, that is based on a system of symbols.

infinite generativity The ability to produce an endless number of meaningful sentences using a finite set of words and rules.

phonology The sound system of a language, which includes the sounds used and rules about how they may be combined.

Arabic these two sounds are separate phonemes. However, this variation is not distinguished in English, and the /k/ sound is therefore a single phoneme.

Morphology

morphology The rule system that governs how words are formed in a language.

Morphology **Morphology** is the rule system that governs how words are formed in a language. A *morpheme* is a minimal unit of meaning; it is a word or a part of a word that cannot be broken into smaller meaningful parts. Every word in the English language is made up of one or more morphemes. Some words consist of a single morpheme (for example, *help*), whereas others are made up of more than one morpheme (for example, *helper*, which has two morphemes, *help* and *er*, with the morpheme *-er* meaning "one who"—in this case "one who helps"). Thus, not all morphemes are words by themselves; for example, *-pre*, *-tion*, and *-ing* are morphemes.

Just as the rules that govern phonology describe the sound sequences that can occur in a language, the rules of morphology describe the way meaningful units (morphemes) can be combined in words (Stump, 2017). Morphemes have many jobs in grammar, such as marking tense (for example, she *walks* versus she *walked*), number (she *walks* versus they *walk*), and gender in some languages (Stump, 2017).

Syntax

syntax The ways words are combined to form acceptable phrases and sentences.

Syntax **Syntax** involves the way words are combined to form acceptable phrases and sentences. The term *syntax* is often used interchangeably with the term *grammar*. If someone says to you, "Bob slugged Tom" or "Bob was slugged by Tom," you know who did the slugging and who was slugged in each case because you have a syntactic understanding of these sentence structures. You also understand that the sentence, "You didn't stay, did you?" is a grammatical sentence but that "You didn't stay, didn't you?" is unacceptable and ambiguous.

If you learn another language, English syntax will not get you very far. For example, in English an adjective usually precedes a noun (as in *blue sky*), whereas in Spanish the adjective usually follows the noun (*cielo azul*). Despite the differences in their syntactic structures, however, the world's languages have much in common (Lyovin, Kessler, & Leben, 2017). For example, consider the following short sentences:

The cat killed the mouse.
The farmer chased the cat.
The mouse ate the cheese.

In many languages, it is possible to combine these sentences into more complex sentences. For example:

The farmer chased the cat that killed the mouse.
The mouse the cat killed ate the cheese.

However, no language we know of permits sentences like the following one:

The mouse the cat the farmer chased killed ate the cheese.

Can you make sense of this sentence? If you can, you probably can do it only after wrestling with it for several minutes. You likely could not understand it at all if someone uttered it during a conversation. It appears that language users cannot process subjects and objects arranged in too complex a fashion in a sentence. That is good news for language learners, because it means that all syntactic systems have some common ground. Such findings are also considered important by researchers who are interested in the universal properties of syntax (Berman, 2018).

Semantics

semantics The meaning of words and sentences.

Semantics **Semantics** refers to the meaning of words and sentences. Every word has a set of semantic features, or required attributes related to meaning. *Girl* and *woman*, for example, share many semantic features but differ semantically in regard to age.

Words have semantic restrictions on how they can be used in sentences. The sentence *The bicycle talked the boy into buying a candy bar* is syntactically correct but semantically incorrect. The sentence violates our semantic knowledge that bicycles don't talk.

Rule System	Description	Examples
Phonology	The sound system of a language. A phoneme is the smallest sound unit in a language.	The word *chat* has three phonemes or sounds: /ch/ /ã/ /t/. Here is an example of a phonological rule in the English language: While the phoneme /r/ can follow the phonemes /t/ or /d/ in an English consonant cluster (such as *track* or *drab*), the phoneme /l/ cannot follow these letters.
Morphology	The system of meaningful units involved in word formation.	The smallest sound units that have a meaning are called morphemes, or meaning units. The word *girl* is one morpheme, or meaning unit; it cannot be broken down any further and still have meaning. When the inflection *s* is added, the word becomes *girls* and has two morphemes because the *s* changed the meaning of the word, indicating that there is more than one girl.
Syntax	The system that involves the way words are combined to form acceptable phrases and sentences.	Word order is very important in determining meaning in the English language. For example, the sentence "Sebastian pushed the bike" has a different meaning from "The bike pushed Sebastian."
Semantics	The system that involves the meaning of words and sentences.	Knowing the meaning of individual words—that is, vocabulary. For example, semantics includes knowing the meaning of such words as *orange, transportation,* and *intelligent.*
Pragmatics	The system of using appropriate conversation and knowledge of how to effectively use language in context.	An example is using polite language in appropriate situations, such as being mannerly when talking with one's teacher. Taking turns in a conversation involves pragmatics.

FIGURE 1
THE RULE SYSTEMS OF LANGUAGE

Pragmatics A final set of language rules involves **pragmatics,** the appropriate use of language in different contexts. Pragmatics covers a lot of territory (Jaszczolt, 2016). When you take turns speaking in a discussion or use a question to convey a command ("Why is it so noisy in here?" "What is this, Grand Central Station?"), you are demonstrating knowledge of pragmatics. You also apply the pragmatics of English when you use polite language in appropriate situations (for example, when talking to your teacher) or tell stories that are interesting, jokes that are funny, and lies that convince. In each of these cases, you are demonstrating that you understand the rules of your culture for adjusting language to suit the context.

Pragmatic rules can be complex and differ from one culture to another (Jaszczolt, 2016). If you were to study the Japanese language, you would come face-to-face with countless pragmatic rules about conversing with individuals of various social levels and with various relationships to you. Some of these pragmatic rules concern the ways of saying *thank you*. Indeed, the pragmatics of saying *thank you* are complex even in our own culture. Preschoolers' use of the phrase *thank you* varies with sex, socioeconomic status, and the age of the individual they are addressing.

At this point, we have discussed five important rule systems involved in language. An overview of these rule systems is presented in Figure 1.

pragmatics The appropriate use of language in different contexts.

Review Connect Reflect

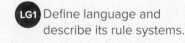 Define language and describe its rule systems.

Review
- What is language?
- What are language's five main rule systems?

Connect
- Describe how the use of dialogue in scaffolding is reflected in the story about Helen Keller and Anne Sullivan at the beginning of this chapter.

Reflect *Your Own Personal Journey of Life*
- How good are your family members and friends at the pragmatics of language? Describe an example in which someone showed pragmatic skills and another in which someone did not.

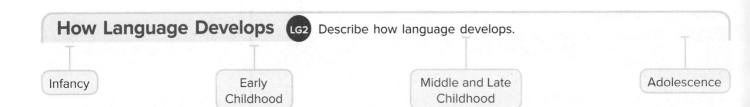
According to a historian of ancient cultures, a thirteenth-century emperor of Germany, Frederick II, had a cruel idea. He wanted to know what language children would speak if no one talked to them. He selected several newborns and threatened their caregivers with death if they ever talked to the infants. Frederick never found out what language the children would speak because they all died. As we move forward in the twenty-first century, we are still curious about infants' development of language, although our experiments and observations are, to say the least, far more humane than the evil Frederick's.

INFANCY

Whatever language they learn, infants all over the world follow a similar path in language development. What are some key milestones in this development?

Babbling and Other Vocalizations   Long before infants speak recognizable words, they produce a number of vocalizations (Lee & others, 2017). The functions of these early vocalizations are to practice making sounds, to communicate, and to attract attention. Babies' sounds go through the following sequence during the first year:

1. *Crying.* Babies cry even at birth. Crying can signal distress, but as we will discuss in the chapter "Emotional Development," different types of cries signal different things.

2. *Cooing.* Babies first coo at about 1 to 2 months. These are gurgling sounds that are made in the back of the throat and usually express pleasure during interaction with the caregiver.

3. *Babbling.* In the middle of the first year babies babble—that is, they produce strings of consonant-vowel combinations, such as *ba, ba, ba, ba.*

When deaf infants are born to deaf parents who use sign language, they babble with their hands and fingers at about the same age that hearing children babble vocally (Wille & others, 2018). Such similarities in timing and structure between manual and vocal babbling indicate that a unified language capacity underlies signed and spoken language.

Gestures   Infants start using gestures, such as showing and pointing, at about 8 to 12 months of age. They may wave bye-bye, nod to mean "yes," show an empty cup to ask for more milk, and point to a dog to draw attention to it. Some early gestures are symbolic, as when an infant smacks her lips to indicate food or drink. Pointing is considered by language experts to be an important index of the social aspects of language, and it follows this developmental sequence: from pointing without checking on adult gaze to pointing while looking back and forth between an object and the adult (Goldin-Meadow, 2018). It is not just sticking the finger out that is important but the point in conjunction with drawing someone's attention to something that is an important communication milestone.

Lack of pointing is a significant indicator of problems in the infant's communication system (Goldin-Meadow, 2018). Pointing is a key aspect of the development of joint attention and an important index of the social aspects of language (Lucca & Wilbourn, 2019). Failure to engage in pointing also characterizes many autistic children.

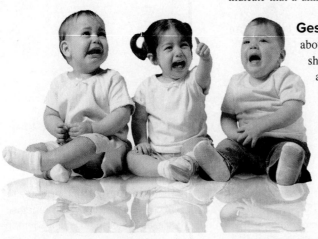

Long before infants speak recognizable words, they communicate by producing a number of vocalizations and gestures. *At approximately what ages do infants begin to produce different types of vocalizations and gestures?*
Don Hammond/Design Pics

---

developmental connection

Emotional Development

Three basic cries that infants display are the basic cry, anger cry, and pain cry. Connect to "Emotional Development."

The ability to use the pointing gesture effectively is enhanced in the second year of life as advances in other aspects of language communication occur (Goldin-Meadow, 2018).

A study of the functions of infants' pointing found that, as when older children ask questions, infants use gestures to obtain information (Lucca & Wilbourn, 2019). When 18-month-olds pointed at novel objects in an experiment and were provided with labels for the objects, they were less likely to persist in pointing than if the experimenter did not label the objects, suggesting that infants were pointing to obtain information.

Recognizing Language Sounds

Long before they begin to learn words, infants can make fine distinctions among the sounds of the language. In Patricia Kuhl's (2017) research, phonemes from languages all over the world are piped through a speaker for infants to hear (see Figure 2). A box with a toy bear in it is placed where the infant can see it. A string of identical syllables is played; then the syllables are changed (for example, *ba ba ba ba*, and then *pa pa pa pa*). If the infant turns its head when the syllables change, the box lights up and the bear dances and drums, rewarding the infant for noticing the change.

Kuhl's (2017) research has demonstrated that from birth to about 6 months of age, infants are "citizens of the world": they recognize when sounds change most of the time, no matter what language the syllables come from. But over the next six months, infants get even better at perceiving the changes in sounds from their "own" language, the one their parents speak, and gradually lose the ability to recognize differences that are not important in their own language.

Infants must fish out individual words from the nonstop stream of sound that makes up ordinary speech (Karaman & Hay, 2018). To do so, they must find the boundaries between words, which is very difficult for infants because adults don't pause between words when they speak. Still, infants begin to detect word boundaries by 8 months of age. In one study, 8-month-olds whose families spoke English were exposed to Italian sentences with four embedded target words (Karaman & Hay, 2018). After an initial familiarization period with the target words, they looked longer at a visual stimulus such as a pinwheel during select test trials. This behavioral change suggested they were able to use features of the words to distinguish them from the surrounding flow of language.

First Words

Infants understand words before they can produce or speak them. For example, many infants recognize their name when someone says it as early as 5 months of age. However, the infant's first spoken word, a milestone eagerly anticipated by every parent, usually doesn't occur until 10 to 15 months of age and at an average of about 13 months. Yet long before babies say their first words, they have been communicating with their parents, often by gesturing and using their own special sounds. The appearance of first words is a continuation of this communication process (Berko Gleason & Ratner, 2017).

A child's first words include those that name important people (*dada*), familiar animals (*kitty*), vehicles (*car*), toys (*ball*), food (*milk*), body parts (*eye*), clothes (*hat*), household items (*clock*), and greeting terms (*bye*). These were the first words of babies 50 years ago. They are the first words of babies today. Children often express various intentions with their single words, so that "cookie" might mean "That's a cookie" or "I want a cookie."

As indicated earlier, children understand their first words earlier than they speak them. On average, infants understand about 50 words at age 13 months, but they can't say this many words until about 18 months (Berko Gleason & Ratner, 2017). Thus, in infancy *receptive vocabulary* (words the child understands) considerably exceeds *spoken vocabulary* (words the child uses). Infants as young as 4 months old can understand that specific words refer to specific body parts when their parents touch their bodies while saying words referring to the body parts (Tincoff & others, 2019).

The infant's spoken vocabulary increases rapidly once the first word is spoken (Berko Gleason & Ratner, 2017). The average 18-month-old can speak about 50 words, but by the age of 2 years a child can speak about 200 words. This rapid increase in vocabulary that begins at approximately 18 months is called the *vocabulary spurt* (Chow & others, 2019).

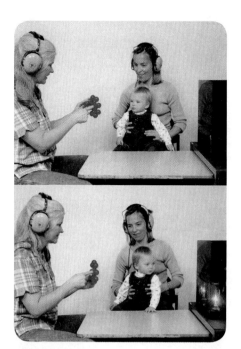

FIGURE 2

FROM UNIVERSAL LINGUIST TO LANGUAGE-SPECIFIC LISTENER. In Patricia Kuhl's research laboratory, babies listen to tape-recorded voices that repeat syllables. When the sounds of the syllables change, the babies quickly learn to look at the bear. Using this technique, Kuhl has demonstrated that babies are universal linguists until about 6 months of age, but in the next six months become language-specific listeners. *What does Kuhl's research suggest about the role of "nature" and "nurture" in language acquisition?*

Courtesy of Dr. Patricia Kuhl, Institute for Learning and Brain Sciences, University of Washington

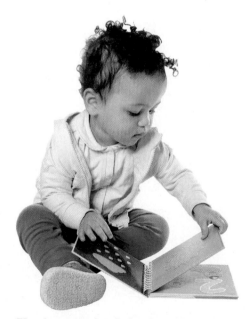

What characterizes the infant's early word learning?
Africa Studio/Shutterstock

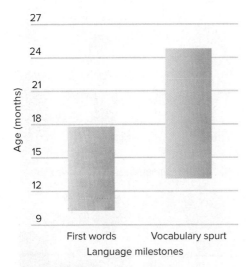

FIGURE 3
VARIATION IN LANGUAGE MILESTONES

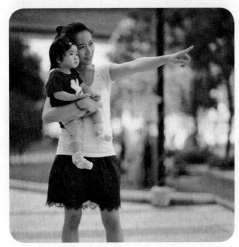

What is a difference in the way children learn Mandarin Chinese and English?
Tang Ming Tung/Getty Images

telegraphic speech The use of short, precise words without grammatical markers such as articles, auxiliary verbs, and other connectives.

Like the timing of a child's first word, the timing of the vocabulary spurt varies. Figure 3 shows the range for these two language milestones in 14 children. On average, these children said their first word at 13 months and had a vocabulary spurt at 19 months. However, the ages for the first word of individual children varied from 10 to 17 months and for their vocabulary spurt from 13 to 25 months.

Cross-linguistic differences occur in word learning. Children learning Mandarin Chinese, Korean, and Japanese acquire more verbs earlier in their development than do children learning English (Tardif, 2016). This cross-linguistic difference reflects the richer variety of verbs in these Asian languages as well as the fact that the use of the subject, which is obligatory in English, often is optional in other languages.

Children sometimes overextend or underextend the meanings of the words they use (Berko Gleason & Ratner, 2017). Overextension is the tendency to apply a word to objects that are inappropriate for the word's meaning. For example, children at first may say "dada" not only for "father" but also for other men, strangers, or boys. Children may overextend word meanings because they don't know the appropriate word or can't recall it. With time, overextensions decrease and eventually disappear. Underextension is the tendency to apply a word too narrowly; it occurs when children fail to use a word to name a relevant event or object. For example, a child might use the word *boy* to describe a 5-year-old neighbor but not apply the word to a male infant or to a 9-year-old male. The most common explanation of underextension is that children have heard a name used only in reference to a small, unrepresentative sample.

Two-Word Utterances By the time children are 18 to 24 months of age, they usually utter two-word messages (Tomasello, 2011). To convey meaning with just two words, the child relies heavily on gesture, tone, and context. The wealth of meaning children can communicate with a two-word utterance includes the following (Slobin, 1972):

- Identification: "See doggie."
- Location: "Book there."
- Repetition: "More milk."
- Possession: "My candy."
- Attribution: "Big car."
- Agent-action: "Mama walk."
- Question: "Where ball?"

These examples are from children whose first language is English, German, Russian, Finnish, Turkish, or Samoan.

Notice that the two-word utterances omit many parts of speech and are remarkably succinct. In fact, in every language, a child's first combinations of words have this economical quality; they are telegraphic. **Telegraphic speech** is the use of short and precise words without grammatical markers such as articles, auxiliary verbs, and other connectives. Telegraphic speech is not limited to two words. "Mommy give ice cream" and "Mommy give Tommy ice cream" also are examples of telegraphic speech.

We have discussed a number of language milestones in infancy. Figure 4 summarizes the ages at which infants typically reach these milestones. Despite these general patterns, there is also variability in the ages at which infants reach each milestone, depending on factors such as socioeconomic status and other environmental inputs as well as infants' abilities such as sustained attention (Brooks, Flynn, & Ober, 2018).

EARLY CHILDHOOD

Toddlers move rather quickly from producing two-word utterances to creating three-, four-, and five-word combinations. Between 2 and 3 years of age they begin the transition from saying simple sentences that express a single proposition to saying complex sentences (Berko Gleason & Ratner, 2017).

Young children's understanding sometimes goes far beyond their speech. One 3-year-old, laughing with delight as an abrupt summer breeze stirred his hair and tickled his skin, commented, "I got breezed!" Many of the oddities of young children's language sound like mistakes to adult listeners. However, from the children's point of view, they are not mistakes. They represent the way young children perceive and understand their world. As children go through their early childhood years, their grasp of the rule systems that govern language increases.

As young children learn the special features of their own language, there are extensive regularities in how they acquire that particular language (Berko Gleason & Ratner, 2017). For example, children in English-speaking families learn the prepositions *on* and *in* before other prepositions. Children learning other languages, such as Russian or Chinese, also acquire the particular features of those languages in a consistent order.

However, some children develop language problems, including speech and hearing problems. To read about the work of one individual who helps children who have speech/language and hearing problems, see *Connecting with Careers*.

Understanding Phonology and Morphology

During the preschool years, most children gradually become more sensitive to the sounds of spoken words and become increasingly capable of producing all the sounds of their language. By the time children are 3 years of age, they can produce all the vowel sounds and most of the consonant sounds (Prelock & Hutchins, 2018).

Young children can even produce complex consonant clusters such as *str-* and *mpt* in languages such as English where consonant clusters are common. They notice rhymes, enjoy poems, make up silly names for things by substituting one sound for another (such as bubblegum, bubblebum, bubbleyum), and clap along with each syllable in a phrase.

By the time children move beyond two-word utterances, they demonstrate a knowledge of morphology rules (Stump, 2017). Children begin using the plural and possessive forms of nouns (such as *dogs* and *dog's*). They put appropriate endings on verbs (such as *-s* when the subject is third-person singular and *-ed* for the past tense). They use prepositions (such as *in* and *on*), articles (such as *a* and *the*), and various forms of the verb *to be* (such as "I was going to the store"). Some of the best evidence for changes in children's use of morphological rules occurs in their overgeneralization of the rules, as when a preschool child says "foots" instead of "feet," or "goed" instead of "went."

In a classic experiment that was designed to study children's knowledge of morphological rules, such as how to make a plural, Jean Berko (1958) presented preschool children and first-grade children with cards such as the one shown in Figure 5. Children were asked to look at the card while the experimenter read aloud the words on the card. Then the children were asked to supply the missing word. This might sound easy, but Berko was interested in the children's ability to apply the appropriate morphological rule—in this case, to say "wugs" with the *z* sound that indicates the plural.

Although the children's answers were not perfect, they were much better than they could have been by chance. What makes Berko's study impressive is that most of the words were made up for the experiment. Thus, the children could not base their responses on remembering past instances of hearing the words. Since they could make the plurals or past tenses of words they had never heard before, this was evidence that they knew the morphological rules.

Changes in Syntax and Semantics

Preschool children also learn and apply rules of syntax (Messenger & Fisher, 2018). They show a growing mastery of complex rules for how words should be ordered.

Consider *wh-* questions, such as "Where is Daddy going?" or "What is that boy doing?" To ask these questions properly, the child must know two important differences between *wh-* questions and affirmative statements (for instance, "Daddy is going to work" and "That boy is waiting on the school bus"). First, a *wh-* word must be added at the beginning of the sentence. Second, the auxiliary verb must be inverted—that is, exchanged with the subject of the sentence. Young children learn quite early where to put the *wh-* word, but they take much longer to learn the auxiliary-inversion rule. Thus, preschool children might ask, "Where Daddy is going?" and "What that boy is doing?"

Gains in semantics also characterize early childhood. Vocabulary development is dramatic. Some experts have concluded that between 18 months and 6 years of age, young

Typical Age	Language Milestones
Birth	Crying
2 to 4 months	Cooing begins
5 months	Understands first word
6 months	Babbling begins
7 to 11 months	Change from universal linguist to language-specific listener
8 to 12 months	Uses gestures, such as showing and pointing Comprehension of words appears
13 months	First word spoken
18 months	Vocabulary spurt starts
18 to 24 months	Uses two-word utterances Rapid expansion of understanding of words

FIGURE 4

SOME LANGUAGE MILESTONES IN INFANCY. Despite great variations in the language input received by infants, around the world they follow a similar path in learning to speak.

Sharla Peltier, Speech Pathologist

A speech pathologist is a health professional who works with individuals who have a communication disorder. Sharla Peltier is a speech pathologist in Manitoulin, Ontario, Canada. Peltier works with Native American children in the First Nations Schools. She conducts screening for speech/language and hearing problems and assesses infants as young as 6 months of age as well as school-aged children. She works closely with community health nurses to identify hearing problems.

Diagnosing problems is only about half of what Peltier does in her work. She especially enjoys treating speech/language and hearing problems. She conducts parent training sessions to help parents understand and help with their children's language problems. As part of this training, she guides parents in improving their communication skills with their children.

For more information about what speech therapists do, see the Careers in Child Development appendix.

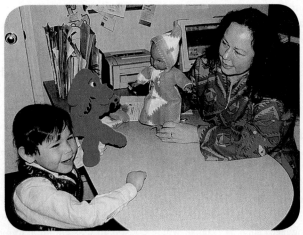

Speech therapist Sharla Peltier helps a young child improve her language and communication skills.
Courtesy of Sharla Peltier

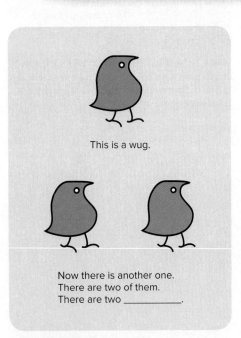

This is a wug.

Now there is another one.
There are two of them.
There are two _____.

FIGURE 5

STIMULI IN BERKO'S STUDY OF YOUNG CHILDREN'S UNDERSTANDING OF MORPHOLOGICAL RULES. In Jean Berko's (1958) study, young children were presented cards, such as this one with a "wug" on it. Then the children were asked to supply the missing word; in supplying the missing word, they had to say it correctly too. "Wugs" is the correct response here.

children learn approximately one new word every waking hour (Carey, 1977; Gelman & Kalish, 2006)! By the time they enter first grade, it is estimated that children know about 14,000 words (Clark, 1993). Children who enter elementary school with a small vocabulary are at risk for developing reading problems (McLeod, Hardy, & Kaiser, 2017).

Why can children learn so many new words so quickly? One possible explanation is **fast mapping,** which involves children's ability to make an initial connection between a word and its referent after only limited exposure to the word (Eviatar & others, 2018). However, fast mapping may have more to do with knowing what a word refers to in the immediate environment than with truly learning the word because children can rarely recall the words they have apparently learned in a fast mapping context (McMurray, Horst, & Samuelson, 2012). Researchers have found that exposure to words on multiple occasions over several days results in more successful word learning than the same number of exposures in a single day (Slone & Sandhofer, 2017).

Language researchers have proposed that young children may use a number of working hypotheses to learn new words. One working hypothesis children use is to give a novel label to a novel object. Parents can be especially helpful in aiding children's learning of novel labels for novel objects. As a mother looks at a picture book with her young child, she knows that the child understands the referent for *car* but not *bus*, so she says, "That's a bus, not a car. A bus is bigger than a car." Another working hypothesis children use is that a word refers to a whole object rather than parts of an object, such as labeling a tiger a *tiger* instead of a *tail* or *paw*. Sometimes children's initial mappings are incorrect. In such cases, they benefit from hearing the words mature speakers use to test and revise their word-referent connections (McMurray, Horst, & Samuelson, 2012).

What are some important aspects of how word learning optimally occurs? Kathy Hirsh-Pasek and Roberta Golinkoff (Harris, Golinkoff, & Hirsh-Pasek, 2012; Hirsh-Pasek & Golinkoff, 2013) emphasize six key principles in young children's vocabulary development:

1. *Children learn the words they hear most often.* They learn the words that they encounter when interacting with parents, teachers, siblings, and peers, and also from books. They especially benefit from encountering words that they do not know.

2. *Children learn words for things and events that interest them.* Parents and teachers can direct young children to experience words in contexts that interest the children; playful peer interactions are especially helpful in this regard.

3. *Children learn words best in responsive and interactive contexts rather than in passive contexts.* Children who experience turn-taking opportunities, joint focusing experiences, and positive, sensitive socializing contexts with adults encounter the scaffolding necessary for optimal word learning. They learn words less effectively when they are passive learners. It is harder for children to learn words from watching television than from interacting with adults.

4. *Children learn words best in contexts that are meaningful.* Young children learn new words more effectively when new words are encountered in integrated contexts rather than as isolated facts.

5. *Children learn words best when they access clear information about word meaning.* Children whose parents and teachers are sensitive to words the children might not understand and provide support and elaboration with hints about word meaning learn words better than children whose parents and teachers quickly state a new word and don't monitor whether children understand its meaning.

6. *Children learn words best when grammar and vocabulary are considered.* Children who experience a large number of words and diversity in verbal stimulation develop a richer vocabulary and better understanding of grammar. In many cases, vocabulary and grammar development are connected.

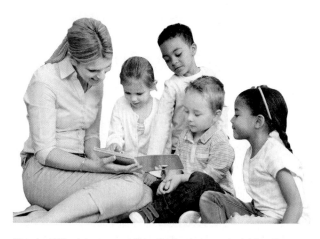

How do children's language abilities develop during early childhood?
Dean Mitchell/Vetta/Getty Images

How parents talk to their children is linked with the children's vocabulary growth and the family's socioeconomic status. To read about how family environment affects children's language development, see *Connecting Through Research.*

Advances in Pragmatics   Changes in pragmatics also characterize young children's language development (Papafragou, 2018). A 6-year-old is simply a much better conversationalist than a 2-year-old is. What are some of the improvements in pragmatics during the preschool years?

Young children begin to engage in extended discourse (Akhtar & Herold, 2017). For example, they learn culturally specific rules of conversation and politeness, and increasingly adapt their speech in different settings. Their developing linguistic skills and improving ability to understand the perspective of others contribute to their use of more competent narratives.

As children get older, they become increasingly able to talk about things that are not here (Grandma's house, for example) and not now (what happened to them yesterday or might happen tomorrow, for example). A preschool child can tell you what she wants for lunch tomorrow, something that would not have been possible at the two-word stage of language development.

At about 4 years of age, children develop a remarkable sensitivity to the needs of others in conversation. One way in which they show such sensitivity is through their use of the articles *the* and *an* (or *a*). When adults tell a story or describe an event, they generally use *an* (or *a*) when they first refer to an animal or an object, and then use *the* when referring to it later. (For example, "Two boys were walking through the jungle when *a* fierce lion appeared. *The* lion lunged at one boy while the other ran for cover.") Even 3-year-olds follow part of this rule; they consistently use the word *the* when referring to previously mentioned things. However, the use of the word *a* when something is initially mentioned develops more slowly. Although 5-year-old children follow this rule on some occasions, they fail to follow it on others.

> Children pick up words as pigeons peas.
>
> —**John Ray**
> *English naturalist, 17th century*

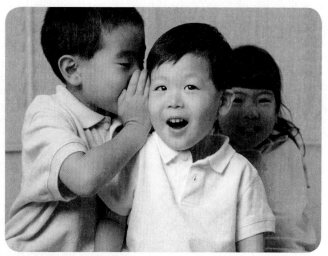

What are some advances in pragmatics that characterize children's development in early childhood?
Hill Street Studios/age fotostock

fast mapping A process that helps to explain how young children learn the connection between a word and its referent so quickly.

How Does Family Environment Affect Young Children's Language Development?

What characteristics of families influence children's language development? Socioeconomic status has been linked with how much parents talk to their children and with young children's vocabulary. Betty Hart and Todd Risley (1995) observed the language environments of children whose parents were professionals and children whose parents were on welfare. Compared with the professional parents, the parents on welfare talked much less to their young children, talked less about past events, and provided less elaboration. As indicated in Figure 6, the children of the professional parents had a much larger vocabulary at 36 months of age than the children whose parents were on welfare.

More recent studies of language to which children are exposed make use of LENA recording technology, which is a small digital audio-recorder that is worn by the child in specialized clothing. The device records all speech that is "near and clear" to the child over a time period of up to 16 hours. The system provides automated word counts of all adult speech, but also automated counts of the number of child vocalizations and conversational (back-and-forth) turns between caregivers and the target child. This recording technology provides a comprehensive picture of the talk that young children hear.

The LENA device can pick up on meaningful differences in the amount of talk that children hear as a function of SES as early as 18 months (Fernald, Marchman, & Weisleder, 2013). In addition, these SES differences are related to children's early skill at processing language in real-time, an important early indicator of children's

early language comprehension that has long-term consequences for later outcomes (Marchman & Fernald, 2008).

Studies using structural and functional MRI to examine the brains of 4- to 6-year-old children have shown that children who engage in more conversational turns have different white matter properties and engage in tasks differently from children who hear fewer conversational turns (Romeo & others, 2018). The amount of talk that children hear between 18 and 24 months is correlated with language and cognitive outcomes in adolescence (Gilkerson & others, 2018).

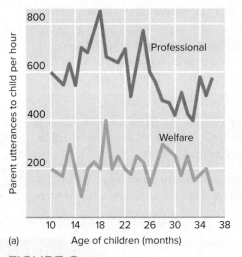

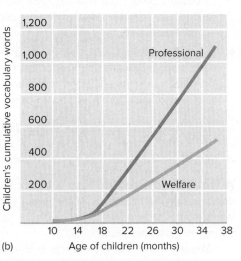

(a) Age of children (months) (b) Age of children (months)

FIGURE 6

LANGUAGE INPUT IN PROFESSIONAL AND WELFARE FAMILIES AND YOUNG CHILDREN'S VOCABULARY DEVELOPMENT. (*a*) In this study (Hart & Risley, 1995), parents who were professionals talked with their young children more than parents from welfare families. (*b*) All of the children learned to talk, but children whose parents were professionals developed vocabularies that were twice as large as those of children from welfare families. Thus, by the time children go to preschool, they already have experienced considerable differences in language input in their families and developed different levels of vocabulary that are linked to their socioeconomic context. *Does this study indicate that poverty caused deficiencies in vocabulary development?*

At around 4 to 5 years of age, children learn to change their speech style to suit the situation. For example, even 4-year-old children speak to a 2-year-old differently from the way they speak to a same-aged peer; they use shorter sentences with the 2-year-old. They also speak to an adult differently from the way they speak to a same-aged peer, using more polite and formal language with the adult (Ikeda, Kobayashi, & Itakura, 2018).

Early Literacy   Concern about U.S. children's reading and writing skills has led to a careful examination of preschool and kindergarten children's educational experiences, in the hope that a positive orientation toward reading and writing can be developed early in life (Dickinson & others, 2019). What should a literacy program for preschool children be like? Instruction should be built on what children already know about oral language, reading, and writing. Further, early precursors of literacy and academic success include language skills, phonological and syntactic knowledge, letter identification, and conceptual knowledge about print and its conventions and functions (Pavelko & others, 2018). Parents and teachers need to provide a supportive environment to help children develop literacy skills (Tamis-LeMonda & others, 2018). Children's emergent literacy skills are highly correlated with their parents' literacy skills (Taylor, Greenberg, & Terry, 2016). One study found that literacy experiences (such as how often the child was read to), the quality of the mother's engagement with her child (such as attempts to cognitively stimulate the child), and provision of learning materials (such as age-appropriate learning materials and books) were important home literacy experiences in low-income families that were linked to the children's language development in positive ways (Wood, Fitton, & Rodriguez, 2018).

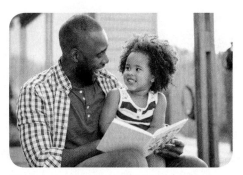

What are some effective strategies for supporting young children's literacy skills?
Monkey Business Images/Shutterstock

What are some strategies for using books effectively with preschool children? Ellen Galinsky (2010) emphasized the following strategies:

- *Use books to initiate conversation with young children.* Ask them to put themselves in the book characters' places and imagine what they might be thinking or feeling.
- *Use what and why questions.* Ask young children what they think is going to happen next in a story and then see if it occurs.
- *Encourage children to ask questions about stories.*
- *Choose some books that play with language.* Creative books on the alphabet, including those with rhymes, often interest young children.

The following longitudinal studies indicate the importance of early language skills to children's school readiness:

- Linguistic input when parents read to toddlers predicts language and literacy outcomes in elementary school, even controlling for parents' other linguistic input, perhaps in part because vocabulary is more diverse and syntax more complex in reading than in everyday conversation (Demir-Lira & others, 2019).
- Mothers' responsiveness and linguistic input during a shared picturebook reading task at 18 months predicted children's pre-academic skills at the age of 4.5 years (Wade & others, 2018).

So far, our discussion of early literacy has focused on U.S. children. However, the extent to which phonological awareness supports learning to read effectively varies across language to some extent (McBride, 2016). Phonological awareness is less important for early reading development in languages that use characters, such as Chinese, rather than alphabets (Ruan & others, 2018). Further, rates of dyslexia differ across countries and are linked with the spelling and phonetic rules that characterize the language (McBride, Wang, & Cheang, 2018). English is one of the more difficult languages to learn because of its irregular spellings and pronunciations. In countries where English is spoken, the rate of dyslexia is higher than it is in countries where the alphabet script is more phonetically pronounced.

MIDDLE AND LATE CHILDHOOD

Children gain new skills as they enter school that make it possible for them to learn to read and write, or to advance the reading and writing skills they have developed in early childhood. These new skills include increasingly using language to talk about things that are not physically present, learning what a word is, and learning how to recognize and talk about sounds (Berko Gleason & Ratner, 2017). They have to learn the alphabetic principle, that the letters of the alphabet represent sounds of the language, in languages that use alphabets, and that characters represent concepts in languages such as Chinese. As children develop during middle and late childhood, changes in their vocabulary and grammar also take place (Suggate & others, 2018).

Vocabulary, Grammar, and Metalinguistic Awareness   During middle and late childhood, changes occur in the way children's mental vocabulary is organized. When asked to say the first word that comes to mind when they hear a word, young children typically provide a word that often follows the word in a sentence. For example, when asked

Stage	Age Range/Grade Level	Descripton
0	Birth to first grade	Children master several prerequisites for reading. Many learn the left-to-right progression and order of reading, how to identify letters of the alphabet, and how to write their names. Some learn to read words that appear on signs. As a result of TV shows like *Sesame Street* and attending preschool and kindergarten programs, many young children today develop greater knowledge about reading earlier than in the past.
1	First and second grades	Many children learn to read at this time. In doing so, they acquire the ability to sound out words (that is, translate letters into sounds and blend sounds into words). They also complete their learning of letter names and sounds.
2	Second and third grades	Children become more fluent at retrieving individual words and other reading skills. However, at this stage reading is still not used much for learning. The demands of reading are so taxing for children at this stage that they have few resources left over to process the content.
3	Fourth through eighth grades	In fourth through eighth grade, children become increasingly able to obtain new information from print. In other words, they read to learn. They still have difficulty understanding information presented from multiple perspectives within the same story. When children don't learn to read, a downward spiral unfolds that leads to serious difficulties in many academic subjects.
4	High school	Many students become fully competent readers. They develop the ability to understand material told from many perspectives. This allows them to engage in sometimes more sophisticated discussions of literature, history, economics, and politics.

FIGURE 7

A MODEL OF DEVELOPMENTAL STAGES IN READING

- - - - - - - - - - - - - - - - →

developmental **connection**

Information Processing

Metacognition is cognition about cognition or knowing about knowing. Connect to "Information Processing."

← - - - - - - - - - - - - - - -

metalinguistic awareness Knowledge about language.

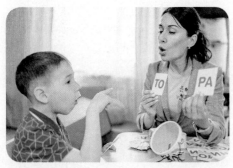

This teacher is helping a student sound out words. Researchers have found that phonics instruction is a key aspect of teaching students to read, especially beginning readers and students with weak reading skills.
Mordolff/Getty Images

to respond to *dog* the young child may say "barks," or to the word *eat* say "lunch." At about 7 years of age, children begin to respond with a word that is the same part of speech as the stimulus word. For example, a child may now respond to the word *dog* with "cat" or "horse." To *eat*, they now might say "drink." This is evidence that at age 7 children have begun to categorize their vocabulary by parts of speech (Berko Gleason & Ratner, 2017).

The process of categorizing becomes easier as children increase their vocabulary (Russell, 2017). Children's vocabulary increases from an average of about 14,000 words at 6 years of age to an average of about 40,000 words by 11 years of age.

Children make similar advances in grammar (Hoff, Quinn, & Giguere, 2018). During the elementary school years, children's improvement in logical reasoning and analytical skills helps them to understand constructions such as the appropriate use of comparatives (shorter, deeper) and subjunctives ("If you were president . . ."). During the elementary school years, children become increasingly able to understand and use complex grammar, such as the following sentence: "The boy who kissed his mother wore a hat." They also learn to use language to produce connected discourse. They become able to relate sentences to one another to produce descriptions, definitions, and narratives that make sense. Children must be able to do these things orally before they can be expected to deal with them in written assignments.

These advances in vocabulary and grammar during the elementary school years are accompanied by the development of **metalinguistic awareness,** which is knowledge about language, such as understanding what a preposition is or being able to discuss the sounds of a language. Metalinguistic awareness allows children "to think about their language, understand what words are, and even define them" (Berko Gleason, 2009, p. 4). This awareness improves considerably during the elementary school years (Winne, 2017). Defining words becomes a regular part of classroom discourse, and children increase their knowledge of syntax as they study and talk about the components of sentences such as subjects and verbs (Crain, 2012).

Children also make progress in understanding how to use language in culturally appropriate ways—pragmatics (Papafragou, 2018). By the time they enter adolescence, most children know the rules for the use of language in everyday contexts—that is, what is appropriate to say and what is inappropriate to say.

Reading One model identifies five stages in the development of reading skills (Chall, 1979) (see Figure 7). The age boundaries are approximate and do not apply to every child, but the stages convey a sense of the developmental changes involved in learning to read.

Before learning to read, children learn to use language to talk about things that are not present; they learn what a word is; and they learn how to recognize sounds and talk about them (Berko Gleason & Ratner, 2017). If they develop a large vocabulary, their path to reading is eased. Children who begin elementary school with a small vocabulary are at risk when it comes to learning to read (Berko Gleason & Ratner, 2017).

Vocabulary development plays an important role in reading comprehension (Reutzel & Cooter, 2018). For example, in one longitudinal study, vocabulary at 19 months predicted reading comprehension at 12 years (Suggate & others, 2018). Having a good vocabulary helps readers access word meaning effortlessly.

Analyses by Rich Mayer (2008) focused on the cognitive processes a child needs to go through in order to read a printed word. In his view, the three processes are (1) being aware of sound units in words, which consists of recognizing phonemes; (2) decoding words, which involves converting printed words into sounds; and (3) accessing word meaning, which consists of finding a mental representation of a word's meaning.

What are the most effective ways to teach children how to read? Education and language experts continue to debate how children should be taught to read. Currently, debate focuses on the phonics approach versus the whole-language approach (Fox, 2012; Reutzel & Cooter, 2013; Vacca & others, 2012).

The **phonics approach** emphasizes that reading instruction should focus on teaching basic rules for translating written symbols into sounds. Early reading instruction should involve simplified materials. Only after children have learned the correspondence rules that relate spoken phonemes to the alphabet letters that represent them should they be given complex reading materials, such as books and poems (Fox, 2012).

By contrast, the **whole-language approach** stresses that reading instruction should parallel children's natural language learning. Reading materials should be whole and meaningful. That is, children should be given material in its complete form, such as stories and poems, so that they learn to understand language's communicative function. Reading should be connected with listening and writing skills. Although there are variations in whole-language programs, most share the premise that reading should be integrated with other skills and subjects, such as science and social studies, and that it should focus on real-world material. Thus, a class might read newspapers, magazines, or books, and then write about and discuss them. In some whole-language classes, beginning readers are taught to recognize whole words or even entire sentences, and to use the context of what they are reading to guess at unfamiliar words.

Which approach is better? Early in development, a strong foundation for oral language (for example, vocabulary) is important for building pre-reading skills. Then phonics becomes important, and later, comprehension and language knowledge become important again as children put things together. It is not that either phonics or whole language is necessarily more important but rather a developmental sequence where one is more important than the other at different times in development.

Beyond the phonics/whole language issue in learning to read, becoming a good reader includes learning to read fluently (Jamshidifarsani & others, 2019). Many beginning or poor readers do not recognize words automatically. Their processing capacity is consumed by the demands of word recognition, so they have less capacity to devote to comprehension of groupings of words as phrases or sentences. As their processing of words and passages becomes more automatic, it is said that their reading becomes more *fluent* (Swain, Leader-Janssen, & Conley, 2017). Metacognitive strategies, such as learning to monitor one's reading progress, getting the gist of what is being read, and summarizing also are important in becoming a good reader (Winne, 2017).

Reading, like other important skills, takes time and effort. In a national assessment, children in the fourth grade had higher scores on a national reading test when they read 11 or more pages daily for school and homework (National Assessment of Educational Progress, 2000) (see Figure 8). Teachers who required students to read a great deal on a daily basis had students who were more proficient at reading than teachers who required little reading by their students.

Writing Children's writing emerges out of their early scribbles, which appear at around 2 to 3 years of age. In early childhood, children's motor skills usually develop to the point that they can begin printing letters. Most 4-year-olds can print their first name. Five-year-olds can reproduce letters and copy several short words. They gradually learn to distinguish the

developmental **connection**

Conditions, Diseases, and Disorders

Dyslexia is a severe impairment in the ability to read and spell; dysgraphia is a severe impairment in handwriting ability. Connect to "Schools and Achievement."

phonics approach An educational approach emphasizing that reading instruction should focus on teaching the basic rules for translating written symbols into sounds.

whole-language approach An educational approach stressing that reading instruction should parallel children's natural language learning. Reading materials should be whole and meaningful.

Children most at risk for reading difficulties in the first grade are those who began school with less verbal skill, less phonological awareness, less letter knowledge, and less familiarity with the basic purposes and mechanisms of reading.

—CATHERINE SNOW
Harvard University

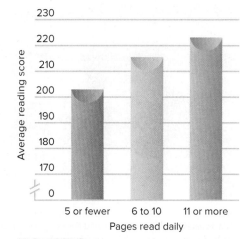

FIGURE **8**

THE RELATION OF READING ACHIEVEMENT TO NUMBER OF PAGES READ DAILY. In the analysis of reading in the fourth grade in the National Assessment of Educational Progress (2000), reading more pages daily in school and as part of homework assignments was related to higher scores on a reading test in which scores ranged from 0 to 500.

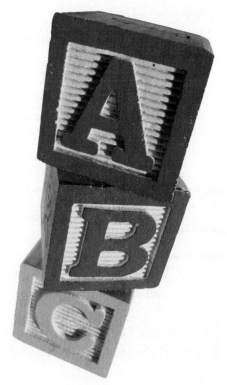

Comstock/PunchStock/Getty Images

distinctive characteristics of letters, such as whether the lines are curved or straight, open or closed. During the early elementary grades, many children continue to reverse letters such as *b* and *d* and *p* and *q* (Feldgus, Cardonick, & Gentry, 2017). At this age, if other aspects of the child's development are normal, letter reversals do not predict literacy problems.

As they begin to write, children often invent spellings. Usually they base these spellings on the sounds of words they hear (Ouellette & Sénéchal, 2017). Parents and teachers should encourage children's early writing but not be overly concerned about letter formation or spelling.

Like becoming a good reader, becoming a good writer takes many years and lots of practice (Feldgus, Cardonick, & Gentry, 2017). Children should be given many writing opportunities in the elementary and secondary school years (Graham, Harris, & Chambers, 2016). As their language and cognitive skills improve with good instruction, so will their writing skills. For example, developing a more sophisticated understanding of syntax and grammar serves as an underpinning for better writing (Graham & Harris, 2018).

Equally important are cognitive skills such as organization and logical reasoning. As they go through elementary, middle, and high school, students develop increasingly sophisticated methods of organizing their ideas. In early elementary school, they narrate and describe or write short poems. In late elementary and middle school, they move to projects such as book reports that combine narration with more reflection and analysis. In high school, they become more skilled at forms of exposition that do not depend on narrative structure (Conley, 2008). A meta-analysis (use of statistical techniques to combine the results of studies) revealed that the following interventions were the most effective in improving fourth- through twelfth-grade students' writing quality: (1) strategy instruction, (2) summarization, (3) peer assistance, and (4) setting goals (Graham & Perin, 2007).

The metacognitive strategies needed to be a competent writer are linked with those required to be a competent reader because the writing process involves competent reading and rereading during composition and revision (Feldgus, Cardonick, & Gentry, 2017). Further, researchers have found that strategy instruction in planning, drafting, revising, and editing improves older elementary school children's metacognitive awareness and writing competence (Graham & Harris, 2018).

As with reading, teachers play a critical role in students' development of writing skills (Adger, Snow, & Christian, 2018). Classroom observations made by Michael Pressley and his colleagues (2007) indicate that students become good writers when teachers spend considerable time on writing instruction and are passionate about teaching students to write. Their observations also indicate that classrooms with students who receive high scores on writing assessments have walls that overflow with examples of effective writing, whereas it is much harder to find such examples on the walls of classrooms that have many students who receive low scores on writing assessments.

Bilingualism and Second-Language Learning   Many different scenarios account for how and when children learn two or more languages. Some people learn a first language and then a second language later in life. Others learn two languages from birth. Are there sensitive periods in learning a second language? That is, if individuals want to learn a second language, how important is the age at which they begin to learn it? For many years, it was claimed that if individuals did not learn a second language prior to puberty, they would never reach native-language-learners' proficiency in the second language (Johnson & Newport, 1991). However, research indicates a more complex conclusion: Sensitive periods likely vary across different language systems (Frankenhuis & Fraley, 2017). Thus, for late language learners, such as adolescents and adults, new vocabulary is easier to learn than new sounds or new grammar (DeKeyser, 2018). For example, children's ability to pronounce words with a native-like accent in a second language typically decreases with age, with an especially sharp drop occurring after the age of about 10 to 12. Also, adults tend to learn a second language faster than children, but their final level of second-language attainment is not as high as children's. And the way children

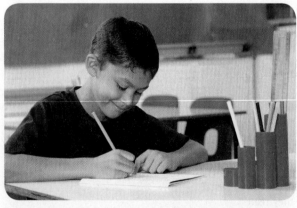

Beverly Gallagher, a third-grade teacher in Princeton, New Jersey, works with students to stimulate their interest in writing. She created the Imagine the Possibilities program, which brings nationally known poets and authors to her school. She phones each student's parents periodically to describe their child's progress and new interests. She invites students from higher grades to work with small groups in her class so that she can spend more one-on-one time with students. Each of her students keeps a writer's notebook to record thoughts, inspirations, and special words that intrigue them. Students get special opportunities to sit in an author's chair, where they read their writing to the class. (*Source: USA Today,* 2000)

Darrin Henry/Shutterstock

and adults learn a second language differs somewhat. Compared with adults, children are less sensitive to feedback, less likely to use explicit strategies, and more likely to learn a second language from a large amount of input (Thomas & Johnson, 2008).

Some aspects of children's ability to learn a second language are transferred more easily to the second language than others (Culpeper, Mackey, & Taguchi, 2018). Children who are fluent in two languages perform better than their single-language counterparts on tests of control of attention, concept formation, analytical reasoning, inhibition, cognitive flexibility, cognitive complexity, and cognitive monitoring (Bialystok, 2018). They also are more conscious of the structure of spoken and written language and better at noticing errors of grammar and meaning, skills that benefit their reading ability (Bialystok, 2018). Vocabulary size in bilingual children is related to a number of factors, including metalinguistic awareness and whether they have a preference for one language over the other (Altman, Goldstein, & Armon-Lotem, 2018).

Students in the United States are far behind their counterparts in many developed countries in learning a second language. For example, schools in Russia have 10 grades, called *forms,* that correspond roughly to the 12 grades in American schools. Children begin school at age 7 in Russia and begin learning English in the third form. Because of this emphasis on teaching English, most Russian citizens under the age of 40 today are able to speak at least some English. The United States is the only technologically advanced Western nation that does not require foreign language study in high school, even for students in rigorous academic programs.

In the United States, many immigrant children go from being monolingual in their home language to bilingual in that language and in English, only to end up monolingual speakers of English. This is called subtractive bilingualism, and it can have negative effects on children if they become ashamed of their home language.

A current controversy related to English Language Learners (ELLs) involves the most effective way of teaching children whose primary language is not English and who are enrolled in U.S. schools (Gonzalez, 2009; Oller & Jarmulowicz, 2010). To read about the work of one teacher of ELLs, see the *Connecting with Careers* profile of Salvador Tamayo, and for a discussion of the debate about teaching ELLs, read the *Connecting with Diversity* interlude that follows.

developmental connection

Cognitive Theory

According to Piaget, at 11 to 15 years of age a new stage—formal operational thought—emerges that is characterized by thinking that is more abstract, idealistic, and logical. Connect to "Cognitive Developmental Approaches."

connecting with careers

Salvador Tamayo, Teacher of English Language Learners

Salvador Tamayo teaches English Language Learners (ELLs) in the fifth grade at Indian Knoll Elementary School in West Chicago. In 2000, he received a National Educator Award from the Milken Family Foundation for his ELL work at Turner Elementary School in West Chicago. Tamayo is especially adept at integrating technology into his ELL classes. He and his students created several award-winning websites about the West Chicago City Museum, the local Latino community, and the history of West Chicago. His students also developed an "I Want to Be an American Citizen" websites to assist family and community members in preparing for the U.S. Citizenship Test. Tamayo also teaches a class in ELL instruction at Wheaton College.

For more information about what elementary school teachers do, see the Careers in Child Development appendix.

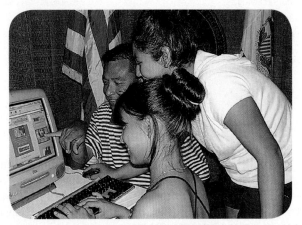

Salvador Tamayo working with English Language Learners.
Courtesy of Salvador Tamayo

English Language Learners

What is the best way to teach English language learners? ELLs have been taught in one of two main ways: (1) instruction in English only, or (2) a *dual-language* (formerly called *bilingual*) approach that involves instruction in their home language and English (Kuo & others, 2017). In a dual-language approach, instruction is given in both the ELL child's home language and English for varying amounts of time at certain grade levels. One of the arguments in favor of the dual-language approach is the research discussed earlier demonstrating that bilingual children have more advanced information-processing skills than monolingual children (Bialystok, 2018).

If a dual-language strategy is used, too often it has been thought that immigrant children need only one or two years of this type of instruction. However, a longitudinal study of immigrant children in the Los Angeles public schools found that most children needed four to seven years to become proficient in a new language and that even after nine years, one-fourth of students were not yet considered fully proficient (Thompson, 2015). Importantly, bilingualism has been found to narrow gaps in executive functioning and self-regulation otherwise found between children from higher versus lower socioeconomic backgrounds (Hartanto, Toh, & Yang, 2018). Thus, especially for immigrant children from low socioeconomic backgrounds, more years of dual-language instruction may be needed than they currently are receiving.

What have researchers found regarding outcomes of ELL programs? Drawing conclusions about the effectiveness of ELL programs is difficult because of variations across programs in the number of years they are in effect, type of instruction, quality of schooling other than ELL instruction, teachers, children, and other factors. In research studies comparing English-only versus dual-language programs, dual-language programs have shown benefits for students' academic achievement above and beyond students' proficiency in English (MacSwan & others, 2017).

Experts generally support the combined home language and English approach because (1) children have difficulty learning a subject when it is taught in a language they do not understand; and (2) when both languages are integrated in the classroom, children learn the second language more readily and participate more actively. Most large-scale studies have found that the academic achievement of ELLs is higher in dual-language programs than English-only programs (MacSwan & others, 2017).

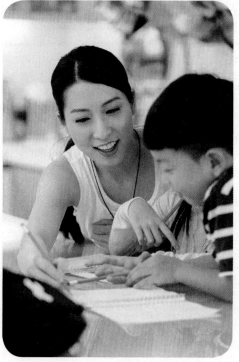

A first- and second-grade English-Cantonese teacher instructing ELL students in Chinese in Oakland, California. *What have researchers found about the effectiveness of ELL instruction?*
RichLegg/E+/Getty Images

You learned that immigrant children who come from lower-socioeconomic-status (SES) backgrounds typically have a more difficult time learning English. What did you learn about SES and vocabulary development in the Connecting Through Research *interlude earlier in this chapter? What research questions are suggested by comparing these findings?*

ADOLESCENCE

Language development during adolescence includes increased sophistication in the use of words (Berman, 2017). With an increase in abstract thinking, adolescents are much better than children at analyzing the function a word performs in a sentence.

Adolescents also develop more subtle abilities with words. They make strides in understanding **metaphor,** which is an implied comparison between unlike things. For example, individuals "draw a line in the sand" to indicate a nonnegotiable position; a political campaign is said to be "a marathon, not a sprint"; a person's faith is "shattered." And adolescents become better able to understand and to use **satire,** which is the use of irony, derision, or wit to expose folly or wickedness. Caricatures are an example of satire. More advanced logical thinking also allows adolescents, from about 15 to 20 years of age, to understand complex literary works.

metaphor An implied comparison between two unlike things.

satire The use of irony, derision, or wit to expose folly or wickedness.

Most adolescents are also much better readers and writers than children are. As indicated in Figure 7, many adolescents increase their understanding of material told from different perspectives, which allows them to engage in more sophisticated discussions of various topics. In terms of writing, they are better at organizing ideas before they write, at distinguishing between general and specific points as they write, at stringing together sentences that make sense, and at organizing their writing into an introduction, body, and concluding remarks.

Everyday speech changes during adolescence, and "part of being a successful teenager is being able to talk like one" (Berko Gleason, 2005, p. 9). Young adolescents often speak a **dialect** with their peers that is characterized by jargon and slang (Cave, 2002). A dialect is a variety of language that is distinguished by its vocabulary, grammar, or pronunciation. For example, when meeting a friend, instead of saying hello, a young adolescent might say, "Hey, dude, 'sup?" Nicknames that are satirical and derisive ("Stilt," "Refrigerator," "Spaz") also characterize the dialect of young adolescents. Such labels might be used to show that one belongs to the group and to reduce the seriousness of a situation (Cave, 2002).

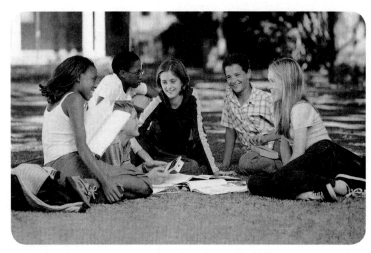

What are some changes in language development in adolescence?
Digital Vision/Flying Colours Ltd/Punchstock/Getty Images

dialect A variety of language that is distinguished by its vocabulary, grammar, or pronunciation.

Review Connect Reflect

LG2 Describe how language develops.

Review

- What are some key milestones of language development during infancy?
- How do language skills change during early childhood?
- How does language develop in middle and late childhood?
- How does language develop in adolescence?

Connect

- Which of the teaching strategies inspired by Vygotsky's theory would you say is related to the whole-language approach discussed in this section?

Reflect *Your Own Personal Journey of Life*

- How many languages can you speak and read? If and when you have children, do you want them to learn more than one language while they are young? Explain.

Biological and Environmental Influences

LG3 Discuss the biological and environmental contributions to language development.

Biological Influences   Environmental Influences   An Interactionist View of Language

We have described how language develops, but we have not explained what makes this amazing development possible. Everyone who uses language in some way "knows" its rules and has the ability to create an infinite number of words and sentences. Where does this knowledge come from? Is it the product of biology? Or is language learned and influenced by experiences?

BIOLOGICAL INFLUENCES

Some language scholars view the remarkable similarities in how children acquire language all over the world, despite the vast variation in language input they receive, as strong

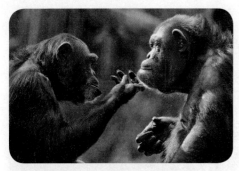

In the wild, chimps communicate through calls, gestures, and expressions, which evolutionary psychologists believe might be the roots of true language.

Patrick Rolands/Shutterstock

Broca's area An area of the brain's left frontal lobe that is involved in speech production and grammatical processing.

Wernicke's area An area of the brain's left hemisphere that is involved in language comprehension.

aphasia A disorder resulting from brain damage to Broca's area or Wernicke's area that involves a loss or impairment of the ability to use or comprehend words.

language acquisition device (LAD) Chomsky's term that describes a biological endowment enabling children to detect the features and rules of language, including phonology, syntax, and semantics.

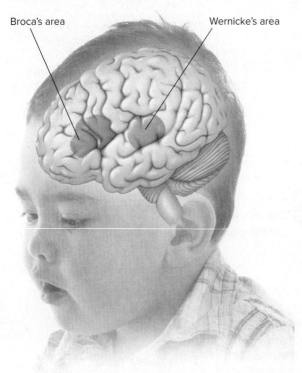

Broca's area   Wernicke's area

FIGURE 9

BROCA'S AREA AND WERNICKE'S AREA. Broca's area is located in the frontal lobe of the brain's left hemisphere, and it is involved in the control of speech. Wernicke's area is a portion of the left hemisphere's temporal lobe that is involved in understanding language. *How does the role of these areas of the brain relate to lateralization?*

Photo: Swissmacky/Shutterstock

evidence that language has a biological basis. What role did evolution play in the biological foundations of language?

Evolution and the Brain's Role in Language   The ability to speak and understand language requires a certain vocal apparatus as well as a nervous system with certain capabilities. The nervous system and vocal apparatus of humanity's predecessors changed over hundreds of thousands or millions of years. With advances in the nervous system and vocal structures, Homo sapiens went beyond the grunting and shrieking of other animals to develop speech. Although estimates vary, many experts believe that humans acquired language about 100,000 years ago, which in evolutionary time represents a very recent acquisition. It gave humans an enormous edge over other animals and increased the chances of human survival (Arbib, 2017).

Brain-imaging studies show that language depends on networks connecting different regions of the brain (Alemi & others, 2018). Two regions involved in language were first discovered in studies of brain-damaged individuals: **Broca's area,** an area in the left frontal lobe of the brain involved in speech production and grammatical processing, and **Wernicke's area,** a region of the brain's left hemisphere involved in language comprehension (see Figure 9). Damage to either of these areas produces types of **aphasia,** which is a loss or impairment of language processing. Individuals with damage to Broca's area have difficulty producing words correctly; individuals with damage to Wernicke's area have poor comprehension and often produce fluent but incomprehensible speech.

Chomsky's Language Acquisition Device (LAD)   Linguist Noam Chomsky (1957) proposed that humans are biologically prewired to learn language at a certain time and in a certain way. He said that children are born into the world with a **language acquisition device (LAD),** a biological endowment that enables the child to detect certain features and rules of language, including phonology, syntax, and semantics. Children are prepared by nature with the ability to detect the sounds of language, for example, and to follow rules such as how to form plurals and ask questions.

Chomsky's LAD is a theoretical construct, not a physical part of the brain. Is there evidence for the existence of a LAD? Supporters of the LAD concept cite the uniformity of language milestones across languages and cultures, evidence that children create language even in the absence of well-formed input, and biological substrates of language. But as we will see, critics argue that even if infants have something like a LAD, it cannot explain the whole story of language acquisition.

ENVIRONMENTAL INFLUENCES

Decades ago, behaviorists opposed Chomsky's hypothesis and argued that language represents nothing more than chains of responses acquired through reinforcement (Skinner, 1957). A baby happens to babble "Ma-ma"; Mama rewards the baby with hugs and smiles; the baby says "Mama" more and more. Bit by bit, said the behaviorists, the baby's language is built up. According to behaviorists, language is a complex, learned skill, much like playing the piano or dancing.

The behavorial view of language learning has several problems. First, it does not explain how people create novel sentences—sentences that people have never heard or spoken before. Second, children learn the syntax of their native language even if they are not reinforced for doing so. Social psychologist Roger Brown (1973) spent long hours observing parents and their young children. He found that parents did not directly or explicitly reward or correct the syntax of most children's utterances. That is, parents did not say "good," "correct," "right," "wrong," and so on. Also, parents did not offer direct corrections such as "You should say two shoes, not two shoe." However, as we will see shortly, many parents do expand on their young children's grammatically incorrect utterances and recast many of those that have grammatical errors (Brito, 2017).

The behavioral view is no longer considered a viable explanation of how children acquire language. But a great deal of research describes ways in which children's environmental experiences influence their language skills (Berko Gleason & Ratner, 2017). Many language experts argue that a child's experiences, the particular language to be learned, and the context in which learning takes place can strongly influence language acquisition (Brito, 2017).

Language is not learned in a social vacuum. Most children are bathed in language from a very early age (Kuhl, 2017). The Wild Boy of Aveyron, who never learned to communicate effectively, had lived in social isolation for years. The support and involvement of caregivers and teachers greatly facilitate a child's language learning (Morgan, 2019). For example, one study found that when mothers immediately smiled and touched their 8-month-old infants after they babbled, the infants subsequently made more complex speech-like sounds than when mothers responded to their infants in a random manner (Goldstein, King, & West, 2003) (see Figure 10). Furthermore, in a study of mother-infant dyads in 11 countries, mothers and infants responded contingently to one another so that infants were more likely to vocalize immediately after their mothers finished speaking to them, and mothers were more likely to speak to their infants immediately after infants finished vocalizing (Bornstein & others, 2015).

Michael Tomasello (2018) stresses that young children are intensely interested in their social world and that early in their development they can understand the intentions of other people. His interaction view of language emphasizes that children learn language in specific contexts. For example, when a toddler and a father are jointly focused on a book, the father might say, "See the birdie." In this case, even a toddler understands that the father intends to name something and knows to look in the direction of the pointing. Through this kind of joint attention, early in their development children are able to use their social skills to acquire language (Moberg & others, 2017).

One intriguing component of the young child's linguistic environment is **child-directed speech,** language spoken in a higher pitch than normal with simple words and sentences (Peter & others, 2016). It is hard to use child-directed speech when not in the presence of a baby. As soon as you start talking to a baby, though, you shift into child-directed speech. Much of this is automatic and something most parents are not aware they are doing. As mentioned previously in this chapter, even 4-year-olds speak in simpler ways to 2-year-olds than to their 4-year-old friends. Child-directed speech has the important function of capturing the infant's attention and maintaining communication (Spinelli, Fasolo, & Mesman, 2017).

Adults often use strategies other than child-directed speech to enhance the child's acquisition of language, including recasting, expanding, and labeling:

- **Recasting** is rephrasing something the child has said, perhaps turning it into a question or restating the child's immature utterance in the form of a fully grammatical sentence. For example, if the child says, "The dog was barking," the adult can respond by asking, "When was the dog barking?" Effective recasting lets the child indicate an interest and then elaborates on that interest.

- **Expanding** is restating, in a linguistically sophisticated form, what a child has said. For example, a child says, "Doggie eat," and the parent replies, "Yes, the doggie is eating."

- **Labeling** is identifying the names of objects. Young children are continually being asked to identify the names of objects. Roger Brown (1958) called this "the original word game" and claimed that much of a child's early vocabulary is motivated by this adult pressure to identify the words associated with objects.

Parents use these strategies naturally and in meaningful conversations. Parents do not (and should not) use any deliberate method to teach their children to talk, even for children who are slow in learning language. Children usually benefit when parents guide their children's discovery of language rather than overloading them with language; "following in order to lead" helps a child learn language. If children are not ready to take in some information, they are likely to tell you (perhaps by turning away). Thus, giving the child more information is not always better. Children's language acquisition also benefits from adults' undivided attention. In an experimental study in which mothers were asked to teach their 2-year-old two new words in a laboratory setting, children did not learn the new word in a condition that was interrupted by a cell phone call placed

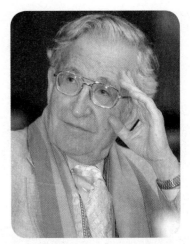

MIT linguist Noam Chomsky. *What is Chomsky's view of language?*
Deshakalyan Chowdhury/AFP/Stringer/Getty Images

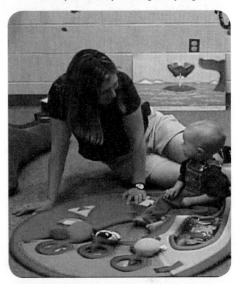

FIGURE **10**

SOCIAL INTERACTION AND BABBLING. One study focused on two groups of mothers and their 8-month-old infants (Goldstein, King, & West, 2003). One group of mothers was instructed to smile and touch their infants immediately after the babies cooed and babbled; the other group was also told to smile and touch their infants but in a random manner, unconnected to sounds the infants made. The infants whose mothers immediately responded in positive ways to their babbling subsequently made more complex, speechlike sounds, such as "da" and "gu." The research setting for this study, which underscores how important caregivers are in the early development of language, is shown here.
Michael Goldstein

child-directed speech Language spoken in a higher pitch than normal, with simple words and sentences.

recasting Rephrasing a statement that a child has said, perhaps turning it into a question, or restating a child's immature utterance in the form of a fully grammatical utterance.

expanding Restating, in a linguistically sophisticated form, what a child has said.

labeling Identifying the names of objects.

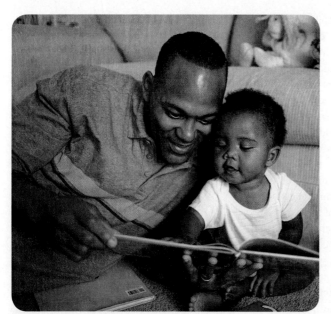

What is shared reading and how might it benefit infants and toddlers?
Elyse Lewin/Brand X Pictures/Getty Images

by the experimenter but did learn the new word in the uninterrupted condition, even though the mothers said the new words the same number of times in both conditions (Reed, Hirsh-Pasek, & Golinkoff, 2017).

Infants, toddlers, and young children benefit when adults read books to and with them (shared reading) (Gilkerson, Richards, & Topping, 2017). Daily reading to infants at 6 months predicts better vocabulary comprehension and production, cognition, and socioemotional competence at 12 months (O'Farrelly & others, 2018). Shared reading is especially beneficial for children's language acquisition because adults use more diverse vocabulary and more complex syntax when reading than in everyday conversation (Demir-Lira & others, 2019).

Although there is debate about the nature of linguistic input to which low-income children are exposed (Sperry, Sperry, & Miller, 2018), the bulk of the research suggests that low-income children are exposed to less language overall as well as to less of the kinds of language that promote school readiness and academic achievement (Golinkoff & others, 2019). To read further about ways that parents can facilitate children's language development, see *Caring Connections.*

Our discussion of environmental influences on language development has mainly focused on parents. However, children interact with many other people who can influence their language development, including teachers and peers. A study of dual-language and English-only learners in kindergarten showed that peers' vocabulary diversity and syntactic complexity influenced the vocabulary diversity and syntactic complexity of their classmates (Gámez & others, 2019).

AN INTERACTIONIST VIEW OF LANGUAGE

If language acquisition depended only on biology, then Genie and the Wild Boy of Aveyron (discussed earlier in the chapter) should have talked without difficulty. A child's experiences influence language acquisition. But we have seen that language does have strong biological foundations (Arbib, 2017). No matter how much you converse with a dog, it won't learn to talk. In contrast, children are biologically prepared to learn language. Children all over the world acquire language milestones at about the same time and in about the same order. However, there are cultural variations in the type of support given to children's language development. For example, caregivers in the Kaluli culture prompt young children to use a loud voice and particular morphemes that direct the speech act performed (calling out) and to refer to names, kinship relations, and places where there has been a shared past experience that indicates a closeness to the person being addressed (Roque & Schieffelin, 2018).

> The linguistics problems children have to solve are always embedded in personal and interpersonal contexts.
>
> —LOIS BLOOM
> *Contemporary psychologist, Columbia University*

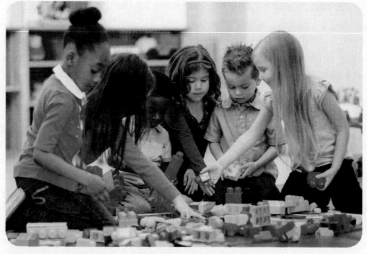

How might peers' language skills influence a child's language development?
FatCamera/E+/Getty Images

How Parents Can Facilitate Infants' and Toddlers' Language Development

Linguist Naomi Baron (1992) in *Growing Up with Language,* and more recently Ellen Galinsky (2010) in *Mind in the Making,* provided ideas to help parents facilitate their infants' and toddlers' language development. A summary of their ideas follows:

- *Be an active conversational partner.* Talk to your baby from the time it is born. Initiate conversation with the baby. If the baby is in a day-long child-care program, ensure that the baby receives adequate language stimulation from adults.

- *Talk in a slowed-down pace and don't worry about how you sound to other adults when you talk to your baby.* Talking in a slowed-down pace helps babies detect words in the sea of sounds they experience. Babies enjoy and attend to the high-pitched sound of child-directed speech.

- *Use parent-look and parent-gesture, and name what you are looking at.* When you want your child to pay attention to something, look at it and point to it. Then name it—for example, by saying "Look, Alex, there's an airplane."

- *When you talk with infants and toddlers, be simple, concrete, and repetitive.* Don't try to talk to them in abstract, high-level ways and think you have to say something new or different all of the time. Using familiar words often will help them remember the words.

- *Play games.* Use word games like peek-a-boo and pat-a-cake to help infants learn words.

- *Remember to listen.* Since toddlers' speech is often slow and laborious, parents are often tempted to supply words and thoughts for them. Be patient and let toddlers express themselves, no matter how painstaking the process is or how great a hurry you are in.

- *Expand and elaborate language abilities and horizons with infants and toddlers.* Ask questions that encourage answers other than "Yes" and "No." Actively repeat, expand, and recast the utterances. Your toddler might say, "Dada." You could follow with, "Where's Dada?", and then you might continue, "Let's go find him."

- *Adjust to your child's idiosyncrasies instead of working against them.* Many toddlers have difficulty pronouncing words and making themselves understood. Whenever possible, make toddlers feel that they are being understood.

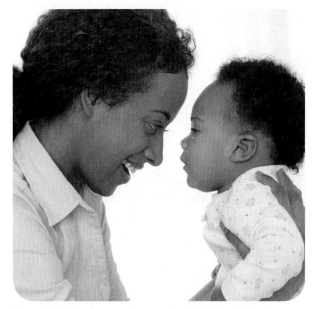

It is a good idea for parents to begin talking to their babies at the start. The best language teaching occurs when the talking is begun before the infant becomes capable of intelligible speech. *What are some other guidelines for parents to follow in helping their infants and toddlers develop their language skills?*
Tetra Images/Getty Images

- *Resist making normative comparisons.* Be aware of the ages at which your child reaches specific milestones (such as the first word, first 50 words), but do not measure this development rigidly against that of other children. Such comparisons can bring about unnecessary anxiety.

Based on what you read earlier in this section of the chapter, would parents be wise to combine these strategies here with deliberate methods to teach their children to talk?

An interactionist view emphasizes that both biology and experience contribute to language development (Sinha, 2017). This interaction of biology and experience can be seen in the variations in the acquisition of language. Children vary in their ability to acquire language, and this variation cannot be readily explained by differences in environmental input alone. However, virtually every child benefits enormously from opportunities to talk and be talked with. Children whose parents and teachers provide them with a rich verbal environment show many positive outcomes (Pace & others, 2017). Parents and teachers who pay attention to what children are trying to say, expand children's utterances, read to them, and label things in the environment, are providing valuable, if unintentional, benefits (Golinkoff & others, 2019).

LG3 Discuss the biological and environmental contributions to language development.

Review

- What are the biological foundations of language?
- What are the behavioral and environmental aspects of language?
- How does an interactionist view describe language?

Connect

- In this section, you learned about two areas in the left hemisphere of the brain that are involved in speech production and recognition. Related to this, what have you learned about hemisphere specialization in infants?

Reflect *Your Own Personal Journey of Life*

- If and when you become a parent, how should you respond to your child's grammatical mistakes when conversing with the child? Will you allow the mistakes to continue and assume that your young child will grow out of them, or will you closely monitor your young child's grammar and correct mistakes whenever you hear them? Explain.

Language and Cognition   Evaluate how language and cognition are linked.

As a teenager, Wendy Verougstraete felt that she was on the road to becoming a professional author. "You are looking at a professional author," she said. "My books will be filled with drama, action, and excitement. And everyone will want to read them. I am going to write books, page after page, stack after stack."

Overhearing her remarks, you might have been impressed not only by Wendy's optimism and determination, but also by her expressive verbal skills. In fact, at a young age Wendy showed a flair for writing and telling stories. Wendy has a rich vocabulary, creates lyrics for love songs, and enjoys telling stories. You probably would not be able to immediately guess that she has an IQ of only 49 and cannot tie her shoes, cross the street by herself, read or print words beyond the first-grade level, or do even simple arithmetic.

Wendy Verougstraete has Williams syndrome, a genetic birth disorder that was first described in 1961 and affects about 1 in 7,500 births (Cashon & others, 2016). Williams syndrome stems from a genetic deletion on chromosome 7 (Lew & others, 2017). The most noticeable features of the syndrome include a unique combination of expressive verbal skills with an extremely low IQ and limited visuospatial skills and motor control (Cashon & others, 2016). Children with Williams syndrome are natural-born storytellers who provide highly expressive narratives (Rossi & Giacheti, 2017). Figure 11 shows the great disparity in the verbal and motor skills of one person with Williams syndrome. Individuals with Williams syndrome often have good emotion recognition and interpersonal skills (Ibernon, Touchet, & Pochon, 2018). One study indicated that children with Williams syndrome performed as well as typically developing children at recognizing six emotions through facial expressions (Ibernon, Touchet, & Pochon, 2018). The syndrome also includes a number of physical characteristics as well, such as heart defects and a pixie-like facial appearance. Despite having excellent verbal skills and competent interpersonal skills, most individuals with Williams syndrome cannot live independent lives (Copes, Pober, & Terilli, 2016). For example, Wendy Verougstraete lives in a group home for adults who are have an intellectual disability.

The verbal abilities of individuals with Williams syndrome are very distinct from those shown by individuals with Down syndrome, an organic intellectual disability (Ibernon, Touchet, & Pochon, 2018). On vocabulary tests, children with Williams syndrome show a liking for unusual words. When asked to name as many animals as they can think of in one minute, Williams children come up with creatures like ibex, chihuahua, saber-toothed tiger, weasel, crane, and newt. Children with Down syndrome give simple examples like dog, cat, and mouse. When children with Williams syndrome tell stories, their voices come alive with drama and emotion, punctuating the dialogue with audience attention-grabbers like "gadzooks" or "lo and behold!" By contrast, children with Down syndrome tell very simple stories with little emotion.

Aside from being an interesting genetic disorder, Williams syndrome offers insights into the normal development of thinking and language (Rossi & Giacheti, 2017). In our society, verbal ability is generally associated with high intelligence. But Williams syndrome raises the possibility that thinking and language might not be so closely related. Williams disorder is due to a defective gene that seems to protect expressive verbal ability but not reading and many other cognitive skills (Rossi & Giacheti, 2017). Thus, cases like Wendy Verougstraete's cast some doubt on the general categorization of intelligence as verbal ability and prompt the question, "What is the relationship between thinking and language?"

Two basic and separate issues characterize connections between language and cognition. The first is whether cognition is necessary for language. Although some researchers have noted that certain aspects of language development typically follow mastery of selected cognitive skills in both typically developing children and children with an intellectual disability, it is not clear that language development depends on any specific aspect of cognitive abilities (Perlovsky & Sakai, 2014). Language and cognitive development may occur in parallel but dissociated fashions.

The second issue is whether spoken language is necessary for (or important to) cognition. This issue is addressed by studies of deaf children. On a variety of thinking and problem-solving skills, deaf children perform at the same level as children of the same age who have no hearing problems. Although study habits and use of particular learning strategies differ for children who are deaf or have normal hearing, cognitive capacities themselves do not (Antoñanzas & Lorente, 2017). Thus, based on studies of deaf children, spoken language is not necessary for cognitive development.

There is, however, evidence of links between the cognitive and language worlds of children (Slot & von Suchodoletz, 2018). In a one-year longitudinal study of 3- and 4-year-old German children, growth in language abilities predicted growth in executive functioning and vice versa, although language was a better predictor of the development of executive functioning abilities than executive functioning was of language abilities (Slot & von Suchodoletz, 2018).

One study explored whether four aspects of information-processing skills—memory, representational competence, processing speed, and attention—were related to infants' and young children's language development (Rose, Feldman, & Jankowski, 2009). In this study, memory and representational competence assessed at 12 months of age predicted language at 36 months of age independently of birth status, 12-month language, and 12-month scores on the Bayley Developmental Scales. The dimensions of memory that best predicted language development were recognition and recall but not short-term memory; the dimensions of representation competence that best predicted language development were cross-modal transfer (matching touch to vision) and object permanence. Other research has found that joint attention in infancy is linked to vocabulary development in childhood (Moberg & others, 2017).

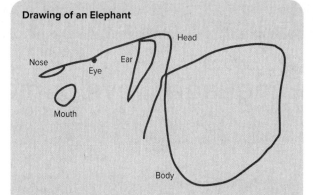

Drawing of an Elephant

Verbal Description of an Elephant

And what an elephant is, it is one of the animals. And what the elephant does, it lives in the jungle. It can also live in the zoo. And what it has, it has long gray ears, fan ears, ears that can blow in the wind. It has a long trunk that can pick up grass, or pick up hay. . . . If they're in a bad mood it can be terrible. . . . If the elephant gets mad it could stomp; it could charge. Sometimes elephants can charge. They have big long tusks. They can damage a car. . . . It could be dangerous. When they're in a pinch, when they're in a bad mood it can be terrible. You don't want an elephant as a pet. You want a cat or a dog or a bird. . . .

FIGURE 11

DISPARITY IN THE VERBAL AND MOTOR SKILLS OF AN INDIVIDUAL WITH WILLIAMS SYNDROME

Review Connect Reflect

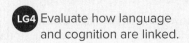 Evaluate how language and cognition are linked.

Review

- What characterizes children with Williams syndrome? To what extent are language and cognition linked? Are they part of a single cognitive system?

Connect

- You have learned that Down syndrome is classified as an intellectual disability. However, Williams syndrome is not classified as an intellectual disability. Why not?

Reflect *Your Own Personal Journey of Life*

- Did you always think in words when you were growing up? Explain.

Language Development

What Is Language?

- Defining Language
- Language's Rule Systems

LG1 Define language and describe its rule systems.

- Language is a form of communication, whether spoken, written, or signed, that is based on a system of symbols. Language consists of all the words used by a community and the rules for varying and combining them. Infinite generativity is the ability to produce an endless number of meaningful sentences using a finite set of words and rules.

- The five main rule systems of language are phonology, morphology, syntax, semantics, and pragmatics. Phonology is the sound system of a language, including the sounds used and the particular sound sequences that may occur in the language. Morphology refers to how words are formed. Syntax is the way words are combined to form acceptable phrases and sentences. Semantics involves the meaning of words and sentences. Pragmatics is the appropriate use of language in different contexts.

How Language Develops

- Infancy
- Early Childhood
- Middle and Late Childhood
- Adolescence

LG2 Describe how language develops.

- Among the milestones in infant language development are crying (birth), cooing (1 to 2 months), babbling (6 months), making the transition from universal linguist to language-specific listener (6 to 12 months), using gestures (8 to 12 months), recognition of their name (as early as 5 months), first word spoken (10 to 15 months), vocabulary spurt (18 months), rapid expansion of understanding words (18 to 24 months), and two-word utterances (18 to 24 months).

- Advances in phonology, morphology, syntax, semantics, and pragmatics continue in early childhood. The transition to complex sentences begins at 2 or 3 years and continues through the elementary school years. Currently, there is considerable interest in the early literacy of children.

- In middle and late childhood, children become more analytical and logical in their approach to words and grammar. One model proposes five stages in reading, ranging from birth/first grade to high school. Current debate involving how to teach children to read focuses on the phonics approach versus the whole-language approach. Researchers have found strong evidence that the phonics approach should be used in teaching children to read, especially in kindergarten and the first grade and with struggling readers, but that children also benefit from the whole-language approach. Children's writing emerges out of scribbling. Advances in children's language and cognitive development provide the underpinnings for improved writing. Strategy instruction is especially effective in improving children's writing. Children who are fluent in two languages have more advanced information-processing skills. Instruction for English language learners (ELLs) has taken one of two main forms: (1) instruction in English only, or (2) dual-language instruction in the child's home language and English. The majority of large-scale research studies have found a higher level of academic achievement when the dual-language approach is used.

- In adolescence, language changes include more effective use of words; improvements in the ability to understand metaphor, satire, and adult literary works; and improvements in writing. Young adolescents often speak a dialect with their peers, using jargon and slang.

Biological and Environmental Influences

 LG3 Discuss the biological and environmental contributions to language development.

Biological Influences

Environmental Influences

An Interactionist View of Language

- In evolution, language clearly gave humans an enormous edge over other animals and increased their chances of survival. A substantial portion of language processing occurs in the brain's left hemisphere, with Broca's area and Wernicke's area being important left-hemisphere locations. Chomsky argues that children are born with the ability to detect basic features and rules of language. In other words, they are biologically equipped to learn language with a prewired language acquisition device (LAD).

- The behavioral view of language acquisition—that children acquire language as a result of reinforcement—is no longer supported. Adults help children acquire language through child-directed speech, recasting, expanding, and labeling. Environmental influences are demonstrated by differences in the language development of children as a consequence of being exposed to different language environments in the home. Parents should talk extensively with an infant, especially about what the baby is attending to.

- An interactionist view emphasizes the contributions of both biology and experience in language.

Language and Cognition

 LG4 Evaluate how language and cognition are linked.

- Children with Williams syndrome have a unique combination of expressive verbal skills with an extremely low IQ and limited visuospatial skills and motor control. Study of these children offers insights into the normal development of thinking and language. Two basic and separate issues are these: (1) Is cognition necessary for language? (2) Is language necessary for cognition? At an extreme, the answer likely is no to these questions, but there is evidence of linkages between language and cognition. Infants' information-processing skills are linked to the growth of language development in early childhood.

key terms

aphasia 262
Broca's area 262
child-directed speech 263
dialect 261
expanding 263
fast mapping 253

infinite generativity 245
labeling 263
language 245
language acquisition device
(LAD) 262
metaphor 260

metalinguistic awareness 256
morphology 246
phonics approach 257
phonology 245
pragmatics 247
recasting 263

satire 260
semantics 246
syntax 246
telegraphic speech 250
Wernicke's area 262
whole-language approach 257

key people

Naomi Baron 265
Jean Berko 251
Roger Brown 262

Noam Chomsky 262
Ellen Galinsky 255
Roberta Golinkoff 252

Betty Hart 254
Kathy Hirsh-Pasek 252
Helen Keller 244

Patricia Kuhl 249
Todd Risley 254

section four

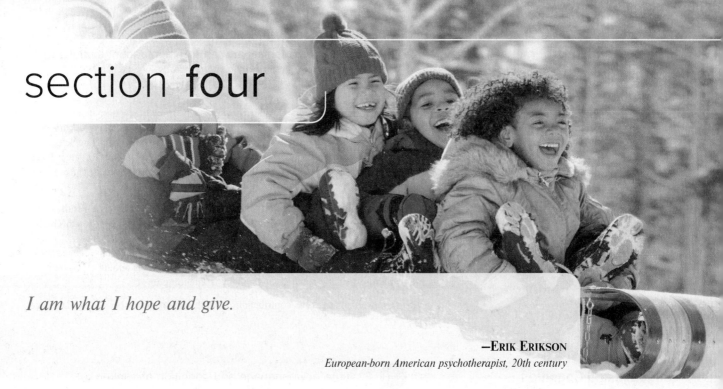

I am what I hope and give.

—**Erik Erikson**
European-born American psychotherapist, 20th century

Ariel Skelley/Blend Images/Getty Images

Socioemotional Development

As children develop, they need the meeting eyes of love. They split the universe into two halves: "me" and "not me." They juggle the need to curb their own will with becoming what they can will freely. They also want to fly but discover that first they have to learn to stand and walk and climb and dance. As they become adolescents, they try on one face after another, looking for a face of their own. In Section 4, you will read four chapters: "Emotional Development," "The Self and Identity," "Gender," and "Moral Development."

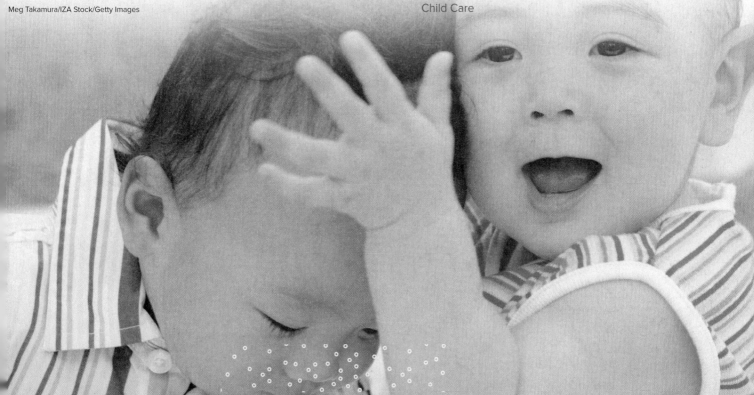

EMOTIONAL DEVELOPMENT

chapter **outline**

Meg Takamura/IZA Stock/Getty Images

Today an increasing number of fathers are staying home to care for their children (Parke & Cookston, 2019). Consider 17-month-old Darius. On weekdays, Darius' father, a writer, cares for him during the day while his mother works full-time as a landscape architect. Darius' father is doing a great job of caring for him. Darius' father keeps Darius nearby while he is writing and spends lots of time talking to him and playing with him. From their interactions, it is clear that they genuinely enjoy each other's company.

Last month, Darius began spending one day a week at a child-care center. His parents carefully selected the center after observing a number of centers and interviewing teachers and center directors. His parents placed him in the center one day a week so Darius could get some experience with peers and his father could have some time out from caregiving.

Darius' father looks to the future and imagines the Little League games Darius will play in and the many other activities he can enjoy with Darius. Remembering how little time his own father spent with him, he is dedicated to making sure that Darius has an involved, nurturing experience with his father.

When Darius' mother comes home in the evening, she spends considerable time with him. Darius has a secure attachment with both his mother and his father.

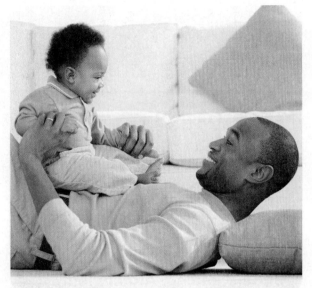

Many fathers are spending more time with their infants today than in the past.
Tetra Images/Getty Images

preview

For many years, emotion was neglected in the study of children's development. Today, emotion is increasingly important in conceptualizations of development. Even infants show different emotional styles, display varying temperaments, and begin to form emotional bonds with their caregivers. In this chapter, we will study the roles of temperament and attachment in development. But first we will examine emotion itself, exploring the functions of emotions in children's lives and the development of emotion from infancy through middle and late childhood.

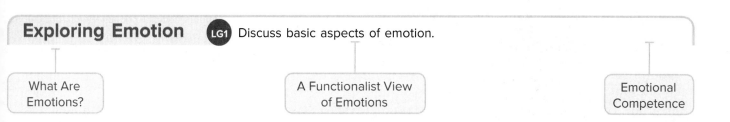

Exploring Emotion **LG1** Discuss basic aspects of emotion.

What Are Emotions?

A Functionalist View of Emotions

Emotional Competence

Imagine your life without emotion. Emotion is the color and music of life, as well as the tie that binds people together. How do psychologists define and classify emotions, and why are they important to development?

WHAT ARE EMOTIONS?

For our purposes, we will define **emotion** as feeling, or affect, that occurs when people are in a state or an interaction that is important to them, especially one that influences their well-being. In many instances emotions involve people's communication with the world. Although emotion consists of more than communication, in infancy the communication aspect is at the forefront of emotion (Walle & others, 2017).

Psychologists classify the broad range of emotions in many ways, but almost all classifications designate an emotion as either positive or negative (Christenfeld & Mandler, 2013; Izard, 2009). Positive emotions include enthusiasm, joy, and love. Negative emotions include anxiety, anger, guilt, and sadness.

Emotions are influenced by biological foundations and experience (Hanford & others, 2018). In evolutionary theory, evolution endowed human beings with a biological foundation for emotion. The biological foundation of emotion involves the development of the nervous system. Emotions are linked with early-developing regions of the human nervous system, including structures of the limbic system and the brain stem (Ng & others, 2018). The capacity of infants to show distress, excitement, and rage reflects the early emergence of these biologically rooted emotional brain systems. Significant advances in emotional responding occur during infancy and childhood as a result of changes in neurobiological systems (including the frontal regions of the cerebral cortex) that can exert control over the more primitive limbic system (Xie, Mallin, & Richards, 2019). As children develop, maturation of the cerebral cortex allows a decrease in unpredictable mood swings and an increase in the self-regulation of emotion. However, such mood swings increase during adolescence, likely as a result of the earlier development of the limbic system, especially the amygdala (which is extensively involved in emotional processing), and the protracted development of the prefrontal cortex (which is heavily involved in reasoning and self-regulation) (Lee, Hollarek, & Krabbendam, 2018).

Social relationships, in turn, provide the setting for the development of a rich variety of emotions (Zachary & others, 2019). When toddlers hear their parents quarreling, they often react with distress and inhibit their play. Members of well-functioning families make each other laugh and may develop a light mood to defuse conflicts.

Blossoms are scattered by the wind And the wind cares nothing, but The blossoms of the heart, No wind can touch.

—YOUSHIDA KENKO
Buddhist monk, 14th century

- - - - - - - - ▶

developmental **connection**

Brain Development

The prefrontal cortex is not as well developed in adolescence as it is in adulthood. For adolescents, it is as if their brain doesn't have the brakes to slow down their emotions. Connect to "Physical Development and Health."

◀ - - - - - - - -

emotion Feeling, or affect, that occurs when people are engaged in an interaction that is important to them, especially one that influences their well-being.

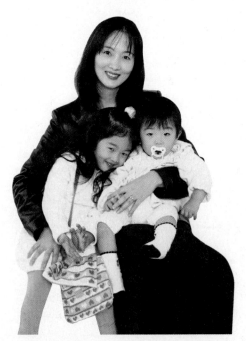

How do Japanese mothers handle their infants' and children's emotional development differently from non-Latino White mothers?

Digital Archive Japan/Alamy Stock Photo

Cultural variations reveal the role of experience in emotion (Savina & Wan, 2017). For example, display rules—when, where, and how emotions should be expressed—are not culturally universal. Researchers have found that East Asian infants display less frequent and less intense positive and negative emotions than non-Latino White infants do (Chen, 2018). Throughout childhood, East Asian parents encourage their children to be emotionally reserved rather than emotionally expressive (Krassner & others, 2017). Further, Japanese parents try to prevent their children from experiencing negative emotions, whereas non-Latino White mothers are more likely to respond after their children become distressed and then help them cope (Cole & Tan, 2007).

Caregivers play a role in the infant's regulation of emotions (Zimmer-Gembeck & others, 2017). For example, by soothing the infant when the infant cries and shows distress, caregivers help infants to modulate their emotion and reduce the level of stress hormones (Gunnar & Hostinar, 2015).

In sum, biological evolution has endowed human beings to be emotional, but culture and relationships with others provide diversity in emotional experiences (Labella, 2018). As we see next, this emphasis on the role of relationships in emotion is at the core of the functionalist view of emotion.

A FUNCTIONALIST VIEW OF EMOTIONS

Many developmentalists today view emotions as the result of individuals' attempts to adapt to specific contextual demands (Raval, Walker, & Daga, 2018). Thus, a child's emotional responses cannot be separated from the situations in which they are evoked. In many instances, emotions are elicited in interpersonal contexts. For example, emotional expressions serve the important functions of signaling to others how one feels, regulating one's own behavior, and playing pivotal roles in social exchange.

One implication of the functionalist view is that emotions are *relational rather than strictly internal, intrapsychic phenomena* (Batki, 2018). Consider just some of the roles of emotion in parent-child relationships. The beginnings of an emotional bond between parents and an infant are based on affectively toned interchanges, as when an infant cries and the caregiver sensitively responds. By the end of the first year, a parent's facial expression—either smiling or fearful—influences whether an infant will explore an unfamiliar environment. When a positive mood has been induced in a child, the child is more likely to comply with a parent's directions.

A second implication of the functionalist view is that emotions are *linked with an individual's goals in a variety of ways* (Tamir, 2016). Regardless of what the goal is, an individual who overcomes an obstacle to attain a goal experiences happiness. By contrast, a person who must relinquish a goal as unattainable experiences sadness. And a person who faces difficult obstacles in pursuing a goal often experiences frustration, which can become anger when the obstacles are perceived as unfair or intentionally put in the way to hinder the individual's goal attainment.

The specific nature of the goal can affect the experience of a given emotion. For example, the avoidance of threat is linked with fear, the desire to atone is related to guilt, and the wish to avoid the scrutiny of others is associated with shame.

EMOTIONAL COMPETENCE

Previously, we briefly described the concept of emotional intelligence. Here we will examine a closely related concept, emotional competence, that focuses on the adaptive nature of emotional experience. Becoming emotionally competent involves developing a number of skills in social contexts (Camras & Halberstadt, 2017). Figure 1 describes these skills and provides examples of each one. As children acquire these emotional competence skills in a variety of contexts, they are more likely to effectively manage their emotions, become resilient in the face of stressful circumstances, and develop more positive relationships.

developmental **connection**

Intelligence

Emotional intelligence involves perceiving and expressing emotions accurately, understanding emotion and possessing emotional knowledge, using feelings to facilitate thought, and managing emotions effectively. Connect to "Intelligence."

Skill	Example
Awareness of one's emotional states	Being able to differentiate whether sad or anxious
Detecting others' emotions	Understanding when another person is sad rather than afraid
Using the vocabulary of emotion terms in socially and culturally appropriate ways	Appropriately describing a social situation in one's culture when a person is feeling distress
Empathic and sympathetic sensitivity to others' emotional experiences	Being sensitive to others when they are feeling distressed
Recognizing that inner emotional states do not have to correspond to outer expressions	Recognizing that one can feel very angry yet manage one's emotional expression so that it appears more neutral
Adaptively coping with negative emotions by using self-regulatory strategies that reduce the intensity or duration of such emotional states	Reducing anger by walking away from an aversive situation and engaging in an activity that takes one's mind off of the aversive situation
Awareness that the expression of emotions plays a major role in a relationship	Knowing that expressing anger toward a friend on a regular basis is likely to harm the friendship
Viewing oneself overall as feeling the way one wants to feel	Feeling like one can cope effectively with the stress in one's life and feeling that one is doing this successfully

FIGURE 1
EMOTIONAL COMPETENCE SKILLS

Review Connect Reflect

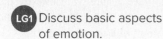 Discuss basic aspects of emotion.

Review
- How is emotion defined?
- What characterizes functionalism in emotion?
- What constitutes emotional competence?

Connect
- How are the competence skills listed in Figure 1 related to the four aspects of emotional intelligence?

Reflect *Your Own Personal Journey of Life*
- Think back to your childhood and adolescent years. How would you describe your emotional competence as a child and adolescent, based on the descriptions in Figure 1?

Development of Emotion

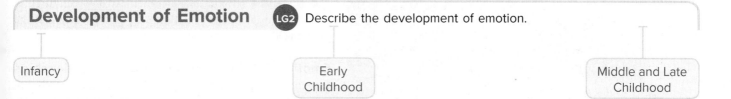 Describe the development of emotion.

Infancy · Early Childhood · Middle and Late Childhood

Does an older child's emotional life differ from a younger child's? Does a young child's emotional life differ from an infant's? Does an infant even have an emotional life? In this section, we will sketch an overview of the changes in emotion from infancy through late childhood, looking not only at changes in emotional experience but also at the development of emotional competence.

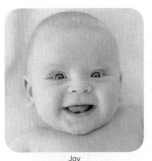
Joy

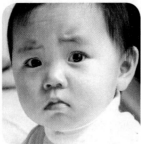
Sadness

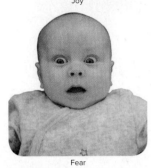
Fear

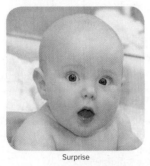
Surprise

FIGURE 2

EXPRESSION OF DIFFERENT EMOTIONS IN INFANTS
(Joy) Kozak_O_O/Shutterstock; (Sadness) Jill Braaten/McGraw Hill Companies (Fear) Stanislav/Shutterstock; (Surprise) Photodisc Collection/EyeWire/Getty Images

primary emotions Emotions that are present in humans and other animals, and emerge early in life; examples are joy, anger, sadness, fear, and disgust.

self-conscious emotions Emotions that require self-awareness, especially consciousness and a sense of "me"; examples include jealousy, empathy, and embarrassment.

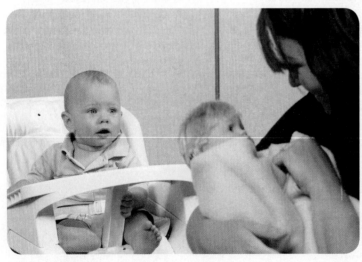

FIGURE 3

IS THIS THE EARLY EXPRESSION OF JEALOUSY? In the study by Hart and Carrington (2002), the researchers concluded that the reactions of the 6-month-old infants who observed their mothers giving attention to a baby doll may indicate the early appearance of jealousy because of the negative emotions—such as anger and sadness— they displayed. However, experts on emotional development, such as Joseph Campos (2009) and Jerome Kagan (2018) argue that emotions such as jealousy don't appear during the first year. *Why do they conclude that jealousy does not occur in the first year?*
Kenny Braun/Braun Photography

INFANCY

What are some early developmental changes in emotions? What functions do infants' cries serve? When do infants begin to smile?

Early Emotions A leading expert on infant emotional development, Michael Lewis (Lewis, 2014) distinguishes between primary emotions and self-conscious emotions. **Primary emotions** are emotions that are present in humans and other animals; these emotions appear in the first six months of the human infant's development. Primary emotions include surprise, interest, joy, anger, sadness, fear, and disgust (see Figure 2 for infants' facial expressions of some of these early emotions). In Lewis' classification, **self-conscious emotions** require self-awareness that involves consciousness and a sense of "me." Self-conscious emotions include jealousy, empathy, embarrassment, pride, shame, and guilt. Lewis argues that these self-conscious emotions occur for the first time at some point in the second half of the first year through the second year. Some experts on emotion call self-conscious emotions such as embarrassment, shame, guilt, and pride *other-conscious emotions* because they involve the emotional reactions of others when they are generated (Saarni & others, 2006). For example, approval from parents is linked to toddlers beginning to show pride when they successfully complete a task.

Leading researchers such as Joseph Campos (2009) and Michael Lewis (2014) debate how early in the infant and toddler years the emotions that we have described first appear and their sequence. As an indication of the controversy regarding when certain emotions first are displayed by infants, consider jealousy. Some researchers argue that jealousy does not emerge until approximately 18 months of age (Lewis, 2014), whereas others emphasize that it is displayed much earlier (Hart, 2018). Consider a research study in which 6-month-old infants observed their mothers giving attention either to a life-like baby doll (hugging or gently rocking it, for example) or to a book (Hart & Carrington, 2002). When mothers directed their attention to the doll, the infants were more likely to display negative emotions, such as anger and sadness, which may have indicated their jealousy (see Figure 3). However, their expressions of anger and sadness may have reflected frustration in not being able to have the novel doll to play with.

Debate about the onset of an emotion such as jealousy illustrates the complexity and difficulty of indexing early emotions. That said, some experts on infant socioemotional development, such as Jerome Kagan (2018), conclude that the structural immaturity of the infant brain makes it unlikely that emotions requiring thought—such as guilt, pride, despair, shame, empathy, and jealousy—can be experienced in the first year. Thus, both Kagan (2018) and Campos (2009) argue that so-called "self-conscious" emotions don't occur until after the first year, which increasingly reflects the view of most developmental psychologists. Thus, in regard to the photograph in Figure 3, it is unlikely that the 6-month-old infant is experiencing jealousy.

Emotional Expression and Social Relationships

Emotional expressions are involved in infants' first relationships. The ability of infants to communicate emotions permits coordinated interactions with their caregivers and the beginning of an emotional bond between them (Broesch & others, 2016). Not only do parents change their emotional expressions in response to infants' emotional expressions, but infants also modify their emotional expressions in response to their parents' emotional expressions. In other words, these interactions are mutually regulated (Kokkinaki & others, 2017). Because of this coordination, the interactions are described as *reciprocal,* or *synchronous,* when all is going well. Sensitive, responsive parents help their infants grow emotionally, whether the infants respond in distressed or happy ways (Zimmer-Gembeck & others, 2017). A meta-analysis of 22 studies found that when parents talked more with young children about mental states, children had a better understanding of emotions (Tompkins & others, 2018).

Crying and smiling are two emotional expressions that infants display when interacting with parents. These are babies' first forms of emotional communication.

Crying Crying is the most important mechanism newborns have for communicating with their world. The first cry verifies that the baby's lungs have filled with air. Cries also may provide information about the health of the newborn's central nervous system. Newborns even tend to respond with cries and negative facial expressions when they hear other newborns cry (Hay, Caplan, & Nash, 2018). Infants as young as 4 months expect unfamiliar adults to respond to a crying baby (Jin & others, 2018).

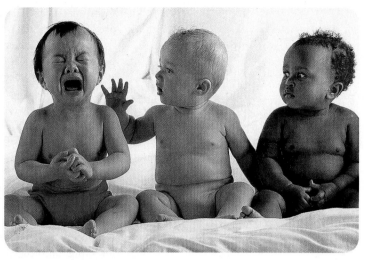

What are some different types of cries?
Andy Cox/The Image Bank/Getty Images

Babies have at least three types of cries:

- **Basic cry:** A rhythmic pattern that usually consists of a cry, followed by a briefer silence, then a shorter whistle that is somewhat higher in pitch than the main cry, then another brief rest before the next cry. Some infancy experts argue that hunger is one of the conditions that incite the basic cry.

- **Anger cry:** A variation of the basic cry in which more excess air is forced through the vocal cords.

- **Pain cry:** A sudden long, initial loud cry followed by breath holding; no preliminary moaning is present. The pain cry is elicited by a high-intensity stimulus.

Most adults can determine whether an infant's cries signify anger or pain (Esposito & others, 2015). Parents can interpret the cries of their own baby better than those of another baby.

Smiling Smiling is critical as a means of developing a new social skill and is a key social signal (Martin & Messinger, 2018). Two types of smiling can be distinguished in infants:

- **Reflexive smile:** A smile that does not occur in response to external stimuli and appears during the first month after birth, usually during sleep.

- **Social smile:** A smile that occurs in response to an external stimulus, typically a face in the case of the young infant. Social smiling occurs as early as 4 to 6 weeks of age in response to a caregiver's voice (Campos, 2005).

Infant smiling follows a predictable developmental course (Martin & Messinger, 2018). From two to six months after birth, infants' social smiling increases considerably, both in self-initiated smiles and smiles in response to others' smiles. At 6 to 12 months of age, smiles that couple what is called the Duchenne marker (eye constriction) and mouth opening occur in the midst of highly enjoyable interactions and play with parents (see Figure 4). In the second year, smiling continues to occur in such positive circumstances with parents, and in many cases an increase in smiling occurs when interacting with peers. Also in the second year, toddlers become increasingly aware of the social meaning of smiles, especially in their relationship with parents.

Infants also engage in *anticipatory smiling,* in which they communicate preexisting positive emotion by smiling at an object and then turning their smile toward an adult. One study revealed that anticipatory smiling at 9 months of age was linked to parents' rating of the child's social competence at 2½ years of age (Parlade & others, 2009).

Fear One of a baby's earliest emotions is fear, which typically first appears at about 6 months of age and peaks at about 18 months. However, abused and neglected infants can show fear as early as 3 months (Witherington & others, 2010). Researchers have

He who binds himself to joy
Does the winged life destroy;
But he who kisses the joy as it
flies; Lives in eternity's sun rise.

—WILLIAM BLAKE
English poet, 19th century

basic cry A rhythmic pattern usually consisting of a cry, a briefer silence, a shorter inspiratory whistle that is higher pitched than the main cry, and then a brief rest before the next cry.

anger cry A cry similar to the basic cry but with more excess air forced through the vocal cords.

pain cry A sudden appearance of loud crying without preliminary moaning, and a long initial cry followed by an extended period of breath holding.

reflexive smile A smile that does not occur in response to external stimuli. It happens during the month after birth, usually during sleep.

social smile A smile in response to an external stimulus, which, early in development, typically is a face.

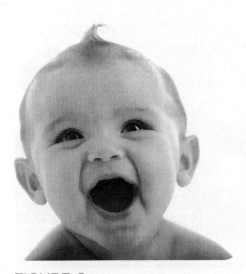

FIGURE 4

A 6-MONTH-OLD'S STRONG SMILE. This strong smile reflects the Duchenne marker (eye constriction) and mouth opening.

JBryson/Getty Images

stranger anxiety An infant's fear of and wariness toward strangers; it tends to appear in the second half of the first year of life.

separation protest Occurs when infants experience a fear of being separated from a caregiver, which results in crying when the caregiver leaves.

found that infant fear is linked to guilt, empathy, and low aggression at 6 to 7 years of age (Rothbart, 2011).

The most frequent expression of an infant's fear involves **stranger anxiety,** in which an infant shows a fear and wariness of strangers. Stranger anxiety usually emerges gradually. It first appears at about 6 months of age in the form of wary reactions. By age 9 months, the fear of strangers is often more intense, and it continues to escalate through the infant's first birthday (Finelli, Zeanah, & Smyke, 2019).

Not all infants show distress when they encounter a stranger. Besides individual variations, whether an infant shows stranger anxiety also depends on the social context, infant temperament, caregiver characteristics, and the characteristics of the stranger (Shapiro, 2018).

Infants show less stranger anxiety when they are in familiar settings. For example, in one study, 10-month-olds showed little stranger anxiety when they met a stranger in their own home but much greater fear when they encountered a stranger in a research laboratory (Sroufe, Waters, & Matas, 1974). Also, infants show less stranger anxiety when they are sitting on their mothers' laps than when they are placed in an infant seat several feet away from their mothers (Bohlin & Hagekull, 1993). Thus, it appears that when infants feel secure, they are less likely to show stranger anxiety.

Who the stranger is and how the stranger behaves also influence stranger anxiety in infants. Infants are less fearful of child strangers than adult strangers. They also are less fearful of friendly, outgoing, smiling strangers than of passive, unsmiling strangers (Bretherton, Stolberg, & Kreye, 1981).

In addition to stranger anxiety, infants experience fear of being separated from their caregivers (Keeton, Schleider, & Walkup, 2017). The result is **separation protest**—crying when the caregiver leaves. Separation protest tends to peak at about 15 months among U.S. infants (Keeton, Schleider, & Walkup, 2017). In fact, one study found that separation protest peaked at about 13 to 15 months in four different cultures (Kagan, Kearsley, & Zelazo, 1978). The percentage of infants who engaged in separation protest varied across cultures, but the infants reached a peak of protest at about the same age—just before the middle of the second year of life.

Emotional Regulation and Coping During the first year of life, the infant gradually develops an ability to inhibit, or minimize, the intensity and duration of emotional reactions (Calkins, 2012). From early in infancy, babies put their thumbs in their mouths to soothe themselves. But at first, infants mainly depend on caregivers to help them soothe their emotions, as when a caregiver rocks an infant to sleep, sings lullabies to the infant, gently strokes the infant, and so on.

The caregivers' actions influence the infant's neurobiological regulation of emotions (Hanford & others, 2018). Infant crying elicits neuropsychological responses in mothers, too, and mothers who are better able to regulate their own emotional responses to their infants' cries are able to respond to infants in more sensitive ways (Firk & others, 2018). A longitudinal study following infants from the age of 10 to 18 months found that infants with mothers who engaged in sensitive caregiving showed better emotion regulation and took longer to become distressed; maternal sensitivity was especially important for infants who showed low or medium levels of sustained attention, suggesting that infants who do not have the internal resources to regulate their emotions especially benefit from external supports (Frick & others, 2018).

In the second year of life, when infants become aroused, they sometimes redirect their attention or distract themselves in order to reduce their arousal (Schoppmann, Schneider, & Seehagen, 2019). By 2 years of age, toddlers can use language to define their feeling states and the context that is upsetting them (Kopp & Neufeld, 2002). A toddler might say, "Feel bad. Dog scare." This type of communication may help caregivers to assist the child in regulating emotion.

Contexts can influence emotional regulation (Easterbrooks & others, 2013). Infants are often affected by fatigue, hunger, time of day, which people are around them, and where they are. Infants must learn to adapt to different contexts that require emotional regulation. Further, new demands appear as the infant becomes older and parents modify their expectations. For example, a parent may take it in stride if a 6-month-old infant screams in a grocery store but may react very differently if a 2-year-old starts screaming.

To soothe or not to soothe—should a crying baby be given attention and soothed, or does this spoil the infant? Many years ago, the behaviorist John Watson (1928) argued that parents spend too much time responding to infant crying. As a consequence, he said, parents reward crying and increase its incidence. However, infancy experts Mary Ainsworth (1979) and John Bowlby (1989) stress the value of responding when infants cry during the first year of life. They argue that a quick, comforting response to the infant's cries is an important ingredient in the development of a strong bond between the infant and caregiver. In one of Ainsworth's studies, infants whose mothers responded quickly when they cried at 3 months of age cried less later in the first year of life (Bell & Ainsworth, 1972).

Controversy still surrounds the question of whether or how parents should respond to an infant's cries, particularly when infants are learning to sleep through the night. However, developmentalists increasingly argue that an infant cannot be spoiled in the first year of life, which suggests that parents should soothe a crying infant. This reaction should help infants develop a sense of trust and secure attachment to the caregiver. When mothers are physiologically aroused and emotionally dysregulated in caregiving situations that are distressing to infants, infants are less likely to develop secure attachment relationships and are at increased risk for developing behavior problems (Leerkes & others, 2017). One study found that problems in infant soothability at 6 months of age were linked to insecure attachment at 12 months of age (Mills-Koonce, Propper, & Barnett, 2012).

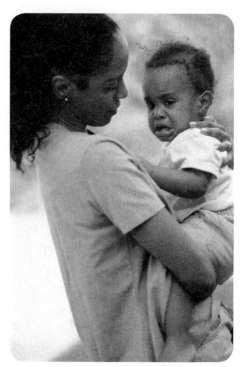

Should a crying baby be given attention and soothed, or does this spoil the infant? Should the infant's age, the type of cry, and the circumstances be considered?
Photodisc Collection/Getty Images

EARLY CHILDHOOD

The young child's growing awareness of self is linked to the ability to feel an expanding range of emotions. Young children, like adults, experience many emotions during the course of a day. At times, they also try to make sense of other people's emotional reactions and to control their own emotions. Parents and peers play important roles in children's emotional development.

Expressing Emotions Recall from our discussion of emotional development in infancy that there is controversy about how early in their development infants experience what Michael Lewis (2014) called *self-conscious emotions.* To experience self-conscious emotions such as pride, shame, embarrassment, and guilt, children must be able to refer to themselves and be aware of themselves as distinct from others (Lewis, 2014). Self-conscious emotions do not appear to develop until self-awareness appears at around 18 months of age.

During the early childhood years, emotions such as pride and guilt become more common. They are especially influenced by parents' responses to children's behavior. For example, a young child may experience shame when a parent says, "You should feel bad about biting your sister." Parents' use of different discipline strategies to invoke shame differs across cultural contexts and is especially common in China (Fung, Li, & Lam, 2017).

Understanding Emotions Among the most important changes in emotional development in early childhood is an increased understanding of emotion (Camras & Halberstadt, 2017). During early childhood, young children increasingly understand that certain situations are likely to evoke particular emotions, that facial expressions indicate specific emotions, that emotions affect behavior, and that emotions can be used to influence others' emotions (Cole & others, 2009). A research meta-analysis revealed that emotion knowledge (such as understanding emotional cues—for example, when a young child understands that a peer feels sad about being left out of a game) was positively related to 3- to 5-year-olds' social competence (such as offering an empathic response to the child left out of a game) and negatively related to their internalizing (high level of anxiety, for example) and externalizing problems (high level of aggressive behavior, for example) (Trentacosta & Fine, 2009). An intervention in which toddlers either participated in conversations about emotions or did not do so after listening to emotion-based stories found that toddlers who participated in the conversations about emotions showed more prosocial behavior following the intervention than did toddlers who did not participate in the emotion conversations (Ornaghi & others, 2017).

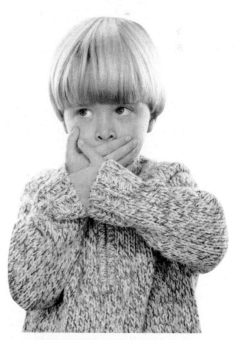

A child expressing the emotion of shame, which occurs when a child evaluates his or her actions as not living up to standards. *Why is shame called a self-conscious emotion?*
James Woodson/Getty Images

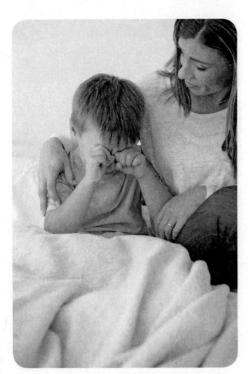

An emotion-coaching parent. *What are some differences between emotion-coaching and emotion-dismissing parents?*
Jamie Grill/Tetra images/Getty Images

Between 2 and 4 years of age, children considerably increase the number of terms they use to describe emotions. During this time, they are also learning about the causes and consequences of feelings (Salmon & others, 2016).

When they are 4 to 5 years of age, children show an increased ability to reflect on emotions. They also begin to understand that the same event can elicit different feelings in different people. Moreover, they show a growing awareness that they need to manage their emotions to meet social standards. And, by 5 years of age, most children can accurately identify emotions that are produced by challenging circumstances and describe strategies they might call on to cope with everyday stress (Cole & others, 2009).

Regulating Emotions   Emotional regulation especially plays a key role in children's ability to manage the demands and conflicts they face in interacting with others (Di Giunta & others, 2017). Many researchers consider the growth of emotional regulation in children to be fundamental to the development of social competence (Camras & Halberstadt, 2017). Emotional regulation can be conceptualized as an important component of self-regulation or of executive function. Recall that executive function is increasingly thought to be a key concept in describing the young child's higher-level cognitive functioning (Merz & others, 2016). Let's explore the roles that parents and peers play in children's emotional regulation.

Parenting and Children's Emotional Development   Parents can play an important role in helping young children regulate their emotions (Zimmer-Gembeck & others, 2017). Depending on how they talk with their children about emotion, parents can be described as taking an *emotion-coaching* or an *emotion-dismissing* approach (Gottman, 2013). The distinction between these approaches is most evident in the way the parent deals with the child's negative emotions (anger, frustration, sadness, and so on). *Emotion-coaching parents* monitor their children's emotions, view their children's negative emotions as opportunities for teaching, assist them in labeling emotions, and coach them in how to deal effectively with emotions. In contrast, *emotion-dismissing parents* view their role as to deny, ignore, or change negative emotions. Emotion-coaching parents interact with their children in a less rejecting manner, use more scaffolding and praise, and are more nurturant than are emotion-dismissing parents (Gottman & DeClaire, 1997). Moreover, the children of emotion-coaching parents are better at soothing themselves when they get upset, more effective in regulating their negative affect, focus their attention better, and have fewer behavior problems than the children of emotion-dismissing parents. Overall, three mechanisms account for how parents influence children's emotions: children's observations of their parents' emotions and emotion regulation, emotion-related parenting practices, and the family's emotional climate (Morris & others, 2017). The pattern of emotion socialization that children receive from both mothers and fathers is related to children's social competence and behavior problems (Miller-Slough & others, 2018).

Parents' knowledge of their children's emotional world can help them to guide their children's emotional development and show them how to cope effectively with problems. Mothers' knowledge about what comforts their children predicts children's ability to cope with distressing situations on their own (Sherman, Grusec, & Almas, 2017).

A problem that parents face is that young children typically don't want to talk about difficult emotional topics, such as being distressed or engaging in negative behaviors. Among the strategies young children use to avoid these conversations is to not talk at all, change the topic, push away, or run away. In one study, Ross Thompson and his colleagues (2009) found that young children were more likely to openly discuss difficult emotional circumstances when they were securely attached to their mother and when their mother conversed with them in a way that validated and accepted the child's views. A number of interventions have been implemented with parents and in early childhood education programs to try to improve children's socioemotional functioning (Britto & others, 2017).

Regulation of Emotion and Peer Relationships   Emotions play a strong role in determining the success of a child's peer relationships (Sette & others, 2018). Specifically, the ability to modulate one's emotions is an important skill that benefits children in their relationships with peers. Moody and emotionally negative children are more likely to experience rejection by their peers, whereas emotionally positive children are more popular (Hernández & others, 2017). Emotional regulation typically increases as children mature. For example, compared with 3-year-olds, 4-year-olds recognize and generate more strategies for controlling their anger (Cole & others, 2009).

MIDDLE AND LATE CHILDHOOD

During middle and late childhood, many children show marked improvement in understanding and managing their emotions (Cole & Jacobs, 2018). However, in some instances, as when they experience stressful circumstances, their coping abilities can be challenged.

Developmental Changes in Emotion   Here are some important developmental changes in emotions during middle and late childhood (Cole & Jacobs, 2018):

- *Improved emotional understanding.* Children in elementary school develop an increased ability to understand complex emotions such as pride and shame. These emotions become less tied to the reactions of other people; they become more self-generated and integrated with a sense of personal responsibility.

- *Increased understanding that more than one emotion can be experienced in a particular situation.* A third-grader, for example, may realize that achieving something might involve both anxiety and joy.

- *Increased tendency to be aware of the events leading to emotional reactions.* A fourth-grader may become aware that her sadness today is influenced by her friend moving to another town last week.

- *Ability to suppress or conceal negative emotional reactions.* A fifth-grader has learned to tone down his anger better than he used to when one of his classmates irritates him.

- *The use of self-initiated strategies for redirecting feelings.* During the elementary school years, children become more reflective about their emotional lives and increasingly use strategies to control their emotions. They become more effective at cognitively managing their emotions, such as by soothing themselves after an upset.

- *A capacity for genuine empathy.* For example, a fourth-grader feels empathy for a distressed person and experiences vicariously the sadness the distressed person is feeling.

Coping with Stress   An important aspect of children's maturation is learning how to cope with stress (Power & Lee, 2018). As children get older, they are able to more accurately appraise a stressful situation and determine how much control they have over it. Older children generate more coping alternatives to stressful conditions and use more cognitive coping strategies (Skinner & Zimmer-Gembeck, 2016). For example, older children are better than younger children at intentionally shifting their thoughts to something that is less stressful. Older children are also better at reframing, or changing their perception of a stressful situation. For example, younger children may be very disappointed that their teacher did not say hello to them when they arrived at school. Older children may reframe this type of situation and think, "She may have been busy with other things and just forgot to say hello."

By 10 years of age, most children are able to use these cognitive strategies to cope with stress (Skinner & Zimmer-Gembeck, 2016). However, in families that have not been supportive or in which children have been exposed to turmoil or trauma, children may be so overwhelmed by stress that they do not use such strategies (Eruyar, Maltby, & Vostanis, 2018).

developmental **connection**

Peers

The combination of being rejected by peers and being aggressive often forecasts problems. Connect to "Peers."

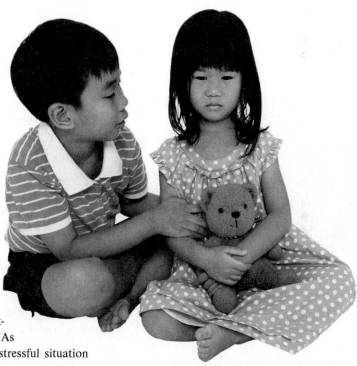

What are some developmental changes in emotion in middle and late childhood?
kdshutterman/Shutterstock

Disasters can especially harm children's development and produce adjustment problems (Acharya, Bhatta, & Assannangkornchai, 2018). Among the outcomes for children who experience disasters are acute stress reactions, depression, panic disorder, and post-traumatic stress disorder (Dorsey & others, 2017). The likelihood that a child will face these problems following a disaster depends on factors such as the nature and severity of the disaster and the type of support available to the child.

Following are descriptions of studies exploring how various aspects of traumatic events and disasters affect children:

- In a study of mothers and their children aged 5 years and younger who were directly exposed to the 9/11 attacks in New York City, the mothers who developed post-traumatic stress disorder (PTSD) and depression were less likely to help their children regulate their emotions and behavior than mothers who were only depressed or only had PTSD (Chemtob & others, 2010). This outcome was linked to their children having anxiety, depression, aggression, and sleep problems.

- A year after the 2015 earthquake in Nepal, 51 percent of children continued to have moderate to severe PTSD symptoms, which were stronger for younger than older children (Acharya, Bhatta, & Assannangkornchai, 2018).

- A research review revealed that children with disabilities are more likely than children without disabilities to live in poverty conditions, which increases their exposure to hazards and disasters (Peek & Stough, 2010). When a disaster occurs, children with disabilities have more difficulty escaping from the disaster.

In research on disasters/trauma, the term *dose-response effects* is often used. A widely supported finding in this research area is that the more severe the disaster/trauma (dose), the worse the adaptation and adjustment (response) following the disaster/trauma (Masten, 2013).

Recommendations for parents, teachers, and other adults caring for children who are involved in disasters and terrorist attacks include the following (Gurwitch & others, 2001, pp. 4-11):

- Reassure children (numerous times, if necessary) of their safety and security.

- Allow children to retell events, and be patient in listening to them.

- Encourage children to talk about any disturbing or confusing feelings, reassuring them that such feelings are normal after a stressful event.

- Protect children from reexposure to frightening situations and reminders of the trauma—for example, by limiting discussion of the event in front of the children.

- Help children make sense of what happened, keeping in mind that children may misunderstand what took place. For example, young children "may blame themselves, believe things happened that did not happen, believe that terrorists are in the school, etc. Gently help children develop a realistic understanding of the event" (p. 10).

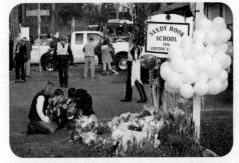

What are some effective strategies to help surviving children cope with traumatic events such as the attack by a gunman at Sandy Hook Elementary School in Connecticut in December 2012, when 26 people—20 of them children—were killed?

Natan Dvir/Polaris/Newscom

Review Connect Reflect

LG2 Describe the development of emotion.

Review

- How does emotion develop in infancy?
- What characterizes emotional development in early childhood?
- What changes take place in emotion during middle and late childhood?

Connect

- In this section, you learned about how children develop the ability to recognize and react appropriately to the emotions of others. How is this ability related to children's theory of mind?

Reflect *Your Own Personal Journey of Life*

- Imagine that you are the parent of an 8-month-old baby and you are having difficulty getting enough sleep because the baby wakes up in the middle of the night crying. How would you deal with this situation?

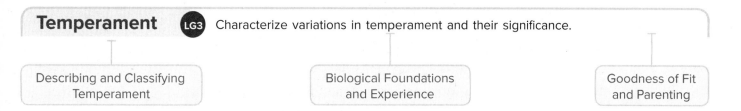
Do you get upset often? Does it take much to get you angry, or to make you laugh? Even at birth, babies seem to have different emotional styles. One infant is cheerful and happy much of the time; another baby seems to cry constantly. These tendencies reflect **temperament,** which involves individual differences in behavioral styles, emotions, and characteristic ways of responding. With regard to its link to emotion, temperament refers to individual differences in how quickly the emotion is shown, how strong it is, how long it lasts, and how quickly it fades away (Campos, 2009).

temperament Involves individual differences in behavioral styles, emotions, and characteristic ways of responding.

DESCRIBING AND CLASSIFYING TEMPERAMENT

How would you describe your temperament or the temperament of a friend? Researchers have described and classified the temperament of individuals in different ways. Here we will examine three of those ways.

Chess and Thomas' Classification   Psychiatrists Alexander Chess and Stella Thomas (Chess & Thomas, 1977; Thomas & Chess, 1991) identified three basic types, or clusters, of temperament:

- An **easy child** is generally in a positive mood, quickly establishes regular routines in infancy, and adapts easily to new experiences.
- A **difficult child** reacts negatively and cries frequently, engages in irregular daily routines, and is slow to accept change.
- A **slow-to-warm-up child** has a low activity level, is somewhat negative, and displays a low intensity of mood.

easy child A temperament style in which the child is generally in a positive mood, quickly establishes regular routines, and adapts easily to new experiences.

difficult child A temperament style in which the child tends to react negatively and cry frequently, engages in irregular daily routines, and is slow to accept new experiences.

slow-to-warm-up child A temperament style in which the child has a low activity level, is somewhat negative, and displays a low intensity of mood.

In their longitudinal investigation, Chess and Thomas found that 40 percent of the children they studied could be classified as easy, 10 percent as difficult, and 15 percent as slow to warm up. Notice that 35 percent did not fit any of the three patterns. Researchers have found that these three basic clusters of temperament are moderately stable across the childhood years. All children benefit from high-quality early child care more than low-quality child care, but child care quality is especially important for children with a difficult temperament (Johnson, Finch, & Phillips, 2019).

Kagan's Behavioral Inhibition   Another way of classifying temperament focuses on the differences between a shy, subdued, timid child and a sociable, extraverted, bold child (Clauss & Blackford, 2012). Jerome Kagan (2002, 2008, 2010, 2013) regards shyness with strangers (peers or adults) as one feature of a broad temperament category called *inhibition to the unfamiliar.* Inhibited children react to many aspects of unfamiliarity with initial avoidance, distress, or subdued affect, beginning at about 7 to 9 months of age.

Kagan has found that inhibition shows considerable stability from infancy through early childhood. One study classified toddlers into extremely inhibited, extremely uninhibited, and intermediate groups (Pfeifer & others, 2002). Follow-up assessments occurred at 4 and 7 years of age. Continuity was demonstrated for both inhibition and lack of inhibition, although a substantial number of the inhibited children moved into the intermediate groups at 7 years of age.

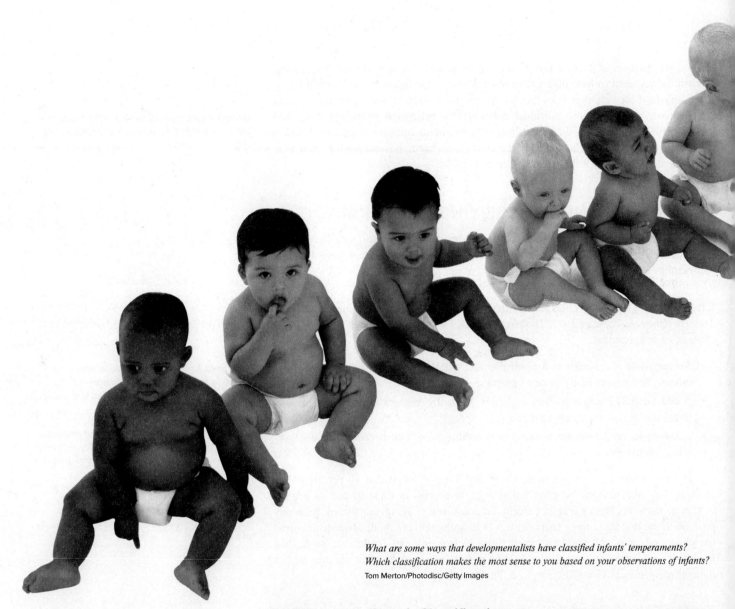

What are some ways that developmentalists have classified infants' temperaments? Which classification makes the most sense to you based on your observations of infants?
Tom Merton/Photodisc/Getty Images

Rothbart and Bates' Classification New classifications of temperament continue to be forged. Mary Rothbart and John Bates (2006) argue that three broad dimensions best represent what researchers have found to characterize the structure of temperament: extraversion/surgency, negative affectivity, and effortful control (self-regulation):

- *Extraversion/surgency* includes "positive anticipation, impulsivity, activity level, and sensation seeking" (Rothbart, 2004, p. 495). Kagan's uninhibited children fit into this category.

- *Negative affectivity* includes "fear, frustration, sadness, and discomfort" (Rothbart, 2004, p. 495). These children are easily distressed; they may fret and cry often. Kagan's inhibited children fit this category. Negative emotional reactivity or irritability reflect the core of Chess and Thomas' category of the difficult child (Bates & Pettit, 2007).

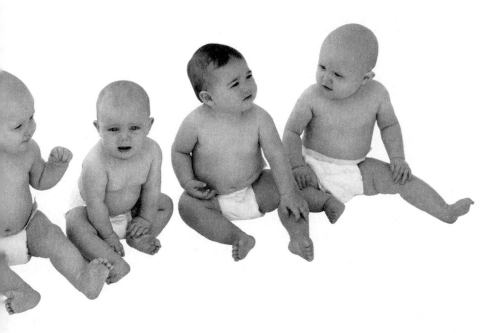

- *Effortful control (self-regulation)* includes "attentional focusing and shifting, inhibitory control, perceptual sensitivity, and low-intensity pleasure" (Rothbart, 2004, p. 495). Infants who are high on effortful control show an ability to keep their arousal from getting too high and have strategies for soothing themselves. By contrast, children low on effortful control are often unable to control their arousal; they become easily agitated and intensely emotional (Bates, McQuillan, & Hoyniak, 2019). Better effortful control at the age of 54 months predicted less externalizing behavior from kindergarten to sixth grade, which was partly accounted for by having fewer conflicts with teachers over that developmental period (Crockett & others, 2018).

In Rothbart's (2004, p. 497) view, "early theoretical models of temperament stressed the way we are moved by our positive and negative emotions or level of arousal, with our actions driven by these tendencies." The more recent emphasis on effortful control, however, underscores the fact that individuals can engage in a more cognitive, flexible approach to stressful circumstances.

An important point about temperament classifications such as those devised by Chess and Thomas and by Rothbart and Bates is that children should not be pigeonholed as having only one temperament dimension, such as "difficult" or "negative affectivity." A good strategy when attempting to classify a child's temperament is to think of temperament as consisting of multiple dimensions (Bates, McQuillan, & Hoyniak, 2019). For example, a child might be extraverted, show little emotional negativity, and have good self-regulation. Another child might be introverted, show little emotional negativity, and have a low level of self-regulation.

Rothbart and Maria Gartstein (2008, p. 323) described the following developmental changes in temperament during infancy. During early infancy, smiling and laughter are emerging as part of the positive affectivity dimension of temperament. Also, by 2 months of age, infants show anger and frustration when their actions don't produce an interesting outcome. During this time, infants often are susceptible to distress and overstimulation. From 4 to 12 months of age fear and irritability become more differentiated, with inhibition (fear) increasingly linked to new and unpredictable experiences. Not all temperament characteristics are in place by the first birthday. Positive emotionality becomes more stable later in infancy, and the characteristics of extraversion/surgency can be determined in the toddler period. Improved attention skills in the toddler and preschool years are related to an increase in effortful control, which serves as a foundation for improved self-regulation.

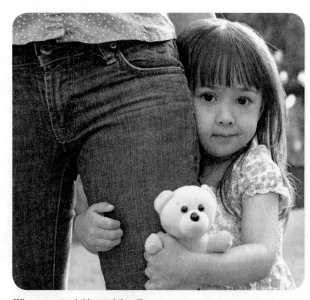

Why are some children inhibited?
Jacqueline Veissid/Getty Images

The developmental changes just described reflect normative capabilities of children, not individual differences in children. The development of these capabilities, such as effortful control, allows individual differences to emerge (Bates, McQuillan, & Hoyniak, 2019). For example, although maturation of the brain's prefrontal lobes must occur for any child's attention to improve and the child to achieve effortful control, some children develop effortful control and others do not. And it is these individual differences in children that are at the heart of what temperament is (Bates, McQuillan, & Hoyniak, 2019).

BIOLOGICAL FOUNDATIONS AND EXPERIENCE

How does a child acquire a certain temperament? Children inherit a physiology that biases them to have a particular type of temperament. However, through experience they may learn to modify their temperament to some degree. For example, children may inherit a physiology that biases them to be fearful and inhibited, but they can learn to reduce their fear and inhibition to some degree.

Biological Influences Physiological characteristics have been linked with different temperaments (Diaz & Bell, 2012; Mize & Jones, 2012). In particular, an inhibited temperament is associated with a unique physiological pattern that includes high and stable heart rate, high level of the hormone cortisol, and high activity in the right frontal lobe of the brain (Kagan, 2003, 2010, 2013). This pattern may be tied to the excitability of the amygdala, a structure of the brain that plays an important role in fear and inhibition (Kagan, 2003, 2010, 2013). An inhibited temperament or negative affectivity may also be linked to low levels of the neurotransmitter serotonin, which may increase an individual's vulnerability to fear and frustration (Brumariu & others, 2016).

What is heredity's role in the biological foundations of temperament? Twin and adoption studies suggest that heredity has a moderate influence on differences in temperament within a group of people (Knopik & others, 2016). The contemporary view is that temperament is a biologically based but evolving aspect of behavior; it evolves as the child's experiences are incorporated into a network of self-perceptions and behavioral preferences that characterize the child's personality (Easterbrooks & others, 2013).

Too often, though, the biological foundations of temperament are interpreted as meaning that temperament cannot develop or change. However, important self-regulatory dimensions of temperament such as adaptability, soothability, and persistence look very different in a 1-year-old and a 5-year-old (Easterbrooks & others, 2013). These temperament dimensions develop and change with the growth of the neurobiological foundations of self-regulation.

Gender, Culture, and Temperament Gender may be an important factor shaping the context that influences the fate of temperament (Hummel & Kiel, 2015). Parents might react differently to an infant's temperament depending on whether the baby is a boy or a girl. For example, in one study, mothers were more responsive to the crying of irritable girls than to the crying of irritable boys (Crockenberg, 1986).

Similarly, the reaction to an infant's temperament may depend in part on culture (Chen & others, 2011; Fung, 2011). For example, an active temperament might be valued in some cultures (such as the United States) but not in other cultures (such as China). And behavioral inhibition is more highly valued in China than in North America (Chen & others, 1998). A comparison of toddler temperament in Chile, Poland, South Korea, and the United States revealed several differences that might be consistent with cultural

developmental **connection**

Research Methods

Twin and adoption studies have been used to sort out hereditary and environmental influences on development. Connect to "Biological Beginnings."

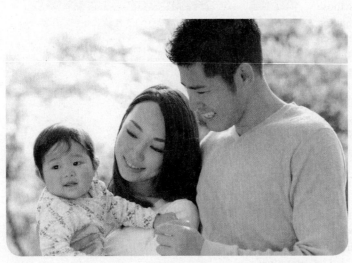

An infant's temperament can vary across cultures. *What do parents need to know about a child's temperament?*

MIXA/Getty Images

values; for example, toddlers in South Korea scored highest on effortful control (Krassner & others, 2017).

Developmental Connections   Do young adults show the same behavioral style and characteristic emotional responses as they did when they were infants or young children? Activity level is an important dimension of temperament. Are children's activity levels linked to their personality in early adulthood? In one longitudinal study, children who were highly active at age 4 were likely to be very outgoing at age 23, which reflects continuity (Franz, 1996). From adolescence into early adulthood, most individuals show fewer emotional mood swings, become more responsible, and engage in less risk-taking behavior, which reflects discontinuity (Shiner, 2019).

Is temperament in childhood linked with adjustment in adulthood? Here is what we know based on the few longitudinal studies that have been conducted on this topic (Shiner, 2019). In one longitudinal study, children who had an easy temperament at 3 to 5 years of age were likely to be well adjusted as young adults (Chess & Thomas, 1977). In contrast, many children who had a difficult temperament at 3 to 5 years of age were not well adjusted as young adults. Also, other researchers have found that boys with a difficult temperament in childhood are less likely as adults to continue their formal education, whereas girls with a difficult temperament in childhood are more likely to experience marital conflict as adults (Wachs, 2000).

Inhibition is another temperament characteristic that has been studied extensively (Bates, McQuillan, & Hoyniak, 2019). A longitudinal study found that greater inhibitory control at 42 months predicted a greater decrease in shyness by the age of 84 months (Eggum-Wilkens & others, 2016). Another study found that fearful inhibition at 2 years of age predicted internalizing behavior problems at age 6, but not if children at age 3 had good inhibitory control or a mother who was low in negative behaviors (Liu, Calkins, & Bell, 2018). And one research study indicated that shy children who had poor cortisol regulation or had mothers who were more likely to endorse non-supportive reactions to their children's behavioral inhibition engaged in more maladaptive play behavior (Davis & Buss, 2012). Also, research indicates that individuals with an inhibited temperament in childhood are less likely as adults to be assertive or to experience social support, and more likely to delay entering a stable job track (Asendorph, 2008). In the Uppsala (Sweden) Longitudinal Study, shyness/inhibition in infancy/childhood was linked to social anxiety at 21 years of age (Bohlin & Hagekull, 2009).

Yet another aspect of temperament involves emotionality and the ability to control one's emotions. In one longitudinal study, when 3-year-old children showed good control of their emotions and were resilient in the face of stress, they were likely to continue to handle emotions effectively as adults (Block, 1993). By contrast, when 3-year-olds had low emotional control and were not very resilient, they were likely to show problems in these areas as young adults.

In sum, these studies reveal some continuity between certain aspects of temperament in childhood and adjustment in early adulthood. However, keep in mind that these connections between childhood temperament and adult adjustment are based on only a small number of studies; more research is needed to verify these linkages (Shiner, 2019).

Developmental Contexts   What accounts for the continuities and discontinuities between a child's temperament and an adult's personality? Physiological and hereditary factors likely are involved in continuity (Kagan, 2008, 2010, 2013). Theodore Wachs (1994, 2000) proposed ways that linkages between temperament in childhood and personality in adulthood might vary depending on the contexts in individuals' experience. Figure 5 summarizes how one characteristic might develop in different ways, depending on the context.

In short, many aspects of a child's environment can encourage or discourage the persistence of temperament characteristics (Bates, McQuillan, & Hoyniak, 2019). One useful way of thinking about these relationships applies the concept of goodness of fit, which we examine next.

developmental **connection**

Culture and Ethnicity

Cross-cultural studies seek to determine culture-universal and culture-specific aspects of development. Connection to "Introduction."

	Child A	Child B
Intervening Context		
Caregivers	Caregivers (parents) who are sensitive and accepting, and who let the child set his or her own pace.	Caregivers who use inappropriate "low-level control" and attempt to force the child into new situations.
Physical Environment	Presence of "stimulus shelters" or "defensible spaces" that the child can retreat to when there is too much stimulation.	Child continually encounters noisy, chaotic environments that allow no escape from stimulation.
Peers	Peer groups include other inhibited children with common interests, so the child feels accepted.	Peer groups consist of athletic extraverts, so the child feels rejected.
Schools	School has sufficient staff, so inhibited children are more likely to be tolerated and feel they can make a contribution.	School is too crowded, so inhibited children are less likely to be tolerated and more likely to feel undervalued.
Personality Outcomes		
	As an adult, individual is closer to extraversion (outgoing, sociable) and is emotionally stable.	As an adult, individual is closer to introversion and has more emotional problems.

FIGURE 5

TEMPERAMENT IN CHILDHOOD, PERSONALITY IN ADULTHOOD, AND INTERVENING CONTEXTS. Varying experiences with caregivers, the physical environment, peers, and schools may modify links between temperament in childhood and personality in adulthood. The example given here is for inhibition.

GOODNESS OF FIT AND PARENTING

goodness of fit The match between a child's temperament and the environmental demands the child must cope with.

Goodness of fit refers to the match between a child's temperament and the environmental demands the child must cope with. Suppose Jason is an active toddler who is made to sit still for long periods of time and Jack is a slow-to-warm-up toddler who is abruptly pushed into new situations on a regular basis. Both Jason and Jack face a lack of fit between their temperament and environmental demands. Lack of fit can produce adjustment problems (Newland & Crnic, 2017).

Some temperament characteristics pose more parenting challenges than others, at least in modern Western societies (Bates, McQuillan, & Hoyniak, 2019). When children are prone to distress, as exhibited by frequent crying and irritability, their parents may eventually respond by ignoring the child's distress or trying to force the child to "behave." In one research study, though, extra support and training for mothers of distress-prone infants improved the quality of mother-infant interaction (van den Boom, 1989). The training led the mothers to alter their demands on the child, improving the fit between the child and the environment. A meta-analysis of 84 studies found that, compared with children with an easy temperament, children with a more difficult temperament were more vulnerable to negative parenting but also benefited more from positive parenting (Slagt & others, 2016).

Many parents don't become believers in temperament's importance until the birth of their second child. They viewed their first child's behavior as a result of how they treated the child. But then they find that some strategies that worked with their first child are not as effective with the second child. Some problems experienced with the first child (such as those involved in feeding, sleeping, and coping with strangers) do not exist with the second child, but new problems arise.

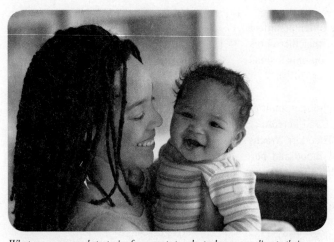

What are some good strategies for parents to adopt when responding to their infant's temperament?
Corbis/age fotostock

Parenting and the Child's Temperament

What are the implications of temperamental variations for parenting? Although answers to this question necessarily are speculative, these conclusions regarding the best parenting strategies to use in relation to children's temperaments were reached by temperament experts Ann Sanson and Mary Rothbart (1995):

- *Attention to and respect for individuality.* One implication is that it is difficult to generate general prescriptions for "good parenting." A goal might be accomplished in one way with one child and in another way with another child, depending on the child's temperament. Parents need to be sensitive to the infant's signals and flexible in adjusting to his or her needs.
- *Structuring the child's environment.* Crowded, noisy environments can pose greater problems for some children (such as a "difficult child") than for others (such as an "easy child"). We might also expect that a fearful, withdrawing child would benefit from slower entry into new contexts.
- *The "difficult child" and packaged parenting programs.* Programs for parents often focus on dealing with children who have "difficult" temperaments, such as children who are irritable, display anger often, and don't follow directions well. Acknowledging that some children are harder than others to parent is often helpful, and advice on how to

handle particular difficult characteristics can be useful. However, whether a particular characteristic is difficult depends on its fit with the environment. To label a child "difficult" has the danger of becoming a self-fulfilling prophecy. If a child is identified as difficult, people may treat the child in a way that actually elicits difficult behavior. One study found that attending publicly funded preschool programs can be especially beneficial for improving school readiness and reducing behavior problems for low-income children with difficult temperaments (Johnson, Finch, & Phillips, 2019).

Too often, we pigeonhole children into categories without examining the context (Bates, McQuillan, & Hoyniak, 2019). Nonetheless, caregivers need to take children's temperaments into account. Research does not yet allow for many highly specific recommendations, but in general, caregivers should (1) be sensitive to the individual characteristics of the child, (2) be flexible in responding to these characteristics, and (3) avoid applying negative labels to the child.

How does the advice to "structure the child's environment" reflect what you learned about the concept of "goodness of fit"?

Such experiences strongly suggest that children differ from each other very early in life, and that these differences have important implications for parent-child interaction (Bates, McQuillan, & Hoyniak, 2019).

To read further about some positive strategies for parenting that take into account the child's temperament, see *Caring Connections.*

Review *Connect* Reflect

 Characterize variations in temperament and their significance.

Review

- How can temperament be described and classified?
- How is temperament influenced by biological foundations and experience?
- What is goodness of fit? What are some positive parenting strategies for dealing with a child's temperament?

Connect

- In this section, you learned that twin and adoption studies suggest that heredity has a moderate influence on

differences in temperament. What have you learned previously about the issues that complicate the interpretation of twin studies?

Reflect *Your Own Personal Journey of Life*

- Consider your own temperament. We described a number of temperament categories. Which one best describes your temperament? Has your temperament changed as you have gotten older? If your temperament has changed, what factors contributed to the changes?

Social Orientation/Understanding, Attachment, and Child Care

LG4 Explain the early development of social orientation/understanding, attachment, and variations in child care.

Social Orientation/Understanding   •   Attachment   •   Fathers and Mothers as Caregivers   •   Child Care

So far, we have discussed how emotions and emotional competence change as children develop. We have also examined the role of emotional style; in effect, we have seen how emotions set the tone of our experiences in life. But emotions also write the lyrics because they are at the core of our interest in the social world and our relationships with others.

SOCIAL ORIENTATION/UNDERSTANDING

As socioemotional beings, infants show a strong interest in their social world and are motivated to orient to it and understand it (Lowe & others, 2016). In earlier chapters, we described many of the biological and cognitive foundations that contribute to the infant's development of social orientation and understanding. We will call attention to relevant biological and cognitive factors as we explore social orientation; locomotion; intention, goal-directed behavior, and cooperation; and social referencing.

Social Orientation   From early in their development, infants are captivated by their social world. As we discussed in our coverage of infant perception, young infants stare intently at faces and are attuned to the sounds of human voices, especially their caregiver's (Lowe & others, 2016). Later, they become adept at interpreting the meaning of facial expressions.

Face-to-face play often begins to characterize caregiver-infant interactions when the infant is about 2 to 3 months of age. The focused social interaction of face-to-face play may include vocalizations, touch, and gestures (Beebe & others (2018). Such play is part of many mothers' motivation to create a positive emotional state in their infants (Thompson, 2013a, d).

In part because of such positive social interchanges between caregivers and infants, by 2 to 3 months of age infants respond to people differently from the way they respond to objects, showing more positive emotion toward people than inanimate objects such as puppets (Legerstee, 1997). At this age, most infants expect people to react positively when the infants initiate a behavior, such as a smile or a vocalization. This finding has been discovered using a method called the still-face paradigm, in which the caregiver alternates between engaging in face-to-face interaction with the infant and remaining still and unresponsive (Qu & Leerkes, 2018). As early as 2 to 3 months of age, infants show more withdrawal, negative emotions, and self-directed behavior when their caregivers are still and unresponsive (Adamson & Frick, 2003). Infants' autonomic nervous system activity changes reliably during both the still-face and recovery period using the still-face paradigm (Jones-Mason & others, 2018). A meta-analysis revealed that infants' higher positive affect and lower negative affect as displayed during the still-face paradigm were linked to secure attachment at 1 year of age (Mesman, van IJzendoorn, & Bakermans-Kranenburg, 2009).

Infants also learn about their social world through contexts other than face-to-face play with a caregiver (Easterbrooks & others, 2013). Even though infants as young as 6 months of age show an interest in each other, their interaction with peers increases considerably in the last half of the second year. Between 18 and 24 months of age, children markedly increase their imitative and reciprocal play, such as imitating nonverbal actions like jumping and running (Kupán & others, 2017). One study involved presenting 1- and 2-year-olds with a simple cooperative task that consisted of pulling handles to activate an attractive musical toy (Brownell, Ramani, & Zerwas, 2006) (see Figure 6). Any coordinated actions of the 1-year-olds appeared to be mostly coincidental rather than cooperative,

developmental connection

Biological, Cognitive, and Socioemotional Processes

Discussing biological, cognitive, and social processes together reminds us of an important aspect of development: These processes are intricately intertwined (Diamond, 2013). Connect to "Introduction."

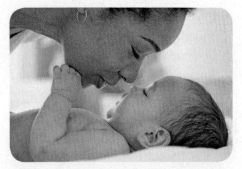

A mother and her baby engaging in face-to-face play. *At what age does face-to-face play usually begin, and when does it typically start decreasing in frequency?*
Tom Grill/JGI/Blend Images/Getty Images

whereas the 2-year-olds' behavior was characterized more as active cooperation to reach a goal. As increasing numbers of U.S. infants experience child care outside the home, they are spending more time in social play with peers (Lamb & Lewis, 2013). Later in the chapter, we will further discuss child care.

Locomotion   Recall from earlier in the chapter how important independence is for infants, especially in the second year of life. As infants develop the ability to crawl, walk, and run, they are able to explore and expand their social world. These newly developed self-produced locomotor skills allow the infant to independently initiate social interchanges on a more frequent basis (Thurman & Corbetta, 2017). The acquisition of these gross motor skills is the result of a number of factors including the development of the nervous system, the goal the infant is motivated to reach, and environmental support for the skill (Adolph & Franchak, 2017).

The infant's and toddler's push for independence also is likely paced by the development of locomotor skills. Locomotion is important for its motivational implications. Once infants have the ability to move in goal-directed pursuits, the reward from these pursuits leads to further efforts to explore and develop skills. In one study, 15-month-olds in a toy-filled room took more steps and covered more ground exploring the room than did infants in a room without toys, who took fewer steps and stayed closer to their caregivers (Hoch, O'Grady, & Adolph, 2018).

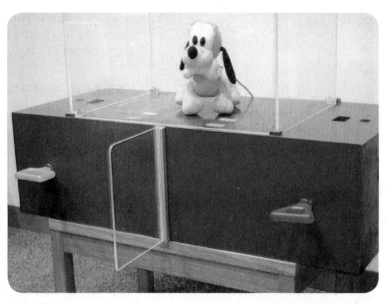

FIGURE 6

THE COOPERATION TASK. The cooperation task consisted of two handles on a box, atop which was an animated musical toy, surreptitiously activated by remote control when both handles were pulled. The handles were placed far enough apart that one child could not pull both handles. The experimenter demonstrated the task, saying, "Watch! If you pull the handles, the doggie will sing" (Brownell, Ramani, & Zerwas, 2006).

Courtesy of Celia A. Brownell, University of Pittsburgh

Intention, Goal-Directed Behavior, and Cooperation   Perceiving people as engaging in intentional and goal-directed behavior is an important social cognitive accomplishment, and this initially occurs toward the end of the first year (Thompson, 2013a, d). Joint attention and gaze following help the infant to understand that other people have intentions (Mateus & others, 2013). Recall that *joint attention* occurs when the caregiver and infant focus on the same object or event. We indicated that emerging aspects of joint attention occur at about 7 to 8 months, but at about 10 to 11 months of age joint attention intensifies and infants begin to follow the caregiver's gaze. By their first birthday, infants have begun to direct the caregiver's attention to objects that capture their interest (Salo, Rowe, & Reeb-Sutherland, 2018).

Social Referencing   Another important social cognitive accomplishment in infancy is developing the ability to "read" the emotions of other people (DeQuinzio & others, 2016). **Social referencing** is the term used to describe "reading" emotional cues in others to help determine how to act in a particular situation. The development of social referencing helps infants to interpret ambiguous situations more accurately, as when they encounter a stranger and need to know whether to fear the person (Walle, Reschke, & Knothe, 2017). By the end of the first year, a mother's facial expression—either smiling or fearful—influences whether an infant will explore an unfamiliar environment.

Infants become better at social referencing in the second year of life. At this age, they tend to "check" with their mother before they act; they look at her to see if she is happy, angry, or fearful. In the second year of life, infants also become more sophisticated in understanding whether adults' emotions are specific to individual attitudes or provide more generalizable information (Hoehl & Striano, 2018).

Infants' Social Sophistication and Insight   In sum, researchers are discovering that infants are more socially sophisticated and insightful at younger ages than was previously envisioned (Thompson, 2013a, d). This sophistication and insight is reflected in infants' perceptions of others' actions as intentionally motivated and goal-directed and

developmental **connection**

Dynamic Systems Theory

Dynamic systems theory is increasingly recognized as an important means of understanding children's development. Connect to "Motor, Sensory and Perceptual Development."

social referencing "Reading" emotional cues in others to help determine how to act in a particular situation.

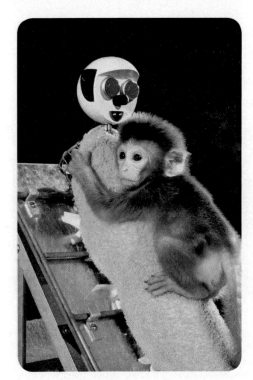

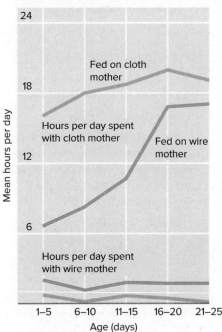

FIGURE 7

CONTACT TIME WITH WIRE AND CLOTH SURROGATE MOTHERS. Regardless of whether the infant monkeys were fed by a wire or a cloth mother, they overwhelmingly preferred to spend contact time with the cloth mother. *How do these results compare with what Freud's theory and Erikson's theory would predict about human infants?*

Martin Rogers/The Image Bank/Getty Images

attachment A close emotional bond between two people.

their motivation to share and participate in that intentionality by their first birthday. The more advanced social cognitive skills of infants could be expected to influence their understanding and awareness of attachment to a caregiver.

ATTACHMENT

What is attachment? **Attachment** is a close emotional bond between two people. Interest in attachment has especially focused on infants and their caregivers.

Theories of Attachment   There is no shortage of theories about why infants become attached to a caregiver. Three theorists—Freud, Erikson, and Bowlby—proposed influential views.

Freud reasoned that infants become attached to the person or object that provides oral satisfaction. For most infants, this is the mother, since she is most likely to feed the infant. Is feeding as important as Freud thought? A classic study by Harry Harlow (1958) reveals that the answer is no (see Figure 7).

Harlow removed infant monkeys from their mothers at birth; for six months they were reared by surrogate (substitute) "mothers." One surrogate mother was made of wire, the other of cloth. Half of the infant monkeys were fed by the wire mother, half by the cloth mother. Periodically, the amount of time the infant monkeys spent with either the wire or the cloth mother was computed. Regardless of which mother fed them, the infant monkeys spent far more time with the cloth mother. Even if the wire mother but not the cloth mother provided nourishment, the infant monkeys spent more time with the cloth mother. And when Harlow frightened the monkeys, those "raised" by the cloth mother ran to the mother and clung to it; those raised by the wire mother did not. Whether the mother provided comfort seemed to determine whether the monkeys associated the mother with security. This study clearly demonstrated that feeding is not the crucial element in the attachment process, and that contact comfort is important. Follow-up studies documented other characteristics of surrogate mothers, such as warm temperature, that could confer comfort and security (Harlow & Suomi, 1970).

Physical comfort also plays a role in Erik Erikson's (1968) view of the infant's development. Recall Erikson's proposal that the first year of life represents the stage of trust versus mistrust. Physical comfort and sensitive care, according to Erikson (1968), are key to establishing a basic trust in infants. The infant's sense of trust, in turn, is the foundation for attachment and sets the stage for a lifelong expectation that the world will be a good and pleasant place to be.

The ethological perspective of British psychiatrist John Bowlby (1969, 1989) also stresses the importance of attachment in the first year of life and the responsiveness of the caregiver. Bowlby points out that both infants and their primary caregivers are biologically predisposed to form attachments. He argues that the newborn is biologically equipped to elicit attachment behavior. The baby cries, clings, coos, and smiles. Later, the infant crawls, walks, and follows the mother. The immediate result is to keep the primary caregiver nearby; the long-term effect is to increase the infant's chances of survival.

Attachment does not emerge suddenly but rather develops in a series of phases, moving from a baby's general preference for human beings to a partnership with primary caregivers. Following are four such phases based on Bowlby's conceptualization of attachment (Schaffer, 1996):

- *Phase 1: From birth to 2 months.* Infants instinctively orient to human figures. Strangers, siblings, and parents are equally likely to elicit smiling or crying from the infant.
- *Phase 2: From 2 to 7 months.* Attachment becomes focused on one figure, usually the primary caregiver, as the baby gradually learns to distinguish familiar from unfamiliar people.
- *Phase 3: From 7 to 24 months.* Specific attachments develop. With increased locomotor skills, babies actively seek contact with regular caregivers, such as the mother or father.

- *Phase 4: From 24 months on.* Children become aware of others' feelings, goals, and plans and begin to take these into account in directing their own actions. Researchers' recent findings that infants are more socially sophisticated and insightful than previously envisioned suggests that some of the characteristics of Bowlby's phase 4, such as understanding the goals and intentions of the attachment figure, appear to be developing in phase 3 as attachment security is taking shape (Thompson, 2008).

Bowlby argued that infants develop an *internal working model* of attachment: a simple mental model of the caregiver, their relationship, and the self as deserving of nurturant care. The infant's internal working model of attachment with the caregiver influences the infant's and later the child's subsequent responses to other people (Fearon & Roisman, 2017). The internal model of attachment also has played a pivotal role in the discovery of links between attachment and subsequent emotion understanding, conscience development, and self-concept (Thompson, 2013a).

In sum, attachment emerges from the social cognitive advances that allow infants to develop expectations for the caregiver's behavior and to determine the affective quality of their relationship (Thompson, 2013a). These social cognitive advances include recognizing the caregiver's face, voice, and other features, as well as developing an internal working model of expecting the caregiver to provide pleasure in social interaction and relief from distress.

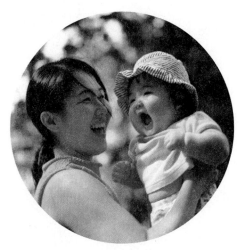

In Bowlby's model, what are the four phases of attachment?
Camille Tokerud/Getty Images

Individual Differences in Attachment   Although attachment to a caregiver intensifies midway through the first year, isn't it likely that the quality of babies' attachment experiences varies? Mary Ainsworth (1979) thought so. Ainsworth created the **Strange Situation,** an observational measure of infant attachment in which the infant experiences a series of introductions, separations, and reunions with the caregiver and an adult stranger in a prescribed order. In using the Strange Situation, researchers hope that their observations will provide information about the infant's motivation to be near the caregiver and the degree to which the caregiver's presence provides the infant with security and confidence.

Based on how babies respond in the Strange Situation, they are described as being securely attached or insecurely attached (in one of three ways) to the caregiver:

- **Securely attached babies** use the caregiver as a secure base from which to explore the environment. When they are in the presence of their caregiver, securely attached infants explore the room and examine toys that have been placed in it. When the caregiver departs, securely attached infants might protest mildly, and when the caregiver returns these infants reestablish positive interaction with her, perhaps by smiling or climbing onto her lap. Subsequently, they often resume playing with the toys in the room.
- **Insecure avoidant babies** show insecurity by avoiding the caregiver. In the Strange Situation, these babies engage in little interaction with the caregiver, are not distressed when she leaves the room, usually do not reestablish contact with her on her return, and may even turn their back on her. If contact is established, the infant usually leans away or looks away.
- **Insecure resistant babies** often cling to the caregiver and then resist her by fighting against the closeness, perhaps by kicking or pushing away. In the Strange Situation, these babies often cling anxiously to the caregiver and don't explore the playroom. When the caregiver leaves, they often cry loudly and push away if she tries to comfort them on her return.
- **Insecure disorganized babies** are disorganized and disoriented. In the Strange Situation, these babies might appear dazed, confused, and fearful. To be classified as disorganized, babies must show strong patterns of avoidance and resistance or display certain specified behaviors, such as extreme fearfulness around the caregiver.

Evaluating the Strange Situation   Does the Strange Situation capture important differences among infants? As a measure of attachment, it may be culturally biased. For example, German and Japanese babies often show patterns of attachment different from those of American infants. As illustrated in Figure 8, German infants are more likely to

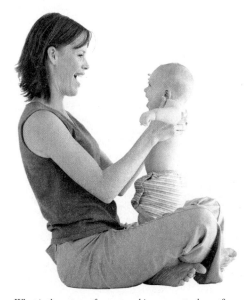

What is the nature of secure and insecure attachment?
George Doyle/Stockbyte/Getty Images

Strange Situation Ainsworth's observational measure of infant attachment to a caregiver, which requires the infant to move through a series of introductions, separations, and reunions with the caregiver and an adult stranger in a prescribed order.

securely attached babies Babies who use the caregiver as a secure base from which to explore the environment.

insecure avoidant babies Babies who show insecurity by avoiding the mother.

insecure resistant babies Babies who might cling to the caregiver, then resist her by fighting against the closeness, perhaps by kicking or pushing away.

insecure disorganized babies Babies who show insecurity by being disorganized and disoriented.

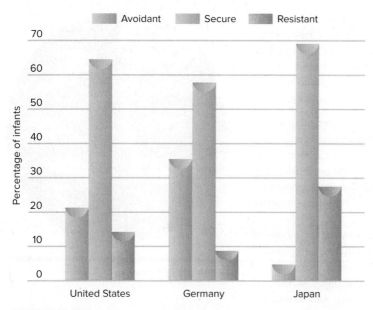

FIGURE 8

CROSS-CULTURAL COMPARISON OF ATTACHMENT. In one study, infant attachment in three countries—the United States, Germany, and Japan—was measured in the Ainsworth Strange Situation (van IJzendoorn & Kroonenberg, 1988). The dominant attachment pattern in all three countries was secure attachment. However, German infants were more avoidant and Japanese infants were less avoidant and more resistant than U.S. infants. *What are some explanations for differences in how German, Japanese, and U.S. infants respond to the Strange Situation?*

Source: van IJzendoorn, M.H., and Kroonenberg, P.M. 1988. Cross-cultural patterns of attachment: A meta-analysis of the Strange Situation. Child Development, 59, 147–156

show an avoidant attachment pattern and Japanese infants are less likely to display this pattern than U.S. infants (van IJzendoorn & Kroonenberg, 1988). The avoidant pattern in German babies likely occurs because their caregivers encourage them to be independent (Grossmann & others, 1985). Also as shown in Figure 8, Japanese babies are more likely than American babies to be categorized as resistant. This may have more to do with the Strange Situation as a measure of attachment than with attachment insecurity itself. Japanese mothers rarely let anyone unfamiliar with their babies care for them. Thus, the Strange Situation might create considerably more stress for Japanese infants than for American infants, who are more accustomed to separation from their mothers (Kondo-Ikemura & others, 2018). Even though there are cultural variations in attachment classification, the most frequent classification in every culture studied so far is secure attachment (Thompson, 2006, 2012; van IJzendoorn & Kroonenberg, 1988).

Some critics stress that behavior in the Strange Situation—like other laboratory assessments—might not indicate what infants would do in a natural environment. But researchers have found that infants' behaviors in the Strange Situation are closely related to how they behave at home in response to separation and reunion with their mothers (Bailey & others, 2017). Thus, many infant researchers conclude that the Strange Situation continues to show merit as a measure of infant attachment.

Interpreting Differences in Attachment   Do individual differences in attachment matter? Ainsworth observes that secure attachment in the first year of life provides an important foundation for psychological development later in life. The securely attached infant moves freely away from the mother but keeps track of where she is through periodic glances. The securely attached infant responds positively to being picked up by others and, when put back down, freely moves away to play. An insecurely attached infant, by contrast, avoids the mother or is ambivalent toward her, fears strangers, and is upset by minor, everyday separations.

If early attachment to a caregiver is important, it should influence a child's social behavior later in development. For many children, early attachments foreshadow later functioning (Woodhouse, 2018). In the extensive longitudinal study conducted by Alan Sroufe and his colleagues (2005; Sroufe, Coffino, & Carlson, 2010), early secure attachment (assessed by the Strange Situation at 12 and 18 months) was linked with positive emotional health, high self-esteem, self-confidence, and socially competent interaction with peers, teachers, camp counselors, and romantic partners through adolescence. Another study found that attachment security at 24 and 36 months was linked to the child's enhanced social problem-solving at 54 months (Raikes & Thompson, 2009). And a meta-analysis revealed that disorganized attachment was more strongly linked to externalizing problems (aggression and hostility, for example) than were avoidant and resistant attachment (Fearon & others, 2010).

Few studies have assessed infants' attachment security to the mother and the father separately. However, one study revealed that infants who were insecurely attached to their mother and father ("double-insecure") at 15 months of age had more externalizing problems (out-of-control behavior, for example) in the elementary school years than their counterparts who were securely attached to at least one parent (Kochanska & Kim, 2013).

An important issue regarding attachment is whether infancy is a critical or sensitive period for development. Many, but not all, research studies reveal the power of infant attachment to predict subsequent development (Fearon & Roisman, 2017). In a meta-analytic review, early attachment predicted social competence with peers, internalizing behaviors such as anxiety, and externalizing behaviors such as aggression, but the researchers suggested that a number of other risk and protective factors could strengthen or attenuate links between early attachment and subsequent development (Groh & others, 2017).

Consistently positive caregiving over a number of years is likely an important factor in connecting early attachment with the child's functioning later in development.

Indeed, researchers have found that early secure attachment and subsequent experiences, especially parental care and life stresses, are linked with children's later behavior and adjustment (Sutton, 2019). For example, a longitudinal study revealed that changes in attachment security/insecurity from infancy to adulthood were linked to stresses and supports in socioemotional contexts (Van Ryzin, Carlson, & Sroufe, 2011). These results suggest that attachment continuity may reflect stable social contexts as much as early working models. The study just described (Van Ryzin, Carlson, & Sroufe, 2011) reflects an increasingly accepted view of the development of attachment and its influence on development. That is, it is important to recognize that attachment security in infancy does not always by itself produce long-term positive outcomes, but rather is linked to later outcomes through connections with the way children and adolescents subsequently experience various social contexts as they develop.

The Van Ryzin, Carlson, and Sroufe (2011) study reflects a **developmental cascade model,** which involves connections across domains over time that influence developmental pathways and outcomes (DePasquale, Handley, & Cicchetti, 2018). Developmental cascades can include connections between a wide range of biological, cognitive, and socioemotional processes (attachment, for example), and also can involve social contexts such as families, peers, schools, and culture. Further, links can produce positive or negative outcomes at different points in development, such as infancy, early childhood, middle and late childhood, adolescence, and adulthood.

Some developmentalists conclude that too much emphasis has been placed on the attachment bond in infancy (Newcombe, 2007). They point out that children can be highly resilient and adaptive, even in the face of wide variations in parenting and other environmental contexts (Masten, 2018). Genetic factors, temperament, and exposure to a wide range of risk and protective factors may play a larger role than attachment in child development. For example, if some infants inherit a low tolerance for stress, this—rather than an insecure attachment bond—may be responsible for an inability to get along with peers. One study found that infants with the short version of the serotonin transporter gene—5-HTTLPR— were prone to distress and wariness but not to insecure attachment (Brumariu & others, 2016).

Another criticism of attachment theory is that it ignores the diversity of socializing agents and contexts that exists in an infant's world. A culture's value system can influence the nature of attachment and what is considered sensitive parenting (Mesman & others, 2016). Mothers' expectations for infants to be independent are high in northern Germany, whereas Japanese mothers are more strongly motivated to keep their infants close to them (Grossmann & others, 1985; Rothbaum & Trommsdorff, 2007). Not surprisingly, northern German infants tend to show less distress than Japanese infants when separated from their mothers. Also, in some cultures, infants show attachments to many people. Among the Hausa (who live in Nigeria), both grandmothers and siblings provide a significant amount of care for infants (Harkness & Super, 1995). Infants in agricultural societies tend to form attachments to older siblings, who are assigned a major responsibility for younger siblings' care. Researchers recognize the importance of competent, nurturant caregivers in an infant's development (Grusec & others, 2013). At issue, though, is whether or not secure attachment, especially to a single caregiver, is critical (Fraley, Roisman, & Haltigan, 2013; Thompson, 2013c, d).

Despite such criticisms, there is ample evidence that security of attachment is important to development (Zimmer-Gembeck & others, 2017). Secure attachment in infancy is important because it reflects a positive parent-infant relationship and provides a foundation that supports healthy socioemotional development in the years that follow.

Caregiving Styles and Attachment   Is the style of caregiving linked with the quality of the infant's attachment? Securely attached babies have caregivers who are sensitive to their signals and are consistently available to respond to their infants' needs (Bohr & others, 2018). These caregivers often let their babies have an active part in determining the onset and pacing of interaction in the first year of life. A review of 687 articles revealed extensive evidence that maternal sensitivity is related to infant attachment and child outcomes (Deans, 2018). Another study found that maternal sensitivity to distress and nondistress when their infant was 6 months old interacted with infant temperament in predicting attachment security at 12 months (Leerkes & Zhou, 2018). Yet another study

developmental cascade model Involves connections across domains over time that influence developmental pathways and outcomes.

developmental **connection**

Nature and Nurture

What is involved in gene-environment (G × E) interaction? Connect to "Biological Beginnings."

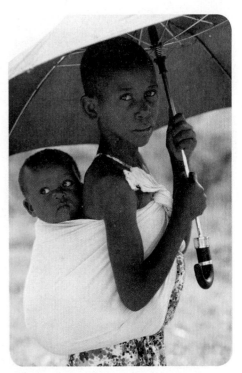

In the Hausa culture, siblings and grandmothers provide a significant amount of care for infants. *How might this practice affect attachment?*
Penny Tweedie/The Image Bank/Getty Images

found that maternal sensitivity in parenting was related to secure attachment in infants in Colombia, Mexico, Peru, and the United States (Posada & others, 2016). Although maternal sensitivity is positively linked to the development of secure attachment in infancy, it is important to note that the link is not especially strong (Campos, 2009).

How do the caregivers of insecurely attached babies interact with them? Caregivers of avoidant babies tend to be unavailable or rejecting (Groh & others, 2019). They often don't respond to their babies' signals and have little physical contact with them. When they do interact with their babies, they may behave in an angry and irritable way. Caregivers of resistant babies tend to be inconsistent; sometimes they respond to their babies' needs, and sometimes they don't. In general, they tend not to be very affectionate with their babies and show little synchrony when interacting with them. Caregivers of disorganized babies often neglect or physically abuse them (Granqvist & others, 2017). In some cases, these caregivers are depressed. In sum, caregivers' interactions with infants influence whether the infants are securely or insecurely attached to them (Leerkes & Zhou, 2018).

So far in our discussion of attachment, we have focused on the importance of secure attachment in infancy and the role of sensitive parenting in attachment (Bohr & others, 2018). Attachment to parents continues to be significantly related to various child outcomes in the middle and late childhood years (Boldt & others, 2016). During middle childhood, children who are securely attached to their parents are better at regulating their emotions (Movahed Abtahi & Kerns, 2017). In addition, secure attachment to parents during middle childhood predicts better school adaptation, social competence with peers, and self-esteem, and fewer behavioral problems (Brumariu & others, 2018). Attachments beyond the immediate family unit also become important during middle and late childhood as children spend more of their time with peers, teachers, and others. In the chapter "Families," you will read about the role of attachment in adolescent development.

Developmental Social Neuroscience and Attachment Earlier, we described the field of developmental social neuroscience that examines connections between socioemotional processes, development, and the brain (Telzer & others, 2018). Attachment is one of the main areas in which theory and research on developmental social neuroscience has focused. These connections of attachment and the brain involve the neuroanatomy of the brain, neurotransmitters, and hormones.

Brain-imaging studies have revealed connections among infants' cues such as crying, mothers' responses, and brain activity (Esposito & others, 2017). In an intervention in which mothers were assigned to either an intervention group to reduce parenting stress or a no-intervention control group, the intervention group showed improvement in areas of the brain involved in social responses, self-awareness, and decision-making (Swain & others, 2017). These brain areas included the precuneus and its functional connectivity with subgenual anterior cingulate cortex and amygdala–temporal pole functional connectivity (Swain & others, 2017).

Research on the role of hormones and neurotransmitters in attachment has emphasized the importance of two neuropeptide hormones—oxytocin and vasopressin—in the formation of the maternal-infant bond (Kohlhoff & others, 2017). Oxytocin, a mammalian hormone that also acts as a neurotransmitter in the brain, is released during breast feeding and by contact and warmth (Bos, 2017). Oxytocin is especially thought to be a likely candidate in the formation of infant-mother attachment (Kohlhoff & others, 2017). Sensitive maternal caregiving is predicted by higher levels of oxytocin, suggesting a biological pathway fostering attachment relationships (Kohlhoff & others, 2017).

The influence of these neuropeptides on the neurotransmitter dopamine in the nucleus accumbens (a collection of neurons in the forebrain that are involved in pleasure) likely is important in motivating approach to the attachment object (Bos, 2017). Figure 9 shows the regions of the brain we have described that are likely to be important in infant-mother attachment.

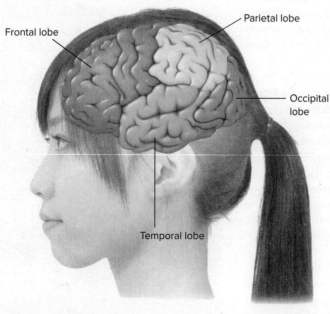

Frontal lobe

Parietal lobe

Occipital lobe

Temporal lobe

FIGURE 9

REGIONS OF THE BRAIN PROPOSED AS LIKELY IMPORTANT IN INFANT-MOTHER ATTACHMENT. This illustration shows the brain's left hemisphere. The corpus callosum is the large bundle of axons that connect the brain's two hemispheres.

Photo: Takayuki/Shutterstock

FATHERS AND MOTHERS AS CAREGIVERS

Much of our discussion of attachment has focused on mothers as caregivers. Do mothers and fathers differ in their caregiving roles?

On average, mothers spend considerably more time in caregiving with infants and children than do fathers (Blakemore, Berenbaum, & Liben, 2009; Shwalb, Shwalb, & Lamb, 2013). Mothers especially are more likely to engage in the managerial role with their children, coordinating their activities, making sure their health care needs are fulfilled, and so on (Parke & Buriel, 2006).

However, an increasing number of U.S. fathers stay home full-time with their children (Livingston, 2018). As indicated in Figure 10, there was a 400-plus percent increase in stay-at-home fathers in the United States from 1996 to 2013. A large proportion of full-time fathers have career-focused wives who provide the main family income. Even when fathers do not stay home with their children full-time, they play many crucial roles in children's development (Cabrera, Volling, & Barr, 2018).

Observations of infants separately interacting with their fathers and their mothers suggest that global measures of attachment security do not differ for fathers and mothers (Fernandes & others, 2018). When fathers are actively involved as caregivers, children are more likely to interact in similar ways with fathers and mothers (McHale & Sirotkin, 2019). Fathers' involvement is predicted by a number of factors including residential status, education, income, beliefs about gender roles, and the quality of the father's relationship with the mother (Macon & others, 2017).

Consider the Aka pygmy culture in Africa, where fathers spend as much time interacting with their infants as do their mothers (Meehan, Hagen, & Hewlett, 2017). Remember, however, that although fathers can be active, nurturant, involved caregivers with their infants as Aka pygmy fathers are, in many cultures men have not chosen to follow this pattern (Lynn, Grych, & Fosco, 2016). As with mothers, if fathers have mental health problems, they may not interact as effectively with their infants. Depressed fathers interact with their infants in ways that are less playful and less engaged, and they touch their infants less than do non-depressed fathers (Sethna & others, 2018).

Do fathers behave differently from mothers with their infants? Maternal interactions usually center on child-care activities—feeding, changing diapers, and bathing. Paternal interactions are more likely to include play (Kuhns & Cabrera, 2018). Fathers engage in more rough-and-tumble play. They bounce infants, throw them up in the air, tickle them, and so on. Mothers do play with infants, but their play is less physical and arousing than that of fathers.

In one study, fathers were interviewed about their caregiving responsibilities when their children were 6, 15, 24, and 36 months of age (NICHD Early Child Care Research Network, 2000). Some of the fathers were videotaped while playing with their children at 6 and 36 months. Fathers were more involved in caregiving—bathing, feeding, dressing the child, taking the child to child care, and so on—when they worked fewer hours and mothers worked more hours, when mothers and fathers were younger, when mothers reported greater marital intimacy, and when the children were boys.

Children benefit when fathers are positively involved in their caregiving. One study of more than 7,000 children who were assessed from infancy to adulthood revealed that those whose fathers were extensively involved in their lives (such as engaging in various activities with them and showing a strong interest in their education) were more successful in school (Flouri & Buchanan, 2004).

CHILD CARE

Many U.S. children today experience multiple caregivers. Most do not have a parent staying home to care for them; instead, the children have some type of care provided by others—"child care." Many parents worry that child care will reduce their infants' emotional attachment to them, interfere with infants' cognitive development, fail to teach them how to control anger, and allow them to be unduly influenced by their peers. How extensive is the use of child care? Are the worries of these parents justified?

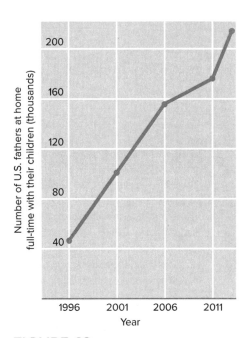

FIGURE **10**

THE INCREASE IN THE NUMBER OF U.S. FATHERS STAYING AT HOME FULL-TIME WITH THEIR CHILDREN

Source: U.S. Government.

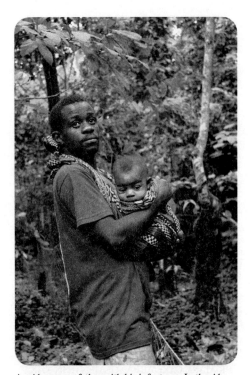

An Aka pygmy father with his infant son. In the Aka culture, fathers were observed to be holding or near their infants 47 percent of the time (Hewlett, 1991).

Nick Greaves/Alamy Stock Photo

Child-Care Policies Around the World

Child-care policies around the world vary (Bartel & others, 2018). Europe led the way in creating new standards of parental leave: The European Union (EU) mandated a paid 14-week maternity leave in 1992. In most European countries today, working parents on leave receive from 70 to 100 percent of their prior wage, and paid leave averages about 16 weeks (Bartel & others, 2018). The United States currently allows workers up to 12 weeks of unpaid leave to care for a newborn, but only if the company has more than 50 employees within a 75-mile radius, which means that many Americans are not eligible for any leave, paid or unpaid.

Most countries restrict eligible benefits to women employed for a minimum time prior to childbirth, but in Denmark, even unemployed mothers are eligible for extended parental leave related to childbirth. In Germany, child-rearing leave is available to almost all parents. The Nordic countries (Denmark, Finland, Iceland, Norway, and Sweden) have extensive gender-equity family leave policies for childbirth that emphasize the contributions of both women and men (Eydal & Rostgaard, 2016). For example, in Sweden, parents can take an 18-month job-protected parental leave with benefits that can be shared by parents and applied to full-time or part-time work.

In light of the data you saw in Figure 11, why might it be helpful if U.S. leave policies were more like those in Scandinavian countries?

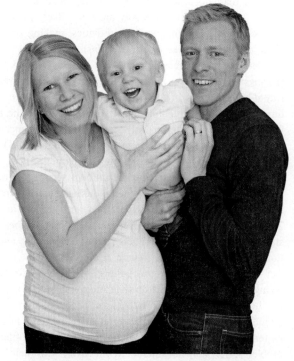

How are child-care policies in many European countries, such as Sweden, different from those in the United States?
Juliana Wiklund/Getty Images

Parental Leave   Today far more young children are in child care than at any other time in history. About 15 million children under the age of 6 years are in child care in the United States (Child Care Aware, 2018). In part, these numbers reflect the fact that U.S. adults cannot receive paid leave from their jobs to care for their young children. However, as described in *Connecting with Diversity,* many countries provide extensive parental leave policies.

Variations in Child Care   Because the United States does not have a comprehensive policy of paid leave for child care, child care in the United States has become a major national concern (Isaacs, Healy, & Peters, 2017). Many factors influence the effects of child care, including the age of the child, the type of child care, how long the child is in child care, and the quality of the program.

Types of child care vary extensively (Bratsch-Hines & others, 2017). Child care is provided in large centers with elaborate facilities and in private homes. Some child-care centers are commercial operations; others are nonprofit centers run by churches, civic groups, and employers. Some child-care providers are professionals; others are untrained adults who want to earn extra money. Figure 11 presents the primary care arrangement for children under 5 years of age with employed mothers (Clarke-Stewart & Miner, 2008).

In the United States, approximately 15 percent of children 5 years of age and younger attend more than one child-care arrangement. Whether and how child-care arrangements are related to children's school readiness and behavioral adjustment

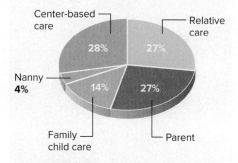

FIGURE **11**

PRIMARY CARE ARRANGEMENTS IN THE UNITED STATES FOR CHILDREN UNDER 5 YEARS OF AGE WITH EMPLOYED MOTHERS

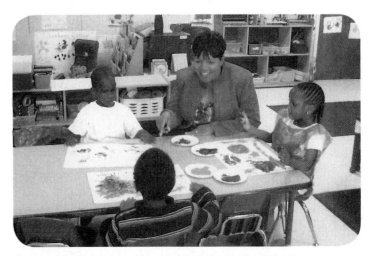
depend on a number of factors, such as the quality and consistency of the care (Dearing & Zachrisson, 2017).

Use of different types of child care varies by ethnicity, socioeconomic status, geographic region, and age of the child. Parents' reports of whether good child-care options are available to them and barriers to finding good child care also vary by these factors. For example, cost is less likely to be a barrier in higher-income families, and lack of available spots is less likely to be a barrier for older children than for infants (U.S. Department of Education, National Center for Education Statistics, 2018).

Child-care quality makes a difference. What constitutes a high-quality child-care program for infants? In high-quality child care (Clarke-Stewart & Miner, 2008, p. 273),

> caregivers encourage the children to be actively engaged in a variety of activities, have frequent, positive interactions that include smiling, touching, holding, and speaking at the child's eye level, respond properly to the child's questions or requests, and encourage children to talk about their experiences, feelings, and ideas.

High-quality child care also involves providing children with a safe environment, access to age-appropriate toys and participation in age-appropriate activities, and a low child-to-caregiver ratio that allows caregivers to spend considerable time with children on an individual basis.

Children are more likely to experience poor-quality child care if they come from families with few resources (psychological, social, and economic) (Krafft, Davis, & Tout, 2017). Many researchers have examined the role of poverty in quality of child care (Carlin & others, 2019). A number of studies have demonstrated that high-quality child care can benefit low-income children. For example, spending more time in child care buffered the otherwise negative effects of household chaos on low-income children's cognitive and social outcomes at age 5 years (Berry & others, 2016).

To read about one individual who provides quality child care to individuals from impoverished backgrounds, see the *Connecting with Careers* profile of Wanda Mitchell. Do children in low-income families get quality care at day care? For the answer to that question, as well as other information on the effects of child care on children's development, see *Connecting Through Research*.

> We have all the knowledge necessary to provide absolutely first-rate child care in the United States. What is missing is the commitment and the will.
>
> —EDWARD ZIGLER
> *Contemporary developmental psychologist, Yale University*

What are some strategies parents can follow in regard to child care? Child-care expert Kathleen McCartney (2003, p. 4) offered this advice:

- Recognize that the quality of your parenting is a key factor in your child's development.
- Make decisions that will improve the likelihood you will be good parents. "For some this will mean working full-time"—for personal fulfillment, income, or both. "For others, this will mean working part-time or not working outside the home."
- Monitor your child's development. "Parents should observe for themselves whether their children seem to be having behavior problems." They need to talk with child-care providers and their pediatrician about their child's behavior.
- Take some time to find the best child care available. Observe different child-care facilities and be certain that you like what you see. Quality child care is expensive, and not all parents can afford the child care they want. However, state subsidies and programs like Head Start are available for families in need.

connecting through research

How Does the Quality and Quantity of Child Care Affect Children?

In 1991, the National Institute of Child Health and Human Development (NICHD) began a comprehensive, longitudinal study of child-care experiences. Data were collected on a diverse sample of almost 1,400 children and their families at 10 locations across the United States over a period of seven years. Researchers used multiple methods (trained observers, interviews, questionnaires, and testing) and measured many facets of children's development, including physical health, cognitive development, and socioemotional development. Following are some of the results of what is now referred to as the NICHD Study of Early Child Care and Youth Development or NICHD SECCYD (NICHD Early Child Care Network, 2001, 2002, 2003, 2004, 2005, 2006, 2010).

- *Patterns of use.* Many families placed their infants in child care very soon after the child's birth, and there was considerable instability in the child-care arrangements. By 4 months of age, nearly three-fourths of the infants had entered some form of nonmaternal child care. Almost half of the infants were cared for by a relative when they first entered care; only 12 percent were enrolled in child-care centers. Socioeconomic factors were linked to the amount and type of care. For example, mothers with higher incomes and families that were more dependent on the mother's income placed their infants in child care at an earlier age. Mothers who believed that maternal employment has positive effects on children were more likely than other mothers to place their infant in nonmaternal care for more hours. Low-income families were more likely than more affluent families to use child care, but infants from low-income families who were in child care averaged as many hours as other income groups. In the preschool years, mothers who were single, those with more education, and families with higher incomes used more hours of center care than other families. Minority families and mothers with less education used more hours of care by relatives.

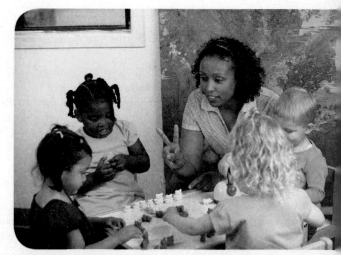

What are some important findings from the National Longitudinal Study of Child Care conducted by the National Institute of Child Health and Human Development?
Christopher Futcher/iStock/Getty Images

- *Quality of care.* Evaluations of quality of care were based on such characteristics as group size, child-adult ratio, physical environment, caregiver characteristics (such as formal education, specialized training, and child-care experience), and caregiver behavior (such as sensitivity to children). An alarming conclusion is that a majority of the child care in the first three years of life was of unacceptably low quality. Positive caregiving by nonparents in child-care settings was infrequent—only 12 percent of the children studied experienced positive nonparental child care (such as positive talk, lack of detachment or flat affect, and language stimulation)! Further, infants from low-income

(continued)

(continued)

families experienced lower-quality child care than infants from higher-income families. When quality of care was high, children performed better on cognitive and language tasks, were more cooperative with their mothers during play, showed more positive and skilled interaction with peers, and had fewer behavior problems. Caregiver training and good child-staff ratios were linked with higher cognitive and social competence when children were 54 months of age.

Higher-quality child care was also related to higher-quality mother-child interaction among the families that used nonmaternal care. Further, poor-quality care was related to an increase in insecure attachment to the mother among infants who were 15 months of age, but only when the mother was low in sensitivity and responsiveness. However, child-care quality was not linked to attachment security at 36 months of age. Higher-quality child care and fewer hours spent in child care predicted better executive functioning in preschoolers, which in turn predicted better academic and social skills in preschool and kindergarten (Son & Chang, 2018). In a long-term longitudinal study, higher-quality early child care predicted better grades in high school and admission to more selective colleges, controlling for a wide variety of family background factors (Vandell, Burchinal, & Pierce, 2016).

- *Amount of child care.* The quantity of child care predicted some child outcomes. When children spent extensive amounts of time in child care beginning in infancy, they experienced less sensitive interactions with their mother, showed more behavior problems, and had higher rates of illness. Many of these comparisons involved children in child care for less than 30 hours a week versus those in child care for more than 45 hours a week. In general, though, when children spent 30 hours or more per week in child care, their development was less than optimal (Ramey, 2005).

- *Family and parenting influences.* The influence of families and parenting was not weakened by extensive child care. Parents played a significant role in helping children to regulate their emotions. Especially important parenting influences were being sensitive to children's needs, being involved with children, and cognitively stimulating them. Indeed, parental sensitivity has been the most consistent predictor of a secure attachment, with child-care experiences being relevant in many cases only when mothers engage in insensitive parenting (Friedman, Melhuish, & Hill, 2010). An important point about the extensive NICHD research is that findings show that family factors are considerably stronger and more consistent predictors of a wide variety of child outcomes than are child-care experiences (such as quality, quantity, type). The worst outcomes for children occur when both home and child-care settings are of poor quality. For example, a recent study involving the NICHD SECCYD data revealed that worse socioemotional outcomes (more problem behavior, low level of prosocial behavior) for children occurred when they experienced both home and child-care environments that conferred risk (Watamura & others, 2011).

This study reinforces the conclusions of other researchers cited earlier in this section of the chapter—it is not the *quantity* as much as the *quality* of child care a child receives that is important. What is also significant is the emphasis on the positive effect families and parents can have on children's child-care experiences.

Review *Connect* Reflect

 LG4 Explain the early development of social orientation/understanding, attachment, and variations in child care.

Review

- What characterizes the early development of social orientation and social understanding?
- How does attachment develop in infancy?
- How do mothers and fathers interact with infants?
- What is the nature of child care?

Connect

- In this section, you learned that maternal sensitive responding was linked to security of infant attachment. What have you learned about maternal sensitivity and children's language development?

Reflect *Your Own Personal Journey of Life*

- Imagine that a friend of yours is getting ready to put her baby in child care. What advice would you give to her? Do you think she should stay home with the baby? Why or why not? What type of child care would you recommend?

Emotional Development

Exploring Emotion   **LG1** Discuss basic aspects of emotion.

What Are Emotions?

- Emotion is feeling, or affect, that occurs when people are engaged in interactions that are important to them, especially those that influence their well-being. Emotions can be classified as positive or negative. Psychologists stress that emotions, especially facial expressions of emotions, have a biological foundation. Facial expressions of emotion are similar across cultures, but display rules are not culturally universal. Biological evolution endowed humans to be emotional, but culture and relationships with others provide diversity in emotional experiences.

A Functionalist View of Emotions

- The functionalist view of emotion emphasizes the importance of contexts and relationships in emotion. For example, when parents induce a positive mood in their child, the child is more likely to follow the parents' directions. In this view, goals are involved in emotions in a variety of ways, and the goal's specific nature can affect the individual's experience of a given emotion.

Emotional Competence

- Becoming emotionally competent involves developing a number of skills such as being aware of one's emotional states, discerning others' emotions, adaptively coping with negative emotions, and understanding the role of emotions in relationships.

Development of Emotion   **LG2** Describe the development of emotion.

Infancy

- Infants display a number of emotions early in their development, although researchers debate the onset and sequence of these emotions. Lewis distinguishes between primary emotions and self-conscious emotions. Primary emotions include joy, anger, and fear, while self-conscious emotions include pride, shame, and guilt. Crying is the most important mechanism newborns have for communicating with their world. Babies have at least three types of cries—basic, anger, and pain cries. Social smiling in response to a caregiver's voice occurs as early as 4 to 6 weeks of age. Two fears that infants develop are stranger anxiety and separation from a caregiver (which is reflected in separation protest). Controversy swirls about whether babies should be soothed when they cry, although increasingly experts recommend immediately responding in a caring way during the first year. Infants gradually develop an ability to inhibit the duration and intensity of their emotional reactions.

Early Childhood

- Advances in young children's emotions involve expressing emotions, understanding emotions, and regulating emotions. Young children's range of emotions expands during early childhood as they increasingly experience self-conscious emotions such as pride, shame, and guilt. Between 2 and 4 years old, children use an increasing number of terms to describe emotion and learn more about the causes and consequences of feelings. At 4 to 5 years of age, children show an increased ability to reflect on emotions and understand that a single event can elicit different emotions in different people. They also show a growing awareness of the need to manage emotions to meet social standards. Emotion-coaching parents have children who engage in more effective self-regulation of their emotions than do the children of emotion-dismissing parents. Young children in a secure attachment relationship with their mother are more willing to engage in conversation about difficult emotional circumstances. Emotion regulation plays an important role in successful peer relationships.

Middle and Late Childhood

- In middle and late childhood, children show a growing awareness of the need to control and manage emotions to meet social standards. Also in this age period, they show increased emotional understanding, markedly improve their ability to suppress or conceal negative emotions, use self-initiated strategies for redirecting feelings, have an increased tendency to take into fuller account the events that lead to emotional reactions, and develop a capacity for genuine empathy.

Temperament

LG3 Characterize variations in temperament and their significance.

Describing and Classifying Temperament

- Temperament involves individual differences in behavioral styles, emotions, and characteristic ways of responding. Developmentalists are especially interested in the temperament of infants. Chess and Thomas classified infants as (1) easy, (2) difficult, or (3) slow to warm up. Kagan argues that inhibition to the unfamiliar is an important temperament category. Rothbart and Bates' view of temperament emphasizes the following classification: (1) extraversion/surgency, (2) negative affectivity, and (3) effortful control (self-regulation).

Biological Foundations and Experience

- Physiological characteristics are associated with different temperaments, and a moderate influence of heredity has been found in twin and adoption studies of the heritability of temperament. Children inherit a physiology that biases them to have a particular type of temperament, but through experience they learn to modify their temperament style to some degree. Very active young children are likely to become outgoing adults. In some cases, a difficult temperament is linked with adjustment problems in early adulthood. The link between childhood temperament and adult personality depends in part on context, which helps shape the reaction to a child and thus the child's experiences. For example, the reaction to a child's temperament depends in part on the child's gender and on the culture.

Goodness of Fit and Parenting

- Goodness of fit refers to the match between a child's temperament and the environmental demands the child must cope with. Goodness of fit can be an important aspect of a child's adjustment. Although research evidence is sketchy at this point, some general recommendations are that caregivers should (1) be sensitive to the individual characteristics of the child, (2) be flexible in responding to these characteristics, and (3) avoid negative labeling of the child.

Social Orientation/Understanding, Attachment, and Child Care

LG4 Explain the early development of social orientation/ understanding, attachment, and variations in child care.

Social Orientation/ Understanding

- Infants show a strong interest in their social world and are motivated to understand it. Infants orient to their social world early in their development. Face-to-face play with a caregiver begins to occur at 2 to 3 months of age. Newly developed self-produced locomotion skills significantly expand infants' ability to initiate social interchanges and explore their social world more independently. Perceiving people as engaging in intentional and goal-directed behavior is an important social cognitive accomplishment that occurs toward the end of the first year. Social referencing increases in the second year of life.

Attachment

- Attachment is a close emotional bond between two people. In infancy, contact comfort and trust are important in the development of attachment. Bowlby's ethological theory stresses that the caregiver and the infant are biologically predisposed to form an attachment. Attachment develops in four phases during infancy. Securely attached babies use the caregiver, usually the mother, as a secure base from which to explore the environment. Three types of insecure attachment are avoidant, resistant, and disorganized. Ainsworth created the Strange Situation, an observational measure of attachment. Ainsworth points out that secure attachment in the first year of life provides an important foundation for psychological development later in life. The strength of the link between early attachment and later development has varied somewhat across studies. Some critics argue that attachment theorists have not given adequate attention to genetics and temperament. Other critics stress that they have not adequately taken into account the diversity of social agents and contexts. Cultural variations in attachment have been found, but in all cultures studied to date, secure attachment is the most common classification. Caregivers of secure babies are sensitive to the babies' signals and are consistently available to meet their needs. Caregivers of avoidant babies tend to be unavailable or rejecting. Caregivers of resistant babies tend to be inconsistently available to their babies and usually are not very affectionate. Caregivers of disorganized babies often neglect or physically abuse their babies. Increased interest has been directed toward the role of the brain in the development of attachment. The hormone oxytocin is a key candidate for influencing the development of maternal-infant attachment. Secure attachment continues to be important in the childhood years.

Fathers and Mothers as Caregivers

Child Care

- In recent years fathers have increased the amount of time they interact with infants, but mothers still spend considerably more time in caregiving with infants than do fathers. In many U.S. families, the mother's primary role when interacting with the infant is caregiving; the father's is playful interaction.

- More U.S. children are in child care now than at any earlier point in history. The quality of child care is uneven, and child care remains a controversial topic. Quality child care can be achieved and seems to have few adverse effects on children. In the NICHD child-care study, infants from low-income families were more likely to receive the lowest quality of care. Also, higher quality of child care was linked to a higher level of children's cognitive development and to fewer childhood problems.

key **terms**

anger cry 277
attachment 292
basic cry 277
developmental cascade model 295
difficult child 283
easy child 283

emotion 273
goodness of fit 288
insecure avoidant babies 293
insecure disorganized babies 293
insecure resistant babies 293
pain cry 277

primary emotions 276
reflexive smile 277
securely attached babies 293
self-conscious emotions 276
separation protest 278
slow-to-warm-up child 283

social referencing 291
social smile 277
stranger anxiety 278
Strange Situation 293
temperament 283

key **people**

Mary Ainsworth 279
John Bowlby 279
Joseph Campos 276
Alexander Chess 283

Erik Erikson 292
Harry Harlow 292
Jerome Kagan 276
Michael Lewis 276

Kathleen McCartney 300
Mary Rothbart 284
Alan Sroufe 294
Stella Thomas 283

Theodore Wachs 287
John Watson 279

THE SELF AND IDENTITY

chapter outline

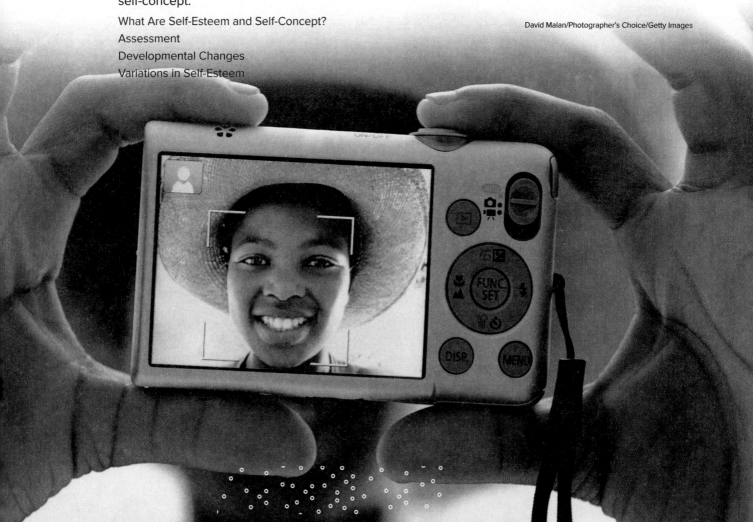

David Malan/Photographer's Choice/Getty Images

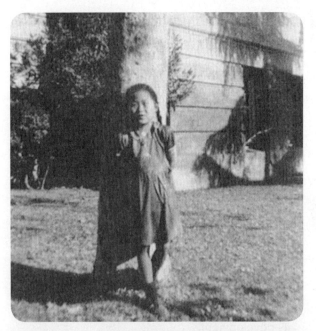

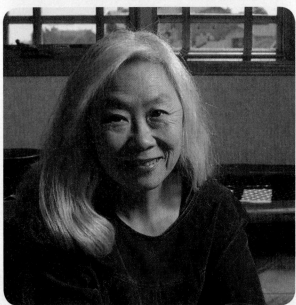

Maxine Hong Kingston's vivid portrayals of her Chinese ancestry and the struggles of Chinese immigrants have made her one of the world's leading Asian American writers. Kingston's parents were Chinese immigrants. Born in California in 1940, she spent many hours working with her parents and five brothers and sisters in the family's laundry. As a youth, Kingston was profoundly influenced by her parents' struggle to adapt to American culture and by their descriptions of their Chinese heritage.

Growing up as she did, Kingston felt the pull of two very different cultures. She was especially intrigued by stories about Chinese women who were perceived as either privileged or degraded.

Her first book was *The Woman Warrior: Memoirs of a Girlhood Among Ghosts* (Kingston, 1976). In *The Woman Warrior,* Kingston described her aunt, who gave birth to an illegitimate child. Because having a child outside of wedlock was taboo and perceived as a threat to the community's stability, the entire Chinese village condemned her, pushing her to kill herself and her child. From then on, even mentioning her name was forbidden. Kingston says she likes to guide people to find meaning in their lives, especially by exploring their cultural backgrounds.

Maxine Hong Kingston as a young girl and as an adult.
(Top) Glenda Hyde; *(bottom)* Eric Risberg/AP Images

preview

Maxine Hong Kingston's life and writings remind us of important aspects of each of our lives as we grew up: our efforts to understand ourselves and to develop an identity that reflects our cultural heritage. This chapter is about the self and identity. As we examine these topics, reflect on how well you understood yourself at different points in your life as you were growing up, and think about how you acquired the stamp of your identity.

Self-Understanding and Understanding Others Discuss the development of self-understanding and understanding others.

- Self-Understanding
- Understanding Others

The **self** consists of all of the characteristics of a person. Theorists and researchers who focus on the self usually argue that the self is the central aspect of the individual's personality and that the self lends an integrative dimension to our understanding of different personality characteristics (Harter, 2012, 2015; Rochat, 2013). Several aspects of the self have been studied more than others. These include self-understanding, self-esteem, and self-concept.

A number of research studies show that young children are more psychologically aware of themselves and others than used to be thought (Thompson, 2013). This psychological awareness reflects young children's expanding psychological sophistication.

SELF-UNDERSTANDING

Self-understanding is a child's cognitive representation of the self—the substance and content of the child's self-conceptions. For example, an 11-year-old boy understands that he is a student, a boy, a football player, a family member, a video game lover, and a rock music fan. A 13-year-old girl understands that she is a middle school student, in the midst of puberty, a girl, a cheerleader, a student council member, and a movie fan. A child's self-understanding is based, in part, on the various roles and membership categories that define who children are (Harter, 2012, 2015). Though not the whole of personal identity, self-understanding provides its rational underpinnings.

Developmental Changes   Children are not just given a self by their parents or culture; rather, they construct selves. As children develop, their self-understanding changes.

Infancy   Studying the self in infancy is difficult mainly because infants cannot tell us how they experience themselves. Infants cannot verbally express their views of the self. They also cannot understand complex instructions from researchers.

A rudimentary form of self-recognition—being attentive and positive toward one's image in a mirror—appears as early as 3 months of age. However, a central, more complete index of self-recognition—the ability to recognize one's physical features—does not emerge until the second year (Filippetti & Tsakiris, 2018; Thompson, 2006).

One ingenious strategy to test infants' visual self-recognition is the use of a mirror technique, in which an infant's mother first puts a dot of rouge on the infant's nose without the infant's awareness. Then an observer watches to see how often the infant touches its nose. Next, the infant is placed in front of a mirror, and observers detect whether nose touching increases. Why does this matter? The idea is that increased nose touching indicates that the infant recognizes the self in the mirror and is trying to touch

> When I say "I," I mean something absolutely unique, not to be confused with any other.
>
> **—UGO BETTI**
> *Italian playwright, 20th century*

self All of the characteristics of a person.

self-understanding A child's cognitive representation of the self—the substance and content of a child's self-conceptions.

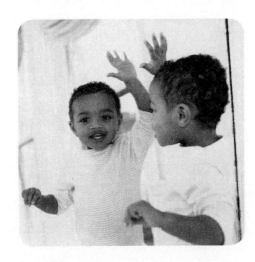

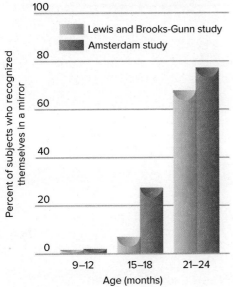

100

Lewis and Brooks-Gunn study
Amsterdam study

80

60

40

20

0

Percent of subjects who recognized themselves in a mirror

9–12   15–18   21–24

Age (months)

FIGURE 1

THE DEVELOPMENT OF SELF-RECOGNITION IN INFANCY. The graph shows the findings of two studies in which infants less than 1 year of age did not recognize themselves in the mirror. A slight increase in the percentage of infant self-recognition occurred around 15 to 18 months of age. By 2 years of age, a majority of children recognized themselves. *Why do researchers study whether infants recognize themselves in a mirror?*
Digital Vision/Getty Images

The living self has one purpose only: to come into its own fullness of being, as a tree comes into full blossom, or a bird into spring beauty, or a tiger into lustre.

—**D. H. LAWRENCE**
English author, 20th century

or rub off the rouge because the rouge violates the infant's perception of what he or she looks like. Increased touching indicates that the infant realizes that it is the self in the mirror but that something is not right since the real self does not have a dot of rouge on it.

Figure 1 displays the results of two early investigations that used the mirror technique. The researchers found that before infants were 1 year old, they did not recognize themselves in the mirror (Amsterdam, 1968; Lewis & Brooks-Gunn, 1979). Signs of self-recognition began to appear among some infants when they were 15 to 18 months old. By the time they were 2 years old, most children recognized themselves in the mirror. In sum, infants begin to develop a self-understanding called visual self-recognition at approximately 18 months of age (Filippetti & Tsakiris, 2018).

Late in the second year and early in the third year (with some small differences in timing being found across cultures), toddlers show other emerging forms of self-awareness that reflect a sense of "me." For example, they refer to themselves by saying "Me big"; they label internal experiences such as emotions; they monitor themselves, as when a toddler says, "Do it myself"; and they say that things are theirs (Davoodi, Nelson, & Blake, 2018; Ross & others, 2017). It is during the second year that infants develop a conscious awareness of their own bodies (Waugh & Brownell, 2015). This developmental change in body awareness marks the beginning of children's representation of their own three-dimensional body shape and appearance, providing an early step in the development of their self-image and identity.

Early Childhood   Because children can communicate verbally, research on self-understanding in childhood is not limited to visual self-recognition, as it is during infancy (Harter, 2012, 2015). Mainly through interviews, researchers have probed many aspects of children's self-understanding (Starmans, 2017; Thompson, 2013). Here are five main characteristics of self-understanding in young children:

- *Confusion of self, mind, and body.* Young children generally confuse self, mind, and body. Most young children conceive of the self as part of the body, which usually means the head. For them, the self can be described along many material dimensions, such as size, shape, and color.

- *Concrete descriptions.* Preschool children mainly think of themselves and define themselves in concrete terms. A young child might say, "I know my ABC's," "I can count," and "I live in a big house" (Harter, 2012). Although young children mainly describe themselves in terms of concrete, observable features and action tendencies, at about 4 to 5 years of age, as they hear others use psychological trait and emotion terms, they begin to include these in their own self-descriptions (Thompson, 2013). Thus, in a self-description, a 4-year-old might say, "I'm not scared. I'm always happy."

- *Physical descriptions.* Young children also distinguish themselves from others through many physical and material attributes. Says 4-year-old Andrea, "I'm different from Saphia because I have brown hair and she has black hair." Says 4-year-old Darren, "I am different from my brother because I am taller, and I am different from my sister because I have a bicycle."

- *Active descriptions.* The *active dimension* is a central component of the self in early childhood. For example, preschool children often describe themselves in terms of activities such as play.

- *Unrealistic positive overestimations.* Self-evaluations during early childhood are often unrealistically positive and represent an overestimation of personal attributes (Harter, 2012). These unrealistic positive overestimations of the self occur because young children (1) have difficulty differentiating between their desired and actual competence, (2) cannot yet generate an ideal self that is distinguished from a real self, and (3) rarely engage in *social comparison*—exploring how they compare with others. This overestimation of one's attributes helps to protect young children against negative self-evaluations.

However, as in virtually all areas of children's development, there are individual variations in young children's self-conceptions, and there is increasing evidence that some children are vulnerable to negative self-beliefs (Müller & others, 2015). For example, one study revealed that preschool children had a lower self-concept if they had insecure attachments with their fathers or mothers, and even more so if they were rejected by their peers (Pinto & others, 2015). This research indicates that young children's generally optimistic self-views do not protect them from adverse, stressful family and peer group conditions.

Middle and Late Childhood   Children's self-evaluation becomes more complex during middle and late childhood (Harter, 2012, 2015). Five key changes characterize the increased complexity:

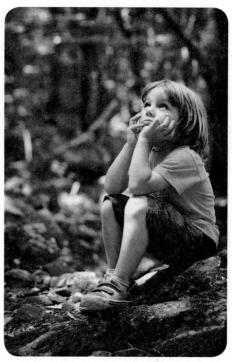

What characterizes young children's self-understanding?
Tatyana Aleksieva Photography/Getty Images

- *Psychological characteristics and traits.* In middle and late childhood, especially from 8 to 11 years of age, children increasingly describe themselves with psychological characteristics and traits in contrast to the more concrete self-descriptions of younger children. Older children are more likely to describe themselves as *popular, nice, helpful, mean, smart,* and *dumb.* Older children also are less likely than younger children to overestimate their abilities or to cite only virtuous aspects of the self. Rather, they now have the cognitive capabilities to realize that they can be both *nice* and *mean, smart* as well as *dumb.*

- *Social descriptions.* In middle and late childhood, children begin to include *social aspects* such as references to social groups in their self-descriptions (Harter, 2012). For example, children in elementary school are increasingly aware of discrimination against groups of people, as well as of power differences that affect their self-understanding and social relationships with others (Killen, Rutland, & Yip, 2016).

- *Social comparison.* Children's self-understanding in middle and late childhood includes increasing reference to social comparison. At this point in development, children are more likely to distinguish themselves from others in comparative rather than in absolute terms. That is, elementary-school-age children are likely to think about what they can do in comparison with others. If they feel that they fall short of others, they are likely to evaluate themselves negatively.

- *Real self and ideal self.* In middle and late childhood, children begin to distinguish between their real and ideal selves. This involves differentiating their actual competencies from those they aspire to have and think are the most important. This discrepancy also can lead to negative self-evaluations.

- *Realistic.* In middle and late childhood, children's self-evaluations become more realistic. This may occur because of increased social comparison and perspective taking.

Adolescence   The development of self-understanding in adolescence is even more complex and involves a number of aspects of the self (Harter, 2012, 2015):

- *Abstract and idealistic.* Remember from our discussion of Piaget's theory of cognitive development that many adolescents begin to think in more *abstract* and *idealistic* ways. When asked to describe themselves, adolescents are more likely than children to use abstract and idealistic labels. Consider 14-year-old Laurie's abstract description of herself: "I am a human being. I am indecisive. I don't know who I am." Also consider her idealistic description of herself: "I am a naturally sensitive person who really cares about people's feelings. I think I'm pretty good looking." Not all adolescents describe themselves in idealistic ways, but most adolescents distinguish between the real self and the ideal self.

- *Self-consciousness.* Adolescents are more likely than children to be *self-conscious* about and *preoccupied* with their self-understanding. This self-consciousness and self-preoccupation reflect adolescent egocentrism.

developmental **connection**

Cognitive Theory

In Piaget's fourth stage of cognitive development, thought becomes more abstract, idealistic, and logical. Connect to "Cognitive Developmental Approaches."

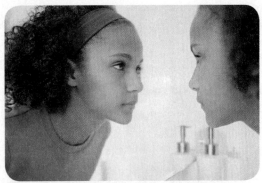

How does self-understanding change in adolescence?
Roy McMahon/Image Source/SuperStock

Know thyself, for once we
know ourselves, we may learn
how to care for ourselves, but
otherwise we never shall.

—SOCRATES
Greek philosopher, 5th century B.C.

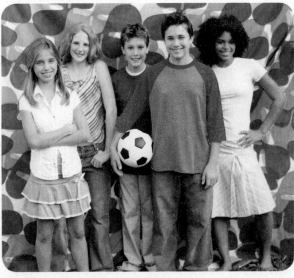

What characterizes adolescents' possible selves?
Stockbyte/Getty Images

- - - - - - - - - - - - - - - - - ➤
developmental **connection**

Attention

Joint attention and gaze following help
the infant to understand that other people
have intentions. Connect to "Emotional
Development."

◄- - - - - - - - - - - - - - - - -

possible self What an individual might become,
would like to become, and is afraid of becoming.

social cognition The processes involved in
understanding the world around us, especially
how we think and reason about other people.

- *Contradictions within the self.* As adolescents begin to differentiate their concept of the self into multiple roles in different relationship contexts, they sense potential contradictions between their differentiated selves. An adolescent might use self-descriptions with contrasts: "I'm tough and easy-going," or "I'm quiet and chatty." These contradictions characterize the self-descriptions of young adolescents more than older adolescents.

- *The fluctuating self.* The adolescent's self-understanding fluctuates across situations and across time. The adolescent's self continues to be characterized by instability until the adolescent constructs a more unified theory of self, usually not until late adolescence or emerging adulthood (Michikyan, Dennis, & Subrahmanyam, 2015).

- *Real and ideal selves.* The adolescent's emerging ability to construct ideal selves in addition to actual ones can be perplexing and agonizing to the adolescent. In one view, an important aspect of the ideal or imagined self is the **possible self**—what individuals might become, what they would like to become, and what they are afraid of becoming (Markus & Kitayama, 2012). The attributes of future positive selves (getting into a good college, being admired, having a successful career) can direct future positive outcomes. And the attributes of future negative selves (being unemployed, being lonely, not getting into a good college) can identify what is to be avoided (Oyserman, Destin, & Novin, 2015).

- *Social comparison.* The tendency to compare themselves with others continues to increase during the adolescent years. However, when asked whether they engage in social comparison, most adolescents deny it because they are aware that it is somewhat socially undesirable to do so. That is, they think that acknowledging their social comparison motives will endanger their popularity. An individual's beliefs about how he or she is viewed by others is referred to as the *looking glass* self.

- *Self-integration.* In late adolescence and emerging adulthood, self–understanding becomes more *integrative* as the disparate parts of the self are more systematically pieced together. Older adolescents are more likely to detect inconsistencies in their earlier self-descriptions as they attempt to construct a stable self and an integrated sense of identity.

UNDERSTANDING OTHERS

Young children are more sophisticated at understanding not only themselves, but others, than used to be thought (Thompson, 2013). The term **social cognition** refers to the processes involved in understanding the world around us, especially how we think and reason about other people. Developmental psychologists study how children develop this understanding of others (Mills, 2013; Slaughter, 2015).

In the chapter "Emotional Development," we described the development of social understanding in infancy. Recall that perceiving people as engaging in intentional and goal-directed behavior is an important social cognitive accomplishment, and this occurs toward the end of the first year. Social referencing, which involves "reading" emotional cues in others to help determine how to act in a particular situation, increases in the second year of life. Here we will describe further changes in social understanding that occur during childhood and adolescence.

Early Childhood   Children also make advances in their understanding of others in early childhood (Mills, 2013). As you saw in the chapter "Information Processing," young children's theory of mind includes understanding that other people have emotions and desires (Lagattuta, Elrod, & Kramer, 2016; Wellman, 2011). And at about 4 to 5 years, children not only start describing themselves in terms of psychological traits but also begin to perceive *others* in terms of psychological traits. Thus, a 4-year-old might say, "My teacher is nice."

An important step in children's development is beginning to understand that people don't always accurately describe their beliefs (Quintanilla, Giménez-Dasí, & Gaviria, 2018). Researchers have found that even 4-year-olds understand that people may make untrue statements to obtain what they want or to avoid trouble (Nancarrow & others, 2018). One illustrative study revealed that 4- and 5-year-olds were increasingly skeptical of another child's claim to be sick when the children were informed that the child was motivated to avoid having to go to camp (Gee & Heyman, 2007).

Both the extensive theory of mind research and the research on young children's social understanding underscore that young children are not always as egocentric as Piaget and others had previously envisioned (Fizke & others, 2017; Slaughter, 2015). The concept of egocentrism has become so ingrained in people's thinking about young children that too often the current research on social awareness in infancy and early childhood has been overlooked. Research increasingly shows that young children are more socially sensitive and perceptive than previously envisioned, suggesting that parents and teachers can help them to better understand and interact in the social world by how they interact with them (Thompson, 2013). If young children are seeking to better understand various mental and emotional states (intentions, goals, feelings, desires) that they know underlie people's actions, then talking with them about these internal states can improve young children's understanding of them (Ruffman & others, 2018). However, debate continues to characterize whether young children are socially sensitive or basically egocentric.

Another important aspect of understanding others involves understanding joint commitments and cooperation (Warneken, 2018). One study revealed that 5-year-olds were more likely than 3-year-olds to understand when they and a partner were committed to the same goal of collaborating in joint activities (Kachel & Tomasello, 2019).

Individual differences characterize young children's social understanding (Laurent & others, 2018). Some young children are better than others at understanding what people are feeling and what they desire, for example. To some degree, these individual differences are linked to conversations caregivers have with young children about other people's feelings and desires, and children's opportunities to observe others talking about people's feelings and desires (Ruffman & others, 2018). For example, a mother might say to a 3-year-old, "I want you to think about Raphael's feelings next time before you hit him."

To understand others, it is necessary to take their perspective. **Perspective taking** is the social cognitive process involved in assuming the perspective of others and understanding their thoughts and feelings. Executive function is at work in perspective taking (Galinsky, 2010). Among the executive functions called on when children engage in perspective taking are cognitive inhibition (controlling one's own thoughts to consider the perspective of others) and cognitive flexibility (seeing situations in different ways).

Middle and Late Childhood

In middle and late childhood, children show an increase in perspective taking and understanding of other people's viewpoints (Lagattuta & others, 2015). In middle childhood, children begin to understand that others may have a different perspective because some people have more access to information than others do. During this developmental period, children become increasingly aware that each individual can make use of the other's perspective and that putting oneself in another person's place is a way of judging the other person's intentions, purposes, and actions.

Perspective taking is especially important in determining whether children develop prosocial or antisocial attitudes and behavior. In terms of prosocial behavior, taking another's perspective improves children's understanding of others and sympathizing with others who are distressed or in need. One study revealed that when 10-year-old children were put in a negative emotional state and presented with stories of someone in need, children who had better emotion regulation were more likely to engage in increased empathy and prosocial behavior (Hein, Röder, & Fingerle, 2018).

developmental **connection**

Cognitive Theory

Theory of mind refers to awareness of one's own mental processes and the mental processes of others. Connect to "Information Processing."

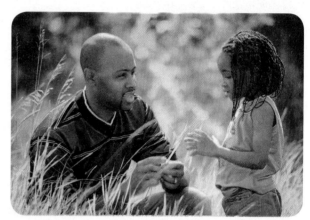

Young children are more psychologically aware of themselves and others than used to be thought. Some children are better than others at understanding people's feelings and desires—and, to some degree, these individual differences are influenced by conversations caregivers have with young children about feelings and desires.
Don Hammond/DesignPics

perspective taking The social cognitive process involved in assuming the perspective of others and understanding their thoughts and feelings.

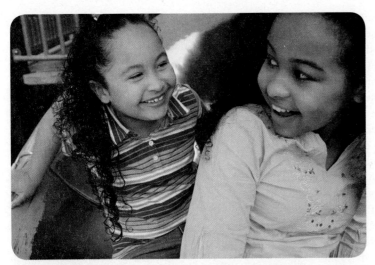

What are some changes in children's understanding of others in middle and late childhood?
Image Source/DigitalVision/Getty Images

Earlier we indicated that even 4-year-old children show some skepticism of others' claims (Gee & Heyman, 2007). In middle and late childhood, children become increasingly skeptical of some sources of information about psychological traits. For example, in one study, 8- to 11-year-olds and adults were less likely than younger children to accept the accuracy or usefulness of another person's boasting (Lockhart, Goddu, & Keil, 2018). Compared with 5- to 7-year-olds, the more psychologically sophisticated 8- to 11-year-olds also showed a better understanding that others' self-reports on socially desirable tendencies should be scrutinized.

Elementary-school-aged children also begin to understand others' motivations and how these fit with culturally bound standards of behavior. For example, children in China are taught to avoid drawing attention to themselves. Across middle childhood, children develop increased understanding of the motivation behind public versus private acts of generosity (Heyman & others, 2016).

Adolescence Becoming a competent adolescent involves not only understanding oneself but also understanding others. Among the key aspects of understanding others that increase during adolescence are perspective taking, perceiving others' traits, and social cognitive monitoring.

Perspective Taking As described above, perspective taking begins with having an egocentric viewpoint in early childhood. It matures and ends with using in-depth perspective taking in adolescence. Following are examples of investigations on this topic:

- Among 13- to 15-year-olds, those who engaged in more empathic distress, which involves taking on their friend's distress as their own, were more likely to experience depressive feelings even while feeling close to their friend (Schwartz-Mette & Smith, 2018).

- In a longitudinal study from ninth to eleventh grade, African American and Latino/a adolescents showed growth in developing a social justice perspective that was increasingly aware of the disparities that exist between vulnerable and less vulnerable social groups in regard to racism and discrimination (Seider & others, 2019).

- A lower level of perspective taking was linked to increased relational aggression (harming someone by using strategies such as spreading vicious rumors) one year later in middle school students (Batanova & Loukas, 2011).

Perceiving Others' Traits One way to study how adolescents perceive others' traits is to ask them about the extent to which others' self-reports are accurate. In one illustrative comparison of 6- and 10-year-olds, the 10-year-olds were much more skeptical about others' self-reports of their intelligence and social skills than the 6-year-olds were (Heyman & Legare, 2005). In this study, the 10-year-olds understood that other people at times may distort the truth about their own traits to make a better impression on others.

As adolescence proceeds, teenagers develop a more sophisticated understanding of others. They come to understand that other people are complex and have public and private faces (Harter, 2012, 2015).

Social Cognitive Monitoring An important cognitive activity in metacognition is cognitive monitoring, which can also be very helpful in social situations (McCormick, Dimmitt, & Sullivan, 2013). As part of their increased awareness of themselves and others, adolescents monitor their social world more

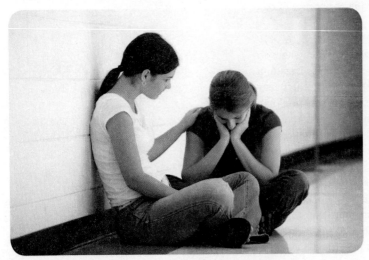

What are some important aspects of social understanding in adolescence?
Thinkstock/Getty Images

extensively than they did when they were children. Adolescents engage in a number of social cognitive monitoring activities on virtually a daily basis. An adolescent might think, "I would like to get to know this guy better, but he is not very open. Maybe I can talk to some other students about what he is like." Another adolescent might check incoming information about a club or a new peer group to determine whether it is consistent with her initial impressions. Yet another adolescent might question someone or paraphrase what the person has just said about her feelings, to make sure that he has accurately understood them. Adolescents' ability to monitor their social cognition may be an important aspect of their social maturity (Bosacki, 2016).

Review Connect Reflect

 LG1 Discuss the development of self-understanding and understanding others.

Review

- What is self-understanding? How does self-understanding change from infancy through adolescence?
- How does understanding of others develop?

Connect

- In this section, you learned that in middle and late childhood, children show an increase in perspective taking. Which spectrum of disorders causes children to have difficulty understanding others' beliefs and emotions?

Reflect *Your Own Personal Journey of Life*

- If a psychologist had interviewed you at 10 and at 16 years of age, how would your self-understanding have changed?

Self-Esteem and Self-Concept

 LG2 Explain self-esteem and self-concept.

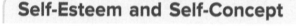

| What Are Self-Esteem and Self-Concept? | Assessment | Developmental Changes | Variations in Self-Esteem |

Self-conception involves more than self-understanding. Not only do children try to define and describe attributes of the self (self-understanding), but they also evaluate these attributes. These evaluations create self-esteem and self-concept, and they have far-reaching implications for children's development.

WHAT ARE SELF-ESTEEM AND SELF-CONCEPT?

Sometimes the terms *self-esteem* and *self-concept* are used interchangeably, or they are not precisely defined (Harter, 2012, 2015). Here we use **self-esteem** to refer to a person's self-worth or self-image, a global evaluation of the self. For example, a child might perceive that she is not merely a person but a good person. (To evaluate your self-esteem, see Figure 2.) We use the term **self-concept** to refer to domain-specific evaluations of the self. Children can make self-evaluations in many domains of their lives—academic, athletic, physical appearance, and so on. In sum, self-esteem refers to global self-evaluations, self-concept to more domain-specific evaluations. Having high self-esteem and a positive self-concept are important aspects of children's well-being (Kadir, Yeung, & Diallo, 2018).

The foundations of self-esteem and self-concept emerge from the quality of parent-child interaction in infancy and early childhood. Thus, if children have low self-esteem in middle and late childhood, they may have experienced neglect or abuse in relationships with their parents earlier in development. Children with high self-esteem are more likely to be securely attached to their parents and have parents who engage in sensitive caregiving (Thompson, 2006, 2013).

self-esteem The global evaluative dimension of the self; also called self-worth or self-image.

self-concept Domain-specific self-evaluations.

These items are from a widely used measure of self-esteem, the Rosenberg Scale of Self-Esteem. The items deal with your general feelings about yourself. Place a check mark in the column that best describes your feelings about yourself:
1 = strongly agree, 2 = agree, 3 = disagree, 4 = strongly disagree.

	1	2	3	4
1. I feel that I am a person of worth, at least on an equal plane with others.				
2. I feel that I have a number of good qualities.				
3. All in all, I am inclined to feel that I am a failure.				
4. I am able to do things as well as most other people.				
5. I feel I do not have much to be proud of.				
6. I take a positive attitude toward myself.				
7. On the whole, I am satisfied with myself.				
8. I wish I could have more respect for myself.				
9. I certainly feel useless at times.				
10. At times I think I am no good at all.				

To obtain your self-esteem score, reverse your scores for items 3, 5, 8, 9, and 10. (That is, on item 3 if you gave yourself a 1, instead give yourself a 4.) Add those scores to your scores for items 1, 2, 4, 6, and 7 for your overall self-esteem score. Scores can range from 10 to 40. If you scored below 20, consider contacting the counseling center at your college or university for help in improving your self-esteem.

FIGURE 2
EVALUATING SELF-ESTEEM

For most children, high self-esteem and a positive self-concept are important aspects of their well-being. However, for some children, self-esteem reflects perceptions that do not always match reality, yet having a clear and consistent self-concept and self-esteem is key to healthy development (Becht & others, 2017). A child's self-esteem might reflect a belief about whether he or she is intelligent and popular with peers, for example, but that belief is not necessarily accurate. Thus, high self-esteem may refer to accurate, justified perceptions of one's worth as a person and one's successes and accomplishments, but it can also refer to an arrogant, grandiose, unwarranted sense of superiority over others (Brummelman, Thomaes, & Sedikides, 2016). In the same manner, low self-esteem may reflect either an accurate perception of one's shortcomings or a distorted, even pathological insecurity and inferiority (Paxton & Damiano, 2017; Stadelmann & others, 2017).

ASSESSMENT

Measuring self-esteem and self-concept hasn't always been easy (Buhrmester, Blanton & Swann, 2011). An example of a useful measure developed to assess self-evaluations by children is Susan Harter's (1985) Self-Perception Profile for Children. It taps general self-worth plus self-concept for five specific domains: scholastic competence, athletic competence, social acceptance, physical appearance, and behavioral conduct.

The Self-Perception Profile for Children is designed to be used with third-grade through sixth-grade children. Harter also developed a separate scale for adolescents, the Self-Perception Profile for Adolescents (Harter, 1989). It assesses global self-worth and the five domains tested for children plus three additional domains—close friendship, romantic appeal, and job competence.

Harter's measures can separate self-evaluations in different domains of one's life. How are these specific self-evaluations related to self-esteem in general? Even children have both a general level of self-esteem and varying levels of self-conceptions in particular domains of their lives (Cvencek & others, 2018; Harter, 2012, 2015). For example, a child might have a moderately high level of general self-esteem but have varying self-conceptions in specific areas: high in athletic competence, high in social acceptance, high in physical appearance, high in behavioral conduct, but low in scholastic competence.

Self-esteem appears to have an especially strong tie with self-perception in one domain in particular: physical appearance. Researchers have found that among adolescents, global self-esteem is correlated more strongly with perceived physical appearance than with scholastic competence, social acceptance, behavioral conduct, or athletic competence (Broc, 2014; Harter, 2012, 2015; Nagai & others, 2018) (see Figure 3). Notice in Figure 3 that the link between perceived physical appearance and self-esteem has been made in many countries. This association between physical appearance and self-esteem is not confined to adolescence; it holds from early childhood through middle age (von Soest, Wichstrom, & Kvalem, 2016; Wichstrøm & von Soest, 2016).

Domain	Harter's U.S. samples	Other countries
Physical Appearance	.65	.62
Scholastic Competence	.48	.41
Social Acceptance	.46	.40
Behavioral Conduct	.45	.45
Athletic Competence	.33	.30

FIGURE 3

CORRELATIONS BETWEEN GLOBAL SELF-ESTEEM AND SELF-EVALUATIONS OF DOMAINS OF COMPETENCE. *Note:* The correlations shown are the average correlations computed across a number of studies. The other countries in this evaluation were England, Ireland, Australia, Canada, Germany, Italy, Greece, the Netherlands, and Japan. Recall that correlation coefficients can range from −1.00 to +1.00. The correlations between physical appearance and global self-esteem (.65 and .62) are moderately high.

DEVELOPMENTAL CHANGES

In the past, researchers have disagreed about the extent to which self-esteem varies with age. One large study found that self-esteem is high in childhood, declines in adolescence, and increases in adulthood until late adulthood, when it declines again (Robins & others, 2002) (see Figure 4). The largest study to date is a meta-analysis of over 300 samples that included more than 160,000 participants around the globe (Orth, Erol, & Luciano, 2018). This study showed that self-esteem increased across childhood, was stable across early adolescence, but increased in late-adolescence and into early adulthood. Self-esteem continued to climb across middle age, then was stable into old age, only to decline slightly in very old age (past 90 years).

Notice in Figure 4 that the self-esteem of males was higher than that of females through most of the life span. One explanation for this gender difference holds that the difference in self-esteem is driven by a negative body image and that girls tend to have more negative body images during pubertal change than boys do. Another explanation emphasizes the greater interest that adolescent girls take in social relationships and society's failure to reward that interest (Peets & Hodges, 2018). But also note in Figure 4 that despite the lower self-esteem among adolescent girls, their average self-esteem score (3.3) was still higher than the neutral point on the scale (3.0). How do adolescents rate different aspects of their self-images, such as their psychological self, social self, coping self, familial self, and sexual self? To find out, see *Connecting Through Research*.

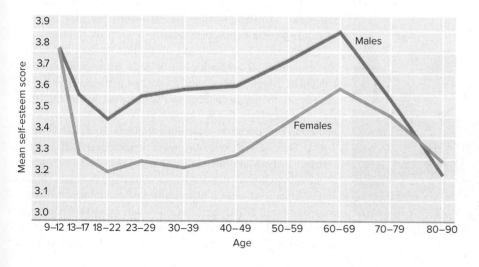

FIGURE 4

SELF-ESTEEM ACROSS THE LIFE SPAN. One large-scale study asked more than 300,000 individuals to rate the extent to which they have high self-esteem on a 5-point scale, with 5 being "Strongly Agree" and 1 being "Strongly Disagree." Self-esteem dropped in adolescence and late adulthood. Self-esteem of females was lower than self-esteem of males through most of the life span.

Source: Robins, R.W., Trzesniewski, K.H., Tracev, J.L., Potter, J., and Gosling, S.D. 2002. Age differences in self-esteem from age 9 to 90. *Psychology and Aging*, 17, 423–434. The American Psychological Association, Inc.

connecting through research

How Do Adolescents Rate Their Self-Images Across Five Different Areas?

One illuminating study examined the self-images of 675 adolescents (289 males and 386 females) ranging from 13 to 19 years of age in Naples, Italy (Bacchini & Magliulo, 2003). Self-image was assessed using the Offer Self-Image Questionnaire, which consists of 130 items grouped into 11 scales that define five different aspects of self-image:

- The psychological self (made up of scales that assess impulse control, emotional tone, and body image)
- The social self (consists of scales that evaluate social relationships, morals, and vocational and educational aspirations)
- The coping self (composed of scales that measure mastery of the world, psychological problems, and adjustment)
- The familial self (made up of only one scale that evaluates how adolescents feel about their parents)
- The sexual self (composed of only one scale that examines adolescents' feelings and attitudes about sexual matters)

The adolescents had positive self-images, with scores higher than a neutral score (3.5) on all 11 scales. For example, the adolescents' average body self-image score was 4.2. The aspect of their lives in which adolescents had the most positive self-image involved their educational and vocational aspirations (average score of 4.8). The lowest self-image score was for impulse control (average score of 3.9). These results support the view that adolescents have a more positive perception of themselves than is commonly believed.

Gender differences were found on a number of the self-image scales, with boys consistently having more positive self-images than did girls. This finding has been replicated in more recent research (for example, Nelson & others, 2018). Keep in mind, though, that as we indicated earlier, even though adolescent girls reported lower self-images than boys, their self-images still were mainly in the positive range.

VARIATIONS IN SELF-ESTEEM

Variations in self-esteem have been linked with many aspects of children's development. However, much of the research is *correlational* rather than *experimental*. Recall that correlation does not equal causation. Thus, if a correlational study finds an association between children's low self-esteem and low academic achievement, low academic achievement could cause the low self-esteem as much as low self-esteem might cause low academic achievement (Scherrer & Preckel, 2018). Studies of youth around the globe show that there are moderate correlations between school performance and self-esteem (Körük, 2017), but these correlations do not necessarily mean that high self-esteem produces better school performance.

Turning to other aspects of development, children with high self-esteem sometimes show greater initiative, but this can produce positive or negative outcomes. Children with high self-esteem may be more likely to show both prosocial and antisocial actions (Barry & others, 2018). For example, they are more likely than children with low self-esteem to defend victims against bullies, but they are also more likely to be bullies themselves.

Researchers have also found strong links between self-esteem and happiness. It seems likely that high self-esteem increases happiness. Many studies have found that individuals with low self-esteem, including children and adolescents, report that they feel more depressed and are more likely to suffer from emotional and behavioral disorders (Masselink & others, 2018; Reed-Fitzke, 2019). One of the longest-running longitudinal studies also revealed that adolescents with low self-esteem had lower levels of life satisfaction at 30 years of age (Birkeland & others, 2012).

Although self-esteem historically has been thought to derive from doing well at activities that individuals believe are important for themselves, cross-cultural research suggests that self-esteem is more closely tied to doing well at activities that one's cultural

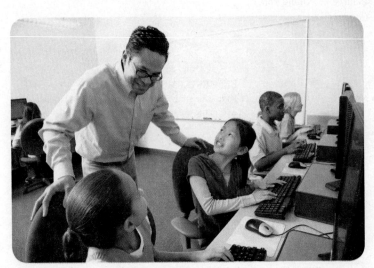

What are some issues involved in understanding children's self-esteem in school?
Inti St Clair/Digital Vision/Getty Images

caring *connections*

Increasing Children's Self-Esteem

A current concern is that too many of today's children and adolescents grow up receiving empty praise and as a consequence develop inflated self-esteem. Inflated praise, although well intended, may cause children with low self-esteem to avoid important learning experiences such as tackling challenging tasks (Brummelman, Thomaes, & Sedikides, 2016). In particular, adults tend to praise the personal qualities (such as intelligence) rather than behavior (such as hard work) of children with low self-esteem. However, person-oriented praise may backfire. Children who had been praised for their personal qualities rather than their behavior were less likely to persist in the face of difficulties. If individuals have been praised for their intelligence but then fail, they may think there is nothing they can do to improve their performance in the future. But, if children have been praised for their hard work and fail, they may think that they need to work harder in the future. Holding an incremental theory of intelligence (believing that intelligence can be improved by working hard) and having learning goals (wanting to learn to understand the material better, rather than just to get a good grade) are both related to better school performance (Gunderson & others, 2018).

It is possible to raise children's self-esteem by (1) identifying the domains of competence important to the child, (2) providing emotional support and social approval, (3) praising achievement, and (4) encouraging coping. Children have the highest self-esteem when they perform competently in domains that are important to them. Therefore, children should be encouraged to identify and to value areas in which they are competent.

Emotional support and social approval also powerfully influence children's self-esteem. Some children with low self-esteem come from conflicted families or experienced abuse or neglect—situations in which emotional support was unavailable. For some children, formal programs such as Big Brothers & Big Sisters can provide alternative sources of emotional support and social approval; for others, support can come informally through the encouragement of a teacher, a coach, or another significant adult. Peer approval becomes increasingly important during adolescence, but adult as well as peer support continues to be an important influence on self-esteem through adolescence.

Achievement also can improve children's self-esteem. The straightforward teaching of real skills to children often results in increased achievement and enhanced self-esteem. When children know what tasks are necessary to achieve goals and have experience performing these or similar tasks, their self-esteem improves.

Self-esteem also is often increased when children face a problem and try to cope with it, rather than avoid it. If coping rather than avoidance prevails, children often face problems realistically, honestly, and nondefensively. This produces favorable self-evaluative thoughts, which lead to the self-generated approval that raises self-esteem. The converse is true of low self-esteem: unfavorable self-evaluations trigger denial, deception, and avoidance, which lead to self-generated disapproval.

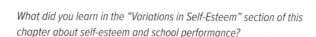

How can parents help children develop higher self-esteem?
Purestock/SuperStock

What did you learn in the "Variations in Self-Esteem" section of this chapter about self-esteem and school performance?

---

group believes are important. In a study of more than 5,000 young people in 19 countries, self-esteem was not related to personal values but rather to fulfilling values of other people in that culture. For example, in Western Europe and parts of South America, self-esteem was related to individual freedom and feeling in control of one's life, whereas in the Middle East, Africa, and Asia, self-esteem was related to perceiving oneself as fulfilling obligations to others and doing one's duty (Becker & others, 2014). In addition, cultures differ in the importance placed on self-esteem. For example, European American mothers often spontaneously mention building children's self-esteem as important for promoting positive adjustment. By contrast, Taiwanese mothers rarely mention self-esteem, and if they do, they describe it as a vulnerability that can lead to rudeness, poor self-control, and stubbornness (Miller & Cho, 2018).

To explore ways that children's low self-esteem might be increased, see *Caring Connections*.

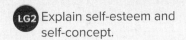
Review

- What are self-esteem and self-concept?
- What are two measures for assessing self-esteem and self-concept?
- How is self-esteem linked with age?
- What are some variations in self-esteem, and how are they linked to children's development? What role do parent-child relationships play in self-esteem?

Connect

- As discussed in the "Regulation of Emotion" section of the chapter

"Emotional Development," which parenting approach might help accomplish the fourth strategy for increasing children's self-esteem mentioned in the *Caring Connections* interlude "Increasing Children's Self-Esteem"?

Reflect *Your Own Personal Journey of Life*

- Review the characteristics of self-understanding in adolescence. Which of these characteristics do you associate most closely with your self-understanding as an adolescent?

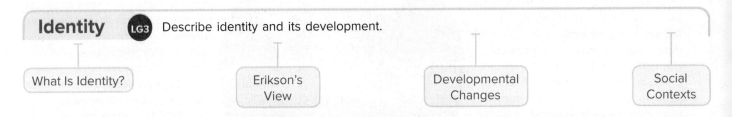

Identity   **LG3**   Describe identity and its development.

| What Is Identity? | Erikson's View | Developmental Changes | Social Contexts |

Who am I? What am I all about? What am I going to do with my life? What is different about me? How can I make it on my own? These questions reflect the search for an identity.

By far the most comprehensive and provocative theory of identity development is Erik Erikson's. In this section, you will explore his views on identity, contemporary research on how identity develops, and how social contexts influence that development.

WHAT IS IDENTITY?

Identity is who a person is, representing a synthesis and integration of self-understanding. Identity is a self-portrait composed of many pieces, including these:

- The career and work path the person wants to follow (vocational/career identity)
- Whether the person is conservative, liberal, or middle-of-the-road (political identity)
- The person's spiritual beliefs (religious identity)
- Whether the person is single, married, divorced, and so on (relationship identity)
- The extent to which the person is motivated to achieve and is intellectually oriented (achievement, intellectual identity)
- Whether the person is heterosexual, homosexual, bisexual, or transgendered (sexual identity)
- Which part of the world or country a person is from and how intensely the person identifies with his or her cultural heritage (cultural/ethnic identity)
- The things a person likes to do, which can include sports, music, hobbies, and so on (interests)
- The individual's personality characteristics, such as being introverted or extraverted, anxious or calm, friendly or hostile, and so on (personality)
- The individual's body image (physical identity)

We put these pieces together to form a sense of ourselves continuing through time within a social world. Synthesizing the identity components can be a long and complex process,. with many negations and affirmations of various roles and faces. Identity

"Who are you?" said the caterpillar. Alice replied rather shyly, "I—I hardly know, sir, just at present—at least I know who I was when I got up this morning, but I must have changed several times since then."

—LEWIS CARROLL
English writer, 19th century

identity Who a person is, representing a synthesis and integration of self-understanding.

development takes place in bits and pieces. Decisions are not made once and for all, but have to be made again and again. Identity development does not happen neatly, nor does it happen cataclysmically (Arnold, 2017; Negru-Subtirica, Pop, & Crocetti, 2017).

ERIKSON'S VIEW

Questions about identity surface as common, virtually universal, concerns during adolescence. It was Erik Erikson (1968) who first understood how central such questions are to understanding adolescent development. Identity is now believed to be a key aspect of adolescent development. In fact, Erikson's fifth developmental stage, which individuals experience during adolescence, is **identity versus identity confusion.** Adolescents face an overwhelming number of choices. As they gradually come to realize that they will be responsible for themselves and their own lives, adolescents try to determine what those lives are going to be like.

During adolescence, society generally permits trying out different identities—something Erikson called the **psychosocial moratorium.** Adolescents in effect search their culture's identity files, experimenting with different roles and personalities. They may want to pursue one career one month (lawyer, for example) and another career the next month (doctor, actor, teacher, social worker, or astronaut, for example). They may dress neatly one day, sloppily the next. This experimentation is a deliberate effort on the part of adolescents to find out where they fit in the world.

Youth who successfully cope with these conflicting identities emerge with a new sense of self that is both refreshing and acceptable. Adolescents who do not successfully resolve this identity crisis suffer what Erikson calls *identity confusion*. The confusion takes one of two courses: individuals withdraw, isolating themselves from peers and family, or they immerse themselves in the world of peers and lose their identity in the crowd.

There are hundreds of roles for adolescents to try out, and probably just as many ways to pursue each role. Erikson stresses that, by late adolescence, vocational roles are central to identity development, especially in the highly technological societies found throughout industrialized and emerging economies in many countries around the globe. Youth who are on track to enter higher education so they can prepare to enter a vocation that offers the potential of reasonably high self-esteem will experience the least stress during this phase of identity development. Adolescents also have much to contribute to their families, peers, schools and communities; this need to contribute is a key element of adolescents' emerging identity as they approach adulthood (Fuligni, 2019).

Over the past few decades, many societies have extended adolescence into the twenties, as expectations of prolonged training and education have grown (Stetka, 2017). One concern arising from this trend is that too many of today's youth aren't moving toward any identity resolution. For example, Damon (2008) proposed that too many youth are left to their own devices in dealing with some of life's biggest questions: "What is my calling? What can I contribute to the world? What am I here for?" Damon acknowledges that adults can't make youths' decisions for them, but he emphasizes that it is very important for parents, teachers, mentors, and other adults to provide guidance, feedback, and contexts that will improve the likelihood that youth will develop a positive identity. Youth need a cultural climate that inspires rather than demoralizes them and supports their chances of reaching their aspirations. This can be accomplished in part by viewing adolescent and young adult development as a period of flexibility, learning, and building on strengths (Lerner, 2017).

DEVELOPMENTAL CHANGES

Although questions about identity are particularly likely to emerge during adolescence, identity formation neither begins nor ends during these years (McLean & others, 2018; Syed & Mitchell, 2016). It begins with the appearance of attachment, the development of the sense of self, and the emergence of independence in infancy; the process reaches its final phase with a life review and integration in old age. The most important aspect of

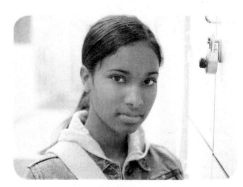

What are some important dimensions of identity?
L. Mouton/PhotoAlto

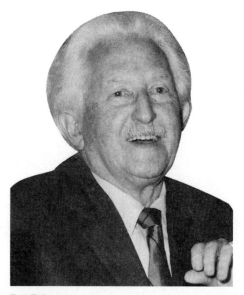

Erik Erikson.
Bettmann/Getty Images

identity versus identity confusion Erikson's fifth developmental stage, which individuals experience during the adolescent years. At this time, adolescents examine who they are, what they are all about, and where they are going in life.

psychosocial moratorium Erikson's term for the gap between childhood security and adult autonomy that adolescents experience as part of their identity exploration.

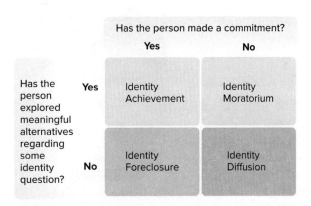

Has the person made a commitment?

	Yes	No
Has the person explored meaningful alternatives regarding some identity question? **Yes**	Identity Achievement	Identity Moratorium
No	Identity Foreclosure	Identity Diffusion

FIGURE 5

MARCIA'S FOUR STATUSES OF IDENTITY

crisis A period of identity development during which the adolescent is choosing among meaningful alternatives.

commitment Personal investment in identity.

identity diffusion Marcia's term for the status of individuals who have not yet experienced a crisis (that is, they have not yet explored meaningful alternatives) or made any commitments.

identity foreclosure Marcia's term for the status of individuals who have made a commitment but have not experienced a crisis.

identity moratorium Marcia's term for the status of individuals who are in the midst of a crisis but whose commitments either are absent or are only vaguely defined.

identity achievement Marcia's term for the status of individuals who have undergone a crisis and made a commitment.

identity development in adolescence, especially late adolescence, is that for the first time, physical development, cognitive development, and socioemotional development advance to the point at which the individual can begin to sort through and synthesize childhood identities and identifications to construct a viable path toward adult maturity.

Some decisions made during adolescence might seem trivial: whom to date, whether or not to break up, which major to study, whether to study or play, whether or not to be politically active, and so on. Over the years of adolescence, however, such decisions begin to form the core of what the individual is all about as a human being—what is called his or her identity.

Systematic reviews of longitudinal and cross-sectional studies show that adolescents who have a mature identity show high levels of adjustment and a positive personality profile. For example, adolescents who are highly committed in their identity development are characterized by higher levels of conscientiousness and emotional stability (Meeus, 2018).

As individuals mature from early adolescence to emerging adulthood, they increasingly pursue in-depth exploration of their identity (Klimstra & others, 2010). One way that researchers are examining identity changes in depth is to use a *narrative approach,* which involves asking individuals to tell their life stories and then evaluating the extent to which their stories are meaningful and integrated (Fivush, 2019; McAdams & McLean, 2013; McLean & Lilgendahl, 2019). For example, a study using the narrative identity approach revealed that from age 11 to 18, boys increasingly engaged in thinking about the meaningfulness of their lives, especially meaning related to the self as changing (McLean, Breen, & Fournier, 2010).

Identity Statuses How do individual adolescents go about the process of forming an identity? Eriksonian researcher James Marcia (1993, 1994) proposes that Erikson's theory of identity development contains four statuses of identity, or ways of resolving the identity crisis: identity diffusion, identity foreclosure, identity moratorium, and identity achievement. What determines an individual's identity status? Marcia classifies individuals based on the existence or extent of their crisis or commitment (see Figure 5). **Crisis** is defined as a period of identity development during which the individual is exploring alternatives. Most researchers use the term *exploration* rather than *crisis.* **Commitment** is personal investment in identity.

The four statuses of identity are as follows:

- **Identity diffusion** is the status of individuals who have not yet experienced a crisis or made any commitments. Not only are they undecided about occupational and ideological choices, they are also likely to show little interest in such matters.
- **Identity foreclosure** is the status of individuals who have made a commitment but not experienced a crisis. This occurs most often when parents hand down commitments to their adolescents, usually in an authoritarian way, before adolescents have had a chance to explore different approaches, ideologies, and vocations on their own.
- **Identity moratorium** is the status of individuals who are in the midst of a crisis but whose commitments are either absent or are only vaguely defined.
- **Identity achievement** is the status of individuals who have undergone a crisis and made a commitment.

To evaluate your identity in different areas of development, see Figure 6. Let's explore some examples of Marcia's identity statuses. Thirteen-year-old Mia has neither begun to explore her identity in any meaningful way nor made an identity commitment; she is identity diffused. Eighteen-year-old Oliver's parents want him to be a medical doctor, so he is planning on majoring in premedicine in college and has not explored other options; he is identity foreclosed. Nineteen-year-old Sasha is not quite sure what life paths she wants to follow, but she recently went to the counseling center at her college to find out about different careers; she is in identity moratorium status. Twenty-one-year-old Marcelo

Think deeply about your exploration and commitment in the areas listed here. For each area, check whether your identity status is diffused, foreclosed, moratorium, or achieved.

Identity Component	Identity Status			
	Diffused	Foreclosed	Moratorium	Achieved
Vocational (career)				
Political				
Religious				
Relationships				
Achievement				
Sexual				
Gender				
Ethnic/Cultural				
Interests				
Personality				
Physical				

FIGURE 6

EXPLORING YOUR IDENTITY. If you checked diffused or foreclosed for any areas, take some time to think about what you need to do to move into a moratorium identity status in those areas.

extensively explored several career options in college, eventually getting his degree in science education, and is looking forward to his first year of teaching high school students; his status is identity achieved. These examples focused on the career dimension, but remember that identity has a number of dimensions.

According to Marcia's theory, young adolescents are primarily in the identity statuses of diffusion, foreclosure, or moratorium. To move to the status of identity achievement, young adolescents need three things: (1) they must be confident that they have parental support, (2) they must have an established sense of industry, and (3) they must be able to adopt a self-reflective stance toward the future.

The identity status approach has been criticized by some researchers and theoreticians because it places too much emphasis on completing identity development by making decisions in adolescence and early adulthood. Contemporary views have adapted Erikson's theory to consider identity development as a lifelong, ongoing process involving continuous identity commitment, exploration, and reconsideration of identity commitment (Crocetti, 2017).

Emerging Adulthood and Beyond A consensus is developing that the key changes in identity are taking place in emerging adulthood (18 to 25 years of age) or later than in adolescence (Schwartz, Luyckx, & Crocetti, 2015; Syed & Mitchell, 2016). One of the key transitions from adolescence to emerging adulthood is attending college. Why might college produce some key changes in identity? Increased complexity in the reasoning skills of college students, combined with a wide range of new experiences that highlight contrasts between home and college and between themselves and others, stimulates them to reach a higher level of integrating various dimensions of their identity (Murray & Arnett, 2019). As already noted, identity development is facilitated by challenging new tasks and transitions, but it is an ongoing process that continues into and through young adulthood (Crocetti, 2017).

Identity is more stable in adulthood than in adolescence (Meeus, 2018), but resolution of the identity issue during adolescence and emerging adulthood does not mean that identity will be stable through the remainder of life. Many individuals who develop positive identities follow what are called "MAMA" cycles; that is, their identity status changes from *m*oratorium to *a*chievement to *m*oratorium to *a*chievement. These cycles may be repeated throughout life. Marcia (2002) points out that the first identity is just that—it is not, and should not be expected to be, the final product.

As long as one keeps searching, the answers come.

—Joan Baez
American folk singer, 20th century

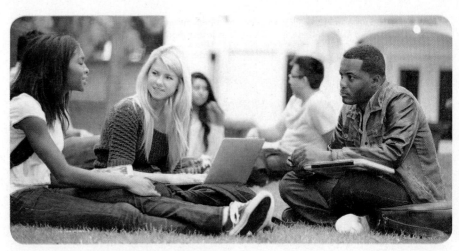

How does identity change in emerging adulthood?
Monkey Business Images/Shutterstock

SOCIAL CONTEXTS

Social contexts play important roles in identity. Let's examine how family, culture, and ethnicity are linked to identity development.

Family Influences   Parents are important figures in the adolescent's development of identity (Cooper & Seginer, 2018). It is during adolescence that the search for balance between the need for autonomy and the need for connectedness becomes especially important to identity. Developmentalists Catherine Cooper and Harold Grotevant (Grotevant & Cooper, 1998) established that the presence of a family atmosphere that promotes both individuality and connectedness is important for the adolescent's identity development:

- **Individuality** consists of two dimensions: self-assertion—the ability to have and communicate a point of view, and separateness—the use of communication patterns to express how one is different from others.
- **Connectedness** also consists of two dimensions: mutuality, which involves sensitivity to and respect for others' views, and permeability, which involves openness to others' views.

In general, Cooper's research indicates that identity formation is enhanced by family relationships that are both individuated, which encourages adolescents to develop their own point of view, and connected, which provides a secure base from which to explore the widening social worlds of adolescence. When connectedness is strong and individuation weak, adolescents often have an identity-foreclosure status. When connectedness is weak, adolescents often reveal identity confusion.

Research interest also has increased regarding the role that attachment to parents might play in identity development. A meta-analysis found weak to moderate correlations between attachment to parents in adolescence and identity development (Arseth & others, 2009). A large cross-cultural study including youth in Japan, Italy, and Lithuania confirmed this overall finding in a diverse international sample of adolescents (Sugimura & others, 2018).

Peer/Romantic Relationships   Researchers have found that the capacity to explore one's identity during adolescence and emerging adulthood is linked to the quality of friendships and romantic relationships. For example, a study of Jamaicans spanning emerging adulthood found that identity achievement was associated with greater openness to and less fear of intimacy with partners and friends (Strudwick-Alexander, 2017). Another study found that an open, active exploration of identity when adolescents are comfortable with close friends contributes to the positive quality of the friendship

developmental **connection**

Attachment

Even while adolescents seek autonomy, attachment to parents is important; secure attachment in adolescence is linked to a number of positive outcomes. Connect to "Families."

individuality Consists of two dimensions: self-assertion, the ability to have and communicate a point of view; and separateness, the use of communication patterns to express how one is different from others.

connectedness Consists of two dimensions: mutuality, sensitivity to and respect for others' views; and permeability, openness to others' views.

(Deamen & others, 2012). It is within close personal friendships that individuals can explore their identities through dialogue and emotional closeness (Albarello, Crocetti, & Rubini, 2018).

In terms of links between identity and romantic relationships in adolescence and emerging adulthood, two individuals in a romantic relationship are both in the process of constructing their own identities and each person provides the other with a context for identity exploration. The extent of their secure attachment with each other can influence how each partner constructs his or her own identity (Kerpelman & Pittman, 2018).

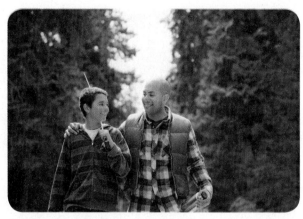

How is an adolescent's identity development influenced by parents?
Hero Images/Getty Images

Culture and Ethnicity   Much of the prior research on identity development has been based on data obtained from adolescents and emerging adults in the United States and Canada, most of whom were non-Latino Whites (Schwartz, Luyckx, & Crocetti, 2015). Many of these individuals have grown up with a cultural identity that emphasizes the individual. However, the research is shifting rapidly to address what is already known about the rich diversity of cultures and experiences that also influence identity. In many countries around the world, adolescents and emerging adults have grown up influenced by a collectivist emphasis on fitting in with the group and connecting with others. The collectivist emphasis is especially prevalent in Asian countries such as Japan (Sugimura & others, 2018). Researchers have found that self-oriented identity exploration may not be the main process through which identity achievement is attained in Asian cultures. Rather, adolescents and emerging adults in those cultural contexts may develop their identity through developing their independence as well as commitment to others in their cultural group (Hatano & Sugimura, 2017; McCabe & Dinh, 2016). This emphasis on interdependence in Asian and Latino cultures includes an expectation that adolescents and emerging adults will accept and embrace social and family roles. Thus, some patterns of identity development, such as the foreclosed status, may be more adaptive in non-Western cultures (Cheng & Berman, 2013; Hassan, Vignoles, & Schwartz, 2018; Stein & others, 2015).

Adolescents and emerging adults who are part of the cultural majority are unlikely to view their majority status as part of their identity. However, for many adolescents and emerging adults who have emigrated or grown up as members of an ethnic minority group in their country and community, cultural dimensions likely are an important aspect of their identity. For example, researchers have found that at both the high school and college level, Latino students were more likely to indicate that their cultural identity was an important dimension of their overall self-concept than were non-Latino White students (Urdan, 2012).

Ethnic identity is an enduring aspect of the self that includes a sense of membership in an ethnic group, along with the attitudes and feelings related to that membership (Phinney, 2006; Verkuyten, 2018). Throughout the world, ethnic minority groups face a challenge: to maintain their ethnic identities while also being part of the dominant culture. Many adolescents develop a **bicultural identity.** That is, they identify in some ways with their ethnic group and in other ways with the majority culture (Cooper & Seginer, 2018; Feliciano & Rumbaut, 2018; Vietze & others, 2018). A study of U.S.-born Mexican American college students found that they identified both with the American mainstream culture and with their culture of origin, and that individual differences in the strength of their Mexican identity were associated with political and social attitudes (Naumann, Benet-Martínez, & Espinoza, 2017).

Many aspects of sociocultural contexts may influence ethnic identity (Lilgendahl & others, 2018; Verkuyten, 2018). Ethnic identity tends to be stronger among members of minority groups than among members of mainstream groups. For example, in one early study, the exploration of ethnic identity was higher among ethnic minority college students than among White non-Latino college students (Phinney & Alipuria, 1990).

Time is another aspect of the sociocultural context that influences ethnic identity. The indicators of identity often differ for each succeeding generation of immigrants (Huynh, Benet-Martínez, & Nguyen, 2018; Phinney & Ong, 2007). For example, consider

ethnic identity An enduring aspect of the self that includes a sense of membership in an ethnic group, along with the attitudes and feelings related to that membership.

bicultural identity Identity formation that occurs when adolescents identify in some ways with their ethnic group and in other ways with the majority culture.

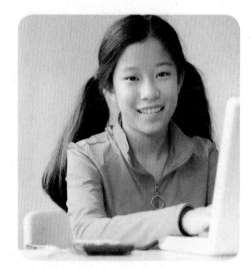

One adolescent girl, 16-year-old Michelle Chin, made these comments about ethnic identity development: "My parents do not understand that teenagers need to find out who they are, which means a lot of experimenting, a lot of mood swings, a lot of emotions and awkwardness. Like any teenager, I am facing an identity crisis. I am still trying to figure out whether I am a Chinese American or an American with Asian eyes." *What are some other aspects of developing an ethnic identity in adolescence?*
Red Chopsticks/Getty Images

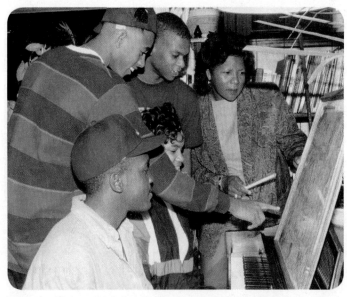

Researcher Margaret Beale Spencer, shown here talking with adolescents, stresses that adolescence is often a critical juncture in the identity development of ethnic minority individuals. Most ethnic minority individuals consciously confront their ethnicity for the first time in adolescence.

Courtesy of Margaret Beale Spencer

the generational differences among those who emigrated to the United States. First-generation immigrants are likely to be secure in their identities and unlikely to change much; they may or may not develop a new identity. The degree to which they begin to feel "American" appears to be related to whether or not they learn English, develop social networks beyond their ethnic group, and become culturally competent in their new country. Second-generation immigrants are more likely to think of themselves as "American," possibly because citizenship is granted at birth. Maxine Hong Kingston, a Chinese American author who was introduced in the opening of this chapter, noted, "I have been in America all of my life; Chinese is a foreign culture to me" (Powellsbooks.blog, 2006). For second-generation immigrants, ethnic identity is likely to be linked to retention of their ethnic language and social networks. In the third and later generations, the issues become more complex. Broad social factors may affect the extent to which members of this generation retain their ethnic identities. For example, media images may encourage members of an ethnic group to identify with their group or retain parts of its culture. Discrimination may force people to see themselves as cut off from the majority group and encourage them to seek support from their own ethnic culture. This acculturation stress can have implications for identity and health (Cavanaugh & others, 2018; Romero & Piña-Watson, 2017).

Researchers also are increasingly finding that a positive ethnic identity is related to positive outcomes for ethnic minority adolescents (Neblett, Rivas-Drake, & Umana-Taylor, 2011; Umaña-Taylor & others, 2018). One study indicated that Native American adolescents' positive ethnic identity was derived from parents' and community members' socialization of ethnicity and ways of coping with discrimination. This preparation protected the youth from experiencing depressive symptoms (Yasui & others, 2015). Also, an intervention study of ethnic majority and minority youth indicated that growth in identity exploration was linked with heightened self-esteem and fewer symptoms of depression (Umaña-Taylor & others, 2018). And another study revealed that having a positive ethnic identity among Latino youth was influenced by the neighborhood context (for example, whether there were other Latino families in the area) and parents' ethnic socialization in the family (White & others, 2018).

To read about one individual who guides Latino adolescents in developing a positive identity, see the *Connecting with Careers* profile of Armando Ronquillo.

Jean Phinney (2006) described how ethnic identity may change in emerging adulthood, especially highlighting how certain experiences of ethnic minority individuals may shorten or lengthen emerging adulthood. For ethnic minority individuals who must take on family responsibilities and cannot go to college, identity formation may occur earlier. By contrast, especially for ethnic minority individuals who go to college, identity formation may take longer because of the complexity of exploring and understanding a bicultural identity. The cognitive challenges of higher education likely stimulate ethnic minority individuals to reflect on their identity and examine changes in the way they want to identify themselves. This increased reflection may focus on integrating parts of one's ethnic minority culture with elements of the mainstream culture. For example, some emerging adults have to come to grips with resolving a conflict between the family loyalty and interdependence emphasized in their ethnic minority culture and the values of independence and self-assertion emphasized by the mainstream culture found in most industrialized, technological societies and cultures (Arnett, 2015). To read further about ethnic identity development in adolescence, see *Connecting with Diversity*.

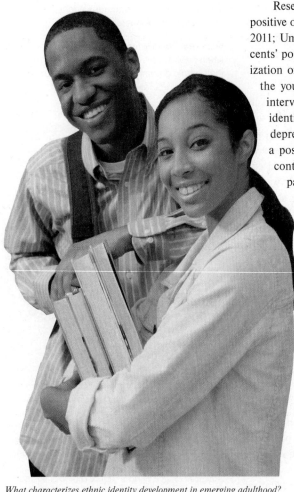

What characterizes ethnic identity development in emerging adulthood?

Mark Edward Atkinson/Blend Images/Getty Images

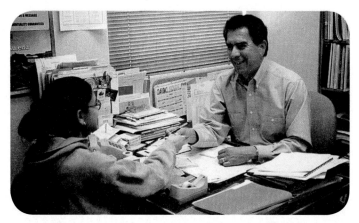
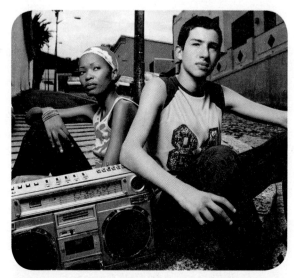

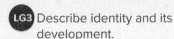

Review Connect Reflect

LG3 Describe identity and its development.

Review

- What is identity?
- What is Erikson's view of identity?
- How do individuals develop their identity? What identity statuses can be used to classify individuals?
- How do the social contexts of family, peers/romantic relationships, culture, and ethnicity influence identity?

Connect

- Identity versus identity confusion is the fifth stage of Erikson's theory of development. What crisis should a child have resolved in the fourth stage to be able to successfully move on to confront the identity versus identity confusion crisis?

Reflect *Your Own Personal Journey of Life*

- How did your identity change as you developed through adolescence? How does your current identity differ from your identity as an adolescent? To guide your self-evaluation of your identity changes, revisit Figure 6 and reflect on what are likely some of the key aspects of your identity.

reach your **learning goals**

The Self and Identity

Self-Understanding and Understanding Others

 LG1 Discuss the development of self-understanding and understanding others.

Self-Understanding

- Self-understanding is a child's cognitive representation of the self—the substance and content of the child's self-conceptions. It provides the rational underpinnings for personal identity. Infants develop a rudimentary form of self-recognition as early as 3 months of age and a more complete form of self-understanding at approximately 18 months of age. Self-understanding in early childhood is characterized by confusion of self, mind, and body; concrete, physical, and active descriptions; and unrealistic positive overestimations. Self-understanding in middle and late childhood involves an increased use of psychological characteristics and traits, social descriptions, and social comparison; distinction between the real and ideal self; and increasingly realistic self-evaluations. Adolescents develop abstract and idealistic conceptions of themselves, become more self-conscious about their self-understanding, and engage in more social comparison than when they were children. Their self-understanding often fluctuates and they construct multiple selves, including possible selves.

Understanding Others

- Young children display more sophisticated self-understanding and understanding of others than was previously thought. Even 4-year-olds understand that people make statements that aren't true to obtain what they want or to avoid trouble. Children increase their perspective taking in middle and late childhood, and they become even more skeptical of others' claims. Three important aspects of understanding others in adolescence are perspective taking, perceiving others' traits, and social cognitive monitoring.

Self-Esteem and Self-Concept

 LG2 Explain self-esteem and self-concept.

What Are Self-Esteem and Self-Concept?

- Self-esteem, also referred to as self-worth or self-image, is the global, evaluative dimension of the self. Self-concept refers to domain-specific evaluations of the self.

- Harter's Self-Perception Profile for Children is used with third-grade through sixth-grade children to assess general self-worth and self-concept in five skill domains. Harter's Self-Perception Profile for Adolescents assesses global self-worth in five skill domains, plus additional domains dealing with friendship, romance, and job competence.

- Some researchers have found that self-esteem drops in adolescence, more so for girls than boys, but there is controversy about how extensively self-esteem varies with age.

- Researchers have found only moderate correlations between self-esteem and school performance. Individuals with high self-esteem have greater initiative than those with low self-esteem, and this can produce positive or negative outcomes. Self-esteem is related to perceived physical appearance and happiness. Low self-esteem is linked with depression, suicide attempts, and anorexia nervosa.

Identity

LG3 Describe identity and its development.

- Identity development is complex and takes place in bits and pieces. At a bare minimum, identity involves commitment to a vocational direction, an ideological stance, and a sexual orientation. Synthesizing identity components can be a long, complex process.

- Erikson argues that identity versus identity confusion is the fifth stage of the human life span, which individuals experience during adolescence. This stage involves entering a psychosocial moratorium between the security of childhood and the autonomy of adulthood. Personality and role experimentation are important aspects of identity development. In technological societies like those in North America, the vocational role is especially important.

- Identity development begins during infancy and continues through old age. James Marcia proposed four identity statuses—identity diffusion, foreclosure, moratorium, and achievement—that are based on crisis (exploration) and commitment. Some experts argue the main changes in identity occur in emerging adulthood rather than adolescence. Individuals often follow moratorium-achievement-moratorium-achievement (MAMA) cycles in their lives.

- Parents are important figures in adolescents' identity development. Both individuality and connectedness in family relations are related to identity development. Peer and romantic relationships also provide social contexts that influence adolescents' identity development. Throughout the world, ethnic minority groups have struggled to maintain their identities while blending into the majority culture. A positive ethnic identity is linked to positive outcomes for ethnic minority adolescents.

key terms

bicultural identity 323	identity achievement 320	individuality 322	self-esteem 313
commitment 320	identity diffusion 320	perspective taking 311	self-understanding 307
connectedness 322	identity foreclosure 320	possible self 310	social cognition 310
crisis 320	identity moratorium 320	psychosocial moratorium 319	
ethnic identity 323	identity versus identity	self 307	
identity 318	confusion 319	self-concept 313	

key people

Catherine Cooper 322	Harold Grotevant 322	James Marcia 320
Erik Erikson 319	Susan Harter 314	Jean Phinney 324

GENDER

chapter **outline**

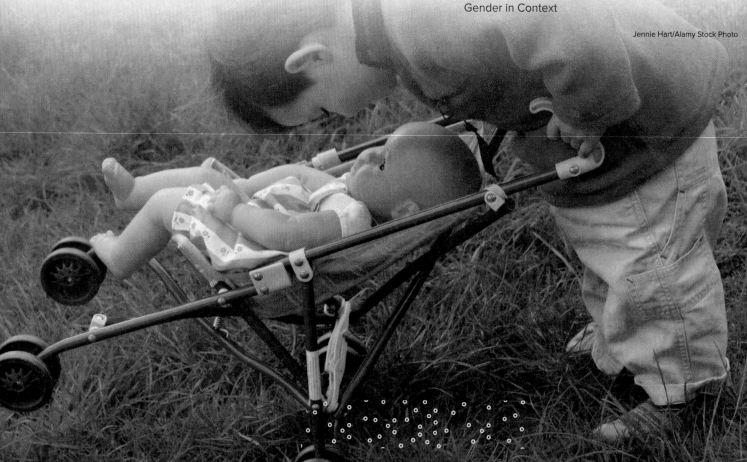

Jennie Hart/Alamy Stock Photo

Consider popular Disney princess movies from previous decades: *Snow White and the Seven Dwarfs* (1937), *Cinderella* (1950), *Sleeping Beauty* (1959), and *The Little Mermaid* (1989). All portray the princesses in gender-stereotyped ways, with each princess being rescued and ending up in a romantic relationship with the prince. By contrast, consider more recent Disney princess movies: *The Princess and the Frog* (2009), *Brave* (2012), *Frozen* (2013), and *Moana* (2016). These later movies portray the princesses in less gender-stereotyped ways, with the princesses being more likely to engage in rescue behaviors and to remain single (Hine & others, 2018).

Contemporary movies geared for older audiences also reflect societal changes in gender roles by portraying female characters who are strong and male characters who are more willing to show their emotions than was typical in movies in the past. Consider Katniss Everdeen in *The Hunger Games*, who is brave, determined, and a skilled hunter, and Peeta Mellark, a boy who is more open with his emotions than Katniss is with hers. As we will see later in this chapter, gender experts have examined the extent to which gender stereotypes are borne out in males' and females' actual beliefs and behaviors.

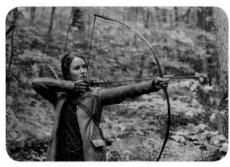

How are gender, emotion, and caring portrayed in the movie Hunger Games?
PictureLux/The Hollywood Archive/Alamy Stock Photo

preview

We begin this chapter by examining what gender involves, then turn our attention to various influences on gender development—biological, social, and cognitive. Next, we explore gender stereotypes, similarities, and differences. Our final discussion focuses on how gender roles are classified.

What Is Gender? Summarize what gender involves.

> To be meek, patient, tactful, modest, honorable, brave, is not to be either manly or womanly; it is to be humane.
>
> —JANE HARRISON
> *English writer, 20th century*

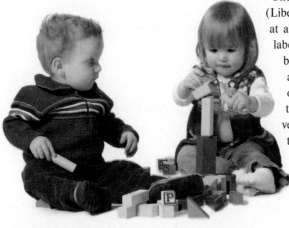

At what age do children know whether they are male or female?
Rubberball/Getty Images

Gender refers to the characteristics of people as males and females. **Gender identity** involves a sense of one's own gender, including knowledge, understanding, and acceptance of being male or female (Liben, 2017). **Gender roles** are sets of expectations that prescribe how females or males should think, act, and feel. During the preschool years, most children increasingly act in ways that match their culture's gender roles. **Gender typing** refers to acquisition of a traditional masculine or feminine role. For example, fighting is more characteristic of a traditional masculine role and crying is more characteristic of a traditional feminine role.

One aspect of gender identity involves knowing whether you are a boy or a girl (Liben, 2017). Until recently, it was thought that this aspect of gender identity emerged at about 2½ years. However, a study that examined use and recognition of gender labels and gender-typed appearance revealed that gender identity likely emerges before 2 years of age (Halim & others, 2018). In this study, mothers' gender role attitudes were not related to their 2-year-olds' gender-typed appearance, but 2-year-olds' own ability to recognize and use gender labels was related to their gender-typed appearance. The study suggests that children are aware of gender from a very early age and motivated to adhere to gender stereotypes by dressing in traditionally masculine or feminine ways.

One study revealed that sex-typed toy play (boys playing with cars and girls with dolls, for example) during the preschool years predicted sex-typed behaviors five years later, regardless of whether children were being reared by lesbian, gay, or heterosexual parents (Li, Kung, & Hines, 2017).

Review Connect Reflect

 Summarize what gender involves.

Review

- What is gender? What are some components of gender?

Connect

- What have you learned about gender and research that you should keep in mind as you read more about research in the area of gender and development in the following sections of this chapter?

Reflect *Your Own Personal Journey of Life*

- As you begin this chapter, think about the role of gender in your life as you were growing up. What are some examples of how your behavior as a child reflected a masculine or feminine role?

Influences on Gender Development **LG2** Discuss the main biological, social, and cognitive influences on gender.

Biological Influences	Social Influences	Cognitive Influences

How is gender influenced by biology? By children's social experiences? By cognitive factors?

BIOLOGICAL INFLUENCES

It was not until the 1920s that researchers confirmed the existence of human sex chromosomes, the genetic material that determines our sex. Humans normally have 46 chromosomes, arranged in pairs. A 23rd pair with two X-shaped chromosomes produces a female. A 23rd pair with an X chromosome and a Y chromosome produces a male.

Hormones Two classes of hormones have the greatest influence on gender: estrogens and androgens. Estrogens and androgens occur in both females and males, but in very different concentrations.

Estrogens primarily influence the development of female physical sex characteristics and help regulate the menstrual cycle. Estrogens are a general class of hormones. An example of an important estrogen is estradiol. In females, estrogens are produced mainly by the ovaries.

Androgens primarily promote the development of male genitals and secondary sex characteristics. One important androgen is testosterone. Androgens are produced by the adrenal glands in males and females, and by the testes in males.

In the first few weeks of gestation, female and male embryos look alike. Male sex organs start to differ from female sex organs when a gene on the Y chromosome directs a small piece of tissue in the embryo to turn into testes. Once the tissue has turned into testes, they begin to secrete testosterone. Because females have no Y chromosome, the tissue turns into ovaries. To explore biological influences on gender, researchers have studied individuals who are exposed to unusual levels of sex hormones early in development (Eme, 2015). Here are four examples of problems that may occur as a result (Lippa, 2005, pp. 122–124, 136–137):

- *Congenital adrenal hyperplasia (CAH).* Some girls have this condition, which is caused by a genetic defect. Their adrenal glands enlarge, resulting in abnormally high levels of androgens. Although CAH girls are XX females, they vary in how much their genitals look like male or female genitals. Their genitals may be surgically altered to look more like those of a typical female. Girls with CAH have been found to prefer toys and activities more stereotypically preferred by boys and to have stronger cross-gender identity than girls without CAH (Pasterski & others, 2015). In addition, girls with CAH have higher levels of aggression than girls without CAH (Spencer & others, 2017).

- *Androgen-insensitive males.* Because of a genetic error, a small number of XY males don't have androgen cells in their bodies. Their bodies look female, they develop a female gender identity, and they usually are sexually attracted to males.

- *Pelvic field defect.* A small number of newborns have a disorder called pelvic field defect. XX girls with pelvic field defect generally have a vagina but no clitoris and are raised as females. In boys, pelvic field defect involves a missing penis. These XY boys have normal amounts of testosterone prenatally but usually have been castrated just after being born and raised as females. One study revealed that despite the efforts by parents to rear them as girls, most of the XY children insisted that they were boys (Reiner & Gearhart, 2004). Apparently, normal

developmental **connection**

Biological Processes

Hormones are powerful chemical substances secreted by the endocrine glands and carried through the body by the bloodstream. Connect to "Physical Development and Health."

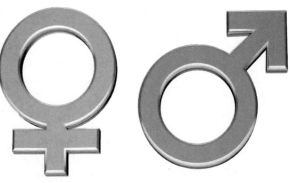

gender The characteristics of people as males and females.

gender identity The sense of being male or female, which most children acquire by the time they are 3 years old.

gender role A set of expectations that prescribes how females or males should think, act, and feel.

gender typing Acquisition of a traditional masculine or feminine role.

estrogens Hormones, the most important of which is estradiol, that influence the development of female physical sex characteristics and help regulate the menstrual cycle.

androgens Hormones, the most important of which is testosterone, that promote the development of male genitals and secondary sex characteristics.

developmental connection

Theories

Evolutionary psychology emphasizes the importance of adaptation, reproduction, and "survival of the fittest" in shaping behavior. Connect to "Biological Beginnings."

exposure to androgens prenatally had a stronger influence on their gender identity than being castrated and raised as girls.

- In an unusual and ultimately tragic case, one of two identical twin boys lost his penis during a botched circumcision. The twin who lost his penis, Bruce Reimer, was castrated, given female hormones, renamed "Brenda," and raised as a girl. Initially John Money (1975), the psychologist who handled the Reimer case, reported that the sex reassignment had produced positive outcomes, but later it became clear that "Brenda" had not adjusted well to life as a girl and was bullied and ostracized by classmates (Diamond & Sigmundson, 1997). As an adolescent, "Brenda" was told about the sex reassignment and decided to live as a male and take the name David. He underwent hormonal and surgical treatment, got married, and adopted his wife's children (Colapinto, 2000). In 2004, when David was 38 years old and his marriage was disintegrating, he committed suicide.

Although sex hormones alone do not determine behavior, researchers have found links between sex hormone levels and certain behaviors (McEwen & Milner, 2017). The most established effects of testosterone on humans involve aggressive behavior and sexual behavior (Hyde & Else-Quest, 2013). Levels of testosterone are correlated with sexual behavior in boys during puberty (Geniole & Carré, 2018). Higher fetal testosterone levels measured from amniotic fluid predict more male-typical play in preschool (Jones, 2018).

The Evolutionary Psychology View   Evolutionary psychology emphasizes that adaptation during the evolution of humans produced psychological differences between males and females (Buss, 2016). Evolutionary psychologists argue that primarily because of their differing roles in reproduction, males and females faced different pressures in primeval environments when the human species was evolving. In particular, because having multiple sexual liaisons improves the likelihood that males will pass on their genes, natural selection favored males who adopted short-term mating strategies. These males competed with other males to acquire more resources in order to access females. Therefore, say evolutionary psychologists, males evolved dispositions that favor violence, competition, and risk taking.

In contrast, according to evolutionary psychologists, females' contributions to the gene pool were enhanced by securing resources for their offspring, which was promoted by obtaining long-term mates who could support a family. As a consequence, natural selection favored females who devoted effort to parenting and chose mates who could provide their offspring with resources and protection. Females developed preferences for successful, ambitious men who could provide these resources (Buss, 2016).

Critics of evolutionary psychology argue that its hypotheses are backed by speculations about prehistory, not evidence, and that in any event people are not locked into behavior that was adaptive in the evolutionary past. Critics also claim that the evolutionary view pays little attention to cultural and individual variations in gender differences (Brannon, 2017).

SOCIAL INFLUENCES

Social scientists recognize that psychological gender differences are not due only to dispositions but also to social experiences. Two theories that reflect this view have been influential—social role theory and social cognitive theory.

Alice Eagly proposed **social role theory,** which states that gender differences result from the contrasting roles of women and men (Eagly & Wood, 2016). In most cultures around the world, women have less power and status than men do and they control fewer resources (OECD, 2017). Compared with men, women perform more domestic work, spend fewer hours in paid employment, receive lower pay, and are more thinly represented in the highest levels of organizations. In Eagly's view, as women adapted to roles with less power and less status in society, they showed more cooperative,

social role theory A theory stating that gender differences result from the contrasting roles of women and men—social hierarchy and division of labor strongly influence gender differences in power, assertiveness, and nurture.

social cognitive theory of gender This theory emphasizes that children's gender development occurs through observation and imitation of gender behavior, and through rewards and punishments they experience for gender-appropriate and gender-inappropriate behavior.

Theory	Processes	Outcome
Social role theory	Observation and adaptation to gendered social roles that are common within a particular cultural context	Gender behavior conforms to expectations for roles within social hierarchies
Social cognitive theory	Rewards and punishments of gender-appropriate and -inappropriate behavior by adults and peers; observation and imitation of models' masculine and feminine behavior	Gender behavior that is rewarded within a cultural context becomes more common

FIGURE 1

PARENTS INFLUENCE THEIR CHILDREN'S GENDER DEVELOPMENT BY ACTION AND EXAMPLE

less dominant profiles than men. Thus, the social hierarchy and division of labor are important causes of gender differences in power, assertiveness, and nurture (Eagly & Wood, 2016).

The social cognitive approach provides an alternative explanation of how children develop gender-typed behavior (see Figure 1). According to the **social cognitive theory of gender,** children's gender development occurs through observation and imitation, and through the rewards and punishments children experience for gender-appropriate and gender-inappropriate behavior (Spinner, Cameron, & Calogero, 2018). Social cognitive theory emphasizes the importance of social contexts—such as parenting, peer relationships, schools, and the media—in gender development.

Parental Influences   Parents, by action and example, influence their children's and adolescents' gender development (Liben, 2017). As soon as the label *girl* or *boy* is assigned, virtually everyone, from parents to siblings to strangers, begins treating the infant in gender-specific ways (see Figure 2). Parents often use rewards and punishments to teach their daughters to be feminine ("Karen, you are such a good mommy with your dolls") and their sons to be masculine ("C'mon now, Keith, big boys don't cry").

Mothers and fathers often interact differently with their children and adolescents. Mothers are more involved with their children and adolescents than are fathers, although fathers increase the time they spend in parenting when they have sons and are less likely to become divorced when they have sons (Galambos, Berenbaum, & McHale, 2009). Historically, mothers' interactions with their children and adolescents often have centered on caregiving and teaching activities, while fathers' interactions often have involved leisure activities (Galambos, Berenbaum, & McHale, 2009).

Mothers and fathers often interact differently with sons and daughters, and these gendered interactions that begin in infancy usually continue through childhood and adolescence. In reviewing research on this topic, Phyllis Bronstein (2006) provided these conclusions:

- *Mothers' socialization strategies.* In many cultures mothers socialize their daughters to be more obedient and responsible than their sons. They also place more restrictions on daughters' autonomy.

- *Fathers' socialization strategies.* Fathers show more attention to sons than daughters, engage in more activities with sons, and put forth more effort to promote sons' intellectual development.

Thus, according to Bronstein (2006, pp. 269–270), "Despite an increased awareness in the United States and other Western cultures of the detrimental effects of gender stereotyping, many parents continue to foster behaviors and perceptions that are consonant with traditional gender role norms."

Peers   As children get older, peers become increasingly important. Peers extensively reward and punish gender behavior (Leaper, 2018). For example, when children play in ways that the culture views as sex-appropriate, they tend to be rewarded by their peers. Those who engage in activities that are considered sex-inappropriate tend to be criticized or abandoned by their peers. It is generally more accepted for girls to act more like boys than it is for boys to act more like girls; thus, use of the term *tomboy* to describe masculine

developmental **connection**

Social Cognitive Theory

Social cognitive theory holds that behavior, environment, and person/cognitive factors are the key aspects of development. Connect to "Introduction."

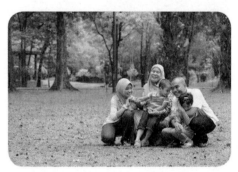

How do mothers and fathers interact differently with their children and adolescents?
Wong Sze Fei/EyeEm/Getty Images

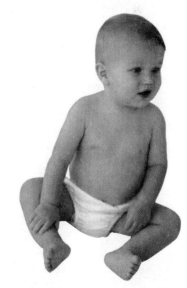

FIGURE 2

EXPECTATIONS FOR BOYS AND GIRLS. First imagine that this is a photograph of a baby girl. *What expectations would you have for her?* Then imagine that this is a photograph of a baby boy. *What expectations would you have for him?*
Kwame Zikomo/Purestock/SuperStock

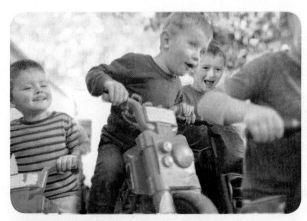

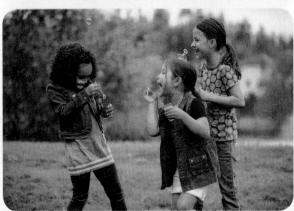

What are some developmental changes that characterize the gender makeup of children's peer relations?

(top): Zero Creatives/Getty Images; (bottom): FatCamera/E+/Getty Images

girls is often thought of as less derogatory than the term *sissy* to describe feminine boys (Pasterski, Golombok, & Hines, 2011).

Children show a clear preference for being with and liking same-sex peers, and this tendency usually becomes stronger during the middle and late childhood years (Maccoby, 2002) (see Figure 3). What kind of socialization takes place in these same-sex play groups? In one study, researchers observed preschoolers over a period of six months (Martin & Fabes, 2001). The more time boys spent interacting with other boys, the more their activity level, rough-and-tumble play, and sex-typed choice of toys and games increased, and the less time boys spent near adults. By contrast, the more time preschool girls spent interacting with other girls, the more their activity level and aggression decreased, and the more their girl-type play activities and time spent near adults increased. The preference for interacting in same-gender dyads is more pronounced for girls than for boys (Gasparini & others, 2015).

In adolescence, peer approval or disapproval is a powerful influence on gender attitudes and behavior (Shin, 2017). Peer groups in adolescence are more likely to be a mix of boys and girls than they were in childhood. However, even into adolescence and adulthood, gender segregation continues to characterize some aspects of social life (Mehta & Smith, 2019). In this study, even adults reported preferring and feeling closer to their same-gender friends than their cross-gender friends.

Schools and Teachers   Some observers have expressed concerns that schools and teachers have biases against both boys and girls (Glock & Kleen, 2017). What evidence might indicate that the classroom is biased against boys? Here are some factors to consider (DeZolt & Hull, 2001):

- Compliance, following rules, and being neat and orderly are valued and reinforced in many classrooms. These are behaviors that usually characterize girls more than boys.
- A large majority of teachers are female, especially in elementary schools. This trend may make it more difficult for boys than for girls to identify with their teachers and model their teachers' behavior. One study revealed that male teachers perceived boys more positively and saw them as being more educationally competent than did female teachers (Mullola & others, 2012).
- Boys are more likely than girls to have a learning disability or ADHD and to drop out of school.
- Boys are more likely than girls to be criticized.
- School personnel tend to ignore the fact that many boys are clearly having academic problems, especially in the language arts.
- School personnel tend to stereotype boys' behavior as problematic.

What evidence suggests that the classroom is biased against girls? Consider the following (Sadker & Sadker, 2005):

- In a typical classroom, girls are more compliant, boys more rambunctious. Boys demand more attention, girls are more likely to quietly wait their turn. Teachers are more likely to scold and reprimand boys, as well as send boys to school authorities for disciplinary action. Educators worry that girls' tendency to be compliant and quiet comes at a cost: diminished assertiveness.
- In many classrooms, teachers spend more time watching and interacting with boys, whereas girls work and play quietly on their own. Most teachers don't intentionally favor boys by spending more time with them, yet somehow the classroom frequently ends up with this type of gendered profile.
- Boys get more instruction than girls and more help when they have trouble with a question. Teachers often give boys more time to answer a question, provide

FIGURE 3

DEVELOPMENTAL CHANGES IN PERCENTAGE OF TIME SPENT IN SAME-SEX AND MIXED-GROUP SETTINGS. Observations of children show that they are more likely to play in same-sex than mixed-sex groups. This tendency increases between 4 and 6 years of age.

more hints regarding the correct answer, and allow further tries if they give the wrong answer.

- Boys are more likely than girls to get lower grades and to be grade repeaters, yet girls are less likely to believe that they will be successful in college work.
- Girls and boys enter first grade with roughly equal levels of self-esteem. Yet by the middle school years, girls' self-esteem is lower than boys'.
- When elementary school children are asked to list what they want to do when they grow up, boys describe more career options than girls do.

Thus, there is evidence of gender bias against both males and females in schools. Many school personnel are not aware of their gender-biased attitudes. These attitudes are deeply entrenched in and supported by the general culture. Increasing awareness of gender bias in schools is clearly an important strategy for reducing such bias.

Might single-sex education be better for children than coed schooling? An argument in favor of single-sex education is that it eliminates distraction from the other sex and reduces sexual harassment. Single-sex public education has increased dramatically in recent decades. In 2002, only 12 public schools in the United States provided same-sex education; in the 2014–2015 school year, there were 170 public schools for boys and 113 for girls, with 21,000 girls and 17,000 boys enrolled (Mitchell & others, 2017).

Despite the increase in single-sex education, a review of 184 studies that included 1.6 million students from 21 countries concluded that the highest-quality studies showed that same-sex education did not provide benefits absent from mixed-sex education (Pahlke & others, 2014). In one review, titled "The Pseudoscience of Single-Sex Schooling," Diane Halpern and her colleagues (2011) concluded that same-sex education is highly misguided, misconstrued, and unsupported by any valid scientific evidence. They emphasize that among the many arguments against same-sex education, the strongest is its reduction of opportunities for boys and girls to work together in a supervised, purposeful environment.

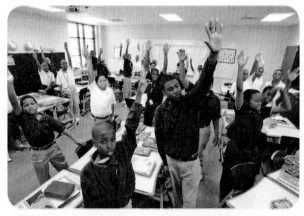

What are some changes in single-sex education in the United States? What does research say about whether same-sex education is beneficial?
Tammy Ljungblad/KRT/Newscom

There has been a special call for same-sex public education for one group of adolescents—African American boys—because of their historically poor academic achievement and high dropout rate from school (Mitchell & Stewart, 2013). In 2010, the Urban Prep Academy for Young Men became the first all-male, all African American public charter school. Every year since 2010, 100 percent of graduating seniors have been accepted into four-year colleges and universities. Currently Urban Prep Academies operates three open-enrollment public charter high schools in high-need communities in Chicago. Students are admitted via random lottery, and the three campuses have a total capacity of 2,000 students.

Media Influences   The messages about gender roles carried by the mass media also are important influences on children's and adolescents' gender development (Coyne & others, 2016). Men are portrayed as more powerful than women on many TV shows. A review of 135 studies found that in laboratory settings as well as in everyday life, exposure to media portrayals that sexually objectify women are related to men's and women's views of women as being less competent and less moral and to increased tolerance of sexual violence against women (Ward, 2016). The media influence adolescents' body images, and some studies reveal gender differences in this area (Tatangelo & Ricciardelli, 2017). For example, two studies of 10- to 15-year-old girls found that the more they internalized sexualized images from the media, the more likely they were to wear sexualized clothing, to feel shame about their bodies, and to regard their bodies as objects to be looked at and evaluated by others (McKenney & Bigler, 2016). Another study revealed that the more time that adolescent girls and boys spent using social media, the more negative their body images were (Fardouly & Vartanian, 2016). Adolescent boys are exposed to a highly muscular body ideal for males in media outlets, especially in advertisements that include professional athletes and in video games (Near, 2013).

How Do Young Children Use Gender Schemas to Make Judgments About Occupations?

In one study, researchers interviewed children 3 to 7 years old about 10 traditionally masculine occupations (airplane pilot, car mechanic) and feminine occupations (clothes designer, secretary), using questions such as the following (Levy, Sadovsky, & Troseth, 2000):

- *Example of a traditionally masculine occupation item:* An airplane pilot is a person who "flies airplanes for people." Who do you think would do the best job as an airplane pilot, a man or a woman?

- *Example of a traditionally feminine occupation item:* A clothes designer is a person "who draws up and makes clothes for people." Who do you think would do the best job as a clothes designer, a man or a woman?

As indicated in Figure 4, the children had well-developed gender schemas, in this case reflected in stereotypes of occupations. They "viewed men as more competent than women in masculine occupations, and rated women as more competent than men in feminine occupations" (p. 993). Also, "girls' ratings of women's competence at feminine occupations were substantially higher than their ratings of men's competence at masculine occupations. Conversely, boys' ratings of men's competence at masculine occupations were considerably greater than their ratings of women's competence at feminine occupations" (p. 1002). These findings demonstrate that most children as young as 3 to 4 years of age tend to have strong gender schemas regarding the perceived competencies of men and women in gender-typed occupations.

The researchers also asked the children to select from a list of emotions how they would feel if they grew up to have each of the 10 occupations. Girls said they would be happy with the feminine occupations and angry or disgusted with the masculine occupations. As expected, boys said they would be happy if they grew up to have the masculine occupations but

	Boy	Girl
"Masculine Occupations"		
Percentage who judged men more competent	87	70
Percentage who judged women more competent	13	30
"Feminine Occupations"		
Percentage who judged men more competent	35	8
Percentage who judged women more competent	64	92

FIGURE **4**

CHILDREN'S JUDGMENTS ABOUT THE COMPETENCE OF MEN AND WOMEN IN GENDER-STEREOTYPED OCCUPATIONS

angry and disgusted with the feminine occupations. However, the boys' emotions were more intense (more angry and disgusted) in desiring to avoid the feminine occupations than girls in wanting to avoid the masculine occupations. An analysis of whether gender stereotypes changed between the early 1980s and 2014 in the United States indicated that males' and females' descriptions of typical traits, role behaviors, occupations, and physical characteristics that men and women would have were as stereotyped in 2014 as in the 1980s (Haines, Deaux, & Lofaro, 2016).

Children in this study were at the height of gender stereotyping. Most older children, adolescents, and adults become more flexible about occupational roles (Barth & others, 2018). What does our understanding of this flexibility suggest about the role of education in reducing gender-based stereotypes?

COGNITIVE INFLUENCES

Observation, imitation, rewards, and punishment—these are the mechanisms by which gender develops, according to social cognitive theory. Interactions between the child and the social environment are the main keys to gender development in this view. Some critics argue that this explanation pays too little attention to the child's own mind and understanding by depicting the child as passively acquiring gender roles (Martin, Ruble, & Szkrybalo, 2002).

gender schema theory According to this theory, gender typing emerges as children gradually develop schemas of what is gender-appropriate and gender-inappropriate in their culture.

One influential cognitive theory is **gender schema theory,** which states that gender typing emerges as children gradually develop gender schemas of what is gender-appropriate and gender-inappropriate in their culture (Starr & Zurbriggen, 2017). A *schema* is a cognitive structure, a network of associations that guide an individual's perceptions. A *gender schema* organizes the world in terms of female and male. Children are internally motivated to perceive the world and to act in accordance with their developing schemas. Bit by bit, children pick up what is gender-appropriate and gender-inappropriate in their culture, and develop gender schemas that shape how they perceive the world and what they remember (Conry-Murray, Kim, & Turiel, 2015). Children are motivated to act in ways that conform with these gender schemas. Thus, gender schemas fuel gender typing.

How do young children use gender schemas to make judgments about occupations? To find out, see the *Connecting Through Research* interlude.

In sum, cognitive factors contribute to the way children think and act as males and females. Through biological, social, and cognitive processes, children develop their gender attitudes and behaviors (Liben, 2017).

Review Connect Reflect

 LG2 Discuss the main biological, social, and cognitive influences on gender.

Review

- What are some ways that biology may influence gender?
- What are two social theories of gender, and how might social contexts influence gender development?
- How does a cognitive view explain gender development?

Connect

- In this section, you learned that in most cultures around the world, women have less power and status than men do and they control fewer resources. How might this be related to what you read about gender and education in the *Connecting with Diversity* interlude in the chapter "Introduction"?

Reflect *Your Own Personal Journey of Life*

- How do you think your parents influenced your gender development? How do you think your peers influenced your gender development?

Gender Stereotypes, Similarities, and Differences

 LG3 Describe gender stereotypes, similarities, and differences.

```
Gender
Stereotyping

Gender Similarities
and Differences
```

How pervasive is gender stereotyping? What are the real differences between boys and girls?

GENDER STEREOTYPING

Gender stereotypes are general impressions and beliefs about females and males. For example, men are powerful; women are weak. Men make good mechanics; women make good nurses. Men are good with numbers; women are good with words. Women are emotional; men are not. All of these are stereotypes. They are generalizations about a group that reflect widely held beliefs (Miller & others, 2018). Researchers have found that boys' gender stereotypes are more rigid than girls' (Spinner, Cameron, & Calogero, 2018).

gender stereotypes Broad categories that reflect impressions and widely held beliefs about what behavior is appropriate for females and males.

Traditional Masculinity and Femininity A classic study in the early 1970s assessed which traits and behaviors college students believed were characteristic of females and which they believed were characteristic of males (Broverman & others, 1972). The traits associated with males were labeled *instrumental:* They included characteristics such as being independent, aggressive, and power oriented. The traits associated with females were labeled *expressive:* They included characteristics such as being warm and sensitive.

Thus, the instrumental traits associated with males suited them for the traditional masculine role of going out into the world as the breadwinner. The expressive traits associated with females paralleled the traditional feminine role of being the sensitive, nurturing caregiver in the home. These roles and traits, however, are not just different; they also are unequal in terms of social status and power. The traditional feminine characteristics are childlike, suitable for someone who is dependent upon and subordinate to others. The traditional masculine characteristics equip a person to deal competently with the wider world and to wield authority.

If you are going to generalize about women, you will find yourself up to here in exceptions.

—Dolores Hitchens
American mystery writer, 20th century

Stereotyping and Culture How widespread is gender stereotyping? In a far-ranging study of college students in 30 countries, stereotyping of females and males was pervasive

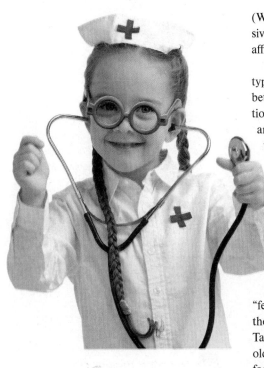

(Williams & Best, 1982). Males were widely believed to be dominant, independent, aggressive, achievement oriented, and enduring. Females were widely believed to be nurturant, affiliative, less esteemed, and more helpful in times of distress.

Of course, in the decades since this study was conducted, traditional gender stereotypes and gender roles have been challenged in many societies, and social inequalities between men and women have diminished. Do gender stereotypes change when the relationship between men and women changes? At a societal level, there is evidence that men and women in countries higher in gender equality (as indicated by education, representation at high levels of government, and the like) have less stereotypical gender roles within the family and that children interact more similarly with their mothers and fathers (Bartel & others, 2018). However, in a study of eighth-grade students in 36 countries, in every country girls had more egalitarian attitudes about gender roles than boys did (Dotti Sani & Quaranta, 2017). In this study, girls had the most egalitarian gender attitudes in countries with higher levels of societal gender equality.

Developmental Changes in Gender Stereotyping Earlier we described how young children stereotype occupations as being "masculine" or "feminine." When do children begin to engage in gender stereotyping? One study examined the extent to which children and their mothers engage in gender stereotyping (Gelman, Taylor, & Nguyen, 2004). The researchers videotaped mothers and their 2-, 4-, and 6-year-old sons and daughters as they discussed a picture book with stereotyped (a boy playing football, for example) and nonstereotyped (a female race car driver, for example) gender activities. Children engaged in more gender stereotyping than did their mothers. However, mothers expressed gender concepts to their children by referencing categories of gender ("Why do you think only *men* can be firefighters?" for example), labeling gender ("That looks like a daddy," for example), and contrasting males and females ("Is that a girl job or a boy job?" for example). Gender stereotyping by children was present even in the 2-year-olds, but increased considerably by 4 years of age. This study demonstrated that even when adults don't explicitly engage in gender stereotyping when talking with children, they provide children with information about gender by categorizing gender, labeling gender, and contrasting males and females. Children use these cues to construct an understanding of gender and to guide their behavior (Halim & others, 2018).

Gender stereotyping continues to change during middle and late childhood and adolescence (Brannon, 2017). Five-year-old boys and girls are equally likely to say that boys and girls are "really, really smart," but by the age of 6, girls are likely to say that more boys than girls are "really, really smart" and to avoid activities that are described as being for children who are "really, really smart" (Bian, Leslie, & Cimpian, 2017). In a review of 78 studies in which students in kindergarten through twelfth grade were asked to draw a scientist, cohort differences were found and children in more recent decades were more likely to draw female scientists than were children in previous decades (Miller & others, 2018). However, even children in recent decades were more likely to draw male than female scientists, particularly at older ages, suggesting continuing stereotypes associating science with men. Five-year-olds who were more engaged with Disney princess media and products showed more female gender stereotypical behavior one year later, even after statistically accounting for their earlier gender stereotypical behavior (Coyne & others, 2016). To study children's ability to resist gender stereotypes, children were told about gender stereotype conforming groups (girls doing ballet, boys playing football) and gender stereotype nonconforming groups (girls playing football, boys doing ballet). Children believed it would be easier for girls than boys to challenge gender stereotypes and that exclusion from the peer group was a possible consequence of challenging gender stereotypes, but they also believed themselves to be personally able to resist gender stereotypes (Mulvey & Killen, 2015).

GENDER SIMILARITIES AND DIFFERENCES

What is the reality behind gender stereotypes? Let's examine some of the differences between the sexes, keeping in mind that (1) the differences are averages and do not apply

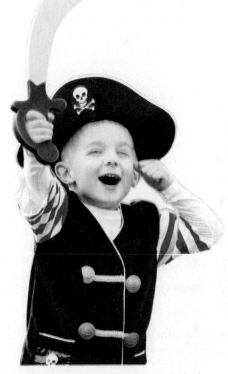

What are some developmental changes in children's gender stereotyping?

(Top): Anna.danilkova/Shutterstock; (Botttom): Rebecca Nelson/Getty Images

to all females or all males; (2) even when gender differences occur, there often is considerable overlap between males and females; and (3) the differences may be due primarily to biological factors, sociocultural factors, or both.

Physical Similarities and Differences We could devote pages to describing physical differences between the average man and woman. For example, women have about twice the body fat of men, with most of it concentrated around their breasts and hips. In males, fat is more likely to go to the abdomen. On average, males grow to be 10 percent taller than females. Androgens (the "male" hormones) promote the growth of long bones; estrogens (the "female" hormones) stop such growth at puberty.

Many physical differences between men and women are tied to health. From conception on, females have a longer life expectancy than males, and females are less likely than males to develop physical or mental disorders. Females are more resistant to infection, and their blood vessels are more elastic than males'. Males have higher levels of stress hormones, which cause faster clotting and higher blood pressure.

Does gender matter when it comes to brain structure and activity? Human brains are much more alike than different, whether the brain belongs to a male or a female (Ruigrok & others, 2014). However, researchers have found some brain differences between females and males. Among the differences that have been discovered are the following:

- On average, not correcting for overall body size, female brains are approximately 10 percent smaller than male brains. However, differences in brain size are typically found during adulthood rather than childhood.
- Some specific regions of the brain are larger in males, whereas other specific regions of the brain are larger in females.
- Portions of the corpus callosum—the band of tissues through which the brain's two hemispheres communicate—may be larger in females than in males, although some studies have found this not to be the case (Shiino & others, 2017).
- The average gender differences in specific brain regions map onto gender differences in functions controlled by those regions.

Although some differences in brain structure and function have been found, many of these differences are either small or inconsistently supported by research. Also, when sex differences in the brain have been revealed, in many cases they have not been directly linked to psychological differences (Blakemore, Berenbaum, & Liben, 2009). Overall, it appears that there are far more similarities than differences in the brains of females and males. A further point is worth noting: Anatomical sex differences in the brain may be due to the biological origins of these differences, behavioral experiences (demonstrating the brain's ongoing plasticity), or a combination of these factors.

developmental **connection**

Brain Development

The human brain has two hemispheres (left and right). To some extent the type of information processed by neurons depends on whether they are in the left or right hemisphere of the brain. Connect to "Physical Development and Health."

Cognitive and Socioemotional Similarities and Differences In the largest synthesis of research to date regarding gender differences and similarities in cognitive and socioemotional development, data from over 20,000 individual studies and 12 million participants were used to examine whether gender differences are found in a number of psychological domains (Zell, Krizan, & Teeter, 2015). Overall, when gender differences were found, 46 percent were characterized as being small and 39 percent as very small. Across all of the cognitive and socioemotional domains examined, 84 percent of the distributions of the variables overlapped between males and females. Gender differences were consistent across ages, generations, and cultural contexts.

Despite this overall pattern suggesting more gender similarities than differences, there were 10 areas that showed moderate to large differences between males and females (Zell, Krizan, & Teeter, 2015). Males scored higher than females in aggression, masculinity, spatial rotation ability, attention to physical attractiveness in mate selection, confidence in physical abilities, and performance in same-sex groups. Females scored higher than males in reactions to painful stimuli, fear, attachment to peers, and interest in people rather than things.

One area that emerged in the research synthesis as a domain with moderate to large differences between males and females is visuospatial skills, which include being able to

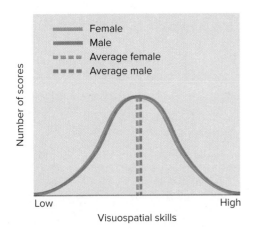

Female
Male
Average female
Average male

Number of scores

Low   High
Visuospatial skills

FIGURE 5

VISUOSPATIAL SKILLS OF MALES AND

FEMALES. Notice that, although an average male's visuospatial skills are higher than an average female's, scores for the two sexes almost entirely overlap. Not all males have better visuospatial skills than all females—the overlap indicates that, although the average male score is higher, many females outperform most males on such tasks.

rotate objects mentally and determine what they would look like when rotated. These types of skills are important in courses such as plane and solid geometry and geography. However, even when gender differences are found, most of the distribution of males' and females' visuospatial skills overlaps (Hyde, 2014) (see Figure 5).

Are there gender differences in reading and writing skills? There is strong evidence that females outperform males in reading and writing. In national studies, girls have shown higher reading achievement than boys (National Assessment of Educational Progress, 2018). Girls also have consistently outperformed boys in writing skills in the National Assessment of Educational Progress in fourth-, eighth-, and twelfth-grade assessments.

Let's further explore gender differences related to schooling and achievement. In the United States, school dropout rates do not differ for males and females (National Center for Education Statistics, 2018). Boys predominate in the academic bottom half of high school classes. Half a century ago in 1961, less than 40 percent of women who graduated from high school went on to attend college. Beginning in 1996, women were more likely to enroll in college than men. Currently, about 56 percent of college students in the United States are women, but the gender discrepancy favoring women is more pronounced in some ethnic and racial groups than others (National Center for Education Statistics, 2018).

Piecing together the information about school dropouts, the percentage of males in the bottom half of their high school classes, and the percentage of males in college classes, we can conclude that currently females show greater overall academic interest and achievement than do males in the United States. Females are more likely to be engaged with academic material, to pay attention in class, to put forth more academic effort, and to participate more in class than boys are (DeZolt & Hull, 2001). A large-scale study revealed that girls had more positive attitudes about school than boys did (Orr, 2011). And further, girls' positive attitudes about school were linked to their higher grades; boys' negative attitudes about school were related to their lower grades.

Despite these positive characteristics of girls, increasing evidence of similarity in the math and science skills of girls and boys, and legislative efforts to attain gender equality in recent years, gender differences in science, technology, and math careers continue to favor males (Lawton, 2018). Toward the end of high school, girls are less likely to take high-level math courses and less likely to plan to enter the so-called "STEM" fields of science, technology, engineering, and math. A research review concluded that girls have more negative math attitudes and that parents' and teachers' expectancies for children's math competence are often gender-biased in favor of boys (Gunderson & others, 2012).

Four areas of socioemotional development in which gender similarities and differences have been studied extensively are aggression, relationship communication, emotion, and prosocial behavior.

Aggression One of the most consistent gender differences is that boys are more physically aggressive than girls (Dayton & Malone, 2017). The difference occurs in all cultures and appears very early in children's development. The physical aggression difference is especially pronounced when children are provoked. Both biological and environmental factors have been proposed to account for gender differences in aggression. Biological factors include heredity and hormones. Environmental factors include cultural expectations, adult and peer models, and social agents that reward aggression in boys and punish aggression in girls.

Although boys are consistently more physically aggressive than girls, might girls show at least as much verbal aggression (such as yelling) as boys? When verbal aggression is examined, gender differences typically disappear (Björkqvist, 2018).

Recently, increased interest has been shown in relational, social, and indirect aggression, which involves harming someone by manipulating a relationship (Casper & Card, 2017; Underwood, 2011). Relational aggression includes such behaviors as

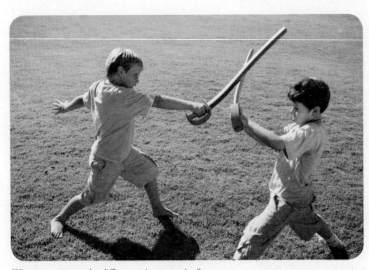

What are some gender differences in aggression?
Fuse/Corbis RF/Getty Images

trying to make others dislike a certain individual by spreading malicious rumors about the person. Relational aggression increases in middle and late childhood (Murray-Close & others, 2016). Mixed findings have characterized research on whether girls show more relational aggression than boys, but one consistency in findings is that relational aggression comprises a greater percentage of girls' overall aggression than is the case for boys (Björkqvist, 2018).

Relationship Communication   Are males and females so dramatically different that "men are from Mars" and "women are from Venus," as was proposed in a best-selling book many years ago (Gray, 1992)? Perhaps the gender differences that fascinate people most involve how males and females communicate with each other.

In relationship communication, sociolinguist Deborah Tannen (1990) distinguishes between rapport talk and report talk:

- **Rapport talk** is the language of conversation and a way of establishing connections and negotiating relationships. Girls enjoy rapport talk and conversation that is relationship oriented more than boys do.
- **Report talk** is talk that gives information. Public speaking is an example of report talk. Males hold center stage through report talk with verbal performances such as storytelling, joking, and lecturing with information.

rapport talk The language of conversation and a way of establishing connections and negotiating relationships; more characteristic of females than of males.

report talk Talk that conveys information; more characteristic of males than females.

Tannen says that boys and girls grow up in different worlds of talk—parents, siblings, peers, teachers, and others talk to boys and girls differently. The play of boys and girls is also different. Boys tend to play in large groups that are hierarchically structured, and their groups usually have a leader who tells the others what to do and how to do it. Boys' games have winners and losers and often are the subject of arguments. And boys often boast of their skill and argue about who is best at what. In contrast, girls are more likely to play in small groups or pairs, and at the center of a girl's world is often a best friend. In girls' friendships and peer groups, intimacy is pervasive. Turn-taking is more characteristic of girls' games than of boys' games. And much of the time, girls simply like to sit and talk with each other, concerned more about being liked by others than jockeying for status in some obvious way.

In sum, Tannen concludes that females are more relationship oriented than males—and that this relationship orientation should be prized as a skill in our culture more than it currently is. Note, however, that some researchers criticize Tannen's ideas as being overly simplified and suggest that communication between males and females is more complex than Tannen indicates (Palczewski, DeFrancisco, & McGeough, 2017). An analysis of recorded conversations between same-sex and mixed-sex pairs of undergraduates found several gender differences in self-disclosure and negotiation (Leaper, 2019).

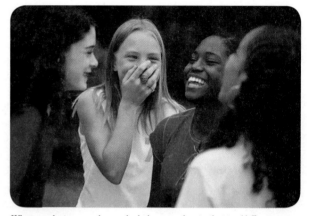

What conclusions can be reached about gender similarities/differences in relationship communication?
Tom Grill/Getty Images

For example, during negotiations, females were more likely to use affiliative strategies such as making requests and indirect suggestions, whereas males were more likely to make direct suggestions; women were more likely to self-disclose and to respond with elaborations in response to others' self-disclosures, whereas men were more likely to make negative comments in response to others' disclosure. However, all of these differences were small.

Researchers have found that girls are more "people oriented" and boys are more "things oriented" (Hyde, 2014). In a research review on gender and adolescent development, this conclusion was supported by findings that girls spend more time in relationships, while boys spend more time alone, playing video games, and playing sports; that girls work at part-time jobs that are people-oriented such as waitressing and baby-sitting, while boys are more likely to take part-time jobs that involve manual labor and using tools; and that girls are interested in careers that are more people-oriented, such as teaching and social work, while boys are more likely to be interested in object-oriented careers, such as mechanics and engineering (Perry & Pauletti, 2011). Also, in support of Tannen's view, researchers have found that adolescent girls engage in more self-disclosure (communication of intimate details about themselves) in close relationships and are better at actively listening in a conversation than are boys (Leaper, 2019).

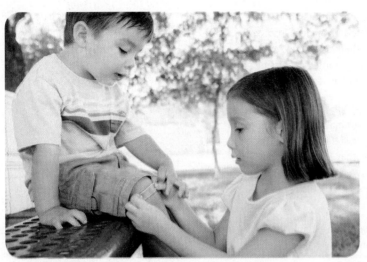

What gender differences characterize children's prosocial behavior?
Fuse/Corbis/Getty Images

- - - - - - - - - - - - - ➤

developmental connection

Moral Development

Prosocial behavior involves behavior intended to benefit other people. Connect to "Moral Development."

◀ - - - - - - - - - - - - -

Emotion and Its Regulation   Gender differences occur in some aspects of emotion (Deng & others, 2016). Females express emotion more than males do, are better than males at decoding emotion, smile more, cry more, and are happier (Chaplin, 2015). Males report experiencing and expressing more anger than do females (Kring, 2000). One meta-analysis found that overall gender differences in children's emotional expression were small, with girls showing more positive emotion (sympathy, for example) and more internalized emotions (sadness and anxiety, for example) than boys (Chaplin & Aldao, 2013). In this analysis, the gender difference in positive emotions became more pronounced with age as girls more strongly expressed positive emotions than boys in middle and late childhood and in adolescence.

An important skill is to be able to regulate and control one's emotions and behavior (Di Giunta & others, 2018). Boys usually develop self-regulation later and more slowly than girls do (Montroy & others, 2016). This low self-control can translate into behavior problems.

Prosocial Behavior   Are there gender differences in prosocial behavior? Females view themselves as more prosocial and empathic than males (Eisenberg & Spinrad, 2016). Across childhood and adolescence, females engage in more prosocial behavior (Eisenberg & Spinrad, 2016). The biggest gender difference occurs for kind and considerate behavior, with a smaller difference in sharing.

Gender Controversy   There is ongoing controversy about the extent of gender differences and what might cause them (Liben, 2017). As we saw earlier, evolutionary psychologists such as David Buss (2016) argue that gender differences are extensive and caused by the adaptive problems humans have faced across their evolutionary history. Alice Eagly also concludes that gender differences are substantial, but she reaches a very different conclusion about their cause (Eagly & Wood, 2016). She emphasizes that gender differences are due to social conditions that have resulted in women having less power and controlling fewer resources than men.

By contrast, Janet Shibley Hyde (Hyde & others, 2019) concludes that gender differences have been greatly exaggerated, with this perspective being especially fueled by popular books such as John Gray's (1992) *Men Are from Mars, Women Are from Venus* and Deborah Tannen's (1990) *You Just Don't Understand.* She argues that the research indicates females and males are similar on most psychological factors, and she provides examples from five domains of psychological research suggesting that binary distinctions between men and women are not well supported by the research evidence. In a research review, Hyde (2005) summarized the results of 44 meta-analyses of gender differences and similarities. A *meta-analysis* is a statistical analysis that combines the results of many different studies. In most areas, including math ability and communication, gender differences either were nonexistent or small. Gender differences in physical aggression were moderate. The largest difference occurred in motor skills (favoring males), followed by sexuality (males masturbate more and are more likely to endorse sex in a casual, uncommitted relationship), and physical aggression (males are more physically aggressive than are females). A research review also concluded that gender differences are small in most areas of functioning (Zell, Krizan, & Teeter, 2015).

Hyde's summary of meta-analyses is still not likely to quiet the controversy about gender differences and similarities, but further research should continue to provide a basis for more accurate judgments about this topic.

At this point, we have discussed many aspects of gender stereotypes, similarities, differences, and controversies in children's development. The following *Caring Connections* interlude provides some recommendations for parents and teachers in regard to children's gender development.

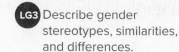

caring *connections*

Guiding Children's Gender Development

Boys

1. ***Encourage boys to be sensitive in relationships and engage in more prosocial behavior.*** An important socialization task is to help boys become more interested in having positive close relationships and become more caring. Fathers can play an especially important role for boys in this regard by being a model of a male who is sensitive and caring.

2. ***Encourage boys to be less physically aggressive.*** Too often, boys are encouraged to be tough and physically aggressive. A positive strategy is to encourage them to be self-assertive but not physically aggressive.

3. ***Encourage boys to handle their emotions more effectively.*** This involves helping boys not only to regulate their emotions, as in controlling their anger, but also to express their anxieties and concerns rather than keeping them bottled up.

4. ***Work with boys to improve their school performance.*** Girls get better grades, put forth more academic effort, and are less likely than boys to be assigned to special/remedial classes. Parents and teachers can help boys by emphasizing the importance of school and expecting better academic effort.

Girls

1. ***Encourage girls to be proud of their relationship skills and caring.*** The strong interest that girls show in relationships and caring should be supported by parents and teachers.

2. ***Encourage girls to develop their self-competencies.*** While guiding girls to retain their relationship strengths, adults also can help girls to develop their ambition and achievement.

3. ***Encourage girls to be more self-assertive.*** Girls tend to be more passive than boys and can benefit from being encouraged to be more self-assertive.

4. ***Encourage girls' achievement.*** This can involve encouraging girls to have higher academic expectations and exposing them to a wider range of career options.

Boys and Girls

1. ***Help children to reduce gender stereotyping and discrimination.*** Don't engage in gender stereotyping and discrimination yourself; otherwise, you will be providing a model of gender stereotyping and discrimination for children.

The second piece of advice for guiding boys' gender development is to encourage them to be less physically aggressive. Near the beginning of this chapter, what did you learn about hormones and boys' aggression?

Review *Connect* Reflect

LG3 Describe gender stereotypes, similarities, and differences.

Review

- What are gender stereotypes? How extensive is gender stereotyping?
- What are some gender similarities and differences in the areas of biological, cognitive, and socioemotional development?

Connect

- In this section, you learned about the ways in which parents may purposefully or unwittingly engage in gender stereotyping of their children. Earlier, you learned that parents have

to deal with being gender stereotyped too. For instance, what did you learn about mothers' and fathers' roles within families?

Reflect *Your Own Personal Journey of Life*

- How is your gender behavior and thinking similar to or different from your mother's and grandmothers' if you are a female? How is your gender behavior and thinking similar to or different from your father's and grandfathers' if you are a male?

Not long ago, it was accepted that boys should grow up to be masculine and girls to be feminine, that boys are made of "snips and snails and puppy dogs' tails" and girls are made of "sugar and spice and everything nice." Let's further explore gender classifications of boys and girls as "masculine" and "feminine."

WHAT IS GENDER-ROLE CLASSIFICATION?

In the past, a well-adjusted boy was expected to be independent, aggressive, and powerful. A well-adjusted girl was expected to be dependent, non-aggressive, and uninterested in power. The masculine characteristics were valued more highly by society than the feminine ones.

In the 1970s, as both females and males became dissatisfied with the burdens imposed by their stereotypic roles, alternatives to femininity and masculinity were proposed. Instead of describing masculinity and femininity as a continuum in which more of one means less of the other, it was proposed that individuals could have both masculine and feminine traits. This thinking led to the development of the concept of **androgyny,** the presence of masculine and feminine characteristics in the same person (Bem, 1977; Spence & Helmreich, 1978). For example, the androgynous boy might be assertive (masculine) and nurturant (feminine). The androgynous girl might be powerful (masculine) and sensitive to others' feelings (feminine). Between 1974 and 2012, college women's reports of their femininity decreased and androgyny increased, although men's reports of their masculinity and androgyny did not change over this time period (Donnelly & Twenge, 2017).

Measures have been developed to assess androgyny. One of the most widely used measures is the Bem Sex-Role Inventory. To find out whether your gender-role classification is masculine, feminine, or androgynous, see Figure 6.

Gender experts such as Sandra Bem argue that androgynous individuals are more flexible, competent, and mentally healthy than their masculine or feminine counterparts. To some degree, though, deciding which gender-role classification is best depends on the context involved (Mustafa & Nazir, 2018). For example, in close relationships, feminine and androgynous orientations might be more desirable because of the expressive nature of such relationships. However, masculine and androgynous orientations might be more desirable in traditional academic and work settings because of the achievement demands in these contexts. For example, one study found that masculine and androgynous individuals had higher expectations for being able to control the outcomes of their academic efforts than feminine or undifferentiated (neither masculine nor feminine) individuals (Choi, 2004).

GENDER IDENTITY IN CHILDHOOD AND ADOLESCENCE

Gender identity encompasses children's understanding of themselves in terms of cultural definitions of what it means to be male or female. Gender identity becomes more salient during adolescence but has precursors in childhood. Some of the most important issues in the study of gender identity involve understanding children who identify with the gender associated with their biological sex at birth (cisgender children) and those who identify with the gender not consistent with their biological sex at birth (transgender children). Prevalence rates are difficult to obtain accurately because of barriers to disclosure, but it is estimated that approximately 0.7 percent of youth ages 13–17 years identify as transgender (Herman & others, 2017).

In studies of socially transitioned transgender children (children who refer to themselves using pronouns of the gender with which they identify rather than their sex at birth,

androgyny The presence of masculine and feminine characteristics in the same person.

Examples of masculine items

Defends own beliefs

Forceful

Willing to take risks

Dominant

Aggressive

Examples of feminine items

Does not use harsh language

Affectionate

Loves children

Understanding

Gentle

Scoring: The items are scored on independent dimensions of masculinity and femininity as well as androgyny and undifferentiated classifications.

FIGURE 6

THE BEM SEX-ROLE INVENTORY. These items are from the Bem Sex-Role Inventory (BSRI). When taking the BSRI, an individual is asked to indicate on a 7-point scale how well each of the 60 characteristics describes herself or himself. The scale ranges from 1 (never or almost never true) to 7 (always or almost always true). The items are scored on independent dimensions of masculinity and femininity. Individuals who score high on the masculine items and low on the feminine items are categorized as masculine; those who score high on the feminine items and low on the masculine items are categorized as feminine; and those who score high on both the masculine and feminine items are categorized as androgynous.

but with no hormonal or surgical interventions involved), children report that by the age of 3 years, they identified with their current gender (Olson & Gülgöz, 2018). In a study of 5- to 12-year-old transgender children, transgender boys and girls had cognitive patterns more consistent with their expressed gender than their natal sex (Olson, Key, & Eaton, 2015). In terms of expressed preferences related to clothes, toys, and other gender-stereotypical items and activities, transgender children were indistinguishable from cisgender children who had the same gender identity. Transgender children and their siblings are less likely than unrelated children to endorse gender stereotypes and more likely to befriend peers who are gender non-conforming (Olson & Enright, 2018).

Prejudice, discrimination, bullying, family rejection, and lack of self-acceptance are all concerns for transgender children (Adelson, Stroeh, & Ng, 2016). Family support is especially important for transgender children's mental health. Socially transitioned transgender children have been found to have markedly lower levels of anxiety and depression than transgender children who continue to live as their natal sex (Olson & others, 2016).

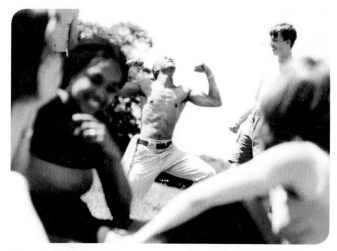

What are some concerns about adolescent males adopting a strong masculine role?
Corbis/VCG/Getty Images

GENDER-ROLE TRANSCENDENCE

Some critics of androgyny say that there has been too much talk about gender and that androgyny is less of a panacea than originally envisioned. An alternative is *gender-role transcendence*, the view that when an individual's competence is at issue, it should be conceptualized on a personal basis rather than on the basis of masculinity, femininity, or androgyny (Pleck, 2018). That is, we should think about ourselves as people first, not as being masculine, feminine, or androgynous. Parents should rear their children to be competent boys and girls, not masculine, feminine, or androgynous, say the gender-role critics. They stress that such gender-role classification leads to too much stereotyping.

GENDER IN CONTEXT

The concept of gender-role classification involves categorization of a person in terms of personality traits. However, it may be helpful to think of personality in terms of person-situation interaction rather than traits alone (Cloninger, 2013). Thus, in our discussion of gender-role classification, we described how some gender roles might be more appropriate than others, depending on the context or setting involved.

To understand the importance of considering gender in context, let's examine helping behavior and emotion. The stereotype is that females are better than males at helping. However, the difference depends on the situation. For example, girls are more likely than boys to notice when bullying is occurring, react with empathy, and intervene (Jenkins & Nickerson, 2019). However, in situations in which males feel a sense of competence, especially circumstances that involve danger, males are more likely than females to help (Eagly & Crowley, 1986). For example, a male is more likely than a female to stop and help a person who is stranded by the roadside with a flat tire.

"She is emotional; he is not"—that is the master emotional stereotype. However, like differences in helping behavior, emotional differences in males and females depend on the particular emotion involved and the context in which it is displayed (Chaplin & Aldao, 2013). Males are more likely to show anger toward strangers, especially male strangers, when they feel they have been challenged. Males also are more likely to turn their anger into aggressive action. Emotional differences between females and males often show up in contexts that highlight social roles and relationships. For example, females are more likely than males to discuss emotions in terms of relationships, and they are more likely to express fear and sadness.

The importance of considering gender in context is nowhere more apparent than when examining what is culturally prescribed behavior for females and males in various countries around the world (Best, 2010; Matsumoto & Juang, 2013). To read further about cross-cultural variations in gender, see *Connecting with Diversity*.

---

developmental **connection**

Theories

Bronfenbrenner's ecological theory emphasizes the importance of contexts; in his theory, the macrosystem includes cross-cultural comparisons. Connect to "Introduction."

Gender Roles Across Cultures

In recent decades, roles assumed by males and females in the United States have become increasingly similar—that is, more androgynous. In many countries, though, gender roles have remained more gender-specific (UNICEF, 2018). For example, in a number of Middle Eastern countries, the division of labor between males and females is dramatic: males are socialized to work in the public sphere, females in the private world of home and child rearing; a man's duty is to provide for his family, the woman's to care for her family and household. Any deviations from this traditional gender-role orientation receive severe disapproval.

Access to education for girls has improved somewhat around the world, but girls' education still lags behind boys' education. For example, although most countries have achieved gender parity in primary school education, gender gaps widen in secondary school (UNESCO, 2016). In lower secondary school (middle or junior high school), 54 percent of countries have not yet reached gender parity, and in upper secondary school (high school), 77 percent of countries have not yet reached gender parity. Gender disparities are wider among poorer children

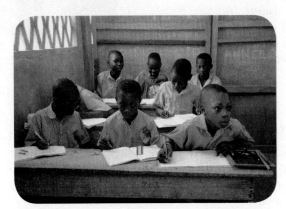

Although access to education for girls has improved, boys still receive approximately 4.4 years more education around the world than girls do. Shown here is a private school for boys in Africa.
Owen Franken/Corbis Documentary/Getty Images

than richer children. Lack of education reduces many girls' chances of developing their full potential.

Although most countries still have gender gaps that favor males, evidence of increasing gender equality is appearing (United Nations, 2019). The Nordic countries are exemplars of gender equality both within and outside the home (Eydal & Rostgaard, 2016). Rates of employment and career opportunities for women are expanding in many countries. Restrictions on adolescent girls' social relationships, especially sexual and romantic relationships, are decreasing in some countries.

Cultural and ethnic backgrounds also influence how boys and girls are socialized in the United States (Sanchez & others, 2017). For example, Latino and Latina children and adolescents are socialized differently (Tyrell & others, 2016). Latinas experienced far greater restrictions than Latinos in curfews, interacting with members of the other sex, getting a driver's license, getting a job, and participating in after-school activities.

The last study mentioned above focused on adolescents. What have you already learned about differences between adolescent girls' and boys' perceptions of their bodies?

Review Connect Reflect

 Identify how gender roles can be classified.

Review

- What is gender-role classification?
- How consistent is gender identity from childhood through adolescence?
- What is gender-role transcendence?
- How can gender be conceptualized in terms of context?

Connect

- How might early or late maturation affect gender identity?

Reflect *Your Own Personal Journey of Life*

- If and when you have a child, how attentive will you likely be to rearing your child to be masculine, feminine, or androgynous? Explain.

Gender

What Is Gender?
LG1 Summarize what gender involves.

- Gender refers to the characteristics of people as males and females. Among the components of gender are gender identity, gender roles, and gender stereotyping. Research indicates that most children know whether they are a boy or a girl by 2 years of age.

Influences on Gender Development
LG2 Discuss the main biological, social, and cognitive influences on gender.

Biological Influences

- The 23rd pair of chromosomes determines our sex. Ordinarily, females have two X chromosomes, and males have one X and one Y. Males and females also produce different concentrations of the hormones known as androgens and estrogens. Early hormonal production is linked with later gender development. In the evolutionary psychology view, evolutionary adaptations produced psychological sex differences that are especially present in sexual behavior and mating strategies. Chromosomes determine anatomical sex differences, but culture and society strongly influence gender.

Social Influences

- In social role theory, gender differences result from men's and women's contrasting roles; in most cultures, women have less power and status than men and control fewer resources. This gender hierarchy and sexual division of labor are important causes of sex-differentiated behavior. Social cognitive theory emphasizes gender models and rewards and punishments for gender-appropriate and gender-inappropriate behavior. Peers are especially adept at rewarding gender-appropriate behavior. Schools and teachers, as well as the media, influence children's gender development.

Cognitive Influences

- Gender schema theories emphasize the role of cognition in gender development. In gender schema theory, gender typing emerges gradually as children develop gender schemas of what their culture considers to be gender-appropriate and gender-inappropriate.

Gender Stereotypes, Similarities, and Differences
LG3 Describe gender stereotypes, similarities, and differences.

Gender Stereotyping

- Gender stereotypes are general impressions and beliefs about males and females. Gender stereotypes are widespread. Gender stereotyping changes developmentally; it is present even at 2 years of age but increases considerably in early childhood. In middle and late childhood, children become more flexible in their gender attitudes, but gender stereotyping may increase again in early adolescence. By late adolescence, gender attitudes are often more flexible.

Gender Similarities and Differences

- Physical and biological differences between males and females are substantial. Women have about twice the body fat of men, are less likely to develop physical or mental disorders, and have a longer life expectancy. Boys and girls show similar achievement in math, although boys have slightly better visuospatial skills. Girls perform better in writing and reading. Some experts, such as Hyde, argue that cognitive differences between males and females have been exaggerated. Males are more physically aggressive than females, while females are more likely to show stronger affiliative interests in adolescence, express their emotions openly and intensely, have better emotional control, and engage in more prosocial behavior. There is considerable controversy about how similar or different females and males are in a number of areas.

Gender-Role Classification

 LG4 Identify how gender roles can be classified.

What Is Gender-Role Classification?

Gender Identity in Childhood and Adolescence

Gender-Role Transcendence

Gender in Context

- In the past, the well-adjusted male was supposed to show masculine traits; the well-adjusted female, feminine traits. During the 1970s, alternatives to traditional gender roles were introduced. It was proposed that competent individuals could show both masculine and feminine traits. This thinking led to the development of the concept of androgyny, the presence of masculine and feminine traits in one individual. Gender-role measures often categorize individuals as masculine, feminine, androgynous, or undifferentiated. Most androgynous individuals are flexible and mentally healthy, although the particular context and the individual's culture also determine the adaptiveness of a gender-role orientation.

- Gender identity becomes more salient in adolescence but has its roots in childhood. Transgender children have been found to have cognitive patterns and preferences that are indistinguishable from cisgender children who share their gender identity.

- One alternative to androgyny is gender-role transcendence, a theory that states that there has been too much emphasis on gender and that a better strategy is to think about competence in terms of individual characteristics rather than gender.

- In thinking about gender, it is important to keep in mind the context in which gender behavior is displayed. In many countries, traditional gender roles remain dominant.

key terms

androgens 331
androgyny 344
estrogens 331
gender 331

gender identity 331
gender role 331
gender schema theory 336
gender stereotypes 337

gender typing 331
rapport talk 341
report talk 341

social cognitive theory of gender 332
social role theory 332

key people

Sandra Bem 344
Phyllis Bronstein 333

David Buss 342
Alice Eagly 332

Diane Halpern 335
Janet Shibley Hyde 342

Deborah Tannen 341

chapter 13

MORAL DEVELOPMENT

chapter outline

1 Domains of Moral Development

Learning Goal 1 Discuss theory and research on the domains of moral development.

What Is Moral Development?
Moral Thought
Moral Behavior
Moral Feeling
Moral Personality
Social-Cognitive Domain Theory

2 Contexts of Moral Development

Learning Goal 2 Explain how parenting and schools influence moral development.

Parenting
Schools

3 Prosocial and Antisocial Behavior

Learning Goal 3 Describe the development of prosocial and antisocial behavior.

Prosocial Behavior
Antisocial Behavior

4 Religious and Spiritual Development

Learning Goal 4 Summarize the nature of children's and adolescents' religious and spiritual development.

Childhood
Adolescence

Lordn/iStock/Getty Images

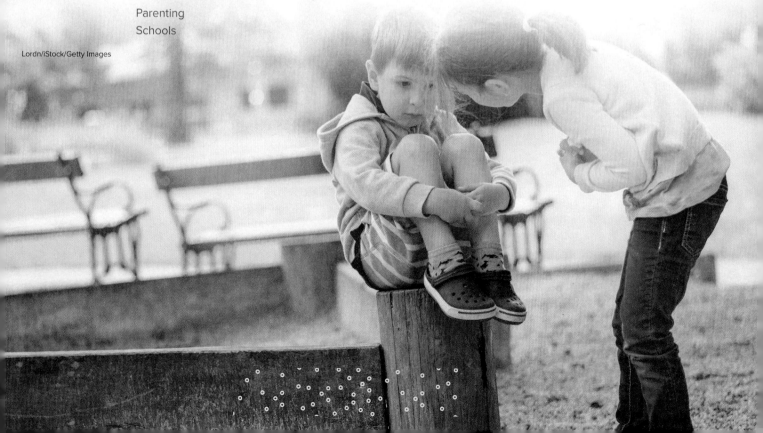

Jewel Cash is a young professional in the Boston area. The mayor of Boston once said that this young woman was "everywhere." At the age of 16, Jewel persuaded the city's school committee to consider ending the practice of locking tardy students out of their classrooms. She also swayed a neighborhood group to support her proposal for a winter jobs program. According to one city councilman at the time, "People are just impressed with the power of her arguments and the sophistication of the argument" (Silva, 2005, pp. B1, B4).

Jewel was raised in one of Boston's housing projects by her mother, a single parent. As a high school student she belonged to the Boston Student Advisory Council, mentored children, volunteered at a women's shelter, managed and danced in two troupes, and volunteered with a neighborhood watch group—among other activities.

Jewel once told an interviewer from the *Boston Globe*:

> I see a problem and I say, "How can I make a difference?" . . . I can't take on the world, even though I can try. . . . I'm moving forward but I want to make sure I'm bringing people with me (Silva, 2005, pp. B1, B4).

Jewel is far from typical, but her motivation to help others—as an adult today and as a teenager previously—illustrates the positive side of moral development.

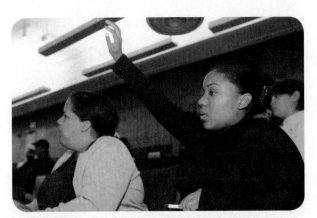

Jewel Cash as a teenager, seated next to her mother, participating in a crimewatch meeting at a community center. She exemplifies positive teenage community involvement.

Matthew J. Lee/The Boston Globe/Getty Images

preview

Most people have strong opinions not only about moral and immoral behavior but also about how moral behavior should be fostered in children. We will begin our coverage of moral development by exploring its main domains and then examine some important contexts that influence moral development. Next, we discuss children's prosocial and anti-social behavior. The chapter concludes with an overview of children's religious and spiritual development.

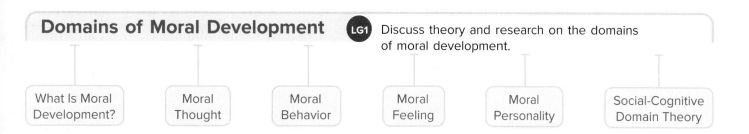

Domains of Moral Development — LG1 Discuss theory and research on the domains of moral development.

- What Is Moral Development?
- Moral Thought
- Moral Behavior
- Moral Feeling
- Moral Personality
- Social-Cognitive Domain Theory

What is moral development? What are its main domains?

WHAT IS MORAL DEVELOPMENT?

Moral development involves changes in thoughts, feelings, and behaviors regarding standards of right and wrong. Moral development has an *intrapersonal* dimension, which pertains to a person's activities when she or he is not engaged in social interaction, and an *interpersonal* dimension, which pertains to social interactions, including cooperation and conflict (Walker, 2006). To understand moral development, consider these five basic questions:

First, how do children and adolescents reason*, or think, about rules for ethical conduct?* For example, we might present them with a story in which someone has a conflict about whether or not to cheat on a test in school. Then they are asked to decide what is appropriate for the character to do and why. The focus is placed on the reasoning the children and adolescents use to justify their moral decisions.

Second, how do children and adolescents actually behave *in moral circumstances?* For example, with regard to cheating, we might observe whether they resist the temptation to cheat and the circumstances that produced the resistance or cheating. We could conduct our study by discreetly observing them as they are taking a test. We might note whether they take out "cheat" notes, look at another student's answers, and so on.

Third, how do children and adolescents feel *about moral issues?* In the example of cheating, do they feel enough guilt to resist temptation? If they do cheat, do feelings of guilt afterwards keep them from cheating the next time they face temptation?

Fourth, what comprises children's and adolescents' personality *with respect to morality?* Continuing with the example of cheating, do they have a moral identity and character that is so strong they resist the temptation to cheat?

Fifth, how is the moral domain *different from social conventional and personal domains?* In **social-cognitive domain theory** (discussed later in this chapter), cheating resides in the moral domain, along with lying, stealing, and harming another person. Behaviors such as cutting in a line or speaking out of turn are in the social conventional rather than the moral domain. Choosing friends is in the personal domain.

Let's now discuss the major aspects of moral development. We begin with the cognitive aspect involving thoughts.

moral development Changes in thoughts, feelings, and behaviors regarding standards of right and wrong.

social-cognitive domain theory Theory stating that there are different domains of social knowledge and reasoning, including moral, social conventional, and personal domains. These domains arise from children's and adolescents' attempts to understand and deal with different forms of social experience.

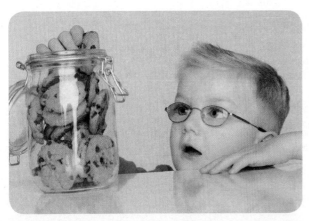

How is this child's moral thinking likely to be different about stealing a cookie, depending on whether he is in Piaget's heteronomous or autonomous stage?
Fuse/Getty Images

MORAL THOUGHT

How do individuals think about what is right and wrong? Are children able to evaluate moral questions in the same way that adults can? Piaget had some answers to these questions. So did Lawrence Kohlberg.

Piaget's Theory   Jean Piaget (1932) watched children play marbles to learn how they used and thought about the game's rules. He also asked children about ethical issues—theft, lies, punishment, and justice, for example. Piaget concluded that children go through two distinct stages of moral development, separated by a transition period:

- From 4 to 7 years of age, children display **heteronomous morality,** the first stage of moral development in Piaget's theory. Children think of justice and rules as unchangeable properties of the world, removed from the control of people. From 7 to 10 years, children transition gradually into the next stage.

- From about 10 years of age and older, children show **autonomous morality,** Piaget's second stage of moral development. They become aware that rules and laws are created by people, and in judging an action, they consider the actor's intentions as well as the consequences.

Because young children are "heteronomous moralists," they judge the rightness or goodness of behavior by considering its consequences, not the intentions of the actor. For example, to the heteronomous moralist, breaking twelve cups accidentally is worse than breaking one cup intentionally. As children develop into moral autonomists, intentions become more important.

The heteronomous thinker also believes that rules are unchangeable and are handed down by all-powerful authorities. By contrast, older children—moral autonomists—accept change and recognize that rules are conventions, subject to change. The heteronomous thinker also believes in **immanent justice,** the concept that if a rule is broken, punishment will be delivered immediately. The young child believes that a violation is connected automatically to its punishment. Thus, young children often look around worriedly after doing something wrong, expecting inevitable punishment. Older children, who are moral autonomists, recognize that punishment occurs only if someone witnesses the wrongdoing and that, even then, punishment is not inevitable. They also begin to realize that bad things can happen to innocent people.

How do these changes in moral reasoning occur? Piaget argued that, as children develop, they become more sophisticated in thinking about social matters, especially about the possibilities and conditions of cooperation. Piaget reasoned that this social understanding comes about through the mutual give-and-take of peer relations. In the peer group, where others have power and status similar to the child's, plans are negotiated and coordinated, and disagreements are reasoned about and eventually settled. Parent-child relations, in which parents have power and children do not, are less likely to advance moral reasoning because rules are often handed down through the parent's authority.

However, young children are not as egocentric as Piaget once envisioned. Thompson (2012) argued that recent research indicates young children often show a non-egocentric awareness of others' goals, feelings, and desires and how such internal states are influenced by the actions of others. These ties between advances in moral understanding and theory of mind indicate that young children possess cognitive resources that allow them to be aware of others' intentions and to know when someone violates a moral prohibition. One study of 3- and 5-year-olds found that they were less likely to offer rewards to a puppet character they had previously observed being selfish to another individual (Vogelsang & Tomasello, 2016).

However, because of limitations in their self-control skills, social understanding, and cognitive flexibility, young children's moral advancements often are inconsistent and vary

------------➤

developmental **connection**

Cognitive Theory

In which of Piaget's cognitive developmental stages is a 5-year-old heteronomous thinker likely to be? Connect to "Cognitive Developmental Approaches."

◄------------

heteronomous morality The first stage of moral development in Piaget's theory, occurring from 4 to 7 years of age. Justice and rules are conceived of as unchangeable properties of the world, beyond the control of people.

autonomous morality The second stage of moral development in Piaget's theory, displayed by older children (about 10 years of age and older). The child becomes aware that rules and laws are created by people and that, in judging an action, one should consider the actor's intentions as well as the consequences.

immanent justice Piaget's concept of the childhood expectation that if a rule is broken, punishment will be meted out immediately.

across situations. They still have a long way to go before they have the capacity to develop a consistent moral character and make ethical judgments.

Kohlberg's Theory A second major perspective on moral development was proposed by Lawrence Kohlberg (1958, 1986). Based partly on Piaget's theory, Kohlberg suggested that there are six stages of moral development. These stages, he argued, are universal. Development from one stage to another, said Kohlberg, was fostered by taking the perspective of others and experiencing a conflict between one's current moral thinking and a more advanced level of moral reasoning.

Kohlberg arrived at his view after 20 years of using a unique interview with children. In the interview, children were presented with stories in which characters faced moral dilemmas. The following is the most famous example:

> In Europe a woman was near death from a special kind of cancer. There was one drug that the doctors thought might save her. It was a form of radium that a druggist [pharmacist] in the same town had recently discovered. The drug was expensive to make, but the druggist was charging ten times what the drug cost him to make. He paid $200 for the radium and charged $2,000 for a small dose of the drug. The sick woman's husband, Heinz, went to everyone he knew to borrow the money, but he could only get together $1,000, which is half of what it cost. He told the druggist that his wife was dying and asked him to sell it cheaper or let him pay later. But the druggist said, "No, I discovered the drug, and I am going to make money from it." So Heinz got desperate and broke into the man's store to steal the drug for his wife. (Kohlberg, 1969, p. 379)

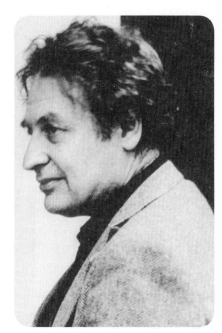

Lawrence Kohlberg.
UAV 605.295.8 Box 7, Harvard University Archives.

After reading the story, the interviewee answers a series of questions about the moral dilemma. Should Heinz have stolen the drug? Was stealing it right or wrong? Why? Is it a husband's duty to steal the drug for his wife if he can get it no other way? Would a good husband steal? Did the pharmacist have the right to charge that much when there was no law setting a limit on the price? Why or why not?

The Kohlberg Stages Based on the answers, three levels of moral thinking (each with two stages) could be defined (see Figure 1). The progression through the levels and stages involves the person's morality gradually becoming more internal rather than being based on external or superficial reasons they would have given when they were younger.

- *Kohlberg's Level 1: Preconventional Reasoning* **Preconventional reasoning** is the lowest level and consists of two stages: punishment and obedience orientation (stage 1) and individualism, instrumental purpose, and exchange (stage 2).

  Stage 1. Punishment and obedience orientation is the first stage, in which moral thinking is often tied to punishment. For example, children and adolescents obey adults because adults tell them to obey.

  Stage 2. Individualism, instrumental purpose, and exchange is the second stage, when individuals pursue their own interests but also let others do the same. Thus, what is right involves an equal exchange. People are nice to others so that others will be nice to them in return.

- *Kohlberg's Level 2: Conventional Reasoning* **Conventional reasoning** is the second, or intermediate, level. Individuals have certain standards (internal), but they are the same standards held by others (external), such as parents or the laws of society. The conventional reasoning level consists of two stages: mutual interpersonal expectations, relationships, and interpersonal conformity (stage 3) and social systems morality (stage 4).

  Stage 3. Mutual interpersonal expectations, relationships, and interpersonal conformity is the third stage when individuals value trust, caring, and loyalty to others as a basis of moral judgments. Children and adolescents often adopt their parents' moral standards at this stage, seeking to be thought of by their parents as being "good."

preconventional reasoning The lowest level in Kohlberg's theory. At this level, morality is often focused on reward and punishment. The two stages in preconventional reasoning are punishment and obedience orientation (stage 1) and individualism, instrumental purpose, and exchange (stage 2).

conventional reasoning The second, or intermediate, level in Kohlberg's theory of moral development. At this level, individuals abide by certain standards (internal), but they are the standards of others such as parents or the laws of society (external). The conventional level consists of two stages: mutual interpersonal expectations, relationships, and interpersonal conformity (stage 3) and social systems morality (stage 4).

FIGURE 1
KOHLBERG'S THREE LEVELS AND SIX STAGES OF MORAL DEVELOPMENT

postconventional reasoning The third and highest level in Kohlberg's theory of moral development. At this level, morality is more internal. The postconventional level consists of two stages: social contract or utility and individual rights (stage 5) and universal ethical principles (stage 6).

Stage 4. Social systems morality is the fourth stage, in which moral judgments are based on understanding the social order, law, justice, and duty. For example, adolescents may say that, for a community to work effectively, it needs to be protected by laws that everyone follows.

- *Kohlberg's Level 3: Postconventional Reasoning* **Postconventional** reasoning is the third and highest level in Kohlberg's theory. At this level, morality is more internal. The postconventional level of morality consists of two stages: social contract or utility and individual rights (stage 5) and universal ethical principles (stage 6).

Stage 5. Social contract or utility and individual rights is the fifth stage, when individuals reason that values, rights, and principles undergird or transcend the law. A person evaluates the validity of actual laws and examines social systems in terms of the degree to which they preserve and protect fundamental human rights and values.

Stage 6. Universal ethical principles is the sixth and highest stage, in which the person has developed a moral standard based on universal human rights. When faced with a conflict between law and conscience, the person will follow her or his own conscience, even when it involves personal risk.

Kohlberg observed that before age 9, most children used stage 1, preconventional reasoning based on external rewards and punishments, when they consider moral choices. By early adolescence, their moral reasoning was increasingly based on the application of standards set by others. Most adolescents reasoned at stage 3, with some signs of stages 2 and 4. By early adulthood, a small number of individuals began reasoning in postconventional ways.

A classic 20-year longitudinal investigation of boys and men found that use of stages 1 and 2 decreased with age (Colby & others, 1983) (see Figure 2). Stage 4, which did not appear at all in the moral reasoning of 10-year-olds, was reflected in the moral thinking of 62 percent of 36-year-olds. Stage 5 did not appear until age 20 to 22 and never characterized more than 10 percent of individuals.

This study showed that the moral stages appeared somewhat later than Kohlberg initially envisioned, and reasoning at the higher stages, especially stage 6, was rare. Although stage 6 has been removed from the interview scoring manual, it still is considered to be theoretically important by some developmentalists.

Influences on the Kohlberg Stages Moral reasoning at each stage is based on the individual's level of cognitive development, but Kohlberg argued that advances in children's cognitive development did not ensure development of moral reasoning. Instead, moral reasoning also reflects children's experiences in dealing with moral questions and moral conflict.

Several investigators have tried to advance individuals' levels of moral development by having a person present arguments that reflect moral thinking one stage above the individuals' established levels—or by observing whether a child's parents essentially do this when discussing moral conflicts. This approach applies the concepts of equilibrium and conflict that Piaget used to explain cognitive development. By presenting arguments slightly beyond the children's level of moral reasoning, the researchers created a disequilibrium that motivated the children to restructure their moral thought. The upshot of studies using this approach is that virtually any plus-stage discussion, for any length of time, seems to promote more advanced moral reasoning (Walker, 1982; Walker & Taylor, 1991).

Kohlberg emphasized that peer interaction and perspective taking are critical aspects of the social stimulation that challenges children to change their moral reasoning. Whereas adults characteristically impose rules and regulations on children, the give-and-take among peers gives children an opportunity to take the perspective of another person and to generate rules democratically. Kohlberg stressed that in principle, encounters with any peers can produce perspective-taking opportunities that may advance a child's moral reasoning. Comprehensive reviews of cross-cultural studies involving Kohlberg's theory and similar types of measures have revealed strong support for a link between perspective-taking skills and more advanced moral judgments (Gibbs, 2019).

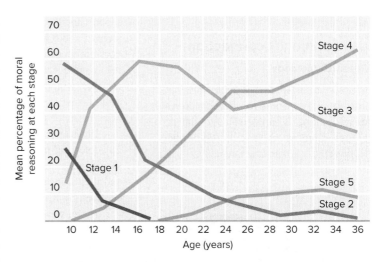

FIGURE 2

AGE AND THE PERCENTAGE OF INDIVIDUALS AT EACH KOHLBERG STAGE. In a classic longitudinal study of males from 10 to 36 years of age, at age 10 most moral reasoning was at stage 2 (Colby & others, 1983). At 16 to 18 years of age, stage 3 became the most frequent type of moral reasoning, and it was not until the mid-twenties that stage 4 became the most frequent. Stage 5 did not appear until 20 to 22 years of age and it never characterized more than 10 percent of the individuals. In this study, the moral stages appeared somewhat later than Kohlberg envisioned, and stage 6 was absent.

Kohlberg's Critics   Kohlberg's theory has provoked debate, research, and criticism (Gray & Graham, 2018; Hoover & others, 2018; Killen & Dahl, 2018; Narváez, 2018; Railton, 2016; Turiel & Gingo, 2017).

Moral Thought and Moral Behavior   Kohlberg's theory has been criticized for placing too much emphasis on moral thought and not enough emphasis on moral behavior. Moral reasons can sometimes be a shelter for immoral behavior. Corrupt CEOs and politicians endorse the loftiest of moral virtues in public until their own behavior is exposed. Whatever the latest public scandal, you will probably find that the culprits displayed virtuous thoughts but engaged in immoral behavior. No one wants a nation of cheaters and thieves who can reason at the postconventional level. The cheaters and thieves may know what is right yet still do what is wrong. Heinous actions can be cloaked in a mantle of moral virtue.

Moral disengagement is a psychological process that allows the individual to distinguish the self from harmful effects of behaviors (Bandura, 2016). By blaming victims and diffusing responsibility, individuals can continue to feel good about themselves while doing immoral things.

Culture and Moral Reasoning   Culture influences moral development more than Kohlberg thought. Kohlberg emphasized that his stages of moral reasoning are universal, but some critics claim his theory is culturally biased (Christen, Narváez, & Gutzwiller, 2017; Graham & Valdesolo, 2017; Gray & Graham, 2018). Both Kohlberg and his critics may be partially correct.

One review of 45 studies in 27 cultures around the world, mostly non-European, provided support for the universality of Kohlberg's first four stages (Snarey, 1987). Individuals in diverse cultures developed through these four stages in sequence as Kohlberg predicted. More recent research suggests

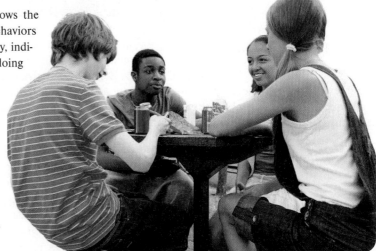

Why did Piaget and Kohlberg think peer relations are so important in moral development?
Alys Tomlinson/Image Source

developmental **connection**

Research Methods

Cross-cultural studies provide information about the degree to which children's development is universal, or similar, across cultures or is culture-specific. Connect to "Culture and Diversity."

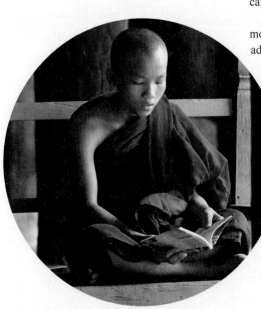

In a unique study of 20 adolescent male Buddhist monks in Nepal, the issue of justice, a basic theme in Kohlberg's theory, was not evident in the monks' moral views (Huebner & Garrod, 1993). Also, the monks' concerns about prevention of suffering and the importance of compassion are not mentioned in Kohlberg's theory.
Thierry Falise/LightRocket/Getty Images

developmental **connection**

Gender

Janet Shibley Hyde concluded that many views and studies of gender exaggerate differences. Connect to "Gender."

support for the qualitative shift from stage 2 to stage 3 across cultures, but the shifts to stages 5 and 6 have not been found in all cultures. Furthermore, Kohlberg's scoring system does not recognize the higher-level moral reasoning of certain cultures—thus, moral reasoning is more culture-specific than Kohlberg envisioned (Gibbs, 2019; Snarey, 1987). For example, it appears that notions of morality in personal domains (for example, lying to avoid taking credit for a good deed) vary across cultures, depending on whether self-benefiting behavior is encouraged or discouraged in the culture (Helwig, 2017).

Illustrative results occurred in a study that assessed the moral development of 20 adolescent male Buddhist monks in Nepal (Huebner & Garrod, 1993). Justice, a basic theme in Kohlberg's theory, was not of paramount importance in the monks' moral views, and their concerns about the prevention of suffering and the role of compassion are not captured by Kohlberg's theory.

In the view of John Gibbs (2019), most young adolescents around the world use the moral judgment of mutuality (stage 3) that makes intimate friendships possible. And by late adolescence, many individuals also are beginning to grasp the importance of agreed-upon standards and institutions for the common good (stage 4). A main exception, though, is the delayed moral judgment of adolescents who regularly engage in delinquency.

Another study explored links between culture, mindset, and moral judgment (Narváez & Hill, 2010). In this study, higher levels of multicultural experience were linked to lower levels of closed mindedness (being cognitively inflexible), a growth mindset (perceiving that one's qualities can change and improve through effort), and higher moral judgment. Narváez and her colleagues (Christen, Narváez, & Gutzwiller, 2017) stress that we need to make better progress in dealing with an increasing array of temptations and possible wrongdoings in a human social world in which complexity is accumulating over time.

In sum, although Kohlberg's approach does capture much of the moral reasoning voiced in various cultures around the world, his approach misses or misconstrues some important moral concepts in particular cultures (Gibbs, 2019). To read further about cultural variations in moral reasoning, see *Connecting with Diversity*.

The Role of Emotion Kohlberg argued that emotion has negative effects on moral reasoning. However, emotions play an important role in moral thinking (Gui, Gan, & Liu, 2016; Schalkwijk & others, 2016). People who have damage to a particular region in the brain's prefrontal cortex find it difficult to integrate emotions into their moral judgments (Damasio, 1994). After losing their intuitive feelings about what is right or wrong, they struggle to make choices involving moral issues. Also, studies with healthy individuals have shown that moral decisions are linked to the intensity and activation of emotion in the same prefrontal brain region, as well as in the amygdala (Shenhav & Greene, 2014).

Conscious/Deliberative Reasoning Versus Unconscious/Automatic Responses Social psychologist Jonathan Haidt (2013, 2017) argues that a major flaw in Kohlberg's theory is the assumption that moral thinking is deliberative—that we frequently reason and contemplate our moral decisions. According to Haidt, moral thinking is usually an intuitive "gut reaction"; the deliberative contemplation usually occurs after the fact. Accordingly, morality begins with rapid judgments of others rather than with slow, strategic reasoning (Graham & Valdesolo, 2017).

Families and Moral Development Kohlberg argued that family processes are essentially unimportant in children's moral development. As noted earlier, he argued that parent-child relationships usually provide children with little opportunity for give-and-take or perspective taking. Rather, Kohlberg said that such opportunities are more likely to be provided by children's peer relations.

Did Kohlberg underestimate the contribution of family relationships to moral development? Many developmentalists emphasize that children's conversations with parents about moral dilemmas in daily life are important to children's moral development, and that parents' basic moral attitudes influence children's moral thinking (Carlo & others, 2018; Eisenberg, Spinrad, & Knafo-Noam, 2015; Wainryb & Recchia, 2014). Conversations about

Moral Reasoning in the United States and India

Cultural meaning systems vary around the world, and these systems shape children's morality (Gibbs, 2019; Shiraev & Levy, 2016). Consider the cultural context of Indian Hindu Brahman children (Choudhuri & Basu, 2013). Like people in many other non-Western societies, Indian Hindus view moral rules as part of the natural world order. This means that they do not necessarily distinguish between physical, moral, and social regulation, as Americans do. For example, in India, violations of food taboos and marital restrictions can be just as serious as acts intended to cause harm to others. In India, social rules are seen as inevitable, like laws of nature.

According to William Damon in a classic text (1988), in places where culturally specific practices take on profound moral and religious significance, as in India, the moral development of children focuses extensively on their adherence to custom and convention. In contrast, Western moral doctrine tends to elevate abstract principles, such as justice and welfare, as having high moral status. As in India, socialization practices in many countries actively instill in children a great respect for their culture's traditional codes and practices.

How would you revise Kohlberg's stages of moral development to better accommodate other cultures?

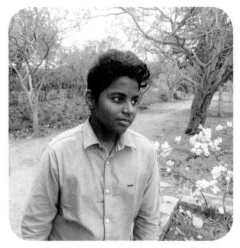

How might Asian Indian children and American children reason differently about moral issues?
Mohamed Aswir/EyeEm/Getty Images

moral dilemmas may be most effective when they draw the child's focus to the consequences of their actions for others (Grusec & others, 2014). In addition, families connect children with religious organizations, community service opportunities, and other experiences that can foster moral development and reduce antisocial behaviors (Guo, 2018).

Gender and the Care Perspective The most publicized criticism of Kohlberg's theory has come from Carol Gilligan (Gilligan, 1992; Jorgensen, 2007), who argues that Kohlberg's theory reflects a gender bias. According to Gilligan, Kohlberg's theory is based on a male norm that puts abstract principles above relationships and concern for others and sees the individual as standing alone and independently making moral decisions. It puts justice at the heart of morality. In contrast to Kohlberg's **justice perspective,** which focuses on the rights of the individual, Gilligan argues for a **care perspective,** a moral perspective that views people in terms of their connectedness with others and emphasizes interpersonal communication, relationships with others, and concern for others. According to Gilligan, Kohlberg greatly underplayed the care perspective, perhaps because he was a male, because most of his research was with males rather than females, and because he used male responses as a model for his theory.

In extensive interviews with girls from 6 to 18 years of age, Gilligan and her colleagues found that girls consistently interpret moral dilemmas in terms of human relationships and base these interpretations on watching and listening to other people (Gilligan, 1992). However, a meta-analysis (a statistical analysis that combines the results of many different studies) casts doubt on Gilligan's claim of substantial gender differences in moral judgment (Jaffee & Hyde, 2000). In this study, overall, only a small sex difference in care-based reasoning favored females, but this sex difference was greater in adolescence than childhood. When differences occurred, they were better explained by the nature of

justice perspective A moral perspective that focuses on the rights of the individual; individuals independently make moral decisions.

care perspective The moral perspective of Carol Gilligan, in which people are assessed in terms of their connectedness with others and the quality of their interpersonal communication, relationships with others, and concern for others.

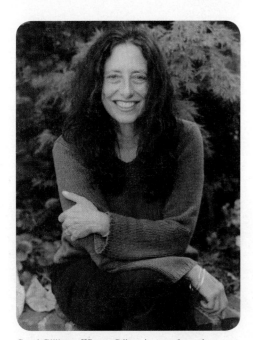

Carol Gilligan. *What is Gilligan's view of moral development?*

Courtesy of Dr. Carol Gilligan

the dilemma than by gender (for example, both males and females tended to use care-based reasoning to deal with interpersonal dilemmas and justice reasoning to handle societal dilemmas). A review concluded that girls' moral orientations are "somewhat more likely to focus on care for others than on abstract principles of justice, but they can use both moral orientations when needed (as can boys . . .)" (Blakemore, Berenbaum, & Liben, 2009, p. 132).

MORAL BEHAVIOR

What are the basic processes responsible for moral behavior? What is the nature of self-control and resistance to temptation? How does social cognitive theory view moral development?

Basic Processes The processes of reinforcement, punishment, and imitation have been invoked to explain how individuals learn certain responses and why their responses differ from those of other persons (Grusec, 2017). When individuals are reinforced for behavior that is consistent with laws and social conventions, they are likely to repeat that behavior. When provided with models who behave morally, individuals are likely to adopt their actions. Finally, when individuals are punished for immoral behaviors, those behaviors can be eliminated, but at the expense of sanctioning punishment by its very use and of causing negative emotional effects for the individual.

These general conclusions come with some important qualifiers. The effectiveness of reward and punishment depends on their consistency and timing. For example, it is generally more effective to reward moral behavior soon after the event occurs than to do so later. The effectiveness of modeling depends on the characteristics of the model and the cognitive skills of the observer. For example, if a parent models giving a donation to a charity, her child must be old enough to understand this behavior in order for it to have an impact on the child's moral development.

Another qualifier is that behavior is situationally dependent. Individuals do not consistently behave morally in different situations. In a classic investigation of moral behavior, Hugh Hartshorne and Mark May (1928–1930) observed the moral responses of 11,000 children who were given the opportunity to lie, cheat, and steal in a variety of circumstances—at home, at school, at social events, and in athletics. A completely honest or a completely dishonest child was rare. Situation-specific behavior was the rule. Children were more likely to cheat when there was peer pressure and the odds of being caught were slim. Nevertheless, although moral behavior is influenced by situational determinants, some individuals are more likely than others to cheat, lie, and steal (Hertz & Krettenauer, 2016).

In further support of situational influences on moral behavior, one study found that very few 7-year-olds were willing to donate any money after watching a UNICEF film on children suffering from poverty (van IJzendoorn & others, 2010). However, after gentle probing by an adult, most children were willing to donate some of their money.

social cognitive theory of morality The theory that distinguishes between moral competence—the ability to produce moral behaviors—and moral performance—use of those behaviors in specific situations.

developmental **connection**

Social Cognitive Theory

What are the main themes of Bandura's social cognitive theory? Connect to "Introduction."

Social Cognitive Theory The **social cognitive theory of morality** emphasizes a distinction between an individual's *ability* to perform moral behaviors and the actual performance of those behaviors in specific situations. *Moral competencies* include what individuals are capable of doing, what they know, their skills, their awareness of moral rules and regulations, and their cognitive ability to construct behaviors. *Moral performance*, or behavior, however, is determined by motivation and the rewards and incentives to act in a specific moral way. Studies of children have shown that having the social and cognitive skills to behave morally often does not predict who will behave in morally acceptable or unacceptable ways (Gasser & Keller, 2009).

Albert Bandura (2002, 2016) also has stressed that moral development reflects a combination of social and cognitive factors, especially those involving self-control. In developing a moral self, individuals adopt standards of right and wrong that serve as guides and deterrents for conduct. In this self-regulatory process, people monitor their conduct and the conditions under which it occurs, judge it in relation to moral standards, and control their actions by the consequences they apply to themselves. They do things that provide them with satisfaction and a sense of self-worth. They refrain from behaving in ways that violate their moral standards because such conduct will bring self-condemnation. Self-sanctions keep conduct in line with internal standards. Thus, in Bandura's view, self-regulation rather than abstract moral reasoning is the key to moral development and behavior.

MORAL FEELING

Think about how you feel when you do something you sense is wrong. Does it affect you emotionally? Maybe you get a twinge of guilt. And when you give someone a gift, you might feel joy. What role do emotions play in moral development, and how do these emotions develop?

According to Sigmund Freud, guilt and the desire to avoid feeling guilty are the foundation of moral behavior. Researchers have examined the extent to which children *feel guilty* when they misbehave. Grazyna Kochanska and her colleagues (Kochanska & others, 2009; Kim & Kochanska, 2017) have conducted a number of studies that explore children's conscience development. In a comprehensive research review of children's guilt and conscience, the evidence from these and other researchers' studies showed that young children are aware of right and wrong, have the capacity to show empathy and prosocial behavior toward others, experience guilt, indicate discomfort following a transgression, and are sensitive to violating rules (Malti, 2016). In one illustrative study, Kochanska and her colleagues (2002) observed 106 preschool children in laboratory situations in which they were led to believe that they had damaged valuable objects. In these mishaps, the behavioral indicators of guilt that were coded by observers included avoiding gaze (looking away or down), body tension (squirming, backing away, hanging head down, covering face with hands), and distress (looking uncomfortable, crying). Girls expressed more guilt than boys, and those with a more fearful temperament also expressed more guilt. In contrast, children of mothers who used power-oriented discipline (such as spanking, slapping, and yelling) displayed less guilt.

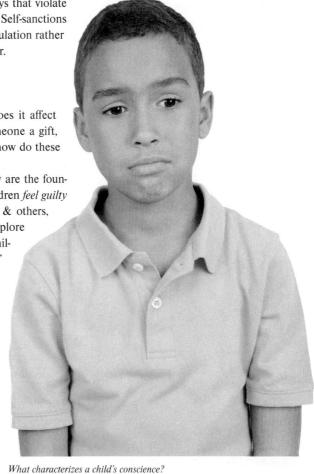

What characterizes a child's conscience?
Holly Curry/McGraw-Hill Education

Empathy   Guilt is an obvious aspect of moral feelings and their development. However, positive feelings such as empathy also contribute to the child's moral development (Eisenberg, Spinrad, & Sadovsky, 2014). Feeling **empathy** means reacting to another's feelings with an emotional response that is similar to the other's feelings. To empathize is not just to sympathize; it is to put oneself in another's place emotionally.

Although empathy is an emotional state, it has a cognitive component—the discerning of another's inner psychological states, or what we have previously called *perspective taking* (Decety, Meidenbauer, & Cowell, 2018). Infants have the capacity for some purely empathic responses, but for effective moral action, children must learn to identify a wide range of emotional states in others and to anticipate what kinds of actions will improve another person's emotional state.

What are the milestones in children's development of empathy? According to a classic analysis by William Damon (1988), changes in empathy take place in early infancy, at 1 to 2 years of age, in early childhood, and at 10 to 12 years of age.

Global empathy is the young infant's empathic response in which clear boundaries between the feelings and needs of the self and those of another have not yet been established. For example, one 11-month-old infant fought off her own tears, sucked her thumb, and buried her head in her mother's lap after she had seen another child fall and hurt himself. Not all infants cry every time someone else is hurt, though. Many times, an infant will stare at another's pain with curiosity. Although global empathy is observed in some infants, it does not consistently characterize all infants' behavior.

When they are 1 to 2 years of age, infants may feel genuine concern for the distress of other people, but only when they reach early childhood can they respond appropriately to another person's distress. This ability depends on children's new awareness that people have different reactions to situations. By late childhood, they may begin to feel empathy for the unfortunate.

empathy Reacting to another's feelings with an emotional response that is similar to the other's feelings.

- - - - - - - - - - - →
developmental **connection**

Social Cognition

In Robert Selman's view, perspective taking is a key aspect of whether children develop prosocial or antisocial attitudes and behavior. Connect to "The Self and Identity."
← - - - - - - - - - - -

FIGURE **3**

DAMON'S DESCRIPTION OF
DEVELOPMENTAL CHANGES IN EMPATHY

Age Period	Nature of Empathy
Early infancy	Characterized by global empathy, the young infant's empathic response does not distinguish between feelings and needs of self and others.
1 to 2 years of age	Undifferentiated feelings of discomfort at another's distress grow into more genuine feelings of concern, but infants cannot translate realization of another person's unhappy feelings into effective action.
Early childhood	Children become aware that every person's perspective is unique and that someone else may have a different reaction to a situation. This awareness allows the child to respond more appropriately to another person's distress.
10 to 12 years of age	Children develop an emergent orientation of empathy for people who live in unfortunate circumstances—the poor, the disabled, and the socially outcast. In adolescence, this newfound sensitivity may advance the individual's ideological and political views.

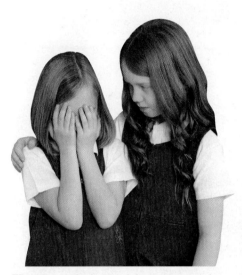

What are some developmental changes in empathy?
Image Source/Getty Images

At about 10 to 12 years of age, individuals develop an empathy for people who live in unfortunate circumstances. Children's concerns are no longer limited to the feelings of specific persons in situations they directly observe. Instead, 10- to 12-year-olds expand their concerns to the general problems of people in unfortunate circumstances—those who are poor, disabled, social outcasts, and so forth. This newfound sensitivity may lead older children to behave altruistically, and later to advance adolescents' development of ideological and political views. To read further about Damon's description of the developmental changes in empathy from infancy through adolescence, see Figure 3.

Although every individual may be capable of responding with empathy, not all do so. Empathic behavior varies considerably between individuals. For example, in older children and adolescents, empathic deficits can contribute to antisocial behavior. Some delinquents convicted of violent crimes show a lack of feeling for their victims' distress. A 13-year-old boy convicted of violently mugging a number of older adults, when asked about the pain he had caused one blind woman, said, "What do I care? I'm not her" (Damon, 1988).

The Contemporary Perspective on the Role of Emotion in Moral Development   We have seen that foundational theories emphasize the role of guilt in moral development but that other theorists, such as Damon, emphasize the role of empathy. Today, many developmentalists conclude that both positive feelings—such as empathy, sympathy, admiration, and self-esteem—and negative feelings—such as anger, outrage, shame, and guilt—contribute to children's moral development (Eisenberg, Spinrad, & Sadovsky, 2014; Thompson, 2015). When strongly experienced, these emotions influence children to act in accord with standards of right and wrong (Malti & others, 2017).

MORAL PERSONALITY

So far we have examined three key dimensions of moral development: thoughts, behavior, and feelings. Recently, there has been a surge of interest in a fourth dimension: personality (Meindl & others, 2015; Walker, 2014). Three aspects of moral personality that have recently been emphasized are (1) moral identity, (2) moral character, and (3) moral exemplars.

Moral Identity   A central aspect of the recent interest in the role of personality in moral development focuses on **moral identity.** Individuals have a moral identity when moral notions and commitments are central to their life. In this view, behaving in a manner that violates this moral commitment places the integrity of the self at risk (Matsuba, Murazyn, & Hart, 2014; Walker, 2014).

Darcia Narváez (2010) has concluded that a mature moral individual cares about morality and being a moral person. For these individuals, moral responsibility is central to their identity. Mature moral individuals engage in moral metacognition, including moral self-monitoring and moral self-reflection. Moral self-monitoring involves monitoring one's thoughts and actions related to moral situations, and engaging in self-control when it is needed. Moral self-reflection encompasses critical evaluations of one's self-judgments and

- - - - - - - - ->

developmental **connection**

Identity

According to James Marcia, what are the four statuses of identity development? Connect to "The Self and Identity."

<- - - - - - - - - - - -

moral identity The aspect of personality that is present when individuals have moral notions and commitments that are central to their lives.

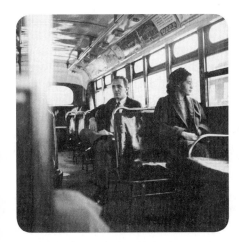

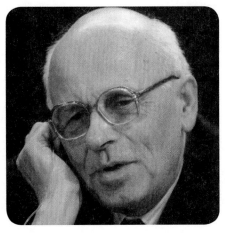

Rosa Parks (*left photo*, sitting in the front of a bus after the U.S. Supreme Court ruled that segregation was illegal on her city's bus system) and Andrei Sakharov (*right photo*) are moral exemplars. Parks (1913–2005), an African American seamstress in Montgomery, Alabama, became famous for her quiet, revolutionary act of not giving up her bus seat to a non-Latino White man in 1955. Her heroic act is cited by many historians as the beginning of the modern civil rights movement in the United States. Across the next four decades, Parks continued to work for progress in civil rights. Sakharov (1921–1989) was a Soviet physicist who spent several decades designing nuclear weapons for the former Soviet Union and came to be known as the father of the Russian hydrogen bomb. However, later in his life he became one of his country's most outspoken critics and worked tirelessly to promote human rights and democracy there and throughout the world.

(left) Bettmann/Getty Images; (right) Alain Nogues/Sygma/Getty Images

efforts to minimize bias and self-deception. A strong moral identity predicts behaving in moral ways in many situations (Hertz & Krettenauer, 2016).

Moral Character   *Moral character* involves having strong convictions, persisting, and overcoming distractions and obstacles. If individuals don't have moral character, they may wilt under pressure or fatigue, fail to follow through, or become distracted and discouraged, and fail to behave morally. Moral character presupposes that the person has set moral goals and that achieving those goals involves the commitment to act in accord with those goals (Cohen & Morse, 2014).

Lawrence Walker (2014) has studied moral character by examining people's conceptions of moral excellence. Among the moral virtues people emphasize are "honesty, truthfulness, and trustworthiness, as well as those of care, compassion, thoughtfulness, and considerateness. Other salient traits revolve around virtues of dependability, loyalty, and conscientiousness" (Walker, 2002, p. 74).

Moral Exemplars   **Moral exemplars** are people who have lived exemplary lives. Moral exemplars have a moral personality, identity, character, and set of virtues that reflect moral excellence and commitment (Vos, 2018; Walker, 2014).

In one study, three different exemplars of morality were examined—brave, caring, and just (Walker & Hennig, 2004). Different personality profiles emerged for the three exemplars. The brave exemplar was characterized by being dominant and extraverted, the caring exemplar by being nurturant and agreeable, and the just exemplar by being conscientious and open to experience. However, a number of traits characterized all three moral exemplars, considered by the researchers to reflect a possible core of moral functioning. This core included being honest and dependable.

SOCIAL-COGNITIVE DOMAIN THEORY

Judith Smetana (Jambon & Smetana, 2018; Smetana, Jambon, & Ball, 2014) has proposed social-cognitive domain theory, which states that there are different domains of social knowledge and reasoning, including moral, social conventional, and personal domains. In social-cognitive domain theory, children's and adolescents' moral, social conventional, and personal knowledge and reasoning emerge from their attempts to understand and deal with different forms of social experience (Killen & Dahl, 2018; Turiel, 2015).

Social conventional reasoning focuses on conventional rules that have been established by social consensus in order to control behavior and maintain the social system. The rules themselves are arbitrary, such as raising your hand in class before speaking, using one staircase at school to go up and the other to go down, not cutting in front of someone standing in line to buy movie tickets, and stopping at a stop sign when driving. There are sanctions if we violate these conventions, although the rules can be changed by consensus.

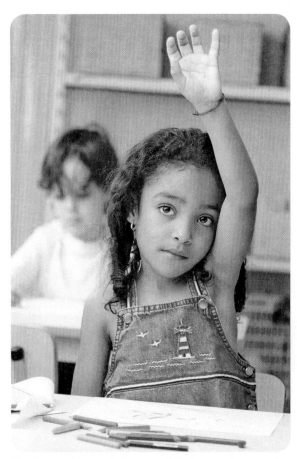

How does social conventional reasoning differ from moral reasoning? What are some examples of social conventional reasoning?
Glow Images

moral exemplars People who have lived extraordinary lives, having developed their personality, identity, character, and virtue to a level that reflects moral excellence and commitment.

social conventional reasoning Focuses on conventional rules established by social consensus, as opposed to moral reasoning that stresses ethical issues.

In contrast, moral reasoning focuses on ethical issues and rules of morality. Unlike conventional rules, moral rules are not arbitrary. They are obligatory, widely accepted, and somewhat impersonal (Killen & Dahl, 2018; Turiel & Gingo, 2017). Rules pertaining to lying, cheating, stealing, and physically harming another person are moral rules because violation of these rules affronts ethical standards that exist apart from social consensus and convention. Moral judgments involve concepts of justice, whereas social conventional judgments are concepts of social organization. Violating moral rules is usually more serious than violating conventional rules. As exemplified in one study of 2- to 5-year-olds, children distinguished moral from conventional transgressions on many criteria, but older preschoolers were much clearer in distinguishing their judgments of and preferences for conventional versus moral transgressors (Smetana & others, 2018).

The social conventional approach is a serious challenge to Kohlberg's approach because Kohlberg argued that social conventions are a stopover on the road to higher moral sophistication. For social conventional reasoning advocates, social conventional reasoning is not lower than postconventional reasoning but rather something that needs to be disentangled from the moral thread (Dahl & Killen, 2018; Smetana, Jambon, & Ball, 2014; Turiel & Gingo, 2017).

Recently, a distinction also has been made between moral and conventional issues, which are viewed as legitimately subject to adult social regulation, and personal issues, which are more likely subject to the child's or adolescent's independent decision making and personal discretion (Dahl & Killen, 2018; Turiel & Gingo, 2017). Personal issues include control over one's body, privacy, and choice of friends and activities. Thus, some actions belong to a *personal* domain not governed by moral strictures or social norms.

Review Connect Reflect

LG1 Discuss theory and research on the domains of moral development.

Review

- What is moral development?
- What are Piaget's and Kohlberg's theories of moral development? What are some criticisms of Kohlberg's theory? What is social conventional reasoning?
- What processes are involved in moral behavior? What is the social cognitive theory of moral development?
- How are moral feelings related to moral development?
- What characterizes moral personality?
- What characterizes the social-cognitive domain theory of moral development?

Connect

- In this section, you learned that, according to Piaget, children from 7 to 10 years of age are in a transition period between the heteronomous morality and autonomous morality stages of development. Which stage of cognitive development would these children be in, according to Piaget?

Reflect *Your Own Personal Journey of Life*

- Which of the five approaches—cognitive, psychoanalytic, behavioral/social cognitive, personality, and social-cognitive domain—do you think best describes the way you developed morally? Explain.

Contexts of Moral Development

LG2 Explain how parenting and schools influence moral development.

Parenting

Schools

What other contexts play a role in moral development? In particular, what are the roles of parents and schools?

PARENTING

Both Piaget and Kohlberg held that parents do not provide unique or essential inputs to children's moral development. Parents, in their view, are responsible for providing role-taking opportunities and cognitive challenges, but peers play the primary role in moral development. Research reveals that both parents and peers contribute to children's moral maturity (Walker, Hennig, & Krettenauer, 2000). One study found that Italian 3- to 6-year-olds' moral disengagement, along with their parents' moral disengagement, predicted individual differences in the children's aggressive and oppositional behavioral problems (Camodeca & Taraschi, 2015). Also, features of authoritative parenting (such as a combination of responsiveness, autonomy-granting, and demandingness) have been linked with stronger moral identity among adolescents (Rote & Smetana, 2015).

In Ross Thompson's (2014, 2015) view, young children are moral apprentices, striving to understand what is moral. They can be assisted in this quest by adult mentors in the home who communicate lessons about morality in everyday experiences. Among the most important aspects of the relationship between parents and children that contribute to children's moral development are relational quality, parental discipline, and proactive strategies to prevent child misbehavior.

Relational Quality   Parent-child relationships introduce children to the mutual obligations of close relationships (Thompson, 2014, 2015). Parents' obligations include engaging in positive caregiving and guiding children to become competent human beings. Children's obligations include responding appropriately to parents' initiatives and maintaining a positive relationship with parents.

In terms of relationship quality, secure attachment may play an important role in children's and adolescents' moral development. A secure attachment can place children on a positive path for internalizing parents' socializing goals and family values. In one longitudinal study, early secure attachment defused a maladaptive trajectory toward antisocial behavior (Kochanska & others, 2010). In another study, securely attached children's willing, cooperative stance was linked to positive future socialization outcomes such as a lower incidence of parent-child conflict, noncompliance, and aggressive behavior problems (Goffin, Boldt, & Kochanska, 2018).

Parental Discipline   Discipline techniques used by parents can be classified in a variety of ways, depending on the theory. One classic approach distinguishes three dimensions: love withdrawal, power assertion, and induction (Hoffman, 1988):

- **Love withdrawal** is a discipline technique in which a parent withholds attention or love from the child, as when the parent refuses to talk to the child or states a dislike for the child. For example, the parent might say, "I'm going to leave you if you do that again" or "I don't like you when you do that."
- **Power assertion** is a discipline technique in which a parent attempts to gain control over the child or the child's resources. Examples include spanking, threatening, or removing privileges.
- **Induction** is a discipline technique in which a parent uses reasoning and explains how the child's actions are likely to affect other people. Examples of induction include, "Don't hit him. He was only trying to help" and "Why are you yelling at her? She didn't mean to trip you."

Among these three discipline techniques, induction is the most likely to produce a moderate level of arousal in children, a level that permits them to attend to the explanations and rationale parents offer. Furthermore, induction focuses the child's attention on the action's consequences for others, not on the child's own potential shortcomings. In contrast, love withdrawal and power assertive discipline can be highly arousing and upsetting to the child and interfere with any explanations or rationale that the child might have received during the discipline episode. Thus, child developmentalists recommend induction over power assertion and love withdrawal in disciplining children. One illustrative study explored the role of inductive discipline in the moral development

> Both theory and empirical data support the conclusion that parents play an important role in children's moral development.
>
> **—Nancy Eisenberg**
> *Contemporary psychologist, Arizona State University*

love withdrawal A discipline technique in which a parent withholds attention or love from the child in an effort to control the child's behavior.

power assertion A discipline technique in which a parent attempts to gain control over the child or the child's resources.

induction A discipline technique in which a parent uses reasoning and explains how the child's actions are likely to affect others.

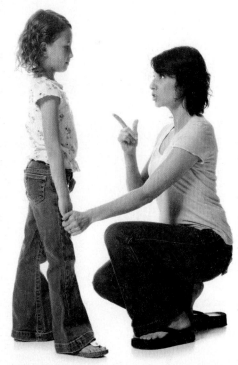

How are parents' discipline techniques linked to children's moral development? What are some proactive strategies parents can use to avert potential misbehavior by children before it happens?
Mike Kemp/Rubberball/Getty Images

Parenting Recommendations for Raising a Moral Child

A comprehensive and influential review of the research (Eisenberg & Valiente, 2002, p. 134) concluded that, in general, children who behave morally tend to have parents who:

- "are warm and supportive rather than punitive;
- use inductive discipline;
- provide opportunities for the children to learn about others' perspectives and feelings;
- involve children in family decision making and in the process of thinking about moral decisions;
- model moral behaviors and thinking themselves, and provide opportunities for their children to do so;
- provide information about what behaviors are expected and why; and
- foster an internal rather than an external sense of morality."

Parents who show this configuration of behaviors likely foster concern and caring about others in their children, and create a positive parent-child relationship. In addition, parenting recommendations based on Ross Thompson's (2014) analysis of parent-child relations suggest that children's conscience and moral development benefits when there are mutual parent-child obligations involving warmth and responsibility, and when

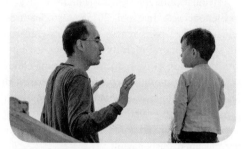

What are some good strategies parents can adopt to foster their child's moral development?
Anna Pekunova/Getty Images

parents use proactive strategies instead of punitive reactions, when disciplining for misbehavior.

One of the strategies above suggests modeling moral behaviors and thinking. According to the research cited in the Moral Exemplars section of this chapter, which two traits were common to moral exemplars?

of adolescents (Patrick & Gibbs, 2012). In this study, adolescents considered parental induction and expression of disappointed expectations as more appropriate than power assertion and love withdrawal and responded with more positive emotion, as well as guilt, to parental induction than to the other parenting techniques. Further, parental induction was linked to a higher moral identity among the youth. Nevertheless, if parents are using induction of guilt regularly or in an extreme way, it can be counterproductive for promoting moral development and behavior among children and adolescents (Rote & Smetana, 2017).

Proactive Strategies   An important parenting strategy is to proactively avert potential misbehavior by children before it takes place (Chang & others, 2015; Wainryb & Recchia, 2017). With younger children, being proactive means using diversion, such as distracting their attention or engaging them in alternative activities. With older children, being proactive may involve talking with them about values that the parents deem important, prior to a misbehavior taking place. Transmitting these values can help older children and adolescents to resist the temptations that inevitably emerge in contexts such as peer relations and the media that can be outside the scope of direct parental monitoring.

To read further about strategies parents can adopt to promote their children's moral development, see *Caring Connections*.

SCHOOLS

No matter how parents treat their children at home, they may feel that they have little control over a great deal of their children's moral education. This is because children and adolescents spend extensive time away from their parents at school, and the time spent in that environment can influence children's moral development (Berkowitz & others, 2006; Narváez & Lapsley, 2009; Nucci, 2014).

The Hidden Curriculum

Many years ago, educator John Dewey (1933) recognized that even when schools do not have specific programs in moral education, they provide moral education through a "hidden curriculum." The **hidden curriculum** is conveyed by the moral atmosphere that is a part of every school. The moral atmosphere is created by school and classroom rules, the moral orientation of teachers and school administrators, and text materials. Teachers serve as models of ethical or unethical behavior. Classroom rules and peer relations at school transmit attitudes about cheating, lying, stealing, and consideration for others. And by creating and enforcing rules and regulations, the school administration infuses the school with a value system.

Character Education

Yet another approach to moral education is **character education,** a direct education approach that involves teaching students a basic "moral literacy" to prevent them from engaging in immoral behavior and doing harm to themselves or others (Arthur & others, 2016). The argument is that behaviors such as lying, stealing, and cheating are wrong, and students should be taught this throughout their education (Berkowitz & others, 2006; Pattaro, 2016).

Every school should have an explicit moral code that is clearly communicated to students. Any violations of the code should be met with sanctions. Instruction in specified moral concepts, such as cheating, can take the form of example and definition, class discussions and role playing, or rewarding students for proper behavior. More recently, an emphasis on the importance of encouraging students to develop a care perspective has been accepted as a relevant aspect of character education. Rather than just instructing adolescents to refrain from engaging in morally deviant behavior, a care perspective advocates educating students in the importance of engaging in prosocial behaviors, such as considering others' feelings, being sensitive to others, and helping others through a semester-long course covering a number of moral issues. The hope is that students will develop more advanced notions of concepts such as cooperation, trust, responsibility, and community (McCarty & others, 2016). Currently, nearly 20 states have mandates to include character education in children's education, although there is no federal education guideline requiring it (O'Conner, Peterson, & Fluke, 2014).

Cognitive Moral Education

Another approach to moral education, **cognitive moral education,** is based on the belief that students should learn to value such things as democracy and justice as their moral reasoning develops. Kohlberg's theory has served as the foundation for a number of cognitive moral education programs. In a typical program, high school students meet in a semester-long course to discuss a number of moral issues. The instructor acts as a facilitator rather than as a director of the class. The hope is that students will develop more advanced notions of concepts such as cooperation, trust, responsibility, and community (Power & Higgins-D'Alessandro, 2008).

Service Learning

At the beginning of the chapter you read about Jewel Cash, who is strongly motivated to make a positive difference in her community. Jewel Cash has a sense of social responsibility that a number of educational programs seek to promote in students through **service learning,** a form of education that promotes social responsibility through service to the community. In service learning, adolescents engage in activities such as tutoring, helping older adults, working in a hospital, assisting at a child-care center, or cleaning up a vacant lot to make a play area. Much of the effort to get students involved in service learning is orchestrated through the Corporation for National and Community Service. Examples of large programs include Americorps and Senior Corps. For program descriptions and opportunities to volunteer, go to www.nationalservice.gov.

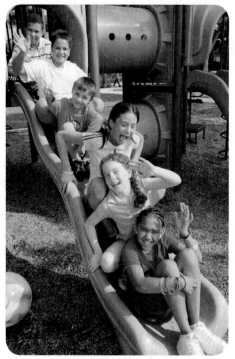

More than just about anything else, 12-year-old Katie Bell wanted a playground in her New Jersey town. She knew that other kids also wanted one, so she put together a group that generated fundraising ideas for the playground. They presented their ideas to the town council. Her group got more youth involved. They helped raise money by selling candy and sandwiches door-to-door. Katie says, "We learned to work as a community. This will be an important place for people to go and have picnics and make new friends." Katie's advice: "You won't get anywhere if you don't try."
Golden Pixels LLC/Alamy Stock Photo

hidden curriculum The pervasive moral atmosphere that characterizes each school.

character education A direct moral education approach that involves teaching students a basic "moral literacy" to prevent them from engaging in immoral behavior or doing harm to themselves or others.

cognitive moral education Education based on the belief that students should learn to value things like democracy and justice as their moral reasoning develops; Kohlberg's theory has been the basis for many of the cognitive moral education approaches.

service learning A form of education that promotes social responsibility and service to the community.

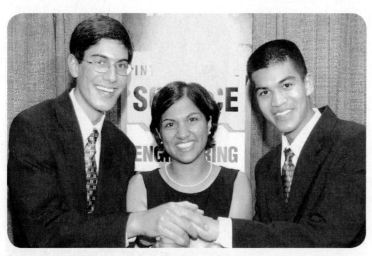

As an adolescent, Nina Vasan, MD (center) founded ACS Teens, a nationwide group of adolescent volunteers who supported the efforts of the American Cancer Society (ACS). Nina's organization raised hundreds of thousands of dollars for cancer research, helped change state tobacco laws, and conducted a number of cancer control programs. She created a national letter-writing campaign to obtain volunteers, established a website and set up an e-mail network, started a newsletter, and arranged monthly phone calls to communicate ideas and plan projects. Today, Nina is a psychiatrist and advocate for social change.

Feature Photo Service/Newscom

An important goal of service learning is to help adolescents become less self-centered and more strongly motivated to help others (Chung & McBride, 2015; Schmidt, Shumow, & Kackar, 2012). Service learning takes education out into the community. Adolescent volunteers tend to be extraverted, be committed to others, and have a high level of self-understanding (Eisenberg & others, 2009). Also, some research suggests there may be complex gender differences in adolescents' service learning and community service activities and what they take away from these experiences (Flanagan & others, 2015).

Researchers have found that service learning benefits adolescents in a number of ways (Hart & Wandeler, 2018). Improvements in adolescent development attributed to service learning include higher grades in school, increased goal-setting, higher self-esteem, an improved sense of empowerment to make a difference for others, and an increased likelihood of serving as volunteers in the future. A study of more than 4,000 high school students revealed that those who worked directly with individuals in need were better adjusted academically, while those who worked for organizations had better civic outcomes (Schmidt, Shumow, & Kackar, 2007). And in another study, 74 percent of African American and 70 percent of Latino adolescents said that service learning programs could have a "fairly or very big effect" on keeping students from dropping out of school (Bridgeland, Dilulio, & Wulsin, 2008).

Civic engagement might play a role in adolescents' identity and moral development (Malin, Ballard, & Damon, 2015). One study found that compared with adolescents who have a diffused identity status, those who were identity achieved were more involved in volunteering in their community (Crocetti, Jahromi, & Meeus, 2012). In this study, adolescents' volunteer activity also was linked to their values, such as social responsibility, and the view that they, along with others, could make an impact on their community. Another study of more than 5,000 adolescents in Chile showed distinct profiles reflecting different levels and types of subjective civic engagement. School programs had a major effect on adolescents' community engagement (Martínez & others, 2019).

The benefits of service learning, both for the volunteer and the recipient, suggest that more adolescents should be required to participate in such programs (Enfield & Collins, 2008). However, the most rigorously conducted longitudinal studies show that engagement must be voluntary and supported in adolescence for it to have lasting effects. Forcing teenagers to volunteer increases participation in the short term but has no lasting effects into adulthood (Henderson, Brown, & Pancer, 2019; Kim & Morgül, 2017).

Cheating A moral education concern is whether students cheat and how to handle the cheating if teachers discover it (Ramberg & Modin, 2019). Academic cheating can take many forms, including plagiarism, using "cheat sheets" during an exam, copying from a neighbor during a test, purchasing papers, and falsifying lab results. A foundational 2008 survey of almost 30,000 high school students in the United States revealed that 64 percent of the students said they had cheated on a test in school during the past year and 36 percent of the students reported that they had plagiarized information from the Internet for an assignment in the past year (Josephson Institute of Ethics, 2008). Over the past decade, evidence has mounted in many countries showing similarly concerning levels of academic dishonesty (Pan & others, 2019).

Why do students cheat? Among the reasons students give for cheating include pressure to get high grades, compressed schedules, poor teaching, and lack of interest. A growing body of international and cross-cultural research shows some consistent patterns: cheating is least likely among adolescents or young adults who are morally focused on honesty, believe that cheating is wrong, and have a sense of control over their decisions and actions (Chudzicka-Czupała & others, 2016).

The context affects whether or not students cheat (McCabe, 2016). For example, students are more likely to cheat when they are not being closely monitored during a test, when they know their peers are cheating, when they know whether another student has been caught cheating, and when student scores are made public. More broadly, the culture of the school has a major impact. A large study of high schoolers in Stockholm, Sweden, revealed that cheating was least common in schools that had a culture emphasizing fairness and honesty, and in which administrators and teachers were engaged with the students (Ramberg & Modin, 2019).

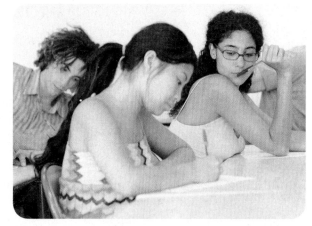

Why do students cheat? What are some strategies teachers can adopt to prevent cheating?
Eric Audras/PhotoAlto/Getty Images

Among the strategies for decreasing academic cheating are preventive measures such as making sure students are aware of what constitutes cheating and what the consequences will be if they cheat; closely monitoring students' behavior while they are taking tests; and emphasizing the importance of being a moral, responsible individual who engages in academic integrity. In promoting academic integrity, many colleges have instituted an honor code policy that emphasizes self-responsibility, fairness, trust, and scholarship. However, few secondary schools have developed honor code policies. The Center for Academic Integrity (www.academicintegrity.org/) has made extensive materials available to help schools develop academic integrity policies. To be most effective, Darcia Narváez (2010, 2018; Lee, 2018) emphasizes an *integrative approach* to moral education. This approach would encompass both the reflective moral thinking and commitment to justice advocated in Kohlberg's approach, and the process of developing a particular moral character emphasized in the character education approach.

Review *Connect* Reflect

LG2 Explain how parenting and schools influence moral development.

Review

- How does parental discipline affect moral development? What are some effective parenting strategies for advancing children's moral development?
- What is the hidden curriculum? What are some contemporary approaches to moral education?

Connect

- In this section, you learned that secure attachment in infancy was linked to early development of conscience. What characterizes secure attachment?

Reflect *Your Own Personal Journey of Life*

- What type of discipline did your parents use with you? What effect do you think this approach has had on your moral development?

Prosocial and Antisocial Behavior

LG3 Describe the development of prosocial and antisocial behavior.

Prosocial Behavior

Antisocial Behavior

Service learning encourages positive moral behavior. This behavior is not just moral behavior but behavior that is intended to benefit other people, and psychologists call it *prosocial behavior* (Caprara & others, 2015; Eisenberg, Spinrad, & Sadovsky, 2014). Jewel Cash, whose story was introduced at the beginning of the chapter, is an exemplary model of someone committed to prosocial behavior. Of course, people have always engaged in antisocial behavior as well. In this section, we will take a closer look at prosocial and antisocial behavior, focusing on how each type of behavior develops.

We only have what we give.

ISABEL ALLENDE
Chilean author, 20th to 21st century

PROSOCIAL BEHAVIOR

Caring about the welfare and rights of others, feeling concern and empathy for them, and acting in a way that benefits others are all components of prosocial behavior. The purest forms of prosocial behavior are motivated by **altruism,** an unselfish interest in helping another person (Dahl & Brownell, 2019). As we see next, learning to share is an important aspect of prosocial behavior.

altruism An unselfish interest in helping another person.

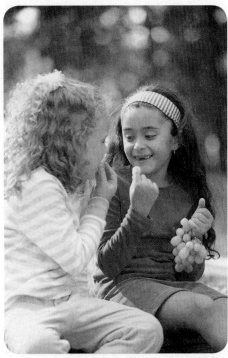

How does children's sharing change from the preschool to the elementary school years?
Ariel Skelley/age fotostock

William Damon (1988) once described a developmental sequence by which sharing develops in children. Most sharing during the first three years of life is done for non-empathic reasons, such as for the fun of the social play ritual or out of imitation. Then, at about 4 years of age, a combination of empathic awareness and adult encouragement produces a sense of obligation on the part of the child to share with others. Most 4-year-olds are not selfless saints, however. Children believe they have an obligation to share but do not necessarily think they should be as generous to others as they are to themselves. Neither do their actions always support their beliefs, especially when they covet an object. What is important developmentally is that the child has developed a belief that sharing is an obligatory part of a social relationship and involves a question of right and wrong. These early ideas about sharing set the stage for giant strides that children make in the years that follow. An extensive body of research in many diverse cultures indicates fairly similar patterns of development in early childhood (Callaghan & Corbit, 2018).

By the start of the elementary school years, children begin to express more complicated notions of what is fair. Throughout history, varied definitions of fairness have been used as the basis for distributing goods and resolving conflicts. These definitions involve the principles of equality, merit, and benevolence: *Equality* means that everyone is treated the same; *merit* means giving extra rewards for hard work, skillful performance, or other laudatory behavior; *benevolence* means giving special consideration to individuals in a disadvantaged condition.

Equality is the first of these principles used regularly by elementary school children. It is common to hear 6-year-old children use the word *fair* as synonymous with *equal* or *same.* By the middle to late elementary school years, children also believe that equity means special treatment for those who deserve it—a belief that applies the principles of merit and benevolence. Extensive cross-cultural observations and analyses have revealed consistent patterns across cultures. However, there are also important differences in the age at which these shifts occur, based on the degree to which the culture values individualism or collectivism (Huppert & others, 2019).

Parental advice and prodding certainly foster standards of sharing, but the give-and-take of peer requests and arguments provide the most immediate stimulation of sharing. Parents can set examples that children carry into their interactions and communication with peers, but parents are not present during all of their children's peer exchanges. The day-to-day construction of fairness standards is often done by children in collaboration and negotiation with each other. One study found that authoritative parenting by mothers, but not fathers, contributed to adolescents' subsequent engagement in prosocial behavior one year later (Padilla-Walker & others, 2012). Other research also suggests that mothers are more likely to influence adolescents' prosocial behavior than are fathers (Carlo & others, 2011).

How does prosocial behavior change through childhood and adolescence? Prosocial behavior occurs more often in adolescence than in childhood, although examples of caring for others and comforting someone in distress occur even during the preschool years (Ball, Smetana, & Sturge-Apple, 2017). One study of 5- to 13-year-olds found that with increasing age children attribute more positive emotions to people who sacrifice their own desires to help others who are needy; they also become more aware of situations that call for altruistic action (Weller & Lagattuta, 2013). Also, keep in mind gender differences in prosocial behavior. Females view themselves as more prosocial and empathic, and they also engage in more prosocial behavior than males (Van der Graaff & others, 2018).

Are there different types of prosocial behavior? Gustavo Carlo and his colleagues (2010) explored this topic and confirmed the presence of six types of prosocial behavior in young adolescents in Mexican American and European American families:

- altruism ("One of the best things about doing charity work is that it looks good.")
- public ("Helping others while I'm being watched is when I work best.")
- emotional ("I usually help others when they are very upset.")
- dire ("I tend to help people who are hurt badly.")
- anonymous ("I prefer to donate money without anyone knowing.")
- compliant ("I never wait to help others when they ask for it.")

In this study, adolescent girls reported more emotional, dire, compliant, and altruistic behavior than did boys, while boys engaged in more public prosocial behavior. Parental monitoring was positively related to emotional, dire, and compliant behavior but not to the other types of behavior. Compliant, anonymous, and altruistic prosocial behavior were positively related to religiosity.

Most research on prosocial behavior depicts the concept in a global and unidimensional manner. Studies conducted by Carlo and colleagues, as well as by other researchers, illustrate the important point that in thinking about and studying prosocial behavior, it is important to consider multiple dimensions (Mesurado, Richaud, & Rodriguez, 2018). Two other important aspects of prosocial behavior are forgiveness and gratitude. **Forgiveness** is an aspect of prosocial behavior that occurs when the injured person releases the injurer from possible behavioral retaliation. An overview of the research literature on development of forgiveness showed that a number of factors are involved, including personal characteristics and peer and family influences (van der Wal, Karremans, & Cillessen, 2017). One study revealed that when adolescents encountered hurtful experiences in school settings if they disliked the transgressor they had more hostile thoughts, feelings of anger, and avoidance/revenge tendencies than when they liked the transgressing peer (Peets, Hodges, & Salmivalli, 2013).

Gratitude is a feeling of thankfulness and appreciation, especially in response to someone doing something kind or helpful (Tudge & Frietas, 2018). Interest in studying adolescents' gratitude or lack thereof is increasing. Consider the following evidence:

- Gratitude is linked to a number of positive aspects of development in young adolescents, including satisfaction with one's family, optimism, and prosocial behavior (Bausert & others, 2018).
- Adolescents' expression of gratitude is linked to having fewer depressive and anxious symptoms (Rey, Sánchez-Álvarez, & Extremera, 2018).
- Chinese adolescents who have a higher level of gratitude may be less likely to engage in suicidal ideation and suicide attempts (Li & others, 2012).
- A longitudinal study assessed the gratitude of adolescents from middle to high school in the United States (Bono & others, 2019). Across this period of adolescent development, growth in gratitude was both a predictor of, and an outcome of, decreases in antisocial behavior and increases in prosocial behavior. These links were explained, in part, by improvements in overall life satisfaction that were associated with growth in gratitude.

Compared with antisocial behavior such as juvenile delinquency (described in detail next), less attention has been given to research on prosocial behavior in adolescence. Although the research literature is growing, we still do not have adequate research information about such topics as how youth perceive prosocial norms and how school policies and peers influence prosocial behavior (Dijkstra & Gest, 2015).

ANTISOCIAL BEHAVIOR

Most children and adolescents at one time or another "act out" or do things that are destructive or troublesome for themselves or others. If these behaviors occur often, clinical psychologists and psychiatrists diagnose them as conduct disorders. If these behaviors result in

forgiveness An aspect of prosocial behavior that occurs when an injured person releases the injurer from possible behavioral retaliation.

gratitude A feeling of thankfulness and appreciation, especially in response to someone doing something kind or helpful.

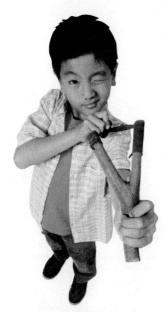

What are some characteristics of conduct disorder?
Stockdisc/Getty Images

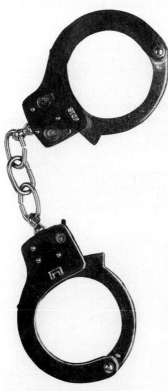

Comstock Images/Alamy Stock Photo

conduct disorder Age-inappropriate actions and attitudes that violate family expectations, society's norms, and the personal or property rights of others.

juvenile delinquency Refers to a great variety of behaviors by an adolescent, ranging from unacceptable behavior to breaking the law.

index offenses Criminal acts, such as robbery, rape, and homicide, whether they are committed by juveniles or adults.

illegal acts by juveniles, society labels them delinquents; if these behaviors continue or escalate into adulthood, they cross the line into being considered criminals. Antisocial behavior problems are more common in males than in females (Choy & others, 2017).

Conduct Disorder   **Conduct disorder** refers to age-inappropriate actions and attitudes that violate family expectations, society's norms, and the personal or property rights of others. Children with conduct problems show a wide range of rule-violating behaviors, from swearing and temper tantrums to severe vandalism, theft, and assault (Freitag & others, 2018). Conduct disorder is much more common among boys than girls (Mohan & Ray, 2019).

An estimated 5 percent of children show serious conduct problems. These children are often described as showing an *externalizing,* or *undercontrolled,* pattern of behavior. Children who show this pattern often are impulsive, overactive, and aggressive and engage in delinquent actions.

Conduct problems in children are best explained by a confluence of causes, or risk factors, operating over time (Thio, Taylor, & Schwartz, 2018). These include possible genetic inheritance of a difficult temperament, ineffective parenting, living in a neighborhood where violence is common, and ineffective schools. A comprehensive meta-analysis of studies revealed that young adolescents' school connectedness or "belonging" serves as a protective factor against growth in adolescent conduct problems (Allen & others, 2018).

Despite considerable efforts to help children with conduct problems, effective treatment is challenging and requires addressing multiple individual, family, and peer factors to reduce exposure to the causes of the antisocial behaviors (Mohan & Ray, 2019). Sometimes recommended is a multisystem treatment carried out with all family members, school personnel, juvenile justice staff, and other individuals in the child's life.

Juvenile Delinquency   What is a juvenile delinquent? What are the antecedents of delinquency? What types of interventions have been used to prevent or reduce delinquency?

What Is Juvenile Delinquency?   The term **juvenile delinquency** refers to a broad range of behaviors, from socially unacceptable behavior (such as acting out in school) to status offenses (such as running away) to criminal acts (such as burglary) (Mallett & Tedor, 2019). For legal purposes, a distinction is made between index offenses and status offenses:

- **Index offenses** are criminal acts regardless of whether they are committed by juveniles or adults. They include acts such as robbery, aggravated assault, rape, and homicide.
- **Status offenses,** such as running away, truancy, underage drinking, sexual promiscuity, and uncontrollability, are less serious acts. They are performed by youth under a specified age, which classifies them as juvenile offenses.

One issue in juvenile justice is whether an adolescent who commits a crime should be tried as an adult. Some psychologists have proposed that individuals 12 and under should not be evaluated under adult criminal laws and that those 17 and older should be (Steinberg, 2009). They also recommend that individuals 13 to 16 years of age be given some type of individualized assessment in terms of whether they ought to be tried in a juvenile court or an adult criminal court. This framework argues strongly against court placement based solely on the nature of an offense and takes into account the offender's developmental maturity. Note that it was not until 2005 (in *Roper vs. Simmons*), that the U.S. Supreme Court ruled that juveniles cannot be executed. Internationally, the vast majority of countries have signed onto the United Nation's International Covenant on Civil and Political Rights (ICCPR), which bans execution of minors. Enforcement of this standard varies widely across countries, however (DPIC, 2019).

Juvenile court delinquency caseloads in the United States increased dramatically from 1960 to 1996 and then decreased dramatically through 2016 (see Figure 4) (Hockenberry, 2019). Note that this figure does not include those who were arrested but not assigned to caseloads, or those who committed offenses but were not caught.

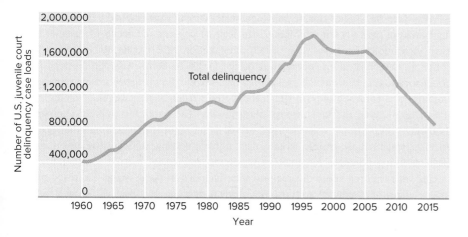

FIGURE **4**

INCREASE IN U.S. JUVENILE COURT DELINQUENCY CASELOADS FROM 1960 TO 2016

Source: Hockenberry, S. (March, 2019). Juvenile justice statistics: National report series fact sheet. Washington DC: US Department of Justice. https://www.ojjdp.gov/pubs/252473.pdf.

Males are more likely to engage in delinquency than are females (Thio, Taylor, & Schwartz, 2018). However, U.S. government statistics revealed that the percentage of delinquency caseloads involving females increased from 19 percent in 1985 to 27 percent in 2005, but then decreased at the same rate as males through 2016 (Hockenberry, 2019).

As adolescents reach adulthood, do their rates of delinquency and crime change? Recent analyses indicate that theft, property damage, and physical aggression peak at 18 years. The peak for property damage is 16 to 18 years of age for males, and 15 to 17 years of age for females. However, the peak for violence is 18 to 19 years of age for males and 19 to 21 years of age for females (Farrington, 2009; Hockenberry, 2019).

A distinction is made between early-onset (before age 11) and late-onset (11 and older) antisocial behavior. Early-onset antisocial behavior is associated with more negative developmental outcomes than late-onset antisocial behavior. Early-onset antisocial behavior is more likely to persist into emerging adulthood and is associated with increased problems involving mental health and relationships (McGee & Moffitt, 2019).

Predictors of Juvenile Delinquency Predictors of delinquency include conflict with authority, minor secretive acts that are followed by property damage and other more serious acts; minor aggression followed by fighting and violence; a negative sense of self and identity; poor self-control; self-centered cognitions; starting younger; being male; having low expectations for education; poor school performance in earlier grades; having delinquent peers and older siblings; belonging to a lower-socioeconomic-status family; exposure to harsh, ineffective, and unengaged parenting; and living in a high-crime urban neighborhood.

Family support systems are also associated with increasing or decreasing levels of adolescent delinquency (Farrington, 2009; Nkuba, Hermenau, & Hecker, 2019). Parental monitoring of adolescents is especially important in determining whether an adolescent becomes a delinquent. For example, a large international longitudinal study of young adolescents in low- and middle-income countries (for example, Colombia, the Philippines, Kenya) found that low levels of monitoring, along with harsh rejecting parenting, played a key role in linking exposure to dangerous and chaotic homes and neighborhoods to growth in delinquent behavior problems (Deater-Deckard & others, 2019). Another illustrative study found that early parental monitoring in adolescence and ongoing parental support were linked to a lower incidence of criminal behavior in emerging adulthood (Johnson & others, 2011). A comprehensive review of the international literature showed that authoritative parenting (warm but firm, with limit setting) was most effective at deterring delinquent behavior, in part because of its impact on adolescents' interpretation of this type of parenting as an indicator of adults' legitimate authority (Ruiz-Hernández & others, 2019).

A growing research base indicates that family therapy is often effective in reducing delinquency (Henderson, Hogue, & Dauber, 2019). A meta-analysis found that of five program types (case management, individual treatment, youth court, restorative justice, and family treatment), family treatment was the only one that was linked to a reduction in repeated offending (recidivism) for juvenile offenders (Schwalbe & others, 2012).

status offenses Juvenile offenses, performed by youth under a specified age, that are not as serious as index offenses. These offenses may include acts such as underage drinking, truancy, and sexual promiscuity.

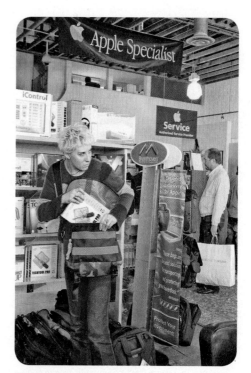

What are some factors that influence whether adolescents will become delinquents?
Bill Aron/PhotoEdit

developmental **connection**

Parenting

A neglectful parenting style is linked with a low level of self-control in children. Connect to "Families."

Rare are the studies that actually demonstrate in an experimental design that changing parenting practices in childhood can lead to a lower incidence of juvenile delinquency in adolescence. However, family intervention experiments are becoming more common. One illustration (Forgatch & others, 2009) randomly assigned divorced mothers of sons to an experimental group (in which the mothers received extensive parenting training) or a control group (in which the mothers received no parenting training) when their sons were in the first through third grades. The parenting training consisted of 14 parent group meetings that focused primarily on improving parenting practices (skill encouragement, limit setting, monitoring, problem solving, and positive involvement). Best parenting practices for emotion regulation, managing interparental conflict, and talking with children about divorce also were included in the sessions. Improved parenting practices and reduced contact with deviant peers were linked with lower rates of delinquency in the experimental group compared with the control group at a 9-year follow-up assessment.

An increasing number of studies have found that siblings can have a strong influence on delinquency. In the largest and longest-running longitudinal study on this topic, having an older sibling who engaged in delinquent behavior was predictive of the target adolescent's growth in delinquent behavior, even after controlling for other competing predictors (Huijsmans & others, 2018).

An even larger body of research studies has shown that having delinquent peers increases the risk of becoming delinquent. For example, researchers found that peer rejection and having delinquent friends at 7 to 13 years of age were linked with increased delinquency at 14 to 15 years of age (Vitaro, Pedersen, & Brendgen, 2007). An exhaustive review of this and other studies, involving low- to high-SES families and youth of various races and ethnicities, reported that having peers who exhibit these behaviors is a consistent and powerful predictor, especially for males (McCoy & others, 2019).

Although delinquency can occur at all levels of family and neighborhood socioeconomic status, some characteristics of lower-SES settings appear to be particularly influential in promoting delinquency. The norms of many low-SES peer groups and gangs are antisocial, or counterproductive to the goals and norms of society at large. Getting into and staying out of trouble are prominent features of life for some adolescents in low-income neighborhoods. Adolescents from low-income backgrounds may sense that they can gain attention and status by performing antisocial actions. Being "tough" and

connecting with careers

Rodney Hammond, Health Psychologist

In describing his college experiences, Rodney Hammond recalls, "When I started as an undergraduate at the University of Illinois at Champaign-Urbana, I hadn't decided on my major. But to help finance my education, I took a part-time job in a child development research program sponsored by the psychology department. There, I observed inner-city children in settings designed to enhance their learning. I saw firsthand the contribution psychology can make, and I knew I wanted to be a psychologist" (American Psychological Association, 2003, p. 26).

Rodney Hammond went on to obtain a doctorate in school and community psychology with a focus on children's development. For a number of years, he trained clinical psychologists at Wright State University in Ohio and directed a program to reduce violence in ethnic minority youth. There, he and his associates taught at-risk youth how to use social skills to effectively manage conflict and to recognize situations that could lead to violence. For nearly two decades, Hammond has served as Director of Violence Prevention at the Centers for Disease Control and Prevention in Atlanta. Hammond's career shows that if you are interested in people and problem solving, psychology is a wonderful way to put these together.

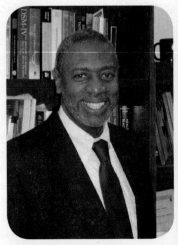

Rodney Hammond.
Courtesy of Rodney Hammond

"masculine" are high-status traits for low-SES boys, and these traits are often measured by the adolescent's success in performing and getting away with delinquent acts. One study revealed that engaged parenting and mothers' social network support were linked to a lower level of delinquency in low-income families (Ghazarian & Roche, 2010). A summary of the literature indicates that chronic poverty in particular is a robust predictor of growth in delinquency, in part due to its harmful effects on parenting and family environments, including increased levels of stress (Wadsworth & others, 2016).

The nature of a community can contribute to delinquency (Howell & Griffiths, 2019). A community with a high crime rate allows adolescents to observe many models who engage in criminal activities and might be rewarded for their criminal accomplishments. Such communities often are characterized by poverty, unemployment, and feelings of alienation. Poor-quality schools, lack of funding for education, and the absence of organized neighborhood activities are other community factors that might be related to delinquency. Turning to school settings, lack of academic success also is associated with delinquency. A thorough review of the research indicates that early patterns of academic failure and resulting disengagement from learning predict higher levels of delinquent behavior. These effects can be worse in school contexts that are punitive and remove troubled adolescents from school environments (Hirschfield, 2018).

Cognitive factors such as low self-control, low intelligence, and lack of sustained attention also are implicated in delinquency. For example, data from the long-running Adolescent to Adult Health (Add Health) longitudinal study in the United States has shown that low levels of self-control not only predict growth in delinquency across adolescence but also persist with criminal and antisocial behavior into adulthood (Bekbolatkyzy & others, 2019). A different study that followed more than a thousand children with documented maltreatment histories found that having lower intelligence and executive function increased the odds that individuals would commit delinquent and criminal acts in adolescence and adulthood (Nikulina & Widom, 2019).

One individual whose personal and career goal has been to reduce juvenile delinquency and help adolescents cope more effectively with the challenges in their lives is Rodney Hammond. To read about his work, see *Connecting with Careers*. Next, read *Connecting Through Research* to find out whether intervening in the lives of children who show early conduct problems can reduce their delinquency risk in adolescence.

connecting through research

Can Intervention in Childhood Reduce Delinquency in Adolescence?

Fast Track is an intervention that attempts to reduce the incidence of juvenile delinquency and other problems (Conduct Problems Prevention Research Group, 2011, 2013). Schools in four areas (Durham, North Carolina; Nashville, Tennessee; Seattle, Washington; and rural central Pennsylvania) were identified as high-risk based on neighborhood crime and poverty data. Researchers screened more than 9,000 kindergarten children in the four schools and randomly assigned 891 of the highest-risk and moderate–risk children to intervention or control conditions. The average age of the children when the intervention began was 6.5 years of age. The 10-year intervention consisted of behavior management training of parents, social cognitive skills training of children, reading tutoring, home visitations, mentoring, and a revised classroom curriculum that was designed to increase socioemotional competence and decrease aggression.

The extensive intervention was most successful for children and adolescents who were identified as the highest risk in kindergarten, lowering their incidence of conduct disorder, attention deficit hyperactivity disorder, any externalized disorder, and antisocial behavior. Positive outcomes for the intervention occurred as early as the third grade and continued through the ninth grade. For example, in the ninth grade the intervention reduced the likelihood that the highest-risk kindergarten children would develop conduct disorder by 75 percent, attention deficit hyperactivity disorder by 53 percent, and any externalized disorder by 43 percent. The longest follow-up evidence (up to age 25 years) indicates that the comprehensive Fast Track intervention was successful in reducing rates of arrests, criminal convictions, and psychiatric disorder diagnoses (Dodge & others, 2015). Most of the effects appear to be due to positive effects of the intervention on children's and adolescents' social skills and self-regulation capabilities (Sorensen & others, 2016).

Review Connect Reflect

 LG3 Describe the development of prosocial and antisocial behavior.

Review

- How is altruism defined? How does prosocial behavior develop?
- What is juvenile delinquency? What is conduct disorder? What are key factors in the development of juvenile delinquency?

Connect

- In this section, you learned that being "tough" and "masculine" are high-status traits for low-SES boys and that this can lead to delinquent acts. What are some ways that masculine traits might lead to increases in delinquency across adolescence?

Reflect *Your Own Personal Journey of Life*

- Did you commit acts of delinquency as an adolescent? Most adolescents commit one or more acts of juvenile delinquency without becoming habitual juvenile delinquents. Reflect on your experiences of either committing juvenile offenses or not committing them, then review the discussion of factors that are likely causes of juvenile delinquency and apply them to your development.

Religious and Spiritual Development

 LG4 Summarize the nature of children's and adolescents' religious and spiritual development.

Childhood

Adolescence

> Irrespective of whether we are believers or agnostics, whether we believe in God or karma, moral ethics is a code which everyone is able to pursue.
>
> **DALAI LAMA XIV**
> *Contemporary holy spiritual leader of Buddhism, Tibet*

Can religion, religiousness, and spirituality be differentiated? Analysis of theory and prior research studies has been conducted by Pamela King and her colleagues (King, Ramos, & Clardy, 2012; King & others, 2017). They make the following distinctions:

- **Religion** is an organized set of beliefs, practices, rituals, and symbols that increases an individual's connection to a sacred or transcendent other (God, higher power, or ultimate truth).
- **Religiousness** refers to the degree of affiliation with an organized religion, participation in its prescribed rituals and practices, connection with its beliefs, and involvement in a community of believers.
- **Spirituality** involves experiencing something beyond oneself in a transcendent manner and living in a way that benefits others and society.

CHILDHOOD

How do parents influence children's religious thought and behavior? Societies use many methods—such as religious schools, parochial education, and parental teaching—to ensure that people will carry on a religious tradition. In the United States, about two-thirds of adults who profess a belief in God or Gods also are parents of children or teenagers; many participate in religious practices and education experiences on a regular basis (Pew Research Center, 2019). Does this religious socialization work? In many cases it does, and children usually adopt the religious beliefs of their parents. One study revealed that parents' religiousness assessed during youths' adolescence was positively related to youths' own religiousness during adolescence, which in turn was linked to their religiousness following the transition to adulthood (Spilman & others, 2013). The largest study to date examined over 40,000 individuals raised in two-parent families in 37 countries and showed that religious beliefs and participation were most prevalent for those who had experienced their religion in childhood; the effect was weaker if only one of the parents was observant (McPhail, 2019).

religion An organized set of beliefs, practices, rituals, and symbols that increases an individual's connection to a sacred or transcendent other (God, higher power, or higher truth).

religiousness The degree of affiliation with an organized religion, participation in prescribed rituals and practices, connection with its beliefs, and involvement in a community of believers.

spirituality Experiencing something beyond oneself in a transcendent manner and living in a way that benefits others and society.

ADOLESCENCE

Religious issues are important to many adolescents and emerging adults around the globe (King & others, 2017; Sugimura & others, 2019). However, in the twenty-first century, a decrease in religious interest among millennials has occurred. In the United States, by 2015 there was about a 15 percent difference in religious service participation between middle-aged adults and young adults, and this gap continues to grow. However, there are vast differences between regions of the world, with religious participation across generations remaining high in equatorial and southern-hemisphere countries (Pew Research Center, 2018).

One illustrative longitudinal study revealed that religiousness declined among adolescents between age 14 and age 20 in the United States (Koenig, McGue, & Iacono, 2008) (see Figure 5). In this study, religiousness was assessed with items such as frequency of prayer, frequency of discussing religious teachings, frequency of deciding moral actions for religious reasons, and the overall importance of religion in everyday life. As indicated in Figure 5, a greater change in religiousness occurred from 14 to 18 years of age than from 20 to 25 years of age. Also, reported frequency of attending religious services was highest at 14 years of age, declining from 14 to 18 years of age and increasing at 20 years of age. More change occurred in attending religious services than in religiousness.

Researchers have found that in Australia and New Zealand, China, the southern tip of Africa, much of Europe, and nearly all of South and North America, females are more religious than males—a difference that emerges in adolescence (Pew Research Center, 2016). When it comes to regularity of attendance in religious services, however, clear distinctions arise. In predominantly Muslim or Jewish countries, males attend more regularly; in predominantly Christian countries, females attend more often (Pew Research Center, 2016). Much less is known about gender and age differences in religious participation in Buddhist and Hindu areas of the globe.

Further analysis of the factors that can influence religiosity among youth and adults points to factors that include poverty, health risks, and life expectancy. The Pew Research Center (2018) data indicate that a baby born in 2015 in Nigeria (where 89 percent are religiously affiliated) has a life expectancy of 52 years, while a baby born the same year in Denmark (where only about 5 percent are affiliated) has a life expectancy of 81 years.

Religion and Cognitive Development Adolescence and emerging adulthood can be especially important developmental periods in religious identity and behavior (Good & Willoughby, 2008; Lerner, Roeser, & Phelps, 2009). Even if children have been indoctrinated into a religion by their parents, because of advances in their cognitive development adolescents and emerging adults may question what their own religious beliefs truly are.

Many of the cognitive changes thought to influence religious development involve Piaget's stages of cognitive development. More so than in childhood, adolescents think abstractly, idealistically, and logically. The increase in abstract thinking lets adolescents consider various ideas about religious and spiritual concepts. For example, an adolescent might ask how a loving God can possibly exist given the extensive suffering of many people in the world. Adolescents' increasingly idealistic thinking provides a foundation for questioning whether religion provides the best route to a better, more ideal world. And adolescents' increased logical reasoning gives them the ability to develop hypotheses and systematically sort through different answers to spiritual questions (Good & Willoughby, 2008).

Religion and Identity Development During adolescence and especially emerging adulthood, identity development becomes a central focus (Erikson, 1968; Schwartz & others, 2015). Adolescents and emerging adults are looking for answers to questions such as "Who am I?" "What am I all about as a person?" "What kind of life do I want to lead?" As part of their search for identity, adolescents and emerging adults begin to grapple in more sophisticated, logical ways with questions such as "Why am I on this planet?" "Is there really a God or higher spiritual being, or have I just been believing what my parents and culture embedded in my mind?" "What are my own religious views?" It is during the transition to adulthood that these questions begin to get answered as individuals become more autonomous and their identities solidify.

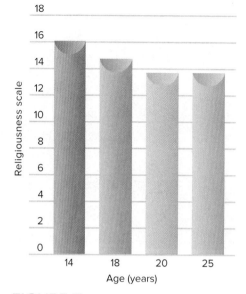

FIGURE 5

DEVELOPMENTAL CHANGES IN RELIGIOUSNESS FROM 14 TO 25 YEARS OF AGE. *Note:* The religiousness scale ranged from 0 to 32, with higher scores indicating stronger religiousness.

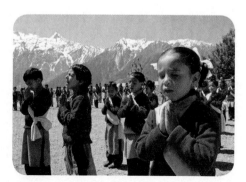

What are some cognitive developmental changes that could influence religious development?
Eitan Simanor/Photodisc/Getty Images

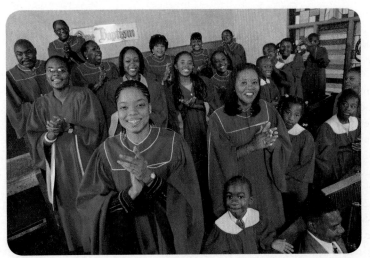

Adolescents participating in a church choir. *What are some positive aspects of religion in adolescents' lives?*
Digital Vision/Getty Images

The Positive Role of Religion in Adolescents' Lives

Researchers have found that various aspects of religion are linked with positive outcomes for adolescents and adults alike (Chen & VanderWeele, 2018; Harakeh & others, 2012). One study revealed that women in late adolescence who had been exposed to maltreatment when they were children had higher self-esteem and better interpersonal relationships if they held views of God as benevolent rather than punishing (Waldron, Scarpa, & Kim-Spoon, 2018).

Religion also plays a role in adolescents' health and well-being, influencing the degree to which they experience troubled emotions or engage in problem behaviors (Eskin & others, 2019). In a national random sample of more than 17,000 12- to 17-year-olds, those who believed their religious views influenced their thinking and the lives of their friends in positive ways were less likely to experience major depressive disorder (King, Topalian, & Vidourek, 2019).

A meta-analysis found that spirituality/religiosity was positively related to well-being, self-esteem, and three of the Big Five factors of personality (conscientiousness, agreeableness, openness) (Yonker, Schnabelrauch, & DeHaan, 2012). In this meta-analysis, spirituality/-religion was negatively associated with risky behavior and depression.

Review Connect Reflect

LG4 Summarize the nature of children's and adolescents' religious and spiritual development.

Review

- How does religious and spiritual interest and understanding develop in childhood?
- What characterizes religious and spiritual development in adolescence?

Connect

- In this section, you learned that many of the cognitive changes thought to influence adolescents' religious development reflect Piaget's stages of cognitive development. What is the adolescent stage of Piaget's theory called, and what else characterizes it?

Reflect *Your Own Personal Journey of Life*

- Reflect on your religious/spiritual upbringing. How have your religious/spiritual views changed or stayed the same as you developed through childhood and adolescence? Have your religious/spiritual views changed since adolescence? Explain.

---

reach your **learning goals**

Moral Development

Domains of Moral Development

What Is Moral Development?

Moral Thought

LG1 Discuss theory and research on the four domains of moral development.

- Moral development involves changes in thoughts, feelings, and behaviors regarding right and wrong. Moral development includes intrapersonal and interpersonal dimensions.

- Piaget distinguished between the heteronomous morality of younger children and the autonomous morality of older children. Kohlberg developed a provocative theory of moral reasoning. He argued that development of moral reasoning consists of three levels—preconventional, conventional, and postconventional—and six stages (two at each level). Kohlberg reasoned that these stages were age related. Influences on the Kohlberg stages include cognitive development, dealing with moral questions and moral conflict, peer relations, and perspective taking. Criticisms of Kohlberg's theory have been made, especially by Gilligan, who advocates a stronger care perspective. Other criticisms focus on the inadequacy of moral reasoning to predict moral behavior, to account for the influences of culture and family, and to assess moral reasoning.

| Moral Behavior |

- The processes of reinforcement, punishment, and imitation have been used to explain the acquisition of moral behavior, but they provide only a partial explanation. Situational variability is stressed by behaviorists. Social cognitive theory emphasizes a distinction between moral competence and moral performance.

| Moral Feeling |

- According to some theorists, guilt is the foundation of children's moral behavior. Empathy is an important aspect of moral feelings, and it changes developmentally. In the contemporary perspective, both positive and negative feelings contribute to moral development.

| Moral Personality |

- Recently, there has been a surge of interest in studying moral personality. This interest has focused on moral identity, moral character, and moral exemplars. Moral character involves having strong convictions; persisting; overcoming distractions and obstacles; and having virtues such as honesty, truthfulness, loyalty, and compassion. Moral exemplars have a moral character, identity, personality, and a set of virtues reflecting excellence and commitment; they are honest and dependable.

| Social-Cognitive Domain Theory |

- Social-cognitive domain theory states that there are different domains of social knowledge and reasoning, including moral, social conventional, and personal domains.

Contexts of Moral Development

 Explain how parenting and schools influence moral development.

| Parenting |

- Warmth and responsibility in mutual obligations of parent-child relationships provide important foundations for the child's positive moral growth. Love withdrawal, power assertion, and induction are discipline techniques. Induction is most likely to be linked with positive moral development. Moral development can be advanced by parenting strategies such as being warm and supportive rather than punitive; using inductive discipline; providing opportunities to learn about others' perspectives and feelings; involving children in family decision making; modeling moral behaviors; and averting misbehavior before it takes place.

| Schools |

- The hidden curriculum, initially described by Dewey, is the moral atmosphere of each school. Contemporary approaches to moral education include character education, cognitive moral education, service learning, and integrative ethical education. Cheating is a moral education concern that can take many forms. Various aspects of the school situation influence whether students will cheat or not.

Prosocial and Antisocial Behavior

 Describe the development of prosocial and antisocial behavior.

| Prosocial Behavior |

- An important aspect of prosocial behavior is altruism, an unselfish interest in helping others. Damon described a sequence by which children develop their understanding of fairness and become willing to share more consistently. Peers play a key role in this development. Forgiveness and gratitude are two additional aspects of prosocial behavior.

| Antisocial Behavior |

- Conduct disorder is a psychiatric diagnostic category used to describe multiple delinquent-type behaviors occurring over a six-month period. Juvenile delinquency consists of a broad range of behaviors, from socially undesirable behavior to status offenses. For legal purposes, a distinction is made between index and status offenses. Predictors of juvenile delinquency include authority conflict, minor covert acts such as lying, overt acts of aggression, a negative identity, cognitive distortions, low self-control, early initiation of delinquency, being a male, low expectations for education and school grades, low parental monitoring, low parental support and ineffective discipline, having an older delinquent sibling, heavy peer influence and low resistance to peers, low socioeconomic status, and living in a high-crime, urban area. Effective juvenile delinquency prevention and intervention programs have been identified.

Religious and Spiritual Development   Summarize the nature of children's and adolescents' religious and spiritual development.

- Childhood
- Adolescence

- Many children and adolescents show an interest in religion. Many children adopt their parents' religious beliefs.

- The twenty-first century has shown a downturn in adolescents' religious interest. Emerging adults from less-developed countries are more likely to be religious than those from more-developed countries. Cognitive changes in adolescence—such as increases in abstract, idealistic, and logical thinking—increase the likelihood that adolescents will seek a better understanding of religion and spirituality. As part of their search for identity, many adolescents and emerging adults begin to grapple with more complex aspects of religion. Various aspects of religion are linked with positive outcomes in adolescent development.

key **terms**

altruism 368
autonomous morality 352
care perspective 357
character education 365
cognitive moral education 365
conduct disorder 370
conventional reasoning 353
empathy 359
forgiveness 369

gratitude 369
heteronomous morality
  (Piaget) 352
hidden curriculum 365
immanent justice 352
index offenses 370
induction 363
justice perspective 357
juvenile delinquency 370

love withdrawal 363
moral development 351
moral exemplars 361
moral identity 360
postconventional reasoning 354
power assertion 363
preconventional reasoning 353
religion 374
religiousness 374

service learning 365
social-cognitive domain
  theory 351
social cognitive theory of
  morality 358
social conventional reasoning 361
spirituality 374
status offenses 371

key **people**

Albert Bandura 358
Gustavo Carlo 369
William Damon 359
John Dewey 365

Carol Gilligan 357
Hugh Hartshorne 358
Pamela King 374
Grazyna Kochanska 359

Lawrence Kohlberg 353
Mark May 358
Darcia Narváez 360
Jean Piaget 352

Judith Smetana 361
Ross Thompson 363
Lawrence Walker 361

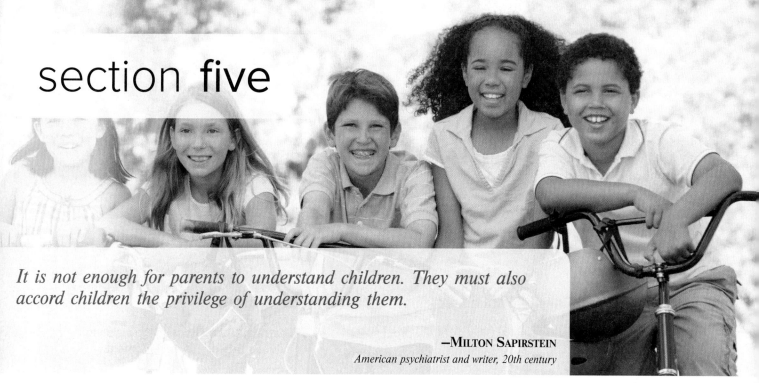

It is not enough for parents to understand children. They must also accord children the privilege of understanding them.

—**MILTON SAPIRSTEIN**
American psychiatrist and writer, 20th century

Monkey Business Images/Getty Images

Social Contexts of Development

Parents cradle children's lives, but children's growth is also shaped by successive choirs of siblings, peers, friends, and teachers. Children's small worlds widen as they discover new refuges and new people. In the end, there are but two lasting bequests that parents can leave children, one being roots, the other wings. In this section, we will study four chapters: "Families," "Peers," "Schools and Achievement," and "Culture and Diversity."

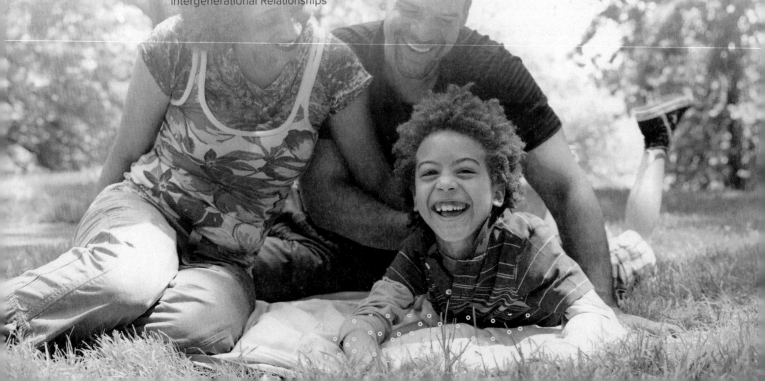

FAMILIES

chapter outline

Jasper Cole/Getty Images

When Shelley Peterman Schwarz (2004) and her husband, David, had been married four years, they decided to have children. They had two children, Jamie and Andrew. When the children were 3 and 5 years old, Shelley was diagnosed with multiple sclerosis. Two years later, she had to quit her job as a teacher of hearing-impaired children because of her worsening condition.

By the time the children were 7 and 9 years old, it was more difficult for Shelley to prepare meals for the family by herself, so David began taking over that responsibility. They also enlisted the children's help in preparing meals.

Despite her multiple sclerosis, Shelley participated in parenting classes and workshops at her children's school. She even initiated a "Mothers of 10-year-olds" support group. But parenting with multiple sclerosis had its frustrations for Shelley. In her words,

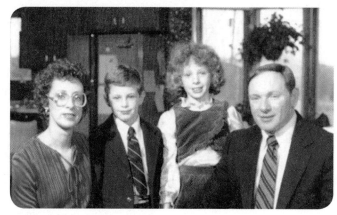

Shelley Peterman Schwarz (*left*) with her family.
Shelley Peterman Schwarz, Making Life Easier

attending school functions, teacher's conferences, and athletic events often presented problems because the facilities weren't always easily wheelchair accessible. I felt guilty if I didn't at least "try" to attend. I didn't want my children to think I didn't care enough to try. . . .

When Jamie was 19 and Andrew was 17, I started to relax a little. I could see how capable and independent they were becoming. My having a disability hadn't ruined their lives. In fact, in some ways, they are better off because of it. They learned to trust themselves and to face personal challenges head-on. When the time came for them to leave the nest and head off to college, I knew they were ready.

As for me, I now understand that having a disability wasn't the worst thing in the world that could happen to a parent. What would be a tragedy is letting your disability cripple your ability to stay in your children's lives. Parenting is so much more than driving car pools, attending gymnastic meets, or baking cookies for an open house. It's loving, caring, listening, guiding, and supporting your child. It's consoling a child crying because her friends thought her haircut was ugly. It's counseling a child worried because his 12-year-old friend is drinking. It's helping a child understand relationships and what it's like to "be in love." (Schwarz, 2004, p. 5)

preview

This chapter is about the many aspects of children's development in families from many different cultures. We will explore how families work, ways to parent children, relationships among siblings, and the changing family in a changing social world. Along the way, we will examine topics such as child maltreatment, working parents, children in divorced families, stepfamilies, and many others.

Family Processes **LG1** Discuss family processes.

| Interactions in the Family System | Cognition and Emotion in Family Processes | Multiple Developmental Trajectories | Domain-Specific Socialization | Sociocultural and Historical Changes |

As we examine the family and other social contexts of development, it will be helpful to keep in mind Urie Bronfenbrenner's (2000, 2004) ecological theory. Recall that Bronfenbrenner analyzes the social contexts of development in terms of five environmental systems:

- The *microsystem* or the setting in which the individual lives, such as a family, the world of peers, schools, work, and so on
- The *mesosystem*, which consists of links between microsystems, such as the connection between family processes and peer relations
- The *exosystem,* which consists of influences from another setting that the individual does not experience directly, such as how parents' experiences at work might affect their parenting at home
- The *macrosystem* or the culture in which the individual lives, such as a nation or an ethnic group
- The *chronosystem* or sociohistorical circumstances, such as increased numbers of working mothers, divorced parents, and stepparent families in the United States in the last 30 to 40 years

Let's begin our examination of the family at the level of the microsystem.

INTERACTIONS IN THE FAMILY SYSTEM

Every family is a *system*—a complex whole made up of interrelated and interacting parts. The relationships never go in just one direction. For example, the interaction of mothers and their infants is sometimes symbolized as a dance in which successive actions of the partners are closely coordinated. This coordinated dance can assume the form of *mutual synchrony,* which means that each person's behavior depends on the partner's previous behavior. Or the interaction can be *reciprocal* in a precise sense, which means that the actions of the partners can be matched, as when one partner imitates the other or when there is mutual smiling (Cohn & Tronick, 1988)—a pattern seen in many ethnic and cultural groups (Kuchirko, Tafuro, & Tamis-LeMonda, 2018). An important example of early synchronized interaction is mutual gaze or eye contact. This "paired behavior" actually reflects reciprocity in mother-infant brain activity during face-to-face communication (Leong & others, 2017).

Another example of synchronization occurs in **scaffolding,** which means adjusting the level of guidance to fit the child's performance (Melzi, Schick, & Kennedy, 2011). The parent responds to the child's behavior with scaffolding, which in turn affects the child's behavior. Scaffolding can be used to support children's efforts at any age. A study of Hmong families living in the United States revealed that maternal scaffolding, especially in the form of cognitive support, of young children's problem solving the summer before kindergarten predicted the children's reasoning skills in kindergarten (Stright, Herr, & Neitzel, 2009). Another study found that low-income U.S. Latino caregivers' elaborated speech during scaffolding predicted more growth in young children's language skills (Schick, Melzi, & Obregon, 2017).

developmental **connection**

Theories

An important contribution of Bronfenbrenner's ecological theory is its focus on a range of social contexts that influence the child's development. Connect to "Introduction."

scaffolding Adjusting the level of parental guidance to fit the child's efforts, allowing children to be more skillful than they would be if they relied only on their own abilities.

reciprocal socialization The bidirectional process by which children socialize parents just as parents socialize them.

The game of peek-a-boo, in which parents initially cover their babies, then remove the covering, and finally register "surprise" at the babies' reappearance, reflects the concept of scaffolding. As infants become more skilled at peek-a-boo, infants gradually do some of the covering and uncovering. Parents try to time their actions in such a way that the infant takes turns with the parent.

In addition to peek-a-boo, patty-cake and so-big are other caregiver games that exemplify scaffolding and turn-taking sequences. In one classic study, infants who had more extensive scaffolding experiences with their parents, especially in the form of turn taking, were more likely to engage in turn taking as they interacted with their peers (Vandell & Wilson, 1988). Engaging in turn taking and games like peek-a-boo reflect the development of joint attention by the caregiver and infant (Tomasello, 2009).

The mutual influence that parents and children exert on each other goes beyond specific interactions in games such as peek-a-boo; it extends to the whole process of socialization (Crouter & Booth, 2013; Grusec, 2017). Socialization between parents and children is not a one-way process. Parents do socialize children, but socialization in families is reciprocal (Capaldi, 2013; McHale & Crouter, 2013). **Reciprocal socialization** is socialization that is bidirectional; children socialize parents just as parents socialize children. These reciprocal interchanges and mutual influence processes are sometimes referred to as *transactional* (Sameroff, 2009).

While parents are interacting with their children, often they are also interacting with each other. To understand these interactions and relationships, it helps to think of the family as a constellation of subsystems defined in terms of generation, gender, and role. Each family member participates in several subsystems—some *dyadic* (involving two people) and some *polyadic* (involving more than two people). The father and child represent one dyadic subsystem, the mother and father another; the mother-father-child represent one polyadic subsystem, the mother and two siblings another (Fiese, Jones, & Saltsman, 2018).

These subsystems interact and influence one another (Carlson & others, 2011). Thus, as Figure 1 illustrates, the marital relationship, parenting, and infant/child behavior can have both direct and indirect effects on one another (Belsky, 1981; Berryhill & others, 2016). The link between marital relationships and parenting has received a great deal of attention. The most consistent findings are that compared with unhappily married parents, happily married parents are more sensitive, responsive, warm, and affectionate toward their children (Grych, 2002), and their children have fewer adjustment problems (Knopp & others, 2017).

Researchers have found that promoting marital satisfaction often leads to good parenting. The marital relationship provides an important support for parenting (Cowan & others, 2013; Cummings & others, 2012). When parents report more intimacy and better communication in their marriage, they are more affectionate toward their children (Grych, 2002). Thus, marriage-enhancement programs may end up improving parenting and helping children. Programs that focus on enhancing parenting skills might also benefit from including attention to the participants' marriages.

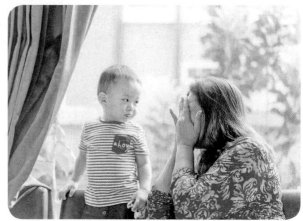

How does the game of peek-a-boo reflect the concept of scaffolding?
MIA Studio/Shutterstock

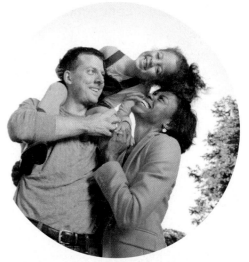

Children socialize parents just as parents socialize children.

Katrina Wittkamp/Photodisc/Getty Images

COGNITION AND EMOTION IN FAMILY PROCESSES

Both cognition and emotion are central to understanding how family processes work (Crockenberg & Leerkes, 2013; Thompson, 2015a, b). The role of cognition in family socialization takes many forms, including parents' thoughts, beliefs, and values about their parental role, as well as how parents perceive, organize, and understand their children's behaviors and beliefs. For example, one study found a link between mothers' beliefs and their preschool children's social problem-solving skills (Rubin, Mills, & Rose-Krasnor, 1989). Mothers who placed a higher value on skills such as making friends, sharing with others, and leading or influencing other children had children who were more assertive, prosocial, and competent problem solvers than mothers who valued these skills less.

Children's social competence is also linked to the emotional lives of their parents (Ablow, 2013). For example, one study found that parents who expressed positive emotions had children who were high in competence (Eisenberg & others, 2001). Through interaction with parents, children learn to express their emotions in appropriate ways.

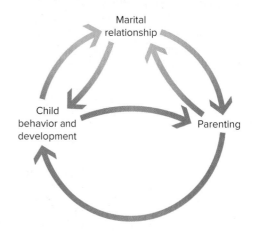

FIGURE 1

INTERACTION BETWEEN CHILDREN AND THEIR PARENTS: DIRECT AND INDIRECT EFFECTS

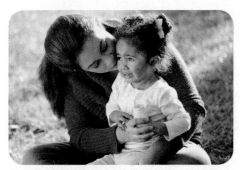

How are cognition and emotion involved in understanding family processes in children's development?

kali9/E+/Getty Images

developmental **connection**

Attention

Joint attention can play an important role in interchanges between a caregiver and an infant. Connect to "Information Processing."

developmental **connection**

Parenting

Emotion-coaching parents use more scaffolding and praise when interacting with their children than do emotion-dismissing parents. Connect to "Emotional Development."

multiple developmental trajectories Concept that adults follow one trajectory and children and adolescents another one; understanding how these trajectories mesh is important.

Researchers are also finding that parental sensitivity to children's emotions is related to children's ability to manage their emotions in positive ways (Thompson, 2015a, b). Recall the distinction between emotion-coaching and emotion-dismissing parents (Gottman, 2012). *Emotion-coaching parents* monitor their children's emotions, view their children's negative emotions as opportunities for teaching, assist them in labeling emotions, and coach them in how to deal effectively with emotions. In contrast, *emotion-dismissing parents* view their role as to deny, ignore, or change negative emotions.

MULTIPLE DEVELOPMENTAL TRAJECTORIES

The concept of **multiple developmental trajectories** refers to the idea that adults follow one trajectory and children and adolescents follow another (Parke & Buriel, 2006; Parke & Clarke-Stewart, 2011). Tracing how adult and child/adolescent developmental trajectories mesh is important for understanding the timing of entry into various family tasks. Adult developmental trajectories include timing of entry into marriage, cohabitation, or parenthood; child developmental trajectories include timing of child care and entry into middle school. The timing of some family tasks and changes are planned, such as reentry into the workforce or delaying parenthood, whereas others are not, such as job loss or divorce (Parke & Buriel, 2006).

Consider the developmental period of adolescence. Most adolescents' parents either are in middle adulthood or are rapidly approaching this period of life. However, in the last two decades, the timing of parenthood in the United States has undergone some dramatic shifts (Beal, Crockett, & Peugh, 2016). Parenthood is taking place earlier for some, and later for others, than in previous decades. First, the number of adolescent pregnancies in the United States increased considerably in the 1970s and 1980s. Although the adolescent pregnancy rate has decreased since then, the U.S. adolescent pregnancy rate remains one of the highest in the developed world. Second, the number of women who postpone childbearing until their thirties and early forties simultaneously has increased.

What are some advantages of having children early or late? Some of the advantages of having children early (in the twenties) are these: (1) the parents are likely to have more physical energy—for example, they can cope better with such matters as getting up in the middle of the night with infants and waiting up until adolescents come home at night; (2) the mother is likely to have fewer medical problems with pregnancy and childbirth; and (3) the parents may be less likely to build up expectations for their children, as do many couples who have waited many years to have children.

There are also advantages to having children later (in the thirties): (1) the parents will have had more time to consider their goals in life, such as what they want from their family and career roles; (2) the parents will be more mature and will be able to benefit from their experiences to engage in more competent parenting; and (3) the parents will be better established in their careers and have more income for child-rearing expenses.

DOMAIN-SPECIFIC SOCIALIZATION

When discussion turns to how parents socialize children, it has been common to describe the socialization process and child outcomes in general terms, such as "Parents who are warm, sensitive, and involved with their children have children who are socially competent." In such broad descriptions, too often the complexity and specificity of parental socialization and child outcomes are lost.

Researchers' interest in the domain specificity of socializing children has increased. Joan Grusec and Marilyn Davidov (2010) proposed a domain-specific view of parenting that emphasizes how parents often operate in different domains characterized by different types of relationships. The five domains are described below:

- *Protection.* Many species, including *homo sapiens,* have evolved so that their young maintain proximity to a caregiver, especially when they are in stressful or dangerous circumstances. In this domain, effective parenting involves responding in such a manner that the child develops a sense of security and perceives being comforted. Child outcomes of appropriate parental protection include the ability to respond appropriately to danger and to engage in self-regulation of distress.

- *Reciprocity.* This domain is not involved when the child is distressed but rather when the parent and child are interacting on an equal basis as partners, as in the context of play. Child outcomes in the reciprocity domain include the development of cooperativeness and a desire to comply with parental requests.

- *Control.* In the control domain, interactions between parents and children typically involve conflict because parents want one thing and children another. The control domain is often activated when children misbehave. In such circumstances, parents can use their power advantage to discourage the misbehavior through various means such as reasoning, social isolation, and physical punishment. Child outcomes in the control domain include the development of moral and principled behavior.

- *Guided Learning.* In this domain, parents guide children's learning of skills through the use of effective strategies and feedback. In the guided learning domain, parents function as teachers and their children as students. Children's outcomes in the guided learning domain include acquiring knowledge and skills.

- *Group Participation.* In this domain, socialization involves increasing children's participation in cultural practices. Child outcomes include conformity to cultural group practices and values that provide the child with a sense of social identity.

Grusec and Davidov (2010) acknowledge that real-life interactions in families often overlap across these domains, but the extent of this overlap has not yet been identified (Dunn, 2010). Also, it is not yet known how the different domains might play out at different points in children's development.

developmental **connection**

Moral Development

The domain view of moral development emphasizes different domains of social knowledge and reasoning, including moral, social conventional, and personal. Connect to "Moral Development."

SOCIOCULTURAL AND HISTORICAL CHANGES

Family development does not occur in a social vacuum. Important sociocultural and historical influences affect family processes, reflecting Bronfenbrenner's concepts of the macrosystem and chronosystem (Bronfenbrenner & Morris, 2006). Great upheavals such as war, famine, or massive immigration, as well as subtle transitions in ways of life, may stimulate changes in families (Fuligni, 2012). One example is the effect on U.S. families of the Great Depression of the 1930s. During its height, the Depression produced economic deprivation, adult discontent, and widespread unemployment. It also increased marital conflict, inconsistent child rearing, and unhealthy lifestyles—heavy drinking, demoralized attitudes, and health impairments—especially in fathers (Elder & Shanahan, 2006). Very similar effects have been seen in recent major economic recessions in the United States, Canada, South Korea, and nearly all of the countries in Europe (Brooks-Gunn, Schneider, & Waldfogel, 2013; Solantaus, Leinonen, & Punamäki, 2004; UNICEF, 2014).

Families are also affected by subtle and gradual changes in society and culture (Mistry & Dutta, 2015). These changes are occurring in nearly all countries in the world. The shifts include increased longevity of older adults, movement from rural to urban and suburban areas, technological advances, and many other aspects of living.

For instance, consider that in the first part of the twentieth century, individuals who survived infancy were usually hardy and still closely linked to the family, often helping to maintain the family's existence for their entire lives. Today, individuals live longer, which means that middle-aged adults are often pressed into a caregiving role for their aging parents, or the elderly parents may be placed in a nursing home (Fingerman, Secrest, & Birditt, 2013). Older parents may have lost some of their socializing role in the family during the twentieth century as many of their children moved great distances away. However, in the twenty-first century, an increasing number of grandparents are raising their grandchildren (Hayslip, Fruhauf, & Dolbin-MacNab, 2017).

Many of the family moves in the last 100 years have been away from farms and small towns to urban and suburban settings. In the small towns and farms, individuals were surrounded by lifelong neighbors, relatives, and friends. Today, neighborhood and extended-family support systems are not nearly as prevalent. In most industrialized countries in the world, such as the United States, Canada, Australia, and many countries in Europe, families move frequently, often uprooting children from a school and peer group where they

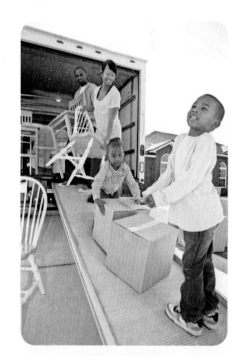

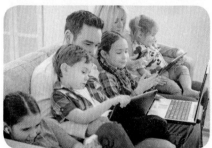

Two important changes in families are the increased mobility of families and the increase in screen time. *What are some other changes?*
(Top) Kali9/E+/Getty Images; (Bottom) Jamie Grill/JGI/Getty Images

developmental **connection**

Media

In the twenty-first century, children and adolescents have dramatically increased the amount of time they spend with media and the number of hours they engage in multitasking that involves media. Connect to "Culture and Diversity."

have spent a considerable length of time. It is not unusual for this type of move to occur multiple times in childhood and adolescence as one or both parents' employment changes (Hanushek, Kain, & Rivkin, 2004).

The media and technology also play a major role in the changing family (Blumberg & Brooks, 2017). Many children who watch television or online video programs find that parents are too busy working to share this experience with them. Children increasingly experience a world in which their parents are not participants. Instead of interacting in neighborhood peer groups, children come home after school and engage in social media, watch programs, and play video games online.

Another change in families has been an increase in family structural changes, reflecting cultural, religious, and legal shifts in society. In many parts of the globe, societies have a hodgepodge of family structures. For example, in western industrial countries such as the United States, Canada, Australia, Sweden, and the United Kingdom, there are far greater numbers of divorced and remarried families than ever before in history (Lansford, 2009; Ganong & Coleman, 2017).

Indeed, many of the changes we have described in this section apply not only to U.S. families but also to families in many countries around the world. Later in this chapter, we discuss aspects of the changing social world of the child and the family in greater detail.

Review Connect Reflect

 LG1 Discuss family processes.

Review

- How can the family be viewed as a system? What is reciprocal socialization?
- How are cognition and emotion involved in family processes?
- What characterizes multiple developmental trajectories?
- What are five domain-specific socialization practices?
- What are some sociocultural and historical changes that have influenced the family?

Connect

- In this section, scaffolding was mentioned as an example of synchronization. Which concept of Vygotsky's is scaffolding also linked to?

Reflect *Your Own Personal Journey of Life*

- Reflect on your experiences with your own family as you were growing up, and give examples of the family processes discussed in this section as you experienced them in your own family.

Parenting **LG2** Explain how parenting is linked to children's and adolescents' development.

| Parental Roles and the Timing of Parenthood | Adapting Parenting to Developmental Changes in Children | Parents as Managers of Children's Lives | Parenting Styles and Discipline | Parent-Adolescent Relationships | Intergenerational Relationships |

Parenting is a very important profession, but no test of fitness for it is ever imposed in the interest of children.

—GEORGE BERNARD SHAW

Irish playwright, 20th century

Parenting calls on numerous interpersonal skills and makes intense emotional demands, yet there is little in the way of formal education for this task. Most parents learn parenting practices from their own parents. Some of these practices they accept, and others they discard. Fathers and mothers may bring different views of parenting to their relationship.

Unfortunately, when parents' methods are passed on from one generation to the next, both desirable and undesirable practices are perpetuated. What have developmentalists learned about parenting? How should parents adapt their practices to developmental changes in their children? How important is it for parents to be effective managers of their children's lives? And how do various parenting styles and methods of discipline influence children's development?

PARENTAL ROLES AND THE TIMING OF PARENTHOOD

Many adults decide when they would like to become parents and consider how parenting will fit with their economic situation. For others, the discovery that they are about to become parents is a startling surprise. In either event, the prospective parents may have mixed emotions and romantic illusions about having a child. The needs and expectations of parents have stimulated many myths about parenting.

Currently, there is a tendency to have fewer children, and the number of one-child families is increasing (Carl, 2012). Is there a best time to have children? What are some of the restrictions individuals face when they become parents? These are some of the questions we now consider.

Like the age when people marry for the first time, the age at which individuals have children has been increasing (Lauer & Lauer, 2012). In 2014, the average age at which women gave birth for the first time was 27, up from 21 years of age in 1970 (Mathews & Hamilton, 2016).

As birth control has become common practice, many individuals choose when they will have children and how many children they will raise. Couples are not only moving in together and marrying later but also having children later or not at all. For instance, the percentage of 40- to 44-year-old U.S. women who were childless increased from 10 percent in 1976 to 24 percent in 2006-2010, and 45 percent of 15- to 44-year-old women were childless in 2015—an all-time high (Martinez & others, 2018).

ADAPTING PARENTING TO DEVELOPMENTAL CHANGES IN CHILDREN

Children change dramatically as they grow from infancy to early childhood and on through middle and late childhood and across adolescence. The 5-year-old and the 2-year-old have different needs and abilities. Researchers and practitioners have long known that a competent parent adapts to the child's developmental changes (Maccoby, 1984). However, perhaps the largest adaptation is required in making the transition to parenthood.

The Transition to Parenthood   Whether people become parents through pregnancy, adoption, or stepparenting, they face disequilibrium and must adapt (Maas & others, 2018). Parents want to develop a strong attachment with their infant, but they also want to maintain strong attachments to their spouse and friends, and possibly continue their careers. Parents ask themselves how this new being will change their lives. A baby places new restrictions on partners; no longer will they be able to rush out to a movie on a moment's notice, and money may not be readily available for vacations and other luxuries. Dual-career parents ask, "Will it harm the baby to place her in child care? Will we be able to find responsible babysitters?"

In an influential longitudinal study of couples from late pregnancy until 3½ years after the baby was born, couples enjoyed more positive marital relations before the baby was born than after (Cowan & Cowan, 2000, 2009; Cowan, Cowan, & Barry, 2011; Cowan & others, 2005). Still, almost one-third showed an increase in marital satisfaction after the birth. Some couples said that the baby had both brought them closer together and moved them farther apart; being parents enhanced their sense of themselves and gave them a new, more stable identity as a couple. Babies opened men up to having concerns with intimate relationships, and the demands of juggling work and family roles stimulated women to manage family tasks more efficiently and pay attention to their own personal growth. Subsequent research has shown that lower levels of satisfaction with relationships are often linked to reductions in quality time spent together and perceived unfairness in dividing up household tasks (Dew & Wilcox, 2011; Maas & others, 2018).

We never know the love of our parents until we have become parents.

—HENRY WARD BEECHER
American clergyman, 19th century

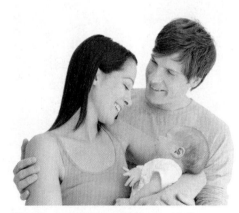

What characterizes the transition to parenting?
Chris Ryan/OJO Images/Getty Images

The Bringing Home Baby project is a workshop that helps new parents strengthen their relationship with their partner, understand and become acquainted with their baby, resolve conflict, and develop parenting skills. Evaluations of the project revealed that parents who participated improved their ability to work together as parents, fathers were more involved with their baby and sensitive to the baby's behavior, mothers had a lower incidence of postpartum depression symptoms, and babies showed better overall development than babies of participants in a control group (Gottman, 2013; Gottman Relationship Institute, 2009; Gottman, Gottman, & Shapiro, 2009; Shapiro & Gottman, 2005).

Other studies have explored the transition to parenthood (Brown, Feinberg, & Kan, 2012). Several studies have found similar negative and positive changes in relationship satisfaction for married and cohabiting women who stayed with the father during and after the transition to parenthood (Carlson & Van Orman, 2017; Mortensen & others, 2012). Other research has revealed that mothers experience unmet expectations in the transition to parenting, with fathers doing less than their partners anticipate (Biehle & Mickelson, 2012)—and that fathers experience perceived unfairness too (Newkirk, Perry-Jenkins, & Sayer, 2017).

Infancy   During the first year, parent-child interaction moves from a heavy focus on routine caregiving—feeding, changing diapers, bathing, and soothing—to gradually include more noncaregiving activities, such as play, visual-vocal exchanges, and managing the infant's behavior (Bornstein, 2002).

Early Childhood   Parent-child interactions during early childhood focus on such matters as modesty and compliance, bedtime regularities, control of temper, fighting with siblings and peers, eating behavior and manners, autonomy in dressing, and attention seeking (Edwards & Liu, 2002). Although some of these issues—fighting with siblings, for example—are carried forward into the elementary school years, many new issues appear by the age of 7. These include whether children should be made to perform chores and if so, whether they should be paid for them, how to help children learn to entertain themselves rather than relying on parents for everything, and how to monitor children's lives outside the family in school and peer settings.

Middle and Late Childhood   As children move into the middle and late childhood years, parents spend less time with them. In one study, parents spent less than half as much time with their children aged 5 to 12 in caregiving, instruction, reading, talking, and playing than they did when the children were younger (Del Giudice, 2014). Although parents spend less time with their children in middle and late childhood than in early childhood, parents continue to be extremely important in their children's lives. In a detailed analysis of the contributions of parents during middle and late childhood, the following conclusion was reached: "Parents serve as gatekeepers and provide scaffolding as children assume more responsibility for themselves and . . . regulate their own lives" (Huston & Ripke, 2006, p. 422).

Parents play an especially important role in supporting and stimulating children's academic achievement in middle and late childhood (Cowan & Heming, 2013; Huston & Ripke, 2006). The value parents place on education can determine whether children do well in school. Parents not only influence children's in-school achievement, but they also make decisions about children's out-of-school activities (Eccles & Roeser, 2013). Whether children participate in sports, music, and other activities is heavily influenced by the extent to which parents sign up children for such activities and encourage their participation (Simoncini & Caltabiono, 2012).

In middle and late childhood, youth receive less physical discipline than they did as preschoolers. Instead of spanking or coercive holding, their parents are more likely to use removal of privileges, appeals to the child's self-esteem, comments designed to increase the child's sense of guilt, and statements that the child is responsible for his or her actions—a developmental pattern seen in many cultures in countries as different from each other as the United States, Kenya, and China (Gershoff & others, 2010).

During middle and late childhood, some control is transferred from parent to child. The process is gradual, and it produces *coregulation* rather than control by either the child

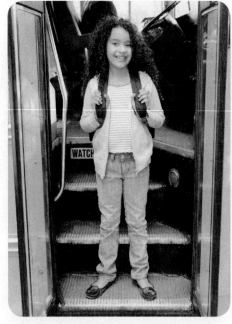

What are some changes in the focus of parent-child relationships in middle and late childhood?
Jamie Grill/JGI/Getty Images

or the parent alone. Parents continue to exercise general supervision and control, and children can engage in moment-to-moment self-regulation (Koehn & Kerns, 2017). The major shift to autonomy does not occur until early adolescence. A key developmental task as children move toward autonomy is learning to relate to adults outside the family on a regular basis—adults such as teachers who interact with children differently from the ways their parents interact with them.

In sum, considerable adaptation in parenting is required as children develop. Later in the chapter, we will further examine adaptations in parenting when discussing family influences on adolescents' development.

PARENTS AS MANAGERS OF CHILDREN'S LIVES

Parents can play important roles as managers of children's opportunities, as monitors of their lives, and as social initiators and arrangers (Bradley & Corwyn, 2013; Parke & Buriel, 2006; Parke & Clarke-Stewart, 2011). An important task of childhood and adolescence is to develop the ability to make competent decisions in an increasingly independent manner. To help children and adolescents reach their full potential, a parent needs to be an effective manager—one who finds information, makes contacts, helps structure choices, and provides guidance. Parents who fulfill this important managerial role help children and adolescents to avoid pitfalls and to work their way through a myriad of choices and decisions (Beckmeyer & Russell, 2018). Mothers are more likely than fathers to engage in a managerial role in parenting.

From infancy through adolescence, parents can play important roles in managing their children's experiences and opportunities. In infancy this might involve taking a child to a doctor and arranging for child care; in early childhood it might involve selecting the preschool that the child will attend; in middle and late childhood it might include directing the child to take a bath, to match their clothes and wear clean clothes, and to put away toys; in adolescence it could involve participating in a parent-teacher conference and subsequently managing the adolescent's homework and free time activities.

Managing and Guiding Infants' Behavior In addition to sensitive parenting involving warmth and caring that can result in infants being securely attached to their parents, other important aspects of parenting infants involve managing and guiding their behavior in an attempt to reduce or eliminate undesirable behaviors (Holden, Vittrup, & Rosen, 2011). This management process includes (1) being proactive and childproofing the environment so infants will not encounter potentially dangerous objects or situations, and (2) using corrective methods when infants engage in undesirable behaviors, such as excessive fussing and crying, biting others, or throwing objects.

In one very detailed study, investigators assessed discipline and corrective methods that parents had used by the time their infants were 12 and 24 months old (Vittrup, Holden, & Buck, 2006) (see Figure 2). The figure shows that the main corrective method at 12 months old was diverting the infant's attention, followed by reasoning, ignoring, and negotiating. However, more than one-third of parents had yelled at their infant, one-fifth had slapped the infant's hands or threatened the infant, and approximately one-sixth had spanked the infant by 12 months.

As infants move into the second year of life and become toddlers who are mobile and capable of exploring a wider range of environments, parental management of behavior often involves increased corrective feedback and discipline. As indicated in Figure 2, yelling increased dramatically from 36 percent at 12 months to 81 percent by 24 months of age; slapping the infant's hands increased from 21 percent to 31 percent; and spanking increased from 14 percent to 45 percent.

A special concern is that these and other corrective discipline tactics not become abusive. Too often what starts out as mild to moderately intense discipline on the part of parents can move into highly intense anger. Later in this chapter,

There's no vocabulary for love within a family, love that's lived in but not looked at, love within the light of which all else is seen, the love within which all other love finds speech. That love is silent.

—T. S. ELIOT
American-born English poet, 20th century

Method	12 Months	24 Months
Spank with hand	14	45
Slap infant's hand	21	31
Yell in anger	36	81
Threaten	19	63
Withdraw privileges	18	52
Time-out	12	60
Reason	85	100
Divert attention	100	100
Negotiate	50	90
Ignore	64	90

FIGURE 2

PARENTS' METHODS FOR MANAGING AND CORRECTING INFANTS' UNDESIRABLE BEHAVIOR.
Shown here are the percentages of parents who had used various corrective methods by the time their infant was 12 and 24 months old. *Source:* Based on data presented in Table 1 in Vittrup, Holden, & Buck (2006).

Janis Keyser, Parent Educator

Janis Keyser is a parent educator who also teaches in the Department of Early Childhood Education at Cabrillo College in California. In addition to teaching college classes and conducting parenting workshops, she coauthored a book with Laura Davis (1997), *Becoming the Parent You Want to Be: A Sourcebook of Strategies for the First Five Years.*

Keyser also has written as an expert on parenting websites, and she was a coauthor of a nationally syndicated parenting column, "Growing Up, Growing Together."

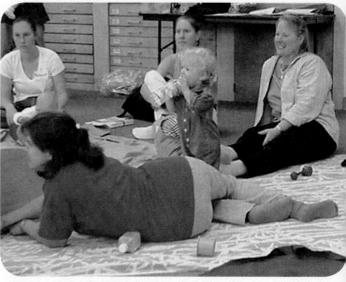

Janis Keyser *(right) conducts* a parenting workshop.
Courtesy of Janis Keyser

you will read more extensively about the use of punishment with children and links with child maltreatment.

Parental Monitoring in Childhood and Adolescence   A key aspect of the managerial role of parenting is effective monitoring, which becomes especially important as children move into the adolescent years (Bradley & Corwyn, 2013). Monitoring includes supervising an adolescent's choices of social settings, activities, and friends. The largest study to date (more than 36,000 eighth- and tenth-grade adolescents) revealed that a higher level of parental monitoring was associated with lower rates of alcohol and marijuana use, with stronger effects for girls and adolescents who were most likely to take risks (Dever & others, 2013). Further, a research review of the influence of family functioning on African American students' academic achievement found that when African American parents monitored their son's academic achievement by ensuring that homework was completed, restricted time spent on nonproductive distractions (such as video games and TV), and participated in a consistent, positive dialogue with teachers and school officials, their son's academic achievement benefited (Mandara, 2006). Similar effects are seen in Latino cultural groups in the United States and for daughters as well as sons (Jeynes, 2017).

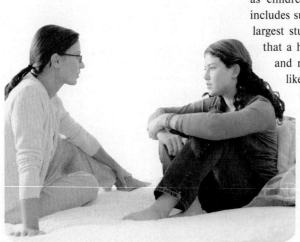

What factors are involved in whether adolescents will voluntarily disclose information to their parents?
Ryan McVay/Getty Images

A current interest in research involves ways that adolescents control their parents' access to information, especially the extent to which adolescents disclose or conceal strategies about their activities (Chan, Brown, & Von Bank, 2015; Rote & others, 2012). Researchers have found that adolescents' disclosure to parents about their whereabouts, activities, and friends is linked to positive adolescent adjustment and achievement (Laird & Marrero, 2011; Smetana, 2011a, b). These effects may operate similarly across cultures. For example, one study of U.S. and Chinese young adolescents found that adolescents' disclosure to parents was linked to a higher level of academic competence (better learning strategies, autonomous motivation, and better grades) over time (Cheung, Pomerantz, & Dong, 2013).

To read about one individual who helps parents become more effective in managing their children's lives, see *Connecting with Careers.*

Researchers also have found that family management practices are related positively to students' grades and self-responsibility, and negatively to school-related problems

(Degol & others, 2017; Eccles & Roeser, 2013). Among the most important family management practices in this regard are maintaining a structured and organized family environment, such as establishing routines for homework, chores, bedtime, and so on, and effectively monitoring the adolescent's behavior.

PARENTING STYLES AND DISCIPLINE

Good parenting takes time and effort. You cannot do it in a minute here and a minute there, or with online videos. Of course, it's not just the quantity of time parents spend with children that is important for development—the quality of the parenting is clearly important (Grusec, 2013; Grusec & others, 2013). To understand variations in parenting, let's consider the styles parents use when they interact with their children, how they discipline their children, and coparenting.

Baumrind's Parenting Styles Diana Baumrind (1971, 2013) emphasizes that parents should be neither punitive nor aloof. Rather, they should develop rules for their children and be affectionate with them. She has described four types of parenting styles that have been examined in thousands of studies in many cultures and countries spanning the globe (Larzalere, Morris, & Harrist, 2013):

- **Authoritarian parenting** is a restrictive, punitive style in which parents exhort the child to follow their directions and respect their work and effort. The authoritarian parent places firm limits and controls on the child and allows little verbal exchange. For example, an authoritarian parent might say, "You will do it my way or else." Authoritarian parents also might spank the child frequently, enforce rules rigidly but not explain them, and show rage toward the child. Children of authoritarian parents are often unhappy, fearful, and anxious about comparing themselves with others, fail to initiate activity, and have weak communication skills. Sons of authoritarian parents may behave aggressively.
- **Authoritative parenting** encourages children to be independent but still places limits and controls on their actions. Extensive verbal give-and-take is allowed, and parents are warm and nurturant toward the child. An authoritative parent might put his arm around the child in a comforting way and say, "You know you should not have done that. Let's talk about how you can handle the situation better next time." Authoritative parents show pleasure and support in response to children's constructive behavior. They also expect mature, independent, and age-appropriate behavior by children. Children whose parents are authoritative are often cheerful, self-controlled and self-reliant, and achievement oriented; they tend to maintain friendly relations with peers, cooperate with adults, and cope well with stress.
- **Neglectful parenting** is a style in which the parent is very uninvolved in the child's life. Children whose parents are neglectful develop the sense that other aspects of the parents' lives are more important than they are. These children tend to be socially incompetent. Many have poor self-control and don't handle independence well. They frequently have low self-esteem, are immature, and may be alienated from the family. In adolescence, they may show patterns of truancy and delinquency.
- **Indulgent parenting** is a style in which parents are highly involved with their children but place few demands or controls on them. Such parents let their children do what they want. The result is that the children never learn to control their own behavior and always expect to get their way. Some parents deliberately rear their children in this way because they believe the combination of warm involvement and few restraints will produce a creative, confident child. However, children whose parents are indulgent rarely learn respect for others and have difficulty controlling their behavior. They might be domineering, egocentric, noncompliant, and have difficulties in peer relations.

These four classifications of parenting involve combinations of acceptance and responsiveness on the one hand and demand and control on the other (Larzalere, Morris, &

authoritarian parenting A restrictive, punitive style in which the parent exhorts the child to follow the parent's directions and to respect their work and effort. Firm limits and controls are placed on the child, and little verbal exchange is allowed. This style is associated with children's social incompetence, including a lack of initiative and weak communication skills.

authoritative parenting This style encourages children to be independent but still places limits and controls on their actions. Extensive verbal give-and-take is allowed, and parents are warm and nurturant toward the child. This style is associated with children's social competence, achievement orientation, and self-reliance.

neglectful parenting A style in which the parent is very uninvolved in the child's life. It is associated with children's social incompetence, especially a lack of self-control and poor self-esteem.

indulgent parenting A style in which parents are highly involved with their children but place few demands or controls on them. This is associated with children's social incompetence, especially a lack of self-control and a lack of respect for others.

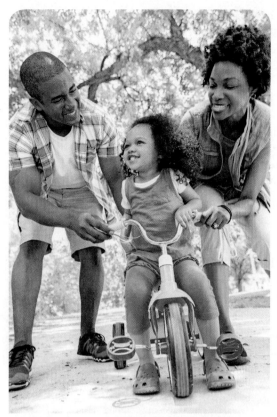

	Accepting, responsive	Rejecting, unresponsive
Demanding, controlling	Authoritative	Authoritarian
Undemanding, uncontrolling	Indulgent	Neglectful

FIGURE 3

CLASSIFICATION OF PARENTING STYLES. The four types of parenting styles (authoritative, authoritarian, indulgent, and neglectful) involve the dimensions of acceptance and responsiveness, on the one hand, and demand and control on the other. For example, authoritative parenting involves being both accepting/responsive and demanding/controlling.

Steve Debenport/Getty Images

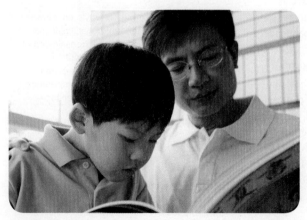

According to Ruth Chao, what type of parenting style do many Asian American parents use?

James Hardy/PhotoAlto/Getty Images

Harrist, 2013). How these dimensions combine to produce authoritarian, authoritative, neglectful, and indulgent parenting is shown in Figure 3.

Parenting Styles in Context Do the benefits of authoritative parenting transcend the boundaries of ethnicity, socioeconomic status (SES), and household composition? Although occasional exceptions have been found, evidence linking authoritative parenting with competence on the part of the child occurs in research across a wide range of ethnic groups, social strata, cultures, and family structures (Low, Snyder, & Shortt, 2012; Morris, Cui, & Steinberg, 2013; Prevoo & Tamis-LeMonda, 2017; Steinberg & Silk, 2002).

Nonetheless, researchers have found that in some ethnic groups, aspects of the authoritarian style may be associated with more positive child outcomes than Baumrind predicts (Parke & Buriel, 2006). Elements of the authoritarian style may take on different meanings and have different effects depending on the context.

For example, Asian American parents often continue aspects of traditional Asian child-rearing practices that have sometimes been described as authoritarian. The parents exert considerable control over their children's lives. However, Ruth Chao (2001; Chao & Otsuki-Clutter, 2011; Chao & Tseng, 2002) argues that the style of parenting used by many Asian American parents is distinct from the domineering control of the authoritarian style. Instead, Chao argues that the control reflects parental concern and involvement in their children's lives and is best conceptualized as a type of training. The high academic achievement of Asian American children may be a consequence of their "training" parents (Stevenson & Zusho, 2002). In research involving Chinese American adolescents and their parents, parental control was endorsed as were the Confucian parental goals of perseverance, working hard in school, obedience, and being sensitive to parents' wishes (Russell, Crockett, & Chao, 2010). Similar patterns have been observed in research with mainland Chinese families (Zhang & others, 2017).

An emphasis on requiring respect and obedience is also associated with the authoritarian style, but in Latino child rearing this focus may be positive rather than punitive. Rather than suppressing the child's development, it may encourage the development of a self and an identity that are embedded in the family and require respect and obedience (Harwood & others, 2002; Prevoo & Tamis-LeMonda, 2017).

Even physical punishment, another characteristic of the authoritarian style, may have varying effects in different contexts. African American parents are more likely than non-Latino White parents to use physical punishment (Deater-Deckard, Dodge, & Sorbring, 2005). The use of physical punishment has been linked with increased externalized child problems (such as acting out and high levels of aggression) in non-Latino White families, but these outcomes are not always found in African American families. One explanation of this finding points to the need for African American parents to enforce rules in the dangerous environments in which they are more likely to live (Harrison-Hale, McLoyd, & Smedley, 2004). In this context, requiring obedience to parental authority may be an adaptive strategy to keep children from engaging in antisocial behavior that can have serious consequences for their development (McElhaney & Allen, 2012).

Further Thoughts on Parenting Styles Several caveats about parenting styles are in order. First, the parenting styles do not capture the important themes of reciprocal socialization and synchrony (Crouter & Booth, 2013). Keep in mind that children socialize parents, just as parents socialize children (Capaldi, 2013; Shanahan & Sobolewski, 2013). Second, many parents use a combination of techniques rather than a single technique, although one technique may be dominant. Although consistent parenting is usually recommended, the wise parent may sense the importance of being more permissive in certain situations, more authoritarian under different circumstances, and more authoritative in others. Also, some critics argue that the concept of parenting style is too broad and that more research needs to be conducted to "unpack" parenting styles by studying various components of the styles (Grusec, 2011; Maccoby, 2007). For example, is parental monitoring more important than warmth in predicting child and adolescent outcomes?

Punishment   For centuries, corporal (physical) punishment, such as spanking, has been considered a necessary and even desirable method of disciplining children. Use of corporal punishment is legal in every state in America. A national survey of U.S. parents with 3- and 4-year-old children found that 26 percent of parents reported spanking their children frequently, and 67 percent of the parents reported yelling at their children frequently (Regalado & others, 2004). An international comparison found that individuals in the United States and Canada were among those with the most favorable attitudes toward corporal punishment and were the most likely to remember it being used by their parents (Curran & others, 2001) (see Figure 4). Yet in many countries, attitudes supporting physical punishment are decreasing. Research has shown decreases in places as diverse from each other as Sierra Leone, Montenegro, Macedonia, and the Ukraine (Lansford & others, 2017).

An increasing number of studies have examined the outcomes of physically punishing children, although those that have been conducted are correlational. Clearly, it would be highly unethical to randomly assign parents to either spank or not spank their children in an experimental study. Recall that cause and effect cannot be determined in a correlational study. In one correlational study, spanking by parents was linked with children's antisocial behavior, including cheating, telling lies, being mean to others, bullying, getting into fights, and being disobedient (Strauss, Sugarman, & Giles-Sims, 1997).

A research review concluded that corporal punishment by parents is associated with higher levels of immediate compliance and aggression by the children (Gershoff, 2002). The review also found that corporal punishment is linked to lower levels of moral internalization and mental health. A large study in eight countries (China, Colombia, Italy, Jordan, Kenya, Philippines, Thailand, and the United States) revealed that parental use of physical punishment was linked to highest rates of aggressive and nonaggressive behavior problems in their children and adolescents (Alampay & others, 2017). Numerous longitudinal studies also have found that physical punishment of young children is associated with higher levels of aggression later in childhood and adolescence (Berlin & others, 2009; Gershoff & others, 2012; Lansford & others, 2011; Taylor & others, 2010; see Pinquart, 2017, for an overview).

What are some reasons to avoid spanking or similar punishments? The reasons include the following:

- When adults punish a child by yelling, screaming, or spanking, they are presenting children with out-of-control models for handling stressful situations. Children may imitate this aggressive, out-of-control behavior.

- Punishment can instill fear, rage, or avoidance. For example, spanking the child may cause the child to avoid being around the parent and to fear the parent.

- Punishment tells children what not to do rather than what to do. Children should be given feedback, such as "Why don't you try this?"

- Punishment can be abusive. Parents might unintentionally become so emotional when they are punishing the child that they become abusive (Durrant, 2008; Knox, 2010).

Most child psychologists recommend handling misbehavior by reasoning with the child, especially explaining the consequences of the child's actions for others. *Time out,* in which the child is removed from a setting that offers positive reinforcement, can also be effective. For example, when the child has misbehaved, a parent might take away TV viewing for a specified time.

A final point about the use of punishment with children is that there is ongoing debate about its effects on children's development (Gershoff & others, 2012; Grusec, 2011; Lansford & Deater-Deckard, 2012). Some experts (including Diana Baumrind) argue that

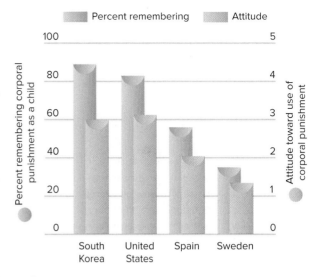

FIGURE 4

CORPORAL PUNISHMENT IN DIFFERENT COUNTRIES.
A 5-point scale was used to assess attitudes toward corporal punishment, with scores closer to 1 indicating an attitude against its use and scores closer to 5 suggesting an attitude favoring its use. *Why are studies of corporal punishment correlational studies, and how does that affect their interpretation?*

Do Marital Conflict and Individual Hostility Predict the Use of Physical Punishment in Parenting?

A longitudinal study assessed couples across the transition to parenting to investigate possible links between marital conflict, individual adult hostility, and the use of physical punishment with young children (Kanoy & others, 2003). Before the birth of the first child, the level of marital conflict was observed in a marital problem-solving discussion; answers to questionnaires regarding individual characteristics were also obtained. Thus, these characteristics of the couples were not influenced by characteristics of the child. When the children were 2 and 5 years old, the couples were interviewed about the frequency and intensity of

their physical punishment of the children. On both occasions, the parents' level of marital conflict was again observed in a marital problem-solving discussion.

The researchers found that both hostility and marital conflict were linked with the use of physical punishment. Individuals with high rates of hostility on the prenatal measures used more frequent and more severe physical punishment with their children. The same was evident for marital conflict—when marital conflict was high, both mothers and fathers were more likely to use physical punishment in disciplining their young children.

much of the evidence for the negative effects of physical punishment has been based on studies in which parents acted in an abusive manner (Baumrind, Larzelere, & Cowan, 2002). She concludes from her research that when parents used punishment in a calm, reasoned manner (which she says characterized most of the authoritative parents in her studies), children's development benefitted. Thus, she emphasizes that physical punishment does not need to present children with an out-of-control adult who is yelling and screaming, as well as spanking. A detailed analysis of many studies concluded that only severe or predominant use of spanking, not mild spanking, compared unfavorably with alternative practices for disciplining children (Larzelere & Kuhn, 2005).

Indeed, there are few longitudinal studies that distinguish adequately between moderate and heavy use of punishment. Thus, in the view of some experts, available research evidence makes it difficult to tell whether the effects of physical punishment are harmful to children's development, even though such a view might be distasteful to some individuals (Grusec, 2009).

In addition to considering whether physical punishment is mild or out of control, another factor in evaluating effects on children's development involves cultural contexts. Research has indicated that in countries such as Kenya in which physical punishment is considered normal and necessary for handling children's transgressions, the effects of physical punishment are less harmful than in countries such as Thailand in which physical punishment is perceived as more harmful to children's development (Lansford & others, 2005, 2013). However, evidence of these culture-specific effects is mixed (see Gershoff & Grogan-Kaylor, 2016).

One thing that is clear regarding research on punishment of children is that if physical punishment is used, it needs to be mild, infrequent, age-appropriate, and used in the context of a positive parent-child relationship (Grusec, 2011). It is also clear that when physical punishment involves abuse, it can be very harmful to children's development (Cicchetti, 2013; Garcia, McKee, & Forehand, 2012).

Earlier in this chapter, we described the family as a system and discussed possible links between marital relationships and parenting practices (Cox & others, 2004). Do marital conflict and individual hostility predict the use of physical punishment in parenting? To find out, read *Connecting Through Research*.

coparenting Support parents provide for each other in jointly raising children.

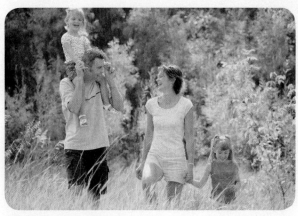

What characterizes coparenting?
Don Hammond/Design Pics

Coparenting   The relationship between marital conflict and the use of punishment highlights the importance of **coparenting**, which is the support

Darla Botkin, Marriage and Family Therapist

Darla Botkin is a marriage and family therapist who teaches, conducts research, and engages in marriage and family therapy. She is on the faculty of the University of Kentucky. Botkin obtained a bachelor's degree in elementary education with a concentration in special education and then went on to receive a master's degree in early childhood education. She spent the next six years working with children and their families in a variety of settings, including child care, elementary school, and Head Start. These experiences led Botkin to recognize the interdependence of the developmental settings that children and their parents experience (such as home, school, and work). She returned to graduate school and obtained a Ph.D. in family studies from the University of Tennessee. She then became a faculty member in the Family Studies program at the University of Kentucky. Completing further coursework and clinical training in marriage and family therapy, she became certified as a marriage and family therapist.

Botkin's current interests include working with young children in family therapy, addressing gender and ethnic issues in family therapy, and exploring the role of spirituality in family wellness.

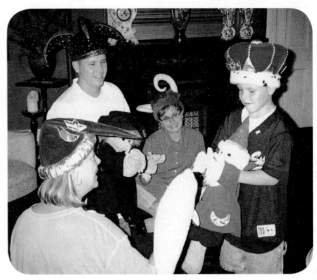

Darla Botkin *(left)* conducts a family therapy session.
Courtesy of Dr. Darla Botkin

For more information about what marriage and family therapists do, see the Careers in Child Development appendix.

that parents provide one another in jointly raising a child. Poor coordination between parents, undermining of the other parent, lack of cooperation and warmth, and disconnection by one parent are conditions that place children at risk for problems (Padilla & others, 2017; Young, Riggs, & Kaminski, 2017). For example, one study revealed that coparenting influenced young children's effortful self-control above and beyond maternal and paternal parenting by themselves (Karreman & others, 2008). And another study found that greater father involvement in young children's play was linked to an increase in supportive coparenting (Jia & Schoppe-Sullivan, 2011).

Parents who do not spend enough time with their children or who have problems in child rearing can benefit from counseling and therapy. To read about the work of marriage and family counselor Darla Botkin, see *Connecting with Careers*.

Child Maltreatment Unfortunately, punishment or neglect sometimes leads to the abuse of infants and children (Cicchetti, 2011, 2013). In 2015, approximately 683,000 U.S. children were found to be victims of child abuse at least once during that year (U.S. Department of Health and Human Services, 2017). The vast majority of these children were abused by a parent or parents. Laws in many states now require physicians and teachers to report suspected cases of child abuse, yet many cases go unreported, especially those involving battered infants.

Whereas the public and many professionals use the term *child abuse* to refer to both abuse and neglect, developmentalists increasingly use the term *child maltreatment* (Cicchetti, 2011, 2013; Cicchetti & Toth, 2011). This term does not have quite the emotional impact of the term *abuse* and acknowledges that maltreatment includes diverse conditions.

Child maltreatment involves grossly inadequate and destructive aspects of parenting.

—DANTE CICCHETTI

Contemporary developmental psychologist, University of Minnesota

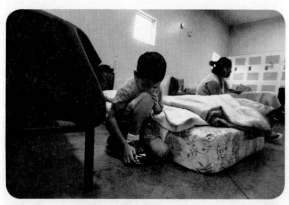

This family of four children are having dinner in a cramped motel room that's handling shelter overflow. Homeless advocates say many families are being denied shelter. *What are some different types of child abuse?*

John Moore/Getty Images

Types of Child Maltreatment

The four main types of child maltreatment are physical abuse, child neglect, sexual abuse, and emotional abuse (Child Welfare Information Gateway, 2016):

- *Physical abuse* is characterized by the infliction of physical injury as a result of punching, beating, kicking, biting, burning, shaking, or otherwise harming a child. The parent or other person may not have intended to hurt the child; the injury may have resulted from excessive physical punishment (Milot & others, 2010).

- *Child neglect* is characterized by failure to provide for the child's basic needs (Newton & Vandeven, 2010). Neglect can be physical (abandonment, for example), educational (allowing chronic truancy, for example), or emotional (marked inattention to the child's needs, for example). Child neglect is by far the most common form of child maltreatment. In every country where relevant data have been collected, neglect occurs up to three times as often as abuse (Benoit, Coolbear, & Crawford, 2008).

- *Sexual abuse* includes fondling a child's genitals, intercourse, incest, rape, sodomy, exhibitionism, and commercial exploitation through prostitution or the production of pornographic materials (Bahali & others, 2010).

- *Emotional abuse (psychological/verbal abuse/mental injury)* includes acts or failures to act by parents or other caregivers that have caused, or could cause, serious behavioral, cognitive, or emotional problems (van Harmelen & others, 2010).

Although any of these forms of child maltreatment may be found separately, they often occur in combination. Emotional abuse is almost always present when other forms are identified.

The Context of Abuse

No single factor causes child maltreatment (Cicchetti, 2011, 2013). A combination of factors, including the culture, family, and developmental characteristics of the child, likely contribute to child maltreatment (Cicchetti & Toth, 2011).

The extensive violence that takes place in the American culture, including TV violence, is reflected in the occurrence of violence in the family (Durrant, 2008). The family itself is obviously a key part of the context of abuse. Research in many countries, including the United States, Australia, and other nations as diverse from each other as Nigeria, Laos, Chile, and Vietnam, shows that family and family-associated characteristics contribute to child maltreatment. These include substance use, parenting stress, social isolation, single parenting, and socioeconomic difficulties (especially poverty) (Cicchetti, 2013; Laslett & others, 2017). The interactions of all family members need to be considered, regardless of who performs the violent acts against the child. For example, even though the father may be the one who physically abuses the child, the behavior of the mother, the child, and siblings also should be evaluated.

Were abusive parents abused by their own parents? About one-third of parents who were abused when they were young go on to abuse their own children (Guild, Alto, & Toth, 2017). Thus, some, but not a majority, of abusive parents are involved in an intergenerational transmission of abuse.

Developmental Consequences of Abuse

Among the consequences of child maltreatment in childhood and adolescence are poor emotional regulation, attachment problems, problems in peer relations, difficulty in adapting to school, and other psychological problems such as depression and delinquency. These effects occur because the maltreatment alters psychological development in ways that increases risk for disordered emotions, thoughts, and behaviors (Jaffee, 2017). For instance, one longitudinal study found that early maltreatment was linked to emotional negativity (age 7) that increased poor emotional regulation (age 8), which in turn predicted an increase in internalizing symptoms (from age 8 to 9) (Kim-Spoon, Cicchetti, & Rogosch, 2013). As shown in Figure 5, another study found that maltreated young children in foster care were more likely to show abnormal stress hormone levels than middle-SES young children living with their birth family (Gunnar, Fisher, & The Early Experience, Stress, and Prevention Network, 2006). In that study, the abnormal stress

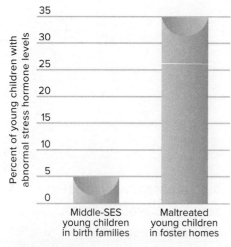

FIGURE 5

ABNORMAL STRESS HORMONE LEVELS IN YOUNG CHILDREN IN DIFFERENT TYPES OF REARING CONDITIONS

hormone levels were mainly present in the foster children who had been neglected, best described as "institutional neglect" (Fisher, 2005). Subsequent research has shown that adolescents who experienced abuse or neglect as children are more likely than adolescents who were not maltreated as children to engage in violent romantic relationships, delinquency, sexual risk taking, and substance abuse (Kaufman-Parks & others, 2017; Shin, Hong, & Hazen, 2010). Repeated exposure to abuse in childhood even has been linked with subsequent suicide attempts before age 18 (Jonson-Reid, Kohl, & Drake, 2012).

Later, during the adult years, individuals who were maltreated as children are more likely to experience problems with physical health, mental health, and sexual function (Lacelle & others, 2012). A groundbreaking 30-year longitudinal study found that middle-aged adults who had experienced child maltreatment had increased risk for diabetes, lung disease, malnutrition, and vision problems (Widom & others, 2012). A comprehensive analysis of many studies revealed that child maltreatment was linked to depression in adulthood and to unfavorable outcomes for treatment of depression (Nanni, Uher, & Danese, 2012). Further, adults who were maltreated as children often have difficulty in establishing and maintaining healthy intimate relationships (Dozier, Stovall-McClough, & Albus, 2009). As adults, maltreated children are also at higher risk for violent behavior toward other adults—especially dating partners and marital partners—as well as for substance abuse, anxiety, and depression (Miller-Perrin, Perrin, & Kocur, 2009).

A critically important agenda is to discover how to prevent child maltreatment in high-risk settings and families or to intervene in children's lives as soon as possible after they have been maltreated (Guild, Alto, & Toth, 2017; Jaffee, 2017). This may best be accomplished by taking a "public health" approach toward expanding supports for positive, enriching parenting and toward minimizing harsh abusive child rearing. In "Triple P," the most widely used parenting prevention and intervention program in the world, emphasis is placed on strengthening positive parenting by building parents' self-control and sense of competency and self-worth in the parenting role (M. Sanders, 2008; Shapiro, Prinz, & Sanders, 2012).

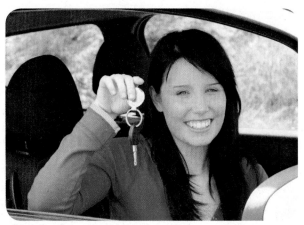
What are strategies that parents can use to guide adolescents in effectively handling their increased motivation for autonomy?
Wavebreakmedia Ltd/Getty Images

PARENT-ADOLESCENT RELATIONSHIPS

Even the best parents may find their relationship with their child strained during adolescence. Important aspects of parent-adolescent relationships include autonomy/attachment and conflict.

Autonomy and Attachment With most adolescents, parents are likely to find themselves engaged in a delicate balancing act, weighing competing needs for autonomy and control, for independence and connection.

The Push for Autonomy The typical adolescent's push for autonomy and responsibility puzzles and angers many parents. Most parents anticipate that their teenager will have some difficulty adjusting to the changes that adolescence brings, but few parents imagine and predict just how strong an adolescent's desires will be to spend time with peers or how intensely adolescents will want to show that it is they—not their parents—who are responsible for their successes and failures.

Adolescents' ability to attain autonomy and gain control over their behavior is acquired through appropriate adult reactions to their desire for control (Laursen & Collins, 2009; McElhaney & Allen, 2012). At the onset of adolescence, the average individual does not have the knowledge to make appropriate or mature decisions in all areas of life. As the adolescent pushes for autonomy, the wise adult relinquishes control in those areas where the adolescent can make reasonable decisions, but continues to guide the adolescent to make reasonable decisions in areas in which the adolescent's knowledge is more limited. Gradually, adolescents acquire the ability to make mature decisions on their own. In two longitudinal studies of multiple ethnic groups in the United States, young adolescents with parents who promoted more psychological autonomy and less psychological control had fewer depressive symptoms in adolescence and later in development, although the

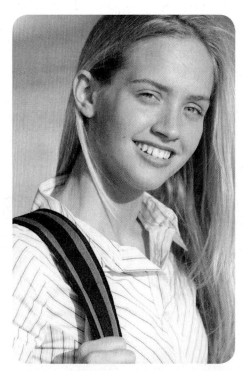
According to one adolescent, Stacey Christensen, age 16: "I am lucky enough to have open communication with my parents. Whenever I am in need or just need to talk, my parents are there for me. My advice to parents is to let your teens grow at their own pace, be open with them so that you can be there for them. We need guidance; our parents need to help but not be too overwhelming."
Stockbyte/Getty Images

effects varied by ethnicity, suggesting important cultural factors in this process (Eagleton, Williams, & Merten, 2016; Sher-Censor, Parke, & Coltrane, 2011).

Gender differences characterize autonomy-granting in adolescence. Some studies show that boys are given more independence than girls. In one older study, this was especially true in U.S. families with a traditional gender-role orientation (Bumpus, Crouter, & McHale, 2001). However, a meta-analysis of many studies suggested these gender differences are small (Endendijk & others, 2016). Also, Latino parents protect and monitor their daughters more closely than is the case for non-Latino White parents (McElhaney & Allen, 2012; Updegraff & others, 2010). Although Latino cultures may place a stronger emphasis on parental authority and restrict adolescent autonomy, one study revealed that regardless of where they were born, Mexican-origin adolescent girls living in the United States had expectations for autonomy at an earlier age than their mothers preferred (Bamaca-Colbert & others, 2012).

The Role of Attachment   Recall that one of the most widely discussed aspects of socioemotional development in infancy is secure attachment to caregivers. In the past decade, researchers have explored whether secure attachment also might be an important aspect of adolescents' relationships with their parents (Laursen & Collins, 2009). For example, Joseph Allen and his colleagues have reported that adolescents who were securely attached at 14 years of age were more likely to report that they were in an exclusive relationship, comfortable with intimacy in relationships, and achieving increased financial independence at 21 years of age (Szwedo & others, 2017). A detailed analysis shows that the most consistent outcomes of secure attachment in adolescence involve positive peer relations and development of the adolescent's emotion-regulation capacities (Allen & Miga, 2010).

Balancing Freedom and Control   We have seen that parents play very important roles in adolescent development (McKinney & Renk, 2011). Although adolescents are moving toward independence, they still need to stay connected with families (McElhaney & Allen, 2012). For example, the National Longitudinal Study on Adolescent Health surveyed more than 12,000 adolescents and found that those who ate dinner with a parent multiple times each week had lower rates of smoking, drinking, marijuana use, depressive symptoms, aggression, and other delinquent activities—effects that were strongest in families with close relationships (Meier & Musick, 2014).

Parent-Adolescent Conflict   Although parent-adolescent conflict increases in early adolescence, it does not reach the tumultuous proportions G. Stanley Hall envisioned at the beginning of the twentieth century (Laursen & Collins, 2009). Rather, much of the conflict involves the everyday events of family life, such as keeping a bedroom clean, dressing neatly, getting home by a certain time, and not talking or text messaging for hours at a time. The conflicts rarely involve major issues such as drugs or delinquency.

Conflict with parents often escalates during early adolescence, remains somewhat stable during the high school years, and then lessens as the adolescent reaches 17 to 20 years of age. Parent-adolescent relationships become more positive if adolescents go away to college than if they attend college while living at home (Sullivan & Sullivan, 1980).

The everyday conflicts that characterize parent-adolescent relationships may actually serve a positive developmental function. These minor disputes and negotiations facilitate the adolescent's transition from being dependent on parents to being an autonomous individual. Recognizing that conflict and negotiation can serve a positive developmental function can tone down parental hostility.

The old model of parent-adolescent relationships suggested that as adolescents mature they detach themselves from parents and move into a world of autonomy apart from parents. The old model also suggested that parent-adolescent conflict is intense and stressful throughout adolescence. The new model emphasizes that parents serve as important attachment figures and support systems while adolescents explore a wider, more complex social world. The new model also emphasizes that, in most families, parent-adolescent conflict is moderate rather than severe and that the everyday negotiations and minor disputes not only are normal but also

When I was a boy of 14, my father was so ignorant I could hardly stand to have the man around. But when I got to be 21, I was astonished at how much he had learnt in seven years.

—MARK TWAIN
American writer and humorist, 19th century

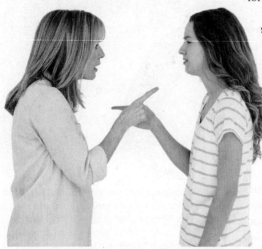

Conflict with parents increases in early adolescence. *What is the nature of this conflict in a majority of American families?*
Wavebreak Media/age fotostock

Old Model	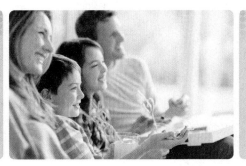	New Model
Autonomy, detachment from parents; parent and peer worlds are isolated		Attachment and autonomy; parents are important support systems and attachment figures; adolescent-parent and adolescent-peer worlds have some important connections
Intense, stressful conflict throughout adolescence; parent-adolescent relationships are filled with storm and stress on virtually a daily basis		Moderate parent-adolescent conflict is common and can serve a positive developmental function; conflict greater in early adolescence

FIGURE 6

OLD AND NEW MODELS OF PARENT-ADOLESCENT RELATIONSHIPS

Martin Barraud/Caia Image/Glow Images

can serve the positive developmental function of helping the adolescent make the transition from childhood dependency to adult independence (see Figure 6).

Still, a high degree of conflict characterizes some parent-adolescent relationships. Researchers established long ago that this prolonged, intense conflict is associated with various adolescent problems: movement out of the home, juvenile delinquency, school dropout, pregnancy and early marriage, membership in religious cults, and drug abuse (Brook & others, 1990). A more recent study revealed that a higher level of parent-adolescent conflict was related to peer-reported aggression and delinquency (Ehrlich, Dykas, & Cassidy, 2012).

Cross-cultural studies reveal that parent-adolescent conflict is lower in some countries than in the United States, but higher in others. In the largest international longitudinal study to date of changes in youth-parent positive and negative relationship features as children enter early adolescence, researchers identified substantial differences in hostility across nine countries spanning five continents. The highest to lowest levels of hostility were reported in Jordan, Kenya, China, Philippines, Thailand, Colombia, Sweden, Italy, and the United States (Deater-Deckard & others, 2018; Putnick & others, 2012).

When families immigrate into another country, children and adolescents typically acculturate more quickly to the norms and values of their new home faster than do their parents (Fuligni, 2012). This likely occurs because of immigrant children's and adolescents' exposure to school and the language of the host country (Titzmann & Gniewosz, 2017). The norms and values immigrant children and adolescents experience are especially likely to diverge from their parents in areas such as autonomy and romantic relationships. Such divergences are likely to increase parent-adolescent conflict in immigrant families. Andrew Fuligni (2012) argues that these conflicts aren't always expressed in open conflict but are often present in underlying, internal feelings. For example, immigrant adolescents may feel that their parents want them to give up their personal interests for the sake of the family, and the adolescents don't think this is fair. Such acculturation-based conflict focuses on issues related to core cultural values and is likely to occur in immigrant families, such as Latino and Asian American families, who come to the United States to live (Gassman-Pines & Skinner, 2018; Juang & Umana-Taylor, 2012).

INTERGENERATIONAL RELATIONSHIPS

Connections between generations play important roles in development through the life span (Antonucci, Birditt, & Ajrouch, 2013; Fingerman & others, 2012). With each new generation, personality characteristics, attitudes, and values are replicated or changed through relationships, stories, and shared memories (Pratt & others, 2008; Shore & Kauko, 2017). As older family members die, their biological, intellectual, emotional, and personal legacies are carried on in the next generation. Their children become the oldest generation and their grandchildren the second generation. In many families, females' relationships across generations are closer and more intimate than are males' relationships (Etaugh & Bridges, 2010).

The generations of living things pass in a short time, and like runners hand on the torch of life.

—LUCRETIUS
Roman poet, 1st century BC

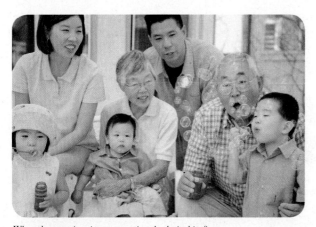

What characterizes intergenerational relationships?
Hill Street Studios/Blend Images LLC

The following studies provide evidence of the importance of intergenerational relationships in children's development:

• Supportive family environments and parenting in childhood (assessed when the children were 3 to 15 years of age) were linked with more positive relationships (in terms of contact, closeness, conflict, and reciprocal assistance) between the children and their middle-aged parents when the children were 26 years of age (Belsky & others, 2001).

• Children of divorce were disproportionately likely to end their own marriage than were children from intact, never-divorced families. Although the transmission of divorce across generations has declined in recent decades (Wolfinger, 2011), the effect persists when nonmarital cohabitation is included (Amato & Patterson, 2017).

• Parents who smoked early and often, and persisted in becoming regular smokers, were more likely to have adolescents who became smokers (Chassin & others, 2008), even when ill health effects such as asthma were present (Clawson & others, 2018).

• Evidence was found for the intergenerational transmission of conduct disorder (multiple delinquent activities) across three generations, with the connection stronger for males than females (D'Onofrio & others, 2007).

Review Connect Reflect

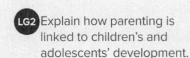 Explain how parenting is linked to children's and adolescents' development.

Review

• What characterizes parental roles and the timing of parenthood?
• In what ways do parents need to adapt their behavior to developmental changes in their children?
• How can parents be effective managers of children's lives?
• What are the main parenting styles and variations in discipline?
• What are some important aspects of parenting adolescents?
• How do intergenerational relationships influence children's development?

Connect

• In this section, we learned about Baumrind's four parenting styles.

Earlier, we learned about three types of discipline techniques. Which techniques are more likely to be used by parents from each parenting style?

Reflect *Your Own Personal Journey of Life*

• What was the nature of your relationship with your parents during middle school and high school? Has your relationship with your parents changed since then? Does it involve less conflict today? What do you think are the most important characteristics of a competent parent of adolescents?

Siblings Identify how siblings influence children's development.

Sibling Relationships

Birth Order

What are sibling relationships like? How extensively does birth order influence behavior?

SIBLING RELATIONSHIPS

Approximately 77 percent of American children have one or more siblings—that is, sisters and brothers (Dunn, 2007). If you grew up with siblings, you probably have a rich memory of aggressive, hostile interchanges. Siblings in the presence of each other when they are 2 to 4 years of age, on average, have a conflict once every 10 minutes. The conflicts go down somewhat from 5 to 7 years of age (Kramer, 2006). One study revealed that higher sibling conflict was linked to increased depressive and delinquency symptoms, whereas higher sibling intimacy was related to positive, prosocial behavior (Harper, Padilla-Walker, & Jensen, 2016). A research review concluded that sibling relationships in adolescence are not as close, are not as intense, and are more egalitarian than in childhood (East, 2009).

Issues of equality and fairness, as well as invasion of one's personal domain, are common in sibling relationships. A study of young adolescents revealed that sibling conflicts involving equality and fairness were associated with an increase in depressed mood one year later, while conflicts associated with invasion of one's personal domain were linked to higher anxiety and lower self-esteem one year later (Campione-Barr, Bassett Greer, & Kruse, 2013).

What do parents do when they encounter siblings in the midst of a verbal or physical confrontation? Several studies have shown that they do one of three things: (1) most commonly, parents will intervene and try to help them resolve the conflict by encouraging resolution through communication, followed by (2) ignoring and intentionally not intervening so that they work it out on their own, or (3) least commonly, admonishing them or telling them to physically stand up to each other (Kramer & Perozynski, 1999; Tucker & Kazura, 2013). Many parents believe that siblings should learn to resolve conflict on their own.

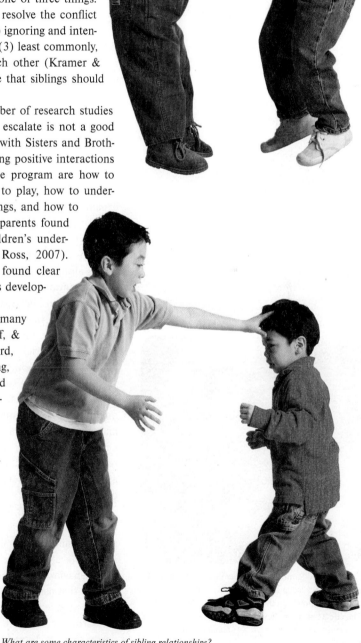

However, Laurie Kramer (2006), who has conducted a number of research studies on siblings, says that not intervening and letting sibling conflict escalate is not a good strategy. She developed a now classic program titled "More Fun with Sisters and Brothers" that teaches 4- to 8-year-old siblings social skills for developing positive interactions (Kramer & Radey, 1997). Among the social skills taught in the program are how to appropriately initiate play, how to accept and refuse invitations to play, how to understand another person's perspective, how to deal with angry feelings, and how to manage conflict. A study of 5- to 10-year-old siblings and their parents found that training parents to mediate sibling disputes increased children's understanding of conflicts and reduced sibling conflict (Smith & Ross, 2007). A comprehensive review of these types of family interventions found clear evidence of positive effects on sibling relationships and children's development (Tucker & Finkelhor, 2017).

As intense as it can be, however, conflict is only one of the many dimensions of sibling relations (Dunn, 2013; McHale, Updegraff, & Whiteman, 2011; Milevsky, 2011; Whiteman, Jensen, & Bernard, 2012). Sibling relations include helping, sharing, teaching, fighting, and playing, and siblings can act as emotional supports, rivals, and communication partners (East, 2009)—dimensions that also influence relationships with peers (Smorti & Ponti, 2018).

Judy Dunn (2007), a leading expert on sibling relationships, described three important characteristics of sibling relationships that have been evident for many years and across diverse family and cultural contexts:

- *Emotional quality of the relationship.* Both intensive positive and negative emotions are often expressed by siblings toward each other. Many children and adolescents have mixed feelings toward their siblings.

- *Familiarity and intimacy of the relationship.* Siblings typically know each other very well, and this intimacy suggests that they can either provide support or tease and undermine each other, depending on the situation.

- *Variation in sibling relationships.* Some siblings describe their relationships more positively than others. Thus, there

What are some characteristics of sibling relationships?
(Top) RubberBall Productions/Getty Images; (Bottom) RubberBall Productions/Getty Images

is considerable variation in sibling relationships. We previously indicated that many siblings have mixed feelings about each other, but some children and adolescents mainly describe their sibling in warm, affectionate ways, whereas others primarily talk about how irritating and mean a sibling is.

Negative aspects of sibling relationships, such as high conflict, are linked to negative outcomes for adolescents. The negative outcomes can develop not only through conflict but also through direct modeling of a sibling's behavior, as when a younger sibling has an older sibling who has poor study habits and engages in delinquent behavior. By contrast, close and supportive sibling relationships can buffer the negative effects of stressful circumstances in an adolescent's life (East, 2009; Hollifield & Conger, 2015). Studies in multiple cultures and of different-aged siblings consistently show the positive role that siblings play in each others' lives, with youth in non-Western nations and cultures taking on more formal caregiving and teaching roles compared with their Western counterparts (Hughes, McHarg, & White, 2018).

BIRTH ORDER

Whether a child has older or younger siblings has been linked to development of certain personality characteristics. For example, a thorough review of the research concluded that "firstborns are the most intelligent, achieving, and conscientious, while later-borns are the most rebellious, liberal, and agreeable" (Paulhus, 2008, p. 210). Compared with later-born children, firstborn children have also been described as more adult oriented, helpful, conforming, and self-controlled. However, when such birth order differences are reported, they often are small. Indeed, the most extensive large-scale rigorous analysis of multiple datasets showed only a small effect, and only for intelligence (Rohrer, Egloff, & Schmukle, 2015).

When birth order effects are found, what accounts for these differences? Proposed explanations usually point to variations in interactions with parents and siblings associated with being in a particular position in the family. This is especially true in the case of the firstborn child (Teti, 2001). The oldest child is the only one who does not have to share parental love and affection with other siblings—until another sibling comes along (on average, two to three years after the firstborn child). An infant requires more attention than an older child; this means that the firstborn sibling receives less attention after the newborn arrives. Does this result in conflict between parents and the firstborn? In one classic research study, mothers became more negative, coercive, and restraining and played less with the firstborn following the birth of a second child (Dunn & Kendrick, 1982).

What is the only child like? The popular conception is that the only child is a "spoiled brat," with such undesirable characteristics as dependency, lack of self-control, and self-centered behavior. But researchers present a more positive portrayal of the only child. Classic studies showed that only children often are achievement oriented and display a desirable personality, especially in comparison with later-borns and children from large families (Falbo & Poston, 1993; Jiao, Ji, & Jing, 1996). More recently, researchers noted potential brain-based differences corresponding to cognitive and behavioral differences between only children and those with siblings (Yang & others, 2017).

Still, as popular as the ideas about birth order might be, researchers have concluded that when all of the factors that influence behavior are considered, birth order and being an only child show limited ability to predict behavior.

Think about some of the other important factors in children's lives that influence their behavior beyond birth order. They include heredity, models of competency or incompetency that parents present to children on a daily basis, peer influences, school influences, socioeconomic factors, sociohistorical factors, and cultural variations. When someone says firstborns are always like this but last-borns are always like that, the person is making overly simplistic statements that do not adequately take into account the complexity of influences on a child's development.

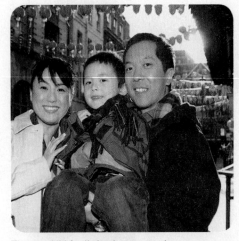

The one-child family has become much more common in China because of the strong motivation to limit population growth in the People's Republic of China. The effects of this policy are currently being examined. *In general, what have researchers found the only child to be like?*

Image Source/Getty Images

Review Connect Reflect

LG3 Identify how siblings influence children's development.

Review

- How can sibling relationships be characterized?
- What role does birth order play in children's development?

Connect

- In this section, you learned that parents typically respond in one of three ways to sibling conflict. How do these three ways align with Baumrind's parenting styles discussed earlier in this chapter?

Reflect *Your Own Personal Journey of Life*

- If you grew up with a sibling, you likely showed some jealousy of your sibling and vice versa. If you had one or more siblings, how did your parents handle sibling conflict? If and when you become a parent and have two or more children, what strategies will you use to reduce sibling conflict?

The Changing Family in a Changing Social World

LG4 Characterize the changing family in a changing social world.

Working Parents | Children in Divorced Families | Stepfamilies | Gay and Lesbian Parents | Cultural, Ethnic, and Socioeconomic Variations in Families

U.S. children are growing up in a greater variety of family contexts than ever before and are experiencing many sorts of caregiving—not only from stay-at-home mothers but also from stay-at-home fathers, from various types of child-care programs, and from after-school programs. The structure of American families also varies. As shown in Figure 7, the United States has a higher percentage of single-parent families than other countries with similar levels of economic and technological development. And many U.S. children are being raised in stepfamilies formed after a divorce and by gay or lesbian parents. How are these and other variations in family life affecting children?

WORKING PARENTS

The increased number of mothers in the labor force represents one source of change in families and society in the United States (Goodman & others, 2011; Grzywacz & Demerouti, 2013). Many mothers spend the greatest part of their day away from their children, even their infants. More than one of every two mothers with a child under the age of 5 is in the labor force; more than two of every three mothers with a child from 6 to 17 years of age work outside the home. How have these changes influenced children's development?

> ### developmental **connection**
>
> **Family Processes**
>
> Research consistently shows that family factors are considerably better at predicting children's developmental outcomes than are child-care experiences. Connect to "Emotional Development."

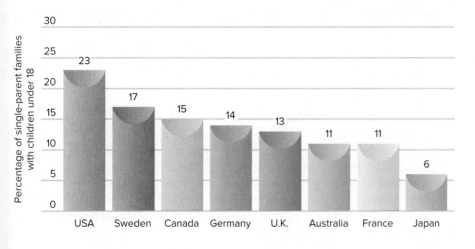

FIGURE 7

SINGLE-PARENT FAMILIES IN DIFFERENT COUNTRIES

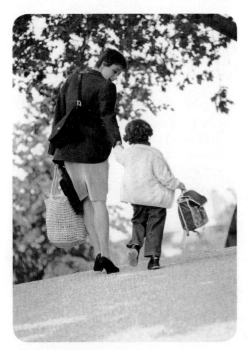

How does work affect parenting?
Eric Audras/Photoalto/Getty Images

Most research on parental work has focused on young children and the mother's employment (Brooks-Gunn, Han, & Waldfogel, 2010). Research on maternal employment and children's development usually reveals few links between the mother's work status and children's cognitive and socioemotional development (Goldberg & Lucas-Thompson, 2008). However, maternal employment may be especially influential in the first several years of the child's life. For example, a study of low-income families found that 7-year-old children whose mothers were employed early, especially in the first 8 months, had better socioemotional functioning than their peers whose mothers had remained unemployed (Coley & Lombardi, 2013). Most recently, this evidence has been seen in large studies conducted in numerous industrialized countries including the United States, Canada, Australia, and the United Kingdom (Lightbody & Williamson, 2017; Lombardi & Coley, 2017).

However, it is important to recognize that the effects of parental work outside the home involve the father as well as the mother when such matters as work schedules and work-family stress are considered (O'Brien & Moss, 2010; Parke & Clarke-Stewart, 2011; Peeters & others, 2013). Extensive research indicates that children's development is affected more strongly by the qualities of parents' work (for example, stressfulness and lack of control in scheduling and hours) than by the employment of one or both parents outside the home (Goodman & others, 2011; Han, 2009; Parke & Clarke-Stewart, 2011). Importantly, the "conflict" parents experience between meeting the demands of their work, and taking care of their partners and children at home, is more similar than different when fathers and mothers are compared across all published studies (Shockley & others, 2017).

Ann Crouter (2006), a researcher who has studied working couples and parenting for decades, described how parents bring their experiences at work into their homes. She concluded that parents who have poor working conditions, such as long hours, overtime work, stressful work, and lack of autonomy on the job, are likely to be more irritable at home and engage in less effective parenting than their counterparts who enjoy better working conditions. One important finding is the children (especially girls) of working mothers engage in less gender stereotyping and have more egalitarian views of gender (Goldberg & Lucas-Thompson, 2008). Interestingly, recent evidence from research on government-mandated family and work policy changes in Scandinavia, in which fathers and mothers are required to take similar amounts of time off from work to care for family members, has shown positive effects on children's academic and social-emotional functioning (Cools, Fiva, & Kirkebøen, 2015).

CHILDREN IN DIVORCED FAMILIES

Divorce rates rose significantly in the United States and many countries around the world during the late twentieth century (Amato & Dorius, 2010). The U.S. divorce rate increased dramatically in the 1960s and 1970s but has declined since the 1980s. However, the divorce rate in the United States is still much higher than in most other countries—even when compared with nations in Europe and South America that have similar economies and family policies (OECD, 2016).

When divorce rates were at their highest level, it was estimated that around 40 percent of children born to married parents in the United States would experience their parents' divorce (Hetherington & Stanley-Hagan, 2002). This percentage has increased slightly in recent decades, in part because more children have parents who live together but do not marry (which means it is legally easier to separate than if they were married). Let's examine some important questions about children in divorced families:

- *Are children better adjusted in intact, never-divorced families than in divorced families?* Most researchers agree that children from divorced families show poorer adjustment than their counterparts in nondivorced families (Amato & Dorius, 2010; Hetherington, 2006; Lansford, 2009, 2012; Wallerstein, 2008) (see Figure 8). Those who have experienced multiple divorces are at greater risk. Children in divorced families are more likely than children in nondivorced families to have academic problems, to show externalized problems (such as

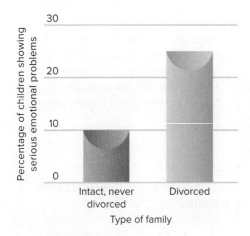

FIGURE **8**

DIVORCE AND CHILDREN'S EMOTIONAL PROBLEMS. In Hetherington's classic studies, 25 percent of children from divorced families showed serious emotional problems compared with only 10 percent of children from intact, never-divorced families. However, keep in mind that a substantial majority (75 percent) of the children from divorced families did not show serious emotional problems.

acting out and delinquency) and internalized problems (such as anxiety and depression), to be less socially responsible, to have less competent intimate relationships, to drop out of school, to become sexually active at an early age, to take drugs, to associate with antisocial peers, to have low self-esteem, and to be less securely attached as young adults (Lansford, 2009). For example, one study revealed that adolescent girls with divorced parents were especially vulnerable to developing depressive symptoms (Oldehinkel & others, 2008). Another study found that experiencing a divorce in childhood was associated with insecure attachment in early adulthood (Brockmeyer, Treboux, & Crowell, 2005). And a subsequent study found that adolescent girls from divorced families displayed lower levels of romantic competence (Shulman & others, 2012). More recently, a comprehensive meta-analysis of many published studies has shown impacts of divorce on children's subsequent risk for depression (Sands, Thompson, & Gaysina, 2017). Nonetheless, it is important to remember that most of the children in divorced families do *not* have significant adjustment problems and that the statistical effects of divorce are usually small.

- *Should parents stay together for the sake of the children?* Whether parents should stay in an unhappy or conflicted marriage for the sake of their children is one of the most commonly asked questions about divorce (Deutsch & Pruett, 2009; Hetherington, 2006; Ziol-Guest, 2009). If the stresses and disruptions in family relationships associated with an unhappy, conflictual marriage that erode the well-being of children are reduced by the move to a divorced, single-parent family, divorce can be advantageous. However, if the diminished resources and increased risks associated with divorce also are accompanied by inept parenting and sustained or increased conflict, not only between the divorced couple but also among the parents, children, and siblings, the best choice for the children would be for an unhappy marriage to be retained (Hetherington & Stanley-Hagan, 2002). It is difficult to determine how these "ifs" will play out when parents either remain together in an acrimonious marriage or become divorced.

  Note that marital conflict has negative consequences for children in the context of marriage or divorce (Cummings & Davies, 2010; Kleinsorge & Covitz, 2012). A longitudinal study revealed that conflict in nondivorced families was associated with emotional problems in children (Amato, 2006). Indeed, many of the problems that children from divorced homes experience begin during the predivorce period, a time when parents are often in active conflict with each other. This conflict increases risks of adjustment problems in part through cascading effects on other social relationships as children move through adolescence (Davies, Martin, & Cummings, 2018). Thus, when children from divorced homes show problems, the problems may be due not only to the divorce but to the marital conflict that led to it.

  E. Mark Cummings and his colleagues (Cummings & Davies, 2010; Cummings, El-Sheikh, & Kouros, 2009; Cummings & Kouros, 2008; Davies & others, 2019) have proposed emotional security theory, which has its roots in attachment theory and states that children appraise marital conflict in terms of their sense of security and safety in the family. These researchers make a distinction between marital conflict that is negative for children (such as hostile emotional displays and destructive conflict tactics) and marital conflict that can be positive for children (such as marital disagreement that involves a calm discussion of each person's perspective and working together to reach a solution). In one such study, Cummings and his colleagues (2018) found that parental conflict during the kindergarten year was linked to children's emotional insecurity later in childhood, which in turn was associated with adolescent adjustment, including higher levels of depression and anxiety.

- *How much do family processes matter in divorced families?* In divorced families, family processes matter a great deal (Hetherington, 2006; Lansford, 2009, 2012; Parke & Clarke-Stewart, 2011; Sigal & others, 2011). When the divorced

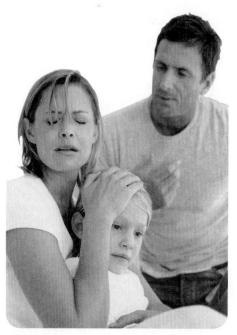

What concerns are involved in whether parents should stay together for the sake of the children or become divorced?
Zoey/Image Source/Getty Images

parents have a harmonious relationship and use authoritative parenting, the adjustment of adolescents is improved (Hetherington, 2006). When the divorced parents can agree on child-rearing strategies and can maintain a cordial relationship with each other, frequent visits by the noncustodial parent usually benefit the child (Fabricius & others, 2010). Following a divorce, father involvement with children drops off more than mother involvement, especially for fathers of girls. Also, one experiment conducted with divorced families revealed that an intervention focused on improving the mother-child relationship was linked to improvements in relationship quality that increased children's coping skills over the short term (6 months) and long term (6 years) (Velez & others, 2011).

- *What factors influence an individual child's vulnerability to suffering negative consequences as a result of living in a divorced family?* Among the factors influencing the child's risk and vulnerability are the child's adjustment prior to the divorce as well as the child's personality and temperament, gender, and custody situation (Hetherington, 2005, 2006). Children whose parents later divorce show poorer adjustment even *before* the breakup (Amato & Booth, 1996; Lansford, 2009), probably due to the conflict that is occurring. Children who are socially mature and responsible, who show few behavioral problems, and who have an easy temperament are better able to cope with their parents' divorce. Children with a difficult temperament often have problems coping with their parents' divorce (Hetherington, 2005).

  Early studies by Hetherington and others reported gender differences in response to divorce, with divorce being more negative for girls than boys in mother-custody families. However, subsequent studies have shown that gender differences are less pronounced and consistent than was previously believed. Some of the inconsistency may be due to the rise in father custody, joint custody, and increased involvement of noncustodial fathers, especially in their sons' lives (Ziol-Guest, 2009). One analysis of studies found that children in joint-custody families were better adjusted than children in sole-custody families (Bauserman, 2002). This effect, though small in size, has been seen across numerous studies in comprehensive analyses of published reports (Baude, Pearson, & Drapeau, 2016). Most importantly, however, joint custody works best for children when the parents can get along with each other (Parke & Clarke-Stewart, 2011). Some studies have shown that boys adjust better in father-custody families, girls in mother-custody families, whereas other studies have not seen this effect (Maccoby & Mnookin, 1992; Santrock & Warshak, 1979).

- *What role does socioeconomic status play in the lives of children in divorced families?* It was shown a few decades ago, and is still true today, that custodial mothers experience a much more substantial loss of their predivorce income, in comparison with the income loss for custodial fathers (Emery, 1994). However, with shifts in marriage, divorce, custody arrangements and employment patterns, this difference is getting smaller (Tamborini, Couch, & Reznik, 2015). Nevertheless, the income loss for divorced mothers is accompanied by increased workloads, high rates of job instability, and residential moves to less desirable neighborhoods with inferior schools (Lansford, 2009).

In sum, many factors are involved in determining how divorce influences a child's development (Amato & Dorius, 2010; Lansford, 2012). To read about some strategies for helping children cope with the divorce of their parents, see *Caring Connections*.

STEPFAMILIES

Not only has divorce become commonplace in the United States, so has getting remarried (Ganong, Coleman, & Jamison, 2011). It takes time for parents to marry, have children, get divorced, and then remarry. Consequently, there are far more elementary and secondary school children than infant or preschool children living in stepfamilies.

Communicating with Children About Divorce

More than thirty years ago Ellen Galinsky and Judy David (1988) developed a number of guidelines for communicating with children about divorce that are still helpful today.

Explain the Separation

As soon as daily activities in the home make it obvious that one parent is leaving, tell the children. If possible, both parents should be present when children are told about the separation to come. The reasons for the separation are very difficult for young children to understand. No matter what parents tell children, children can find reasons to argue against the separation. It is extremely important for parents to tell the children who will take care of them and to describe the specific arrangements for seeing the other parent.

Explain That the Separation Is Not the Child's Fault

Young children often believe their parents' separation or divorce is their own fault. Therefore, it is important to tell children that they are not the cause of the separation. Parents need to repeat this a number of times.

Explain That It May Take Time to Feel Better

Tell young children that it's normal to not feel good about what is happening and that many other children feel this way when their parents become separated. It is also okay for divorced parents to share some of their emotions with children, by saying something like "I'm having a hard time since the separation just like you, but I know it's going to get better after a while." Such statements are best kept brief and should not criticize the other parent.

Keep the Door Open for Further Discussion

Tell your children to come to you anytime they want to talk about the separation. It is healthy for children to express their pent-up emotions in discussions with their parents and to learn that the parents are willing to listen to their feelings and fears.

Provide as Much Continuity as Possible

The less children's worlds are disrupted by the separation, the easier their transition to a single-parent family will be. This means maintaining the rules already in place as much as possible. Children need parents who care enough to not only give them warmth and nurturance but also set reasonable limits.

Provide Support for Your Children and Yourself

After a divorce or separation, parents are as important to children as before the divorce or separation. Divorced parents need to provide children with as much support as possible. Parents function best when other people are available to give them support as adults and as parents. Divorced parents can find people who provide practical help and with whom they can talk about their problems.

How does the third piece of advice above correspond to what you have learned about emotion coaching?

As divorce and remarriage have become more acceptable in some cultures and legally less complicated in many locations, the number of remarriages involving children has grown steadily. Divorces occur at a much higher rate in remarriages than in first marriages (Cherlin & Furstenberg, 1994). Over half of all children whose parents divorce will have a stepparent within four years of the separation. More recent trends in the United States show that older adults are far more likely to remarry than younger adults, men remarry more often than women (although that gap is narrowing), and divorced non-Latino White adults are more likely to remarry than those with other racial and ethnic backgrounds (Livingston, 2014).

Remarried parents face some unique tasks. The couple must define and strengthen their marriage and at the same time renegotiate the biological parent-child relationships and establish stepparent-stepchild and stepsibling relationships (Ganong & Coleman, 2017). The complex histories and multiple relationships make adjustment difficult in a stepfamily (Goldscheider & Sassler, 2006). A majority of stepfamily couples do not stay remarried. And some remarried individuals are more adult-focused, responding more to the concerns of their partner, while

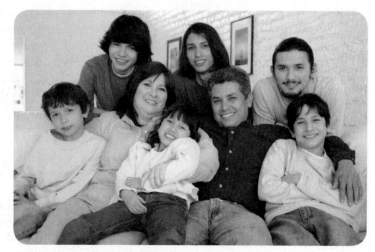

How does living in a stepfamily influence a child's development?
Todd Wright/Blend Images/Getty Images

others are more child-focused, responding more to the concerns of the children (Anderson & Greene, 2011).

In some cases, the stepfamily may have been preceded by the death of a spouse. However, by far the largest number of stepfamilies are preceded by divorce rather than death, and remarriage following divorce happens more quickly than after the death of a spouse—especially for men (Watkins & Waldron, 2017). Three common types of stepfamily structure are (1) stepfather, (2) stepmother, and (3) blended or complex. In stepfather families, the mother typically had custody of the children and remarried, introducing a stepfather into her children's lives. In stepmother families, the father usually had custody and remarried, introducing a stepmother into his children's lives. In a blended or complex stepfamily, both parents bring children from previous marriages to live in the newly formed stepfamily.

In E. Mavis Hetherington's (2006) classic longitudinal study, children and adolescents who had been in a simple stepfamily (stepfather or stepmother) for a number of years were adjusting better than in the early years of the remarried family and were functioning well in comparison with children and adolescents in conflicted nondivorced families and children and adolescents in complex (blended) stepfamilies. More than 75 percent of the adolescents in long-established simple stepfamilies described their relationships with their stepparents as "close" or "very close." Hetherington (2006) concluded that in long-established simple stepfamilies adolescents seem to eventually benefit from the presence of a stepparent and the resources provided by the stepparent.

Long-standing evidence has shown that children often have better relationships with their custodial parents (mothers in stepfather families, fathers in stepmother families) than with stepparents (Santrock, Sitterle, & Warshak, 1988). Also, children in simple families (stepmother, stepfather) often show better adjustment than their counterparts in complex (blended) families (Anderson & others, 1999; Hetherington & Kelly, 2002)—a pattern that still holds today, as shown in a review of over 100 published studies (Saint-Jacques & others, 2018).

A substantial research base shows that, as in divorced families, children in stepfamilies show more adjustment problems than children in nondivorced families. The adjustment problems are similar to those found among children of divorced parents—academic problems and lower self-esteem, for example (Anderson & others, 1999). However, it is important to recognize that a majority of children in stepfamilies do not have problems. In one analysis, 25 percent of children in stepfamilies showed adjustment problems compared with 10 percent in intact, never-divorced families (Hetherington & Kelly, 2002). Large comprehensive reviews of the literature similarly show small differences, on average (Saint-Jacques & others, 2018).

GAY AND LESBIAN PARENTS

Increasingly, gay and lesbian couples are creating families that include children (Patterson & D'Augelli, 2013; Patterson & Farr, 2012) (see Figure 9). Just over one-third of all lesbian and gay couples are parents (Gates, 2013; Patterson, 2004). Today, as many as 6 million children and adults may have an LGBT parent.

In 2015, same-sex marriage became legal everywhere in the United States, and today it is legal or permitted through "civil unions" in nearly 40 countries spanning North and South America, Oceania, and Europe, but not in Africa and Asia. Although these cultural and legal changes have occurred rapidly over the past decade, gay and lesbian parents vary greatly from each other—just like opposite-sex coparents. They may be single or they may have same-gender partners. Many lesbian mothers and gay fathers are noncustodial parents because they lost custody of their children to heterosexual spouses after a divorce. In addition, LGBT individuals are increasingly choosing parenthood through donor insemination or adoption. Researchers have found that the children conceived through new reproductive technologies—such as in vitro fertilization—are as well adjusted as their counterparts conceived by natural means (Golombok, 2017).

Researchers have found few differences in children growing up with gay fathers and lesbian mothers in comparison with adolescents growing up with heterosexual

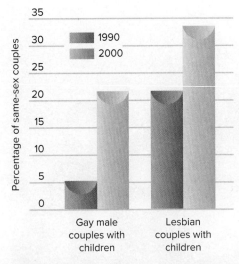

FIGURE 9

PERCENTAGE OF GAY MALE AND LESBIAN COUPLES WITH CHILDREN, 1990 AND 2000.
Why do you think more lesbian couples have children than gay male couples?

parents (Patterson, 2013). For example, children growing up in gay or lesbian families are just as popular with their peers, and there are no differences in the adjustment and mental health of children living in these families in comparison with children in heterosexual families (Hyde & DeLamater, 2011). The majority of children growing up in a gay or lesbian family have a heterosexual orientation (Golombok & Tasker, 2010).

CULTURAL, ETHNIC, AND SOCIOECONOMIC VARIATIONS IN FAMILIES

Parenting can be influenced by culture, ethnicity, and socioeconomic status. In Bronfenbrenner's theory, these influences are described as part of the macrosystem.

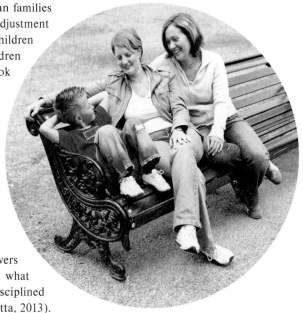

What are the research findings regarding the development and psychological well-being of children raised by gay and lesbian couples?
Creatas/Getty Images

Cross-Cultural Studies Different cultures often give different answers to such basic questions as what the father's role in the family should be, what support systems are available to families, and how children should be disciplined (Conger & others, 2012; Hewlett & McFarlen, 2010; Mistry, Contreras, & Dutta, 2013). There are important cross-cultural variations in parenting (Bornstein & Lansford, 2010). In some countries, authoritarian parenting is widespread. For example, in the Arab world, many families today are very authoritarian, dominated by the father's rule, and children are taught strict codes of conduct and family loyalty (Booth, 2002). In one study, Chinese mothers of preschool children reported that they used more physical coercion, more encouragement of modesty, more shaming and love withdrawal, less warmth, and less democratic participation than U.S. mothers of preschool children (Wu & others, 2002). In a subsequent study describing results from the largest cross-cultural longitudinal study of parenting and adolescent development, investigators reported noteworthy national and cultural differences in various aspects of parenting—especially with respect to firm control and emphasis on authority (Deater-Deckard & others, 2018).

What type of parenting is most frequent? In one classic study of parenting behavior in 186 cultures around the world, the most common pattern was a warm and controlling style, one that was neither permissive nor restrictive (Rohner & Rohner, 1981). The investigators commented that the majority of cultures have discovered, over many centuries, that children's healthy social development is most effectively promoted by love and at least moderate parental control.

Cultural change is coming to families in many countries around the world (Pieterse, 2020). There are trends toward greater family mobility, migration to urban areas, separation as some family members work in cities or countries far from their homes, smaller families, fewer extended-family households, and increases in maternal employment (Abela & Walker, 2013). These trends can change the resources that are available to children. For example, when several generations no longer live near each other, children may lose support and guidance from grandparents, aunts, and uncles. Also, smaller families may produce more openness and communication between parents and children.

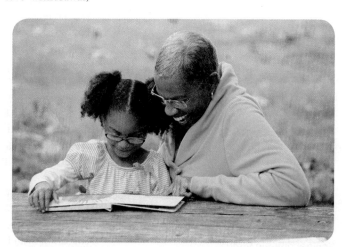

What are some characteristics of families in different ethnic groups?
Ronnie Kaufman/Larry Hirshowitz/Tetra Images, LLC/Alamy Stock Photo

Ethnicity Families within different ethnic groups in the United States differ in their typical size, structure, composition, reliance on kinship networks, and levels of income and education (Conger & others, 2012; Livas-Dlott & others, 2010). These differences reflect complex effects arising from cultural and socioeconomic forces. Large and extended families are more common among minority groups than among the non-Latino White majority (Wright & others, 2012). For example, in 2013 in

developmental **connection**

Culture and Ethnicity

Many families that have immigrated to the United States in recent decades, such as Mexican Americans and Asian Americans, come from collectivist cultures in which family obligation is strong. Connect to "Culture and Diversity."

the United States, 26 percent of Hispanic (the term used by the Census Bureau) individuals had families with five or more people (usually with three or more children), as compared with 14 percent of African American and 10 percent of non-Latino White families (Pew Research Center, 2015). African American and Latino children interact more with grandparents, aunts, uncles, cousins, and more-distant relatives than do non-Latino White children.

Single-parent families are more common among African Americans and Latinos than among White Americans (Zeiders, Roosa, & Tein, 2011). In 2017, 49 percent of African American youth under 18 years of age lived with their mother only, compared with 25 percent of Latino youth and 19 percent of non-Latino White youth (U.S. Census Bureau, 2018). In comparison with two-parent households, single parents often have more limited resources of time, money, and energy (Wright & others, 2012). Ethnic minority parents have less access to higher education and are more likely to live in low-income circumstances than their non-Latino White counterparts. Still, regardless of ethnicity, many impoverished families raise healthy, well-functioning children (Masten, 2018; McLoyd & others, 2009).

Some aspects of home life can help protect ethnic minority children from injustice and the harmful effects of discrimination. The family can filter out destructive racist messages, and parents can present alternative frames of reference to counter those presented by the majority. For example, popular media may present stories and images that emphasize racially charged and biased representations of non-White individuals. However, families and other social contexts in children's lives can show children and adolescents that those messages need not apply to them. The immediate and extended family also can serve as an important buffer to stress that is disproportionately experienced by youth in ethnic minority groups (McAdoo, 2006; Sanders, Munford, & Boden, 2017).

Of course, individual families vary in how they deal with stress—and ethnic majority and minority families are no different in this respect (Nieto & Bode, 2012; Schaefer, 2013; Urdan, 2012). Whether the parents are native-born or immigrants, how long the family has been in this country, their socioeconomic status, and their national origin all make a difference (Cooper, 2011). The characteristics of the family's social context also influence its adaptation. What are the attitudes toward the family's ethnic group within its neighborhood or city? Can the family's children attend good schools? Are there community groups that welcome people from the family's ethnic group? Do members of the family's ethnic group form community groups of their own? To read further about ethnic minority parenting, see *Connecting with Diversity*.

Socioeconomic Status   Low-income families have less access to resources than higher-income families do (Duncan, 2012; Duncan & others, 2013). The differential access to resources includes nutrition, health care, protection from danger, and enriching educational and socialization opportunities, such as tutoring and lessons in various activities. These differences are compounded in low-income families characterized by long-term poverty (Santiago & others, 2012).

In America and most Western cultures, differences also have been found in child rearing among different socioeconomic-status (SES) groups. These were noted nearly two decades ago (Hoff, Laursen, & Tardif, 2002, p. 246), and they persist today:

- "Lower-SES parents (1) are more concerned that their children conform to society's expectations, (2) create a home atmosphere in which it is clear that parents have authority over children," (3) use physical punishment more in disciplining their children, and (4) are more directive and less conversational with their children.
- "Higher-SES parents (1) are more concerned with developing children's initiative" and delay of gratification, "(2) create a home atmosphere in which children are more nearly equal participants and in which rules are discussed as opposed to being laid down" in an authoritarian manner, (3) are less likely to

developmental **connection**

Socioeconomic Status

Living in poverty has many psychological effects on both parents and children. Connect to "Culture and Diversity."

Acculturation and Ethnic Minority Parenting

Ethnic minority children and their parents "are expected to transcend their own cultural background and to incorporate aspects of the dominant culture" into children's development (Garcia Coll & Pachter, 2002, p. 7). They undergo varying degrees of **acculturation,** which refers to cultural changes that occur when one culture comes in contact with another. Asian American parents, for example, may feel pressed to modify the traditional training style of parental control discussed earlier as they encounter the more permissive parenting typical of the dominant culture.

The level of family acculturation can affect parenting style by influencing expectations for children's development, parent-child interactions, and the role of the extended family (Cooper, 2011; Fuligni, 2012). For example, in one study, the level of acculturation and maternal education were the strongest predictors of maternal-infant interaction patterns in Latino families (Perez-Febles, 1992).

The family's level of acculturation also influences important decisions about child care and early childhood education. For example, "an African American mother might prefer to leave her children with extended family while she is at work because the kinship network is seen as a natural way to cope with maternal absence. This well-intentioned, culturally appropriate decision might, however, put the child at an educational and social disadvantage relative to other children of similar age who have the benefit of important preschool experiences that may ease the transition into early school years" (Garcia Coll & Pachter, 2002, pp. 7–8). Less acculturated and more acculturated family members may disagree about the appropriateness of various caregiving practices, possibly creating conflict or confusion.

The opportunities for acculturation that young children experience depend mainly on their parents and extended family. If parents send the children to a child-care center, school, church, or other community setting, the children are likely to learn about the values and behaviors of the dominant culture, and they may be expected to adapt to that culture's norms. Thus, Latino children raised in a traditional

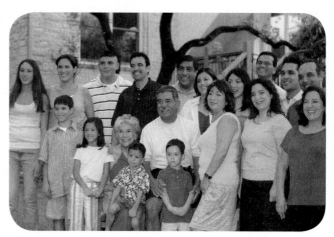

How is acculturation involved in ethnic minority parenting?
Jack Hollingsworth/Getty Images

family in which the family's well-being is considered more important than the individual's interests may attend a preschool in which children are rewarded for asserting themselves. Chinese American children, whose traditional parents value behavioral inhibition, may be rewarded outside the home for being active and emotionally expressive. Over time, the differences in the level of acculturation experienced by children and by their parents and extended family may grow (Garcia Coll & Pachter, 2002).

In this interlude you learned that preschools may encourage behavior that is at odds with some ethnic groups' parenting styles. Is this common worldwide? Which type of parenting is most frequently found worldwide?

use physical punishment, and (4) "are less directive and more conversational" with their children.

Parents in different socioeconomic groups also tend to think differently about education (Brazil, 2016; Huston & Ripke, 2006). Middle- and upper-income parents more often think of education as something that should be mutually encouraged by parents and teachers. By contrast, low-income parents are more likely to view education as the teacher's job. Thus, increased school-family linkages especially can benefit students from low-income families. In later chapters, we will have much more to say about socioeconomic variations in families, especially the negative ramifications of poverty for children's development, as well as other aspects of culture and its role in parenting and children's development.

acculturation Cultural changes that occur when one culture comes in contact with another culture.

Review

- How are children influenced by working parents?
- What characterizes the effects of divorce on children's development?
- How does living in a stepfamily influence children's development?
- How does growing up in a family with same-sex parents influence children's development?
- In what ways is children's development affected by their family's culture, ethnicity, and socioeconomic status?

Connect

- In this section, you learned that low-income families have less access to nutrition, health care, protection from danger, and enriching educational and socialization opportunities. What have you already learned regarding the specific health outcomes for children living in poverty?

Reflect *Your Own Personal Journey of Life*

- Now that you have studied many aspects of families in this chapter, imagine that you have decided to write a book on some aspect of your own family. What aspect of your family would you focus on? What would be the title of your book? What would be the major theme of the book?

reach your **learning goals**

Families

Family Processes

LG1 Discuss family processes.

Interactions in the Family System

Cognition and Emotion in Family Processes

Multiple Developmental Trajectories

Domain-Specific Socialization

Sociocultural and Historical Changes

- The family is a system of interrelated and interacting individuals with different subsystems—some dyadic, some polyadic. The subsystems have both direct and indirect effects on one another. Positive marital relations can have a positive influence on parenting. Reciprocal socialization is the bidirectional process in which children socialize parents just as parents socialize them.

- Cognition and emotion are central to understanding how family processes work. The role of cognition includes parents' cognitions, beliefs, and values about their parental role, as well as the way they perceive, organize, and understand their children's behaviors and beliefs. The role of emotion includes the regulation of emotion in children, understanding emotion in children, and emotion in carrying out the parenting role. Children learn to express and manage emotions appropriately through interaction with emotion-coaching parents and have fewer behavior problems than children of emotion-dismissing parents.

- Adults follow one developmental trajectory and children and adolescents another one. Comprehending how these trajectories mesh is important for understanding the effects of timing of entry into various family tasks.

- Increasingly a domain-specific approach to socialization is being emphasized. One proposal focuses on five domains, each linked to specific child outcomes. The five domains are protection, reciprocity, control, guided learning, and group participation.

- Changes in families may be due to great upheavals, such as war, or more subtle changes, such as technological advances and greater mobility of families. Today there are more divorced and remarried families than in previous centuries.

Parenting

Parental Roles and the Timing of Parenthood

Adapting Parenting to Developmental Changes in Children

Parents as Managers of Children's Lives

Parenting Styles and Discipline

Parent-Adolescent Relationships

Intergenerational Relationships

 LG2 Explain how parenting is linked to children's and adolescents' development.

- Currently, there is a trend toward having fewer children and choosing when to have children. Many adults are waiting longer to having children or not having children at all. Differences have been found between the parenting styles of older and younger parents.

- The transition to parenthood requires considerable adaptation and adjustment on the part of parents. As children grow older, parents increasingly turn to reasoning or withholding privileges in disciplining children. Parents spend less time with children in middle and late childhood, a time when parents play an especially important role in their children's academic achievement. Control is more coregulatory in middle and late childhood.

- A recent trend is to conceptualize parents as managers of children's lives. An important aspect of parenting infants involves managing and guiding infants' behavior. Parents play important roles as managers of children's opportunities, effectively monitoring children's relationships and acting as social initiators and arrangers. Parental monitoring is linked to lower levels of juvenile delinquency, and effective parental management is related to children's higher academic achievement.

- Authoritarian, authoritative, neglectful, and indulgent are the four main parenting styles. Authoritative parenting is associated with socially competent child behavior more than the other styles. However, ethnic variations in parenting styles indicate that in African American and Asian American families, some aspects of authoritarian parenting may benefit children. Latino parents often emphasize connectedness with the family and respect and obedience in their child rearing. There are a number of reasons not to use physical punishment in disciplining children. Intense punishment presents the child with an out-of-control model. Punishment can instill fear, rage, or avoidance in children. Punishment tells children what not to do rather than what to do. Punishment can be abusive. Coparenting has positive outcomes for children. Child maltreatment is a multifaceted problem that involves the cultural context and family influences. Child maltreatment places the child at risk for a number of developmental problems.

- Many parents have a difficult time when their adolescents push for autonomy. Secure attachment to parents increases the likelihood that adolescents will be socially competent. Conflict with parents often increases in early adolescence, but this conflict is generally moderate rather than severe. The increase in conflict probably serves the positive developmental functions of facilitating adolescent autonomy and identity. A subset of adolescents experience high parent-adolescent conflict, and this is linked with negative outcomes for adolescents.

- Connections between parents play important roles in development through the life span. An increasing number of studies indicate that intergenerational relationships influence children's development. Marital interaction, a supportive family environment, divorce, and conduct disorder in the child's family of origin are among the factors that are linked to the child's development.

Siblings

Sibling Relationships

Birth Order

LG3 Identify how siblings influence children's development.

- Three important aspects of sibling relationships involve (1) emotional quality of the relationship, (2) familiarity and intimacy of the relationship, and (3) variation in sibling relationships. Sibling relationships include not only conflict and fighting but also helping, teaching, sharing, and playing—and siblings can function as rivals, emotional supports, and communication partners.

- Birth order is related in certain ways to child characteristics. Firstborn children are more self-controlled, conforming, and argumentative; have more guilt and anxiety; and excel academically and professionally compared with later-born children. However, some critics argue that the influence of birth order has been overestimated as a predictor of child behavior.

The Changing Family in a Changing Social World

 LG4 Characterize the changing family in a changing social world.

Working Parents

Children in Divorced Families

Stepfamilies

Gay and Lesbian Parents

Cultural, Ethnic, and Socioeconomic Variations in Families

- In general, having both parents employed full-time outside the home has not been shown to have negative effects on children. However, depending on the circumstances, work can produce positive or negative effects on parenting. If parents experience poor working conditions, they frequently become inattentive to their children, who show more behavioral problems and do more poorly at school than children whose parents have better working conditions.

- Children in divorced families show more adjustment problems than their counterparts in nondivorced families. Whether parents should stay in an unhappy or conflicted marriage for the sake of the children is difficult to determine. Children show better adjustment in divorced families when parents' relationships with each other are harmonious and authoritative parenting is used. Factors to be considered regarding the adjustment of children in divorced families are adjustment prior to the divorce, personality and temperament, developmental status, gender, and custody arrangements. Income loss for divorced mothers may be linked with a number of stresses that can affect the child's adjustment.

- As in divorced families, children in stepfamilies have more problems than their counterparts in nondivorced families. Restabilization often takes longer in stepfamilies than in divorced families. Children often have better relationships with their biological parents than with their stepparents and show more problems in complex, blended families than simple ones.

- Just over one-third of all lesbian and gay couples are parents. There is considerable diversity among lesbian mothers, gay fathers, and their children. Researchers have found few differences between children growing up with gay or lesbian parents and children growing up with heterosexual parents.

- Cultures vary on a number of issues regarding families. African American and Latino children are more likely than White American children to live in single-parent families, larger families, and families with extended connections. Higher-SES families tend to avoid using physical discipline, strive to create a home atmosphere in which rules are discussed, and are concerned with developing children's initiative and delay of gratification. Lower-SES families are more likely to use physical punishment in disciplining their children, are more directive and less conversational, and want their children to conform to society's expectations.

key **terms**

acculturation 411
authoritarian parenting 391
authoritative parenting 391

coparenting 394
indulgent parenting 391
multiple developmental
   trajectories 384

neglectful parenting 391
reciprocal socialization 382
scaffolding 382

key **people**

Joseph Allen 398
Diana Baumrind 391
Urie Bronfenbrenner 382

Ruth Chao 392
Ann Crouter 404
Marilyn Davidov 384

Judy Dunn 401
Andrew Fuligni 399
Joan Grusec 384

E. Mavis Hetherington 408
Laurie Kramer 401

chapter **outline**

1 Peer Relations

Learning Goal 1 Discuss peer relations in childhood.

Exploring Peer Relations

The Developmental Course of Peer Relations in Childhood

The Distinct but Coordinated Worlds of Parent-Child and Peer Relations

Social Cognition and Emotion

Peer Statuses

Bullying

2 Play

Learning Goal 2 Describe children's play.

Play's Functions

Types of Play

Trends in Play

3 Friendship

Learning Goal 3 Explain friendship.

Friendship's Functions

Similarity and Intimacy

Gender and Friendship

Mixed-Age Friendships

Other-Sex Friendships

4 Peer Relations in Adolescence

Learning Goal 4 Characterize peer relations in adolescence.

Peer Pressure and Conformity

Cliques and Crowds

Romantic Relationships

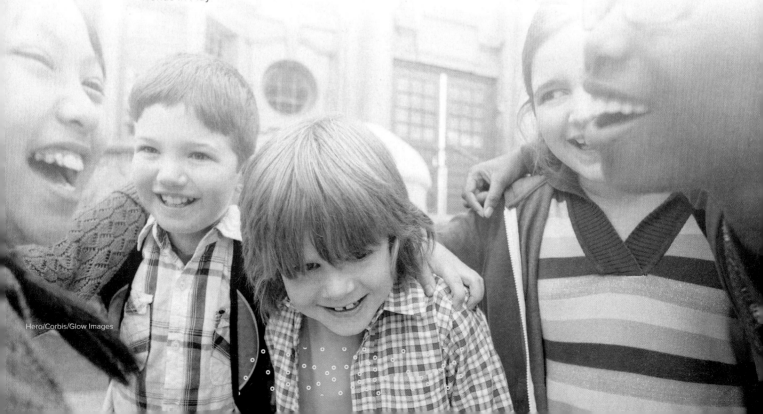

Hero/Corbis/Glow Images

Lynn Brown and Carol Gilligan conducted in-depth interviews of one hundred 10- to 13-year-old girls who were making the transition to adolescence. They listened to what these girls were saying.

A number of the girls talked about how many girls say nice things to be polite but often don't really mean them. The girls know the benefits of being perceived as the perfect, happy girl. Judy spoke about her interest in romantic relationships. Although she and her girlfriends were only 13, they wanted to be romantic, and she talked about her lengthy private conversations with her girlfriends about boys. Noura said that she learned how very painful it is to be the person everyone doesn't like.

Cliques figured largely in these girls' lives. They provided emotional support for girls who were striving to be perfect but knew they were not. Victoria commented that sometimes girls like her, who weren't very popular, nonetheless were accepted into a "club" with three other girls. Now when she was sad or depressed she could count on the "club" for support. Though they were "leftovers" and did not get into the most popular cliques, these four girls knew they were liked.

Through these interviews, we see the girls' curiosity about the social world they lived in. They kept track of what was happening to their peers and friends. The girls spoke at length about the pleasure they derived from the intimacy and fun of human connection, about the potential for hurt in relationships, and about the importance of friends (Brown & Gilligan, 1992).

preview

This chapter is about peers, who clearly are very important in the lives of the adolescent girls just described. They also are very important in the lives of children. We begin this chapter by examining a number of ideas about children's peer relations, including their functions and variations. Then we turn to children's play and the roles of friends in children's development. We conclude by discussing peer relationships in adolescence.

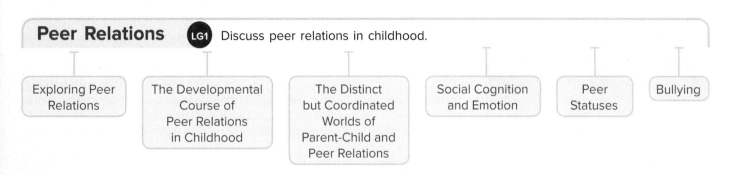

Peer Relations **LG1** Discuss peer relations in childhood.

- Exploring Peer Relations
- The Developmental Course of Peer Relations in Childhood
- The Distinct but Coordinated Worlds of Parent-Child and Peer Relations
- Social Cognition and Emotion
- Peer Statuses
- Bullying

As children grow up, they spend increasing amounts of time with their peers. What are some key aspects of peer relations?

EXPLORING PEER RELATIONS

Peers are children who share the same age or maturity level. They fill a unique role in the child's development. One of their most important functions is to provide a source of information and comparison about the world outside the family. Children receive feedback about their abilities from their peer group. They evaluate what they do in terms of whether it is better than, as good as, or worse than what other children do. It is hard to do this with siblings because they are usually older or younger.

Are Peers Necessary for Development? Good peer relations may be necessary for normal social development (Bukowski, Laursen, & Rubin, 2018; Brown & Larson, 2009; Rubin & others, 2013). Social isolation, or the inability to "plug in" to a social network, is linked with problems and disorders ranging from delinquency and problem drinking to depression (Benner, Hou, & Jackson, 2019; Bornstein, Jager, & Steinberg, 2013; Yearwood & others, 2019).

Positive and Negative Peer Relations Peer influences can be both positive and negative (Bauman & Bellmore, 2015; Rubin & others, 2013; Wentzel, 2018). For example, one study found that in early adolescence, the cognitive skills—or deficits—of our peers and close friends may play a key role in the development of our own skills and deficits (Boutwell, Meldrum, & Petkovsek, 2017). Children and adolescents explore the principles of fairness and justice by working through disagreements with peers. They also learn to be keen observers of peers' interests and perspectives in order to smoothly integrate themselves into ongoing peer activities. And children and adolescents learn to be skilled and sensitive partners in relationships by forging close friendships with selected peers. They carry these intimacy skills forward to help form the foundation of later romantic relationships.

Some researchers have emphasized the negative influences of peers on adolescents' development (McGloin & Thomas, 2019). Being rejected or overlooked by peers leads some adolescents to feel lonely or hostile. Further, such rejection and neglect by peers are related to an individual's subsequent mental health (Hymel & Espelage, 2018). For some adolescents, the peer culture is a corrupt influence that undermines parental values and control. Further, peer relations are linked to adolescents' patterns of drug use, delinquency, and depression. A growing body of research has found that low parental control is linked to higher delinquency

You are troubled at seeing him spend his early years in doing nothing. What! Is it nothing to be happy? Is it nothing to skip, to play, to run about all day long? Never in his life will he be so busy as now.

—JEAN-JACQUES ROUSSEAU
Swiss-born French philosopher, 18th century

peers Children who share the same age or maturity level.

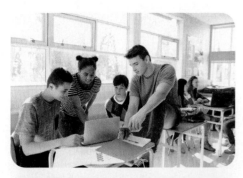

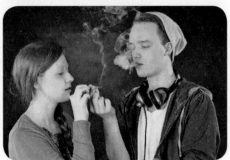

In what ways can peer relations be positive and negative?
(top) Hero Images/Getty Images; (bottom) KatarzynaBialasiewicz/ Getty Images

and substance use in adolescence through its association with deviant peer affiliation as well as through transmitted genetic factors (Deutsch, Wood, & Slutske, 2016).

As you read further about peers, keep in mind that findings about the influence of peers vary according to the way peer experience is defined and measured (Marks & others, 2019). "Peers" and "peer group" are global concepts. A "peer group" of an adolescent might refer to a neighborhood crowd, reference crowd, religious crowd, sports team, friendship group, and friends (Crosnoe, Pivnick, & Benner, 2018).

Peer Contexts   Peer interaction is influenced by contexts, which can include the type of peer the child or adolescent interacts with—such as an acquaintance, a crowd, a clique, a friend, or a romantic partner—and the situation or location—such as a school, neighborhood, community center, dance, religious setting, sporting event, and so on, as well as the culture in which the child or adolescent lives (Crosnoe, Pivnick, & Benner, 2018; Rubin & others, 2013). As they interact with peers in these various contexts, children and adolescents are likely to encounter different messages and different opportunities to engage in adaptive and maladaptive behavior that can influence their development (Milledge & others, 2018).

In terms of contexts, peers play an important role in the development of individuals in all cultures. However, as indicated in *Connecting with Diversity,* cultures vary in the significance of the socializing role of peers (Persike & Seiffge-Krenke, 2016; Way & Silverman, 2012).

Individual Difference Factors   Individual differences among peers also are important to consider in understanding peer relations (Cipra, 2019; Kulig & others, 2019). Among the wide range of individual differences that can affect peer relations are personality traits such as how shy or outgoing children are. For example, a very shy child is more likely than a sociable child to be neglected by peers and have anxiety about introducing himself or herself to new peers. Another individual difference factor that impairs peer relations is the trait of negative emotionality, which involves a relatively low threshold for experiencing anger, fear, anxiety, and irritation. For example, one study revealed that toddlers characterized by anger and tantrums tended to have poorer peer relations and social skills in elementary school, which in turn predicted poorer school success and adjustment in early adolescence (Dollar & others, 2018).

THE DEVELOPMENTAL COURSE OF PEER RELATIONS IN CHILDHOOD

Some researchers argue that the quality of peer interaction in infancy provides valuable information about socioemotional development (Hay, Kaplan, & Nash, 2018). For example, in one investigation, 8-month-old infants were not only found to show concern for a crying peer, but their behavioral responses sometimes helped calm the distressed infant (Liddle, Bradley, & McGrath, 2015). As increasing numbers of infants attend child care, peer interaction in infancy takes on a more important developmental role.

Around the age of 3, children already prefer to spend time with same-sex rather than opposite-sex playmates, and this preference increases in early childhood. One study of 4-year-olds found that gender was a strong influence on who children selected as playmates (Martin & others, 2013). In this study, young children selected playmates of the same sex with similar levels of gender-typed activities, with the child's sex being a more powerful influence than the child's activities.

During the preschool years the frequency of peer interaction, both positive and negative, increases considerably (Bukowski. Laursen, & Rubin, 2018; Rubin & others, 2013). Although aggressive interaction and rough-and-tumble play increase, the proportion of aggressive exchanges, compared with friendly exchanges, decreases gradually. Many preschool children spend considerable time in peer interaction just conversing with playmates about such matters as "negotiating roles and rules in play, arguing, and agreeing" (Rubin, Bukowski, & Parker, 2006).

In early childhood, children also distinguish between friends and non-friends (Howes, 2009). For most young children, a friend is someone to play with. Young

Cross-Cultural Comparisons of Peer Relations

In some countries, adults restrict adolescents' access to peers. For example, in many areas of rural India and in Arab countries, opportunities for peer relations in adolescence are restricted, especially for girls (Makhlouf Obermeyer, 2015). Many of the schools are sex-segregated. In these contexts, interaction with the other sex or opportunities for romantic relationships are less frequent (Gibbons & Poelker, 2019).

In an 18-country cross-cultural analysis, researchers surveyed nearly 5,000 youth around the globe to find out how they experienced stress and enjoyment in their relationships with their peers, friends, and their parents (Persike & Seiffge-Krenke, 2016). Overall, parents were perceived as a greater source of stress than peers. However, there were distinct regional patterns of differences in stress and coping

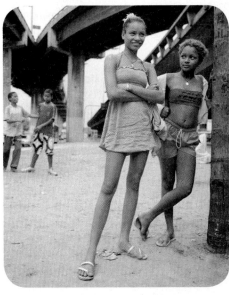

Street youth in Rio de Janeiro.
Tom Stoddart/Hulton Archive/Getty Images

perceptions; by comparison, gender differences were fairly small.

In some cultures, children are placed in peer groups for much greater lengths of time at an earlier age than they are in Western industrialized cultures like the United States. For example, in the Murian culture of eastern India, both male and female children live in a dormitory from the age of 6 until they get married (Barnouw, 1975). The dormitory is a religious haven where members are devoted to work and spiritual harmony. Children work for their parents, and the parents arrange the children's marriages.

In some cultural settings, peers even assume responsibilities usually handled by parents (Way & Silverman, 2012). For example, street youth in Brazil rely on networks of peers to help them negotiate survival in urban environments (Ursin, 2015).

Cross-cultural studies compare aspects of two or more cultures, and the comparison provides information about the degree to which development is similar—or universal—across cultures or is culture-specific.

---

preschool children are more likely than older children to have friends who are of a different gender or ethnicity (Howes, 2009).

As children enter the elementary school years, reciprocity becomes especially important in peer interchanges. Children play games, participate in groups, and cultivate friendships. The amount of time children spend in peer interaction also rises during middle and late childhood and adolescence. Researchers estimate that the percentage of time spent in social interaction with peers increases from approximately 10 percent at 2 years of age to more than 30 percent in middle and late childhood; there also is an increase in the size of the peer group and an increase in the amount of peer interaction that is not supervised by adults (Rubin, Bukowski, & Parker, 2006). These developmental changes have been enhanced by technology, with the dramatic growth of "online" interactions through social media among older children and teenagers (Pew Research Center, 2018a).

Peer interactions take varied forms—cooperative and competitive, boisterous and quiet, joyous and humiliating. There is increasing evidence that gender plays an important role in these interactions. Gender influences not only the composition of children's groups but also their size and the types of interactions within them (Corsaro, 2018). From about 5 years of age onward, boys tend to associate in large clusters more than girls do; girls are more likely than boys to play in groups of two or three. Boys' groups and girls' groups also tend to favor different types of activities. Boys' groups are more likely to engage in rough-and-tumble play, competition, conflict, ego displays, risk taking, and dominance seeking. By contrast, girls' groups are more likely to engage in collaborative discourse and activity (Mehta & Strough, 2009).

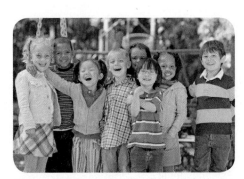

What are some developmental changes in peer relations?
Ariel Skelley/Blend Images

THE DISTINCT BUT COORDINATED WORLDS OF PARENT-CHILD AND PEER RELATIONS

Parents may influence their children's peer relations in many ways, both direct and indirect (Updegraff & others, 2010). Parents affect their children's peer relations through their interactions with their children, how they manage their children's lives, and the opportunities they provide their children (Brown & Bakken, 2011). For example, in an analysis of 10 longitudinal studies, parenting that was supportive and involved was not only associated with better peer relations but also these parenting and peer factors in combination predicted lower levels of antisocial behavior in adolescence (Walters, 2019).

Basic lifestyle decisions by parents—their choices of neighborhoods, religious organizations, schools, and their own friends—largely determine the pool from which their children select possible friends. These choices in turn affect which children their children meet, their purpose in interacting, and eventually which children become their friends.

Do these results indicate that children's peer relations always are determined by their parent-child relationships? Although parent-child relationships influence children's subsequent peer relations, children also learn other modes of interacting through their relationships with peers. For example, rough-and-tumble play occurs mainly with other children, not in parent-child interaction. In times of stress, children often turn to parents rather than peers for support. In parent-child relationships, children learn how to relate to authority figures. With their peers, children are likely to interact on a much more equal basis and to learn a mode of relating based on mutual influence. In these and other ways, peers provide unique opportunities for relationships that are distinct from family relationships.

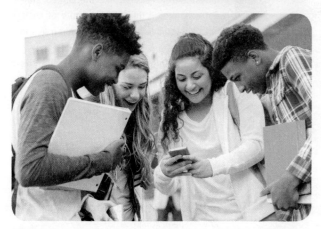

What are some links between relationships with parents and relationships with peers?

(top) Juanmonino/iStock/Getty Images; (bottom) Asiseeit/E+/Getty Images

One of the most consistent findings of attachment research involving adolescents is that secure attachment to parents is linked to positive peer relations (Allen & others, 2018). A large meta-analysis found that the link between mother and peer attachment was much stronger than the relation between father and peer attachment (Gorrese & Ruggieri, 2012).

However, whereas adolescent-parent attachments are correlated with adolescent outcomes, the correlations are not particularly strong, an indication that the success or failure of parent-adolescent attachments does not necessarily guarantee success or failure in peer relationships. Clearly, secure attachment with parents can be an asset for the adolescent, fostering the trust to engage in close relationships with others and lay down the foundation for close relationship skills. Nonetheless, some adolescents from strong, supportive families struggle in peer relations for a variety of reasons, such as being physically unattractive, maturing late, and experiencing cultural and socioeconomic-status (SES) discrepancies. On the other hand, some adolescents from troubled families find a positive, fresh start with peer relations that can compensate for their problematic family environments.

SOCIAL COGNITION AND EMOTION

Peer relations are not just about emotions and behaviors. Social relationships also are affected by *social cognition*, which involves thoughts about social situations (Carpendale & Lewis, 2015; Dodge, 2011a, b). For example, a young child named Mariana expects all her playmates to let her play with their toys whenever she asks. In another example, when Josh isn't picked for a team on the playground, he thinks his friends have turned against him. How might children's social cognitions contribute to their peer relations? Possible influences include children's perspective-taking ability, social information-processing skills, social knowledge, and emotional regulation.

Perspective Taking As children enter the elementary school years, both their peer interaction and their perspective-taking ability increase. *Perspective taking* involves

developmental **connection**

Attachment

Securely attached infants use the caregiver as a secure base from which to explore their environment. Connect to "Emotional Development."

developmental **connection**

Social Cognition

Social cognition refers to the processes involved in understanding the world around us, especially how we think and reason about others. Connect to "The Self and Identity."

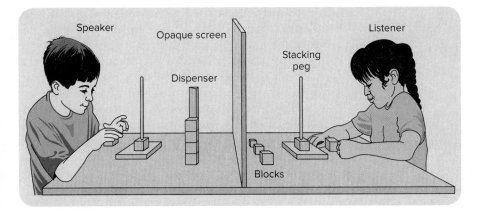

FIGURE **1**

THE DEVELOPMENT OF COMMUNICATION SKILLS. This experimental arrangement of speaker and listener has been used to investigate the development of communication skills.

perceiving another's point of view. Researchers have documented a link between perspective-taking skills and the quality of peer relations, especially in the elementary school years (Slaughter & others, 2015).

Perspective taking is important in part because it helps children communicate effectively. In one classic investigation, the communication exchanges among peers at kindergarten, first-, third-, and fifth-grade levels were evaluated (Krauss & Glucksberg, 1969). Children were asked to instruct a peer in how to stack a set of blocks. The peer sat behind a screen with blocks similar to those the other child was stacking (see Figure 1). The kindergarten children made numerous errors in telling the peer how to duplicate the novel block stack. The older children, especially the fifth-graders, were much more efficient in communicating to a peer how to stack the blocks. They were far superior at perspective taking and figuring out how to talk to a peer so that the peer could understand them. During the elementary school years, children also become more efficient at understanding complex messages, so the listening skills of the peer in this experiment probably helped the communicating peer as well.

Social Information-Processing Skills   How children process information about peer relationships also influences those relationships (Dodge, 2011a, b; Thomas, Connor, & Scott, 2018). For example, suppose Andrew accidentally trips and knocks Alex's soft drink out of his hand. Alex misinterprets the encounter as hostile, which leads him to retaliate aggressively against Andrew. Through repeated encounters of this kind, other peers come to perceive Alex as habitually acting inappropriately.

Peer relations researcher Kenneth Dodge (1993) argues that children go through five steps in processing information about their social world: decoding social cues, interpreting, searching for a response, selecting an optimal response, and enacting it. Dodge has found that aggressive boys are more likely to perceive another child's actions as hostile when the child's intention is ambiguous—and when aggressive boys search for clues to determine a peer's intention, they respond more rapidly, less efficiently, and less reflectively than nonaggressive children. These effects appear to be robust across cultural contexts. In a large nine-country international longitudinal study, biases in children's social information processing predicted aggressive behavior in the transition to early adolescence (Dodge & others, 2015).

Social Knowledge   As children and adolescents develop, they acquire more social knowledge (also sometimes referred to as social intelligence), and there is considerable individual variation in how much one child or adolescent knows about what it takes to make friends, to get peers to like him or her, and so forth (Knopp, 2019). A meta-analysis of studies involving a total of nearly 7,000 3- to-12-year-olds showed clear associations between stronger social knowledge and better social and academic adjustment in school (Voltmer & von Salisch, 2017).

Emotional Regulation   Not only does cognition play an important role in peer relations, so does emotion (Calkins, 2012; Lindsey, 2019). The ability to regulate emotion is linked to successful peer relations, and emotion dysregulation is a major contributing

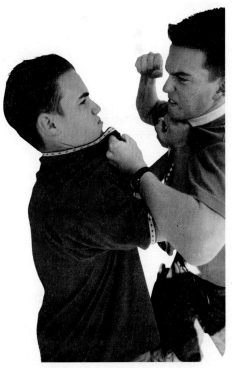

How do aggressive children process information about their social world?

SW Productions/Photodisc/Getty Images

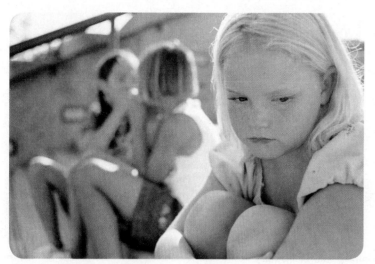

What are some statuses that children have with their peers?
BananaStock/Getty Images

factor to social problems and emerging behavioral and emotional problems (Thompson, 2019). For example, in one study, preschool children who showed high levels of aggressive peer interactions also displayed low levels of self-regulation (Olson & others, 2011). Moody and emotionally reactive individuals experience greater rejection by peers, whereas emotionally positive individuals are more popular (Riley & others, 2019). As early as the preschool years and by the time they begin elementary school, children who have effective self-regulatory skills can modulate their emotional expressiveness in contexts that evoke intense emotions, as when a peer is being aggressive or mean (Denham & Bassett, 2019).

PEER STATUSES

Which types of children are likely to be popular with their peers, and which ones tend to be disliked? Developmentalists address this and similar questions by examining *sociometric status,* a term that describes the extent to which children are liked or disliked by their peer group (Cillessen & van den Berg, 2012; van der Wilt & others, 2018). Sociometric status is typically assessed by asking children to rate how much they like or dislike each of their classmates. Or it may be assessed by asking children to name the children they like the most and those they like the least.

Developmentalists have distinguished five peer statuses (Wentzel & Asher, 1995):

- **Popular children** are frequently nominated as a best friend and are rarely disliked by their peers.
- **Average children** receive an average number of both positive and negative nominations from their peers.
- **Neglected children** are infrequently nominated as a best friend but are not disliked by their peers.
- **Rejected children** are rarely nominated as someone's best friend and are actively disliked by their peers.
- **Controversial children** are frequently nominated both as someone's best friend and as being disliked.

Popular children have a number of social skills that contribute to their being well liked. Researchers have found that popular children give out reinforcements, listen carefully, maintain open lines of communication with peers, are happy, control their negative emotions, act like themselves, show enthusiasm and concern for others, and are self-confident without being conceited. These patterns have been observed in youth and schools in the United States, Canada, China, throughout Europe, and elsewhere (Rytioja, Lappalainen, & Savolainen, 2019; Zhang & others, 2018). One study revealed that the importance of being popular in comparison with other priorities (such as friendship, achievement, and romantic interests) peaked in early adolescence (LaFontana & Cillessen, 2010). Across adolescence, youth become more adept at striking a balance between popularity and other priorities, including how they use social media in their online presence (Yau & Reich, 2019).

Neglected children engage in low rates of interaction with their peers and are often described as shy by peers. Rejected children often have more serious adjustment problems than those who are neglected (McDonald & Asher, 2018). One classic longitudinal study evaluated 112 boys over a period of seven years from fifth grade until the end of high school (Kupersmidt & Coie, 1990). The best predictor of whether rejected children would engage in delinquent behavior or drop out of school later during adolescence was aggression toward peers in elementary school. Another longitudinal study of boys and girls that followed them from kindergarten through the end of high school found that rejection and victimization from peers was a strong, consistent predictor of decreases in school engagement and academic achievement (Ladd, Ettekal, & Kochenderfer-Ladd, 2017).

popular children Children who are frequently identified as a best friend and are rarely disliked by their peers.

average children Children who receive an average number of both positive and negative nominations from their peers.

neglected children Children who are infrequently identified as a best friend but are not disliked by their peers.

rejected children Children who are infrequently identified as a best friend and are actively disliked by their peers.

controversial children Children who are frequently identified both as someone's best friend and as being disliked.

Peer rejection contributes to subsequent problems of adaptation, including antisocial behavior.

—JOHN COIE
Contemporary psychologist, Duke University

Peer Rejection and Aggression   The combination of being rejected by peers and being aggressive especially forecasts problems (Vitaro, Boivin, & Poulin, 2018). A number of studies have shown that for boys and girls alike, and in multiple cultural groups and subgroups, the combination of being rejected and aggressive is linked to higher levels of psychological and academic problems.

This combination of peer rejection and overt, physical aggressiveness is far more common in boys than girls. A key analysis by John Coie (2004, pp. 252–253) provided three reasons why aggressive peer-rejected boys have problems in social relationships:

- First, they are more impulsive and have problems sustaining attention. As a result, they are more likely to be disruptive of ongoing activities in the classroom and in focused group play.

- Second, they are more emotionally reactive. They are aroused to anger more easily and probably have more difficulty calming down once aroused. Because of this they are more prone to become angry at peers and to attack them verbally and physically.

- Third, they have fewer social skills for making friends and maintaining positive relationships with peers.

Not all rejected children are aggressive (Rubin & others, 2018). Although aggression and its related characteristics of impulsiveness and disruptiveness underlie rejection about half the time, approximately 10 to 20 percent of rejected children are shy.

What are the precursors of peer rejection? According to Gerald Patterson, Tom Dishion, and their colleagues (Dishion & Snyder, 2016; Patterson, 2016), poor parenting skills in early childhood and the elementary school years are at the root of children being rejected by their peers. These researchers especially argue that inadequate monitoring and harsh punishment, in some instances provoked by a child's difficult temperament, produce a child with aggressive, antisocial tendencies. The child carries these feelings and behaviors to the world of peers, where the child is rejected by peers who are less reactive and are better self-regulated and have experienced more positive parenting (such as authoritative parenting).

How can rejected children be taught to interact more effectively with their peers? Rejected children may be shown how to accurately assess whether the intentions of their peers are hostile. They can be asked to engage in role playing or to discuss hypothetical situations involving negative encounters with peers, such as times when a peer cuts into a line ahead of them. In some programs, children are shown examples of appropriate peer interaction and asked to draw lessons from what they have seen. Today, there are a variety of social skills training tools and interventions that can be implemented with individuals, small groups, or even whole schools (DiPerna & others, 2018).

Despite the positive outcomes of some programs that attempt to improve social skills, researchers have often found that, by adolescence, it is difficult to improve skills of youth who are actively disliked and rejected. Many of these adolescents are rejected because they are aggressive or impulsive and lack the self-control to keep these behaviors in check. Still, some intervention programs have been successful in improving social behaviors, even among adolescents (Yeager, Dahl, & Dweck, 2018).

Nevertheless, peer group reputations become more fixed as cliques and peer groups become more salient in adolescence. Once an adolescent gains a negative reputation among peers as being "mean," "weird," or a "loner," the peer group's attitude is often slow to change, even after the adolescent's problem behavior has been corrected. Thus, the most effective interventions are those that also include peer group (classroom or school) programs that increase awareness and understanding of their role in supporting each other (Taylor & others, 2017).

BULLYING

Many studies have been conducted (primarily in North America and Europe, but also in Asia, Africa, and South America), showing that significant numbers of students are victimized by bullies (Chen & others, 2017). In the latest available data for a national sample of 6- to 17-year-olds in the United States (Lebrun-Harris & others, 2018), nearly one in four youth reported being a victim of bullying; in contrast, only one in sixteen reported being a bully. Victimization was somewhat more common among children than among adolescents.

What characterizes bullying? Bullies report that their parents tend to be authoritarian, physically punish them, lack warmth, and show indifference to their children (Espelage & Holt, 2012). Bullies often display anger and hostility, and in many cases are morally disengaged (Chen & others, 2018).

Who is likely to be bullied? A number of studies have indicated some general patterns (Green, Collingwood, & Ross, 2010; Smith, Shu, & Madsen, 2001). Victimization is more common among boys, particularly during the early middle school years. Children who are bullied report more loneliness and difficulty in making friends, while those who bully others are more likely to have low grades and to behave delinquently. Researchers also have found that anxious, socially withdrawn, and aggressive children are often the victims of bullying. Anxious and socially withdrawn children may be victimized because they are nonthreatening and unlikely to retaliate if bullied, whereas aggressive children may be the targets of bullying because their behavior is irritating to bullies (Rubin & others, 2018). One study revealed that having supportive friends was linked to a lower level of bullying and victimization (Kendrick, Jutengren, & Stattin, 2012).

Social contexts also influence bullying. Seventy to 80 percent of victims and their bullies are in the same school classroom (Salmivalli & Peets, 2009). Classmates are often aware of bullying incidents and in many cases witness bullying. The larger social context of the peer group and school plays an important role in bullying (Zych, Farrington, & Ttofi, 2018). The massive increase in use of social media has also increased exposure to, and witnessing of, cyberbullying (Bauman & Bellmore, 2015; Zych, Farrington, & Ttofi, 2018). In many cases, bullies torment victims to gain higher status in the peer group, and bullies need others to witness their power displays. Many bullies are not rejected by the peer group (Pouwels, Lansu, & Cillessen, 2018). In one study, bullies were only rejected by peers to whom they were a potential threat (Veenstra & others, 2010). In another study, collaborative behavior and liking one another occurs even between two aggressive youth who first meet each other, suggesting why some bullies affiliate with each other (Andrews & others, 2019).

What are the outcomes of bullying? Researchers have found that children who are bullied are more likely to experience depression, to engage in suicidal ideation, and to attempt suicide than their counterparts who have not been the victims of bullying (Brunstein-Klomek & others, 2019; Green, Collingwood, & Ross, 2010). A longitudinal study of more than 6,000 children in England found that children who were the victims of peer bullying from 4 to 10 years of age were more likely to engage in suicidal ideation at 11 years of age (Winsper & others, 2012). Another analysis of the same sample of youth revealed that 11-year-olds who were victims of peer bullying were more likely to show borderline personality disorder symptoms (a pervasive pattern of unstable interpersonal relationships, low self-image, and emotional difficulties) (Wolke & others, 2012). Several meta-analyses of many studies have revealed a small but significant link between peer victimization and lower academic achievement (Nakamoto & Schwartz, 2010; Schoeler & others, 2018). A large study of over 27,000 Australian adolescents revealed that victims had more health problems (such as headaches, dizziness, sleep problems, and anxiety) than their peers (Agostini, Lushington, & Dorrian, 2019).

Another study asked 18-year-olds who were former victims of bullying to explain what had actually made the bullying stop (Frisen, Hasselblad, & Holmqvist, 2012). The most common reason given was intervention by school personnel, followed by transitioning to a new school level. A third reason is that they changed the way they coped with the bullying, especially by being more assertive or ignoring the bullying. Researchers have found that many victims cope poorly in bullying situations, reacting by crying and withdrawal in many cases, so teaching them to cope in more effective ways might help to reduce the bullying. What kinds of perspective taking and moral motivation skills do bullies, bully-victims, and prosocial children tend to exhibit? To find out, see *Connecting Through Research*.

developmental **connection**

Technology

The Internet and proliferation of social networking on digital devices has created many opportunities for cyberbullying. Connect with "Culture and Diversity."

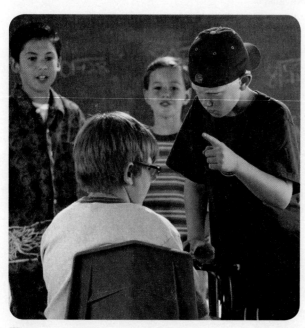

What are some strategies to reduce bullying?
Photodisc/Getty Images

connecting through research

What Are the Perspective Taking and Moral Motivation of Bullies, Bully-Victims, Victims, and Prosocial Children?

The following results were obtained in one illustrative study exploring the roles that perspective taking and moral motivation play in the lives of bullies, bully-victims, victims, and prosocial children (Gasser & Keller, 2009):

- *Bullies* are highly aggressive toward other children but are not victims of bullying.
- *Bully-victims* not only are highly aggressive toward other children but also are the targets of other children's bullying.
- *Victims* are passive, non-aggressive respondents to bullying.
- *Prosocial children* engage in such positive behaviors as sharing, helping, comforting, and empathizing.

Teacher and peer ratings in 34 classrooms of 7- and 8-year-old students were used to classify 212 boys and girls into the aforementioned four categories. On a five-point scale (from "never" to "several times a week"), teachers rated (1) how often the child bullied others, and (2) how often the child was bullied. The ratings focused on three types of bullying and being victimized: physical actions, verbal abuse, and excluding others. On a four-point scale (from not applicable to very clearly applicable), teachers also rated children's prosocial behavior on three items: "willingly shares with others," "comforts others if necessary," and "empathizes with others." Peer ratings assessed children's nominations of which children in the classroom acted as bullies, were victimized by bullies, and engaged in prosocial behavior. Combining the teacher and peer ratings after eliminating those that did not agree regarding which children were bullies, victims, or prosocial children, the final sample consisted of 49 bullies, 80 bully-victims, 33 victims, and 50 prosocial children.

Children's perspective-taking skills were assessed using theory of mind tasks, and moral motivation was examined by interviewing children about aspects of right and wrong in stories about children's transgressions. In one theory of mind task, children were tested to see whether they understood that people may have false beliefs about another individual. In another theory of mind task, children were assessed to determine whether they understood that people sometimes hide their emotions by showing emotions that differ from what they really feel. A moral interview also was conducted in which children were told four moral transgression stories (with content about being unwilling to share with a classmate, stealing candy from a classmate, hiding a victim's shoes, and verbally bullying a victim) and then asked to judge whether the acts were right or wrong and how the participants in the stories likely felt.

The results of the study indicated that only bully-victims—but not bullies—were deficient in perspective taking. Further analysis revealed that both aggressive groups of children—bullies and bully-victims—had a deficiency in moral motivation. The analyses were consistent with a portrait of bullies as socially competent and knowledgeable in terms of perspective-taking skills and ability to effectively interact with peers. However, bullies use this social knowledge for their own manipulative purposes. The analysis also confirmed the picture of the bully as being morally insensitive. Subsequent research in multiple countries has made clear that moral disengagement plays a key role in victimizing others (Chen & others, 2018).

How can researchers ensure that results that might help prevent bullying are properly applied in school settings (and not used instead to label potential bullies or isolate potential victims)?

Extensive attention is being directed to finding ways to prevent and treat bullying and victimization (Smith, 2019). School-based interventions vary greatly, ranging from involving the whole school in an antibullying campaign to providing individualized social skills training (Divecha & Brackett, 2019; Huang & others, 2019). One of the most promising bullying intervention programs has been created by Dan Olweus. This program focuses on 6- to 15-year-olds with the goal of decreasing opportunities and rewards for bullying. School staff are instructed in ways to improve peer relations and make schools safer. When properly implemented, the program reduces bullying by 30 to 70 percent (Olweus, Limber, & Breivik, 2019).

To reduce bullying, schools can adopt the following strategies (Cohn & Canter, 2003; Hyman & others, 2006; Limber, 2004):

- Get older peers to serve as monitors for bullying and intervene when they see it taking place.
- Develop school-wide rules and sanctions against bullying and post them throughout the school.
- Form friendship groups for adolescents who are regularly bullied by peers.
- Incorporate the message of the antibullying program into places of worship, schools, and other community activity areas where adolescents are involved.

- Encourage parents to reinforce their adolescent's positive behaviors and model appropriate interpersonal interactions.
- Identify bullies and victims early and use social skills training to improve their behavior.
- Encourage parents to contact the school's psychologist, counselor, or social worker and ask for help with concerns involving bullying or victimization.

Review Connect Reflect

LG1 Discuss peer relations in childhood.

Review

- What are some key aspects of peer relations?
- What is the developmental course of peer relations in childhood?
- In what ways are the worlds of parents and peers distinct but coordinated?
- How is social cognition involved in peer relations? How is emotion involved in peer relations?
- What are the five peer statuses of children?
- What is the nature of bullying?

Connect

- Earlier in this chapter, you learned that most developmentalists agree that peers play an important role in children's development of moral reasoning. Of the five peer status groups you learned about in this section, in which group do you think children would have the least opportunity to fully develop their moral reasoning capacities? Why?

Reflect *Your Own Personal Journey of Life*

- Think back to your middle school/ junior high and high school years. What kind of relationship did you have with your parents? Were you securely attached or insecurely attached to them? How do you think your relationship with your parents affected your friendships and peer relations?

Play 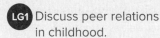 **LG2** Describe children's play.

Play's Functions   Types of Play   Trends in Play

Much of the time when children, especially young children, are interacting with their peers, they are playing. **Play** is a pleasurable activity that is engaged in for its own sake, and social play is just one type of play.

PLAY'S FUNCTIONS

Play makes important contributions to young children's cognitive and socioemotional development (Fromberg & Bergen, 2015). Theorists have focused on different aspects of play and highlighted a long list of functions.

According to Freud and Erikson, play helps the child master anxieties and conflicts. Play permits children to work off excess physical energy and to release pent-up tensions. Because tensions are relieved in play, the child can cope more effectively with life's problems. Therapists use **play therapy** both to allow the child to work off frustrations and to analyze the child's conflicts and ways of coping with them (Ariel, 2019). Children may feel less threatened and be more likely to express their true feelings in the context of play.

Play also is an important context for cognitive development (Hirsh-Pasek & Golinkoff, 2013). Both Piaget and Vygotsky concluded that play is the child's work. Piaget (1962) maintained that play advances children's cognitive development. At the same time, he said that children's cognitive development *constrains* the way they play. Play permits children to practice their competencies and acquired skills in a relaxed, pleasurable way. Piaget

play A pleasurable activity that is engaged in for its own sake.

play therapy Therapy that allows the child to work off frustrations and is a medium through which the therapist can analyze the child's conflicts and ways of coping with them. Children may feel less threatened and be more likely to express their true feelings in the context of play.

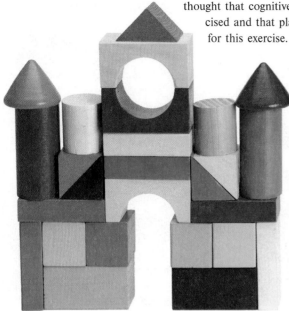

Ken Karp/McGraw-Hill Education

thought that cognitive structures needed to be exercised and that play provided the perfect setting for this exercise.

Vygotsky (1962) also considered play to be an excellent setting for cognitive development. He was especially interested in the symbolic and make-believe aspects of play, as when a child substitutes a stick for a horse and rides the stick as if it were a horse. For young children, the imaginary situation is real. Parents should encourage such imaginary play, because it advances the child's cognitive development, especially creative thought.

Another classic theoretical foundation for play was provided by Daniel Berlyne (1960), who described play as exciting and pleasurable in itself because it satisfies our exploratory drive. This drive involves curiosity and a desire for information about something new or unusual. Play encourages exploratory behavior by offering children the possibilities of novelty, complexity, uncertainty, surprise, and incongruity.

In contemporary developmental science, play has been described as an important context for the development of language and communication skills (Hirsh-Pasek & Golinkoff, 2013) through discussions and negotiations regarding roles and rules in play. These types of social interactions during play can benefit young children's literacy skills (Germeroth & others, 2019; Theodotou, 2019). Play is a central focus of the child-centered kindergarten and thought to be an essential aspect of early childhood education (Lillard, 2018; Neuman, 2019).

An increasing concern is that the large number of hours children spend with electronic media, such as television and tablets, takes time away from play (Fromberg & Bergen, 2015). An important priority for parents should be to include ample time for play in their children's lives.

developmental **connection**

Cognitive Theory

Vygotsky emphasized that children mainly develop their ways of thinking and understanding through social interaction. Connect to "Cognitive Developmental Approaches."

developmental **connection**

Education

The child-centered kindergarten emphasizes the education of the whole child, not just his or her cognitive development, because play is extremely important in the child's development. Connect to "Schools and Achievement."

TYPES OF PLAY

The contemporary perspective on play emphasizes both the cognitive and the social aspects of play (Riede & others, 2018; Tunçgenç & Cohen, 2018). Among the most widely studied types of children's play today are sensorimotor and practice play, pretense/symbolic play, social play, constructive play, and games (Fromberg & Bergen, 2015).

Sensorimotor and Practice Play **Sensorimotor play** is behavior that allows infants to derive pleasure from exercising their sensorimotor schemes. The development of sensorimotor play follows Piaget's description of sensorimotor thought. Infants initially engage in exploratory and playful visual and motor transactions during the second quarter of the first year of life. At 9 months of age, infants begin to select novel objects for exploration and play, especially those that are responsive, such as toys that make noise or bounce. At 12 months of age, infants enjoy making things work and exploring cause and effect.

Practice play involves repeating behavior when new skills are being learned or when physical or mental mastery and coordination of skills are required for games or sports. Sensorimotor play, which often involves practice play, is primarily confined to infancy, whereas practice play can be engaged in throughout life. During the preschool years, children often engage in play that involves practicing various skills. Although practice play declines during the elementary school years, practice play activities such as running,

sensorimotor play Behavior that allows infants to derive pleasure from exercising their existing sensorimotor schemes.

practice play Play that involves repetition of behavior when new skills are being learned or when physical or mental mastery and coordination of skills are required for games or sports. Practice play can be engaged in throughout life.

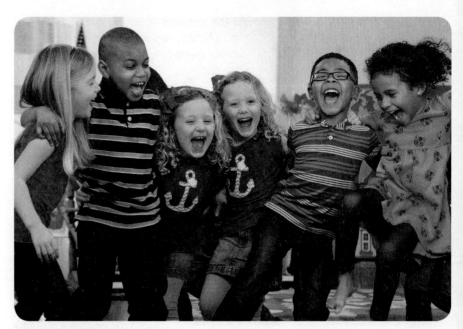

What are some different types of play?
Ariel Skelley/Getty Images

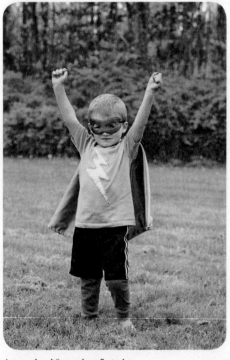

A preschool "superhero" at play.
Michelle D. Milliman/Shutterstock

pretense/symbolic play Play that occurs when a child transforms the physical environment into a symbol.

social play Play that involves interactions with peers.

constructive play Play that combines sensorimotor/practice play with symbolic representation of ideas. Constructive play occurs when children engage in self-regulated creation or construction of a product or a solution.

jumping, sliding, twirling, and throwing balls or other objects are frequently observed on the playgrounds at elementary schools.

Pretense/Symbolic Play **Pretense/symbolic play** occurs when the child transforms the physical environment into a symbol. Between 9 and 30 months of age, children increase their use of objects in symbolic play (Lillard & Taggart, 2019). They learn to transform objects, substituting them for other objects and acting toward them as if they were those other objects (Hopkins & others, 2016). For example, a preschool child treats a table as if it were a car and says, "I'm fixing the car," as he grabs a leg of the table.

Many experts on play view the preschool years as the "golden age" of symbolic/pretense play that is dramatic or sociodramatic in nature (Rubin, Bukowski, & Parker, 2006). This type of make-believe play often appears at about 18 months of age and reaches a peak at 4 to 5 years of age, then gradually declines. Some child psychologists conclude that pretend play is an important aspect of young children's development and often reflects advances in their cognitive development, especially their capacity for symbolic understanding (Lillard & Taggart, 2019). Hidden in young children's pretend play narratives are remarkable capacities for role-taking, balancing of social roles, metacognition (thinking about thinking), testing of the reality-pretense distinction, and numerous nonegocentric capacities that reveal the remarkable cognitive skills of young children. In one analysis, a major accomplishment in early childhood is the development of children's ability to share their pretend play with peers and create a "culture" of play in their group (Breathnach, Danby, & O'Gorman, 2018).

Social Play **Social play** is play that involves interaction with peers; it may or may not involve pretending or imagination. Social play increases dramatically during the preschool years and includes varied interchanges such as turn taking, conversations about numerous topics, social games and routines, and physical play. Social play often evokes a high degree of pleasure on the part of the participants (Sumaroka & Bornstein, 2008).

Constructive Play **Constructive play** combines sensorimotor/practice play with symbolic representation of ideas. Constructive play occurs when children engage in the self-regulated creation of a product or a solution. Constructive play increases in the preschool years as symbolic play increases and sensorimotor play decreases. During the preschool years, some practice play is replaced by constructive play. For example, instead of moving their fingers around and around in finger paint (practice play), children are more likely to draw the outline of a house or a person in the paint (constructive play). Constructive play is also a frequent form of play in the elementary school years, both within and outside the classroom. Constructive play is one of the few playlike activities allowed in academic-centered classrooms. For example, if children create a skit about a social studies topic, they are engaging in constructive play.

Games   **Games** are activities that are engaged in for pleasure and are governed by rules. Often they involve competition between two or more individuals. Preschool children may begin to participate in social game play that involves simple rules of reciprocity and turn taking. However, games take on a much more prominent role in the lives of elementary school children. Game playing increases in prevalence across middle childhood (Fromberg & Bergen, 2015). With the advent of digital games on mobile devices, game playing has become widely available and used by older children, adolescents, and adults (Pew Research Center, 2018a).

games Activities engaged in for pleasure that include rules and often competition with one or more individuals.

In sum, play ranges from an infant's simple exercise of a new sensorimotor talent to a preschool child's riding a tricycle to an older child's participation in organized games. It is also important to note that children's play can involve a combination of the play categories we have described. For example, social play can be sensorimotor (rough-and-tumble), symbolic, and constructive.

TRENDS IN PLAY

Kathy Hirsh-Pasek, Roberta Golinkoff, and Dorothy Singer (Singer, Golinkoff, & Hirsh-Pasek, 2006) are concerned about the decline in the amount of free play time that young children have, reporting that it has declined considerably in recent decades. They especially are worried about young children's playtime being restricted at home and school so they can spend more time on academic subjects. They also point out that many schools have eliminated recess, a trend that has expanded throughout many school systems in industrialized countries (American Academy of Pediatrics, 2013). And it is not just the decline in time allotted to free play that bothers them. They underscore that learning in playful contexts captivates children's minds in ways that enhance their cognitive and socioemotional development—Singer, Golinkoff, and Hirsh-Pasek's (2006) first book on play was titled: *Play = Learning*. Among the cognitive benefits of play they described are creative; abstract thinking; imagination; attention, concentration, and persistence; problem-solving; social cognition, empathy, and perspective taking; language; and mastering new concepts. Among the socioemotional experiences and development they believe play promotes are enjoyment, relaxation, and self-expression; cooperation, sharing, and turn-taking; anxiety reduction; and self-confidence. With so many positive cognitive and socioemotional outcomes of play, clearly it is important that we find more time for play in young children's lives. (Yogman & others, 2018).

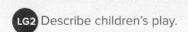

Review *Connect* **Reflect**

LG2 Describe children's play.

Review

- What are the functions of play?
- What are the different types of play?
- What are some trends in play?

Connect

- Pretense/symbolic play takes place during what Piaget called the symbolic function substage of the preoperational stage. According to Piaget, what are two important limitations of children's thought during this substage?

Reflect *Your Own Personal Journey of Life*

- Do you think most young children's lives today are too structured? If and when you become a parent, how will you manage your children's development to provide enough time for play?

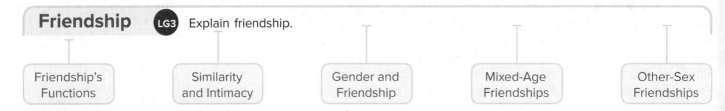

Friendship (LG3) Explain friendship.

Friendship's Functions | Similarity and Intimacy | Gender and Friendship | Mixed-Age Friendships | Other-Sex Friendships

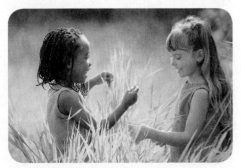

What are some functions of children's friendships?
Don Hammond/Design Pics

Children play with a variety of acquaintances. They interact with some children they barely know, and with others they know well, for hours every day. It is to the latter type—friends—that we now turn.

FRIENDSHIP'S FUNCTIONS

Friendships serve six functions, according to a now classic analysis of these close relationships (Gottman & Parker, 1987):

1. *Companionship:* a familiar partner, someone who is willing to spend time with them and join in collaborative activities
2. *Stimulation:* interesting information, excitement, and amusement
3. *Physical support:* resources and assistance
4. *Ego support:* the expectation of support, encouragement, and feedback that helps children to maintain an impression of themselves as competent, attractive, and worthwhile individuals
5. *Social comparison:* information about where children stand compared with others and whether children are "doing okay"
6. *Intimacy/affection:* a warm, close, trusting relationship with another individual, a relationship that involves self-disclosure

Although having friends can be a developmental advantage, not all friendships are alike and the quality of friendship is also important to consider (Wentzel, 2013). People differ in the company they keep—that is, who their friends are.

Positive friendships in adolescence are associated with a host of positive outcomes, including lower rates of delinquency, substance abuse, risky sexual behavior, and bullying victimization, and a higher level of academic achievement (Heinze & others, 2018; Kendrick, Jutengren, & Stattin, 2012; Way & Silverman, 2012; Wentzel, 2013). Not having a close relationship with a best friend, having less contact with friends, having friends who are depressed, and experiencing peer rejection all increase depressive tendencies in adolescents (Brendgen, 2018a; Schwartz-Mette & Smith, 2018). Researchers have found that interacting with delinquent peers and friends greatly increases the risk of becoming delinquent (McGloin & Thomas, 2019).

Harry Stack Sullivan (1953) was the most influential early theorist to discuss the importance of friendships. In contrast with other theorists' narrow emphasis on the importance of parent-child relationships, Sullivan contended that friends also played important roles in shaping children's and adolescents' well-being and development.

According to Sullivan, all people have a number of basic social needs, including tenderness (secure attachment), playful companionship, social acceptance, intimacy, and sexual relations. Whether or not these needs are fulfilled largely determines our emotional well-being (Whisman, 2017). For example, if the need for playful companionship goes unmet, then we become bored and depressed; if the need for social acceptance is not met, we suffer a diminished sense of self-worth. Sullivan stressed that the need for intimacy intensifies during early adolescence, motivating teenagers to seek close friends.

Research findings support many of Sullivan's ideas. For example, in a classic set of studies, adolescents reported disclosing intimate and personal

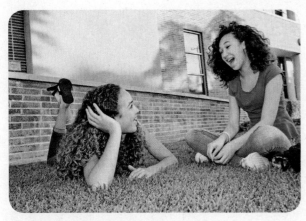

How did Sullivan think friendship changes in adolescence?
Peathegee Inc/Blend Images LLC

430   CHAPTER 15   Peers

information to their friends more often than did younger children (Buhrmester, 1990; Buhrmester & Furman, 1987) (see Figure 2). Adolescents also said they relied more on friends than on parents to satisfy their needs for companionship, reassurance of worth, and intimacy.

Friendships are often important sources of support (Holder & Coleman, 2015; Wentzel, 2013). Sullivan described how adolescent friends support one another's sense of personal worth. When close friends disclose their mutual insecurities and fears about themselves, they discover that they are not "abnormal" and that they have nothing to be ashamed of. Friends also act as important confidants who help children and adolescents work through upsetting problems (such as difficulties with parents or the breakup of romantic relationships) by providing both emotional support and informational advice.

To read about appropriate and inappropriate strategies for making friends, see *Caring Connections.*

SIMILARITY AND INTIMACY

What characteristics do children and adolescents look for in their friends? The answers change somewhat as children grow up, but one characteristic of friends is found throughout the childhood and adolescent years: Friends are generally similar—in terms of age, sex, ethnicity, and many other factors. Similarity is referred to as *homophily,* the tendency to associate with similar others (Laninga-Wijnen & others, 2019; Richmond, Laursen, & Stattin, 2019).

Friends often have similar attitudes toward school, similar educational aspirations, and closely aligned achievement orientations. Friends like the same music, wear the same kinds of clothes, and prefer the same leisure activities. Differences may lead to conflicts

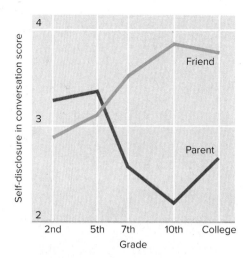

FIGURE **2**

DEVELOPMENTAL CHANGES IN SELF-DISCLOSING CONVERSATIONS. Self-disclosing conversations with friends increased dramatically in adolescence while declining in an equally dramatic fashion with parents. However, self-disclosing conversations with parents began to pick up somewhat during the college years. The measure of self-disclosure involved a 5-point rating scale completed by the children and youth, with a higher score representing greater self-disclosure. The data shown represent the means for each age group.

caring *connections*

Making Friends

Here are some strategies that adults can recommend to children and adolescents for making friends:

- *Initiate interaction.* Learn about a friend: Ask for his or her name, age, favorite activities. Use these prosocial overtures: introduce yourself, start a conversation, and invite him or her to do things.
- *Be nice.* Show kindness, be considerate, and compliment the other person.
- *Engage in prosocial behavior.* Be honest and trustworthy: tell the truth, keep promises. Be generous, share, and be cooperative.
- *Show respect for yourself and others.* Have good manners, be polite and courteous, and listen to what others have to say. Have a positive attitude and personality.
- *Provide social support.* Show you care.

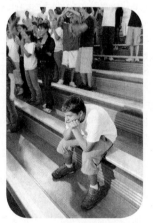

What are some appropriate and inappropriate strategies for making friends?

Thinkstock Images/Stockbyte/Getty Images

And here are some inappropriate strategies for making friends that adults can recommend that children and adolescents avoid using:

- *Be psychologically aggressive.* Show disrespect and have bad manners. Use others, be uncooperative, don't share, ignore others, gossip, and spread rumors.
- *Present yourself negatively.* Be self-centered, snobby, conceited, and jealous; show off, care only about yourself. Be mean, have a bad attitude, be angry, throw temper tantrums, and start trouble.
- *Behave antisocially.* Be physically aggressive, yell at others, pick on them, make fun of them, be dishonest, tell secrets, and break promises.

These recommendations are from a key review of the research literature (Wentzel, 1997). Based on what you read here and earlier in this chapter, what might you recommend to an adolescent about approaching someone as a potential friend?

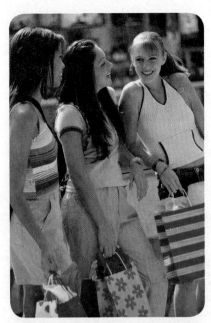

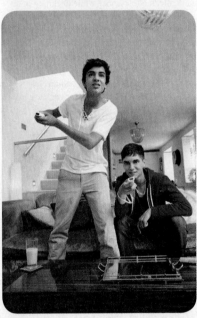

What are some gender differences in peer relations and friendships in adolescence?

(Top) Valueline/Getty Images; (Bottom) Image Source/ Getty Images

intimacy in friendship Self-disclosure or the sharing of private thoughts.

that weaken the friendship. For example, if two friends have differing attitudes toward school, one may repeatedly want to play basketball or go to the mall while the other insists on completing homework, and the two may drift apart (Flynn, 2018).

Priorities change as the child reaches adolescence. The most consistent finding in the last several decades of research on adolescent friendships is that intimacy is an important feature of friendship (Hall, 2011; van Rijsewijk & others, 2019). In most research studies, **intimacy in friendship** is defined narrowly as self-disclosure or sharing of private thoughts; private or personal knowledge about a friend has been used as a measure of intimacy. When young adolescents are asked what they want from a friend or how they can tell someone is their best friend, they frequently say that a best friend will share problems with them, understand them, and listen when they talk about their own thoughts or feelings. When young children talk about their friendships, they rarely comment about intimate self-disclosure or mutual understanding. Recall from the results of studies presented in Figure 2 that friendship intimacy was more prominent among 13- to 16-year-olds than among 10- to 13-year-olds (Buhrmester, 1990).

GENDER AND FRIENDSHIP

Are the friendships of girls different from the friendships of boys? An increasing number of studies indicate that they are different—from late childhood into adolescence, adulthood, and even old age (Dunbar, 2018). Are the friendships of adolescent girls more intimate than the friendships of adolescent boys? A meta-analysis concluded that research indicates girls' friendships are more intimate (Gorrese & Ruggieri, 2012). In this meta-analysis, girls' friendships were deeper, more interdependent, showed more empathy, revealed a greater need for nurturance, and involved a greater desire to sustain intimate relationships. In contrast, boys gave more importance to having a congenial friend with whom they could share their interests in such activities as hobbies and sports, and boys showed more cooperativeness than girls in their friendships. Also in this meta-analysis, adolescent girls showed higher peer attachment, especially related to trust and communication, than did adolescent boys (Gorrese & Ruggieri, 2012). These differences aside, it matters for both girls and boys that they have close friendships and a network of peers that support them (Flynn, Felmlee, & Conger, 2017).

Let's further examine gender differences in the intimacy aspect of friendship. When asked to describe their best friends, girls refer to intimate conversations and faithfulness more than boys do (Rose & others, 2012). For example, girls are more likely to describe their best friend as being trustworthy, sensitive, and responsive like themselves. When problems are present, girls are more likely to talk about them in a positive and supportive way, but boys are more likely to engage in humorous exchanges when discussing problems (Rose & others, 2016). Although girls' friendships in adolescence are more likely to focus on intimacy, boys' friendships tend to emphasize power and excitement (Rose & Smith, 2009). Boys may discourage one another from openly disclosing their problems because self-disclosure is not viewed as masculine (Pollastri & others, 2018). Boys make themselves vulnerable to being called "wimps" if they can't handle their own problems and insecurities. These gender differences are generally assumed to reflect a greater orientation toward interpersonal relationships among girls than boys.

As indicated in the *Caring Connections* interlude, friendship often provides social support. However, researchers have found that some aspects of friendships (especially for girls) may be linked to adolescent emotional problems (Carlucci & others, 2018). For example, an illustrative longitudinal study of third- through ninth-graders revealed that girls' co-rumination (as reflected in excessively discussing problems) predicted not only an increase in positive friendship quality but also an increase in further co-rumination as well as an increase in depressive and anxiety symptoms (Rose, Carlson, & Waller, 2007). One implication of the research is that some girls who are vulnerable to developing anxious and depressive symptoms may go undetected because they have supportive friendships.

MIXED-AGE FRIENDSHIPS

Although most adolescents develop friendships with individuals who are close to their own age, some adolescents become best friends with younger or older individuals. A common fear, especially among parents, is that adolescents who have older friends will be encouraged to engage in delinquent behavior or early sexual behavior. Researchers have found that adolescents who interact with older youth do engage in these behaviors more frequently, but it is not known whether the older youth guide younger adolescents toward deviant behavior or whether the younger adolescents were already prone to deviant behavior before they developed the friendship with the older youth (Jaccard, Blanton, & Dodge, 2005). One longitudinal study also revealed that over time, from the sixth through tenth grades, girls were more likely to have older male friends, which places some girls on a developmental trajectory for engaging in problem behavior (Poulin & Pedersen, 2007). However, another study of young adolescents found that mixed-age friends may protect same-age friendless girls from feelings of loneliness and same-age friendless and anxious-withdrawn boys from victimization (Bowker & Spencer, 2010).

OTHER-SEX FRIENDSHIPS

Although adolescents are more likely to have same-sex friends, associations with other-sex friends also are fairly common (Weger, Cole, & Akbulut, 2019; Wilson & Jamison, 2019). The number of other-sex friendships increases in the transition to and across adolescence, with girls reporting more other-sex friends than boys (Grard & others, 2018). Other-sex friendships and participation in mixed-sex groups provide a context for adolescents to learn how to communicate with the other sex and reduce anxiety in social and dating heterosexual interactions.

However, researchers have found that other-sex friendships are sometimes linked to negative behaviors such as earlier sexual intercourse, as well as increases in alcohol use and delinquency (Grard & others, 2018; Jacobs & others, 2016; Mrug, Borch, & Cillessen, 2011). Parents likely monitor their daughters' other-sex friendships more closely than their sons' because they perceive boys as having a more negative influence, especially in initiating problem behavior. This is exemplified in one study that found that a higher level of parental monitoring led to fewer other-sex friendships, which in turn was associated with a lower level of subsequent alcohol use (Poulin & Denault, 2012).

Review Connect Reflect

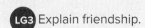 Explain friendship.

Review

- What are six functions of friendship? What is Sullivan's view of friendship?
- What roles do similarity and intimacy play in friendship?
- How does gender influence friendship?
- What is the developmental outcome of mixed-age friendship?
- What characterizes other-sex friendships in adolescence?

Connect

- Relational aggression was discussed in this chapter. In what ways might parenting influence development of relational aggression?

Reflect *Your Own Personal Journey of Life*

- Examine the list of six functions of friendships at the beginning of this section. Rank the six functions from most (1) to least (6) important to you as you were developing in three different time frames: early childhood, middle and late childhood, and adolescence.

Peer Pressure
and Conformity

Cliques and
Crowds

Romantic
Relationships

*I didn't belong as a kid, and
that always bothered me. If
only I'd known that one day
my differentness would be an
asset, then my early life would
have been much easier.*

—Bette Midler
Contemporary American actress

We already have discussed a number of changes in adolescents' peer relations, including the increasing importance of friendships compared with childhood. Peer relations play such a powerful role in the lives of adolescents that we further consider additional aspects in this section.

Peer relations undergo important changes in adolescence (Flynn, 2018; Gibbons & Poelker, 2019). In childhood, the focus of peer relations is on being liked by classmates and being included in games or lunchroom conversations. Being overlooked or, worse yet, being rejected can have damaging effects on children's development that sometimes are carried forward to adolescence. Beginning in early adolescence, teenagers typically prefer to have a smaller number of friendships that are more intense and intimate than those of young children. Cliques are formed and shape the social lives of adolescents as they begin to "hang out" together. Finally, romantic relationships become a more central aspect of adolescents' lives.

PEER PRESSURE AND CONFORMITY

Young adolescents conform more to peer standards than children do. Around the eighth and ninth grades, conformity to peers—especially to their antisocial standards—peaks (Closson, Hart, & Hogg, 2017). At this point, adolescents are most likely to go along with a peer to steal hubcaps off a car, draw graffiti on a wall, or steal cosmetics from a store counter. Several studies have revealed that 14 to 18 years of age is an especially important time for developing the ability to stand up for what one believes and resist peer pressure to do otherwise (Goliath & Pretorius, 2016; Steinberg & Monahan, 2007).

Which adolescents are most likely to conform to peers? Mitchell Prinstein and his colleagues (Brechwald & Prinstein, 2011; Prinstein & Dodge, 2008; Teunissen & others, 2012) have conducted research and analysis addressing this question. They conclude that adolescents who are uncertain about their social identity, which can appear in the form of low self-esteem and high social anxiety, are most likely to conform to peers. This uncertainty often increases during times of transition, such as school and family transitions. Also, peers are more likely to conform when they are in the presence of someone they perceive to have higher status than themselves.

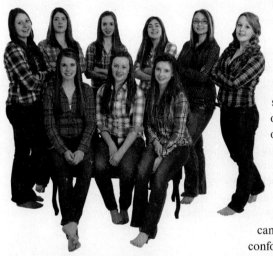

What characterizes peer pressure in adolescence?
The Catcher Photography/Getty Images

CLIQUES AND CROWDS

Cliques and crowds assume more important roles in adolescence than in childhood (Jordan & others, 2019). **Cliques** are small groups that range from 2 to about 12 individuals and average about 5 or 6 individuals. The clique members are usually of the same sex and about the same age. Cliques can form because adolescents engage in similar activities, such as being in a club or on a sports team. Some cliques also form because of friendship. Several adolescents may form a clique because they have spent time with each other and enjoy each other's company. Not necessarily friends, they often develop a friendship if they stay in the clique.

cliques Small groups that range from 2 to about 12 individuals and average about 5 or 6 individuals. Cliques can form because of friendship or because individuals engage in similar activities, and members usually are of the same sex and about the same age.

What do adolescents do in cliques? They share ideas, hang out together, and often develop an in-group identity in which they believe that their clique is better than other cliques. Being a member of a tight-knit group often has benefits as well as costs. Cliques establish and reinforce group norms for attitudes and behavior that can be either antisocial or prosocial. Adolescents must develop skills to conform enough to maintain these friendships but also to hone their individuality and to not conform when the clique's values violate personal standards (Ellis & Zarbatany, 2017).

Dexter Dunphy (1963) documented the increase in mixed-sex groups in a classic observational study. Figure 3 outlines his view of how these mixed-sex groups develop. In late childhood, boys and girls participate in small, same-sex cliques. As they move into the early adolescent years, the same-sex cliques begin to interact with each other. Gradually, the leaders and high-status members form further cliques based on mixed-sex relationships. Eventually, the newly created mixed-sex cliques replace the same-sex cliques. The mixed-sex cliques interact with each other in large crowd activities, too—at dances and athletic events, for example. In late adolescence, the crowd begins to dissolve as couples develop more serious relationships and make long-range plans that may include engagement and marriage.

Crowds are a larger group structure than cliques. Adolescents are usually members of a crowd based on reputation and may or may not spend much time together. Crowds are less personal than cliques. Many crowds are defined by the activities adolescents engage in (such as "jocks" who are good at sports or "nerds" who are bookish and focused on schoolwork) (Brown, 2011; Moran & others, 2017).

Crowds and being a member of a crowd sometimes can have serious consequences in development. In one study, researchers investigated middle-school students' perceptions of and membership in antisocial crowds across one school year in an urban area with heavy gang activity (Schwartz & others, 2017). The young adolescents very clearly perceived this crowd as having gang-like features. Effects of crowd membership were complex; although youth who were in the antisocial crowd were aggressive and not doing well in school, they gained popularity over the school year.

crowds The crowd is a larger group structure than a clique. Adolescents usually are members of a crowd based on reputation and may or may not spend much time together. Many crowds are defined by the activities in which adolescents engage.

ROMANTIC RELATIONSHIPS

Adolescents spend considerable time engaged in romantic relationships or thinking about doing so (Flynn, Felmlee, & Conger, 2017; Lantagne & Furman, 2017). "Dating" can be a form of recreation, a source of status, or a setting for learning about close relationships, as well as a way of finding a mate.

Types of Dating and Developmental Changes   A number of dating variations and developmental changes characterize dating and romantic relationships. First, we examine heterosexual romantic relationships and then turn to romantic relationships among gay, lesbian, and bisexual youth.

Heterosexual Romantic Relationships   Three stages characterize the development of romantic relationships in adolescence, in many but certainly not all national and cultural groups (Connolly & McIsaac, 2009):

1. *Entry into romantic attractions and affiliations at about 11 to 13 years of age.* This initial stage is triggered by puberty. From 11 to 13, adolescents become intensely interested in romance, and the topic dominates many conversations with same-sex friends. Developing a crush on someone is common, and the crush often is shared with a same-sex friend. Young adolescents may or may not interact with the individual who is the object of their infatuation. When dating occurs, it usually takes place in a group setting.

2. *Exploring romantic relationships at approximately 14 to 16 years of age.* At this point in adolescence, two types of romantic involvement occur: (1) *Casual dating* emerges between individuals who are mutually attracted. These dating experiences are often short-lived, last a few months at best, and usually only endure for a few weeks. (2) *Dating in groups* is common and reflects embeddedness in the peer context. Friends often act as a third-party facilitator of a potential dating relationship by communicating their friend's romantic interest and determining whether this attraction is reciprocated.

3. *Consolidating dyadic romantic bonds at about 17 to 19 years of age.* At the end of the high school years, more serious romantic relationships develop. This is characterized by strong emotional bonds more closely resembling those in adult romantic relationships. These bonds often are more stable and enduring than earlier bonds, typically lasting one year or more.

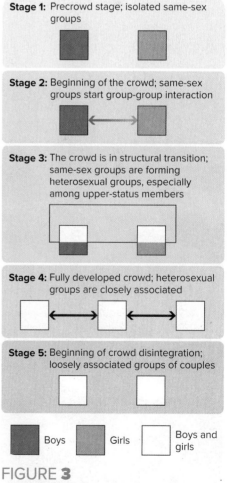

Stage 1: Precrowd stage; isolated same-sex groups

Stage 2: Beginning of the crowd; same-sex groups start group-group interaction

Stage 3: The crowd is in structural transition; same-sex groups are forming heterosexual groups, especially among upper-status members

Stage 4: Fully developed crowd; heterosexual groups are closely associated

Stage 5: Beginning of crowd disintegration; loosely associated groups of couples

Boys   Girls   Boys and girls

FIGURE **3**

DUNPHY'S CLASSIC PROGRESSION OF PEER GROUP RELATIONS IN ADOLESCENCE

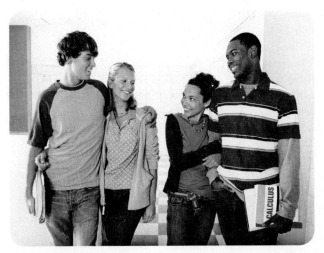

What are some developmental changes in romantic relationships in adolescence?
Digital Vision/Getty Images

Two variations on these stages in the development of romantic relationships in adolescence involve early and late bloomers (Connolly & McIsaac, 2009). *Early bloomers* include 15 to 20 percent of 11- to 13-year-olds who say that they currently are in a romantic relationship and 35 percent who indicate that they have had some prior experience in romantic relationships. *Late bloomers* comprise approximately 10 percent of 17- to 19-year-olds who say that they have had no experience with romantic relationships and another 15 percent who report that they have not engaged in any romantic relationships that lasted more than 4 months.

In their early romantic relationships, today's adolescents are not motivated to fulfill attachment or even sexual needs. Rather, early romantic relationships serve as a context for adolescents to explore how attractive they are, how to interact romantically, and how all of these aspects look to the peer group. After young adolescents acquire some basic competencies in interacting with romantic partners, in later adolescence through early adulthood romantic relationships shift to provide fulfillment of attachment and sexual needs as they do in adulthood (Birnbaum & Ries, 2019; van de Bongardt & others, 2015). A special concern in early dating and "going with" someone is the associated risk for adolescent pregnancy and problems at home and school (Low & Shortt, 2017).

Romantic Relationships in Gay, Lesbian, and Bisexual Youth

Most research on romantic relationships in adolescence has focused on heterosexual relationships, but there has been growth in research on romantic relationships in gay, lesbian, and bisexual youth (Kaestle, 2019; Rosario, 2019).

The average age of the initial same-sex activity for females ranges from 14 to 18 years of age and for males from 13 to 15 (Diamond, 2013a, b). The most common initial same-sex partner is a close friend. More lesbian adolescent girls have sexual encounters with boys before same-sex activity, whereas gay adolescent boys are more likely to show the opposite sequence (Savin-Williams, 2013).

In a large longitudinal study of a national sample of over 6,000 youth in the United States, sexual attraction preceded sexual contact and romantic relationship formation (Kaestle, 2019). Overall, patterns were similar for girls and boys, though girls reported higher levels of same-sex contact and relationships than did boys. The youth were followed through their twenties, and it also was apparent that sexual orientation and identity formation continued to shift and develop in adulthood.

Most gay, lesbian, and bisexual youth have same-sex sexual experience, but relatively few have same-sex romantic relationships because of limited opportunities and the social disapproval such relationships may generate from families or heterosexual peers (Flores & others, 2018). Large international surveys show that attitudes against same-sex romantic feelings and relationships are common, especially in countries and cultural groups that are highly religious or traditional (van den Akker & others, 2013). There is a dramatic generational shift in many countries, however. For example, the first country to legalize same-sex marriage was the Netherlands in 2001. As of 2019, same-sex marriage was legal in over 30 countries, while nearly 20 more permit civil unions or registered partnerships.

The romantic relationship development of gay, lesbian, and bisexual youth is complex and distinct in some ways from trajectories for heterosexual youth. To adequately study romantic relationship development, we can't generalize from heterosexual youth and simply switch the labels. Instead, we need to consider the full range of variation in youths' sexual desires, hopes, and fears involving romantic relationships with same- and other-sex partners (Clarke, Cover, & Aggleton, 2018).

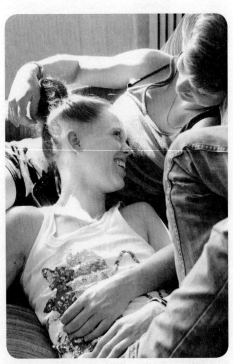

What characterizes romantic relationships in sexual minority youth?
Johner Images/Getty Images

Romantic Relationships and Adjustment Researchers have linked dating and romantic relationships with various measures of how well adjusted adolescents are (Golden, Furman, & Collibee, 2018). Dating and romantic relationships at an early age can be especially problematic (Chen, Rothman, & Jaffee, 2017; Connolly & McIsaac, 2009). These researchers and others (for example, Garthe, Sullivan, & Behrhorst, 2018) have found that early dating and "going with" someone are linked with adolescent pregnancy, delinquency, problems with parents and peers, academic problems, and exposure to partner violence.

Consider also the following studies that link romantic relationships and adjustment in adolescence:

- Adolescents who are more socially anxious (for example, those who avoid social situations and worry about their relationships), also tend to withdraw from romantic and non-romantic friendships; if withdrawal becomes chronic, this can intensify social anxiety (Starr & Davila, 2015).
- Adolescent girls who engaged in co-rumination (excessive discussion of problems with friends) were more likely to be involved in a romantic relationship, and together co-rumination and romantic involvement predicted depressive symptoms in early adolescent girls (Starr & others, 2013).
- Across adolescence into young adulthood, romantic relationships that include jealousy and conflict are more likely to increase exposure to violence and substance abuse (Collibee, Furman, & Shoop, 2019).
- Adolescents with a stronger romantic involvement were more likely to engage in delinquency than their counterparts with a lower level of romantic involvement (Cui & others, 2012).

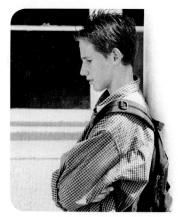
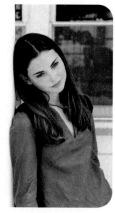

How are romantic relationships linked to adolescent adjustment?
Stockbyte/Getty Images

Relationships with Parents and Adolescent Romantic Relationships

Adolescents' relationships with their parents influence their dating and romantic relationships (Cheshire, Kaestle, & Miyazaki, 2019; Ivanova, Veenstra, & Mills, 2012; Low & Shortt, 2017). Attachment history is linked to couple relationships in adolescence and emerging adulthood (Sroufe, Coffino, & Carlson, 2010). For example, infants who have an anxious attachment with their caregivers in infancy are less likely to develop positive romantic relationships in adolescence than are their securely attached counterparts. It might be that adolescents with a history of secure attachment are better able to control their emotions and more comfortable self-disclosing in romantic relationships. One study of adolescent gay males showed that changes occurred in closeness and conflict in the parent-adolescent relationship after coming out, and these relationship dynamics influenced the boys' attitudes and behaviors around romantic relationships and dating (Feinstein & others, 2018). In another study, Spanish adolescents who had secure and close attachment relationships with their parents also tended to have more positive and rewarding friend and romantic partner relationships (Viejo & others, 2018).

Adolescents' observations of their parents' marital relationship also contribute to their own construction of dating relationships. One illustrative study of 17-year-old Israeli girls and their mothers revealed that mothers who reported a higher level of marital satisfaction had daughters who were more romantically competent (based on multiple dimensions, such as maturity, coherence, and realistic perception of the romantic relationship) (Shulman, Davila, & Shachar-Shapira, 2011).

Marital conflict and divorce also are linked to adolescents' and emerging adults' dating and romantic relationships. Adolescents whose mothers have had more marital and other romantic relationship changes (including divorce and remarriage) are themselves more likely to have more romantic partnership changes. This effect is accounted for, in part, by the overall quality of the mother-adolescent relationship (Cui, Gordon, & Wickrama, 2016). Another study revealed that an adolescent's first romantic relationship occurred earlier in divorced than non-divorced intact families, but only when the divorce occurred in early adolescence (Ivanova, Veenstra, & Mills, 2012).

One longitudinal study examined how youths' personality traits and beliefs about marriage are related to romantic relationships in early adulthood (Masarik & others, 2013). In this study, a higher level of emotional instability in the ninth grade was linked with the belief in late adolescence/early adulthood that marriage is not likely to lead to fulfillment in life and happiness as an adult. And less endorsement of the marriage/fulfillment belief, in turn, predicted fewer observed positive interactions with a romantic partner and lower perceived relationship quality in early adulthood. This "intergenerational transmission" of

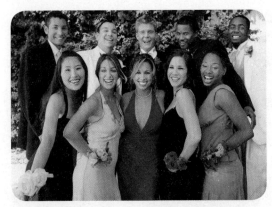

What are some ethnic variations in dating during adolescence?
Mike Watson Images/Moodboard/Getty Images

conflict in romantic relationships and marriages reflects complex interactions between experiences and genetic factors (Salvatore & others, 2018).

Sociocultural Contexts and Dating   The sociocultural context exerts a powerful influence on adolescents' dating patterns (Stein & others, 2018). This influence may be seen in differences in dating patterns among geographic, socioeconomic, and ethnic groups within diverse countries. For example, in the largest study to date in the United States, researchers found that older adolescents are more likely to engage in dating and other "adult-like" behaviors if they are from lower-SES, larger families (Twenge & Park, 2019). In another study comparing low-income urban areas in five cities around the world—Baltimore (United States), Cuenca (Ecuador), Edinburgh (Scotland), Ghent (Belgium), and Nairobi (Kenya)—researchers found consistency in 11- to 13-year-olds' views of romantic relationships and gender roles. However, there were some distinctions, such as a stronger emphasis on concern about dating violence in Nairobi, and emphasis on not being allowed to date among youth in Ghent, Baltimore, and Nairobi (De Meyer & others, 2017).

Values, religious beliefs, and traditions often dictate the age at which dating begins, how much freedom in dating is allowed, whether dates must be chaperoned by adults or parents, and the roles of males and females in dating (Taggart & others, 2018). For example, in the United States, Latino and Asian American cultures have more conservative standards regarding adolescent dating than do the African American and Anglo-American cultures. Dating may become a source of conflict within a family if the parents have immigrated from cultures in which dating begins at a late age, little freedom in dating is allowed, dates are chaperoned, and dating by adolescent girls is especially restricted. When immigrant adolescents choose to adopt the ways of the dominant culture (such as unchaperoned dating), they often clash with parents and extended-family members who hold more traditional values (Shenhav, Campos, & Goldberg, 2017).

Review *Connect* Reflect

LG4 Characterize peer relations in adolescence.

Review
- How are peer pressure and conformity shown in adolescence?
- How are cliques and crowds involved in adolescent development?
- What characterizes adolescents' dating and romantic relationships?

Connect
- In the *Connecting with Diversity* interlude in this chapter, you learned about the Murian culture of eastern India. Based on the information in this

last section, how do you think Murian immigrants in the United States might react to their adolescents' dating?

Reflect *Your Own Personal Journey of Life*
- What were your peer relationships like during adolescence? What peer groups were you involved in? How did they influence your development? If you could change anything about the way you experienced peer relations in adolescence, what would it be?

reach your **learning goals**

Peers

Peer Relations

LG1 Discuss peer relations in childhood.

Exploring Peer Relations

- Peers are children who share the same age or maturity level. Peers provide a means of social comparison and a source of information about the world outside the family. Good peer relations may be necessary for normal social development. The inability to "plug in" to a social network is associated with a number of problems. Peer relations can be both positive and negative. Piaget and Sullivan stressed that peer relations provide the context for learning important aspects of relationships, such as observing others' interests and perspectives and exploring fairness and justice by working through disagreements. Peer relations vary according to the way peer experience is measured, the outcomes specified, and the developmental trajectories traversed. Contexts and individual differences influence peer relations.

The Developmental Course of Peer Relations in Childhood

- Some researchers argue that the quality of social interaction with peers in infancy provides valuable information about socioemotional development. As increasing numbers of infants spend time in child care, infant peer relations have increased. The frequency of peer interaction, both positive and negative, increases during the preschool years. Children spend even more time with peers in the elementary and secondary school years, and their preference for same-sex groups increases. Boys' groups are larger than girls', and they participate in more organized games than girls do. Girls engage in more collaborative discourse in peer groups than boys do.

The Distinct but Coordinated Worlds of Parent-Child and Peer Relations

- Healthy family relations usually promote healthy peer relations. Parents can model or coach their children in ways of relating to peers. Parents' choices of neighborhoods, religious organizations, schools, and their own friends influence the pool from which their children might select possible friends. Rough-and-tumble play occurs mainly in peer relations rather than in parent-child relations. In times of stress, children usually turn to parents rather than peers. Peer relations have a more equal basis than parent-child relations.

Social Cognition and Emotion

- Perspective taking and social information-processing skills are important dimensions of social cognition in peer relations. Perspective taking helps children communicate effectively. Self-regulation of emotion is associated with positive peer relations.

Peer Statuses

- Popular children are frequently identified as a best friend by other children and are rarely disliked by their peers. Average children receive an average number of both positive and negative nominations from their peers. Neglected children are infrequently identified as a best friend but are not disliked by their peers. Rejected children are infrequently identified as a best friend and are disliked by their peers. Rejected children often have more serious adjustment problems than neglected children do. Controversial children are frequently identified both as a best friend and as being disliked by peers.

Bullying

- Bullying is physical or verbal behavior meant to disturb a less powerful individual. Significant numbers of students are bullied, and this is linked to adjustment problems for the victim, the bully, or the individual who is both a bully and a victim.

Play

LG2 Describe children's play.

Play's Functions

- The functions of play include affiliation with peers, tension release, advances in cognitive development, and exploration.

Types of Play

- The contemporary perspective emphasizes both social and cognitive aspects of play. The most widely studied types of play include sensorimotor and practice play, pretense/symbolic play, social play, constructive play, and games.

Trends in Play

- Children's free play time has declined considerably over the years. This change is significant because children often learn best when they are in playful contexts. Play promotes numerous aspects of socioemotional development.

Friendship

LG3 Explain friendship.

Friendship's Functions

- The functions of friendship include companionship, stimulation, physical support, ego support, social comparison, and intimacy/affection. Sullivan pointed out that whether or not these functions of friendship are fulfilled largely determines our emotional well-being. Sullivan argued that there is a dramatic increase in the psychological importance and intimacy of close friends in early adolescence. Research findings support his view.

Similarity and Intimacy

- Similarity and intimacy are two of the most common characteristics of friendships. Friends often have similar attitudes toward school, similar educational aspirations, and so on. Intimacy in friendship is much more common among adolescents than children.

Gender and Friendship

- An increasing number of studies indicate that the friendships of girls differ from the friendships of boys. The influence of friendship, both positive and negative, may be stronger for girls. Intimacy plays a powerful role in girls' friendships, and power, excitement, and control play important roles in boys' friendships.

Mixed-Age Friendships

- Children and adolescents who become friends with older individuals engage in more deviant behaviors than do their counterparts with same-age friends. Adolescent girls who have older male friends may be more likely to engage in problem behavior.

Other-Sex Friendships

- The number of other-sex friendships increases as adolescence proceeds. Other-sex friendships provide a context for learning how to communicate with the other sex and reduce anxiety in social and dating contexts. However, some aspects of other-sex friendships are linked to negative outcomes, such as earlier sexual intercourse and drug use.

Peer Relations in Adolescence

 LG4 Characterize peer relations in adolescence.

Peer Pressure and Conformity

- The pressure to conform to peers is strong during adolescence, especially in eighth and ninth grades, and can have positive or negative effects.

Cliques and Crowds

- Cliques and crowds assume more importance in the lives of adolescents than in the lives of children. Cliques become increasingly mixed-sex in adolescence. Membership in certain crowds is associated with increased self-esteem.

Romantic Relationships

- Three stages characterize the development of romantic relationships in adolescence, although there are cultural variations in adolescent dating: (1) entry into romantic attractions and affiliations at about 11 to 13 years of age, (2) exploring romantic relationships at approximately 14 to 16 years of age, and (3) consolidating dyadic romantic bonds at about 17 to 19 years of age. A special concern is early dating, which is associated with a number of problems. Most gay, lesbian, and bisexual youth have same-sex sexual experience, but same-sex romantic relationships are less common. Many date other-sex peers, which can help them to clarify their sexual orientation or disguise it from others. Adolescents who date have more problems, such as substance abuse, than those who do not date, but they also have more acceptance with peers. Parent-adolescent relationships are linked to adolescents' and emerging adults' dating and romantic relationships. Culture can exert a powerful influence on dating. Many adolescents from immigrant families face conflicts with their parents about dating.

key terms

average children 422	games 429	play therapy 426	rejected children 422
cliques 434	intimacy in friendship 432	popular children 422	sensorimotor play 427
constructive play 428	neglected children 422	practice play 427	social play 428
controversial children 422	peers 417	pretense/symbolic play 428	
crowds 435	play 426		

key people

Daniel Berlyne 427	Erik Erikson 426	Kathy Hirsh-Pasek 429	Dorothy Singer 429
Kenneth Dodge 421	Sigmund Freud 426	Jean Piaget 426	Harry Stack Sullivan 430
Dexter Dunphy 435	Roberta Golinkoff 429	Mitchell Prinstein 434	Lev Vygotsky 426

chapter 16

SCHOOLS AND ACHIEVEMENT

chapter outline

1 Exploring Children's Schooling

Learning Goal 1 Discuss approaches to schooling and development.

Contemporary Approaches to Student Learning and Assessment

Early Childhood Education

Elementary School

Educating Adolescents

Socioeconomic Status and Ethnicity

2 Children with Disabilities

Learning Goal 2 Characterize children with disabilities and their education.

The Scope of Disabilities

Educational Issues

3 Achievement

Learning Goal 3 Explain the development of achievement in children.

Extrinsic and Intrinsic Motivation

Cognitive Processes

Ethnicity and Culture

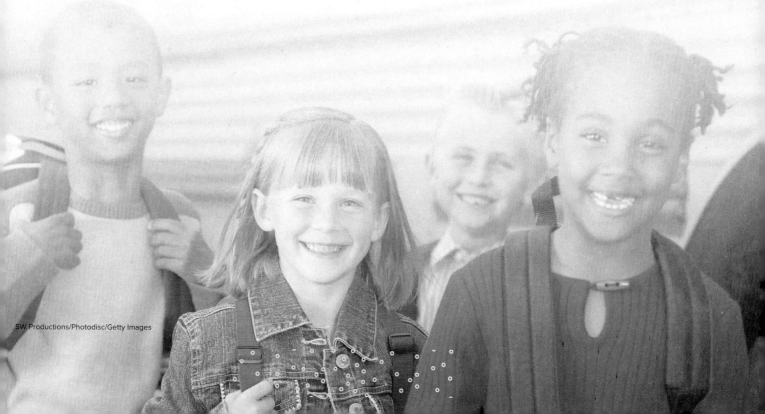

SW Productions/Photodisc/Getty Images

The Reggio Emilia approach is an educational program for young children that was developed in the northern Italian city of Reggio Emilia. Children of single parents and children with disabilities have priority in admission; other children are admitted according to a scale of needs. Parents pay on a sliding scale based on income.

The children are encouraged to learn by investigating and exploring topics that interest them. A wide range of stimulating media and materials is available for children to use as they learn—music, movement, drawing, painting, sculpting, collages, puppets and disguises, and photography, for example (Edwards & Gandini, 2018).

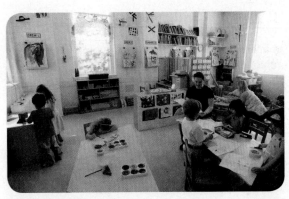

A Reggio Emilia classroom in which young children explore topics that interest them.

Ruby Washington/The New York Times/Redux Pictures

In this program, children often explore topics in a group, which fosters a sense of community, respect for diversity, and a collaborative approach to problem solving (Edwards & Gandini, 2018). Two co-teachers are present to serve as guides for children. The Reggio Emilia teachers view a project as an adventure, which can start from an adult's suggestion, from a child's idea, or from an event, such as a snowfall or something else unexpected. Every project is based on what the children say and do. The teachers allow children enough time to think and to craft a project.

At the core of the Reggio Emilia approach is the image of children who are competent and have rights, especially the right to outstanding care and education. Parent participation is considered essential, and cooperation is a major theme in the schools. Many early childhood education experts believe the Reggio Emilia approach provides a supportive, stimulating context in which children are motivated to explore their world in a competent and confident manner (Edwards & Gandini, 2018).

preview

This chapter is about becoming educated and achieving. We will explore topics such as contemporary approaches to student learning, school transitions, the roles that socioeconomic status and ethnicity play in schools, educational issues involving children with disabilities, and motivation to achieve goals.

Exploring Children's Schooling Discuss approaches to schooling and development.

| Contemporary Approaches to Student Learning and Assessment | Early Childhood Education | Elementary School | Educating Adolescents | Socioeconomic Status and Ethnicity |

You already have read about many aspects of schools throughout this edition, especially in the section "Cognition and Language." Recall our coverage of applications of Piaget's and Vygotsky's theories to education, strategies for encouraging children's critical thinking in schools, applications of Gardner's and Sternberg's theories of intelligence to education, and bilingual education. Here you will take a closer look at contemporary approaches to student learning in U.S. schools, variations in schooling from early childhood education through high school, and the influence of socioeconomic status and ethnicity on children's education.

For most children, entering the first grade signals new obligations. They form new relationships and develop new standards by which to judge themselves. School provides children with a rich source of new ideas to shape their sense of self. They will spend many years in schools as members of small societies in which there are tasks to be accomplished, people to be socialized and to be socialized by, and rules that define and limit behavior, feelings, and attitudes. By the time students graduate from high school, they will have spent 12,000 hours in the classroom.

CONTEMPORARY APPROACHES TO STUDENT LEARNING AND ASSESSMENT

Controversy surrounds questions about the best ways to teach children and how to hold schools and teachers accountable for whether children are learning (Borich, 2017).

Constructivist and Direct Instruction Approaches The **constructivist approach** is a learner-centered approach to teaching that emphasizes the importance of individuals actively constructing their knowledge and understanding with guidance from the teacher. In the constructivist view, teachers should not attempt to simply pour information into children's minds. Rather, children should be encouraged to explore their world, discover knowledge, reflect, and think critically, with careful monitoring and meaningful guidance from the teacher (Kauchak & Eggen, 2017). The constructivists believe that for too long in American education children have been required to sit still, be passive learners, and rotely memorize irrelevant as well as relevant information (Johnson & others, 2018).

Today, constructivism may include an emphasis on collaboration—children working together in their efforts to know and understand (Daniels, 2017). A teacher with a constructivist instructional philosophy would not have children memorize information but instead would give them opportunities to meaningfully construct their knowledge and understand the material while guiding their learning (Cruikshank, Jenkins, & Metcalf, 2012).

developmental **connection**

Cognitive Theory

Piaget's and Vygotsky's theories can be applied to children's education. Connect to "Cognitive Developmental Approaches."

The whole art of teaching is the art of awakening the natural curiosity of young minds.

—ANATOLE FRANCE
French novelist, 20th century

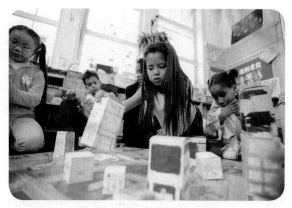

Is the teaching philosophy in this classroom more likely constructivist or direct instruction? Explain.
Stretch Photography/Getty Images

constructivist approach A learner-centered approach that emphasizes the importance of individuals actively constructing their knowledge and understanding, with guidance from the teacher.

direct instruction approach A teacher-centered approach characterized by teacher direction and control, mastery of academic material, high expectations for students' progress, and maximum time spent on learning tasks.

Education is the transmission of civilization.

—Ariel and Will Durant
American authors and philosophers, 20th century

By contrast, the **direct instruction approach** is a structured, teacher-centered approach that is characterized by teacher direction and control, high teacher expectations for students' progress, maximum time spent by students on academic tasks, and efforts by the teacher to keep negative affect to a minimum. An important goal in the direct instruction approach is maximizing student learning time (Parkay, 2016).

Advocates of the constructivist approach argue that the direct instruction approach turns children into passive learners and does not adequately challenge them to think in critical and creative ways (Borich, 2017). The direct instruction enthusiasts say that the constructivist approaches do not give enough attention to the content of a discipline, such as history or science. They also believe that the constructivist approaches are too relativistic and vague.

Some experts in educational psychology believe that many effective teachers use both a constructivist *and* a direct instruction approach rather than relying exclusively on either one (Johnson & others, 2018). Further, some circumstances may call more for a constructivist approach and others for a direct instruction approach. For example, experts increasingly recommend an explicit, intellectually engaging direct instruction approach when teaching students with a reading or a writing disability (Temple & others, 2018).

Accountability   Since the 1990s, the U.S. public and governments at every level have demanded increased accountability from schools. One result was the spread of state-mandated testing to measure what students had or had not learned (Popham, 2017). Many states identified objectives for students in their state and created tests to measure whether students were meeting those objectives. This approach became national policy in 2002 when the No Child Left Behind (NCLB) legislation was signed into law and has continued through the 2015 Every Student Succeeds Act, which scales back but does not eliminate standardized testing.

In 2009, the Common Core State Standards Initiative was endorsed by the National Governors Association in an effort to implement more rigorous state guidelines for educating students. The Common Core State Standards specify what students should know and the skills they should develop at each grade level in various content areas (Common Core State Standards Initiative, 2019). A large majority of states have agreed to implement the Standards, but they have generated considerable controversy. Critics argue that they are simply a further effort by the federal government to control education and that they emphasize a "one-size-fits-all" approach that pays little attention to individual variations in students. Supporters say that the Standards provide much-needed detailed guidelines and important milestones for students to achieve.

Advocates of these initiatives argue that statewide standardized testing will have a number of positive effects. These include improved student performance; more time devoted to teaching the subjects that are tested; high expectations for all students; identification of poorly performing schools, teachers, and administrators; and improved confidence in schools as test scores rise.

Standardized tests can help educators identify students who are struggling as well as content areas in need of more instruction. For example, on the most recent national tests available in the United States, only 37 percent of fourth-grade students and 36 percent of eighth-grade students were identified as proficient or better in reading, and 40 percent of fourth-grade students and 34 percent of eighth-grade students were identified as proficient or better in math (McFarland & others, 2018). These numbers represent an increase from previous years but still indicate gaps in knowledge.

Critics of these programs argue that standardized tests do more harm than good (Ladd, 2017). One criticism stresses that using a single test as the sole indicator of students' progress and competence presents a very narrow view of students' skills (Lewis, 2007). This criticism is similar to the one leveled at IQ tests. To assess student progress and achievement, many psychologists and educators emphasize that a number of measures should be used, including tests, quizzes, projects, portfolios, classroom observations, and so on. Also, standardized tests don't measure creativity, motivation, persistence, flexible thinking, and social skills (Stiggins, 2008). Critics point out that

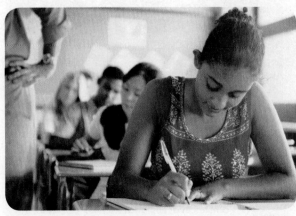

What characterizes the Every Student Succeeds legislation? What are some criticisms of the legislation?

teachers end up spending far too much class time "teaching to the test" by drilling students and having them memorize isolated facts at the expense of teaching that focuses on thinking skills, which students need for success in life (Ladd, 2017). Also, there is concern that students who are gifted are being neglected in the effort to raise the achievement level of students who are not doing well on standardized tests (Ballou & Springer, 2017).

In addition to keeping schools accountable for student achievement, standardized tests often are used to compare how students in different countries perform relative to one another in math, science, and other subjects. For example, the Program for International Student Assessment (PISA) and Trends in International Math and Science Study (TIMSS) have been used to create country rankings of students' performance on benchmark tests at certain grade levels (McFarland & others, 2018). Fourth-grade students in the United States rank 15th in science and 20th in math out of 54 countries that participated in the 2015 TIMSS. Education methods in countries that perform well on international tests have been adopted in other countries in an effort to improve learning and boost student achievement. For example, because Singapore consistently is at the top of the rankings in students' math and science scores, educators in some other countries have adjusted their course content and instructional practices to incorporate the national math curriculum used in elementary schools in Singapore (Jaciw & others, 2016).

Let's now explore what schools are like for different developmental levels of students. We will begin with early childhood education.

developmental **connection**

Cognitive Theory

Both Piaget and Vygotsky believed that play is an excellent setting for young children's cognitive development. Connect to "Peers."

EARLY CHILDHOOD EDUCATION

To the teachers in a Reggio Emilia program (described at the beginning of this chapter), preschool children are active learners, exploring the world with their peers, constructing their knowledge of the world in collaboration with their community, aided but not directed by their teachers. In many ways, the Reggio Emilia approach applies ideas consistent with the views of Piaget and Vygotsky discussed in the chapter "Cognitive Developmental Approaches." Our exploration of early childhood education focuses on variations in programs, educational strategies for young children who are disadvantaged, and some controversies in early childhood education.

Variations in Early Childhood Education   Attending preschool has become the norm for U.S. children. There are many variations in the way young children are educated (Feeney, Moravcik, & Nolte, 2018). The foundation of early childhood education has been the child-centered kindergarten.

The Child-Centered Kindergarten   Nurturing is a key aspect of the **child-centered kindergarten,** which emphasizes the education of the whole child and concern for his or her physical, cognitive, and socioemotional development (Segal & others, 2012). Instruction is organized around children's needs, interests, and learning styles. Emphasis is placed on the process of learning, rather than what is learned (Richards, 2017). The child-centered kindergarten honors three principles: (1) each child follows a unique developmental pattern; (2) young children learn best through firsthand experiences with people and materials; and (3) play is extremely important in the child's total development. Experimenting, exploring, discovering, trying out, restructuring, speaking, and listening are frequent activities in excellent kindergarten programs. Such programs are closely attuned to the developmental status of 5-year-old children.

The Montessori Approach   Montessori schools are patterned after the educational philosophy of Maria Montessori (1870–1952), an Italian physician-turned-educator who crafted a revolutionary approach to young children's education at the beginning of the twentieth century. The **Montessori approach** is a philosophy of education in which children are given considerable freedom and spontaneity in choosing activities. They are allowed to move from one activity to another as they desire. The teacher acts as a facilitator rather than a director. The teacher shows the child how to perform intellectual activities, demonstrates interesting ways to explore curriculum materials, and offers help when the child requests it (Marshall, 2017). The Montessori approach encourages independent problem

child-centered kindergarten Education that involves the whole child by considering both the child's physical, cognitive, and socioemotional development and the child's needs, interests, and learning styles.

Montessori approach An educational philosophy in which children are given considerable freedom and spontaneity in choosing activities and are allowed to move from one activity to another as they desire.

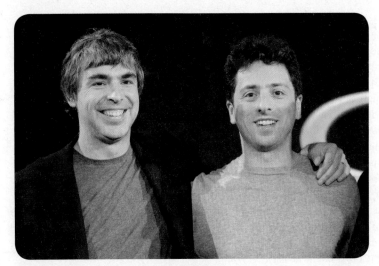

Larry Page and Sergey Brin, founders of the highly successful Internet search engine, Google, said that their early years at Montessori schools were a major factor in their success (International Montessori Council, 2006). During an interview with Barbara Walters, they said they learned how to be self-directed learners and self-starters at Montessori (ABC News, 2005). They commented that Montessori experiences encouraged them to think for themselves and allowed them the freedom to develop their own interests.

James Leynse/Corbis Historical/Getty Images

developmentally appropriate practice Education that focuses on the typical developmental patterns of children (age-appropriateness) and the uniqueness of each child (individual-appropriateness). Such practice contrasts with developmentally inappropriate practice, which relies on abstract paper-and-pencil activities presented to large groups of young children.

Project Head Start Compensatory education designed to provide children from low-income families the opportunity to acquire the skills and experiences important for school success.

solving and effective time management by giving children freedom to make their own decisions from an early age. The number of Montessori schools in the United States has expanded dramatically in recent years, from one school in 1959 to 355 schools in 1970 to more than 4,000 today. Worldwide, there are about 7,000 Montessori schools.

Some developmentalists favor the Montessori approach, but others conclude that it neglects children's socioemotional development. For example, although Montessori fosters independence and the development of cognitive skills, it deemphasizes verbal interaction between the teacher and child and between the children themselves. Montessori's critics also argue that it restricts imaginative play and that its heavy reliance on self-corrective materials may not adequately allow for creativity or accommodate a variety of learning styles.

Developmentally Appropriate and Inappropriate Education   Many educators and psychologists conclude that preschool and young elementary school children learn best through active, hands-on teaching methods such as games and dramatic play. They know that children develop at varying rates and that schools need to allow for these individual differences. They also argue that schools should focus on facilitating children's socioemotional development as well as their cognitive development. Educators refer to this type of schooling as **developmentally appropriate practice (DAP),** which is based on knowledge of the typical development of children within an age span (age-appropriateness), as well as the uniqueness of the child (individual-appropriateness) (Cobanoglu, Capa-Aydin, & Yildirim, 2019). In contrast, developmentally inappropriate practice for young children relies on abstract paper-and-pencil activities presented to large groups. Desired outcomes for DAP include thinking critically, working cooperatively, solving problems, developing self-regulatory skills, and enjoying learning. The emphasis in DAP is on the process of learning rather than its content (Cobanoglu, Capa-Aydin, & Yildirim, 2019). Figure 1 provides recommendations from the National Association for the Education of Young Children (NAEYC) for developmentally appropriate education in a number of areas (NAEYC, 2009).

Many but not all studies show significant positive benefits for developmentally appropriate education (Sanders & Farago, 2018). Among the reasons it is difficult to generalize about research on developmentally appropriate education is that individual programs often vary, and developmentally appropriate education is an evolving concept. Recent changes in the concept have focused more attention on sociocultural factors, the teacher's active involvement and implementation of systematic intentions, as well as the degree to which academic skills should be emphasized and how they should be taught.

Education for Young Children Who Are Disadvantaged   For many years, U.S. children from low-income families did not receive any education before entering the first grade. Often, they began first grade already several steps behind their classmates in their readiness to learn. In the summer of 1965, the federal government began an effort to break the cycle of poverty and poor education for young children in the United States through **Project Head Start.** It is a compensatory program designed to provide children from low-income families the opportunity to acquire the skills and experiences important for success in school (Morris & others, 2018). After more than half a century, Head Start continues to be the largest federally funded program for U.S. children, with almost 1 million children enrolled annually (Administration for Children and Families, 2019). In 2018, 1 percent of Head Start children were 5 years old or older, 38 percent were 4 years old, 35 percent

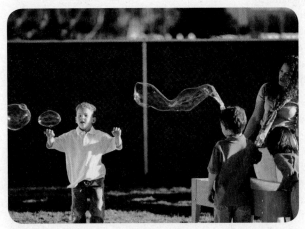

What are some key features of developmentally appropriate education?
Image100/Getty Images

Core Considerations in Developmentally Appropriate Practice

1 Knowledge to Consider in Making Decisions

In all aspects of working with children, early childhood practitioners need to consider these three areas of knowledge: 1) What is known about child development and learning, especially age-related characteristics; 2) What is known about each child as an individual; and 3) What is known about the social and cultural contexts in which children live.

2 Challenging and Achieveable Goals

Keeping in mind desired goals and what is known about the children as a group and individually, teachers plan experiences to promote children's learning and development.

Principles of Child Development and Learning that Inform Practice

1 All the domains of development and learning—physical, cognitive, emotional, and social—are important, and they are linked.

2 Many aspects of children's learning and development follow well-documented sequences, with later abilities, skills, and knowledge building on those already acquired.

3 Development and learning proceed at varying rates from child to child, and at uneven rates across different areas of a child's individual functioning.

4 Development and learning result from the interaction of biological maturation and experience.

5 Early experiences have strong effects—both cumulative and delayed—on children's development and learning; optimal periods exist for certain types of development and learning.

6 Development proceeds toward greater complexity, self-regulation, and symbolic or representational capacities.

7 Children develop best when they have secure, consistent relationships with responsive adults and opportunities for positive peer relations.

8 Development and learning occur in and are influenced by multiple social and cultural contexts.

9 Always mentally active in seeking to understand the world around them, children learn in a variety of ways; a wide range of teaching strategies can be effective in guiding children's learning.

10 Play is an important context for developing self-regulation and for promoting language, cognition, and social competence.

11 Development and learning advance when children are challenged to achieve at a level just beyond their current mastery and when they are given opportunities to practice newly acquired skills.

12 Children's experiences shape their motivation and approaches to learning, such as persistence, initiative, and flexibility; in turn, these characteristics influence their learning and development.

Selected Guidelines for Developmentally Appropriate Practice

1 Creating a Caring Community of Learners

Each member of the community should be valued by the others; relationships are an important context through which children learn; practitioners ensure that members of the community respected.

2 Teaching to Enhance Development and Learning

The teacher takes responsibility for stimulating, directing, and supporting children's learning by providing the experiences that each child needs.

3 Planning Curriculum to Achieve Important Goals

The curriculum is planned to help children achieve goals that are developmentally appropriate and educationally significant.

4 Assessing Children's Development and Learning

In developmentally appropriate practice, assessments are linked to the program's goals for children.

5 Establishing Reciprocal Relationships with Families

A positive partnership between teachers and families benefits children's learning and development.

FIGURE 1

RECOMMENDATIONS BY NAEYC FOR DEVELOPMENTALLY APPROPRIATE PRACTICE IN EARLY CHILDHOOD PROGRAMS SERVING CHILDREN FROM BIRTH THROUGH AGE 8. Source: Adapted from NAEYC (2009). Developmentally appropriate practice in early childhood programs serving children from birth through age 8.

were 3 years old, and the remainder were under 3 years of age (Administration for Children and Families, 2019).

Early Head Start was established in 1995 to serve children from birth to 3 years of age. In 2007, half of all new funds appropriated for Head Start programs were used for the expansion of Early Head Start. Researchers have found positive effects for Early Head Start and indications that Early Head Start can serve as a buffer to protect children from risk factors in the family by offering supports to both parents and children (Paschall, Mastergeorge, & Ayoub, 2019).

Head Start programs are not all created equal. Variations in the effectiveness of Head Start are found as a function of the types of services offered as part of the program, the characteristics of the participating children, and alternative care options that may be available (Morris & others, 2018). More attention needs to be given to developing consistently high-quality Head Start programs (Berlin, Martoccio, & Jones Harden, 2018). One individual who is strongly motivated to make Head Start a valuable learning experience for young children from disadvantaged backgrounds is Yolanda Garcia. To read about her work, see *Connecting with Careers.*

Yolanda Garcia, Director of Children's Services/Head Start

Yolanda Garcia has been the Director of the Children's Services Department for the Santa Clara, California, County Office of Education since 1980. As director, she is responsible for managing child development programs for 2,500 3- to 5-year-old children in 127 classrooms. Her training includes two master's degrees—one in public policy and child welfare from the University of Chicago and the other in education administration from San Jose State University.

Garcia has served on many national advisory committees that have brought about improvements in the staffing of Head Start programs. Most notably, she served on the Head Start Quality Committee that recommended the development of Early Head Start and revised performance standards for Head Start programs. Garcia currently is a member of the American Academy of Science Committee on the Integration of Science and Early Childhood Education.

Evaluations support the positive influence of quality early childhood programs on both the cognitive and social worlds of disadvantaged young children (Yazejian & others, 2017). A national evaluation of Head Start revealed that the program had a positive influence on the language and cognitive development of the 3- and 4-year-olds who participated (National Head Start Association, 2016). However, by the end of the first grade, there were few lasting outcomes, except for a larger vocabulary for those who went to Head Start as 4-year-olds and better oral comprehension for those who went to Head Start as 3-year-olds. Also, in many early childhood educational programs that do not show differences in test scores later in elementary school, program participants show delayed benefits in terms of higher earnings in adulthood, perhaps because programs like Head Start improve socioemotional functioning and other factors that can have long-term benefits even if they are not captured in test scores (National Head Start Association, 2016).

One high-quality early childhood education program (although not a Head Start program) was the Perry Preschool program in Ypsilanti, Michigan, a two-year preschool program that included weekly home visits from program personnel. In analyses of the long-term effects of the program, adults who had been in the Perry Preschool program were compared with a control group of adults from the same background who had not received the enriched early childhood education (Schweinhart, 2019). Those who had been in the Perry Preschool program had fewer teen pregnancies and higher high school graduation rates, and at age 40 they were more likely to be in the workforce, to own their own homes, and to have a savings account, and they were less likely to have been arrested.

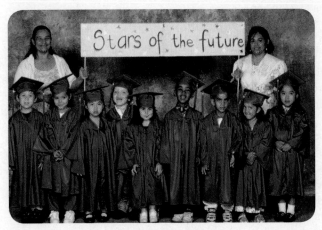

What are two controversies in early childhood education?
Ronnie Kaufman/Corbis/Getty Images

Controversies in Early Childhood Education   Two current controversies in early childhood education involve (1) what the curriculum for early childhood education should be (Auld & Morris, 2019), and (2) whether preschool education should be universal in the United States (Greenberg, 2018).

Curriculum Controversy   A current curriculum controversy in early childhood involves on one side those who advocate a child-centered, constructivist approach much like that emphasized by the NAEYC along the lines of developmentally appropriate practice. On the other side are those who endorse an academic, direct instruction approach.

In reality, many high-quality early childhood education programs include both academic and constructivist approaches. For example, many education experts worry about academic approaches that place too much pressure on young children to achieve and don't provide any opportunities to actively construct knowledge (Faas, Wu, & Geiger, 2017). These experts also point out that effective early childhood programs should focus on both cognitive development and socioemotional development, not exclusively on cognitive development (Tager, 2017).

Universal Preschool Education Another early childhood education controversy focuses on whether preschool education should be instituted for all 4-year-old children in the United States. Proponents of universal preschool education emphasize that quality preschools prepare children for success in school (Cascio, 2017). For example, quality preschool programs increase the likelihood that once children go to elementary and secondary school they will be less likely to be retained in a grade or to drop out of school. Proponents also point to analyses indicating that universal preschool would bring considerable cost savings on the order of billions of dollars because of a diminished need for remedial and justice services (van Huizen, Dumhs, & Plantenga, 2019).

Critics of universal preschool education argue that the gains attributed to preschool and kindergarten education are often overstated. They especially stress that research has not proven that nondisadvantaged children benefit from attending a preschool. Thus, the critics say it is more important to improve preschool education for young children who are disadvantaged than to mandate preschool education for all 4-year-old children. Some critics, especially homeschooling advocates, emphasize that young children should be educated by their parents, not by schools. Thus, controversy continues to surround the issue of universal preschool education.

In many countries, some of the goals of early childhood education are quite different from those of American programs. To read about the differences, see *Connecting with Diversity*.

ELEMENTARY SCHOOL

For many children, entering the first grade signals a change from being a "home-child" to being a "school-child"—a situation in which new roles and obligations are experienced. Children take up the new role of being a student, interact with peers and teachers, develop new relationships, adopt new reference groups, and discover new standards by which to judge themselves. School provides children with a rich source of new ideas to shape their sense of self.

Too often early schooling proceeds mainly on the basis of negative feedback. A meta-analysis of 107 studies found that self-esteem and motivation variables decreased over the course of schooling, with the sharpest declines for intrinsic motivation, math and language academic self-concepts, mastery achievement goals, and performance-approach achievement goals (Scherrer & Preckel, 2019).

EDUCATING ADOLESCENTS

What is the transition from elementary to middle or junior high school like? What are the characteristics of effective schools for young adolescents? How can adolescents be encouraged to stay in school?

The Transition to Middle or Junior High School The first year of middle school or junior high school can be difficult for many students (Coelho, Marchante, & Jimerson, 2017). For example, students' academic motivation and engagement often drop during school transitions, especially if students perceive themselves as lacking control and efficacy to meet new academic challenges (Anderson & others, 2019). School transitions are less stressful for students who have relationships with teachers characterized by high levels of warmth and low levels of conflict (Hughes & Cao, 2018). More than 90 percent of American students also report that their parents are helpful during the transition to middle school (Fite & others, 2019). One reason that school transitions can be difficult is that they tend to disrupt friendships. For example, in a longitudinal study in 26 middle schools in the United States, more than two-thirds of friendships were either gained or lost in the first year of middle school; greater instability in friendships was predictive of less school engagement and lower grades (Lessard & Juvonen, 2018).

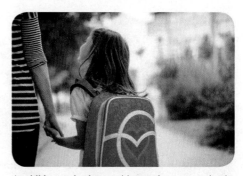

As children make the transition to elementary school, they interact and develop relationships with new and significant others. School provides them with a rich source of new ideas to shape their sense of self.
Damircudic/E+/Getty Images

Early Childhood Education in Japan and Developing Countries

As in America, there is diversity in Japanese early childhood education. Some Japanese kindergartens have specific aims, such as early musical training or the practice of Montessori strategies. In large cities, some kindergartens are attached to universities that have elementary and secondary schools. In most Japanese preschools, however, little emphasis is put on academic instruction.

In one study, 300 Japanese and 210 American preschool teachers, child development specialists, and parents were asked about various aspects of early childhood education (Tobin, Wu, & Davidson, 1989). Only 2 percent of the Japanese respondents listed "to give children a good start academically" as one of their top three reasons for a society to have preschools. In contrast, over half the American respondents chose this as one of their top three reasons. Japanese preschools do not teach reading, writing, and mathematics but focus on the development of skills like persistence, concentration, and the ability to function as a member of a group. The vast majority of young Japanese children are taught to read at home by their parents.

In the comparison of Japanese and American parents, more than 60 percent of the Japanese parents said that the purpose of preschool is to give children experience being a member of the group, as compared with about 20 percent of the U.S. parents (Tobin, Wu, & Davidson, 1989) (see Figure 2). Lessons in living and working together grow naturally out of the Japanese culture. In many Japanese kindergartens, children wear the same uniforms, including caps in different colors to indicate the classrooms to which they belong. They have identical sets of equipment, kept in identical drawers and shelves. This is not intended to turn the young children into robots, as some Americans have commented, but to impress on them that other people, just like themselves, have needs and desires that are equally important (Hendry, 1995).

Japan is a highly advanced industrialized country. What about early childhood education in low- and middle-income countries? Globally, almost half of preschool-age children are not enrolled in any preschool programs (UNICEF, 2019). In low-income countries, only about 20 percent of preschool-aged children are enrolled in preschool, and those who are enrolled often are in crowded classrooms without trained teachers or stimulating curricula. According to UNICEF, universal access to preschool education should be a priority because it sets the stage for early learning, helps students succeed in school, and, eventually promotes economic growth by keeping students in school to prepare for eventual participation in the labor market. The Sustainable Development Goals guiding the international development agenda through 2030 call for universal access to at least one year of preschool for all children globally.

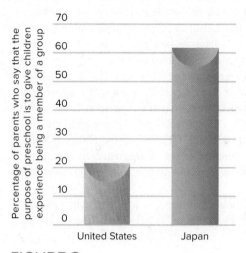

Percentage of parents who say that the purpose of preschool is to give children experience being a member of a group

United States — Japan

FIGURE **2**

COMPARISON OF JAPANESE AND U.S. PARENTS' VIEWS ON THE PURPOSE OF PRESCHOOL

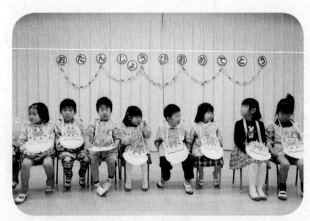

What characterizes early childhood education in Japan?
Andreas Meichsner/Laif/Redux Pictures

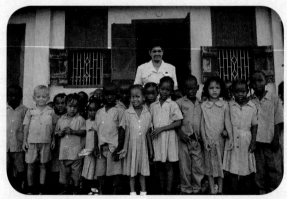

What characterizes early childhood education in many low- and middle-income countries like Jamaica (shown here)?
Nik Wheeler/Corbis NX/Getty Images

The transition to middle or junior high school takes place at a time when many changes—in the individual, in the family, and in school—are occurring simultaneously (Gazelle & Faldowski, 2019). These changes include puberty and related concerns about body image; the emergence of at least some aspects of formal operational thought, including accompanying changes in social cognition; increased responsibility and decreased dependency on parents; change to a larger, more impersonal school structure; change from one teacher to many teachers and from a small, homogeneous set of peers to a larger, more heterogeneous set of peers; and an increased focus on achievement and performance. Moreover, when students make the transition to middle or junior high school, they experience the **top-dog phenomenon** of moving from being the oldest, biggest, and most powerful students in elementary school to being the youngest, smallest, and least powerful students in middle or junior high school.

There can also be positive aspects to the transition to middle or junior high school. Students are more likely to feel grown up, have more subjects from which to select, have more opportunities to spend time with peers and locate compatible friends, and enjoy increased independence from direct parental monitoring. They also may be more challenged intellectually by academic work.

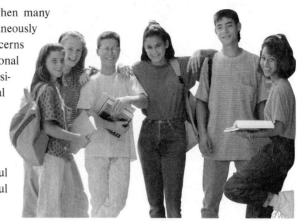

The transition from elementary to middle or junior high school occurs at the same time as a number of other developmental changes. *What are some of these other developmental changes?*

Comstock/SuperStock

Effective Schools for Young Adolescents

Critics argue that middle and junior high schools should offer activities that reflect a wide range of individual differences in biological and psychological development among young adolescents. In 1989 the Carnegie Corporation issued an extremely negative evaluation of U.S. middle schools. It concluded that most young adolescents attended massive, impersonal schools; were taught from irrelevant curricula; trusted few adults in school; and lacked access to health care and counseling. It recommended that the nation develop smaller "communities" or "houses" to lessen the impersonal nature of large middle schools, have lower student-to-counselor ratios (10 to 1 instead of several hundred to 1), involve parents and community leaders in schools, develop new curricula, have teachers team teach in more flexibly designed curriculum blocks that integrate several disciplines, boost students' health and fitness with more in-school programs, and help students who need public health care to get it. Three decades later, experts are still finding that middle schools throughout the United States need a major redesign if they are to be effective in educating adolescents (Yeager, Dahl, & Dweck, 2018).

High School

Just as there are concerns about U.S. middle school education, so are there concerns about U.S. high school education (Roundfield, Sánchez, & McMahon, 2018). Critics stress that in many high schools expectations for success and standards for learning are too low. Critics also argue that too often high schools foster passivity and that schools should create a variety of pathways for students to achieve an identity. Many students graduate from high school with inadequate reading, writing, and mathematical skills—including many who go on to college and have to enroll in remediation classes there. Other students drop out of high school and do not have skills that will allow them to obtain decent jobs, much less to be informed citizens (Lee-St. John & others, 2018).

Another major problem with U.S. high schools is that the negative social aspects of adolescents' lives undermine their academic achievement. For example, some adolescents become immersed in complex peer group cultures that demand conformity (Crosnoe, Pivnick, & Benner, 2018). High school is supposed to be about getting an education, but the reality for many youth is that high school is as much about navigating the social worlds of peer relations that may or may not value education and academic achievement. Adolescents who don't fit in with their peers may become stigmatized.

In the last half of the twentieth century and the first several years of the twenty-first century, U.S. high school dropout rates declined (National Center for Education Statistics, 2018). In the 1940s, more than half of U.S. 16- to 24-year-olds had dropped out of school; by 2016, this figure had decreased to 6.1 percent. The dropout rate of Latino adolescents remains high, although it has been decreasing in the twenty-first century (from 28 percent

top-dog phenomenon The circumstance of moving from the top position in elementary school to the lowest position in middle or junior high school.

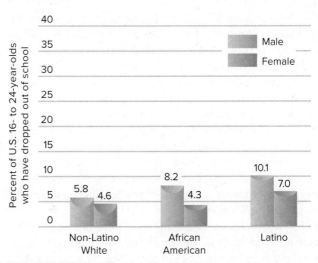

FIGURE **3**

SCHOOL DROPOUT RATES OF U.S. 16- TO 24-YEAR-OLDS BY GENDER AND ETHNICITY

in 2000 to 8.6 percent in 2016). The lowest dropout rate in 2016 occurred for Asian American adolescents (2.0 percent), followed by non-Latino White adolescents (5.2 percent), African American adolescents (6.2 percent), Latino adolescents (8.6 percent), and Native American adolescents (11.0 percent).

Gender differences characterize U.S. dropout rates, with males more likely to drop out than females (7.1 versus 5.1 percent; data for 2016) (National Center for Education Statistics, 2018). Figure 3 shows the dropout rates of 16- to 24-year-olds by ethnicity and gender in 2016.

The average U.S. high school dropout rates just described mask some very high dropout rates in low-income areas of inner cities. For example, in cities such as Detroit, Cleveland, and Chicago, dropout rates are above 50 percent. Also, the percentages cited in Figure 3 are for 16- to 24-year-olds. When dropout rates include students who take longer than four years to complete high school, the percentage of students is also much higher than in Figure 3. Thus, in considering high school dropout rates, it is important to examine age, the number of years it takes to complete high school, and various contexts including ethnicity, gender, and school location.

Students drop out of school for many reasons. In one study, almost 50 percent of the dropouts cited school-related reasons for leaving school, such as not liking school or being expelled or suspended (Rumberger, 1995). Twenty percent of the dropouts (but 40 percent of the Latino students) cited economic reasons for leaving school. One-third of the female students dropped out for personal reasons such as pregnancy or marriage. Students who dropped out of high school were three times as likely to have experienced a major recent stressful life event in comparison with average students as well as high-risk students who stayed in school (Dupéré & others, 2018).

A number of interventions have been developed to prevent students from dropping out of high school; programs that involve regular check-ins with trusted adults and mentoring programs have been found to be particularly effective. High schools that are effective in reducing dropout rates also emphasize the creation of caring environments and relationships, use block scheduling, and offer community-service opportunities.

Early detection of children's school-related difficulties, and getting children engaged with school in positive ways, are important strategies for reducing the dropout rate. The Bill and Melinda Gates Foundation has funded efforts to reduce the dropout rate in schools where dropout rates are high. One strategy that is being emphasized in the Gates' funding is

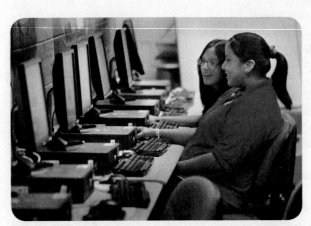

Students at the Ahfachkee School located on the Seminole Tribe's Big Cypress Reservation in Florida. An important educational goal is to increase the high school graduation rate of Native American adolescents.
J. Albert Diaz/Miami Herald/MCT/Tribune News Service/Getty Images

"I Have a Dream"

"I Have a Dream" (IHAD) is an innovative, comprehensive, long-term dropout prevention program administered by the national "I Have a Dream" Foundation in New York. Since the national IHAD Foundation was created in 1986, it has grown to support more than 5,000 students from kindergarten through post-secondary education in nine states and New Zealand ("I Have a Dream" Foundation, 2019). Local IHAD projects around the country "adopt" entire grades (usually the third or fourth) from public elementary schools, or corresponding age cohorts from public housing developments. These children are then provided with a program of academic, social, cultural, and recreational activities throughout their elementary, middle school, and high school years. An important part of this program is that it is personal rather than institutional: IHAD sponsors and staff develop close, long-term relationships with the children. When participants complete high school, IHAD provides the tuition assistance necessary for them to attend a state or local college or vocational school.

The IHAD program was created in 1981, when philanthropist Eugene Lang made an impromptu offer of college tuition to a class of graduating sixth-graders at P.S. 121 in East Harlem. Evaluations of IHAD programs have found dramatic improvements in grades, test scores, and school attendance, as well as a reduction of behavioral problems among participants. Ninety percent of "I Have a Dream" program participants graduate from high school, compared with 74 percent of their low-income peers who do

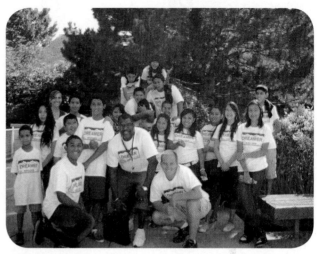

These adolescents participate in the "I Have a Dream" (IHAD) program, a comprehensive, long-term dropout prevention program that has been very successful. *What are some other strategies for reducing high school dropout rates?*
Courtesy of "I Have a Dream" Foundation of Boulder County (www.ihadboulder.org)

not participate in the program. In addition, participants are three times more likely than their nonparticipant peers to earn a bachelor's degree ("I Have a Dream" Foundation, 2019).

keeping students who are at risk for dropping out of school with the same teachers throughout their high school years. The hope is that the teachers will get to know these students much better, their relationship with the students will improve, and teachers will be able to monitor and guide the students toward graduating from high school. To read about one program that attempts to reduce the school dropout rate, see *Caring Connections*.

Extracurricular Activities   Adolescents in U.S. schools usually can choose from a wide array of extracurricular activities in addition to their academic courses. These adult-sanctioned activities typically occur in the after-school hours and can be sponsored either by the school or the community. They include such diverse activities as sports, academic clubs, band, drama, and art clubs. Researchers have found that participation in extracurricular activities is linked to higher grades, increased school engagement, reduced likelihood of dropping out of school, improved probability of going to college, higher self-esteem, and lower rates of depression, delinquency, and substance abuse (Knifsend & others, 2018). Adolescents benefit from a breadth of extracurricular activities more than focusing on a single extracurricular activity.

Of course, the quality of the extracurricular activities matters (Knifsend & others, 2018). High-quality extracurricular activities that are likely to promote positive adolescent development provide competent and supportive adult mentors, opportunities for increasing school connectedness, challenging and meaningful activities, and opportunities for improving skills.

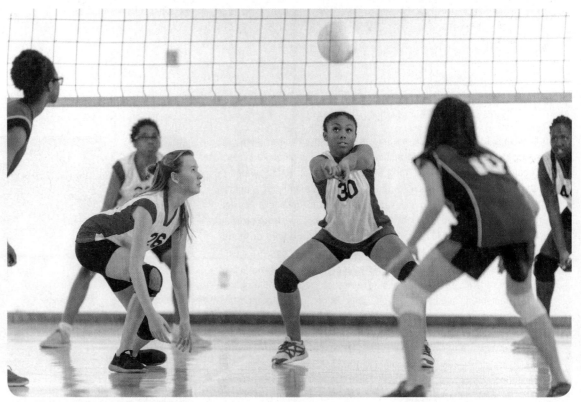

How does participation in extracurricular activities influence development in adolescence and emerging adulthood?
FatCamera/E+/Getty Images

------>

developmental **connection**

Socioeconomic Status

Socioeconomic differences are a proxy for material, human, and social capital within and beyond the family (Pascoe & others, 2016). Connect to "Culture and Diversity."

<------

SOCIOECONOMIC STATUS AND ETHNICITY

Children from low-income, ethnic minority backgrounds have more difficulties in school than do their middle-socioeconomic-status, White counterparts (Koppleman, 2017). Why? Critics argue that schools are not doing a good job of educating low-income or ethnic minority students (Troppe & others, 2017). Let's further explore the roles of socioeconomic status and ethnicity in schools.

Educating Students from Low-Income Backgrounds Many children living in poverty face problems that present barriers to their learning (Gardner, Brooks-Gunn, & Chase-Lansdale, 2016). They might have parents who don't set high educational standards for them, who are incapable of reading to them, or who don't have enough money to pay for educational materials and experiences, such as books and trips to zoos and museums. They might be malnourished or live in areas where crime and violence are a way of life. One study revealed that children born into poverty had lower test scores at 3, 5, and 7 years of age and that children who lived in poverty continuously had cognitive development scores at age 7 that were nearly 20 percentile ranks lower than children who had never lived in poverty, even after statistically controlling for a wide variety of other factors that can affect children's cognitive development (Dickerson & Popli, 2016).

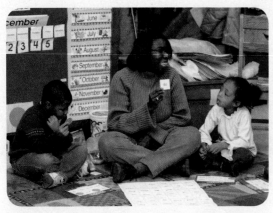

In *The Shame of the Nation,* Jonathan Kozol (2005) criticized the inadequate quality and lack of resources in many U.S. schools, especially those in the poverty areas of inner cities that have high concentrations of ethnic minority children. Kozol praises teachers like Angela Lively (above), who keeps a box of shoes in her Indianapolis classroom for students in need.
Michael Conroy/AP Images

The schools that children from impoverished backgrounds attend often have fewer resources than schools in higher-income neighborhoods (Curtis & Bandy, 2016). In low-income areas, schools are more likely to be staffed by young teachers with less experience than are schools in higher-income neighborhoods (Gollnick & Chinn, 2017). Schools in low-income areas also are more likely to encourage rote learning, whereas schools in higher-income areas are more likely to work with children to improve their thinking skills (Gollnick & Chinn, 2017). In sum, far too many schools in low-income neighborhoods provide students with environments that are not conducive to effective learning (Duncan, Magnuson, & Votruba-Drzal, 2017).

Ethnicity in Schools   More than one-third of all African American and almost one-third of all Latino students attend schools in the 47 largest city school districts in the United States, compared with only 5 percent of all White and 22 percent of all Asian American students. Many of these inner-city schools are still segregated, are grossly underfunded, and do not provide adequate opportunities for children to learn effectively. Thus, the effects of SES and the effects of ethnicity are often intertwined (Chaudry & others, 2017).

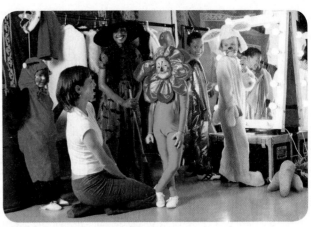

What are some features of a jigsaw classroom?
Richard Lewisohn/Alamy Stock Photo

Even outside of inner-city schools, school segregation remains a factor in U.S. education (Gollnick & Chinn, 2017). Almost one-third of all African American and Latino students attend schools in which 90 percent or more of the students are from minority groups (Banks, 2018).

The school experiences of students from different ethnic groups vary considerably (Koppleman, 2017). African American and Latino students are much less likely than non-Latino White or Asian American students to be enrolled in academic, college preparatory programs and are much more likely to be enrolled in remedial and special education programs. Asian American students are far more likely than other ethnic minority groups to take advanced math and science courses in high school. African American students are twice as likely as Latinos, Native Americans, or Whites to be suspended from school.

Following are some strategies for improving interaction among ethnically diverse students:

- *Turn the class into a jigsaw classroom.* When Elliot Aronson was a professor at the University of Texas at Austin, the school system contacted him for ideas on how to reduce the increasing racial tension in classrooms. Aronson (1986) developed the concept of a "jigsaw classroom" in which students from different cultural backgrounds are placed in a cooperative group where they are required to construct different parts of a project to reach a common goal. Aronson used the term *jigsaw* because he saw the technique as much like a group of students cooperating to put different pieces together to complete a jigsaw puzzle. How might this work? Team sports, drama productions, and music performances are examples of contexts in which students participate cooperatively to reach a common goal; however, the jigsaw technique also lends itself to group science projects, history reports, and other learning experiences involving a variety of subject matter.

- *Encourage students to have positive personal contact with diverse other students.* Mere contact does not do the job of improving relationships with diverse others. For example, busing ethnic minority students to predominantly White schools, or vice versa, has not reduced prejudice or improved interethnic relations. What matters is what happens after children get to school. Especially beneficial in improving interethnic relations is sharing one's worries, successes, failures, coping strategies, interests, and other personal information with people of other ethnicities. When this happens, people tend to look at others as individuals rather than as members of a homogeneous group.

- *Reduce bias.* Teachers can reduce bias by displaying images of children from diverse ethnic and cultural groups, selecting play materials and classroom activities that encourage cultural understanding, helping students resist stereotyping, and working with parents to reduce children's exposure to bias and prejudice at home.

- *Be a competent cultural mediator.* Teachers can play a powerful role as cultural mediators by being sensitive to biased content in curriculum materials and classroom interactions, learning more about different ethnic groups, being sensitive to children's ethnic attitudes, viewing students of color positively, and thinking of positive ways to get parents of color more involved as partners with teachers in educating children (Cushner, McClelland, & Safford, 2019).

- *View the school and community as a team.* James Comer (2010) advocates a community-wide, team-oriented approach as the best way to educate children. Three important aspects of the Comer Project for Change are (1) a governance and management team that develops a comprehensive school plan, assessment

James Comer, Child Psychiatrist

James Comer grew up in a low-income neighborhood in East Chicago, Indiana, and credits his parents with leaving no doubt about the importance of education. He obtained a bachelor's degree from Indiana University. He went on to obtain a medical degree from Howard University College of Medicine, a Master of Public Health degree from the University of Michigan School of Public Health, and psychiatry training at the Yale University School of Medicine's Child Study Center. He currently is the Maurice Falk professor of Child Psychiatry at the Yale University Child Study Center and an associate dean at the Yale University Medical School. During his years at Yale, Comer has concentrated on promoting a focus on child development as a way of improving schools. His efforts in support of healthy development of young people are known internationally.

Comer is, perhaps, best known for the founding of the School Development Program in 1968, which promotes the collaboration of parents, educators, and the surrounding community to improve social, emotional, and academic outcomes for children.

For more information about what psychiatrists do, see the Careers in Child Development appendix.

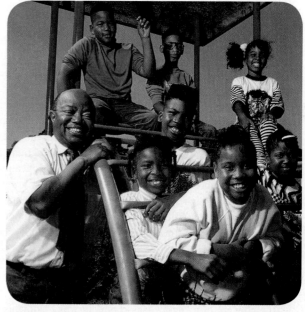

James Comer is shown with some of the inner-city children who attend a school that became a better learning environment because of Comer's intervention.
John S. Abbott

strategy, and staff development plan; (2) a mental health or school support team; and (3) a program for parents. Comer believes that the entire school community should have a cooperative rather than an adversarial attitude. The Comer program is currently operating in more than 1,000 schools in 26 states, Washington, DC, Trinidad and Tobago, South Africa, England, and Ireland. Read further about James Comer's work in the *Connecting with Careers* profile.

Review *Connect* Reflect

 Discuss approaches to schooling and development.

Review

- What are some contemporary approaches to student learning?
- What are some variations in early childhood education?
- What are some characteristics of elementary education?
- How are U.S. adolescents educated, and what are the challenges in educating adolescents?
- How do socioeconomic status and ethnicity affect children's education?

Connect

- In this section, you learned about socioeconomic status (SES) and education. What did you learn earlier about SES and how parents think about education? How does that tie into the importance of programs like IHAD and those sponsored by the Bill and Melinda Gates Foundation?

Reflect *Your Own Personal Journey of Life*

- How would you characterize the approach of the schools that you attended as a child and as an adolescent? Do you think your schools were effective? Explain.

What are some of the disabilities that children have? What characterizes the education of children with disabilities?

THE SCOPE OF DISABILITIES

Of all children from 3 to 21 years of age in the United States, 13.1 percent received special education or related services in 2015–2016, an increase of 3 percent since 1980–1981 (Condition of Education, 2018). Figure 4 shows the four largest groups of students with a disability who were served by federal programs during the 2015–2016 school year (Condition of Education, 2018).

As indicated in Figure 4, students with a learning disability were by far the largest group of students with a disability to be given special education, followed by children with speech or language impairments, other health impairments, and autism. The U.S. government's assessments of the prevalence of students with a disability includes attention deficit hyperactivity disorder (ADHD) in the category of learning disabilities.

Learning Disabilities The U.S. government created a definition of learning disabilities in 1997 and then reauthorized the definition with a few minor changes in 2004. Following is a description of the government's definition of what determined whether a child should be classified as having a learning disability. A child with a **learning disability** has difficulty in learning that involves understanding or using spoken or written language, and the difficulty can appear in listening, thinking, reading, writing, and spelling. A learning disability also may involve difficulty in doing mathematics (Werner, Berg, & Höhr, 2019). To be classified as a learning disability, the learning problem is not primarily the result of visual, hearing, or motor disabilities; intellectual disability; emotional disorders; or due to environmental, cultural, or economic disadvantage.

About three times as many boys as girls are classified as having a learning disability. Among the explanations for this gender difference are a greater biological vulnerability among boys and *referral bias.* That is, boys are more likely to be referred by teachers for treatment because of troublesome behavior.

Approximately 80 percent of children with a learning disability have a reading problem (Shaywitz, Gruen, & Shaywitz, 2007). Three types of learning disabilities are dyslexia, dysgraphia, and dyscalculia:

- **Dyslexia** is a category reserved for individuals who have a severe impairment in their ability to read and spell (Gelbar & others, 2018).
- **Dysgraphia** is a learning disability that involves difficulty in handwriting (Berninger & others, 2017). Children with dysgraphia may write very slowly, their writing products may be virtually illegible, and they may make numerous spelling errors because of their inability to match up sounds and letters (Hayes & Berninger, 2013).
- **Dyscalculia,** also known as developmental arithmetic disorder, is a learning disability that involves difficulty in math computation (Fuchs & others, 2013).

The precise causes of learning disabilities have not yet been determined, but a number of effective approaches can be used to improve educational outcomes of students with learning disabilities (Alquraini & Rao, 2019). Researchers have used brain-imaging techniques, such as magnetic resonance imaging, to reveal any regions of the brain that might be involved in learning disabilities (Jagger-Rickels, Kibby, & Constance, 2018)

Disability	Percentage Distribution of Students with Disabilities by Disability Type
Learning disabilities	34
Speech and language impairments	20
Other health impairments	14
Autism	9

FIGURE 4

U.S. CHILDREN WITH A DISABILITY WHO RECEIVE SPECIAL EDUCATION SERVICES. Figures are for the 2015–2016 school year and represent the four categories with the highest numbers and percentages of children. Both learning disability and attention deficit hyperactivity disorder are combined in the learning disabilities category (Condition of Education, 2018).

learning disabilities Disabilities involving understanding or using spoken or written language. The difficulty can appear in listening, thinking, reading, writing, spelling, or mathematics. To be classified as a learning disability, the problem must not be primarily the result of visual, hearing, or motor disabilities; intellectual disability; emotional disorders; or environmental, cultural, or economic disadvantage.

dyslexia A category of learning disabilities involving a severe impairment in the ability to read and spell.

dysgraphia A learning disability that involves difficulty in handwriting.

dyscalculia Also known as developmental arithmetic disorder; a learning disability that involves difficulty in math computation.

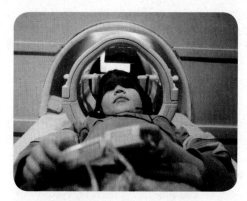

FIGURE 5

BRAIN SCANS AND LEARNING DISABILITIES.
An increasing number of studies are using MRI brain scans to examine the brain pathways involved in learning disabilities. Shown here is 9-year-old Patrick Price, who has dyslexia. Patrick is going through an MRI scanner disguised by drapes to look like a child-friendly castle. Inside the scanner, children must lie virtually motionless as words and symbols flash on a screen, and they are asked to identify them by clicking different buttons.
Manuel Balce Ceneta/AP Images

developmental connection

Attention

Attention, which involves the focusing of mental resources, improves cognitive processing on many tasks. Connect to "Information Processing."

Many children with ADHD show impulsive behavior. *How would you handle this situation if you were a teacher and this were to happen in your classroom?*
Nicole Hill/Rubberball/Getty Images

attention deficit hyperactivity disorder (ADHD)
A disability in which children consistently show one or more of the following characteristics: (1) inattention, (2) hyperactivity, and (3) impulsivity.

(see Figure 5). This research indicates that it is unlikely learning disabilities reside in a single, specific brain location. More likely, learning disabilities are due to problems in integrating information from multiple brain regions or subtle abnormalities in brain structures and functions.

Interventions with children who have a learning disability often focus on improving reading ability (Fletcher & others, 2018). Intensive instruction over a period of time by a competent teacher can help many children (Swanson & Berninger, 2018).

Attention Deficit Hyperactivity Disorder (ADHD) **Attention deficit hyperactivity disorder (ADHD)** is a disability in which children consistently show one or more of the following characteristics over a period of time: (1) inattention, (2) hyperactivity, and (3) impulsivity. Children who are inattentive have so much difficulty focusing on any one thing that they may get bored with a task after only a few minutes—or even seconds. Children who are hyperactive show high levels of physical activity, seeming to be almost constantly in motion. Children who are impulsive have difficulty curbing their reactions; they do not do a good job of thinking before they act. Depending on the characteristics that children with ADHD display, they can be diagnosed as (1) ADHD with predominantly inattention, (2) ADHD with predominantly hyperactivity/impulsivity, or (3) ADHD with both inattention and hyperactivity/impulsivity.

The number of children diagnosed and treated for ADHD has increased substantially in recent decades. The disorder occurs as much as four to nine times more frequently in boys than in girls. There is controversy, however, about the increased diagnosis of ADHD (Friend, 2018). Some experts attribute the increase mainly to heightened awareness of the disorder; others are concerned that many children are being incorrectly diagnosed (Friend, 2018).

One study examined the possible misdiagnosis of ADHD (Bruchmiller, Margraf, & Schneider, 2012). In this study, child psychologists, psychiatrists, and social workers were given vignettes of children with ADHD (some vignettes matched the diagnostic criteria for the disorder, while others did not). Whether each child was male or female varied. The researchers assessed whether the mental health professionals gave a diagnosis of ADHD to the child described in the vignette. The professionals overdiagnosed ADHD almost 20 percent of the time, and regardless of the symptoms described, boys were twice as likely as girls to be given a diagnosis of ADHD.

Definitive causes of ADHD have not been found. However, a number of genetic and environmental causes have been proposed. Some children likely inherit a tendency to develop ADHD from their parents (Huang & others, 2019). Other children likely develop ADHD because of damage to their brain during prenatal or postnatal development (Van den Bergh, Dahnke, & Mennes, 2018). Among early possible contributors to ADHD are cigarette and alcohol exposure during prenatal development, as well as a high level of maternal stress and low birth weight (He & others, 2017). For example, a meta-analysis of 88 studies found a small but significant association between lower birth weight and greater risk for ADHD (Momany, Kamradt, & Nikolas, 2018).

As with learning disabilities, the development of brain-imaging techniques is leading to a better understanding of ADHD (Bessette & Stevens, 2019). One study revealed that peak thickness of the cerebral cortex occurred three years later (10.5 years) in children with ADHD than in children without ADHD (peak at 7.5 years) (Shaw & others, 2007). The delay was more prominent in the prefrontal regions of the brain that are especially important in attention and planning (see Figure 6). Another recent study also found delayed development of the brain's frontal lobes in children with ADHD, likely due to delayed or decreased myelination (Bouziane & others, 2018). Researchers also are exploring the roles that various neurotransmitters, such as serotonin and dopamine, might play in ADHD (Wiers & others, 2018).

The delays in brain development just described are in areas linked to executive function. An increasing focus of interest in the study of children and adolescents with ADHD is their difficulty with executive function tasks, such as inhibiting behavior when necessary, use of working memory, and effective planning (Kofler & others, 2019). Researchers also have found deficits in theory of mind in children with ADHD (Pineda-Alhucema & others, 2018).

Adjustment and optimal development also are difficult for children who have ADHD, so it is important that the diagnosis be accurate. Children diagnosed with ADHD have an increased risk of school dropout, adolescent pregnancy, substance use problems, and antisocial behavior (Adisetiyo & Gray, 2017).

Stimulant medication such as Ritalin or Adderall (which has fewer side effects than Ritalin) is effective in improving the attention of many children with ADHD, but it usually does not improve their attention to the same level as children who do not have ADHD (Cortese & others, 2018). Behavioral interventions can also be effective in reducing behavior problems among children with ADHD (Papadopoulos & others, 2019). Researchers have often found that a combination of medication (such as Ritalin) and behavior management tends to improve the behavior of children with ADHD better than medication alone or behavior management alone, although this is not true in all cases (Caye & others, 2019).

Yoga, mindfulness training, and meditation have been used with some success with children with ADHD, although these approaches are not recommended as the first treatment of choice. A meta-analysis of 11 studies suggested that ADHD symptoms, hyperactivity, inattention, executive function, and on-task behavior of children with ADHD can be improved through yoga, mindfulness, and meditation (Chimiklis & others, 2018).

Emotional and Behavioral Disorders   Most children have minor emotional difficulties at some point during their school years. A small percentage have problems so serious and persistent that they are classified as having an emotional or a behavioral disorder (La Salle & others, 2018).

Emotional and behavioral disorders consist of serious, persistent problems that involve relationships, aggression, depression, and fears associated with personal or school matters, as well as other inappropriate socioemotional characteristics. Approximately 8 percent of children who have a disability and require an individualized education program (discussed later in this chapter) fall into this classification. Boys are three times as likely as girls to have these disorders.

Autism Spectrum Disorders   **Autism spectrum disorders (ASD),** also called pervasive developmental disorders, range from the severe disorder labeled autistic disorder to the milder disorder called Asperger syndrome. Autism spectrum disorders are characterized by problems in social interaction, problems in verbal and nonverbal communication, and repetitive behaviors (Klinger & Dudley, 2019). Children with these disorders may also show atypical responses to sensory experiences (Klinger & Dudley, 2019). Autism spectrum disorders often can be detected in children as young as 1 to 3 years of age.

Estimates of the prevalence of autism spectrum disorders tracked over time indicate that they are increasing in occurrence or are increasingly being detected and labeled (Centers for Disease Control and Prevention, 2018). Once thought to affect only 1 in 2,500 individuals, autism spectrum disorders were estimated to affect 1 in 59 children in 2014 (Centers for Disease Control & Prevention, 2018).

Autistic disorder is a severe developmental autism spectrum disorder that has its onset in the first three years of life and includes deficiencies in social relationships, abnormalities in communication, and restricted, repetitive, and stereotyped patterns of behavior.

Asperger syndrome is a relatively mild autism spectrum disorder in which the child has relatively good verbal ability, milder nonverbal language problems, and a restricted range of interests and relationships (de Giambattista & others, 2019). Children with Asperger syndrome often engage in obsessive, repetitive routines and preoccupations with a particular subject. For example, a child may be obsessed with baseball scores or railroad timetables.

What causes the autism spectrum disorders? The current consensus is that autism is a brain dysfunction involving abnormalities in brain structure and neurotransmitters (Yu & others, 2016). A lack of connectivity between brain regions may be a key factor

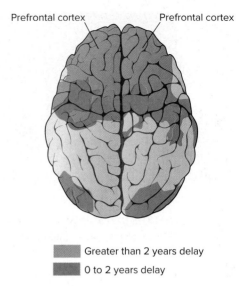

Prefrontal cortex   Prefrontal cortex

■ Greater than 2 years delay
■ 0 to 2 years delay

FIGURE 6

REGIONS OF THE BRAIN IN WHICH CHILDREN WITH ADHD HAD A DELAYED PEAK IN THE THICKNESS OF THE CEREBRAL CORTEX. *Note:* The greatest delays occurred in the prefrontal cortex.

emotional and behavioral disorders Serious, persistent problems that involve relationships, aggression, depression, fears associated with personal or school matters, as well as other inappropriate socioemotional characteristics.

autism spectrum disorders (ASDs) Also called pervasive developmental disorders, they range from the severe disorder labeled autistic disorder to the milder disorder called Asperger syndrome. Children with these disorders are characterized by problems in social interaction, verbal and nonverbal communication, and repetitive behaviors.

autistic disorder A severe developmental autism spectrum disorder that has its onset in the first three years of life and includes deficiencies in social relationships; abnormalities in communication; and restricted, repetitive, and stereotyped patterns of behavior.

Asperger syndrome A relatively mild autism spectrum disorder in which the child has relatively good verbal skills, milder nonverbal language problems, and a restricted range of interests and relationships.

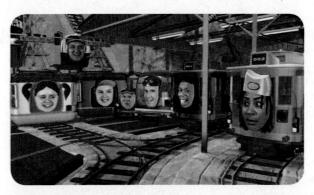

FIGURE 7

A SCENE FROM THE DVD ANIMATIONS USED IN A STUDY BY BARON-COHEN AND OTHERS (2007). *What did they do to improve autistic children's ability to read facial expressions?*

The Autism Research Trust

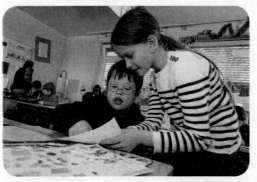

Increasingly, children with disabilities are being taught in the regular classroom, as is this child with a mild intellectual disability.

E.D. Torial/Alamy Stock Photo

individualized education program (IEP) A written statement that spells out a program tailored to the needs of a child with a disability.

least restrictive environment (LRE) The concept that a child with a disability must be educated in a setting that is similar to classrooms in which children without a disability are educated.

inclusion Educating a child with special educational needs full-time in the regular classroom.

in autism (McKinnon & others, 2019). Genetic factors play a role in the development of the autism spectrum disorders (Carrascosa-Romero & De Cabo-De La Vega, 2017). Twin studies document heritability estimates between 80 and 90 percent, but environmental factors also play a role in the manifestation of autism spectrum disorders (Willfors, Tammimies, & Bölte, 2017). There is no evidence that family socialization causes autism. Intellectual disability is present in some children with autism, while others show average or above-average intelligence (Clarke & others, 2016).

It is estimated that boys are four times as likely as girls to have autism spectrum disorders (Centers for Disease Control and Prevention, 2018). Expanding on autism's male linkage, a theory proposed by Simon Baron-Cohen and his colleagues suggests that autism reflects an extreme male brain, especially indicative of males' lesser ability to show empathy and read facial expressions and gestures (Greenberg & others, 2018). In an attempt to improve these skills in 4- to 8-year-old autistic boys, Baron-Cohen and his colleagues (2007) produced a number of animations on a DVD in which faces showing different emotions are placed on toy trains and tractor characters in a boy's bedroom (see Figure 7). (See www.thetransporters.com for a look at a number of the facial expression animations in addition to the one shown in Figure 7.) After the autistic children watched the animations 15 minutes every weekday for one month, their ability to recognize real faces in a different context equaled that of children without autism.

Children with autism benefit from a well-structured classroom, individualized instruction, and small-group instruction. Behavior modification techniques are sometimes effective in helping autistic children learn (Davis & Rispoli, 2018). A research review concluded that when these behavior modifications are intensely provided and used early in the autistic child's life, they are more effective (Howlin, Magiati, & Charman, 2009).

EDUCATIONAL ISSUES

Until the 1970s most U.S. public schools either refused enrollment to children with disabilities or inadequately served them. This changed in 1975, when Public Law 94-142, the Education for All Handicapped Children Act, required that all students with disabilities be given a free, appropriate public education. In 1990, Public Law 94-142 was recast as the Individuals with Disabilities Education Act (IDEA). IDEA was amended in 1997 and then reauthorized in 2004 and renamed the Individuals with Disabilities Education Improvement Act.

IDEA spells out broad mandates for services to children with disabilities of all kinds (U.S. Department of Education, 2019). These services include evaluation and eligibility determination, appropriate education and an individualized education program (IEP), and education in the least restrictive environment (LRE).

An **individualized education program (IEP)** is a written statement that spells out a program that is specifically tailored for the student with a disability. The **least restrictive environment (LRE)** is a setting that is as similar as possible to a classroom in which children who do not have a disability are educated. This provision of the IDEA has given a legal basis to efforts to educate children with a disability in regular classrooms. The term **inclusion** describes educating a child with special educational needs full-time in the regular classroom (U.S. Department of Education, 2019). Figure 8 indicates that in a recent school year, 63.1 percent of U.S. students with a disability spent more than 80 percent of their school day in a general classroom.

Many legal changes regarding children with disabilities have had extremely positive effects (Friend & Bursuck, 2012; McLeskey, Rosenberg, & Westling, 2013). Compared with several decades ago, far more children today are receiving competent, specialized services. For many children, inclusion in the regular classroom, with modifications or supplemental services, is appropriate. However, some leading experts on special education argue that in some cases the effort to educate children with disabilities in the regular classroom has become too extreme. For example, inclusion sometimes involves making accommodations in the regular classroom that do not always benefit children with

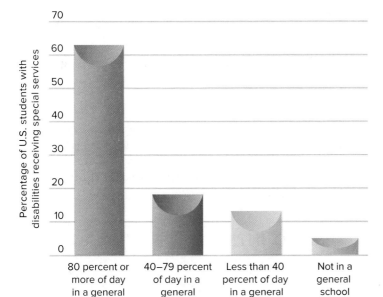

FIGURE 8

PERCENTAGE OF U.S. STUDENTS WITH DISABILITIES 6 TO 21 YEARS OF AGE RECEIVING SPECIAL SERVICES IN THE GENERAL CLASSROOM. Data for 2016–2017 school year, National Center for Education Statistics, 2018

disabilities (Maag, Kauffman, & Simpson, 2019). A more effective alternative might be an individualized approach that does not always involve full inclusion but allows options such as special education outside the regular classroom. James Kauffman and his colleagues (2004, p. 620) acknowledge that children with disabilities "do need the services of specially trained professionals" and "do sometimes need altered curricula or adaptations to make their learning possible." However, "we sell students with disabilities short when we pretend that they are not different from typical students. We make the same error when we pretend that they must not be expected to put forth extra effort if they are to learn to do some things—or learn to do something in a different way." Like general education, special education should challenge students with disabilities "to become all they can be."

Review *Connect* Reflect

 LG2 Characterize children with disabilities and their education.

Review

- Who are children with disabilities? What characterizes children with learning disabilities? How would you describe children with attention deficit hyperactivity disorder? What are emotional and behavioral disorders? What are autism spectrum disorders, what are they caused by, and how are they characterized?
- What are some issues involved in educating children with disabilities?

Connect

- In this section, you learned that exposure to cigarette smoke during prenatal development may be linked

to ADHD. What name is used for agents that can potentially cause a birth defect or negatively alter cognitive and behavioral outcomes?

Reflect *Your Own Personal Journey of Life*

- Think about your own schooling and how children with learning disabilities or ADHD either were or were not diagnosed. Were you aware of such individuals in your classes? Were they helped by specialists? You may know one or more individuals with a learning disability or ADHD. Ask them about their educational experiences and whether they think schools could have done a better job of helping them.

Extrinsic and Intrinsic Motivation	Cognitive Processes	Ethnicity and Culture

Life is a gift . . . Accept it.

Life is an adventure . . . Dare it.

Life is a mystery . . . Unfold it.

Life is a struggle . . . Face it.

Life is a puzzle . . . Solve it.

Life is an opportunity . . . Take it.

Life is a mission . . . Fulfill it.

Life is a goal . . . Achieve it.

—AUTHOR UNKNOWN

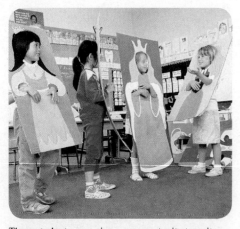

These students were given an opportunity to write and perform their own play. These kinds of self-determining opportunities can enhance students' motivation to achieve.
Elizabeth Crews/The Image Works

extrinsic motivation Response to external incentives such as rewards and punishments.

intrinsic motivation Internal motivational factors such as self-determination, curiosity, challenge, and effort.

In any classroom, no matter who the teacher is or what approach is used, some children achieve more than others (O'Dea & others, 2018). Why? The reasons for variations in achievement include motivation, expectations, goals, and other characteristics of the child as well as sociocultural contexts.

EXTRINSIC AND INTRINSIC MOTIVATION

Extrinsic motivation involves external incentives such as rewards and punishments. **Intrinsic motivation** is based on internal factors such as self-determination, curiosity, challenge, and effort. Cognitive approaches stress the importance of intrinsic motivation in achievement. Some students study hard because they want to make good grades or avoid parental disapproval (extrinsic motivation). Other students work hard because they are internally motivated to achieve high standards in their work (intrinsic motivation).

Current evidence strongly favors establishing a classroom climate in which students are intrinsically motivated to learn (Fong & others, 2019). For example, an experiment in which children were provided with either positive or negative feedback delivered in either a controlling or autonomy-supportive way found that children were most intrinsically motivated to complete a similar task in the future and persisted longer in the face of challenges when adults had provided positive feedback delivered in an autonomy-supportive way on their prior activities (Mabbe & others, 2018). A daily diary study demonstrated links between high school science teachers' autonomy-supportive versus thwarting practices on students' motivation in the classroom (Patall & others, 2018). In particular, students were more internally motivated and engaged in the classroom when teachers provided more choices to students, considered students' preferences and interests, explained why the material was important, and gave students opportunities to ask questions. By contrast, students were less internally motivated when teachers were more controlling, suppressed students' perspectives, and used uninteresting activities.

Students are more motivated to learn when they are given choices, become absorbed in challenges that match their skills, and receive rewards that have informational value but are not used for control. Praise also can enhance students' intrinsic motivation. To see why these things are so, let's first explore three perspectives on intrinsic motivation: (1) self-determination and personal choice, (2) interest, and (3) cognitive engagement and self-responsibility. Then we'll discuss how external rewards can either enhance or undermine intrinsic motivation. Finally, we will offer some concluding thoughts about intrinsic and extrinsic motivation.

Self-Determination and Personal Choice   One view of intrinsic motivation emphasizes self-determination (Deci & Ryan, 2000; Ryan & Deci, 2009). In this view, students want to believe that they are doing something because of their own will, not because of external success or rewards (Vansteenkiste & others, 2009). The architects of self-determination theory, Richard Ryan and Edward Deci (2009), refer to teachers who create circumstances for students to engage in self-determination as *autonomy-supportive teachers.* A recent study of 34 high school classrooms found that students who perceived their classrooms as allowing and encouraging autonomy in the first several weeks of the semester increased their engagement throughout the course (Hafen & others, 2012).

Researchers have found that students' internal motivation and intrinsic interest in school tasks increase when students have some choice and are given opportunities to take personal responsibility for their learning (Li & others, 2018).

Cognitive Engagement and Self-Responsibility Another variation on intrinsic motivation emphasizes the importance of creating learning environments that encourage students to become cognitively engaged and to take responsibility for their learning (Järvelä & others, 2018). The goal is to get students to become motivated to expend the effort to persist and master ideas rather than simply doing enough work to just get by and make passing grades. Especially important in encouraging students to become cognitively engaged and responsible for their learning is to embed subject matter content and skills learning within meaningful contexts, especially real-world situations that mesh with students' interests (Eccles & Roeser, 2011, 2013).

Some Final Thoughts About Intrinsic and Extrinsic Motivation It is important for parents and teachers to encourage students to become intrinsically motivated and to create learning environments that promote students' cognitive engagement and self-responsibility for learning (Good & Lavigne, 2017). That said, the real world is not just one of intrinsic motivation, and too often intrinsic and extrinsic motivation have been pitted against each other as polar opposites. In many aspects of students' lives, both intrinsic and extrinsic motivation are at work (Schunk, 2019). Keep in mind, though, that many psychologists recommend that extrinsic motivation by itself is not a good strategy.

COGNITIVE PROCESSES

Our discussion of extrinsic and intrinsic motivation sets the stage for introducing other cognitive processes involved in motivating students to learn. As we explore these additional cognitive processes, notice how intrinsic and extrinsic motivation continue to be important. The processes are (1) sustained attention, effort, and task persistence; (2) mastery motivation and mindset; (3) self-efficacy; (4) expectations; (5) goal setting, planning, and self–monitoring; and (6) purpose.

Sustained Attention, Effort, and Task Persistence Of course, it is important not only to perceive that effort is an important aspect of achieving, but also to actually engage in sustained attention, effort, and task persistence in school, work, and a career (Moilanen, Padilla-Walker, & Blaacker, 2019). Recall that *sustained attention* is the ability to maintain attention to a selected stimulus for a prolonged period of time. Sustained attention requires effort, and as individuals develop through adolescence, school tasks, projects, and work become more complex and require longer periods of sustained attention, effort, and task persistence than in childhood.

Might the extent to which adolescents persist at tasks be linked to how successful they are in a career as an adult? One study revealed that task persistence at 13 years of age was related to occupational success in middle age (Andersson & Bergman, 2011).

Mastery Motivation and Mindset Becoming cognitively engaged and self-motivated to improve are reflected in adolescents with a mastery motivation. These children also have a growth mindset—a belief that they can produce positive outcomes if they put forth the effort.

Mastery Motivation Developmental psychologist Carol Dweck (2006, 2013) found that children often show two distinct responses to difficult or challenging circumstances. Children who display **mastery motivation** are task oriented; they concentrate on learning strategies and the process of achievement rather than their ability or the outcome. Those with a **helpless orientation** seem trapped by the experience of difficulty, and they attribute their difficulty to lack of ability. They frequently say such things as "I'm not very good at this," even though they might earlier have demonstrated their ability through many successes. And, once they view their behavior as failure, they often feel anxious, and their performance worsens even further. Figure 9 describes some behaviors that might reflect helplessness (Stipek, 2002).

The student:
- Says "I can't"
- Doesn't pay attention to teacher's instructions
- Doesn't ask for help, even when it is needed
- Does nothing (for example, stares out the window)
- Guesses or answers randomly without really trying
- Doesn't show pride in successes
- Appears bored, uninterested
- Is unresponsive to teacher's exhortations to try
- Is easily discouraged
- Doesn't volunteer answers to teacher's questions
- Maneuvers to get out of or to avoid work (for example, has to go to the nurse's office)

FIGURE 9
BEHAVIORS THAT SUGGEST A HELPLESS ORIENTATION

mastery motivation An approach to achievement in which one is task oriented, focusing on learning strategies and the achievement process rather than ability or the outcome.

helpless orientation An orientation in which one seems trapped by the experience of difficulty and attributes one's difficulty to a lack of ability.

performance orientation An orientation in which one focuses on winning rather than achievement outcomes, and happiness is thought to result from winning.

mindset Dweck's concept referring to the cognitive view individuals develop for themselves; individuals have either a fixed or growth mindset.

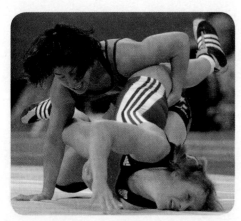

Patricia Miranda (in blue) winning the bronze medal in the 2004 Olympics. *What characterizes her growth mindset and how is it different from someone with a fixed mindset?*

Hasam Sarbakhshian/AP Images

In contrast, mastery-oriented children often instruct themselves to pay attention, to think carefully, and to remember strategies that have worked for them in previous situations. They frequently report feeling challenged and excited by difficult tasks, rather than being threatened by them (Dweck & Yeager, 2018).

Another issue in motivation involves whether to adopt a mastery or a performance orientation. Children with a **performance orientation** are focused on winning, rather than on achievement outcomes and believe that happiness results from winning. Does this mean that mastery-oriented children do not like to win and that performance-oriented children are not motivated to experience the self-efficacy that comes from being able to take credit for one's accomplishments? No. A matter of emphasis or degree is involved, though. For mastery-oriented individuals, winning isn't everything; for performance-oriented individuals, skill development and self-efficacy take a back seat to winning.

A final point needs to be made about mastery and performance goals: They are not always mutually exclusive. Students can be both mastery and performance oriented, and researchers have found that mastery goals combined with performance goals often enhance students' success (Schunk, 2019).

Mindset Carol Dweck's (2006, 2013) analysis of motivation for achievement stresses the importance of children developing a **mindset,** which she defines as the cognitive view individuals develop for themselves. She concludes that individuals have one of two mindsets: (1) a *fixed mindset,* in which they believe that their qualities are carved in stone and cannot change; or (2) a *growth mindset,* in which they believe their qualities can change and improve through their effort. A fixed mindset is similar to a helpless orientation; a growth mindset is much like having mastery motivation (Dweck, 2013).

In her book *Mindset,* Dweck (2006) argued that individuals' mindsets influence whether they will be optimistic or pessimistic, shape their goals and how hard they will strive to reach those goals, and affect many aspects of their lives, including achievement and success in school and sports. Dweck says that mindsets begin to be shaped as children interact with parents, teachers, and coaches, who themselves have either a fixed mindset or a growth mindset. She described the growth mindset of Patricia Miranda:

> [She] was a chubby, unathletic school kid who wanted to wrestle. After a bad beating on the mat, she was told, "You're a joke." First she cried, then she felt: "That really set my resolve. . . . I had to keep going and had to know if effort and focus and belief and training could somehow legitimize me as a wrestler." Where did she get this resolve?
>
> Miranda was raised in a life devoid of challenge. But when her mother died of an aneurysm at age forty, ten-year-old Miranda . . . [thought] "If you only go through life doing stuff that's easy, shame on you." So when wrestling presented a challenge, she was ready to take it on. Her effort paid off. At twenty-four, Miranda was having the last laugh. She won a spot on the U.S. Olympic team and came home from Athens with a bronze medal. And what was next? Yale Law School. People urged her to stay where she was already on top, but Miranda felt it was more exciting to start at the bottom again and see what she could grow into this time. (Dweck, 2006, pp. 22–23)

Related to her emphasis on encouraging students to develop a growth mindset, Dweck and her colleagues (Blackwell & Dweck, 2008; Blackwell, Trzesniewski, & Dweck, 2007; Dweck, 2013) have incorporated information about the brain's plasticity into their effort to improve students' motivation to achieve and succeed. In one study, they assigned two groups of students to eight sessions of either (1) study skills instruction or (2) study skills instruction plus information about the importance of developing a growth mindset (called incremental theory in the research) (Blackwell, Trzesniewski, & Dweck, 2007). One of the exercises in the growth mindset group was titled, "You Can Grow Your Brain," which emphasized that the brain is like a muscle that can change and grow as it gets exercise and develops new connections. Students were informed that the more you challenge your brain to learn, the more your brain cells grow. Both groups had a pattern of declining math scores prior to the intervention. Following the intervention, the group who only received the study skills instruction continued to have declining scores, but the group that received the combination of study skills instruction plus the growth mindset information reversed the downward trend and improved their math achievement.

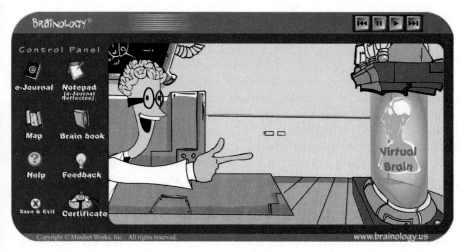

FIGURE **10**

DWECK'S BRAINOLOGY PROGRAM. A screen from Carol Dweck's Brainology program, which is designed to cultivate children's growth mindset.
Courtesy of Carol S. Dweck, Brainology

In other work, Dweck has been creating a computer-based workshop, "Brainology," to teach students that their intelligence can change (Blackwell & Dweck, 2008; Dweck, 2012). Students experience six modules about how the brain works and how they can make their brains improve (see Figure 10). After the program was tested in 20 New York City schools, students strongly endorsed the value of the computer-based brain modules. Said one student, "I will try harder because I know that the more you try the more your brain knows" (Dweck & Master, 2009, p. 137).

Dweck and her colleagues (Good, Rattan, & Dweck, 2012) also have found that a growth mindset can prevent negative stereotypes from undermining achievement. For example, they found that believing math ability can be learned protected women from negative gender stereotyping about math. And other research indicates that people will work and resist temptations more during stressful circumstances if they regard willpower as a virtually unlimited resource (Bernecker & others, 2017).

Self-Efficacy   Like having a growth mindset, **self-efficacy**—the belief that one can master a situation and produce favorable outcomes—is an important cognitive view for children to develop. Albert Bandura (2018), whose social cognitive theory was described earlier, argues that self-efficacy is a critical factor in whether or not children achieve. Self-efficacy has much in common with mastery motivation. Self-efficacy is the belief that "I can"; helplessness is the belief that "I cannot" (Stipek, 2002). Children with high self-efficacy agree with statements such as "I know that I will be able to learn the material in this class" and "I expect to be able to do well at this activity."

Dale Schunk (2019) has applied the concept of self-efficacy to many aspects of students' achievement. In his view, self-efficacy influences a student's choice of activities. Students with low self-efficacy for learning might avoid many learning tasks, especially those that are challenging. In contrast, their high-self-efficacy counterparts eagerly work at learning tasks. High-self-efficacy students are more likely to expend effort and persist longer at a learning task than low-self-efficacy students. Self-efficacy contributes to students' career aspirations. For example, ninth-grade students with high self-efficacy in science are more interested in exploring STEM careers (Mau & Li, 2018).

Children's and adolescents' development is influenced by their parents' self-efficacy. For example, adolescents have higher self-efficacy when their parents also have high self-efficacy (Di Giunta & others, 2018), and adolescents engage in fewer problem behaviors when their parents have higher self-efficacy related to managing behavior problems (Babskie, Powell, & Metzger, 2017).

Expectations   Children's motivation, and likely their performance, are influenced by the expectations that their parents, teachers, and other adults have for their achievement. Children benefit when both parents and teachers have high expectations for them and provide the necessary support for them to meet those expectations. An especially important factor in the lower achievement of students from low-income families is lack of

---

developmental **connection**

Social Cognitive Theory

Social cognitive theory holds that behavior, environment, and person/cognitive factors are the key influences on development. Connect to "Introduction."

They can because they think they can.

—Virgil
Roman poet, 1st century BC

---

self-efficacy The belief that one can master a situation and produce favorable outcomes.

adequate resources, such as an up-to-date computer in the home (or even any computer at all) to support students' learning (Schunk, Pintrich, & Meece, 2008).

Teachers' expectations influence students' motivation and performance (Zhu, Urhahne, & Rubie-Davies, 2018). "When teachers hold high generalized expectations for student achievement and students perceive these expectations, students achieve more, experience a greater sense of self-esteem and competence as learners, and resist involvement in problem behaviors both during childhood and adolescence" (Wigfield & others, 2006, p. 976). In an observational study of 12 classrooms, teachers with high expectations spent more time providing a framework for students' learning, asked higher-level questions, and were more effective in managing students' behavior than teachers with average and low expectations (Rubie-Davies, 2007).

Students', teachers', and parents' expectations are all important to consider in relation to students' motivation and achievement. If teachers or parents have high expectations for students' success in school, these high expectations can serve as a buffer when students' own expectations fall short (Wigfield & Gladstone, 2019). When teachers' and parents' expectations are high, they can provide encouragement and different opportunities to help students achieve.

Teachers often have more positive expectations for high-ability than for low-ability students, and these expectations are likely to influence their behavior toward them (Legette, 2018). For example, teachers require high-ability students to work harder, wait longer for them to respond to questions, respond to them with more information and in a more elaborate fashion, criticize them less often, praise them more often, are more friendly to them, call on them more often, seat them closer to the teacher's desk, and are more likely to give them the benefit of the doubt on close calls in grading than they are for students with low ability (Brophy, 2004). An important strategy for teachers is to monitor their expectations and be sure to have positive expectations for students with low abilities. Fortunately, researchers have found that with support teachers can adapt and raise their expectations for students with low abilities (National Research Council, 2004).

Goal Setting, Planning, and Self-Monitoring

Goal setting, planning, and self-monitoring are important aspects of children's and adolescents' achievement (Won, Wolters, & Mueller, 2018). Researchers have found that self-efficacy and achievement improve when individuals set goals that are specific, proximal, and challenging (DiBenedetto & Schunk, 2018). An example of a nonspecific, fuzzy goal is "I want to be successful." A more concrete, specific goal is "I want to make the honor roll at the end of this semester."

Individuals can set both long-term (distal) and short-term (proximal) goals. It is okay to set some long-term goals, such as "I want to graduate from high school" or "I want to go to college," but it also is important to create short-term goals, which are steps along the way. "Getting an A on the next math test" is an example of a short-term, proximal goal. So is "Doing all of my homework by 4 p.m. Sunday."

Another good strategy is to set challenging goals. A challenging goal is a commitment to self-improvement. Strong interest and involvement in activities is sparked by challenges. Goals that are easy to reach generate little interest or effort. However, goals should be optimally matched to the adolescent's skill level. If goals are unrealistically high, the result will be repeated failures that lower self-efficacy.

Yet another good strategy is to develop personal goals about desired and undesired future circumstances (Höchli, Brügger, & Messner, 2018). Personal goals can be a key aspect of an individual's motivation for coping and dealing with life's challenges and opportunities (Burns, Martin, & Collie, 2019).

It is not enough to simply set goals. It also is important to plan how to reach the goals (Höchli, Brügger, & Messner, 2018). Being a good planner means managing time effectively, setting priorities, and being organized.

Researchers have found that high-achieving individuals often are self-regulatory learners (Winne, 2018). For example, high-achieving students self-monitor their learning

A student and teacher at Langston Hughes Elementary School in Chicago, a school whose teachers have high expectations for students. *How do teachers' expectations influence students' achievement?*

more and systematically evaluate their progress toward a goal more than low-achieving students do. When parents and teachers encourage students to self-monitor their learning, they give them the message that they are responsible for their own behavior and that learning requires their active, dedicated participation (Zimmerman, Bonner, & Kovach, 1996).

One type of self-regulation is *intentional self-regulation,* which involves selecting goals or outcomes, optimizing the means to achieve desired outcomes, and compensating for setbacks along the path to goal achievement (Stefansson & others, 2018). One study found that intentional self-regulation was especially beneficial to young adolescents from low-income backgrounds (Urban, Lewin-Bizan, & Lerner, 2010). In this study, these high self-regulating adolescents were more likely to seek out extracurricular activities, which resulted in more positive developmental outcomes such as academic achievement. Selecting goals or outcomes was assessed by items such as, "When I decide upon a goal, I stick to it"; optimizing the means to achieve desired outcomes was assessed by items such as, "I think exactly about how I can best realize my plans"; and compensating for setbacks was assessed by items such as, "When things don't work the way they used to, I look for other ways to achieve them."

Barry Zimmerman and his colleagues (Zimmerman, 2002, 2012; Zimmerman & Kitsantas, 1997; Zimmerman & Labuhn, 2012) have developed a model of self-regulation in achievement contexts that has three phrases:

- *Forethought.* Adolescents assess task demands, set goals, and estimate their ability to reach the goals.
- *Performance.* Adolescents create self-regulating strategies such as managing time, attentional focusing, help seeking, and metacognition.
- *Self-Reflection.* Adolescents evaluate their performance, including attributions about factors that affected the outcome and how satisfied they are with their behavior.

In addition to planning and self-regulation/monitoring, delaying gratification is an important aspect of reaching goals—especially long-term goals (Rung & Madden, 2018). Delayed gratification involves postponing immediate rewards in order to attain a larger, more valuable reward at a later point in time. While adolescents may find it more appealing to hang out with friends today than to work on a project that is due for a class assignment later in the week, their decision not to delay gratification can have negative consequences for their academic achievement.

Purpose   In the chapter "The Self and Identity," we discussed William Damon's (2008) ideas on the importance of purpose in identity development. Here we explore how purpose is a missing ingredient in many adolescents' and emerging adults' achievement.

For Damon, *purpose* is an intention to accomplish something meaningful to oneself and to contribute something to the world beyond the self. Finding purpose involves answering questions such as "*Why* am I doing this? *Why* does it matter? *Why* is it important for me and the world beyond me? *Why* do I strive to accomplish this end?" (Damon, 2008, pp. 33–34).

In interviews with 12- to 22-year-olds, Damon found that only about 20 percent had a clear vision of where they wanted to go in life, what they wanted to achieve, and why. The largest percentage—about 60 percent—had engaged in some potentially purposeful activities, such as service learning or fruitful discussions with a career counselor, but they still did not have a real commitment or any reasonable plans for reaching their goals.

> developmental **connection**

Identity

William Damon (2008) concludes that too many of today's youth aren't moving toward any identity resolution. Connect to "The Self and Identity."

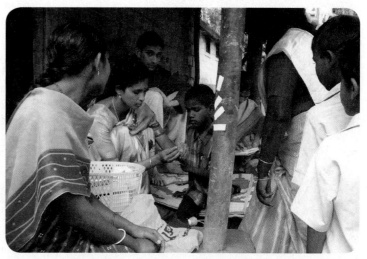

Hari Prabhakar (*in rear*) at a screening camp in India that he created as part of his Tribal India Health Foundation. Hari Prabhakar reflects William Damon's concept of finding a path to purpose. Hari's ambition is to become an international health expert. Hari graduated from Johns Hopkins University in 2006 with a double major in public health and writing. A top student (3.9 GPA), he took the initiative to pursue a number of activities outside the classroom, in the health field. As he made the transition from high school to college, Hari created the Tribal India Health Foundation (www.tihf. org), which provides assistance in bringing low-cost health care to rural areas in India. Juggling his roles as a student and as the foundation's director, Hari spent about 15 hours a week leading Tribal India Health throughout his four undergraduate years.

In describing his work, Hari said (Johns Hopkins University, 2006):

I have found it very challenging to coordinate the international operation. . . . It takes a lot of work, and there's not a lot of free time. But it's worth it when I visit our patients and see how they and the community are getting better.

[*Sources:* Johns Hopkins University (2006); Prabhakar (2007).]

Courtesy of Hari Prabhakar

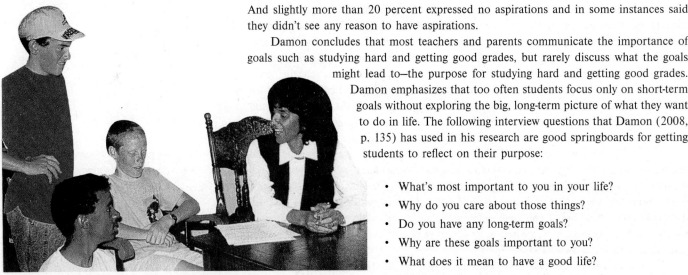

And slightly more than 20 percent expressed no aspirations and in some instances said they didn't see any reason to have aspirations.

Damon concludes that most teachers and parents communicate the importance of goals such as studying hard and getting good grades, but rarely discuss what the goals might lead to—the purpose for studying hard and getting good grades. Damon emphasizes that too often students focus only on short-term goals without exploring the big, long-term picture of what they want to do in life. The following interview questions that Damon (2008, p. 135) has used in his research are good springboards for getting students to reflect on their purpose:

- What's most important to you in your life?
- Why do you care about those things?
- Do you have any long-term goals?
- Why are these goals important to you?
- What does it mean to have a good life?
- What does it mean to be a good person?
- If you were looking back on your life now, how would you like to be remembered?

UCLA educational psychologist Sandra Graham is shown talking with adolescent boys about motivation. She has conducted a number of studies which reveal that middle-socioeconomic-status African American students—like their White counterparts—have high achievement expectations and attribute success to internal factors such as effort rather than external factors such as luck.
Courtesy of Dr. Sandra Graham

Math		Reading	
1. Singapore	564	1. Singapore	535
2. Hong Kong	548	2. Hong Kong	527
3. Macao	544	3. Canada	527
4. Taiwan	542	4. Finland	526
5. Japan	532	5. Ireland	521
6. China	531	6. Estonia	519
7. Korea	524	7. Korea	517
8. Switzerland	521	8. Japan	516
9. Estonia	520	9. Norway	513
10. Canada	516	10. New Zealand	509
11. Netherlands	512	11. Germany	509
12. Denmark	511	12. Macao	509
13. Finland	511	13. Poland	506
14. Slovenia	510	14. Slovenia	505
15. Belgium	507	15. Netherlands	503
16. Germany	506	16. Australia	503
17. Poland	504	17. Sweden	500
18. Ireland	504	18. Denmark	500
19. Norway	502	19. France	499
20. Austria	497	20. Belgium	499
21. New Zealand	495	21. Portugal	498
22. Viet Nam	495	22. United Kingdom	498
23. Russia	494	23. Taiwan	497
24. Sweden	494	**24. United States**	**497**
25. Australia	494	25. Spain	496
26. France	493	26. Russia	495
27. United Kingdom	492	27. China*	494
28. Czech Republic	492	OECD average	493
29. Portugal	492	28. Switzerland	492
OECD average	490	29. Latvia	488
30. Italy	490	30. Czech Republic	487
31. Iceland	488	31. Croatia	487
32. Spain	486	32. Viet Nam	487
33. Luxembourg	486	33. Austria	485
34. Latvia	482	34. Italy	485
35. Malta	479	35. Iceland	482
36. Lithuania	478	36. Luxembourg	481
37. Hungary	477	37. Israel	479
38. Slovak Republic	475	38. Buenos Aires	475
39. Israel	470	39. Lithuania	472
40. United States	**470**	40. Hungary	470

FIGURE 11

INTERNATIONAL COMPARISON OF 15-YEAR-OLDS' READING AND MATH SCORES. Source: OECD (2018). *PISA 2015 results in focus.* Paris, France: OECD.

ETHNICITY AND CULTURE

Americans have been especially concerned about two questions related to ethnicity and culture. First, does their ethnicity deter ethnic minority children from high achievement in school? And second, is there something about American culture that accounts for the poor performance of U.S. children in math and science?

Ethnicity   The diversity that exists among ethnic minority children and adolescents is evident in their achievement (Chen & Graham, 2018). For example, many Asian American students have a strong academic achievement orientation, but some do not.

A special challenge for many ethnic minority students is dealing with negative stereotypes and discrimination. The racial climate of the school as well as teachers' ethnic diversity and cultural competence have implications for biases and expectations encountered by students, which in turn affect students' achievement (Whaley, 2018). Many ethnic minority students living in poverty must also deal with conflict between the values of their neighborhood and those of the majority culture, a lack of high-achieving role models, and as discussed earlier, poor schools (McLoyd, 2019). Even students who are motivated to learn and achieve may find it difficult to perform effectively in such contexts.

Cross-Cultural Comparisons   Since the early 1990s, the poor performance of American children and adolescents in math and science has become well publicized. In a recent large-scale international comparison of 15-year-olds in 73 countries, the top scores in reading, math, and science were held by Singapore, with Asian countries holding the top seven places in math and many of the top places in reading and science (OECD, 2018). In this study, U.S. 15-year-olds placed 24th in reading, 40th in math, and 25th in science. Figure 11 shows international comparisons of reading and math scores in this study.

Why do American students fare so poorly in mathematics? To learn about one researcher's conclusions on the subject, read *Connecting Through Research.*

connecting through research

What Are Some Factors that Influence Children's Math Achievement in Different Countries?

Harold Stevenson conducted research on children's learning for five decades. The research explored the reasons for the poor performance of American students. Stevenson and his colleagues (Stevenson, 1995; Stevenson & others, 1990) completed five cross-cultural comparisons of students in the United States, China, Taiwan, and Japan. In these studies, Asian students consistently outperformed American students. Moreover, the longer the students were in school, the wider the gap became between Asian and American students—the lowest difference was in the first grade, the highest in the eleventh grade (the highest grade studied).

To learn more about the reasons for these large cross-cultural differences, Stevenson and his colleagues spent thousands of hours observing in classrooms, as well as interviewing and surveying teachers, students, and parents. They found that the Asian teachers spent more of their time teaching math than did the American teachers. For example, more than one-fourth of total classroom time in the first grade was spent on math instruction in Japan, compared with only one-tenth of the time in the U.S. first-grade classrooms. Also, the Asian students were in school an average of 240 days a year, compared with 178 days in the United States.

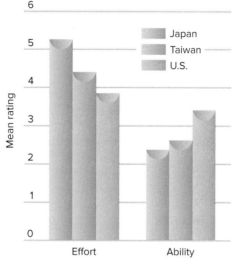

FIGURE 12

MOTHERS' BELIEFS ABOUT THE FACTORS RESPONSIBLE FOR CHILDREN'S MATH ACHIEVEMENT IN THREE COUNTRIES. In one study, mothers in Japan and Taiwan were more likely to believe that their children's math achievement was due to effort rather than innate ability, while U.S. mothers were more likely to believe their children's math achievement was due to innate ability (Stevenson, Lee, & Stigler, 1986). If parents believe that their children's math achievement is due to innate ability and their children are not doing well in math, the implication is that they are less likely to think their children will benefit from putting forth more effort.

In addition, differences were found between the Asian and American parents. The American parents had much lower expectations for their children's education and achievement than did the Asian parents. Also, the American parents were more likely to state that their children's math achievement was due to innate ability; the Asian parents were more likely to say that their children's math achievement was the consequence of effort and training (see Figure 12). The Asian students were more likely to do math homework than were the American students, and the Asian parents were far more likely to help their children with their math homework than were the American parents (Chen & Stevenson, 1989).

Asian and Asian American parenting approaches have been characterized by some experts as an authoritarian style and by others as a "training" style. Those who endorse the training view note that it reflects the parents' concern and involvement in their children's lives and that the high academic achievement of their children may result from this training.

Other research indicates that the more involved parents are in children's learning, particularly in terms of academic socialization, the higher the level of achievement children will attain (Wei & others, 2019). As indicated earlier, East Asian parents spend considerably more time helping their children with homework than

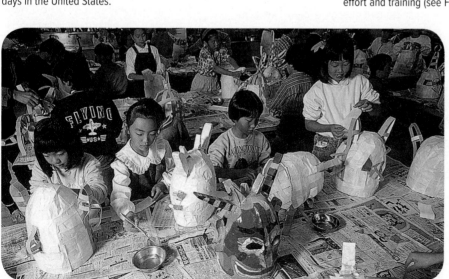

Asian grade schools intersperse studying with frequent periods of activities. This approach helps children maintain their attention and likely makes learning more enjoyable. Shown here are Japanese fourth-graders making wearable masks. *What are some differences in the way children in many Asian countries are taught compared with children in the United States?*
Eiji Miyazawa/Stock Photo/Black Star

(continued)

(continued)

do U.S. parents (Chen & Stevenson, 1989). The greater East Asian parental involvement in children's learning is present as early as the preschool years and continues in the elementary school years (Cheung & Pomerantz, 2012; Siegler & Mu, 2008). In East Asia, children's learning is considered to be a far greater responsibility of parents than in the United States (Pomerantz, Kim, & Cheung, 2012). However, researchers have found that when U.S. parents are more involved in their children's learning, the children's achievement benefits (Cheung & Pomerantz, 2012). In this study, for both U.S. and Chinese children, the more parents were involved in their children's learning, the more motivated the children were to achieve in school for parent-oriented reasons, and this increased motivation was linked to enhanced self-regulated learning and higher grades.

What are some differences in the way children in many Asian countries are taught compared with children in the United States?

Review Connect Reflect

 LG3 Explain the development of achievement in children.

Review

- What are intrinsic and extrinsic motivation? How are they related to achievement?
- What role do mastery motivation and mindset play in children's achievement?
- What is self-efficacy, and how is it related to achievement? How are expectations involved in children's achievement? Why are goal setting, planning, and self-monitoring important in achievement? What is purpose and how is it involved in achievement?
- How do cultural, ethnic, and socioeconomic variations influence achievement?

Connect

- In this section, you learned about the importance of purpose in adolescents' and emerging adults' achievement. In the chapter "The Self and Identity" what did Damon identify as some of the possible negative outcomes of not having purpose?

Reflect *Your Own Personal Journey of Life*

- Think about several of your own past schoolmates who showed low motivation in school. Why do you think they behaved that way? What teaching strategies might have helped them?

---

reach your **learning goals**

Schools and Achievement

Exploring Children's Schooling

 LG1 Discuss approaches to schooling and development.

Contemporary Approaches to Student Learning and Assessment

- Contemporary approaches to student learning include direct instruction, which is a teacher-centered approach, and constructivist instruction, which is learner-centered. Some experts recommend that both a constructivist and direct instruction approach be used, depending on circumstances. Increased concern by the public and government in the United States has produced extensive state-mandated testing, which has both strengths and weaknesses and is controversial.

- The child-centered kindergarten emphasizes the education of the whole child, paying particular attention to individual variation, the process of learning, and the importance of play in development. The Montessori approach is an increasingly popular early childhood education choice. Developmentally appropriate practice focuses on the typical patterns of children (age-appropriateness) and the uniqueness of each child (individual-appropriateness). Such practice contrasts with developmentally inappropriate practice, which relies on pencil-and-paper activities. The U.S. government has tried to break the poverty cycle with programs such as Head Start. Model programs have been shown to have positive effects on children who live in poverty. Controversy surrounds early childhood education curricula. On the one side are the child-centered, constructivist advocates, on the other are those who advocate an instructivist, academic approach. Another controversy focuses on whether universal preschool education should be implemented.

- Children take up the new role of student, interact, develop new relationships, and discover rich sources of new ideas in elementary school. A special concern is that early elementary school education proceeds too much on the basis of providing negative feedback to children.

- The transition to middle or junior high school coincides with many social, familial, and individual changes in the adolescent's life, and this transition is often stressful. One source of stress is the move from the top-dog to the lowest position in school. Some critics argue that a major redesign of U.S. middle schools is needed. Critics say that U.S. high schools foster passivity and do not develop students' academic skills adequately. A number of strategies have been proposed for improving U.S. high schools, including higher expectations and better support. The overall high school dropout rate declined considerably in the last half of the twentieth century, but the dropout rates of Latino and Native American youth remain very high. Participation in extracurricular activities is associated with positive academic and psychological outcomes. Adolescents benefit from participating in a variety of high-quality extracurricular activities.

- Children living in poverty face problems at home and at school that present barriers to learning. Neighborhoods are dangerous, and many schools' buildings are crumbling with age. Teachers are likely to encourage rote learning, and parents often don't set high educational standards. The school experiences of children from different ethnic groups vary considerably. Teachers often have low expectations for children of color. A number of strategies can be adopted to improve relationships with diverse others.

Children with Disabilities

 Characterize children with disabilities and their education.

- Approximately 13 percent of U.S. children from 3 to 21 years of age receive special education or related services. A child with a learning disability has difficulty in learning that involves understanding or using spoken or written language, and the difficulty can appear in listening, thinking, reading, writing, and spelling. A learning disability also may involve difficulty in doing mathematics. To be classified as a learning disability, the learning problem is not primarily the result of visual, hearing, or motor disabilities; intellectual disability; emotional disorders; or due to environmental, cultural, or economic disadvantage. Dyslexia is a category of learning disabilities that involves a severe impairment in the ability to read and spell. Dysgraphia is a learning disability that involves difficulty in expressing thoughts in writing. Dyscalculia is a learning disability that involves difficulties in math computation.

  Attention deficit hyperactivity disorder (ADHD) is a disability in which individuals consistently show problems in one or more of these areas: (1) inattention, (2) hyperactivity, and (3) impulsivity. ADHD has been increasingly diagnosed. Emotional and behavioral disorders consist of serious, persistent problems that involve relationships, aggression, depression, fears associated with personal or school matters, as well as other inappropriate socioemotional characteristics. Autism spectrum disorders (ASD), also called pervasive developmental disorders, range from autistic disorder, a severe developmental disorder, to Asperger syndrome, a relatively mild autism spectrum disorder. The current consensus is that autism is a brain dysfunction involving abnormalities in brain structure and neurotransmitters. Children with autism spectrum disorders are characterized by problems in social interaction, verbal and nonverbal communication, and repetitive behaviors.

- In 1975, Public Law 94-142, the Education for All Handicapped Children Act, required that all children with disabilities be given a free, appropriate public education. This law was renamed the Individuals with Disabilities Education Act (IDEA) in 1990 and updated in 2004. IDEA includes requirements that children with disabilities receive an individualized education program (IEP), which is a written plan that spells out a program tailored to the child, and that children with disabilities be educated in the least restrictive environment (LRE), which is a setting that is as similar as possible to the one in which children without disabilities are educated. Inclusion means educating children with disabilities full-time in the regular classroom.

Achievement

 Explain the development of achievement in children.

Extrinsic and Intrinsic Motivation

- Extrinsic motivation involves external incentives such as rewards and punishment. Intrinsic motivation is based on internal factors such as self-determination, curiosity, challenge, and effort. One view is that giving students some choice and providing opportunities for personal responsibility increase intrinsic motivation. It is important for teachers to create learning environments that encourage students to become cognitively engaged and to develop a responsibility for their learning. Overall, the overwhelming conclusion is that it is a wise strategy to create learning environments that encourage students to become intrinsically motivated. In many real-world situations, both intrinsic and extrinsic motivation are involved, although too often intrinsic and extrinsic motivation have been pitted against each other as polar opposites.

Cognitive Processes

- Children's and adolescents' sustained attention, effort, and task persistence are linked to their achievement. A mastery orientation is preferred over helpless or performance orientations in achievement situations. Mindset is the cognitive view that individuals develop regarding their own potential. Dweck argues that a key aspect of adolescents' development is to guide them in developing a growth mindset. Self-efficacy is the belief that one can master a situation and produce positive outcomes. Bandura points out that self-efficacy is a critical factor in whether students will achieve. Schunk argues that self-efficacy influences a student's choice of tasks, with low-efficacy students avoiding many learning tasks. Students' expectations for success influence their motivation. Children benefit when their parents, teachers, and other adults have high expectations for their achievement. Setting specific, proximal (short-term), and challenging goals benefits students' self-efficacy and achievement. Being a good planner means managing time effectively, setting priorities, and being organized. Self-monitoring is a key aspect of self-regulation that benefits student learning. Damon has proposed that purpose is an especially important aspect of achievement that has been missing from many adolescents' lives. Purpose is the intention to accomplish something meaningful in one's life and to contribute something to the world beyond oneself. Finding one's purpose involves answering a number of questions.

Ethnicity and Culture

- In most investigations, socioeconomic status predicts achievement better than ethnicity. U.S. children receive lower scores on math and science achievement tests than do children in Asian countries such as Singapore, China, and Japan.

key terms

Asperger syndrome 459
attention deficit hyperactivity disorder (ADHD) 458
autism spectrum disorders (ASDs) 459
autistic disorder 459
child-centered kindergarten 444
constructivist approach 443
developmentally appropriate practice 446

direct instruction approach 444
dyscalculia 457
dysgraphia 457
dyslexia 457
emotional and behavioral disorders 459
extrinsic motivation 462
helpless orientation 463

inclusion 460
individualized education program (IEP) 460
intrinsic motivation 462
learning disabilities 457
least restrictive environment (LRE) 460

mastery motivation 463
mindset 464
Montessori approach 444
performance orientation 464
Project Head Start 446
self-efficacy 465
top-dog phenomenon 451

key people

Elliot Aronson 455
Albert Bandura 465

James Comer 455
William Damon 467

Carol Dweck 463
Maria Montessori 445

Dale Schunk 465
Harold Stevenson 469

chapter 17

CULTURE AND DIVERSITY

chapter outline

1 Culture and Children's Development

Learning Goal 1 Discuss the role of culture in children's development.

The Relevance of Culture to the Study of Children

Cross-Cultural Comparisons

2 Socioeconomic Status and Poverty

Learning Goal 2 Describe how socioeconomic status and poverty affect children's lives.

What Is Socioeconomic Status?

Socioeconomic Variations in Families, Neighborhoods, and Schools

Poverty

3 Ethnicity

Learning Goal 3 Explain how ethnicity is linked to children's development.

Immigration

Ethnicity and Socioeconomic Status

Differences and Diversity

Prejudice and Discrimination

4 Technology

Learning Goal 4 Summarize the influence of technology on children's development.

Media Use and Screen Time

Television and Electronic Media

Digital Devices and the Internet

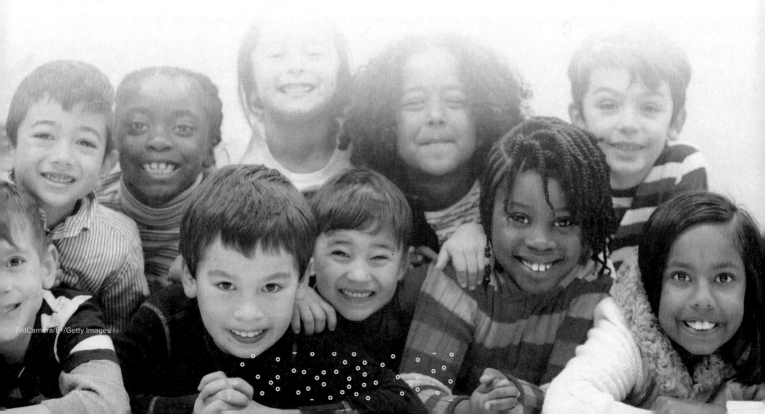

S

onya, a 16-year-old Japanese American girl, was upset over her family's reaction to her White American boyfriend. "Her parents refused to meet him and on several occasions threatened to disown her" (Sue & Morishima, 1982, p. 142). Her older brothers reacted angrily to Sonya's dating a White American, warning that they were going to beat him up. Her parents were also disturbed that Sonya's grades, above average in middle school, were beginning to drop.

Generational issues contributed to the conflict between Sonya and her family (Nagata, 1989). Her parents had experienced strong sanctions against dating Whites when they were growing up and were legally prevented from marrying anyone but a Japanese. As Sonya's older brothers were growing up, they valued ethnic pride and solidarity. The brothers saw her dating a White as "selling out" her own ethnic group. Sonya and the other members of her family obviously had different cultural values.

Michael, a 17-year-old Chinese American high school student, was referred to a therapist by the school counselor because he was depressed and had suicidal tendencies (Huang & Ying, 1989). Michael was failing several classes and frequently was absent from school. Michael's parents, successful professionals, expected Michael to excel in school and go on to become a doctor. They were angered by Michael's school failures, especially since he was the firstborn son, who in Chinese families is expected to achieve the highest standards.

The therapist encouraged the parents to put less academic pressure on Michael and to have more realistic expectations for their son (who had no interest in becoming a doctor). Michael's school attendance changed, and his parents noticed his improved attitude toward school. Michael's case illustrates how expectations that Asian American youth will be "whiz kids" can become destructive.

preview

Culture had a strong influence on the conflicts Sonya and Michael experienced within their families and on their behavior outside the family—in Sonya's case, dating; in Michael's case, school. Of course, a family's cultural background does not always produce conflict between children and other family members, but these two cases underscore the influence of culture in children's development. In this chapter, we will explore many aspects of culture, including cross-cultural comparisons of children's development, the harmful effects of poverty, the role of ethnicity, and the benefits and risks that technology can bring to children's lives.

Culture and Children's Development

 LG1 Discuss the role of culture in children's development.

> The Relevance of Culture to the Study of Children

> Cross-Cultural Comparisons

Culture is defined as the behavior, patterns, beliefs, and all other products of a particular group of people that are passed on from generation to generation. The products result from the interaction between groups of people and their environment over many years. Here we examine the role of culture in children's development.

THE RELEVANCE OF CULTURE TO THE STUDY OF CHILDREN

Culture is relevant to the study of children because of the attitudes that people have and the way they interact with children. For example, culture is manifested in parents' beliefs, values, and goals for their children, and these in turn influence the contexts in which children develop (Bornstein & Lansford, 2018; White, Nair, & Bradley, 2018).

Despite all the differences among cultures, research by American psychologist Donald Campbell and his colleagues (Brewer, 2018; Brewer & Campbell, 1976) revealed that people in all cultures tend to believe that what happens in their culture is "natural" and "correct" and that what happens in other cultures is "unnatural" and "incorrect"; to perceive their cultural customs as universally valid—that is, they believe that what is good for them is good for everyone; and to behave in ways that favor their cultural group and feel hostile toward other cultural groups. In other words, people in all cultures tend to be *ethnocentric*—favoring their own group over others.

The future will bring increasingly extensive contact between people from varied cultural and ethnic backgrounds (Sernau, 2013; Sue & others, 2013; Wright & others, 2012). If the study of child development is to be a relevant discipline in the remainder of the twenty-first century, increased attention will need to be given to culture and ethnicity. Global interdependence is no longer a matter of belief or choice. It is an inescapable reality. Children and their parents are not just citizens of the United States, or Canada, or some other country. They are citizens of the world—a world that, through advances in transportation and technology, has become increasingly interactive.

CROSS-CULTURAL COMPARISONS

Cross-cultural studies compare a culture with one or more other cultures, provide information about other cultures, and examine the role of culture in children's development. This comparison provides information about the degree to which children's development is similar,

> Our most basic common link is that we all inhabit this planet. We all breathe the same air. We all cherish our children's future.
>
> —JOHN F. KENNEDY
> *United States president, 20th century*

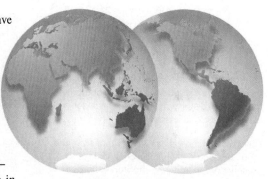

Image Source/Getty Images

---

developmental connection

Theories

In Bronfenbrenner's ecological theory, the macrosystem is the environmental system that involves the influence of culture on children's development. Connect to "Introduction."

---

culture The behavior, patterns, beliefs, and all other products of a particular group of people that are passed on from generation to generation.

cross-cultural studies Research that compares a culture with one or more other cultures, provides information about other cultures, and examines the role of culture in children's development.

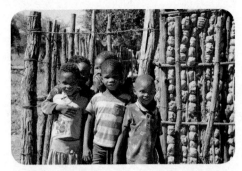

Cross-cultural studies compare a culture with one or more other cultures. Shown here are !Kung children. Delinquency and violence occur much less frequently in the African culture of !Kung than in most cultures around the world.

Franco lucato/Alamy stock Photo

developmental **connection**

Culture and Ethnicity

In the research of Harold Stevenson and his colleagues, the longer students were in school, the wider the gap was between Asian and U.S. students in math achievement. Connect to "Schools and Achievement."

individualism Giving priority to personal goals rather than to group goals; emphasizing values that serve the self, such as feeling good, striving for personal distinction and recognition for achievement, and asserting independence.

collectivism Emphasizing values that serve the group by subordinating personal goals to preserve group integrity, interdependence of members, and harmonious relationships.

or universal, across cultures, or the degree to which it is culture-specific (Deater-Deckard & others, 2018; Molitor & Hsu, 2019). In terms of gender, for example, the experiences of male and female children and adolescents continue to be very different in some cultures (Sernau, 2013). In many countries, males have far greater access to educational opportunities, more freedom to pursue a variety of careers, and fewer restrictions on sexual activity than females (Hyde & Else-Quest, 2018; UNICEF, 2017).

In cross-cultural research, the search for basic dimensions has focused on the dichotomy between individualism and collectivism (Oyserman, 2017; Triandis, 2007):

- **Individualism** involves giving priority to personal goals rather than to group goals; it emphasizes values that serve the self, such as feeling good, seeking personal distinction and recognition for achievement, and asserting independence.
- **Collectivism** emphasizes values that serve the group by subordinating personal goals to preserve group integrity, promote interdependence of the members, and foster harmonious relationships.

Figure 1 summarizes some of the main characteristics of individualistic and collectivistic cultures. Many Western cultures, such as the United States, Canada, Great Britain, and the Netherlands, are described as primarily individualistic; many Eastern cultures, such as China, Japan, India, and Thailand, are described as primarily collectivistic. Mexican culture also is collectivistic. However, there is substantial variation within every nation and many cultures.

Individualistic	Collectivistic
Focuses on individual	Focuses on groups
Self is determined by personal traits independent of groups; self is stable across contexts	Self is defined by in-group terms; self can change with context
Private self is more important	Public self is most important
Personal achievement, competition, power are important	Achievement is for the benefit of the in-group; cooperation is stressed
Cognitive dissonance is frequent	Cognitive dissonance is infrequent
Emotions (such as anger) are self-focused	Emotions (such as anger) are often relationship based
People who are the most liked are self-assured	People who are the most liked are modest, self-effacing
Values: pleasure, achievement, competition, freedom	Values: security, obedience, in-group harmony, personalized relationships
Many casual relationships	Few, close relationships
Save own face	Save own and other's face
Independent behaviors: swimming, sleeping alone in room, privacy	Interdependent behaviors: co-bathing, co-sleeping
Relatively rare mother-child physical contact	Frequent mother-child physical contact (such as hugging, holding)

FIGURE 1

CHARACTERISTICS OF INDIVIDUALISTIC AND COLLECTIVISTIC CULTURES

Researchers have found that self-concepts are related to culture. In one classic study, American and Chinese college students completed 20 sentences beginning with "I am ____" (Trafimow, Triandis, & Goto, 1991). As indicated in Figure 2, the American college students were much more likely to describe themselves with personal traits ("I am assertive"), whereas the Chinese students were more likely to identify themselves by their group affiliations ("I am a member of the math club"). Another study revealed the range of group orientations and collaborative behaviors in distinct cultural groups within Mexico (Correa-Chavez, Mangione, & Mejia-Arauz, 2016). The study focused on the interaction of 8- to 10-year-old children from a more rural indigenous culture and an urban cosmopolitan culture while they played a game. The levels of collaborative play were much higher in the indigenous culture group than the urban group. Furthermore, the more collaborative, group-oriented play included a wider variety of behaviors and strategies for involving players.

Human beings have always lived in groups, whether large or small, and have always needed one another for survival. Critics of the Western notion of psychology argue that the Western emphasis on individualism may undermine the basic need of our species for relatedness (Hitokoto & Uchida, 2018; Sernau, 2013). Some social scientists conclude that many problems in Western cultures are intensified by their emphasis on individualism. Compared with collectivist cultures, individualistic cultures have higher rates of suicide, drug abuse, crime, teenage pregnancy, divorce, child abuse, and mental disorders.

A foundational analysis proposed four values that reflect the beliefs of parents in individualistic cultures about what is required for children's effective development of autonomy: (1) personal choice; (2) intrinsic motivation; (3) self-esteem; and (4) self-maximization, which consists of achieving one's full potential (Tamis-LeMonda & others, 2008). The analysis also proposed that three values reflect the beliefs of parents in collectivistic cultures: (1) connectectness to the family and other close relationships; (2) orientation to the larger group; and (3) respect and obedience. More recent theory has emphasized the ways in which these kinds of cultural distinctions influence the socialization and expression of emotions (Raval & Walker, 2019).

Critics of the concepts of individualistic and collectivistic cultures argue that these terms are too broad and simplistic, especially in an era of increasing globalization (Greenfield, 2018; Vignoles & others, 2016). Regardless of their cultural background, people need a positive sense of self as well as connectedness to others to develop fully as human beings. The analysis by Catherine Tamis-LeMonda and her colleagues (2008) emphasizes that in many families, children are not reared in environments that uniformly endorse individualistic or collectivistic values, thoughts, and actions. Rather, in many families, children are

expected to be quiet, assertive, respectful, curious, humble, self-assured, independent, dependent, affectionate, or reserved depending on the situation, people present, children's age, and social-political and economic circles.

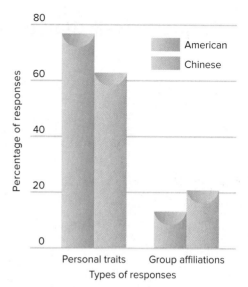

FIGURE 2

AMERICAN AND CHINESE SELF-CONCEPTIONS. College students from the United States and China completed 20 "I am _____" sentences. Both groups filled in personal traits more than group affiliations. However, the U.S. college students more often filled in the blank with personal traits, the Chinese with group affiliations.

Review Connect Reflect

 LG1 Discuss the role of culture in children's development.

Review

- What is the relevance of culture to the study of children?
- What are cross-cultural comparisons?
- What characterizes individualistic and collectivistic cultures? What are some criticisms of the concepts of individualistic and collectivistic cultures?

Connect

- Give examples of individualistic and collectivistic behaviors or beliefs that you read about in previous chapters.

Reflect *Your Own Personal Journey of Life*

- What was the achievement orientation in your family as you grew up? How did the cultural background of your parents influence this orientation?

Socioeconomic Status and Poverty

 Describe how socioeconomic status and poverty affect children's lives.

What Is Socioeconomic Status?

Socioeconomic Variations in Families, Neighborhoods, and Schools

Poverty

Many subcultures exist within countries. For example, Sonya's family, discussed in the opening of the chapter, had beliefs and patterns different from those of Michael's family. Some, but not all, subcultures are tied to ethnicity or socioeconomic characteristics or both. For example, the values and attitudes of children growing up in a crowded city or rural Appalachia may differ from those of children growing up in a wealthy suburb or small town. In any event, children growing up in these different contexts are likely to have different socioeconomic statuses, and this inequality may influence their development (Bradbury, Waldfogel, & Washbrook, 2019; Rivenbark & others, 2019).

WHAT IS SOCIOECONOMIC STATUS?

Socioeconomic status (SES) is the grouping of people with similar occupational, educational, and economic characteristics. Socioeconomic status implies certain inequalities. Generally, members of a society have (1) occupations that vary in prestige, with some individuals having more access than others to higher-status occupations; (2) different levels of educational attainment, with some individuals having more access than others to better education; (3) different economic resources; and (4) different levels of power to influence a community's institutions. These differences in the ability to control resources and to participate in society's rewards produce unequal opportunities (Hurst, Gibbon, & Nurse, 2016; McLoyd, Jocson, & Williams, 2016).

The number of significantly different socioeconomic statuses depends on the community's size and complexity. Most research on socioeconomic status delineates two categories, low and middle, but some research delineates as many as six categories. Sometimes low socioeconomic status is described as low-income, working class, or blue-collar; sometimes the middle category is described as middle-income, managerial, or white-collar. Examples of low-SES occupations are factory worker, manual laborer, and maintenance worker. Examples of middle-SES occupations include skilled worker, manager, and professional, such as a doctor, lawyer, teacher, or accountant (Smith & Son, 2014).

SOCIOECONOMIC VARIATIONS IN FAMILIES, NEIGHBORHOODS, AND SCHOOLS

The families, neighborhoods, and schools of children and adolescents have socioeconomic characteristics. A parent's SES is likely linked to the neighborhoods in which children live and the schools they attend (Hurst, Gibbon, & Nurse, 2016; McLoyd, Jocson, & Williams, 2016). Such variations in neighborhood settings can influence children's adjustment (Manduca & Sampson, 2019). For example, one study of adolescents living in six low- or middle-income countries (for example, China, Colombia, Kenya) found that interconnected levels of neighborhood and household disarray, chaos, and danger were linked with harsher and less supportive parenting, which ultimately predicted poorer social-emotional and academic functioning (Deater-Deckard & others, 2019). Turning to schools, those in low-income neighborhoods not only have fewer resources than those in higher-income areas but also tend to have more students with lower achievement test scores, lower rates of graduation, and smaller percentages of students going to college (Owens & Candipan, 2019).

Let's further examine socioeconomic differences in family life. Research evidence shows that lower-SES parents are more concerned that their children conform to society's expectations, tend to have an authoritarian parenting style, rely on physical punishment more in disciplining their children, and are more directive and less conversational with their children.

---

developmental connection

Socioeconomic Status

Reducing the poverty level and improving the lives of children living in poverty are important goals of U.S. social policy. Connect to "Introduction."

---

socioeconomic status (SES) A grouping of people with similar occupational, educational, and economic characteristics.

By contrast, higher-SES parents tend to be more concerned with developing children's initiative, strive to create a home atmosphere in which children are more nearly equal participants, are less likely to use physical punishment, and are less directive and more conversational with their children (Bornstein & Lansford, 2018; Ramdahl & others, 2018).

Like their parents, children from low-SES backgrounds are at high risk for experiencing mental health problems (Hurst, Gibbon, & Nurse, 2016). Problems such as depression, low self-confidence, peer conflict, and juvenile delinquency are more prevalent among children living in low-SES families than among economically advantaged children (Reiss & others, 2019; Rivenbark & others, 2019).

Of course, children from all SES backgrounds vary considerably in intellectual and psychological functioning. For example, many children from low-SES backgrounds perform well in school; some perform better than many middle-SES students. One study found that high educational aspirations and school engagement among low-income parents were linked to more positive educational outcomes in youth (Day & Dotterer, 2018). When children from low-SES backgrounds are achieving well in school, it is not unusual to find parents, grandparents, and other adults making special sacrifices to provide the living conditions and support that contribute to school success.

So far we have focused on the challenges faced by many children and adolescents from low-income families. However, research by Suniya Luthar and her colleagues (Ebbert, Kumar, & Luthar, 2019; Luthar, Small, & Ciciolla, 2018; Lyman & Luthar, 2014) suggests that adolescents from affluent families also face challenges. In their research, adolescents from affluent families are vulnerable to high rates of substance abuse. Also, in the affluent families studied, males tend to have more adjustment difficulties than females, with affluent female adolescents more likely than male adolescents to attain superior levels of academic success. Another study, though, found that it was neighborhood wealth rather than family affluence per se that was linked to adolescent problems (Lund & Dearing, 2013). In this study, boys in affluent neighborhoods had a higher rate of delinquency and girls in affluent neighborhoods had higher levels of anxiety and depression than youth in middle-class neighborhoods. Family influence did not place these adolescents at risk in these domains; instead, relative differences between peers' affluence within each school were associated with patterns of externalizing and internalizing problems (Coley & others, 2018).

POVERTY

When sixth-graders in a poverty-stricken area of St. Louis were asked to describe a perfect day, one boy said he would erase the world, then he would sit and think (Children's Defense Fund, 1992). Asked if he wouldn't rather go outside and play, the boy responded, "Are you kidding—out *there*?"

As reviewed above, some children are resilient and cope with the challenges of poverty without any major setbacks, but too many struggle unsuccessfully. Each child of poverty who reaches adulthood unhealthy, unskilled, or alienated keeps our nation from being as competent and productive as it can be (Edelman, 2017).

Children and youth who grow up in poverty represent a special concern (Duncan, Kalil, & Ziol-Guest, 2017). In 2017 (the most recent complete data available in the United States), nearly 20 percent of children and adolescents were living in families with incomes below the poverty line (Children's Defense Fund, 2017). The U.S. figure of nearly 20 percent of youth living in poverty is much higher than the rates in other industrialized nations. For example, Canada has a youth poverty rate of 14 percent and Denmark has a rate of 3 percent.

Poverty in the United States is demarcated along family structure and ethnic lines. Over two-thirds of the youth living in poverty are children of color. Income and wealth inequality have intensified, such that White households have seven times the wealth of African American households and five times that of Hispanic households (Children's Defense Fund, 2017).

Persistent and long-standing poverty can have especially damaging effects on children (McLoyd, Jocson, & Williams, 2016; Manduca & Sampson, 2019). A series of studies have revealed that the more years children

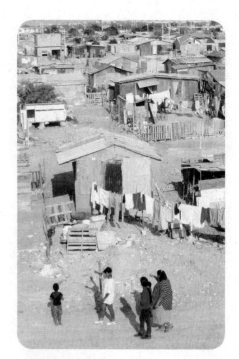

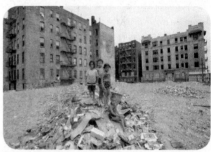

(*Top*) Children playing in Nueva Era, a low-income area on the outskirts of Nuevo Laredo, Mexico. (*Bottom*) Children who live in a poverty section of the South Bronx in New York City. *How does poverty affect the development of children like these?* (*Top*) Paul S. Howell/Liaison/Hulton Archive/Getty Images; (*bottom*) Andy Levin/Science Source

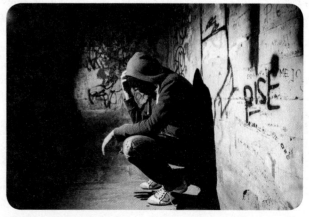

What characterizes socioeconomic variations in neighborhoods? zodebala/Getty Images

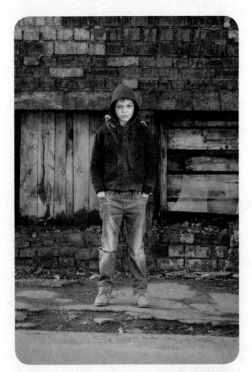

How are the environments that economically more advantaged children and adolescents live in different from the environments that children and adolescents live in that are characterized by poverty?

Bodnarchuk/iStock/Getty Images

spent in poverty, the more their biological indices of stress were elevated or altered in other ways (Kim & others, 2018). Another study found that persistent economic hardship as well as very early poverty was linked to lower cognitive functioning in children at 5 years of age (Schoon & others, 2011). In addition, intermittent poverty arising from income and housing insecurity can have detrimental effects in the long term (Comeau & Boyle, 2018; Pryor & others, 2019).

Psychological Ramifications of Poverty Living in poverty has many psychological effects on both adults and children (Pryor & others, 2019; Reiss & others, 2019). First, the poor are often powerless. In occupations, they rarely are the decision makers. Rules are handed down to them in an authoritarian manner. Second, the poor are often vulnerable to disaster. They are not likely to be given notice before they are laid off from work and usually do not have financial resources to fall back on when problems arise. Third, their range of alternatives is often restricted. Only a limited number of jobs are open to them. Even when alternatives are available, the poor might not know about them or be prepared to choose them, because of inadequate education and inability to read well. Fourth, being poor means having less prestige. This lack of prestige is transmitted to children early in their lives. The child living in poverty observes that many other children wear nicer clothes and live in more attractive houses.

Although positive things occur in the lives of children growing up in poverty, many of their negative experiences are worse than those of their middle-SES counterparts. These adversities involve physical punishment and lack of structure at home, violence in the neighborhood, and domestic violence in their buildings. A foundational research review covering decades of research concluded that compared with their economically more advantaged counterparts, poor children experience widespread environmental inequities that include the following (Evans, 2004, p. 77):

- Exposure to more family turmoil, violence, separation from their families, instability, and chaotic households
- Less social support, and parents who are less responsive and more authoritarian
- Read to relatively infrequently, watch more TV, and have less access to books and computers
- Schools and child-care facilities that are inferior and parents who are less involved in their children's school activities
- Air and water that are more polluted and homes that are more crowded, more noisy, and of lower quality
- More dangerous and physically deteriorating neighborhoods with less adequate municipal services

Do children living in poverty face higher levels of these risks? To find out, see *Connecting Through Research.*

Because of advances in their cognitive growth, adolescents living in poverty likely are more aware of their social disadvantage and the associated stigma than are children (Rivenbark & others, 2019). Combined with the increased sensitivity to peers in adolescence, such awareness may cause them to try to hide their poverty status as much as possible from others.

A special concern is the high percentage of single mothers in poverty (Hurst, 2013). More than one-third of single mothers are in poverty, compared with only one-tenth of single fathers. Vonnie McLoyd and others (2016) have concluded that because poor, single mothers are more distressed than their middle-SES counterparts are, they often show lower levels of support, nurturance, and involvement with their children. Among the reasons for the high poverty rate of single mothers are women's lower incomes, infrequent awarding of alimony payments, and poorly enforced child support by fathers (Hurst, Gibbons, & Nurse, 2016; Nieuwenhuis & Maldonado, 2018).

Countering Poverty's Effects One trend in antipoverty programs is to conduct two-generation interventions (Smith & Coffey, 2015; Sommer & others, 2018). These programs provide services for children (such as educational child care or preschool education) as well as services for parents (such as adult education, literacy training, and job-skill training).

What Risks Are Experienced by Children Living in Poverty?

In a now classic study that explored multiple risks in the lives of children from poverty and middle-income backgrounds (Evans & English, 2002), six risk factors were examined in 287 8- to 10-year-old non-Latino White children living in rural areas of upstate New York: family turmoil, child separation (a close family member being away from home often), exposure to violence, crowding, high noise levels, and inferior housing quality. Family turmoil, child separation, and exposure to violence were assessed by maternal reports of the life events their children had experienced. Crowding was determined by the number of people per room, and noise level was measured by the decibel level in the home. Housing quality (based on structural quality, cleanliness, clutter, resources for children, safety hazards, and climatic conditions) was rated by observers who visited the homes. Each of the six factors was defined as presenting a risk (scored as "1") or no risk (scored as "0"), and then these six scores were summed into an overall risk score. Thus, the multiple risk exposure for children could range from 0 to 6. Families were defined as poor if the household lived at or below the federally defined poverty line. In 2002 when the study was published, the poverty line in the United States was $18,100 per year for a family of four. (In 2019, the poverty level was $25,750 per year.)

Children in poor families experienced greater risks than their middle-income counterparts. As shown in Figure 3, a higher percentage of children in poor families were exposed to each of the six risk factors (family turmoil, child separation, exposure to violence, crowding, excessive noise, and poor quality of housing).

Were there differences in the children's adjustment that might reflect their differing exposure to risk factors? The researchers assessed

Risk factor (stressor)	Poor children exposed (%)	Middle-income children exposed (%)
Family turmoil	45	12
Child separation	45	14
Exposure to violence	73	49
Crowding	16	7
Excessive noise	32	21
Poor housing quality	24	3

FIGURE 3

PERCENTAGE OF POOR AND MIDDLE-INCOME CHILDREN EXPOSED TO EACH OF SIX RISK FACTORS

the children's levels of psychological stress through reports by the children and their mothers. Problems in self-regulation of behavior were determined by whether children chose immediate rather than delayed gratification on a task. Resting blood pressure and overnight neuroendocrine hormones were measured to assess children's levels of psychophysiological stress.

In comparison with children from middle-income backgrounds, poor children had higher levels of psychological stress, more problems in self-regulation of behavior, and elevated psychophysiological stress. Analysis indicated that cumulative exposure to stressors may contribute to difficulties in socioemotional development for children living in poverty.

In an illustrative experimental study, Aletha Huston and her colleagues (Huston & others, 2008) evaluated the effects of New Hope, a program designed to increase parental employment and reduce family poverty, on adolescent development. They randomly assigned families with 6- to 10-year-old children living in poverty to the New Hope program or a control group. New Hope offered benefits to poor adults who were employed at least 30 hours a week: wage supplements ensuring that net income increased as parents earned more; work supports in the form of subsidized child care (for any child under age 13); and health insurance. Management services were provided to New Hope participants to assist them with job searches and other needs. The New Hope program was available to the experimental group families for three years (until the children were 9 to 13 years old). Five years after the program began and two years after it had ended, the program's effects on the children were examined when they were 11 to 16 years old. Compared with adolescents in the control group, New Hope adolescents were more competent at reading, had better school performance, were less likely to be in special education classes, had more positive social skills, and were more likely to be in formal after-school arrangements. New Hope parents reported better psychological well-being and a greater sense of self-efficacy in managing their adolescents than parents in the control group did. In a follow-up assessment, the influence of the New Hope program on adolescents and emerging adults 9 to 19 years after they left the program was evaluated (McLoyd & others, 2011). Positive outcomes especially occurred for African American males, who were more optimistic about their

caring *connections*

The Quantum Opportunities Program

A downward trajectory is not inevitable for youth living in poverty. One potential positive path out of poverty for such youth is to become involved with a caring mentor. The Quantum Opportunities program, funded by the Ford Foundation, was a four-year, year-round mentoring effort (Carnegie Council on Adolescent Development, 1995). The students involved in this program were entering the ninth grade at a high school with high rates of poverty, were members of ethnic minority groups, and came from families that received public assistance. Each day for four years, mentors provided sustained support, guidance, and concrete assistance to these students.

The Quantum program required students to participate in (1) academic-related activities outside school hours, including reading, writing, math, science, and social studies, peer tutoring, and computer skills training; (2) community service projects, including tutoring elementary school students, cleaning up the neighborhood, and volunteering in hospitals, nursing homes, and libraries; and (3) cultural enrichment and personal development activities, including life skills training, college preparation, and job planning. In exchange for their commitment to the program, students were offered financial incentives that encouraged participation, completion, and long-range planning. A stipend of $1.33 was given to students for each hour they participated in these activities. For every 100 hours of education, service, or development activities they completed, students

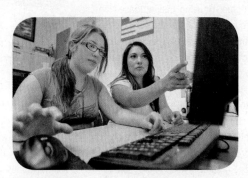

Students working on a computer at the Quantum Opportunities program in St. Petersburg, Florida.
Jim Thompson/Albuquerque/ZUMA Press Inc/Alamy Stock Photo

received a bonus of $100. The average cost per participant was $10,600 for the four years, which is one-half the cost of one year in prison.

An evaluation of the Quantum project compared the mentored students with a nonmentored control group. Sixty-three percent of the mentored students graduated from high school, but only 42 percent of the control group did; 42 percent of the mentored students were enrolled in college, but only 16 percent of the control group were. Furthermore, control-group students were twice as likely as the mentored students to receive food stamps or welfare, and they had more arrests. Such programs clearly have the potential to overcome the intergenerational transmission of poverty and its negative outcomes. The original Quantum Opportunities program has been adapted and expanded nationally by the Eisenhower Foundation, which in 2018 began replicating the Quantum program in Maryland, Ohio, Massachusetts, New Mexico, Wisconsin, and Florida. (Learn more at www. eisenhowerfoundation.org/qop.)

These research results confirm that the most effective programs to discourage dropping out of high school provide tutoring and mentoring, emphasize the creation of caring environments and relationships, and offer community-service opportunities. This research also reinforces the philosophy that goal-setting (such as planning for college and/or a career) is an integral part of achievement.

---

future employment and career prospects. In the most recent assessment of the New Hope Project, the intervention had positive effects on the youths' future orientation eight years after the program began and five years after the benefits ended (Purtell & McLoyd, 2013). In this study, boys' positive educational expectations were linked to improving the intervention's influence on reducing the boys' pessimism about future employment. To read about another program that benefitted youth living in poverty, see *Caring Connections.*

Review *Connect* Reflect

 Describe how socioeconomic status and poverty affect children's lives.

Review
- What is socioeconomic status?
- What are some socioeconomic variations in families, neighborhoods, and schools?
- What characterizes children living in poverty?

Connect
- In this section, you learned about anti-poverty programs that take a two-generation approach to intervention.

How is this similar to efforts to improve the health of children living in poverty?

Reflect *Your Own Personal Journey of Life*
- How would you label the socioeconomic status of your family as you grew up? In what ways do you think the SES status of your family influenced your development?

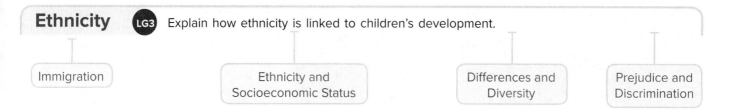

Ethnicity   LG3   Explain how ethnicity is linked to children's development.

Immigration

Ethnicity and Socioeconomic Status

Differences and Diversity

Prejudice and Discrimination

Ethnicity refers to characteristics rooted in cultural heritage, including nationality, race, religion, and language. Many of the largest cities throughout the world, such as Dhaka, Manila, Los Angeles, London, and Hong Kong, have populations in which many (often more than 100) different languages are spoken. With increased diversity have come opportunities for learning, as well as conflict and concerns about the future (Schaefer, 2019).

ethnicity A dimension of culture based on cultural heritage, nationality, race, religion, and language.

IMMIGRATION

In the United States, high rates of immigration are contributing to the growing proportion of ethnic minority adolescents and emerging adults (Frey, 2019). Immigrant families are those in which at least one of the parents is born outside the country of residence. Variations in immigrant families involve whether one or both parents are foreign-born, whether the child was born in the host country, and the ages at which immigration took place for both the parents and the children (Titzmann & Fuligni, 2015).

Different models have been proposed to determine whether children and adolescents in immigrant families are more vulnerable or more successful in relation to the general population of children and adolescents (Zhou & Gonzales, 2019). Historically, an *immigrant risk model* was emphasized, concluding that youth of immigrants had a lower level of well-being and were at risk for more problems. For example, one study found that the longer immigrant youth from the Dominican Republic lived in the United States, the higher their risk for suicide and other mental health problems in comparison with youth residing in the Dominican Republic (Peña & others, 2016).

An *immigrant paradox model* also has been proposed, emphasizing that despite the many cultural, socioeconomic, language, and other obstacles that immigrant families face, their youth show a high level of well-being and fewer problems than native-born youth (Marks & Garcia Coll, 2018). Based on current research, some support exists for each model (Brady & Stevens, 2019). Robert Crosnoe and Andrew Fuligni reached the following conclusion (2012, p. 1473):

> Some children from immigrant families are doing quite well, some less so, depending on the characteristics of migration itself (including the nation of origin) and their families' circumstances in their new country (including their position in socioeconomic and race-ethnic stratification systems.

Today an increasing proportion of the U.S. population consists of ethnic minorities (Frey, 2019), and this growth of ethnic minorities is expected to continue throughout the rest of the twenty-first century. Asian Americans are expected to be the fastest-growing ethnic group of adolescents, with a growth rate of almost 600 percent by 2100. Latino adolescents are projected to increase almost 400 percent by 2100. Figure 4 shows the actual numbers of adolescents in different ethnic groups in the year 2000, as well as the numbers projected through 2100. Notice that by 2100, Latino adolescents are expected to outnumber non-Latino White adolescents.

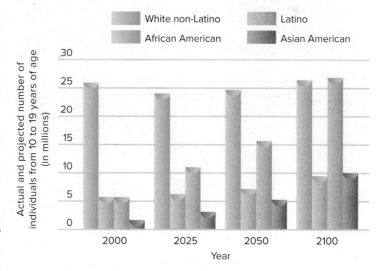

FIGURE **4**

ACTUAL AND PROJECTED NUMBER OF U.S. ADOLESCENTS AGED 10 TO 19, 2000 TO 2100. In 2000, there were more than 25 million White non-Latino adolescents 10 to 19 years of age in the United States, whereas the numbers for ethnic minority groups were substantially lower. However, projections for 2025 through 2100 predict dramatic increases in the numbers of Latino and Asian American adolescents, with more Latino than non-Latino White adolescents and more Asian American than African American adolescents expected to be living in the United States by 2100.

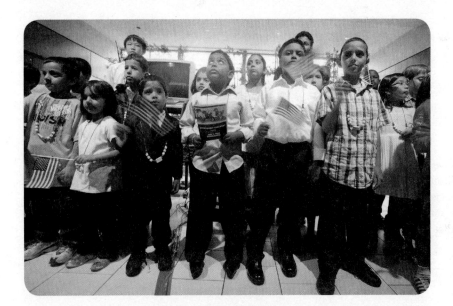

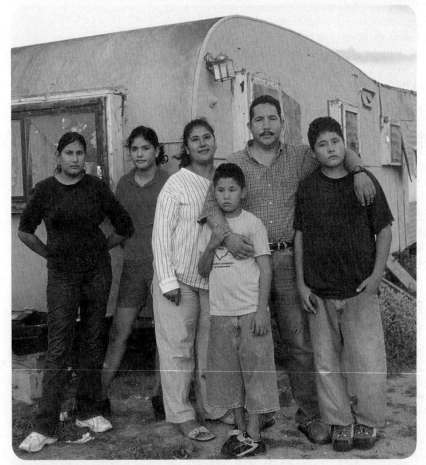

(Top) Immigrant children from 12 countries participating in a U.S. citizenship ceremony in Queens, New York, on June 11, 2009. *(Bottom)* A Latino family who immigrated recently to the Rio Grande Valley in Texas. *What are some characteristics of children and their families who have recently immigrated to the United States?*

(Top) Mario Tama/Getty Images; (Bottom) © Allison Wright/Corbis Documentary/Getty Images

Recently immigrated families may face special problems. Many individuals in immigrant families are dealing with the problems associated with being undocumented. Living in an undocumented family can affect children's developmental outcomes when parents are unwilling to sign up for services for which they are eligible. Also, parents are limited to low-wage jobs with high stress and low benefits, and there is a lack of cognitive stimulation in the home (Kang, 2019; Yoshikawa, 2011).

What are some of the circumstances that immigrants face that challenge their adjustment? Immigrants often experience stressors uncommon to or less prominent among longtime residents. These include language barriers, dislocations and separations from support networks, the dual struggle to preserve identity and to acculturate, and changes in SES (Gollnick & Chinn, 2016; Sheikh & Anderson, 2018). Consequently, when working with adolescents and their immigrant families, counselors need to adapt intervention programs to optimize cultural sensitivity (Suárez-Orozco, Suárez-Orozco, & Qin-Hilliard, 2014; Sue & others, 2016, 2019).

Many members of families that have recently immigrated to the United States adopt a bicultural orientation, selecting characteristics of the U.S. culture that help them to survive and advance, while retaining aspects of their culture of origin (Schwartz & others, 2019; Titzmann & Fuligni, 2015). Immigration also involves cultural "brokering," which has increasingly occurred in the United States as children and adolescents serve as the cultural and linguistic mediators for their immigrant parents (Shen, Kim, & Benner, 2019).

Although many such families adopt a bicultural orientation, parenting in many ethnic minority families also focuses on issues associated with promoting children's ethnic pride, knowledge of their ethnic group, and awareness of discrimination (Liu, Simpkins, & Lin, 2018; Mehta, 2017). In adopting characteristics of the U.S. culture, Latino families are increasingly embracing the importance of education (McDermott, Umaña-Taylor, & Martinez-Fuentes, 2018). Although their school dropout rates have remained higher than for other ethnic groups, this group of youth also have shown the most dramatic reductions in dropout rates over the past two decades (NCES, 2018). Latino families are retaining a strong commitment to family when they immigrate to the United States despite facing challenges advancing economically. For example, divorce rates for Latino families are lower than for non-Latino White families of similar socioeconomic status.

Many of the families that have immigrated in recent decades to the United States, such as those from Mexico, Central America, and various countries throughout Asia,

Carola Suárez-Orozco, Immigration Studies Researcher and Professor

Carola Suárez-Orozco currently is a Professor and Co-director of the Institute for Immigration, Globalization, and Education at UCLA. She formerly served on the faculty at New York University and Harvard. Carola obtained her undergraduate degree (in development studies) and doctoral degree (in clinical psychology) at the University of California at Berkeley.

Suárez-Orozco has worked both in clinical and public school settings in California and Massachusetts. While at Harvard, she conducted a five-year longitudinal study of the adaptation of immigrant adolescents (coming from Central America, China, and the Dominican Republic) to schools and society. She especially advocates more research involving the role of cultural and psychological factors in the adaptation of immigrant and ethnic minority youth (Suárez-Orozco, Suárez-Orozco, & Qin-Hilliard, 2014).

For more information about what researchers and professors do, see the Careers in Child Development appendix.

come from collectivist cultures that emphasize family obligations and duties (Choi & others, 2018; Oyserman, 2017). This family obligation and duty may take the form of adolescents assisting parents in their occupations and contributing to the family's welfare (van Geel & Vedder, 2011). This type of support often occurs in service and manual labor jobs, such as those in construction, gardening, cleaning, and restaurants.

However, there are wide variations in immigrant families' experiences and the degree to which their children and adolescents change as they are exposed to American culture. One illustrative study found that following their immigration, Mexican American adolescents spent less time with their family and identified less with family values (Updegraff & others, 2012). However, in this study, teens with stronger family values in early adolescence were less likely to engage in risky behavior in late adolescence.

Individual families differ, and how ethnic minority families deal with stress depends on many factors (Burnette & others, 2019; Non & others, 2019). Whether the parents are native-born or immigrants, how long the family has been in the United States, its socioeconomic status, and its national origin all make a difference (Gonzales & others, 2012). Research has revealed that parents' education before migrating is linked to their children's academic achievement (Feliciano & Lanuza, 2017).

The characteristics of the family's social context also influence its adaptation. What are the attitudes toward the family's ethnic group within its neighborhood or city? Can the family's children attend good schools? Are there community organizations that welcome people from the family's ethnic group? Do members of the family's ethnic group form community organizations of their own? To read about the work of one individual who studies immigrant adolescents, see *Connecting with Careers*.

ETHNICITY AND SOCIOECONOMIC STATUS

Too often the research on ethnic minority children has failed to tease apart the influences of ethnicity and socioeconomic status (SES). Ethnicity and SES can interact in ways that exaggerate the negative influence of ethnicity because ethnic minority individuals are overrepresented in the lower socioeconomic levels in our societies (Hurst, Gibbon, & Nurse 2016; McLoyd, Jocson, & Williams, 2016). Ethnicity has often defined who will enjoy the privileges of citizenship and to what degree and in what ways. In

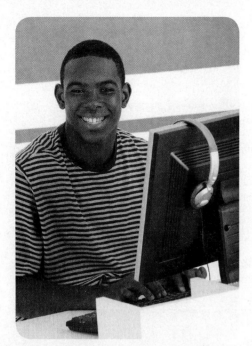

Too often African American male adolescents are negatively stereotyped. As Jason Leonard, age 15 comments, "I want America to know that most of us black teens are not troubled people from broken homes and headed to jail. . . . In my relationships with my parents, we show respect for each other and we have values in our house. We have traditions we celebrate together, including Christmas and Kwanzaa."
Comstock/Getty Images

Consider the flowers of a garden: Though differing in kind, color, form, and shape, yet inasmuch as they are refreshed by the waters of one spring, revived by the breath of one wind, invigorated by the rays of one sun, this diversity increases their charm and adds to their beauty. . . . How unpleasing to the eye if all the flowers and plants, the leaves and blossoms, the fruits, the branches, and the trees of that garden were all of the same shape and color! Diversity of hues, form, and shape enriches and adorns the garden and heightens its effect.

—ABDU'L BAHA
Persian Baha'i religious leader, 19th/20th century

many instances, an individual's ethnic background has determined whether the individual will be alienated or disadvantaged.

In some cases, researchers have given ethnic explanations of child development that were largely based on socioeconomic status rather than ethnicity. For example, decades of research on group differences in self-esteem failed to consider the socioeconomic status of African American and White American children (Hare & Castenell, 1985). When the self-esteem of African American children from low-income backgrounds is compared with that of White American children from middle-class backgrounds, the differences are often large but not informative because of the confounding of ethnicity and SES.

One longitudinal study illustrates the importance of separating the effects of SES from ethnicity. Higher SES predicted greater educational and occupational expectations across ethnic groups among 14- to 26-year-olds (Mello, 2009). Furthermore, after controlling for SES, African American youth reported the highest educational expectations, followed by Latino and Asian American/Pacific Islander, non-Latino White, and American Indian/Alaska Native youth. African American and Asian American/Pacific Islander youth had the highest occupational expectations, followed by Latino, American Indian/Alaska Native, and non-Latino White youth.

Being from a middle-SES background does not entirely protect youth from the problems of minority status (Cushner, McClelland, & Safford, 2019). Middle-SES ethnic minority children still encounter much of the prejudice, discrimination, and bias associated with being a member of an ethnic minority group (Chou & Feagin, 2015).

Poverty contributes to the stressful life experiences of many ethnic minority children. Vonnie McLoyd and her colleagues (McLoyd, 2019) conclude that ethnic minority children experience a disproportionate share of the adverse effects of poverty and unemployment in America today. Thus, many ethnic minority children experience a double disadvantage: prejudice, discrimination, and bias because of their ethnic minority status, accompanied by the stressful effects of poverty.

DIFFERENCES AND DIVERSITY

Historical, economic, and social experiences produce differences between various ethnic minority and majority groups (Bornstein & Lansford, 2018; Molitor & Hsu, 2019). Individuals living in a particular ethnic or cultural group adapt to the values, attitudes, and stresses of that culture. Recognizing and respecting these differences is an important aspect of getting along with others in a diverse, multicultural world. Children, like all of us, need to take the perspective of individuals from ethnic and cultural groups that are different from their own and think, "If I were in their shoes, what kinds of experiences might I have had?" "How would I feel if I were a member of their ethnic or cultural group?" "How would I think and behave if I had grown up in their world?" Such perspective taking often increases empathy and understanding of individuals from ethnic and cultural groups different from one's own.

For too long, differences between any ethnic minority group and the majority culture were conceptualized as deficits or inferior characteristics on the part of the ethnic minority group. Indeed, research on ethnic minority groups often focused only on a group's negative, stressful aspects. For example, in the past, research on African American adolescent girls examined topics such as poverty, unwed motherhood, and dropping out of school; research on the psychological strengths of African American adolescent girls was sorely needed. The self-esteem, achievement, motivation, and self-control of children from different ethnic minority groups deserve considerable study. The current research on ethnic groups underscores the strengths of children and adolescents in minority groups (Raval & Walker, 2019; Updegraff & Umaña-Taylor, 2015). For example, the extended-family support system of relationships that is common in many ethnic minority groups is now recognized as an important factor in coping and thriving.

There is considerable diversity within each ethnic group. Ethnic minority groups have different social, historical, and economic backgrounds (Spring, 2016). For example, Mexican and Cuban immigrants have some shared Latin culture, but these groups had different reasons for migrating, came from varying socioeconomic backgrounds in their native countries, and continue to experience different rates and types of employment in the United States and Canada. The U.S. federal government now recognizes the existence of 511 different Native American tribes, each having a unique ancestral background with differing values and characteristics. Asian Americans include Chinese, Japanese, Filipinos, Koreans, and Southeast Asians (itself a large and very diverse group), with each having a distinct ancestry and language. The diversity of Asian Americans is reflected in educational attainment statistics: Some achieve a high level of education; many others have little education (Hurst, Gibbon, & Nurse, 2016). For example, 90 percent of Korean American males graduate from high school, but only 71 percent of Vietnamese American males do.

No ethnic group is homogeneous. Sometimes well-meaning individuals fail to recognize the diversity within an ethnic group (Sue & others, 2016). In one of the largest studies to date on this topic, investigators examined how much variation there was between youth in a wide range of family environment and psychological outcome variables. The study included over 1,000 young adolescents living in nine countries and representing a wide variety of ethnic and cultural groups. Overall, the vast majority of the variation observed was between youth *within* each cultural group, pointing to very substantial heterogeneity within ethnicities (Deater-Deckard & others, 2018).

developmental **connection**

Identity

Many aspects of sociocultural contexts influence children's and adolescents' ethnic identity. Connect to "The Self and Identity."

prejudice An unjustified negative attitude toward an individual because of her or his membership in a group.

PREJUDICE AND DISCRIMINATION

Prejudice is an unjustified negative attitude toward an individual because of the individual's membership in a group. The group toward which the prejudice is directed can be made up of people of a particular ethnic group, sex, age, religion, or other detectable difference (Brandt & Crawford, 2019). Our current topic is prejudice against members of ethnic minority groups.

Research studies provide insight into the discrimination experienced by ethnic minority children and adolescents (Benner & others, 2018; Hughes & others, 2016; Thakur & others, 2017). Consider the following three studies:

- In one foundational study, discrimination against seventh- to tenth-grade African American students was related to their lower level of psychological functioning, including perceived stress, symptoms of depression, and lower perceived well-being; more positive attitudes toward African Americans were associated with more positive psychological functioning in adolescents (Sellers & others, 2006). Figure 5 shows the percentage of African American adolescents who reported experiencing different types of racial hassles in the past year.

- Second-generation Asian adolescents in the United States were more likely to perceive discrimination than Hispanic and White youth; this was linked with higher rates of depression symptoms (Lo & others, 2017).

- African American and Latino adolescents who encountered more discrimination also experienced increases in depressive symptoms over time. This effect was particularly strong among youth who had low levels of positive feelings about their race or ethnicity (Stein & others, 2016).

Progress has been made in ethnic minority relations, but discrimination and prejudice still exist, and equality has not been achieved. Much remains to be accomplished (Umaña-Taylor, 2016). To read further about diversity and ethnicity, see *Connecting with Diversity*.

Type of Racial Hassle	Percent of Adolescents Who Reported the Racial Hassle in the Past Year
Being accused of something or treated suspiciously	71.0
Being treated as if you were "stupid," being "talked down to"	70.7
Others reacting to you as if they were afraid or intimidated	70.1
Being observed or followed while in public places	68.1
Being treated rudely or disrespectfully	56.4
Being ignored, overlooked, not given service	56.4
Others expecting your work to be inferior	54.1
Being insulted, called a name, or harassed	52.2

FIGURE 5

AFRICAN AMERICAN ADOLESCENTS' REPORTS OF RACIAL HASSLES IN THE PAST YEAR (SELLERS & OTHERS, 2006)

The United States and Canada: Nations with Many Cultures

The United States has been and continues to be a great receiver of ethnic groups. It has embraced new ingredients from many cultures. The cultures often collide and cross-pollinate, mixing their ideologies and identities. Some of the culture of origin is retained, some of it is lost, and some of it is mixed with the broader American culture.

Many nations experience the immigration of varied ethnic groups. Possibly we can learn more about the potential benefits, problems, and varied responses by examining their experiences. Canada is a prominent example. Canada comprises a mixture of cultures that are loosely organized along the lines of economic resources and historical periods. The Canadian cultures include the following (Chavez, 2019; Guo & Wong, 2019):

- Native peoples, or First Nations, who were Canada's original inhabitants;
- Descendants of French settlers who came to Canada during the seventeenth and eighteenth centuries;
- Descendants of British settlers who came to Canada during and after the seventeenth century, or from the United States after the American Revolution in the latter part of the eighteenth century;
- Descendants of immigrants from Asia, mainly China, who settled on the west coast of Canada in the latter part of the nineteenth and early twentieth centuries;
- Descendants of nineteenth-century immigrants from various European countries, who settled in central Canada and the prairie provinces;
- Twentieth-century and current immigrants from countries in economic and political turmoil (in Latin America, the Caribbean, Asia, Africa, the Indian subcontinent, the former Soviet Union, and the Middle East), who have settled in many parts of Canada

Canada has two official languages: English and French. Primarily French-speaking individuals reside mainly in the province of Quebec; primarily English-speaking individuals reside mainly in other Canadian provinces. In addition to its English- and French-speaking populations, Canada has a large multicultural community. This includes hundreds of languages spoken by groups of foreign-born immigrants and their children, as well as a similarly diverse range of native languages and dialects spoken by indigenous people.

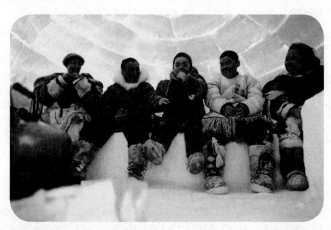

A Canadian Inuit family in Baker Lake, Canada. *What major cultural groups emigrated to Canada and when did they first arrive?*
Wayne R Bilenduke/The Image Bank/Getty Images

Canada has two official languages, based on the nation's two largest ethnic populations. If the United States were to base its official languages on the largest ethnic populations they expect to have in 2100, what might they be? (See Figure 4.)

Review Connect Reflect

 Explain how ethnicity is linked to children's development.

Review

- How does immigration influence children's development?
- How are ethnicity and socioeconomic status related?
- What is important to know about differences and diversity?
- How do prejudice and discrimination affect children's development?

Connect

- In this section, we learned that taking the perspective of individuals from ethnic and cultural groups that are different from one's own can help children (and adults) to better respect and get along with others in a diverse, multicultural world. What do you know about perspective taking and elementary school children's communication skills?

Reflect *Your Own Personal Journey of Life*

- No matter how well intentioned children are, their life circumstances likely have given them some prejudices. If and when you become a parent, how would you attempt to reduce your children's prejudices?

| Media Use and Screen Time | Television and Electronic Media | Digital Devices and the Internet |

Few developments in society over the last 50 years have had a greater impact on children and adolescents than television, digital gaming, and the Internet (Blumberg & others, 2019; Gross, 2013; Roblyer, 2016). The persuasion capabilities of television, gaming apps, and the Internet are staggering. Many of today's adolescents have spent more time since infancy in front of a screen than with their parents or in the classroom. This is now referred to as *screen time,* which encompasses how much time they spend watching/using television, computers, video game systems, and mobile media such as smartphones.

MEDIA USE AND SCREEN TIME

Digital technology is affecting children and adolescents in both positive and negative ways. Technology can provide expansive knowledge and can be used in a constructive way to enhance children's and adolescents' education (Maloy & others, 2016). However, the possible downside of technology was captured in a controversial book, *The Dumbest Generation: How the Digital Age Stupefies Young Americans and Jeopardizes Our Future (Or, Don't Trust Anyone Under 30),* written by Emory University English Professor Mark Bauerlein (2009). Among the book's themes are that many of today's youth are more interested in information retrieval than information formation, don't read books and aren't motivated to read them, can't spell without spellcheck, and have become encapsulated in a world of cell phones, text messaging, YouTube, and social media contexts. Should we be concerned? In terms of cognitive skills such as thinking and reasoning, IQ scores have been rising significantly since the 1930s (Flynn, 2013). Further, there is no consistent research evidence that being immersed in a technological world of gaming and YouTube impairs thinking skills (Blumberg & others, 2019). However, there is evidence suggesting that screen time on social media in particular may be negatively affecting mental and behavioral health of adolescents (Twenge & Campbell, 2019). There are also concerns about negative effects of sedentary behavior during screen time, such as increased risk of obesity and disrupted sleep (Pearson & others, 2014).

If the amount of time spent in an activity is any indication of its importance, there is no doubt that media play important roles in children's and adolescents' lives. To better understand various aspects of media use among U.S. children and adolescents, the Kaiser Family Foundation (KFF) funded three national surveys in 1999, 2004, and 2009. The 2009 survey interviewed more than 2,000 8- to 18-year-olds and documented that media use among children and adolescents had increased dramatically in the preceding decade (Rideout, Foehr, & Roberts, 2010). Today's youth live in a world in which they are encapsulated by media. In this survey, in 2009, 8- to 11-year-olds used media 5 hours and 29 minutes a day, but 11- to 14-year-olds used media an average of 8 hours and 40 minutes a day, and 15- to 18-year-olds an average of 7 hours and 58 minutes a day (see Figure 6). More recent data indicate that these trends have intensified. In 2018 (Pew Research Center, 2018a), 95 percent of adolescents in the United States reported having access to a smartphone, and nearly half were connected to the Internet constantly.

A major trend in the use of technology is the dramatic increase in media multitasking (Aagard, 2019; Wang, Sigerson, & Cheng, 2019). In the 2009 KFF survey, when the amount of time spent multitasking was included in

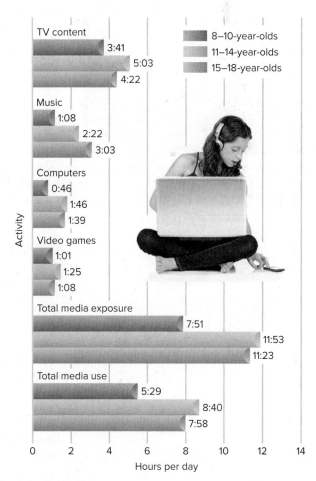

FIGURE 6

AMOUNT OF TIME U.S. 8- TO 18-YEAR-OLDS SPEND PER DAY IN DIFFERENT ACTIVITIES

Alberto Pomares/Apomares/E+/Getty Images

Legend:
- 8–10-year-olds
- 11–14-year-olds
- 15–18-year-olds

Activity / Hours per day:

TV content: 3:41, 5:03, 4:22
Music: 1:08, 2:22, 3:03
Computers: 0:46, 1:46, 1:39
Video games: 1:01, 1:25, 1:08
Total media exposure: 7:51, 11:53, 11:23
Total media use: 5:29, 8:40, 7:58

total media use, 11- to 14-year-olds spent nearly 12 hours a day (compared with almost 9 hours a day when multitasking was not included) exposed to media (Rideout, Foehr, & Roberts, 2010). In this survey, 39 percent of seventh- to twelfth-graders said "most of the time" they use two or more media concurrently, such as surfing the Web while listening to music. In some cases, media multitasking—such as text messaging, listening to music, and updating a YouTube site—is engaged in at the same time as doing homework. It is hard to imagine that this allows a student to do homework efficiently, although there is little research on media multitasking. Several lines of evidence are emerging, however, that suggest negative effects. One longitudinal study of over 2,000 adolescents in the United States found higher multitasking predicted attention problems (Baumgartner & others, 2017). In another, the presence of phones during face-to-face interaction was shown to interfere with, and decrease the enjoyment of, social engagement (Misra & others, 2016). Mobile media, such as cell phones, are driving increased media use and multitasking by adolescents. For example, in the 2004 survey, 39 percent of youth owned a cell phone, a figure that jumped to 66 percent in 2009 (Rideout, Foehr, & Roberts, 2010) and continues to increase today.

TELEVISION AND ELECTRONIC MEDIA

In the previous century, fewer developments had a greater impact on children and teenagers than television (Maloy & others, 2016). And in the last two decades, youth increasingly have played digital games (Blumberg & others, 2019).

Television Many children spend more time in front of a television screen than they spend interacting with their parents. Although it is only one of the many mass media that affect children's behavior, television may be the most influential. The persuasive capabilities of television are staggering. The 20,000 hours of television watched by the time the average American adolescent graduates from high school are greater than the number of hours spent in the classroom.

Television can have positive or negative effects on children's and adolescents' development. Television can have a positive influence by presenting motivating educational programs, increasing children's and adolescents' information about the world beyond their immediate environment, and providing models of prosocial behavior. However, television can have a negative influence on children and adolescents by making them passive learners, distracting them from doing homework, teaching them stereotypes, providing them with violent models of aggression, and presenting them with unrealistic views of the world (Lillard, Li, & Boguszewski, 2015). Further, researchers have found that a high level of TV viewing in early childhood predicts adolescent habits and outcomes years later. One of the largest longitudinal studies from Canada found effects years later on weight, eating habits, and academic engagement (Simonato & others, 2018). A comprehensive review of the literature noted that many of the behavioral and health risks arising from extensive screen viewing reflect impacts on sleep and wake-time habits (LeBourgeois & others, 2017).

A series of research reviews concluded that children and adolescents who experience a heavy media diet of violence are more likely to perceive the world as a dangerous place and to view aggression as more acceptable than their counterparts who see media violence less frequently (Escobar-Chaves & Anderson, 2008; Wilson, 2008). This pattern of effects may be due to the reinforcement of beliefs and attributions about others and can be a source of aggression intent and behavior—an effect that may grow over time with development and prolonged exposure into adulthood (Bushman, 2016). Much of the media violence described above comes from television, but as we see next, exposure also involves violent video games.

Video Games Violent video games, especially those that are highly realistic, also raise concerns about their effects on children and adolescents (Anderson & others, 2017). Correlational studies and meta-analyses of the results indicate that children and adolescents who extensively play violent electronic games are more aggressive than are

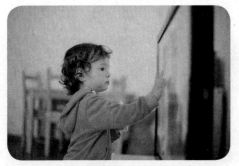

How might watching aggression on TV and playing violent video games be linked to adolescent aggression?
Mayte Torres/Moment/Getty Images

their counterparts who spend less time playing the games or do not play them at all (Calvert & others, 2017). However, there is some controversy in the field about the size and meaning of these effects (for example, Ferguson, 2015).

Are there any positive outcomes when adolescents play video games? Far more studies of video game use by adolescents have focused on possible negative outcomes, but an increasing number of studies are examining possible positive outcomes (Adachi & Willoughby, 2017). Dutch researchers found that elementary and middle-school students who played friendly and competitive but nonviolent video games subsequently behaved in more prosocial ways (Lobel & others, 2019). Another study of elementary and middle-school youth showed that prosocial game playing was associated with more empathy and better social relationships, across a wide SES range of families (Harrington & O'Connell, 2016).

Further, researchers have found that video games requiring exercise (exergames) are linked to weight loss in overweight adolescents (Calvert, Bond, & Staiano, 2014). For example, an experimental study found that overweight adolescents lost more weight when they participated in a 10-week competitive exergame video condition (video games that require gross motor activity–in this study the Ninendo Wii EA Sports Active video game was used) than their overweight counterparts in a cooperative exergame condition or a no-video-game control condition (Staiano, Abraham, & Calvert, 2012). In a subsequent experiment with overweight children, a half-year exergame condition led to noteworthy improvements in metabolic measures of health (Staiano & others, 2018).

Electronic Media, Learning, and Achievement The effects of electronic media on children depend on the child's age and the type of media. A foundational research review reached the following conclusions over a decade ago about infants and young children (Kirkorian, Wartella, & Anderson, 2008):

- *Infancy:* Learning from electronic media is difficult for infants and toddlers, and they learn much more easily from direct experiences with people.
- *Early childhood:* At about 3 years of age, children can learn from electronic media with educational material if the media use effective strategies, such as repeating concepts a number of times, using images and sounds that capture young children's attention, and speaking with the voices of children rather than adults. However, the vast majority of media young children experience is entertainment-oriented rather than educational.

The American Academy of Pediatrics (2016) has recommended that children under 2 years of age should not watch screens (except for live videochatting) because it likely reduces direct interactions with parents. The evidence for this recommendation comes from numerous earlier studies. One study found that the more hours 1- and 3-year-olds watched TV per day, the more likely they were to have attention problems at 7 years of age (Christakis & others, 2004), and another revealed that daily TV exposure at 18 months was linked to increased inattention/hyperactivity at 30 months of age (Cheng & others, 2010). A study of 2- to 48-month-olds indicated that each hour of audible TV was linked to a reduction in child vocalizations (Christakis & others, 2009) and still another study revealed that 8- to 16-month-olds who viewed baby videos had poor language development (Zimmerman, Christakis, & Meltzoff, 2007).

How does television influence children's attention, creativity, and mental ability? Overall, media use has not been found to cause attention deficit hyperactivity disorder, but a small link has been identified between heavy television viewing and nonclinical reduced attention levels in children; the evidence now includes experimental studies of humans and mice (Christakis & others, 2018).

Are media use and screen time linked to children's and adolescents' creativity? Reviews of the literature have concluded that there is a negative association between children's and adolescents' TV viewing and their creativity. An exception, though, occurs when they watch educational TV content that is designed to teach creativity through the use of imaginative characters (Calvert & Valkenberg, 2013). In addition, the versatility of digital media

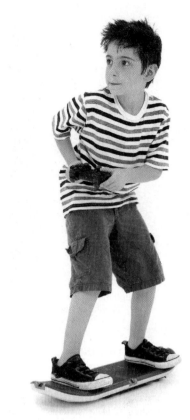

What are some of the ways that researchers are exploring possible positive outcomes of playing some types of video games?
Duplass/Shutterstock

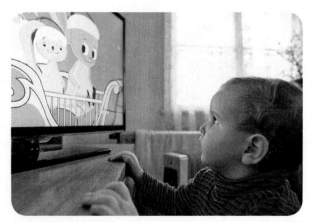

What have researchers found about TV watching by infants?
Deyan Georgiev/Alamy Stock Photo

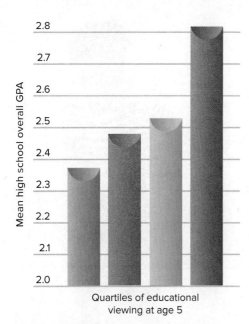

FIGURE 7

EDUCATIONAL TV VIEWING IN EARLY CHILDHOOD AND HIGH SCHOOL GRADE-POINT AVERAGE FOR BOYS. When boys watched more educational television (especially *Sesame Street*) as preschoolers, they had higher grade-point averages in high school. The graph displays the boys' early TV viewing patterns in quartiles and the means of their grade-point averages. The bar on the left is for the lowest 25 percent of boys who viewed educational TV programs, the next bar the next 25 percent, and so on, with the bar on the right for the 25 percent of the boys who watched the most educational TV shows as preschoolers.

options does offer great potential for encouraging and teaching creativity in informal and formal learning settings (Vishkaie, Shively, & Powell, 2018).

The more time children spend watching screens, the lower their school achievement. Why might screen time be negatively linked to children's achievement? Three possibilities involve interference, displacement, and self-defeating tastes/preferences (Comstock & Scharrer, 2006). In terms of interference, having a television on while doing homework can distract children while they are doing cognitive tasks. In terms of displacement, television can take away time and attention from engaging in achievement-related tasks, such as homework, reading, writing, and mathematics. In terms of self-defeating tastes and preferences, television attracts children to entertainment, sports, commercials, and other activities that capture their interest more than school achievement. Children who are heavy screen watchers tend to view books as dull and boring. These effects can create changes that continue into adolescence. A large longitudinal study of German youth showed such effects over time, resulting in lower achievement in school (Poulain & others, 2018).

However, some types of television content—such as educational programming for young children—may enhance achievement. In a classic longitudinal study, individuals who viewed educational programs as preschoolers, such as Sesame Street and Mr. Rogers' Neighborhood, were more likely to experience a number of positive outcomes through high school, including higher grades, reading of more books, and enhanced creativity (Anderson & others, 2001) (see Figure 7). Newer technologies, especially interactive touchscreen games, hold promise for motivating children to learn and become better problem solvers (Blumberg & others, 2019). At the same time, there is mounting evidence that digital training to enhance skills (for example, memory, attention, reaction time) will not have general or long-lasting positive effects on cognitive ability, even if there are short-term effects on some very specific skills (Sala, Tatlidil, & Gobet, 2018).

DIGITAL DEVICES AND THE INTERNET

Culture involves change, and nowhere is that change more apparent than in the technological revolution individuals are experiencing with increased use of digital devices (for example, iPads, laptops, computers, and smartphones) and the Internet (Maloy & others, 2016). Society still relies on some basic nontechnological competencies—for example, good communication skills, positive attitudes, and the ability to solve problems and to think deeply and creatively. But how people pursue these competencies is changing at a speed that few people had to cope with in previous eras. For youth to be adequately prepared for tomorrow's jobs, technology needs to become an integral part of their lives (Edwards, 2013; Gross, 2013; Ikenouye & Clarke, 2018).

The digitally mediated social environment of youth includes email and text messaging, social networking sites such as Instagram and Snapchat, chat rooms, videosharing and photosharing, multiplayer online computer games, and virtual worlds. The remarkable increase in the popularity of social media and texting sites is seen in their popularity in comparison with the most widely used Internet search sites like Google and Bing. Most of these digitally mediated social interactions began on computers but more recently have also shifted to smartphones.

As described earlier in the chapter, there has been a dramatic increase over the past two decades in adolescents' use of smartphones for communicating, playing, and working. Today, nearly all adolescents in the United States, Canada, and a number of other industrialized countries have access to smartphones. Furthermore, the most rapidly growing access is now among young people living in countries with emerging economies (Pew Research Center, 2018a, b).

Special concerns have emerged about children's and adolescents' access to information on the Internet, which has been largely unregulated. Youth can access adult sexual material, instructions for making bombs and weapons, and other information that is inappropriate for them. Another concern is peer bullying and harassment on the Internet (called *cyberbullying*) (Rosa & others, 2019; Selkie, Fales, & Moreno, 2016). A number of surveys and observational

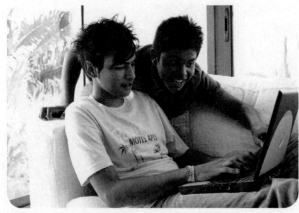

What characterizes the online social environment of adolescents?
Anne Ackermann/Digital Vision/Alamy

studies of youth have now shown that cyberbullying is among the most common forms of peer victimization they experience. A comprehensive review of studies showed that the percentage of youth who perpetrated or were victimized by online bullying varied widely between studies, with estimates as high as 41 percent for perpetration and 72 percent for victimization (Selkie & others, 2016). Information about preventing cyberbullying (and all forms of bullying) can be found at https://www.stopbullying.gov/.

Turning to college students (most of whom are emerging adults in their late teens and early twemties), there is mounting concern based on research evidence that growing up in the age of smartphones and the Internet has created too many opportunities for "cyber-slacking"—such as multitasking with entertainment and communications while taking notes or studying (Flanigan & Kiewra, 2018). If overuse of non-scholastic Internet use is excessive, it can negatively impact social relationships and increase health risk behaviors such as substance use. However, Internet use for academic work can positively impact learning, self-worth, and achievement (Padilla-Walker & others, 2010).

Clearly, adolescents' use of the Internet requires parental monitoring and regulation (Collier & others, 2016; Van Petegem & others, 2019). The following illustrative studies explored the role of parents in guiding adolescents' use of the Internet and other media:

- Parents' tendencies to perceive online dangers were not matched by their willingness to set limits and monitor their adolescents' online activities (Rosen, Cheever, & Carrier, 2008). Also in this study, adolescents who perceived that their parents had an indulgent parenting style (high warmth and involvement but low levels of strictness and supervision) reported engaging in the most risky online behavior, such as meeting someone in person whom they had initially contacted on the Internet. This and other research has led to the recognition that there is a need for parent education regarding ways to communicate effectively with their teenagers about online contact and behavior (Vanwesenbeeck & others, 2018).

- Both maternal and paternal authoritative parenting predicted proactive monitoring of adolescent media use, including restriction of certain media from adolescent use and parent-adolescent discussion of exposure to questionable media content (Padilla-Walker & Coyne, 2011). Subsequent research has replicated these findings and has shown that a supportive relationship in which the parent exercises and enforces control over time online benefits the adolescents' mental health and overall adjustment (Fardouly & others, 2018).

- Problematic mother-adolescent (age 13) relationships (such as insecure attachment and autonomy conflicts) predicted emerging adults' preference for online communication and greater probability of forming a relationship of poor quality with someone they met online (Szwedo, Mikami, & Allen, 2011). Further research has indicated that problematic family relationships can spur not only problematic online relationships but also increase risk for Internet "addiction" and excessive use (Ko & others, 2015).

developmental **connection**

Media Influence

Significant numbers of children are victimized by bullies, and bullying has a number of negative outcomes for children. Connect to "Peers."

Review Connect Reflect

LG4 Summarize the influence of technology on children's development.

Review

- What role do mass media play in the lives of children and adolescents?
- How do television and electronic media influence children's development?
- What roles do computers and the Internet play in children's development?

Connect

- In this section, you learned about cyberbullying. What else have you learned about the outcomes of bullying for those who are bullied?

Reflect Your Own Personal Journey of Life

- How much television and online media did you watch as a child? What effect do you believe this viewing has had on your development?

reach your **learning goals**

Culture and Diversity

Culture and Children's Development

 Discuss the role of culture in children's development.

The Relevance of Culture to the Study of Children

Cross-Cultural Comparisons

- Culture refers to the behavior patterns, beliefs, and all other products of a particular group of people that are passed on from generation to generation. If the study of children is to be a relevant discipline in the decades to come, increased attention must be paid to culture. In future years, children will be citizens of the world, and the more we understand the values of other cultures and others' cultural behaviors, the more effectively we will be able to interact.

- Cross-cultural comparisons contrast one culture with one or more other cultures, which provides information about the degree to which characteristics are universal or culture-specific. The social contexts in which children develop—gender, family, and school—display important differences from one culture to another. One analysis of cross-cultural comparisons suggests that children raised in individualistic cultures are taught different values and self-concepts from those raised in collectivistic cultures. However, critics argue that categorization of cultures as individualist or collectivist is too broad and simplistic, and that in many families, parents expect their children to think and act in ways that reflect both individualistic and collectivistic values.

Socioeconomic Status and Poverty

 Describe how socioeconomic status and poverty affect children's lives.

What Is Socioeconomic Status?

Socioeconomic Variations in Families, Neighborhoods, and Schools

Poverty

- Socioeconomic status (SES) is the grouping of people who share similar occupational, educational, and economic characteristics. SES implies inequalities.

- The families, neighborhoods, and schools of children have SES characteristics that are related to the child's development. Parents from low-SES families are more likely to value conformity and to use physical punishment to a greater extent than their middle-SES counterparts. High-SES children live in more attractive homes and in safer neighborhoods than low-SES children. Low-SES children are more apt to experience problems such as depression, low self-esteem, and delinquency. When low-SES children do well in school, it often is because parents have made sacrifices to improve conditions and provide support that contributes to school success.

- Poverty is defined by economic hardship. The poor often face not only economic hardship but also social and psychological difficulties. Poor children are exposed to more family violence, have less access to books and computers, attend inferior child care and schools, and receive less social support. When poverty is persistent and long-lasting, it has particularly adverse effects on children's development.

Ethnicity

 Explain how ethnicity is linked to children's development.

Immigration

Ethnicity and Socioeconomic Status

- Ethnicity is based on cultural heritage, nationality characteristics, race, religion, and language. The immigration of families to the United States and other countries brings about a number of challenges for helping children adapt to their new culture. Immigrant children often experience language barriers, changes in SES, and separation from support networks in addition to struggling to preserve their ethnic identity while adapting to the majority culture. Parents and children may be at different stages of acculturation, leading to intergenerational conflict.

- Too often researchers have not distinguished between the influences of ethnicity and socioeconomic status when studying ethnic minority children. Many ethnic minority children experience prejudice and discrimination, along with the difficulties caused by poverty. Although not all ethnic minority families are poor, poverty contributes to the stress of many ethnic minority families and to differences between ethnic minority groups and the White majority.

- Recognizing and respecting differences in ethnicity is an important aspect of getting along with others in a diverse, multicultural world. Too often differences have been described as deficits on the part of ethnic minority individuals. Ethnic minority groups are not homogeneous. Failure to recognize this diversity results in stereotyping.

- Prejudice is an unjustified negative attitude toward an individual because of the individual's membership in a group. Despite progress in the treatment of minority groups, children who are members of these groups often face prejudice and discrimination.

Technology

LG4 Summarize the influence of technology on children's development.

- In terms of exposure, a significant increase in media use and screen time has occurred especially among 11- to 14-year-olds. Adolescents are increasing the amount of time they spend in media multitasking. The social environment of adolescents has increasingly become digitally mediated.

- One negative aspect of television is that it involves passive learning. Watching violence on television is linked to higher levels of aggression in children. There also is concern about adolescents playing violent video games. Recently, researchers have found some positive influences of prosocial and exergame videos. Children's cognitive skills and abilities influence their TV viewing experiences. TV viewing is negatively related to children's mental ability and achievement. However, educational TV programming can enhance achievement.

- Today's children and adolescents are experiencing a technology revolution through the use of computers and other digital devices, the Internet, and sophisticated smartphones. The social environment of children and adolescents has increasingly become digitally mediated. The Internet continues to serve as the main focus of digitally mediated social interaction for adolescents but increasingly involves a variety of digital devices. Adolescents' online time can have positive or negative outcomes. Large numbers of adolescents engage in social networking. A special concern is the difficulty parents face in monitoring the information their children and teenagers are accessing.

key terms

collectivism 476	culture 475	individualism 476	socioeconomic status (SES) 478
cross-cultural studies 475	ethnicity 483	prejudice 487	

key people

Donald Campbell 475	Suniya Luthar 479	Catherine Tamis-LeMonda 477
Aletha Huston 481	Vonnie McLoyd 480	

glossary

A

accommodation   Piagetian concept of adjusting schemes to fit new information and experiences.

acculturation   Cultural changes that occur when one culture comes in contact with another culture.

active (niche-picking) genotype-environment correlations   Correlations that exist when children seek out environments they find compatible and stimulating.

adolescence   The developmental period of transition from childhood to early adulthood, entered at approximately 10 to 12 years of age and ending at 18 or 19 years of age.

adolescent egocentrism   The heightened self-consciousness of adolescents, which is reflected in adolescents' beliefs that others are as interested in them as they are in themselves, and in adolescents' sense of personal uniqueness and invulnerability.

adoption study   A study in which investigators seek to discover whether, in behavior and psychological characteristics, adopted children are more like their adoptive parents, who provided a home environment, or more like their biological parents, who contributed their heredity. Another form of the adoption study is one that compares adoptive and biological siblings.

affordances   Opportunities for interaction offered by objects that are necessary to perform activities.

afterbirth   The third stage of birth, when the placenta, umbilical cord, and other membranes are detached and expelled.

altruism   An unselfish interest in helping another person.

amnion   Prenatal life-support system that is a bag or envelope containing a clear fluid in which the developing embryo floats.

amygdala   The seat of emotions in the brain.

androgens   Hormones, the most important of which is testosterone, that promote the development of male genitals and secondary sex characteristics.

androgyny   The presence of masculine and feminine characteristics in the same person.

anger cry   A cry similar to the basic cry but with more excess air forced through the vocal cords.

animism   A facet of preoperational thought: the belief that inanimate objects have lifelike qualities and are capable of action.

A-not-B error   Also called AB error, this occurs when infants make the mistake of selecting the familiar hiding place (A) to locate an object, rather than looking in the new hiding place (B), as they progress into substage 4 in Piaget's sensorimotor stage.

Apgar Scale   A widely used method to assess the health of newborns at one and five minutes after birth. The Apgar Scale evaluates infants' heart rate, respiratory effort, muscle tone, body color, and reflex irritability.

aphasia   A disorder resulting from brain damage to Broca's area or Wernicke's area that involves a loss or impairment of the ability to use or comprehend words.

Asperger syndrome   A relatively mild autism spec-trum disorder in which the child has relatively good verbal skills, milder nonverbal language problems, and a restricted range of interests and relationships.

assimilation   Piagetian concept of the incorporation of new information into existing knowledge.

attachment   A close emotional bond between two people.

attention   Concentrating and focusing mental resources.

attention deficit hyperactivity disorder (ADHD)   A disability in which children consistently show one or more of the following characteristics: (1) inattention, (2) hyperactivity, and (3) impulsivity.

authoritarian parenting   A restrictive, punitive style in which the parent exhorts the child to follow the parent's directions and to respect their work and effort. Firm limits and controls are placed on the child, and little verbal exchange is allowed. This style is associated with children's social incompetence, including a lack of initiative and weak communication skills.

authoritative parenting   This style encourages children to be independent but still places limits and controls on their actions. Extensive verbal give-and-take is allowed, and parents are warm and nurturant toward the child. This style is associated with children's social competence, achievement orientation, and self-reliance.

autism spectrum disorders (ASDs)   Also called pervasive developmental disorders, they range from the severe disorder labeled autistic disorder to the milder disorder called Asperger syndrome. Children with these disorders are characterized by problems in social interaction, verbal and nonverbal communication, and repetitive behaviors.

autistic disorder   A severe developmental autism spectrum disorder that has its onset in the first three years of life and includes deficiencies in social relation-ships; abnormalities in communication; and restricted, repetitive, and stereotyped patterns of behavior.

automaticity   The ability to process information with little or no effort.

autonomous morality   The second stage of moral development in Piaget's theory, displayed by older children (about 10 years of age and older). The child becomes aware that rules and laws are created by people and that, in judging an action, one should consider the actor's intentions as well as the consequences.

average children   Children who receive an average number of both positive and negative nominations from their peers.

B

basic cry   A rhythmic pattern usually consisting of a cry, a briefer silence, a shorter inspiratory whistle that is higher pitched than the main cry, and then a brief rest before the next cry.

Bayley Scales of Infant Development   Initially created by Nancy Bayley, these scales are widely used in assessing infant development. The current version has five scales: cognitive, language, motor, socioemotional, and adaptive.

behavior genetics   The field that seeks to discover the influence of heredity and environment on individual differences in human traits and development.

bicultural identity   Identity formation that occurs when adolescents identify in some ways with their ethnic group and in other ways with the majority culture.

biological processes   Changes in an individual's body.

blastocyst   The inner layer of cells that develops during the germinal period. These cells later develop into the embryo.

bonding   The formation of a close connection, especially a physical bond, between parents and their newborn in the period shortly after birth.

brainstorming   A technique in which children are encouraged to come up with creative ideas in a group, play off one another's ideas, and say practically whatever comes to mind.

Brazelton Neonatal Behavioral Assessment Scale (NBAS)   A measure that is used in the first month of life to assess the newborn's neurological development, reflexes, and reactions to people and objects.

breech position The baby's position in the uterus that causes the buttocks to be the first part to emerge from the vagina.

Broca's area An area of the brain's left frontal lobe that is involved in speech production and grammatical processing.

Bronfenbrenner's ecological theory An environmental systems theory that focuses on five environmental systems: microsystem, mesosystem, exosystem, macrosystem, and chronosystem.

C

care perspective The moral perspective of Carol Gilligan, in which people are assessed in terms of their connectedness with others and the quality of their interpersonal communication, relationships with others, and concern for others.

case study An in-depth look at a single individual.

centration Focusing attention on one characteristic to the exclusion of all others.

cephalocaudal pattern The sequence in which the fastest growth occurs at the top of the body— the head—with physical growth in size, weight, and feature differentiation gradually working from top to bottom.

cesarean delivery Removal of the baby from the mother's uterus through an incision made in her abdomen.

character education A direct moral education approach that involves teaching students a basic "moral literacy" to prevent them from engaging in immoral behavior or doing harm to themselves or others.

child-centered kindergarten Education that involves the whole child by considering both the child's physical, cognitive, and socioemotional development and the child's needs, interests, and learning styles.

child-directed speech Language spoken in a higher pitch than normal, with simple words and sentences.

chromosomes Threadlike structures that come in 23 pairs, with one member of each pair coming from each parent. Chromosomes contain the genetic substance DNA.

cliques Small groups that range from 2 to about 12 individuals and average about 5 or 6 individuals. Cliques can form because of friendship or because individuals engage in similar activities, and members usually are of the same sex and about the same age.

cognitive moral education Education based on the belief that students should learn to value things like democracy and justice as their moral reasoning develops; Kohlberg's theory has been the basis for many of the cognitive moral education approaches.

cognitive processes Changes in an individual's thinking, intelligence, and language skills.

cohort effects Effects due to a person's time of birth, era, or generation but not to actual age.

collectivism Emphasizing values that serve the group by subordinating personal goals to preserve group integrity, interdependence of members, and harmonious relationships.

commitment Personal investment in identity.

concepts Cognitive groupings of similar objects, events, people, or ideas.

concrete operational stage Piaget's third stage, which lasts from approximately 7 to 11 years of age, when children can perform concrete operations, and logical reasoning replaces intuitive reasoning as long as the reasoning can be applied to specific or concrete examples.

conduct disorder Age-inappropriate actions and attitudes that violate family expectations, society's norms, and the personal or property rights of others.

connectedness Consists of two dimensions: mutuality, sensitivity to and respect for others' views; and permeability, openness to others' views.

conservation The realization that altering an object's or substance's appearance does not change its basic properties.

constructive play Play that combines sensorimotor/practice play with symbolic representation of ideas. Constructive play occurs when children engage in self-regulated creation or construction of a product or a solution.

constructivist approach A learner-centered approach that emphasizes the importance of individuals actively constructing their knowledge and understanding, with guidance from the teacher.

context The settings, influenced by historical, economic, social, and cultural factors, in which development occurs.

continuity-discontinuity issue Question about whether development involves gradual, cumulative change (continuity) or distinct stages (discontinuity).

controversial children Children who are frequently identified both as someone's best friend and as being disliked.

conventional reasoning The second, or intermediate, level in Kohlberg's theory of moral development. At this level, individuals abide by certain standards (internal), but they are the standards of others such as parents or the laws of society (external). The conventional level consists of two stages: mutual interpersonal expectations, relationships, and interpersonal conformity (stage 3) and social systems morality (stage 4).

convergent thinking Thinking that produces one correct answer; characteristic of the kind of thinking required on conventional intelligence tests.

coparenting Support parents provide for each other in jointly raising children.

core knowledge approach States that infants are born with domain-specific innate knowledge systems, such as those involving space, number sense, object permanence, and language.

corpus callosum Brain area where fibers connect the brain's left and right hemispheres.

correlational research Research in which the goal is to describe the strength of the relationship between two or more events or characteristics.

correlation coefficient A number based on statistical analysis that is used to describe the degree of association between two variables.

creativity The ability to think in novel and unusual ways and come up with unique solutions to problems.

crisis A period of identity development during which the adolescent is choosing among meaningful alternatives.

critical thinking Thinking reflectively and productively, and evaluating the evidence.

cross-cultural studies Comparisons of one culture with one or more other cultures. These provide information about the degree to which children's development is similar, or universal, across cultures, and the degree to which it is culture-specific.

cross-sectional approach A research strategy in which individuals of different ages are compared at the same point in time.

crowds The crowd is a larger group structure than a clique. Adolescents usually are members of a crowd based on reputation and may or may not spend much time together. Many crowds are defined by the activities in which adolescents engage.

culture The behavior patterns, beliefs, and all other products of a group that are passed on from generation to generation.

culture-fair tests Intelligence tests that aim to avoid cultural bias.

D

descriptive research Research that involves observing and recording behavior.

development The pattern of movement or change that begins at conception and continues through the life span.

developmental cascade model Involves connections across domains over time that influence developmental pathways and outcomes.

developmentally appropriate practice Education that focuses on the typical developmental patterns of children (age-appropriateness) and the uniqueness of each child (individual-appropriateness). Such practice contrasts with developmentally inappropriate practice, which relies on abstract paper-and-pencil activities presented to large groups of young children.

developmental quotient (DQ)   An overall developmental score that combines subscores on motor, language, adaptive, and personal-social domains in the Gesell assessment of infants.

dialect   A variety of language that is distinguished by its vocabulary, grammar, or pronunciation.

difficult child   A temperament style in which the child tends to react negatively and cry frequently, engages in irregular daily routines, and is slow to accept new experiences.

direct instruction approach   A teacher-centered approach characterized by teacher direction and control, mastery of academic material, high expectations for students' progress, and maximum time spent on learning tasks.

dishabituation   The recovery of a habituated response after a change in stimulation.

divergent thinking   Thinking that produces many answers to the same question; characteristic of creativity.

divided attention   Concentrating on more than one activity at the same time.

DNA   A complex molecule that contains genetic information.

doula   A caregiver who provides continuous physical, emotional, and educational support for the mother before, during, and after childbirth.

Down syndrome   A chromosomally transmitted form of intellectual disability, caused by the presence of an extra copy of chromosome 21.

dual-process model   States that decision making is influenced by two systems, one analytical and one experiential, that compete with each other. In this model, it is the experiential system—monitoring and managing actual experiences—that benefits adolescent decision making.

dynamic systems theory   A theory, proposed by Esther Thelen, that seeks to explain how motor behaviors are assembled for perceiving and acting.

dyscalculia   Also known as developmental arithmetic disorder; a learning disability that involves difficulty in math computation.

dysgraphia   A learning disability that involves difficulty in handwriting.

dyslexia   A category of learning disabilities involving a severe impairment in the ability to read and spell.

E

early childhood   The developmental period that extends from the end of infancy to about 5 or 6 years of age, sometimes called the preschool years.

early-later experience issue   Controversy regarding the degree to which early experiences (especially during infancy) or later experiences are the key determinants of children's development.

easy child   A temperament style in which the child is generally in a positive mood, quickly establishes regular routines, and adapts easily to new experiences.

eclectic theoretical orientation   An orientation that does not follow any one theoretical approach but instead selects the best aspects from each theory.

ecological view   The view, proposed by the Gibsons, that people directly perceive information in the world around them. Perception brings people in contact with the environment so that they can interact with and adapt to it.

egocentrism   An important feature of preoperational thought: the inability to distinguish between one's own and someone else's perspective.

embryonic period   The period of prenatal development that occurs from two to eight weeks after conception. During the embryonic period, the rate of cell differentiation intensifies, support systems for the cells form, and organs appear.

emotion   Feeling, or affect, that occurs when people are engaged in an interaction that is important to them, especially one that influences their well-being.

emotional and behavioral disorders   Serious, persistent problems that involve relationships, aggression, depression, fears associated with personal or school matters, as well as other inappropriate socioemotional characteristics.

emotional intelligence   The ability to perceive and express emotion accurately and adaptively, to understand emotion and emotional knowledge, to use feelings to facilitate thought, and to manage emotions in oneself and others.

empathy   Reacting to another's feelings with an emotional response that is similar to the other's feelings.

encoding   The mechanism by which information gets into memory.

epigenetic view   Theory that development is the result of an ongoing, bidirectional interchange between heredity and environment.

equilibration   A mechanism that Piaget proposed to explain how children shift from one stage of thought to the next. The shift occurs as children experience cognitive conflict, or disequilibrium, in trying to understand the world. Eventually, they resolve the conflict and reach a balance, or equilibrium, of thought.

Erikson's theory   Description of eight stages of human development. Each stage consists of a unique developmental task that confronts individuals with a crisis that must be resolved.

estradiol   An estrogen that is a key hormone in girls' pubertal development.

estrogens   Hormones, the most important of which is estradiol, that influence the development of female physical sex characteristics and help regulate the menstrual cycle.

ethnic gloss   Use of an ethnic label such as *African American* or *Latino* in a superficial way that portrays an ethnic group as being more homogeneous than it really is.

ethnic identity   An enduring aspect of the self that includes a sense of membership in an ethnic group, along with the attitudes and feelings related to that membership.

ethnicity   A characteristic based on cultural heritage, nationality, race, religion, and language.

ethology   Stresses that behavior is strongly influenced by biology, is tied to evolution, and is characterized by critical or sensitive periods.

evocative genotype-environment correlations   Correlations that exist when the child's genetically influenced characteristics elicit certain types of environments.

evolutionary psychology   Branch of psychology that emphasizes the importance of adaptation, reproduction, and "survival of the fittest" in shaping behavior.

executive attention   Involves planning actions, allocating attention to goals, detecting and compensating for errors, and monitoring progress on tasks while sometimes dealing with novel or difficult circumstances.

executive function   An umbrella-like concept that consists of a number of higher-level cognitive processes linked to the development of the brain's prefrontal cortex. Executive function involves managing one's thoughts to engage in goal-directed behavior and to exercise self-control.

expanding   Restating, in a linguistically sophisticated form, what a child has said.

experiment   A carefully regulated procedure in which one or more of the factors believed to influence the behavior being studied are manipulated while all other factors are held constant.

explicit memory   Conscious memory of facts and experiences.

extrinsic motivation   Response to external incentives such as rewards and punishments.

F

fast mapping   A process that helps to explain how young children learn the connection between a word and its referent so quickly.

fertilization   A stage in reproduction during which an egg and a sperm fuse to create a single cell, called a zygote.

fetal alcohol spectrum disorders (FASD)   A cluster of abnormalities and problems that appear in the offspring of mothers who drink alcohol heavily during pregnancy.

fetal period   The period from two months after conception until birth, lasting about seven months in typical pregnancies.

fine motor skills   Motor skills that involve more finely tuned movements, such as finger dexterity.

forgiveness An aspect of prosocial behavior that occurs when an injured person releases the injurer from possible behavioral retaliation.

formal operational stage Piaget's fourth and final stage, which occurs between the ages of 11 and 15, when individuals move beyond concrete experiences and think in more abstract and logical ways.

fragile X syndrome A genetic disorder involving an abnormality in the X chromosome, which becomes constricted and often breaks.

fuzzy trace theory States that memory is best understood by considering two types of memory representations: (1) verbatim memory trace; and (2) fuzzy trace, or gist. According to this theory, older children's better memory is attributed to the fuzzy traces created by extracting the gist of information.

G

games Activities engaged in for pleasure that include rules and often competition with one or more individuals.

gender The characteristics of people as males and females.

gender identity The sense of being male or female, which most children acquire by the time they are 3 years old.

gender role A set of expectations that prescribes how females or males should think, act, and feel.

gender schema theory According to this theory, gender typing emerges as children gradually develop schemas of what is gender-appropriate and gender-inappropriate in their culture.

gender stereotypes Broad categories that reflect impressions and widely held beliefs about what behavior is appropriate for females and males.

gender typing Acquisition of a traditional masculine or feminine role.

gene × environment (G × E) interaction The interaction of a specific, measured variation in the DNA and a specific, measured aspect of the environment.

genes Units of hereditary information composed of DNA. Genes help cells to reproduce themselves and manufacture the proteins that maintain life.

genotype A person's genetic heritage; the actual genetic material present in each cell.

germinal period The period of prenatal development that takes place in the first two weeks after conception. It includes the creation of the zygote, continued cell division, and the attachment of the zygote to the uterine wall.

gifted Possession of above-average intelligence (an IQ of 130 or higher) and/or superior talent for something.

goodness of fit The match between a child's temperament and the environmental demands the child must cope with.

grasping reflex A newborn's built-in reaction that occurs when something touches the infant's palms. The infant responds by grasping tightly.

gratitude A feeling of thankfulness and appreciation, especially in response to someone doing something kind or helpful.

gross motor skills Motor skills that involve large-muscle activities, such as moving one's arms and walking.

H

habituation Decreased responsiveness to a stimulus after repeated presentations of the stimulus.

helpless orientation An orientation in which one seems trapped by the experience of difficulty and attributes one's difficulty to a lack of ability.

heritability The fraction of the variance in a population that is attributed to genetics.

heteronomous morality The first stage of moral development in Piaget's theory, occurring from 4 to 7 years of age. Justice and rules are conceived of as unchangeable properties of the world, beyond the control of people.

hidden curriculum The pervasive moral atmosphere that characterizes each school.

horizontal décalage Piaget's concept that similar abilities do not appear at the same time within a stage of development.

hormones Powerful chemical substances secreted by the endocrine glands and carried through the body by the bloodstream.

hypotheses Specific assumptions and predictions that can be tested to determine their accuracy.

hypothetical-deductive reasoning Piaget's formal operational concept that adolescents have the cognitive ability to develop hypotheses about ways to solve problems and can systematically deduce which is the best path to follow in solving the problem.

I

identity Who a person is, representing a synthesis and integration of self-understanding.

identity achievement Marcia's term for the status of individuals who have undergone a crisis and made a commitment.

identity diffusion Marcia's term for the status of individuals who have not yet experienced a crisis (that is, they have not yet explored meaningful alternatives) or made any commitments.

identity foreclosure Marcia's term for the status of individuals who have made a commitment but have not experienced a crisis.

identity moratorium Marcia's term for the status of individuals who are in the midst of a crisis but whose commitments either are absent or are only vaguely defined.

identity versus identity confusion Erikson's fifth developmental stage, which individuals experience during the adolescent years. At this time, adolescents examine who they are, what they are all about, and where they are going in life.

imaginary audience The aspect of adolescent egocentrism that involves attention-getting behavior motivated by a desire to be noticed, visible, and "onstage."

immanent justice Piaget's concept of the childhood expectation that if a rule is broken, punishment will be meted out immediately.

implicit memory Memory without conscious recollection; memory of routine activities that are performed automatically.

inclusion Educating a child with special educational needs full-time in the regular classroom.

index offenses Criminal acts, such as robbery, rape, and homicide, whether they are committed by juveniles or adults.

individualism Giving priority to personal goals rather than to group goals; emphasizing values that serve the self, such as feeling good, striving for personal distinction and recognition for achievement, and asserting independence.

individuality Consists of two dimensions: self-assertion, the ability to have and communicate a point of view; and separateness, the use of communication patterns to express how one is different from others.

individualized education program (IEP) A written statement that spells out a program tailored to the needs of a child with a disability.

induction A discipline technique in which a parent uses reasoning and explains how the child's actions are likely to affect others.

indulgent parenting A style in which parents are highly involved with their children but place few demands or controls on them. This is associated with children's social incompetence, especially a lack of self-control and a lack of respect for others.

infancy The developmental period that extends from birth to about 18 to 24 months.

infinite generativity The ability to produce an endless number of meaningful sentences using a finite set of words and rules.

information-processing approach An approach that focuses on the ways children process information about their world—how they manipulate information, monitor it, and create strategies to deal with it.

information-processing theory Emphasizes that individuals manipulate information, monitor it, and strategize about it. Central to this theory are the processes of memory and thinking.

insecure avoidant babies   Babies who show insecurity by avoiding the mother.

insecure disorganized babies   Babies who show insecurity by being disorganized and disoriented.

insecure resistant babies   Babies who might cling to the caregiver, then resist her by fighting against the closeness, perhaps by kicking or pushing away.

intellectual disability   A condition of limited mental ability in which the individual (1) has a low IQ, usually below 70 on a traditional intelligence test; (2) has difficulty adapting to everyday life; and (3) has an onset of these characteristics by age 18.

intelligence   The ability to solve problems and to adapt to and learn from experiences.

intelligence quotient (IQ)   An individual's mental age divided by chronological age and multiplied by 100; devised in 1912 by William Stern.

intermodal perception   The ability to relate and integrate information about two or more sensory modalities, such as vision and hearing.

intimacy in friendship   Self-disclosure or the sharing of private thoughts.

intrinsic motivation   Internal motivational factors such as self-determination, curiosity, challenge, and effort.

intuitive thought substage   The second substage of preoperational thought, occurring between approximately 4 and 7 years of age, when children begin to use primitive reasoning.

J

joint attention   Individuals focusing on the same object or event; requires the ability to track another's behavior, one person directing another's attention, and reciprocal interaction.

justice perspective   A moral perspective that focuses on the rights of the individual; individuals independently make moral decisions.

juvenile delinquency   Refers to a great variety of behaviors by an adolescent, ranging from unacceptable behavior to breaking the law.

K

kangaroo care   Treatment for preterm infants that involves skin-to-skin contact.

Klinefelter syndrome   A chromosomal disorder in which males have an extra X chromosome, making them XXY instead of XY.

kwashiorkor   Severe malnutrition caused by a protein-deficient diet, causing the feet and abdomen to swell with water.

L

labeling   Identifying the names of objects.

laboratory   A controlled setting from which many of the complex factors of the "real world" have been removed.

language   A form of communication, whether spoken, written, or signed, that is based on a system of symbols.

language acquisition device (LAD)   Chomsky's term that describes a biological endowment enabling children to detect the features and rules of language, including phonology, syntax, and semantics.

lateralization   Specialization of function in one hemisphere of the cerebral cortex or the other.

learning disabilities   Disabilities involving understanding or using spoken or written language. The difficulty can appear in listening, thinking, reading, writing, spelling, or mathematics. To be classified as a learning disability, the problem must not be primarily the result of visual, hearing, or motor disabilities; intellectual disability; emotional disorders; or environmental, cultural, or economic disadvantage.

least restrictive environment (LRE)   The concept that a child with a disability must be educated in a setting that is similar to classrooms in which children without a disability are educated.

longitudinal approach   A research strategy in which the same individuals are studied over a period of time, usually several years.

long-term memory   A relatively permanent and long-lasting type of memory.

love withdrawal   A discipline technique in which a parent withholds attention or love from the child in an effort to control the child's behavior.

low birth weight infant   Infant that weighs less than 5½ pounds at birth.

M

marasmus   Severe malnutrition caused by an insufficient protein-calorie intake, resulting in a shrunken, elderly appearance.

mastery motivation   An approach to achievement in which one is task oriented, focusing on learning strategies and the achievement process rather than ability or the outcome.

meiosis   A specialized form of cell division that forms eggs and sperm (also known as gametes).

memory   Retention of information over time.

menarche   A girl's first menstruation.

mental age (MA)   An individual's level of mental development relative to others.

metacognition   Cognition about cognition, or "knowing about knowing."

metalinguistic awareness   Knowledge about language.

metamemory   Knowledge about memory.

metaphor   An implied comparison between two unlike things.

middle and late childhood   The developmental period that extends from about 6 to 11 years of age, sometimes called the elementary school years.

millennials   The generation born after 1980, the first to come of age and enter emerging adulthood in the new millennium.

mindfulness   Being alert, mentally present, and cognitively flexible while going through life's everyday activities and tasks.

mindset   Dweck's concept referring to the cognitive view individuals develop for themselves; individuals have either a fixed or growth mindset.

mitosis   Cellular reproduction in which the cell's nucleus duplicates itself with two new cells being formed, each containing the same DNA as the parent cell, arranged in the same 23 pairs of chromosomes.

Montessori approach   An educational philosophy in which children are given considerable freedom and spontaneity in choosing activities and are allowed to move from one activity to another as they desire.

moral development   Changes in thoughts, feelings, and behaviors regarding standards of right and wrong.

moral exemplars   People who have lived extraordinary lives, having developed their personality, identity, character, and virtue to a level that reflects moral excellence and commitment.

moral identity   The aspect of personality that is present when individuals have moral notions and commitments that are central to their lives.

Moro reflex   A newborn's startle response that occurs in reaction to a sudden, intense noise or movement. When startled, the newborn arches its back, throws its head back, and flings out its arms and legs. Then the newborn rapidly closes its arms and legs to the center of the body.

morphology   The rule system that governs how words are formed in a language.

multiple developmental trajectories   Concept that adults follow one trajectory and children and adolescents another one; understanding how these trajectories mesh is important.

myelination   The process of encasing axons with a myelin sheath that increases the speed of processing information.

N

natural childbirth   This method attempts to reduce the mother's pain by decreasing her fear through education about childbirth and relaxation techniques during delivery.

naturalistic observation   Behavioral observation that takes place in real-world settings.

nature-nurture issue   Debate about whether development is primarily influenced by nature or nurture. The "nature" proponents claim biological inheritance is the most important influence on development; the "nurture" proponents claim that environmental experiences are the most influential factors.

neglected children   Children who are infrequently identified as a best friend but are not disliked by their peers.

neglectful parenting   A style in which the parent is very uninvolved in the child's life. It is associated with children's social incompetence, especially a lack of self-control and poor self-esteem.

Neonatal Intensive Care Unit Network Neurobehavioral Scale (NNNS)   Based on the NBAS, the NNNS provides an assessment of the "at-risk" newborn's behavior, neurological and stress responses, and regulatory capacities.

neo-Piagetians   Developmentalists who have elaborated on Piaget's theory, believing that children's cognitive development is more specific in many respects than Piaget thought and giving more emphasis to how children use memory, attention, and strategies to process information.

neuroconstructivist view   Theory of brain development emphasizing the following points: (a) biological processes and environmental conditions influence the brain's development, (b) the brain has plasticity and is context dependent, and (c) the development of the brain and the child's cognitive development are closely linked.

neurons   Nerve cells, which handle information processing at the cellular level in the brain.

nonshared environmental experiences   The child's own unique experiences, both within the family and outside the family, that are not shared by another sibling.

normal distribution   A symmetrical distribution with a majority of the cases falling in the middle of the possible range of scores and few scores appearing toward the extremes of the range.

O

object permanence   The Piagetian term for one of an infant's most important accomplishments: understanding that objects and events continue to exist even when they cannot directly be seen, heard, or touched.

operations   Internalized actions that allow children to do mentally what before they had done only physically. Operations also are reversible mental actions.

organization   Piaget's concept of grouping isolated behaviors into a higher-order, more smoothly functioning cognitive system; the grouping or arranging of items into categories.

organogenesis   Organ formation that takes place during the first two months of prenatal development.

P

pain cry   A sudden appearance of loud crying without preliminary moaning, and a long initial cry followed by an extended period of breath holding.

passive genotype-environment correlations   Correlations that exist when the natural parents, who are genetically related to the child, provide a rearing environment for the child.

peers   Children who share the same age or maturity level.

perception   The interpretation of sensation.

performance orientation   An orientation in which one focuses on winning rather than achievement outcomes, and happiness is thought to result from winning.

personal fable   The part of adolescent egocentrism that involves an adolescent's sense of uniqueness and invincibility.

perspective taking   The social cognitive process involved in assuming the perspective of others and understanding their thoughts and feelings.

phenotype   The way an individual's genotype is expressed in observed and measurable characteristics.

phenylketonuria (PKU)   A genetic disorder in which an individual cannot properly metabolize an amino acid. PKU is now easily detected but, if left untreated, results in intellectual disability and hyperactivity.

phonics approach   An educational approach emphasizing that reading instruction should focus on teaching the basic rules for translating written symbols into sounds.

phonology   The sound system of a language, which includes the sounds used and rules about how they may be combined.

Piaget's theory   Theory stating that children actively construct their understanding of the world and go through four stages of cognitive development: sensorimotor, preoperational, concrete operational, and formal operational.

placenta   A life-support system that consists of a disk-shaped group of tissues in which small blood vessels from the mother and offspring intertwine.

play   A pleasurable activity that is engaged in for its own sake.

play therapy   Therapy that allows the child to work off frustrations and is a medium through which the therapist can analyze the child's conflicts and ways of coping with them. Children may feel less threatened and be more likely to express their true feelings in the context of play.

popular children   Children who are frequently identified as a best friend and are rarely disliked by their peers.

possible self   What an individual might become, would like to become, and is afraid of becoming.

postconventional reasoning   The third and highest level in Kohlberg's theory of moral development. At this level, morality is more internal. The postconventional level consists of two stages: social contract or utility and individual rights (stage 5) and universal ethical principles (stage 6).

postpartum depression   Characteristic of women who have such strong feelings of sadness, anxiety, or despair that they have trouble coping with daily tasks during the postpartum period.

postpartum period   The period after childbirth when the mother adjusts, both physically and psychologically, to the process of childbirth. This period lasts about six weeks or until her body has completed its adjustment and returned to a near prepregnant state.

power assertion   A discipline technique in which a parent attempts to gain control over the child or the child's resources.

practice play   Play that involves repetition of behavior when new skills are being learned or when physical or mental mastery and coordination of skills are required for games or sports. Practice play can be engaged in throughout life.

pragmatics   The appropriate use of language in different contexts.

precocious puberty   Very early onset and rapid progression of puberty.

preconventional reasoning   The lowest level in Kohlberg's theory. At this level, morality is often focused on reward and punishment. The two stages in preconventional reasoning are punishment and obedience orientation (stage 1) and individualism, instrumental purpose, and exchange (stage 2).

prefrontal cortex   The highest level of the frontal lobes that is involved in reasoning, decision making, and self-control.

prejudice   An unjustified negative attitude toward an individual because of her or his membership in a group.

prenatal period   The time from conception to birth.

preoperational stage   The second Piagetian developmental stage, which lasts from about 2 to 7 years of age, when children begin to represent the world with words, images, and drawings.

prepared childbirth   Developed by French obstetrician Ferdinand Lamaze, this childbirth strategy is similar to natural childbirth but includes a special breathing technique to control pushing in the final stages of labor and a more detailed anatomy and physiology course.

pretense/symbolic play   Play that occurs when a child transforms the physical environment into a symbol.

preterm infants   Those born before the completion of 37 weeks of gestation (the time between fertilization and birth).

primary emotions Emotions that are present in humans and other animals, and emerge early in life; examples are joy, anger, sadness, fear, and disgust.

Project Head Start Compensatory education designed to provide children from low-income families the opportunity to acquire the skills and experiences important for school success.

proximodistal pattern The sequence in which growth starts at the center of the body and moves toward the extremities.

psychoanalytic theories Theories that describe development as primarily unconscious and heavily colored by emotion. Behavior is merely a surface characteristic, and the symbolic workings of the mind have to be analyzed to understand behavior. Early experiences with parents are emphasized.

psychosocial moratorium Erikson's term for the gap between childhood security and adult autonomy that adolescents experience as part of their identity exploration.

puberty A period of rapid physical maturation involving hormonal and bodily changes that take place primarily in early adolescence.

R

rapport talk The language of conversation and a way of establishing connections and negotiating relationships; more characteristic of females than of males.

recasting Rephrasing a statement that a child has said, perhaps turning it into a question, or restating a child's immature utterance in the form of a fully grammatical utterance.

reciprocal socialization The bidirectional process by which children socialize parents just as parents socialize them.

reflexes Built-in automatic reactions to stimuli.

reflexive smile A smile that does not occur in response to external stimuli. It happens during the month after birth, usually during sleep.

rejected children Children who are infrequently identified as a best friend and are actively disliked by their peers.

religion An organized set of beliefs, practices, rituals, and symbols that increases an individual's connection to a sacred or transcendent other (God, higher power, or higher truth).

religiousness The degree of affiliation with an organized religion, participation in prescribed rituals and practices, connection with its beliefs, and involvement in a community of believers.

report talk Talk that conveys information; more characteristic of males than females.

rooting reflex A newborn's built-in reaction that occurs when the infant's cheek is stroked or the side of the mouth is touched. In response, the infant turns its head toward the side that was touched, in an apparent effort to find something to suck.

S

satire The use of irony, derision, or wit to expose folly or wickedness.

scaffolding In cognitive development, Vygotsky used this term to describe the practice of changing the level of support provided over the course of a teaching session, with the more-skilled person adjusting guidance to fit the child's current performance level.

schemas Mental frameworks that organize concepts and information.

schema theory States that when people reconstruct information, they fit it into information that already exists in their minds.

schemes In Piaget's theory, actions or mental representations that organize knowledge.

scientific method An approach that can be used to obtain accurate information by carrying out four steps: (1) conceptualize the problem, (2) collect data, (3) draw conclusions, and (4) revise research conclusions and theory.

securely attached babies Babies who use the caregiver as a secure base from which to explore the environment.

selective attention Focusing on a specific aspect of experience that is relevant while ignoring others that are irrelevant.

self All of the characteristics of a person.

self-concept Domain-specific self-evaluations.

self-conscious emotions Emotions that require self-awareness, especially consciousness and a sense of "me"; examples include jealousy, empathy, and embarrassment.

self-efficacy The belief that one can master a situation and produce favorable outcomes.

self-esteem The global evaluative dimension of the self; also called self-worth or self-image.

self-understanding A child's cognitive representation of the self—the substance and content of a child's self-conceptions.

semantics The meaning of words and sentences.

sensation Reaction that occurs when information contacts sensory receptors—the eyes, ears, tongue, nostrils, and skin.

sensorimotor play Behavior that allows infants to derive pleasure from exercising their existing sensorimotor schemes.

sensorimotor stage The first of Piaget's stages, which lasts from birth to about 2 years of age, when infants construct an understanding of the world by coordinating sensory experiences (such as seeing and hearing) with motoric actions.

separation protest Occurs when infants experience a fear of being separated from a caregiver, which results in crying when the caregiver leaves.

seriation The concrete operation that involves ordering stimuli along a quantitative dimension (such as length).

service learning A form of education that promotes social responsibility and service to the community.

shape constancy Recognition that an object remains the same even though its orientation to the viewer changes.

shared environmental experiences Siblings' common environmental experiences, such as their parents' personalities and intellectual orientation, the family's socioeconomic status, and the neighborhood in which they live.

short-term memory Limited-capacity memory system in which information is usually retained for up to 30 seconds if there is no rehearsal of the information. Using rehearsal, individuals can keep the information in short-term memory longer.

sickle-cell anemia A genetic disorder that affects the red blood cells and occurs most often in people of African descent.

size constancy Recognition that an object remains the same even though the retinal image of the object changes.

slow-to-warm-up child A temperament style in which the child has a low activity level, is somewhat negative, and displays a low intensity of mood.

small for date infants Also called small for gestational age infants, these infants have birth weights that are below normal when the length of pregnancy is considered. Small for date infants may be preterm or full term.

social cognition The processes involved in understanding the world around us, especially how we think and reason about other people.

social-cognitive domain theory Theory stating that there are different domains of social knowledge and reasoning, including moral, social conventional, and personal domains. These domains arise from children's and adolescents' attempts to understand and deal with different forms of social experience.

social cognitive theory The view of psychologists who emphasize behavior, environment, and cognition as the key factors in development.

social cognitive theory of gender This theory emphasizes that children's gender development occurs through observation and imitation of gender behavior, and through rewards and punishments they experience for gender-appropriate and gender-inappropriate behavior.

social cognitive theory of morality The theory that distinguishes between moral competence—the ability to produce moral behaviors—and moral performance—use of those behaviors in specific situations.

social constructivist approach An emphasis on the social contexts of learning and the construction of knowledge through social interaction. Vygotsky's theory reflects this approach.

social conventional reasoning Focuses on conventional rules established by social consensus, as opposed to moral reasoning that stresses ethical issues.

social play Play that involves interactions with peers.

social policy A government's course of action designed to promote the welfare of its citizens.

social referencing "Reading" emotional cues in others to help determine how to act in a particular situation.

social role theory A theory stating that gender differences result from the contrasting roles of women and men—social hierarchy and division of labor strongly influence gender differences in power, assertiveness, and nurture.

social smile A smile in response to an external stimulus, which, early in development, typically is a face.

socioeconomic status (SES) A grouping of people with similar occupational, educational, and economic characteristics.

socioeconomic status (SES) Categorization based on a person's occupational, educational, and economic characteristics.

socioemotional processes Changes in an individual's interpersonal relationships, emotions, and personality.

spirituality Experiencing something beyond oneself in a transcendent manner and living in a way that benefits others and society.

standardized test A test with uniform procedures for administration and scoring. Many standardized tests allow a person's performance to be compared with the performance of other individuals.

status offenses Juvenile offenses, performed by youth under a specified age, that are not as serious as index offenses. These offenses may include acts such as underage drinking, truancy, and sexual promiscuity.

stereotype threat Anxiety that one's behavior might confirm a stereotype about one's group.

stranger anxiety An infant's fear of and wariness toward strangers; it tends to appear in the second half of the first year of life.

Strange Situation Ainsworth's observational measure of infant attachment to a caregiver, which requires the infant to move through a series of introductions, separations, and reunions with the caregiver and an adult stranger in a prescribed order.

strategy construction Creation of new procedures for processing information.

sucking reflex A newborn's built-in reaction of automatically sucking an object placed in its mouth. The sucking reflex enables the infant to get nourishment before it has associated a nipple with food.

sudden infant death syndrome (SIDS) A condition that occurs when an infant stops breathing, usually during the night, and suddenly dies without an apparent cause.

sustained attention Maintaining attention to a selected stimulus for a prolonged period of time. Sustained attention is also called *focused attention* and *vigilance.*

symbolic function substage The first substage of preoperational thought, occurring roughly between the ages of 2 and 4. In this substage, the young child gains the ability to represent mentally an object that is not present.

syntax The ways words are combined to form acceptable phrases and sentences.

T

telegraphic speech The use of short, precise words without grammatical markers such as articles, auxiliary verbs, and other connectives.

temperament Involves individual differences in behavioral styles, emotions, and characteristic ways of responding.

teratogen From the Greek word *tera,* meaning "monster," this term refers to any agent that causes a birth defect. Teratology is the field of study that investigates the causes of birth defects.

testosterone An androgen that is a key hormone in boys' pubertal development.

theory An interrelated, coherent set of ideas that helps to explain and make predictions.

theory of mind Awareness of one's own mental processes and the mental processes of others.

thinking Transforming and manipulating information in memory. Individuals think in order to reason, reflect, evaluate ideas, solve problems, and make decisions.

top-dog phenomenon The circumstance of moving from the top position in elementary school to the lowest position in middle or junior high school.

transitivity Principle that says if a relation holds between a first object and a second object, and holds between the second object and a third object, then it holds between the first object and the third object. Piaget argued that an understanding of transitivity is characteristic of concrete operational thought.

triarchic theory of intelligence Sternberg's theory that intelligence comes in three forms: analytical, creative, and practical.

trophoblast The outer layer of cells that develops in the germinal period. These cells provide nutrition and support for the embryo.

Turner syndrome A chromosomal disorder in females in which either an X chromosome is missing, making the person XO instead of XX, or the second X chromosome is partially deleted.

twin study A study in which the behavioral similarity of identical twins is compared with the behavioral similarity of fraternal twins.

U

umbilical cord A life-support system that contains two arteries and one vein and connects the baby to the placenta.

V

visual preference method A method developed by Fantz to determine whether infants can distinguish one stimulus from another by measuring the length of time they attend to different stimuli.

Vygotsky's theory A sociocultural cognitive theory that emphasizes how culture and social interaction guide cognitive development.

W

Wernicke's area An area of the brain's left hemisphere that is involved in language comprehension.

whole-language approach An educational approach stressing that reading instruction should parallel children's natural language learning. Reading materials should be whole and meaningful.

working memory A mental "workbench" where individuals actively use memory to manipulate and assemble information when making decisions, solving problems, and comprehending written and spoken language.

X

XYY syndrome A chromosomal disorder in which males have an extra Y chromosome.

Z

zone of proximal development (ZPD) Vygotsky's term for tasks that are too difficult for children to master alone but can be mastered with assistance from adults or more-skilled children.

zygote A single cell formed through fertilization.

references

A

Aagaard, J. (2019). Multitasking as distraction: A conceptual analysis of media multitasking. *Theory and Psychology, 29*(1), 87–99.

ABC News. (2005, December 12). Larry Page and Sergey Brin. Retrieved September 16, 2007, from http://abcnews.go.com?Entertainment/12/8/05

Abela, A., & Walker, J. (2013). Global changes in marriage, parenting and family life. In A. Abela & J. Walker (Eds.). *Contemporary issues in family studies: Global perspectives on partnerships, parenting and support in a changing world.* Oxford UK: John Wiley & Sons.

Ablow, J.C. (2013). When parents conflict or disengage: Children's perception of parents' marital distress predicts school adaptation. In P. A. Cowan & others (Eds.), *The family context of parenting in children's adaptation to elementary school.* New York: Routledge.

Abreu-Villaça, Y., & others (2018). Hyperactivity and memory/learning deficits evoked by developmental exposure to nicotine and/or ethanol are mitigated by cAMP and cGMP signaling cascades activation. *Neurotoxicology, 66,* 150–159.

Acharya, S., Bhatta, D.N., & Assannangkornchai, S. (2018). Post-traumatic stress disorder symptoms among children of Kathmandu 1 year after the 2015 earthquake in Nepal. *Disaster Medicine and Public Health Preparedness, 12,* 486–492.

Ackerman, J.P., Riggins, T., & Black, M.M. (2010). A review of the effects of prenatal cocaine exposure among school-aged children. *Pediatrics, 125,* 554–565.

Adachi, P.J., & Willoughby, T. (2013). Do video games promote positive youth development? *Journal of Adolescent Research, 28*(2), 155–165.

Adachi, P.J., & Willoughby, T. (2017). The link between playing video games and positive youth outcomes. *Child Development Perspectives, 11*(3), 202–206.

Adamson, L., & Frick, J. (2003). The still face: A history of a shared experimental paradigm. *Infancy, 4,* 451–473.

Addabbo, M., Longhi, E., Marchis, I.C., Tagliabue, P., & Turati, C. (2018). Dynamic facial expressions of emotions are discriminated at birth. *PloS One, 13*(3), e0193868.

Adelson, S.L., Stroeh, O.M., & Ng, Y.K.W. (2016). Development and mental health of lesbian, gay, bisexual, or transgender youth in pediatric practice. *Pediatric Clinics, 63,* 971–983.

Adger, C.T., Snow, C.E., & Christian, D. (2018). *What teachers need to know about language.* Bristol, UK: Multilingual Matters.

Adisetiyo, V., & Gray, K.M. (2017). Neuroimaging the neural correlates of increased risk for substance use disorders in attention-deficit/hyperactivity disorder: A systematic review. *The American Journal on Addictions, 26,* 99–111.

Administration for Children and Families (2019). Head Start program facts fiscal year 2018. Retrieved from https://eclkc.ohs.acf.hhs.gov/about-us/article/head-start-program-facts-fiscal-year-2018

Adolph, K.E., & Berger, S.E. (2013). Development of the motor system. In H. Pashler, T. Crane, M. Kinsbourne, F. Ferreira, & R. Zemel (Eds.), *Encyclopedia of the mind.* Thousand Oaks, CA: Sage.

Adolph, K.E., & others (2012). How do you learn to walk? Thousands of steps and dozens of falls per day. *Psychological Science, 23*(11), 1387–1394.

Adolph, K.E., Karasik, L.B., & Tamis-LeMonda, C.S. (2010). Moving between cultures: Cross-cultural research on motor development. In M. Bornstein (Ed.), *Handbook of cross-cultural developmental science, Vol. 1: Domains of development across cultures.* New York: Psychology Press.

Adolph, K.E., & Kretch, K.S. (2012). Infants on the edge: Beyond the visual cliff. In A. Slater & P. Quinn (Eds.), *Developmental psychology: Revisiting the classic studies.* Thousand Oaks, CA: Sage.

Adolph, K.E., Vereijken, B., & Shrout, P.E. (2003). What changes in infant walking and why. *Child Development, 74,* 475–497.

Adolph, K.E. (1997). Learning in the development of infant locomotion. *Monographs of the Society for Research in Child Development, 62* (3, Serial No. 251).

Adolph, K.E., & Franchak, J.M. (2017). The development of motor behavior. *Wiley Interdisciplinary Reviews: Cognitive Science, 8*(1–2), e1430.

Adolph, K.E., & Hoch, J.E. (2018). Motor development: Embodied, embedded, encultured, and enabling. *Annual Review of Psychology, 70,* 26.1–26.24.

Adolph, K.E., Hoch, J.E., & Cole, W.G. (2018). Development (of walking): 15 suggestions. *Trends in Cognitive Sciences, 22*(8), 699–711.

Agency for Healthcare Research and Quality. (2007). *Evidence report/Technology assessment Number 153: Breastfeeding and maternal and health outcomes in developed countries.* Rockville, MD: U.S. Department of Health and Human Services.

Agostini, A., Carskadon, M.A., Dorrian, J., Coussens, S., & Short, M.A. (2017). An experimental study of adolescent sleep restriction during a simulated school week: Changes in phase, sleep staging, performance and sleepiness. *Journal of Sleep Research, 26,* 227–235.

Agostini, A., Lushington, K., & Dorrian, J. (2019). The relationships between bullying, sleep, and health in a large adolescent sample. *Sleep and Biological Rhythms, 17*(2), 173–182.

Agras, W.S., Hammer, L.D., McNicholas, F., & Kraemer, H.C. (2004). Risk factors for childhood overweight: A prospective study from birth to 9.5 years. *Journal of Pediatrics, 145,* 20–25.

Ahmed, M., Mirambo, M.M., Mushi, M.F., Hokororo, A., & Mshana, S.E. (2017). Bacteremia caused by multidrug-resistant bacteria among hospitalized malnourished children in Mwanza, Tanzania: A cross sectional study. *BMC Research Notes, 10*(1), 62.

Ahring, K.K., & others (2018). Comparison of glycomacropeptide with phenylalanine free-synthetic amino acids in test meals to PKU patients: No significant differences in biomarkers, including plasma Phe levels. *Journal of Nutrition and Metabolism,* 2018. Retrieved from https://doi.org/10.1155/2018/6352919

Ainsworth, M.D.S. (1979). Infant-mother attachment. *American Psychologist, 34,* 932–937.

Akhtar, N., & Herold, K. (2017). Pragmatic development. Reference module in *Neuroscience and Biobehavioral Psychology.* doi:10.1016/B978-0-12-809324-5.05868-5

Alampay, L.P., & others (2017). Severity and justness do not moderate the relation between corporal punishment and negative child outcomes: A multicultural and longitudinal study. *International Journal of Behavioral Development, 41*(4), 491–502.

Albarello, F., Crocetti, E., & Rubini, M. (2018). I and us: A longitudinal study on the interplay of personal and social identity in adolescence. *Journal of Youth and Adolescence, 47*(4), 689–702.

Alderman, E.M., & Johnston, B.D. (2018). The teen driver. *Pediatrics, 142*(4), e20182163.

Alemi, R., Batouli, S.A.H., Behzad, E., Ebrahimpoor, M., & Oghabian, M.A. (2018). Not single brain areas but a network is involved in language: Applications in presurgical planning. *Clinical Neurology and Neurosurgery, 165,* 116–128.

Allen, J.P., & Miga, E.M. (2010). Attachment in adolescence: A move to the level of emotion regulation. *Journal of Social and Personal Relationships, 27,* 181–190.

Allen, J.P., Grande, L., Tan, J., & Loeb, E. (2018). Parent and peer predictors of change in attachment security from adolescence to adulthood. *Child Development, 89*(4), 1120–1132.

Allen, K., Kern, M.L., Vella-Brodrick, D., Hattie, J., & Waters, L. (2018). What schools need to know about fostering school belonging: A meta-analysis. *Educational Psychology Review, 30,* 1–34.

Alquraini, T.A., & Rao, S.M. (2019, in press). Developing and sustaining readers with intellectual and multiple disabilities: A systematic review of literature. *International Journal of Developmental Disabilities.*

Altman, C., Goldstein, T., & Armon-Lotem, S. (2018). Vocabulary, metalinguistic awareness and language dominance among bilingual preschool children. *Frontiers in Psychology,* doi:10.3389/fpsyg.2018.01953

Alvarez, O., & others (2012). Effect of hydroxyurea on renal function parameters: Results from the multi-center placebo controlled Baby Hug clinical trial for infants with sickle cell anemia. *Pediatric Blood and Cancer, 59*(4), 668-674.

Amato, P.R., & Booth, A. (1996). A prospective study of divorce and parent-child relationships. *Journal of Marriage and the Family, 58,* 356-365.

Amato, P.R., & Dorius, C. (2010). Fathers, children, and divorce. In M. E. Lamb (Ed.), *The role of the father in child development* (5th ed.). New York: Wiley.

Amato, P.R. (2006). Marital discord, divorce, and children's well-being: Results from a 20-year longitudinal study of two generations. In A. Clarke-Stewart & J. Dunn (Eds.), *Families count.* New York: Cambridge University Press.

Amato, P.R., & Patterson, S.E. (2017). The intergenerational transmission of union instability in early adulthood. *Family Relations, 79,* 723-738.

American Academy of Pediatrics (2013). The crucial role of recess in school. *Pediatrics, 131*(1), 183-188.

American Academy of Pediatrics (2016). Media and young minds. *Pediatrics, 138*(5), e20162591.

American Pregnancy Association (2018). *Mercury levels in fish.* Retrieved November 23, 2018, from www. americanpregnancy.org/pregnancy-health/mercury-levels-in-fish/

American Psychological Association. (2003). *Psychology: Scientific problem solvers.* Washington, DC: Author.

Amso, D., & Johnson, S.P. (2010). Building object knowledge form perceptual input. In B. Hood & L. Santos (Eds.), *The origins of object knowledge.* New York: Oxford University Press.

Amsterdam, B.K. (1968). *Mirror behavior in children under two years of age.* Unpublished doctoral dissertation, University of North Carolina, Chapel Hill.

Anderson, A.J., & Perone, S. (2018). Developmental change in the resting state electroencephalogram: Insights into cognition and the brain. *Brain and Cognition, 126,* 40-52.

Anderson, C.A., & others (2017). Screen violence and youth behavior. *Pediatrics, 140*(Suppl. 2), S142-S147.

Anderson, D.R., Huston, A.C., Schmitt, K., Linebarger, D.L., & Wright, J.C. (2001). Early childhood viewing and adolescent behavior: The recontact study. *Monographs of the Society for Research in Child Development, 66*(1), Serial No. 264.

Anderson, D.R., Lorch, E.P., Field, D.E., Collins, P.A., & Nathan, J.G. (1985, April). *Television viewing at home: Age trends in visual attention and time with TV.* Paper presented at the biennial meeting of the Society of Research in Child Development, Toronto.

Anderson, D.R., & Subrahmanyam, K. (2017). Digital screen media and cognitive development. *Pediatrics, 140*(Suppl. 2), S57-S61.

Anderson, E.R., & Greene, S.M. (2011). "My child and I are a package deal": Balancing adult and child concerns in repartnering after divorce. *Journal of Family Psychology, 25,* 741-750.

Anderson, E., Greene, S.M., Hetherington, E.M., & Clingempeel, W.G. (1999). The dynamics of parental remarriage. In E. M. Hetherington (Ed.), *Coping with divorce, single parenting, and remarriage.* Mahwah, NJ: Erlbaum.

Anderson, E.M., Hespos, S.J., & Rips, L.J. (2018). Five-month-old infants have expectations for the accumulation of nonsolid substances. *Cognition, 175,* 1-10.

Anderson, R.C., & others (2019). Student agency at the crux: Mitigating disengagement in middle and high school. *Contemporary Educational Psychology, 56,* 205-217.

Andersson, H., & Bergman, L.R. (2011). The role of task persistence in young adolescence for successful educational and occupational attainment in middle adulthood. *Developmental Psychology, 47,* 950-960.

Andrews, N.C., Hanish, L.D., Updegraff, K.A., DeLay, D., & Martin, C.L. (2019). Dyadic peer interactions: The impact of aggression on impression formation with new peers. *Journal of Abnormal Child Psychology, 47*(5), 839-850.

Anspaugh, D., & Ezell, G. (2013). *Teaching today's health* (10th ed.). Upper Saddle River, NJ: Pearson.

Antoñanzas, J.L., & Lorente, R. (2017). Study of learning strategies and cognitive capacities in hearing and non-hearing pupils. *Procedia-Social and Behavioral Sciences, 237,* 1196-1200.

Antonopoulos, C., & others (2011). Maternal smoking during pregnancy and childhood lymphoma: A meta-analysis. *International Journal of Cancer, 129,* 2694-2703.

Antonucci, T.C., Birditt, K., & Ajrouch, K. (2013). Social relationships and aging. In I. B. Weiner & others (Eds.), *Handbook of psychology* (2nd ed., Vol. 6). New York: Wiley.

Apperley, L., & others (2018). Mode of clinical presentation and delayed diagnosis of Turner syndrome: A single centre UK study. *International Journal of Pediatric Endocrinology, 4.*

Arbib, M.A. (2017). Toward the language-ready brain: Biological evolution and primate comparisons. *Psychonomic Bulletin & Review, 24,* 142-150.

Arck, P.C., Schepanski, S., Buss, C., & Hanganu-Opatz, I. (2018). Prenatal immune and endocrine modulators of offspring's brain development and cognitive functions later in life. *Frontiers in Immunology, 9,* 2186.

Ariel, S. (2019). *Integrative play therapy with individuals, families, and groups.* London: Routledge.

Arnett, J.J. (2015). Identity development from adolescence to emerging adulthood: What we know and (especially) don't know. In K. McLean & M. Syed (Eds.), *The Oxford handbook of identity development* (pp. 53-64). New York: Oxford University Press.

Arnold, M.E. (2017). Supporting adolescent exploration and commitment: Identity formation, thriving, and positive youth development. *Journal of Youth Development, 12*(4), 1-15.

Aronson, E. (1986, August). *Teaching students things they think they already know about: The case of prejudice and desegregation.* Paper presented at the meeting of the American Psychological Association, Washington, DC.

Arseth, A., Kroger, J., Martinussen, M., & Marcia, J.E. (2009). Meta-analytic studies of identity status and the relational issues of attachment and intimacy. *Identity, 9,* 1-32.

Arterberry, M.E., & Kellman, P.J. (2016). *Development of perception in infancy: The cradle of knowledge revisited.* Oxford, UK: Oxford University Press.

Arthur, J., Kristjánsson, K., Harrison, T., Sanderse, W., & Wright, D. (2016). *Teaching character and virtue in schools.* New York: Routledge.

Arya, S., Mulla, Z.D., & Plavsic, S.K. (2018). Outcomes of women delivering at very advanced maternal age. *Journal of Women's Health, 27,* 1378-1384.

Asarnow, J.R., Kolko, D.J., Miranda, J., & Kazak, A.E. (2017). The pediatric patient-centered medical home: Innovative models for improving behavioral health. *American Psychologist, 72*(1), 13-27.

Asendorph, J.B. (2008). Shyness. In M. M. Haith & J. B. Benson (Eds.), *Encyclopedia of infant and early childhood development.* Oxford, UK: Elsevier.

Ashmead, D.H., & others (1998). Spatial hearing in children with visual disabilities. *Perception, 27,* 105-122.

Aslin, R.N., & Lathrop, A.L. (2008). Visual perception. In M. M. Haith & J. B. Benson (Eds.), *Encyclopedia of infant and early childhood development.* Oxford, UK: Elsevier.

Aslin, R.N. (2009). The role of learning in cognitive development. In A. Woodward & A. Needham (Eds.), *Learning and the infant mind.* New York: Oxford University Press.

Aslin, R.N. (2012). Infant eyes: A window on cognitive development. *Infancy, 17,* 126-140.

Aspen Institute (2018). *Ascend/2Gen.* Retrieved August 24, 2018, from https://ascend.aspeninstitute.org/

Athanasiadis, A.P., & others. (2011). Correlation of second trimester amniotic fluid amino acid profile with gestational age and estimated fetal weight. *Journal of Maternal-Fetal and Neonatal Medicine, 24,* 1033-1038.

Auld, E., & Morris, P. (2019). The OECD and IELS: Redefining early childhood education for the 21st century. *Policy Futures in Education, 17,* 11-26.

Avena-Koenigsberger, A., Misic, B., & Sporns, O. (2017). Communication dynamics in complex brain networks. *Nature Reviews Neuroscience, 19,* 17-33.

Avent, N.D. (2012). Refining noninvasive prenatal diagnosis with single-molecule next generation sequencing. *Clinical Chemistry, 58,* 657-658.

B

Babbar, S., Parks-Savage, A.C., & Chauhan, S.P. (2012). Yoga during pregnancy. *American Journal of Perinatology, 29*(06), 459-464.

Babskie, E., Powell, D.N., & Metzger, A. (2017). Variability in parenting self-efficacy across prudential adolescent behaviors. *Parenting, 17,* 242-261.

Bacchini, D., & Magliulo, F. (2003). Self-image and perceived self-efficacy during adolescence. *Journal of Youth and Adolescence, 32,* 337-349.

Baddeley, A. (2018). *Working memories: Postmen, divers and the cognitive revolution.* London: Routledge.

Bahali, K., Akcan, R., Tahiroglu, A.Y., & Avci, A. (2010). Child sexual abuse: Seven years into practice. *Journal of Forensic Science, 55*(3), 633–636.

Bahrick, L.E., Todd, J.T., & Soska, K.C. (2018). The Multisensory Attention Assessment Protocol (MAAP): Characterizing individual differences in multisensory attention skills in infants and children and relations with language and cognition. *Developmental Psychology, 54*(12), 2207–2225.

Bailey, H.N., & others (2017). Deconstructing maternal sensitivity: Predictive relations to mother-child attachment in home and laboratory settings. *Social Development, 26*, 679–693.

Baillargeon, R., & Carey, S. (2013). Core cognition and beyond: The acquisition of physical and numerical knowledge. In S. Pauen & M. Bornstein (Eds.), *Early childhood development and later achievement.* New York: Cambridge University Press.

Baillargeon, R., & DeJong, G.F. (2017). Explanation-based learning in infancy. *Psychonomic Bulletin & Review, 24*, 1511–1526.

Baillargeon, R., & Devoe, S.J. (1991). Object permanence in young children: Further evidence. *Child Development, 62*, 1227–1246.

Baillargeon, R., & others (2012). Object individuation and physical reasoning in infancy: An integrative account. *Language, Learning, and Development, 8*, 4–46.

Baillargeon, R. (2008). Innate ideas revisited: For a principle of persistence in infants' physical reasoning. *Perspectives on Psychological Science, 3*, 2–13.

Baillargeon, R. (2014). Cognitive development in infancy. *Annual Review of Psychology* (Vol. 65). Palo Alto, CA: Annual Reviews.

Bakeman, R., & Brown, J.V. (1980). Early interaction: Consequences for social and mental development at three years. *Child Development, 51*, 437–447.

Baker-Smith, C.M., & others (2018). Diagnosis, evaluation, and management of high blood pressure in children and adolescents. *Pediatrics, 142*, e20182096.

Ball, C.L., Smetana, J.G., & Sturge-Apple, M.L. (2017). Following my head and my heart: Integrating preschoolers' empathy, theory of mind, and moral judgments. *Child Development, 88*(2), 597–611.

Ballard, S. (2011). Blood tests for investigating maternal well-being. 4. When nausea and vomiting in pregnancy becomes pathological: Hyperemesis gravidarum. *Practicing Midwife, 14*, 37–41.

Ballou, D., & Springer, M.G. (2017). Has NCLB encouraged educational triage? Accountability and the distribution of achievement gains. *Education Finance and Policy, 12*, 77–106.

Bamaca-Colbert, M., Umana-Taylor, A.J., Espinosa-Hernandez, G., & Brown, A.M. (2012). Behavioral autonomy expectations among Mexican-origin mother-daughter dyads: An examination of within-group variability. *Journal of Adolescence, 35*, 691–700.

Bandura, A. (1998, August). *Swimming against the mainstream: Accentuating the positive aspects of humanity.* Paper presented at the meeting of the American Psychological Association, San Francisco.

Bandura, A. (2002). Selective moral disengagement in the exercise of moral agency. *Journal of Moral Education, 31*, 101–119.

Bandura, A. (2012). Social cognitive theory. *Annual Review of Clinical Psychology* (Vol. 8). Palo Alto, CA: Annual Reviews.

Bandura, A. (2016). *Moral disengagement: How people do harm and live with themselves.* New York: Worth.

Bandura, A. (2018). Toward a psychology of human agency: Pathways and reflections. *Perspectives on Psychological Science, 13*(2), 130–136.

Banks, J.A. (2018). *Introduction to multicultural education* (6th ed.). Upper Saddle River, NJ: Pearson.

Barbieri, R.L. (2019). Female infertility. In *Yen and Jaffe's reproductive endocrinology* (8th ed., pp. 556–581). Amsterdam: Elsevier.

Barišić, L.S., Stanojević, M., Kurjak, A., Porović, S., & Gaber, G.(2017). Diagnosis of fetal syndromes by three-and four-dimensional ultrasound: Is there any improvement? *Journal of Perinatal Medicine, 45*, 651–665.

Barnett, S.M., Rindermann, H., Williams, W.M., & Ceci, S.J. (2011). Society and intelligence. In R. J. Sternberg & S. B. Kaufman (Eds.), *Cambridge handbook of intelligence.* New York: Cambridge University Press.

Barnouw, V. (1975). *An introduction to anthropology: Vol. 2. Ethnology.* Homewood, IL: Dorsey Press.

Baron, N.S. (1992). *Growing up with language.* Reading, MA: Addison-Wesley.

Baron-Cohen, S., Golan, O., Chapman, E., & Granader, Y. (2007). Transported to a world of emotions. *The Psychologist, 20*, 76–77.

Barrouillet, P. (2015). Theories of cognitive development: From Piaget to today. *Developmental Review, 38*, 1–12.

Barry, C.T., McDougall, K.H., Anderson, A.C., & Bindon, A.L. (2018). Global and contingent self-esteem as moderators in the relations between adolescent narcissism, callous-unemotional traits, and aggression. *Personality and Individual Differences, 123*, 1–5.

Bartel, A.P., Rossin-Slater, M., Ruhm, C.J., Stearns, J., & Waldfogel, J. (2018). Paid family leave, fathers' leave-taking, and leave-sharing in dual-earner households. *Journal of Policy Analysis and Management, 37*, 10–37.

Bartel, M.A., Weinstein, J.R., & Schaffer, D.V. (2012). Directed evolution of novel adeno-associated viruses for therapeutic gene delivery. *Gene Therapy, 19*, 694–700.

Barth, J.M., Kim, H., Eno, C.A., & Guadagno, R.E. (2018). Matching abilities to careers for others and self: Do gender stereotypes matter to students in advanced math and science classes? *Sex Roles, 79*, 83–97.

Bartsch, K., & Wellman, H.M. (1995). *Children talk about the mind.* Oxford, UK: Oxford University Press.

Baruteau, A.E., Tester, D.J., Kapplinger, J.D., Ackerman, M.J., & Behr, E.R. (2017). Sudden infant death syndrome and inherited cardiac conditions. *Nature Reviews Cardiology, 14*, 715–726.

Basanez, T., Unger, J.B., Soto, D., Crano, W., & Baezconde-Garbanati, L. (2012). Perceived discrimination as a risk factor for depressive symptoms and substance use among Hispanic students in Los Angeles. *Ethnicity and Health, 18*(3), 244–261.

Bascandziev, I., & Harris, P.L. (2011). The role of testimony in young children's solution of a gravity-driven invisible displacement task. *Cognitive Development, 25*, 233–246.

Bassett, H.H., Denham, S.A., Mincic, M.M., & Graling, K. (2012). The structure of preschoolers' relationship knowledge: Model equivalence and validity using an SEM approach. *Early Education and Development, 23*(3), 259–279.

Batanova, M.D., & Loukas, A. (2011). Social anxiety and aggression in early adolescents: Examining the moderating roles of empathic concern and perspective taking. *Journal of Youth and Adolescence, 40*, 1534–1543.

Bates, J.E., & Pettit, G.S. (2007). Temperament, parenting, and socialization. In J. E. Grusec & P. D. Hastings (Eds.), *Handbook of socialization.* New York: Guilford.

Bates, J.E., McQuillan, M.E., & Hoyniak, C.P. (2019). Parenting and temperament. In M.H. Bornstein (Ed.), *Handbook of parenting* (3rd ed.). New York: Taylor and Francis.

Batki, A. (2018). The impact of early institutional care on emotion regulation: Studying the play narratives of post-institutionalized and early adopted children. *Early Child Development and Care, 188*, 1801–1815.

Battista, C., & others (2018). Mechanisms of interactive specialization and emergence of functional brain circuits supporting cognitive development in children. *NPJ Science of Learning, 3*(1), 1.

Baude, A., Pearson, J., & Drapeau, S. (2016). Child adjustment in joint physical custody versus sole custody: A meta-analytic review. *Journal of Divorce & Remarriage, 57*(5), 338–360.

Bauer, P.J., & Fivush, R. (Eds.). (2013). *Wiley-Blackwell handbook of children's memory.* New York: Wiley.

Bauer, P. (2006). *Remembering the times of our lives: Memory in infancy and beyond.* New York: Psychology Press.

Bauer, P. (2009). Learning and memory: Like a horse and carriage. In A. Needham & A. Woodward (Eds.), *Learning and the infant mind.* New York: Oxford University Press.

Bauer, P. (2013). Memory. In P. D. Zelazo (Ed.), *Oxford handbook of developmental psychology.* New York: Oxford University Press.

Bauman, S., & Bellmore, A. (2015). New directions in cyberbullying research. *Journal of School Violence, 14*(1), 1–10.

Baumeister, R.F. (2013). Self-esteem. In E. Anderson (Ed.), *Psychology of classroom learning: An encyclopedia.* Detroit: Macmillan.

Baumgartner, S.E., van der Schuur, W.A., Lemmens, J.S., & te Poel, F. (2017). The relationship between media multitasking and attention problems in adolescents: Results of two longitudinal studies. *Human Communication Research, 44*(1), 3–30.

Baumrind, D., Larzelere, R.E., & Cowan, P.A. (2002). Ordinary physical punishment: Is it harmful? Comment on Gershoff. *Psychological Bulletin, 128,* 590–595.

Baumrind, D. (1971). Current patterns of parental authority. *Developmental Psychology Monographs, 4*(1, Pt. 2).

Baumrind, D. (2013). Authoritative parenting revisited: History and current status. In R. Larzelere, A.S. Morris, & A.W. Harist (Eds.), *Authoritative parenting.* Washington, DC: American Psychological Association.

Bauserman, R. (2002). Child adjustment in joint-custody versus sole-custody arrangements: A meta-analytic review. *Journal of Family Psychology, 16,* 91–102.

Bausert, S., Froh, J.J., Bono, G., Rose-Zornick, R., & Rose, Z. (2018). Gratitude in adolescence. In J. Tudge & L. Freitas (Eds.), *Developing gratitude in children and adolescents.* Cambridge, UK: Cambridge University Press.

Bayley, N. (1969). *Manual for the Bayley Scales of Infant Development.* New York: Psychological Corporation.

Bayley, N. (2006). *Bayley Scales of Infant and Toddler Development* (3rd ed.). San Antonio: Harcourt Assessment.

Beal, S.J., Crockett, L.J., & Peugh, J. (2016). Adolescents' changing future expectations predict the timing of adult role transitions. *Developmental Psychology, 52*(10), 1606–1618.

Becht, A.I., & others (2017). Clear self, better relationships: Adolescents' self-concept clarity and relationship quality with parents and peers across 5 years. *Child Development, 88*(6), 1823–1833.

Becker, M., & others (2014). Cultural bases for self-evaluation: Seeing oneself positively in different cultural contexts. *Personality and Social Psychology Bulletin, 40*(5), 657–675.

Beckmeyer, J.J., & Russell, L.T. (2018). Family structure and family management practices: Associations with positive aspects of youth well-being. *Journal of Family Issues, 39*(7), 2131–2154.

Beebe, B., & others (2018). Family nurture intervention for preterm infants facilitates positive mother–infant face-to-face engagement at 4 months. *Developmental Psychology, 54,* 2016–2031.

Beebe, D.W., Rose, D., & Amin, R. (2010). Attention, learning, and arousal of experimentally sleep-restricted adolescents in a simulated classroom. *Journal of Adolescent Health, 47,* 523–525.

Bekbolatkyzy, D.S., Yerenatovna, D.R., Maratuly, Y.A., Makhatovna, A.G., & Beaver, K.M. (2019). Aging out of adolescent delinquency: Results from a longitudinal sample of youth and young adults. *Journal of Criminal Justice, 60,* 108–116.

Belizán, J.M., & others (2018). An approach to identify a minimum and rational proportion of caesarean sections in resource-poor settings: A global network study. *The Lancet Global Health, 6*(8), e894–e901.

Belk, C., & Maier, V.B. (2013). *Biology* (4th ed.). Upper Saddle River, NJ: Pearson.

Bell, M.A., & Cuevas, K. (2013). Psychobiology of executive function in early development. In J. A. Griffin, L. S. Freund, & P. McCardle (Eds.), *Executive function in preschool children.* Washington, DC: American Psychological Association.

Bell, S.M., & Ainsworth, M.D.S. (1972). Infant crying and maternal responsiveness. *Child Development, 43,* 1171–1190.

Bellieni, C.V., & others (2018). Pain perception in NICU: A pilot questionnaire. *The Journal of Maternal-Fetal & Neonatal Medicine, 31*(14), 1921–1923.

Belsky, J., & Pluess, M. (2009). Beyond diathesis stress: Differential susceptibility to environmental influences. *Psychological Bulletin, 135,* 885–908.

Belsky, J., Jaffe, S., Hsieh, K., & Silva, P. (2001). Child-rearing antecedents of intergenerational relations in young adulthood: A prospective study. *Developmental Psychology, 37,* 801–813.

Belsky, J., Steinberg, L., Houts, R.M., Halpern-Felsher, B.L., & The NICHD Child Care Research Network. (2010). The development of reproductive strategy in females: Early maternal harshness → earlier menarche → increased sexual risk. *Developmental Psychology, 46,* 120–128.

Belsky, J. (1981). Early human experience: A family perspective. *Developmental Psychology, 17,* 3–23.

Belsky, J. (2013). Commentary on perspectives and counter perspectives. In D. Narvaez & others (Eds.), *Evolution, early experience, and development.* New York: Oxford University Press.

Bem, S.L. (1977). On the utility of alternative procedures for assessing psychological androgyny. *Journal of Consulting and Clinical Psychology, 45,* 196–205.

Benner, A.D., & Graham, S. (2013). The antecedents and consequences of racial/ethnic discrimination during adolescence: Does the source of discrimination matter? *Developmental Psychology, 49*(8), 1602–1613.

Benner, A.D. (2011). Latino adolescents' loneliness, academic performance, and the buffering nature of friendships. *Journal of Youth and Adolescence, 5,* 556–567.

Benner, A. (2017). The toll of racial/ethnic discrimination on adolescents' adjustment. *Child Development Perspectives, 11*(4), 251–256.

Benner, A.D., & others (2018). Racial/ethnic discrimination and well-being during adolescence: A meta-analytic review. *American Psychologist, 73*(7), 855.

Benner, A.D., Hou, Y., & Jackson, K.M. (2019, in press). The consequences of friend-related stress across early adolescence. *The Journal of Early Adolescence,* 0272431619833489.

Bennett, C.I. (2018). *Comprehensive multicultural education: Theory and practice* (9th ed.). New York: Pearson.

Benoit, D., Coolbear, J., & Crawford, A. (2008). Abuse, neglect, and maltreatment of infants. In M. M. Haith & J. B. Benson (Eds.), *Encyclopedia of infant and early childhood development.* Oxford, UK: Elsevier.

Benowitz-Fredericks, C.A., Garcia, K., Massey, M., Vassagar, B., & Borzekowski, D.L. (2012). Body image, eating disorders, and the relationship to adolescent media use. *Pediatric Clinics of North America, 59,* 693–704.

Bereczki, E.O., & Kárpáti, A. (2018). Teachers' beliefs about creativity and its nurture: A systematic review of the recent research literature. *Educational Research Review, 23,* 25–56.

Berko Gleason, J., & Ratner, N.B. (Eds.). (2017). *The development of language* (9th ed.). Boston: Pearson.

Berko Gleason, J. (2005). The development of language: An overview and a preview. In J. Berko Gleason (Ed.), *The development of language* (6th ed.). Boston: Allyn & Bacon.

Berko Gleason, J. (2009). The development of language. An overview. In J. Berko Gleason & N. B. Ratner (Eds.), *The development of language* (7th ed.). Boston: Allyn & Bacon.

Berko, J. (1958). The child's learning of English morphology. *Word, 14,* 15–177.

Berkowitz, M.W., Sherblom, S., Bier, M., & Battistich, V. (2006). Educating for positive youth development. In M. Killen & J.G. Smetana (Eds.), *Handbook of moral development.* Mahwah, NJ: Erlbaum.

Berlin, L.J., & others (2009). Correlates and consequences of spanking and verbal punishment for low-income, White, African-American, and Mexican American toddlers. *Child Development, 80,* 1403–1420.

Berlin, L.J., Martoccio, T.L., & Jones Harden, B. (2018). Improving Early Head Start's impacts on parenting through attachment-based intervention: A randomized controlled trial. *Developmental Psychology, 54,* 2316–2327.

Berlyne, D.E. (1960). *Conflict, arousal, and curiosity.* New York: McGraw-Hill.

Berman, R.A. (2017). Language development and literacy. *Encyclopedia of Adolescence,* 1–11.

Berman, R.A. (2018). Development of complex syntax: From early clause-combining to text-embedded syntactic packaging. In A. Bar-On & D. Ravid (Eds.), *Handbook of communication disorders.* Boston: DeGruyter.

Bernecker, K., Herrmann, M., Brandstätter, V., & Job, V. (2017). Implicit theories about willpower predict subjective well-being. *Journal of Personality, 85,* 136–150.

Berninger, V., & Swanson, H.L. (2013). Diagnosing and treating specific learning disabilities in reference to the brain's working memory system. In H. L. Swanson & others (Eds.), *Handbook of learning disabilities* (2nd ed.). New York: Guilford.

Berninger, V., Abbott, R., Cook, C.R., & Nagy, W. (2017). Relationships of attention and executive functions to oral language, reading, and writing skills and systems in middle childhood and early adolescence. *Journal of Learning Disabilities, 50,* 434–449.

Berry, D., & others (2016). Household chaos and children's cognitive and socio-emotional development in early childhood: Does childcare play a buffering role? *Early Childhood Research Quarterly, 34,* 115–127.

Berry, D., Deater-Deckard, K., McCartney, K., Wang, Z., & Petrill, S.A. (2012). Gene-environment interaction between DRD4 7-repeat VNTR and early maternal sensitivity predicts inattention trajectories across middle childhood. *Development and Psychopathology, 56*(3), 373-391.

Berryhill, M., Soloski, K., Durtschi, J., & Adams, R. (2016), Family process: Early child emotionality, parenting stress, and couple relationship quality. *Personal Relationships, 23*, 23-41.

Bertenthal, B.I., Longo, M.R., & Kenny, S. (2007). Phenomenal permanence and the development of predictive tracking in infancy. *Child Development, 78*, 350-363.

Bessette, K.L., & Stevens, M.C. (2019). Neurocognitive pathways in attention-deficit/ hyperactivity disorder and white matter microstructure. *Biological Psychiatry: Cognitive Neuroscience and Neuroimaging, 4*, 233-242.

Best, D.L. (2010). Gender. In M. H. Bornstein (Ed.), *Handbook of cultural developmental science*. New York: Psychology Press.

Bialystok, E. (2018). Bilingualism and executive function: What's the connection? In D. Miller, F. Bayram, J. Rothman, & L. Serratrice (Eds.), *Bilingual cognition and language: The state of the science across its subfields*. Amsterdam: John Benjamins.

Bian, L., Leslie, S.-J., & Cimpian, A. (2017). Gender stereotypes about intellectual ability emerge early and influence children's interests. *Science, 355*, 389-391.

Biehle, S.N., & Mickelson, K.D. (2012). First-time parents' expectations about the division of childcare and play. *Journal of Family Psychology, 26*, 36-45.

Birkeland, M.S., Melkevick, O., Holsen, I., & Wold, B. (2012). Trajectories of global self-esteem development during adolescence. *Journal of Adolescence, 35*, 43-54.

Birnbaum, G.E., & Reis, H.T. (2019). Evolved to be connected: The dynamics of attachment and sex over the course of romantic relationships. *Current Opinion in Psychology, 25*, 11-15.

Björkqvist, K. (2018). Gender differences in aggression. *Current Opinion in Psychology, 19*, 39-42.

Bjorklund, D.F., & Pellegrini, A.D. (2002). *The origins of human nature*. New York: Oxford University Press.

Bjorklund, D.F., & Causey, K.B. (2018). *Children's thinking* (6th ed.). Thousand Oaks, CA: SAGE.

Bjorklund, D.F., Hernández Blasi, C., & Ellis, B.J. (2017). Evolutionary developmental psychology. In D. M. Buss (Ed.), *Handbook of evolutionary psychology* (pp. 904-925). New York: Wiley.

Bjorklund, D.F. (2018). A metatheory for cognitive development (or "Piaget is dead" revisited). *Child Development, 89*, 2288-2302.

Blackwell, L.S., & Dweck, C.S. (2008). *The motivational impact of a computer-based program that teaches how the brain changes with learning*. Unpublished manuscript, Department of Psychology, Stanford University, Palo Alto, CA.

Blackwell, L.S., Trzesniewski, K.H., & Dweck, C.S. (2007). Implicit theories of intelligence predict achievement across an adolescent tradition: A longitudinal study and an intervention. *Child Development, 78*, 246-263.

Blair, C., & Raver, C.C. (2014). Closing the achievement gap through modification of neurocognitive and neuroendocrine function: Results from a cluster randomized controlled trial of an innovative approach to the education of children in kindergarten. *PloS One, 9*(11), e112393.

Blake, M.J., Trinder, J.A., & Allen, N.B. (2018). Mechanisms underlying the association between insomnia, anxiety, and depression in adolescence: Implications for behavioral sleep interventions. *Clinical Psychology Review, 63*, 25-40.

Blakemore, J.E.O., Berenbaum, S.A., & Liben, I.S. (2009). *Gender development*. Clifton, NJ: Psychology Press.

Blakemore, J.E.O., Berenbaum, S.A., & Liben, L.S. (2009). *Gender development*. New York: Psychology Press.

Blakemore, S-J., & Mills, K. (2014). The social brain in adolescence. *Annual Review of Psychology* (Vol. 65). Palo Alto, CA: Annual Reviews.

Block, J. (1993). Studying personality the long way. In D. Funder, R. D. Parke, C. Tomlinson-Keasey, & K. Widaman (Eds.), *Studying lives through time*. Washington, DC: American Psychological Association.

Blumberg, F., & Brooks, P. (Eds.) (2017). *Cognitive development in digital contexts*. New York: Academic Press.

Blumberg, F.C., & others (2019). Digital games as a context for children's cognitive development: Research recommendations and policy considerations. *Social Policy Report, 32*(1), 1-33.

Bodrova, E., & Leong, D.J. (2007). *Tools of the mind* (2nd ed.). Geneva, Switzerland: International Bureau of Education, UNESCO.

Bodrova, E., & Leong, D.J. (2017). The Vygotskian and post-Vygotskian approach: Focusing on "the future child." In L.E. Cohen & S. Waite-Stupiansky (Eds.), *Theories of early childhood education*. New York: Routledge.

Boghossian, N.S., Geraci, M., Edwards, E.M., & Horbar, J.D. (2018). Morbidity and mortality in small for gestational age infants at 22 to 29 weeks' gestation. *Pediatrics, 141*(2), e20172533.

Bohlin, G., & Hagekull, B. (1993). Stranger wariness and sociability in the early years. *Infant Behavior and Development, 16*, 53-67.

Bohlin, G., & Hagekull, B. (2009). Socio-emotional development from infancy to young adulthood. *Scandinavian Journal of Psychology, 50*, 592-601.

Bohr, Y., Putnick, D.L., Lee, Y., & Bornstein, M.H. (2018). Evaluating caregiver sensitivity to infants: Measures matter. *Infancy, 23*, 730-747.

Boldt, L.J., Kochanska, G., Grekin, R., & Brock, R.L. (2016). Attachment in middle childhood: Predictors, correlates, and implications for adaptation. *Attachment & Human Development, 18*, 115-140.

Bolton, S., & Hattie, J. (2017). Cognitive and brain development: Executive function, Piaget, and the prefrontal cortex. *Archives of Psychology, 1*(3).

Bono, G., & others (2019). Gratitude's role in adolescent antisocial and prosocial behavior: A 4-year longitudinal investigation. *The Journal of Positive Psychology, 14*(2), 230-243.

Booth, M. (2002). Arab adolescents facing the future: Enduring ideals and pressures to change. In B. B. Brown, R. W. Larson, & T. S. Saraswathi (Eds.), *The world's youth*. New York: Cambridge University Press.

Borich, G.D. (2017). *Effective teaching methods* (9th ed.). Upper Saddle River, NJ: Pearson.

Borle, K., Morris, E., Inglis, A., & Austin, J. (2018). Risk communication in genetic counseling: Exploring uptake and perception of recurrence numbers, and their impact on patient outcomes. *Clinical Genetics, 94*, 239-245.

Bornstein, M.H., Jager, J., & Steinberg, L. (2013). Adolescents, parents/friends/peers: A relationship model. In I. B. Weiner & others (Eds.), *Handbook of psychology* (2nd ed., Vol. 6). New York: Wiley.

Bornstein, M.H., & Lansford, J.E. (2010). Parenting. In M. H. Bornstein (Ed.), *Handbook of cultural developmental science*. New York: Psychology Press.

Bornstein, M.H. (2002). Parenting infants. In M. H. Bornstein (Ed.), *Handbook of parenting* (2nd ed., Vol. 1). Mahwah, NJ: Erlbaum.

Bornstein, M.H., & Lansford, J.E. (2018). Culture and family functioning. In B. Fiese & others (Eds.), *Handbook of contemporary family psychology*. Washington, DC: American Psychological Association.

Bornstein, M.H., & others (2017). Neurobiology of culturally common maternal responses to infant cry. *Proceedings of the National Academy of Sciences, 114*(45), E9465-E9473.

Bornstein, M.H., Putnick, D.L., Cote, L.R., Haynes, O.M., & Suwalsky, J.T.D. (2015). Mother-infant contingent vocalizations in 11 countries. *Psychological Science, 26*, 1272-1284.

Bornstein, M.H. (2015). Emergence and early development of color vision and color perception. In A.J. Elliott & others (Eds.), *Handbook of color psychology* (pp. 149-179). Cambridge, UK: Cambridge University Press.

Bornstein, M.H. (Ed.) (2018). *The SAGE encyclopedia of lifespan human development*. Thousand Oaks, CA: SAGE.

Bos, P.A. (2017). The endocrinology of human caregiving and its intergenerational transmission. *Development and Psychopathology, 29*, 971-999.

Bosacki, S. (2016). *Social cognition in middle childhood and adolescence: Integrating the personal, social, and educational lives of young people*. New York: Wiley.

Bouchard, T.J., Lykken, D.T., McGue, M., Segal, N.L., & Tellegen, A. (1990). Source of human psychological differences: The Minnesota Study of Twins Reared Apart. *Science, 250*, 223-228.

Boucher, J.M. (2017). *Autism spectrum disorder: Characteristics, causes and practical issues* (2nd ed.). Thousand Oaks, CA: SAGE.

Boutwell, B.B., Meldrum, R.C., & Petkovsek, M.A. (2017). General intelligence in friendship selection:

A study of preadolescent best friend dyads. *Intelligence, 64,* 30-35.

Bouziane, C., & others (2018). ADHD and maturation of brain white matter: A DTI study in medication naive children and adults. *NeuroImage: Clinical, 17,* 53-59.

Bower, T.G.R. (1966). Slant perception and shape constancy in infants. *Science, 151,* 832-834.

Bowker, J.C., Rubin, K., & Coplan, R. (2012). Social withdrawal during adolescence. In J. R. Levesque (Ed.), *Encyclopedia of adolescence.* New York: Springer.

Bowker, J.C., & Spencer, S.V. (2010). Friendship and adjustment: A focus on mixed-grade friendships. *Journal of Youth and Adolescence, 39,* 1318-1329.

Bowlby, J. (1969). *Attachment and loss* (Vol. 1). London: Hogarth Press.

Bowlby, J. (1989). *Secure and insecure attachment.* New York: Basic Books.

Boyer, T.W., Harding, S.M., & Bertenthal, B.I. (2017). Infants' motor simulation of observed actions is modulated by the visibility of the actor's body. *Cognition, 164,* 107-115.

Boyle, J., & Cropley, M. (2004). Children's sleep: Problems and solutions. *Journal of Family Health Care, 14,* 61-63.

Bradbury, B., Waldfogel, J., & Washbrook, E. (2019). Income-related gaps in early child cognitive development: Why are they larger in the United States than in the United Kingdom, Australia, and Canada? *Demography, 56*(1), 367-390.

Bradley, R.H., & Corwyn, R.F. (2013). From parent to child to parent. . . . Paths in and out of problem behavior. *Journal of Abnormal Child Psychology.*

Brady, S.E., & Stevens, M.C. (2019). Is immigration a culture? A qualitative approach to exploring immigrant student experiences within the United States. *Translational Issues in Psychological Science, 5*(1), 17-28.

Brandone, A.C., & Klimek, B. (2018). The developing theory of mental state control: Changes in beliefs about the controllability of emotional experience from elementary school through adulthood. *Journal of Cognition and Development, 19*(5), 509-531.

Brandt, M.J., & Crawford, J.T. (2019, in press). Studying a heterogeneous array of target groups can help us understand prejudice. *Current Directions in Psychological Science.*

Brannon, L. (2017). *Gender.* New York: Routledge.

Bratsberg, B., & Rogeberg, O. (2018). Flynn effect and its reversal are both environmentally caused. *Proceedings of the National Academy of Sciences, 115,* 6674-6678.

Bratsch-Hines, M.E., Mokrova, I., Vernon-Feagans, L., & Family Life Project Key Investigators (2017). Rural families' use of multiple child care arrangements from 6 to 58 months and children's kindergarten behavioral and academic outcomes. *Early Childhood Research Quarterly, 41,* 161-173.

Brazelton, T.B. (1956). Sucking in infancy. *Pediatrics, 17,* 400-404.

Brazil, N. (2016). The effect of social context on youth outcomes: Studying neighborhoods and schools simultaneously. *Teachers College Record, 118*(7).

Breathnach, H., Danby, S., & O'Gorman, L. (2018). 'We're doing a wedding': producing peer cultures in pretend play. *International Journal of Play, 7*(3), 290-307.

Brechwald, W.A., & Prinstein, M.J. (2011). Beyond homophily: A decade of advances in understanding peer influence processes. *Journal of Research on Adolescence, 21,* 166-179.

Breedlove, G., & Fryzelka, D. (2011). Depression screening in pregnancy. *Journal of Midwifery and Women's Health, 56,* 18-25.

Bremner, A.J., & Spence, C. (2017). The development of tactile perception. *Advances in Child Development and Behavior, 52,* 227-268.

Bremner, J.G., Slater, A.M., Mason, U.C., Spring, J., & Johnson, S.P. (2016). Perception of occlusion by young infants: Must the occlusion event be congruent with the occluder? *Infant Behavior and Development, 44,* 240-248.

Brendgen, M. (2018). Peer victimization and adjustment in young adulthood: Introduction to the special section. *Journal of Abnormal Child Psychology, 46*(1), 5-9.

Bretherton, I., Stolberg, U., & Kreye, M. (1981). Engaging strangers in proximal interaction: Infants' social initiative. *Developmental Psychology, 17,* 746-755.

Brewer, M.B., & Campbell, D.T. (1976). *Ethnocentrism and intergroup attitudes.* New York: Wiley.

Brewer, M. (2018). Intergroup discrimination: Ingroup love or outgroup hate? In F. Barlow & C. Sibley (Eds.), *The Cambridge handbook of the psychology of prejudice (Concise Student Edition)* (pp. 15-39). New York: Cambridge University Press.

Bridgeland, J.M., Dilulio, J.J., & Wulsin, S.C. (2008). *Engaged for success.* Washington, DC: Civic Enterprises.

Brion, M., & others. (2012). Sarcomeric gene mutations in sudden infant death syndrome (SIDS). *Forensic Science International, 219*(1-3), 278-281.

Brito, N.H. (2017). Influence of the home linguistic environment on early language development. *Policy Insights from the Behavioral and Brain Sciences, 4,* 155-162.

Britto, P.R., & others (2017). Nurturing care: Promoting early childhood development. *The Lancet, 389,* 91-102.

Broadney, M.M., & others (2018). Effects of interrupting sedentary behavior with short bouts of moderate physical activity on glucose tolerance in children with overweight and obesity: A randomized crossover trial. *Diabetes Care, 41,* 2220-2228.

Broc, M.Á. (2014). Harter's self-perception profile for children: An adaptation and validation of the Spanish version. *Psychological Reports, 115*(2), 444-466.

Brockmeyer, S., Treboux, D., & Crowell, J.A. (2005, April). *Parental divorce and adult children's attachment status and marital relationships.* Paper presented at the meeting of the Society for Research in Child Development, Atlanta.

Brockmeyer, T., & others. (2012). The thinner the better: Self-esteem and low body weight in anorexia nervosa. *Clinical Psychology and Psychotherapy, 20*(5), 394-400.

Brodsky, J.L., Viner-Brown, S., & Handler, A.S. (2009). Change in maternal cigarette smoking among pregnant WIC participants in Rhode Island. *Maternal and Child Health Journal, 13,* 822-831.

Brodzinsky, D.M., & Pinderhughes, E. (2002). Parenting and child development in adoptive families. In M. H. Bornstein (Ed.), *Handbook of parenting* (Vol. 1). Mahwah, NJ: Erlbaum.

Brodzinsky, D.M., & Goldberg, A.E. (2016). Contact with birth family in adoptive families headed by lesbian, gay male, and heterosexual parents. *Children and Youth Services Review, 62,* 9-17.

Broesch, T., Rochat, P., Olah, K., Broesch, J., & Henrich, J. (2016). Similarities and differences in maternal responsiveness in three societies: Evidence from Fiji, Kenya, and the United States. *Child Development, 87,* 700-711.

Bronfenbrenner, U. (1986). Ecology of the family as a context for human development: Research perspectives. *Developmental Psychology, 22,* 723-742.

Bronfenbrenner, U. (2000). Ecological theory. In A. Kazdin (Ed.), *Encyclopedia of psychology.* Washington, DC, & New York: American Psychological Association and Oxford University Press.

Bronfenbrenner, U. (2004). *Making human beings human.* Thousand Oaks, CA: Sage.

Bronfenbrenner, U., & Morris, P.A. (2006). The ecology of developmental processes. In W. Damon & R. Lerner (Eds.), *Handbook of child psychology* (6th ed.). New York: Wiley.

Bronstein, P. (2006). The family environment: Where gender role socialization begins. In J. Worell & C. D. Goodheart (Eds.), *Handbook of girls' and women's psychological health.* New York: Oxford University Press.

Brook, J.S., Brook, D.W., Gordon, A.S., Whiteman, M., & Cohen, P. (1990). The psychological etiology of adolescent drug use: A family interactional approach. *Genetic, Social, and General Psychology Monographs, 116,* 110-267.

Brooker, R.J., Widaier, E.P., Graham, L., & Stiling, P. (2017). *Biology* (4th ed.).

Brooks-Gunn, J., Schneider, W., & Waldfogel, J. (2013). The Great Recession and the risk for child maltreatment. *Child Abuse & Neglect, 37*(10), 721-729.

Brooks, P.J., Flynn, R.M., & Ober, T.M. (2018). Sustained attention in infancy impacts vocabulary acquisition in low-income toddlers. *Proceedings of the 42nd annual Boston University Conference on Language Development.* Somerville, MA: Cascadilla Press.

Brooks.R., & Meltzoff.A.N. (2005). The development of gaze following and its relation to language. *Developmental Science, 8,* 535-543.

Brooks-Gunn, J., Han, W-J., & Waldfogel, J. (2010). First-year maternal employment and child development in the first seven years. *Monographs of the Society for Research in Child Development, 75*(2), 1-147.

Brooks-Gunn, J., & Warren, M.P. (1989). The psychological significance of secondary sexual characteristics in 9- to 11-year-old girls. *Child Development, 59,* 161-169.

Brooks-Gunn, J. (2003). Do you believe in magic?: What we can expect from early childhood programs. *Social Policy Report, Society for Research in Child Development, XVII* (1), 1-13.

Brophy, J. (2004). *Motivating students to learn* (2nd ed.). Mahwah, NJ: Erlbaum.

Broverman, I., Vogel, S., Broverman, D., Clarkson, F., & Rosenkranz, P. (1972). Sex-role stereotypes: A current appraisal. *Journal of Social Issues, 28,* 59-78.

Brown, A.L., & Day, J.D. (1983). Macrorules for summarizing texts: The development of expertise. *Journal of Verbal Learning and Verbal Behavior, 22,* 1-14.

Brown, B.B., & Bakken, J.P. (2011). Parenting and peer relationships: Reinvigorating research on family-peer linkages in adolescence. *Journal of Research on Adolescence, 21,* 153-165.

Brown, B.B., & Larson, J. (2009). Peer relationships in adolescence. In R. L. Lerner & L. Steinberg (Eds.), *Handbook of adolescent psychology* (3rd ed.). New York: Wiley.

Brown, B.B. (1999). Measuring the peer environment of American adolescents. In S. L. Friedman & T. D. Wachs (Eds.), *Measuring environment across the life span.* Washington, DC: American Psychological Association.

Brown, B.B. (2011). Popularity in peer group perspective: The role of status in adolescent peer systems. In A. H. N. Cillessen, D. Schwartz, & L. Mayeux (Eds.), *Popularity in the peer system.* New York: Guilford.

Brown, D. (2013). Morphological typology. In J. J. Song (Ed.), *Oxford handbook of linguistic typology.* New York: Oxford University Press.

Brown, J., & others (2018). Fetal alcohol spectrum disorder (FASD): A beginner's guide for mental health professionals. *Journal of Neurology and Clinical Neuroscience, 2*(1), 13-19.

Brown, L.D., Feinberg, M., & Kan, M.L. (2012). Predicting engagement in a transition to parenthood program for couples. *Evaluation and Program Planning, 35,* 1-8.

Brown, L.M., & Gilligan, C. (1992). *Meeting at the crossroads: Women's and girls' development.* Cambridge, MA: Harvard University Press.

Brown, R. (1958). *Words and things.* Glencoe, IL: Free Press.

Brown, R. (1973). *A first language: The early stage.* Cambridge, MA: Harvard University Press.

Brown, W.H., & others (2009). Social and environmental factors associated with preschoolers' nonsedentary physical activity. *Child Development, 80,* 45-58.

Brownell, C.A., Ramani, G.B., & Zerwas, S. (2006). Becoming a social partner with peers: Cooperation and social understanding in one- and two-year-olds. *Child Development, 77,* 803-821.

Brownell, C.A., Svetlova, M., Anderson, R., Nichols, S.R., & Drummond, J. (2012). Socialization of early prosocial behavior: Parents' talk about emotions is associated with sharing and helping in toddlers. *Infancy, 18*(1), 91-119.

Bruchmiller, K., Margraf, J., & Schneider, S. (2012). Is ADHD diagnosed in accord with diagnostic criteria? Overdiagnosis and influence of client gender on diagnosis. *Journal of Consulting and Clinical Psychology, 80,* 128-138.

Bruck, M., & Ceci, S.J. (2012). Forensic developmental psychology in the courtroom. In D. Faust & M. Ziskin (Eds.), *Coping with psychiatric and psychological testimony.* New York: Cambridge University Press.

Brumariu, L.E., Kerns, K.A., & Siebert, A.C. (2012). Mother-child attachment, emotion regulation, and anxiety symptoms in middle childhood. *Personal Relationships, 19*(3), 569-585.

Brumariu, L.E., Bureau, J.F., Nemoda, Z., Sasvari-Szekely, M., & Lyons-Ruth, K. (2016). Attachment and temperament revisited: Infant distress, attachment disorganisation and the serotonin transporter polymorphism. *Journal of Reproductive and Infant Psychology, 34,* 77-89.

Brumariu, L.E., Madigan, S., Giuseppone, K.R., Movahed Abtahi, M., & Kerns, K.A. (2018). The Security Scale as a measure of attachment: Meta-analytic evidence of validity. *Attachment & Human Development, 20,* 600-625.

Brummelman, E., Thomaes, S., & Sedikides, C. (2016). Separating narcissism from self-esteem. *Current Directions in Psychological Science, 25*(1), 8-13.

Brummelte, S., & Galea, L.A. (2016). Postpartum depression: Etiology, treatment and consequences for maternal care. *Hormones and Behavior, 77,* 153-166.

Brunstein-Klomek, A., & others (2019). Bi-directional longitudinal associations between different types of bullying victimization, suicide ideation/attempts, and depression among a large sample of European adolescents. *Journal of Child Psychology and Psychiatry, 60*(2), 209-215.

Bryck, R.L., & Fisher, P.A. (2012). Training the brain: Practical applications of neural plasticity from the intersection of cognitive neuroscience, developmental psychology, and prevention science. *American Psychologist, 67,* 87-100.

Buckingham-Howes, S., Berger, S.S., Scaletti, L.A., & Black, M.M. (2013). Systematic review of prenatal cocaine exposure and adolescent development. *Pediatrics, 131*(6), e1917-1936.

Budani, M.C., & Tiboni, G.M. (2017). Ovotoxicity of cigarette smoke: A systematic review of the literature. *Reproductive Toxicology, 72,* 164-181.

Buhrmester, D. (1990). Friendship, interpersonal competence, and adjustment in preadolescence and adolescence. *Child Development, 61,* 1101-1111.

Buhrmester, D., & Furman, W. (1987). The development of companionship and intimacy. *Child Development, 58,* 1101-1113.

Buhrmester, M.D., Blanton, H., & Swann Jr, W.B. (2011). Implicit self-esteem: Nature, measurement, and a new way forward. *Journal of Personality and Social Psychology, 100*(2), 365.

Bukasa, A., & others (2018). Rubella infection in pregnancy and congenital rubella in United Kingdom, 2003 to 2016. *Euro surveillance: Bulletin Europeen sur les Maladies Transmissibles (European Communicable Disease Bulletin), 23*(19), 17-00381.

Bukowski, R., & others (2008, January). *Folic acid and preterm birth.* Paper presented at the meeting of the Society for Maternal-Fetal Medicine, Dallas.

Bukowski, W., Laursen, B., & Rubin, K. (2018). *Handbook of peer relationships, interactions, and groups* (2nd ed.). New York: Guilford.

Bulbena-Cabre, A., Nia, A.B., & Perez-Rodriguez, M.M. (2018). Current knowledge on gene-environment interactions in personality disorders: An update. *Current Psychiatry Reports, 20,* 74.

Bumpus, M.F., Crouter, A.C., & McHale, S.M. (2001). Parental autonomy granting during adolescence: Exploring gender differences in context. *Developmental Psychology, 37,* 161-173.

Burge, T. (2018). Do infants and nonhuman animals attribute mental states? *Psychological Review, 125*(3), 409-434.

Burnette, C.E., & others (2019, in press). The Family Resilience Inventory: A culturally grounded measure of current and family-of-origin protective processes in Native American families. *Family Process.*

Burns, C., Dunn, A., Brady, M., Starr, N., & Blosser, C. (2017). *Pediatric primary care* (6th ed.). New York: Elsevier.

Burns, E.C., Martin, A.J., & Collie, R.J. (2019). Understanding the role of personal best (PB) goal setting in students' declining engagement: A latent growth model. *Journal of Educational Psychology, 111*(4), 557-572.

Bushman, B.J. (2016). Violent media and hostile appraisals: A meta-analytic review. *Aggressive Behavior, 42*(6), 605-613.

Buss, A.T., Ross-Sheehy, S., & Reynolds, G.D. (2018). Visual working memory in early development: A developmental cognitive neuroscience perspective. *Journal of Neurophysiology, 120,* 1472-1483.

Buss, D.M. (2018). *Evolutionary psychology* (6th ed.). New York: Routledge.

Butcher, K., Sallis, J.F., Mayer, J.A., & Woodruff, S. (2008). Correlates of physical activity guideline compliance for adolescents in 100 cities. *Journal of Adolescent Health, 42,* 360-368.

Buttermore, E.D., Thaxton, C.L., & Bhat, M.A. (2013). Organization and maintenance of molecular domains in myelinated axons. *Journal of Neuroscience Research, 91,* 603-622.

Byard, R.W. (2018). The autopsy and pathology of Sudden Infant Death Syndrome. In *SIDS Sudden Infant and Early Childhood Death: The Past, the Present and the Future.* Adelaide, Australia: University of Adelaide Press.

Byrou, S., & others (2018). Fast temperature-gradient COLD PCR for the enrichment of the paternally inherited SNPs in cell free fetal DNA: An application to non-invasive prenatal diagnosis of β-thalassaemia. *PLos ONE, 13*(7), e0200348.

C

Cabral, M., & others (2017). Maternal smoking: A life course blood pressure determinant? *Nicotine and Tobacco Research, 20,* 674-680.

Cabrera, N.J., Volling, B.L., & Barr, R. (2018). Fathers are parents, too! Widening the lens on parenting for children's development. *Child Development Perspectives, 12*, 152-157.

Caldwell, S. (2013). *Statistics unplugged* (4th ed.). Boston: Cengage.

Calkins, S.D. (2012). Regulatory competence and early disruptive behavior problems: Role of physiological regulation. In S. L. Olson & A. J. Sameroff (Eds.), *Biopsychosocial regulatory processes in the development of childhood behavioral problems.* New York: Cambridge University Press.

Callaghan, T., & Corbit, J. (2018). Early prosocial development across cultures. *Current Opinion in Psychology, 20*, 102-106.

Calvert, S.L., Bond, B.J., & Staiano, A.E. (2013). Electronic game changers for the obesity crisis. In F. Blumberg (Ed.), *Learning by playing: Frontiers of video gaming in education.* New York: Oxford University Press.

Calvert, S.L., & others (2017). The American Psychological Association Task Force assessment of violent video games: Science in the service of public interest. *American Psychologist, 72*(2), 126-143.

Calvert, S.L., & Valkenburg, P.M. (2013). The influence of television, video games, and the Internet on children's creativity. In M. Taylor (Ed.), *Handbook of the development of imagination.* New York: Oxford University Press.

Calvert, S.L., Bond, B.J., & Staiano, A.E. (2014). Electronic game changers for the obesity crisis. In F. Blumberg (Ed.), *Learning by playing: Frontiers of video gaming in education.* New York: Oxford University Press.

Camodeca, M., & Taraschi, E. (2015). Like father, like son? The link between parents' moral disengagement and children's externalizing behaviors. *Merrill-Palmer Quarterly, 61*(1), 173-191.

Camos, V., & Barrouillet, P. (2018). *Working memory in development.* London: Routledge.

Camos, V., & others (2018). What is attentional refreshing in working memory? *Annals of the New York Academy of Sciences.* doi:142410.1111/nyas.13616

Campagne, D.M. (2018). Antidepressant use in pregnancy: Are we closer to consensus? *Archives of Women's Mental Health,* 1-9.

Campbell-Voytal, K., & others (2017). Evaluation of an evidence-based weight loss trial for urban African American adolescents and caregivers. *Journal of Nutrition and Health, 3*(2), 6.

Campbell, K.L., & others (2018). Factors in the home environment associated with toddler diet: An ecological momentary assessment study. *Public Health Nutrition, 21*, 1855-1864.

Campbell, L., Campbell, B., & Dickinson, D. (2004). *Teaching and learning through multiple intelligences* (3rd ed.). Boston: Allyn & Bacon.

Campione-Barr, N., Bassett- Greer, K., & Kruse, A. (2013). Differential associations domain of sibling conflict and adolescent emotional development. *Child Development, 84*(3), 938-954.

Campolong, K., & others (2018). The association of exercise during pregnancy with trimester-specific and postpartum quality of life and depressive symptoms in a cohort of healthy pregnant women. *Archives of Women's Mental Health, 21*(2), 215-224.

Campos, J.J. (2005). Unpublished review of J. W. Santrock's *Life-span development,* 11th ed. (New York: McGraw-Hill).

Campos, J.J. (2009). Unpublished review of J. W. Santrock's *Life-span development,* 13th ed. (New York: McGraw-Hill).

Campos, J.J., Langer, A., & Krowitz, A. (1970). Cardiac responses on the visual cliff in prelocomotor human infants. *Science, 170,* 196-197.

Camras, L.A., & Halberstadt, A.G. (2017). Emotional development through the lens of affective social competence. *Current Opinion in Psychology, 17,* 113-117.

Capaldi, D.M. (2013). Parental monitoring: A person-environment interaction perspective on this key parenting skill. In A. C. Crouter & A. Booth (Eds.), *Children's influence on family dynamics.* New York: Routledge.

Capogna, G., Camorcia, M., Coccoluto, A., Micaglio, M., & Velardo, M. (2018). Experimental validation of the CompuFlo® Epidural Controlled System to identify the epidural space and its clinical use in difficult obstetric cases. *International Journal of Obstetric Anesthesia, 36,* 28-33.

Caprara, G.V., Kanacri, B.P.L., Zuffianò, A., Gerbino, M., & Pastorelli, C. (2015). Why and how to promote adolescents' prosocial behaviors: Direct, mediated and moderated effects of the CEPIDEA school-based program. *Journal of Youth and Adolescence, 44*(12), 2211-2229.

Cardelle-Elawar, M. (1992). Effects of teaching metacognitive skills to students with low mathematics ability. *Teaching and Teacher Education, 8*(2), 109-121.

Carey, S. (1977). The child as word learner. In M. Halle, J. Bresman, & G. Miller (Eds.), *Linguistic theory and psychological reality.* Cambridge, MA: MIT Press.

Carl, J.D. (2012). *Short introduction to the U.S. Census.* Upper Saddle River, NJ: Pearson.

Carlin, C., Davis, E.E., Krafft, C., & Tout, K. (2019, in press). Parental preferences and patterns of child care use among low-income families: A Bayesian analysis. *Children and Youth Services Review.*

Carlo, G., & others (2018). Longitudinal relations among parenting styles, prosocial behaviors, and academic outcomes in U.S. Mexican adolescents. *Child Development, 89*(2), 577-592.

Carlo, G., Knight, G.P., McGinley, M., Zamboanga, B.L., & Jarvis, L.H. (2010). The multidimensionality of prosocial behaviors and evidence of measurement equivalence in Mexican American and European American early adolescents. *Journal of Research on Adolescence, 20,* 334-358.

Carlo, G., Mestre, M.V., Samper, P., Tur, A., & Armenta, B.E. (2011). The longitudinal relations among dimensions of parenting styles, sympathy, prosocial moral reasoning, and prosocial behaviors. *International Journal of Behavioral Development, 35,* 116-124.

Carlson, M.J., Pilkauskas, N.V., McLanahan, S.S., & Brooks-Gunn, J. (2011). Couples as partners and parents over children's early years. *Journal of Marriage and the Family, 73,* 317-334.

Carlson, M.J., & Van Orman, A.G. (2017). Trajectories of relationship supportiveness after childbirth: Does marriage matter? *Social Science Research, 66,* 102-117.

Carlson, S.M., & White, R. (2013). Executive function and imagination. In M. Taylor (Ed.), *Handbook of imagination.* New York: Oxford University Press.

Carlson, S.M., Zelazo, P.D., & Faja, S. (2013). Executive function. In P. D. Zelazo (Ed.), *Oxford handbook of developmental psychology.* New York: Oxford University Press.

Carlucci, L., D'Ambrosio, I., Innamorati, M., Saggino, A., & Balsamo, M. (2018). Co-rumination, anxiety, and maladaptive cognitive schemas: When friendship can hurt. *Psychology Research and Behavior Management, 11,* 133-144.

Carmina, E., Stanczyk, F.Z., & Lobo, R.A. (2019, in press). In J. Strauss & R. Barbieri (Eds.), *Yen and Jaffe's reproductive endocrinology* (8th ed., pp. 887-914). Amsterdam, The Netherlands: Elsevier.

Carnegie Council on Adolescent Development. (1995). *Great transitions.* New York: Carnegie Foundation.

Carpendale, J.I., & Lewis, C. (2015). The development of social understanding. In W. Damon (Ed.), *Handbook of child psychology and developmental science* (7th ed.). New York: Wiley.

Carpenter, M. (2011). Social cognition and social motivations in infancy. In U. Goswami (Ed.), *Wiley-Blackwell handbook of childhood cognitive development* (2nd ed.). New York: Wiley.

Carrascosa-Romero, M.C., & De Cabo-De La Vega, C. (2017). The genetic and epigenetic basis involved in the pathophysiology of ASD: Therapeutic implications. In M. Fitzgerald & J. Yip (Eds.), *Autism: Paradigms, recent research and clinical applications.* London: IntechOpen.

Carskadon, M.A. (2005). Sleep and circadian rhythms in children and adolescents: Relevance for athletic performance of young people. *Clinical Sports Medicine, 24,* 319-328.

Carsley, D., Khoury, B., & Heath, N.L. (2018). Effectiveness of mindfulness interventions for mental health in schools: A comprehensive meta-analysis. *Mindfulness, 9*(3), 693-707.

Cartwright, R., Agargun, M.Y., Kirkby, J., & Friedman, J.K. (2006). Relation of dreams to waking concerns. *Psychiatry Research, 141,* 261-270.

Cascio, E.U. (2017). *Does universal preschool hit the target? Program access and preschool impacts.* NBER Working Paper No. 23215.

Case, R., Kurland, D.M., & Goldberg, J. (1982). Operational efficiency and the growth of short-term memory span. *Journal of Experimental Child Psychology, 33,* 386-404.

Cashon, C.H., Ha, O.R., Estes, K.G., Saffran, J.R., & Mervis, C.B. (2016). Infants with Williams syndrome detect statistical regularities in continuous speech. *Cognition, 154,* 165-168.

Casper, D.M., & Card, N.A. (2017). Overt and relational victimization: A meta-analytic review of their overlap and associations with social-psychological adjustment. *Child Development, 88,* 466-483.

Caspi, A., & others. (2003). Influence of life stress on depression: Moderation by a polymorphism in the 5-HTT gene. *Science, 301,* 386-389.

Cassoff, J., Knauper, B., Michaelsen, S., & Gruber, R. (2013). School-based sleep promotion programs: Effectiveness, feasibility, and insights for future research. *Sleep Medicine Reviews, 17*(3), 207-214.

Castillo-Gualda, R., & others (2018). A three-year emotional intelligence intervention to reduce adolescent aggression: The mediating role of unpleasant affectivity. *Journal of Research on Adolescence, 28,* 186-198.

Castle, J., & others (2010). Parents' evaluation of adoption success: A follow-up study of intercountry and domestic adoptions. *American Journal of Orthopsychiatry, 79,* 522-531.

Caughey, A.B., Hopkins, L.M., & Norton, M.E. (2006). Chorionic villus sampling compared with amniocentesis and the difference in the rate of pregnancy loss. *Obstetrics and Gynecology, 108,* 612-616.

Causadias, J.M., & Umaña-Taylor, A.J. (2018). Reframing marginalization and youth development: Introduction to the special issue. *American Psychologist, 73*(6), 707.

Cavanagh, S.E. (2009). Puberty. In D. Carr (Ed.), *Encyclopedia of the life course and human development.* Boston: Gale Cengage.

Cavanaugh, A.M., Stein, G.L., Supple, A.J., Gonzalez, L.M., & Kiang, L. (2018). Protective and promotive effects of Latino early adolescents' cultural assets against multiple types of discrimination. *Journal of Research on Adolescence, 28*(2), 310-326.

Cave, R.K. (2002, August). *Early adolescent language: A content analysis of child development and educational psychology textbooks.* Unpublished doctoral dissertation. University of Nevada-Reno, Reno, NV.

Caye, A., Swanson, J.M., Coghill, D., & Rohde, L.A. (2019). Treatment strategies for ADHD: An evidence-based guide to select optimal treatment. *Molecular Psychiatry, 24,* 390-408.

Caylak, E. (2012). Biochemical and genetic analyses of childhood attention deficit/hyperactivity disorder. *American Journal of Medical Genetics B: Neuropsychiatric Genetics, 159*(6), 613-627.

Ceci, S., Hritz, A., & Royer, C. (2016). Understanding suggestibility. In W. O'Donohue & M. Fanetti (Eds.), *Forensic interviews regarding child sexual abuse.* New York: Springer.

Center for Science in the Public Interest. (2008, August). *Kids' meals: Obesity on the menu.* Washington, DC: Author.

Centers for Disease Control and Prevention. (2006, December). *Assisted reproductive success rates.* Atlanta: Author.

Centers for Disease Control and Prevention (2016). *10 leading causes of death by age group, United States - 2016.* Retrieved from https://www.cdc.gov/injury/wisqars/pdf/leading_causes_of_death_by_age_group_2016-508.pdf

Centers for Disease Control and Prevention (2018). *Breastfeeding.* Retrieved from https://www.cdc.gov/breastfeeding/data/facts.html

Centers for Disease Control and Prevention (2018). *Child health.* Retrieved from https://www.cdc.gov/nchs/fastats/child-health.htm

Centers for Disease Control and Prevention (2018). *Defining childhood obesity.* Retrieved from https://www.cdc.gov/obesity/childhood/defining.html

Centers for Disease Control and Prevention (2018). *Lead.* Retrieved from https://www.cdc.gov/nceh/lead/default.htm

Centers for Disease Control and Prevention (2018). *Middle childhood.* Retrieved from https://www.cdc.gov/ncbddd/childdevelopment/positiveparenting/middle.html

Centers for Disease Control and Prevention (2018). Prevalence of autism spectrum disorder among children aged 8 years—Autism and Developmental Disabilities Monitoring Network, 11 sites, United States, 2014. *Surveillance Summaries, 67*(6), 1-23.

Chaillet, N., & others (2014). Nonpharmacologic approaches for pain management during labor compared with usual care: A meta-analysis. *Birth, 41*(2), 122-137.

Chall, J.S. (1979). The great debate: Ten years later with a modest proposal for reading stages. In L. B. Resnick & P. A. Weaver (Eds.), *Theory and practice of early reading.* Hillsdale. NJ: Erlbaum.

Chan, G.J., & others (2016). Kangaroo mother care: A systematic review of barriers and enablers. *Bulletin of the World Health Organization, 94,* 130-141.

Chan, H.Y., Brown, B.B., & Von Bank, H. (2015). Adolescent disclosure of information about peers: The mediating role of perceptions of parents' right to know. *Journal of Youth & Adolescence, 44*(5), 1048-1065.

Chang, H., Shaw, D.S., Dishion, T.J., Gardner, F., & Wilson, M.N. (2015). Proactive parenting and children's effortful control: Mediating role of language and indirect intervention effects. *Social Development, 24*(1), 206-223.

Chang, M., & Gu, X. (2018). The role of executive function in linking fundamental motor skills and reading proficiency in socioeconomically disadvantaged kindergarteners. *Learning and Individual Differences, 61,* 250-255.

Chang, Y.H.A., & Lane, D.M. (2018). It takes more than practice and experience to become a chess master: Evidence from a child prodigy and adult chess players. *Journal of Expertise, 1*(1).

Chang, Z., Lichtenstein, P., Asherson, P.J., & Larsson, H. (2013). Developmental twin study of attention problems: High heritabilities throughout development. *JAMA Psychiatry, 70*(3), 311-318.

Chansakul, T., & Young, G.S. (2017, December). Neuroimaging in pregnant women. *Seminars in Neurology 37*(6), 712-723.

Chao, R.K., & Otsuki-Clutter, M. (2011). Racial and ethnic differences: Sociocultural and contextual explanations. *Journal of Research on Adolescence, 21,* 47-60.

Chao, R., & Tseng, V. (2002). Parenting of Asians. In M. H. Bornstein (Ed.), *Handbook of parenting.* Mahwah, NJ: Erlbaum.

Chao, R. (2001). Extending research on the consequences of parenting style for Chinese Americans and European Americans. *Child Development, 72,* 1832-1843.

Chaplin, T.M., & Aldao, A. (2013). Gender differences in emotion expression in children: A meta-analytic review. *Psychological Bulletin, 139,* 735-765.

Chaplin, T.M. (2015). Gender and emotion expression: A developmental contextual perspective. *Emotion Review, 7,* 14-21.

Charles, C. (2018). Water for labor and birth. In V. Chapman & C. Charles (Eds.), *The midwife's labor and birth handbook* (4th ed.). New York: Wiley.

Charlesworth, B., & Charlesworth, D. (2017). Population genetics from 1966 to 2016. *Heredity, 118,* 2-9.

Chassin, L., & others (2008). Multiple trajectories of cigarette smoking and the intergenerational transmission of smoking: A multigenerational, longitudinal study of a midwestern community sample. *Health Psychology, 27,* 819-828.

Chaudry, A., & others (2017). *Cradle to kindergarten: A new plan to combat inequality.* New York: Russell Sage Foundation.

Chavez, B. (2019). *Immigration and language in Canada, 2011 and 2016.* Ottawa, ON: Statistics Canada.

Chemtob, C.M., & others (2010). Impact of maternal posttraumatic stress disorder and depression following exposure to the September 11 attacks on preschool children's behavior. *Child Development, 81,* 1129-1141.

Chen, C., & Stevenson, H.W. (1989). Homework: A cross-cultural examination. *Child Development, 60,* 551-561.

Chen, F.R., Rothman, E.F., & Jaffee, S.R. (2017). Early puberty, friendship group characteristics, and dating abuse in US girls. *Pediatrics, 139,* e20162847.

Chen, F.R., Rothman, E.F., & Jaffee, S.R. (2017). Early puberty, friendship group characteristics, and dating abuse in US girls. *Pediatrics, 139*(6), e20162847.

Chen, G., Zhang, W., Zhang, W., & Deater-Deckard, K. (2017). A "Defender Protective Effect" in multiple-role combinations of bullying among Chinese adolescents. *Journal of Interpersonal Violence.* doi:10.1177/0886260517698278

Chen, G., Zhao, Q., Dishion, T., & Deater-Deckard, K. (2018). The association between peer network centrality and aggression is moderated by moral disengagement. *Aggressive Behavior, 44,* 571-580.

Chen, J.-Q., & Gardner, H. (2018). Assessment from the perspective of multiple-intelligences theory: Principles, practices, and values. In D.P. Flanagan & E.M. McDonough (Eds.), *Contemporary intellectual assessment: Theories, tests, and issues* (4th ed.). New York: Guilford.

Chen, J., Sperandio, I., & Goodale, M.A. (2018). Proprioceptive distance cues restore perfect size constancy in grasping, but not perception, when vision is limited. *Current Biology, 28*(6), 927–932.

Chen, K.M., White, K., Shabbeer, J., & Schmid, M. (2018). Maternal age trends support uptake of non-invasive prenatal testing (NIPT) in the low-risk population. *The Journal of Maternal-Fetal & Neonatal Medicine, 20*, 1–4.

Chen, S.C., & Chen, C.F. (2018). Antecedents and consequences of nurses' burnout: Leadership effectiveness and emotional intelligence as moderators. *Management Decision, 56*, 777–792.

Chen, W.Y., Corvo, K., Lee, Y., & Hahm, H.C. (2017). Longitudinal trajectory of adolescent exposure to community violence and depressive symptoms among adolescents and young adults: Understanding the effect of mental health service usage. *Community Mental Health Journal, 53*, 39–52.

Chen, X., & Graham, S. (2018). Doing better but feeling worse: An attributional account of achievement–self-esteem disparities in Asian American students. *Social Psychology of Education, 21*, 937–949.

Chen, X., & others (1998). Childrearing attitudes and behavioral inhibition in Chinese and Canadian toddlers: A cross-cultural study. *Developmental Psychology, 34*, 677–686.

Chen, X., Chung, J., Lechccier-Kimel, R., & French, D. (2011). Culture and social development. In P. K. Smith & C. H. Hart (Eds.), *Wiley-Blackwell perspectives on childhood social development* (2nd ed.). New York: Wiley.

Chen, X. (2018). Culture, temperament, and social and psychological adjustment. *Developmental Review, 50*, 42–53.

Chen, Y., & VanderWeele, T.J. (2018). Associations of religious upbringing with subsequent health and well-being from adolescence to young adulthood: An outcome-wide analysis. *American Journal of Epidemiology, 187*(11), 2355–2364.

Chen, Y., Keen, R., Rosancer, K., & von Hosten, C. (2010). Movement planning reflects skill level and age change in toddlers. *Child Development, 81*, 1846–1858.

Cheng, M., & Berman, S.L. (2013). Globalization and identity development: A Chinese perspective. In S. J. Schwartz (Ed.), *Identity around the world: New directions for child and adolescent development.* San Francisco: Jossey-Bass.

Cheng, S., & others (2010). Early television exposure and children's behavioral and social outcomes at age 30 months. *Journal of Epidemiology* (Suppl. 2), S482–S489.

Cherlin, A.J., & Furstenberg, F.F. (1994). Stepfamilies in the United States: A reconsideration. In J. Blake & J. Hagen (Eds.), *Annual Review of Sociology.* Palo Alto, CA: Annual Reviews.

Cheshire, E., Kaestle, C.E., & Miyazaki, Y. (2019). The influence of parent and parent–adolescent relationship characteristics on sexual trajectories into adulthood. *Archives of Sexual Behavior, 48*(3), 893–910.

Chess, S., & Thomas, A. (1977). Temperamental individuality from childhood to adolescence. *Journal of Child Psychiatry, 16*, 218–226.

Cheung, C.S., Pomerantz, E.M., & Dong, W. (2013). Does adolescents' disclosure to their parents matter for their academic adjustment? *Child Development.*

Cheung, C., & Pomerantz, E.M. (2012). Why does parental involvement in children's learning enhance children's achievement? The role of parent-oriented motivation. *Journal of Educational Psychology, 104,* 820–832.

Chi, M.T. (1978). Knowledge structures and memory development. In R. S. Siegler (Ed.), *Children's thinking: What develops?* Hillsdale, NJ: Erlbaum.

Child Care Aware (2018). 2018 fact sheet. Retrieved from http://usa.childcareaware.org/wp-content/uploads/2018/08/2018-state-fact-sheets.pdf

Child Welfare Information Gateway (2016). *Definitions of child abuse and neglect.* Washington, DC: U.S. Department of Health and Human Services, Children's Bureau.

Children's Defense Fund. (1992). *The state of America's children, 1992.* Washington, DC: Author.

Children's Defense Fund (2017). *The state of America's children, 2017.* Washington, DC: Author.

Chilosi, A.M., & others (2019). Hemispheric language organization after congenital left brain lesions: A comparison between functional transcranial Doppler and functional MRI. *Journal of Neuropsychology, 13*(1), 46–66.

Chimiklis, A.L., & others (2018). Yoga, mindfulness, and meditation interventions for youth with ADHD: Systematic review and meta-analysis. *Journal of Child and Family Studies, 27*, 3155–3168.

Chitty, L.S., & others. (2013). Safe, accurate, prenatal diagnosis of thanatophoric dysplasia using ultrasound and free fetal DNA. *Prenatal Diagnosis, 33*(5), 416–423.

Choi, N. (2004). Sex role group differences in specific, academic, and general self-efficacy. *Journal of Psychology, 138*, 149–159.

Choi, S.J. (2017). Use of progesterone supplement therapy for prevention of preterm birth: Review of literatures. *Obstetrics & Gynecology Science, 60*(5), 405–420.

Choi, Y., Kim, T.Y., Noh, S., Lee, J., & Takeuchi, D. (2018). Culture and family process: Measures of familism for Filipino and Korean American parents. *Family Process, 57*(4), 1029–1048.

Chomsky, N. (1957). *Syntactic structures.* The Hague: Mouton.

Chou, R.S., & Feagin, J.R. (2015). *Myth of the model minority: Asian Americans facing racism.* London: Routledge.

Choudhuri, S., & Basu, J. (2013). Rational versus intuitive reasoning in moral judgement: A review of current research trends and new directions. *Journal of the Indian Academy of Applied Psychology, 39*(2), 164.

Chow, J., Aimola Davies, A.M., Fuentes, L.J., & Plunkett, K. (2019, in press). The vocabulary spurt predicts the emergence of backward semantic inhibition in 18-month-old toddlers. *Developmental Science, 22*(2): e12754. doi:10.1111/desc.12754

Choy, O., Raine, A., Venables, P.H., & Farrington, D.P. (2017). Explaining the gender gap in crime: The role of heart rate. *Criminology, 55*(2), 465–487.

Christakis, D.A., Zimmerman, F.J., DiGiuseppe, D.L., & McCarty, C.A. (2004). Early television exposure and subsequent attentional problems in children. *Pediatrics, 113,* 708–713.

Christakis, D.A., Ramirez, J.S.B., Ferguson, S.M., Ravinder, S., & Ramirez, J.M. (2018). How early media exposure may affect cognitive function: A review of results from observations in humans and experiments in mice. *Proceedings of the National Academy of Sciences, 115*(40), 9851–9858.

Christakis, D.A., & others. (2009). Audible television and decreased adult words, infant vocalizations, and conversational turns. *Archives of Pediatrics & Adolescent Medicine, 163,* 554–558.

Christen, M., Narváez, D., & Gutzwiller, E. (2017). Comparing and integrating biological and cultural moral progress. *Ethical Theory and Moral Practice, 20*(1), 55–73.

Christenfeld, N.J.S., & Mandler, G. (2013). Emotion. In I. B. Weiner & others (Eds.), *Handbook of psychology* (2nd ed., Vol. 1). New York: Wiley.

Chu, C.H., & others (2017). Acute exercise and neurocognitive development in preadolescents and young adults: An ERP study. *Neural Plasticity, 2017,* 2631909.

Chudley A.E. (2017). Teratogenic influences on cerebellar development. In H. Marzban (Ed.), *Development of the cerebellum from molecular aspects to diseases* (pp. 275–300). New York: Springer.

Chudzicka-Czupała, A., & others (2016). Application of the theory of planned behavior in academic cheating research: Cross-cultural comparison. *Ethics & Behavior, 26*(8), 638–659.

Chung, S., & McBride, A.M. (2015). Social and emotional learning in middle school curricula: A service learning model based on positive youth development. *Children and Youth Services Review, 53,* 192–200.

Cicchetti, D. (2011). Pathways to resilient functioning in maltreated children: From single to multilevel investigations. In D. Cicchetti & G. I. Roisman (Eds.), *The origins and organization of adaptation and maladaptation: Minnesota Symposia on Child Psychology* (Vol. 36). New York: Wiley.

Cicchetti, D. (2013). Developmental psychopathology. In P. Zelazo (Ed.), *Oxford handbook of developmental psychology.* New York: Oxford University Press.

Cicchetti, D., & Toth, S.L. (2011). Child maltreatment: The research imperative and the exportation of results to clinical contexts. In B. Lester & J. D. Sparrow (Eds.), *Nurturing children and families.* New York: Wiley.

Cicchetti, D., Toth, S.L., Nilsen, W.J., & Manly, J.T. (2013). What do we know and why does it matter? The dissemination of evidence-based interventions for maltreatment. In H. R. Schaffer & K. Durkin (Eds.), *Blackwell handbook of developmental psychology.* Oxford, UK: Blackwell.

Cillessen, A.H.N., & Bellmore, A.D. (2011). Social skills and social competence in interactions with peers. In P. K. Smith & C. H. Hart (Eds.), *Wiley-Blackwell handbook of childhood social development* (2nd ed.). New York: Wiley.

Cillessen, A.H.N., & van den Berg, Y.H.M. (2012). Popularity and school adjustment. In A. M. Ryan & G. W. Ladd (Eds.), *Peer relationships and adjustment at school.* Charlotte, NC: Information Age Publishing.

Cipra, A. (2019). Differential susceptibility and kindergarten peer status. *Child Indicators Research, 12*(2), 689-709.

Clark, E. (1993). *The lexicon in acquisition.* New York: Cambridge University Press.

Clarke, K., Cover, R., & Aggleton, P. (2018). Sex and ambivalence: LGBTQ youth negotiating sexual feelings, desires and attractions. *Journal of LGBT Youth, 15*(3), 227-242.

Clarke, T.K., & others (2016). Common polygenic risk for autism spectrum disorder (ASD) is associated with cognitive ability in the general population. *Molecular Psychiatry, 21*(3), 419-425.

Clarke-Stewart, A.K., & Miner, J.L. (2008). Effects of child and day care. In M. M. Haith & J. B. Benson (Eds.), *Encyclopedia of infant and early childhood development.* Oxford, UK: Elsevier.

Class, Q.A., Lichtenstein, P., Langstrom, N., & D'Onofrio, B.M. (2011). Timing of prenatal maternal exposure to severe life events and adverse pregnancy outcomes: A population study of 2.6 million pregnancies. *Psychosomatic Medicine, 73*, 234-241.

Clauss, J.A., & Blackford, J.U. (2012). Behavioral inhibition and risk for developing social anxiety disorder: A meta-analytic study. *Journal of the American Academy of Child and Adolescent Psychiatry, 51*, 1066-1075.

Clawson, A.H., & others (2018). The longitudinal, bidirectional relationships between parent reports of child secondhand smoke exposure and child smoking trajectories. *Journal of Behavioral Medicine, 41*(2), 221-231.

Clay, R. (2001, February). Fulfilling an unmet need. *Monitor on Psychology,* No. 2.

Cloninger, S.C. (2018). *Theories of personality* (7th ed.). Upper Saddle River, NJ: Pearson.

Closson, L.M., Hart, N.C., & Hogg, L.D. (2017). Does the desire to conform to peers moderate links between popularity and indirect victimization in early adolescence? *Social Development, 26*(3), 489-502.

Cobanoglu, R., Capa-Aydin, Y., & Yildirim, A. (2019). Sources of teacher beliefs about developmentally appropriate practice: A structural equation model of the role of teacher efficacy beliefs. *European Early Childhood Education Research Journal, 27*, 195-207.

Cochet, H., & Byrne, R.W. (2016). Communication in the second and third year of life: Relationships between nonverbal social skills and language. *Infant Behavior and Development, 44*, 189-198.

Coelho, V.A., Marchante, M., & Jimerson, S.R. (2017). Promoting a positive middle school transition: A randomized-controlled treatment study examining self-concept and self-esteem. *Journal of Youth and Adolescence, 46*, 558-569.

CogMed (2016). *CogMed working memory training, v.4.1.* Upper Saddle River, NJ: Pearson.

Cohen, T.R., & Morse, L. (2014). Moral character: What it is and what it does. *Research in Organizational Behavior, 34*, 43-61.

Cohen-Woods, S., Craig, I.W., & McGuffin, P. (2012). The current state of play on the molecular genetics of depression. *Psychological Medicine, 43*(4), 673-687.

Cohn, A., & Canter, A. (2003). *Bullying: Facts for schools and parents.* Washington, DC: National Association of School Psychologists Center.

Cohn, J.F., & Tronick, E.Z. (1988). Mother-infant face-to-face interaction. Influence is bidirectional and unrelated to periodic cycles in either partner's behavior. *Developmental Psychology, 24*, 396-397.

Coie, J. (2004). The impact of negative social experiences on the development of antisocial behavior. In J. B. Kupersmidt & K. A. Dodge (Eds.), *Children's peer relations: From development to intervention.* Washington, DC: American Psychological Association.

Colapinto, J. (2000). *As nature made him.* New York: Simon & Schuster.

Colby, A., Kohlberg, L., Gibbs, J., & Lieberman, M. (1983). A longitudinal study of moral judgment. *Monographs of the Society for Research in Child Development, 48* (21, Serial No. 201).

Cole, P.M., Dennis, T.A., Smith-Simon, K.E., & Cohen, L.H. (2009). Preschoolers' emotion regulation strategy understanding: Relations with emotion socialization and child self-regulation. *Social Development, 18*(2), 324-352.

Cole, P.M., & Tan, P.Z. (2007). Emotion socialization from a cultural perspective. In J. E. Grusec & P. D. Hastings (Eds.), *Handbook of socialization.* New York: Guilford.

Cole, P.M., & Jacobs, A.E. (2018). From children's expressive control to emotion regulation: Looking back, looking ahead. *European Journal of Developmental Psychology, 15*, 658-677.

Coleman-Phox, Odouli, R., & Li, D.K. (2008). Use of a fan during sleep and the risk of sudden infant death syndrome. *Archives of Pediatric and Adolescent Medicine, 162*, 963-968.

Coley, R.L., & Lombardi, C.M. (2013). Does maternal employment following childbirth support or inhibit low-income children's long-term development? *Child Development, 84*(1), 178-197.

Coley, R.L., Votruba-Drzal, E., Miller, P.L., & Koury, A. (2013). Timing, extent, and type of child care and children's functioning in kindergarten. *Developmental Psychology, 49*(10), 1859-1873.

Coley, R.L., Sims, J., Dearing, E., & Spielvogel, B. (2018). Locating economic risks for adolescent mental and behavioral health: Poverty and affluence in families, neighborhoods, and schools. *Child Development, 89*(2), 360-369.

Collett-Solberg, P.F. (2011). Update in growth hormone therapy of children. *Journal of Clinical Endocrinology and Metabolism, 96*, 573-579.

Collibee, C., Furman, W., & Shoop, J. (2019). Risky interactions: Relational and developmental moderators of substance use and dating aggression. *Journal of Youth and Adolescence, 48*(1), 102-113.

Collier, K.M., & others (2016). Does parental mediation of media influence child outcomes? A meta-analysis on media time, aggression, substance use, and sexual behavior. *Developmental Psychology, 52*(5), 798-812.

Colombo, J., Brez, C., & Curtindale, L. (2013). Infant perception and cognition. In I. B. Weiner & others (Eds.), *Handbook of psychology* (2nd ed., Vol. 6). New York: Wiley.

Colombo, J., Shaddy, D.J., Blaga, O.M., Anderson, C.J., & Kannass, K.N. (2009). High cognitive ability in infancy and early childhood. In F. D. Horowitz, R. F. Subotnik, & D. J. Matthews (Eds.), *The development of giftedness and talent across the life span.* Washington, DC: American Psychological Association.

Colombo, J., Shaddy, D.J., Richman, W.A., Maikranz, J.M., & Blaga, O.M. (2004). The developmental course of attention in infancy and preschool cognitive outcome. *Infancy, 4*, 1-38.

Colvin, C.W., & Abdullatif, H. (2012). Anatomy of female puberty: The clinical relevance of developmental changes in the reproductive system. *Clinical Anatomy, 26*(1), 115-129.

Comeau, G., Lu, Y., Swirp, M., & Mielke, S. (2018). Measuring the musical skills of a prodigy: A case study. *Intelligence, 66*, 84-97.

Comeau, J., & Boyle, M.H. (2018). Patterns of poverty exposure and children's trajectories of externalizing and internalizing behaviors. *SSM-Population Health, 4*, 86-94.

Comer, J. (2010). Comer School Development Program. In J. Meece & J. Eccles (Eds.), *Handbook of research on schools, schooling, and human development.* New York: Routledge.

Common Core State Standards Initiative (2019). *Common Core.* Retrieved from www.corestandards.org/

Commoner, B. (2002). Unraveling the DNA myth: The spurious foundation of genetic engineering. *Harper's Magazine, 304*, 39-47.

Comstock, G., & Scharrer, E. (2006). Media and popular culture. In W. Damon & R. Lerner (Eds.), *Handbook of child psychology* (6th ed.). New York: Wiley.

Conde-Agudelo, A., & Diaz-Rossello, J. (2016). Kangaroo mother care to reduce morbidity and mortality in low birthweight infants. *Cochrane Database of Systematic Reviews, 2016*(8).

Condition of Education (2018). *Children and youth with disabilities.* Washington, DC: National Center for Education Statistics.

Conduct Problems Prevention Research Group (2011). The effects of the Fast Track preventive intervention on the development of conduct disorder across childhood. *Child Development, 82*(1), 331-345.

Conduct Problems Prevention Research Group (2013). School outcomes of aggressive disruptive children: Prediction from kindergarten risk factors and impact of the Fast Track prevention program. *Aggressive Behavior, 39*, 114-130.

Cong, X., Ludington-Hoe, S.M., & Walsh, S. (2011). Randomized crossover trial of kangaroo care to reduce biobehavioral pain responses in preterm infants: A pilot study. *Biological Research for Nursing, 13*, 204-216.

Congdon, J.L., & others (2016). A prospective investigation of prenatal mood and childbirth perceptions in an ethnically diverse, low-income sample. *Birth, 43*(2), 159-166.

Conger, R.D., & others. (2012). Resilience and vulnerability of Mexican origin youth and their families: A test of a culturally-informed model of family economic stress. In P. K. Kerig, M. S. Schulz, & S. T. Hauser (Eds.), *Adolescence and beyond.* New York: Oxford University Press.

Conley, M.W. (2008). *Content area literacy: learners in context.* Boston: Allyn & Bacon.

Connolly, J.A., & Mclsaac, C. (2009). Romantic relationships in adolescence. In R. M. Lerner & L. Steinberg (Eds.), *Handbook of adolescent psychology* (3rd ed.). New York: Wiley.

Conry-Murray, C., Kim, J.M., & Turiel, E. (2015). Judgments of gender norm violations in children from the United States and Korea. *Cognitive Development, 35,* 122–136.

Contini, C., & others (2018). Investigation on silent bacterial infections in specimens from pregnant women affected by spontaneous miscarriage. *Journal of Cellular Physiology, 234*(1).

Cools, S., Fiva, J.H., & Kirkebøen, L.J. (2015). Causal effects of paternity leave on children and parents. *The Scandinavian Journal of Economics, 117*(3), 801–828.

Cooper, C.R. (2011). *Bridging multiple worlds.* New York: Oxford University Press.

Cooper, C.R., & Seginer, R. (2018). Introduction: Navigating pathways in multicultural nations: Identities, future orientation, schooling, and careers. *New Directions for Child and Adolescent Development, 2018*(160), 7–13.

Cooper, K., & Stewart, K. (2017). *Does money affect children's outcomes? An update.* CASEpaper no. 203. London: Centre for Analysis of Social Exclusion. Retrieved August 24, 2018 from http://sticerd.lse.ac.uk/dps/case/cp/casepaper203.pdf

Copes, L.E., Pober, B.R., & Terilli, C.A. (2016). Description of common musculoskeletal findings in Williams syndrome and implications for therapies. *Clinical Anatomy, 29,* 578–589.

Coppens, A.D., Alcalá, L., Rogoff, B., & Mejía-Arauz, R. (2018). Children's contributions in family work: Two cultural paradigms. In T. Skelton, S. Punch, & R. Vanderbeck (Eds.), *Families, intergenerationality, and peer group relations.* Singapore: Springer.

Corbetta, D., & Fagard, J. (2017). Infants' understanding and production of goal-directed actions in the context of social and object-related interactions. *Frontiers in Psychology, 8,* 787.

Corbetta, D., Wiener, R.F., Thurman, S.L., & McMahon, E. (2018). The embodied origins of infant reaching: Implications for the emergence of eye-hand coordination. *Kinesiology Review, 7*(1), 10–17.

Cornew, L., & others (2012). Atypical social referencing in infant siblings of children with autism spectrum disorders. *Journal of Autism and Developmental Disorders, 42*(12), 2611–2621.

Correa-Chavez, M., Mangione, H.F., & Mejía-Arauz, R. (2016). Collaboration patterns among Mexican children in an indigenous town and Mexican city. *Journal of Applied Developmental Psychology, 44,* 105–113.

Corsaro, W.A. (2018). *The sociology of childhood* (5th ed.). Thousand Oaks, CA: SAGE.

Cortes, R.A., Weinberger, A.B., Daker, R.J., & Green, A.E. (2019). Re-examining prominent measures of divergent and convergent creativity. *Current Opinion in Behavioral Sciences, 27,* 90–93.

Cortese, S., & others (2018). Comparative efficacy and tolerability of medications for attention-deficit hyperactivity disorder in children, adolescents, and adults: A systematic review and network meta-analysis. The Lancet, 5, 727–738.

Corwin, M.J. (2018). *Patient education: Sudden infant death syndrome.* Retrieved from https://www.uptodate.com/contents/sudden-infant-death-syndrome-sids-beyond-the-basics

Cosmides, L. (2013). Evolutionary psychology. *Annual Review of Psychology* (Vol. 64). Palo Alto, CA: Annual Reviews.

Costigan, S.A., Barnett, L., Plotnikoff, R.C., & Lubans, D.R. (2013). The health indicators associated with screen-based sedentary behavior among adolescent girls: A systematic review. *Journal of Adolescent Health, 52,* 382–392.

Cowan, C.P., Cowan, P.A., & Barry, J. (2011). Couples' groups for parents of preschoolers: Ten-year outcomes of a randomized trial. *Journal of Family Psychology, 25,* 240–250.

Cowan, P.A., & Cowan, C.P. (2000). *When partners become parents: The big life change for couples.* Mahwah, NJ: Erlbaum.

Cowan, P.A., & Cowan, C.P. (2009). How working with couples fosters children's development. In M. S. Schulz, P. K. Kerig, M. K. Pruett, & R. D. Parke (Eds.), *Feathering the nest.* Washington, DC: American Psychological Association.

Cowan, P.A., & Heming, G. (2013). How children and parents fare during transition to school. In P. A. Cowan & others (Eds.), *The family context of parenting in children's adaptation to elementary school.* New York: Routledge.

Cowan, P.A., & others (2013). Family factors in children's adaptation to elementary school: A discussion and integration. In P. A. Cowan & others (Eds.), *The family context of parenting in children's adaptation to elementary school.* New York: Routledge.

Cowan, P.A., Cowan, C.P., Ablow, J., Johnson, V.K., & Measelle, J. (2005). *The family context of parenting in children's adaptation to elementary school.* Mahwah, NJ: Erlbaum.

Cox, M.J., & others (2004). The transition to parenting: Continuity and change in early parenting behavior and attitudes. In R. D. Conger, F. O. Lorenz, & K. A. S. Wickrama (Eds.), *Continuity and change in family relations.* Mahwah, NJ: Erlbaum.

Coyne, S.M., Linder, J.R., Rasmussen, E.E., Nelson, D.A., & Birkbeck, V. (2016). Pretty as a princess: Longitudinal effects of engagement with Disney princesses on gender stereotypes, body esteem, and prosocial behavior in children. *Child Development, 87,* 1909–1925.

Cragg, L. (2016). The development of stimulus and response interference control in mid-childhood. *Developmental Psychology, 52*(2), 242–252.

Craig, M.A., Rucker, J.M., & Richeson, J.A. (2018). The pitfalls and promise of increasing racial diversity: Threat, contact, and race relations in the 21st century. *Current Directions in Psychological Science, 27*(3), 188–193.

Crain, S. (2012). Sentence scope. In E. L. Bavin (Ed.), *Cambridge handbook of child language.* New York: Cambridge University Press.

Creswell, J.W. (2019). *Educational research* (6th ed.). Upper Saddle River, NJ: Pearson.

Crocetti, E., Jahromi, P., & Meeus, W. (2012). Identity and civic engagement in adolescence. *Journal of Adolescence, 35,* 521–532.

Crocetti, E. (2017). Identity formation in adolescence: The dynamic of forming and consolidating identity commitments. *Child Development Perspectives, 11*(2), 145–150.

Crockenberg, S.B. (1986). Are temperamental differences in babies associated with predictable differences in caregiving? In J. V. Lerner & R. M. Lerner (Eds.), *Temperament and social interaction during infancy and childhood.* San Francisco: Jossey-Bass.

Crockenberg, S., & Leerkes, E. (2013). Infant negative emotionality, caregiving, and family relationships. In A.C. Crouter & A. Booth (Eds.), *Children's influence on family dynamics.* New York: Routledge.

Crockett, L.J., Wasserman, A.M., Rudasill, K.M., Hoffman, L., & Kalutskaya, I. (2018). Temperamental anger and effortful control, teacher–child conflict, and externalizing behavior across the elementary school years. *Child Development, 89,* 2176–2195.

Crone, E.A., Peters, S., & Steinbeis, N. (2017). Executive function development in adolescence. In S. Wiebe & J. Karbach (Eds.), *Executive function: Development across the lifespan* (pp. 58–72). New York: Routledge.

Crosnoe, R., & Fuligni, A.J. (2012). Children from immigrant families: Introduction to the special section. *Child Development, 83,* 1471–1476.

Crosnoe, R., Pivnick, L., & Benner, A.D. (2018). The social contexts of high schools. In B. Schneider (Ed.), *Handbook of the sociology of education in the 21st century.* New York: Springer.

Crosnoe, R., Pivnick, L., & Benner, A.D. (2018). The social contexts of high schools. In B. Schneider (Ed.), *Handbook of the sociology of education in the 21st century.* Cham, Switzerland: Springer.

Crouter, A.C. (2006). Mothers and fathers at work. In A. Clarke-Stewart & J. Dunn (Eds.), *Families count.* New York: Cambridge University Press.

Crouter, A.C., & Booth, A. (Eds.). (2013). *Children's influence on family dynamics.* New York: Routledge.

Crowley, K., Callahan, M.A., Tenenbaum, H.R., & Allen, E. (2001). Parents explain more to boys than to girls during shared scientific thinking. *Psychological Science, 12,* 258–261.

Crowley, S.J., Wolfson, A.R., Tarokh, L., & Carskadon, M.A. (2018). An update on adolescent sleep: New evidence informing the perfect storm model. *Journal of Adolescence, 67,* 55–65.

Crugnola, C.R., & others (2013). Maternal attachment influences mother-infant styles of regulation and play with objects at nine months. *Attachment and Human Development, 15*(2), 107–131.

Cruikshank, D.R., Jenkins, D.B., & Metcalf, K.K. (2012). *The act of teaching* (6th ed.). New York: McGraw-Hill.

Cui, M., Gordon, M., & Wickrama, K.A.S. (2016). Romantic relationship experiences of adolescents and young adults: The role of mothers' relationship history. *Journal of Family Issues, 37*(10), 1458-1480.

Cui, M., Ueno, K., Fincham, F.D., Donnellan, M.B., & Wickrama, K.A. (2012). The association between romantic relationships and delinquency in adolescence and young adulthood. *Personal Relationships, 19,* 354-366.

Culpeper, J., Mackey, A., & Taguchi, N. (2018). *Second language pragmatics: From theory to research.* New York: Routledge.

Cummings, E.M., & Davies, P.T. (2010). *Marital conflict and children: An emotional security perspective.* New York: Guilford.

Cummings, E.M., El-Sheikh, M., & Kouros, C.D. (2009). Children and violence: The role of children's regulation in the marital aggression-child adjustment link. *Clinical Child and Family Psychology Review, 12*(1), 3-15.

Cummings, E.M., George, M.R.W., McCoy, K.P., & Davies, P.T. (2012). Interparental conflict in kindergarten and adolescent adjustment: Prospective investigation of emotion security as an explanatory mechanism. *Child Development, 83,* 1703-1715.

Cummings, E.M., & Kouros, C.D. (2008). Stress and coping. In M. M. Haith & J. B. Benson (Eds.), *Encyclopedia of infant and early childhood development, Vol. 3* (pp. 267-281). San Diego: Academic Press.

Curran, K., DuCette, J., Eisenstein, J., & Hyman, I.A. (2001, August). *Statistical analysis of the cross-cultural data: The third year.* Paper presented at the meeting of the American Psychological Association, San Francisco, CA.

Curtis, L.A., & Bandy, T. (2016). *The Quantum Opportunities Program: A randomized controlled evaluation.* Washington, DC: Milton S. Eisenhower Foundation.

Cushner, K.H., McClelland, A., & Safford, P. (2019). *Human diversity in education* (9th ed.). New York: McGraw-Hill.

Cvencek, D., Fryberg, S.A., Covarrubias, R., & Meltzoff, A.N. (2018). Self-concepts, self-esteem, and academic achievement of minority and majority North American elementary school children. *Child Development, 89*(4), 1099-1109.

D

D'Ardenne, K., & others. (2012). Feature article: Role of the prefrontal cortex and the midbrain dopamine system in working memory updating. *Proceedings of the National Academy of Sciences U.S.A., 109,* 19900-19909.

D'Onofrio, B.M., & others. (2007). Intergenerational transmission of childhood conduct problems: A children of twins study. *Archives of General Psychiatry, 64,* 820-829.

da Fonseca, E.B., Celik, E., & others. (2007). Progesterone and the risk of preterm birth among women with a short cervix. *New England Journal of Medicine, 357,* 462-469.

da Silva, S.G., Ricardo, L.I., Evenson, K.R., & Hallal, P.C. (2017). Leisure-time physical activity in pregnancy and maternal-child health: A systematic review and meta-analysis of randomized controlled trials and cohort studies. *Sports Medicine, 47*(2), 295-317.

Dahl, A., & Brownell, C.A. (2019). The social origins of human prosociality. *Current Directions in Psychological Science.* doi:10.1177/0963721419830386

Dahl, A., & Killen, M. (2018). Moral reasoning: Theory and research in developmental science. In S. Ghetti (Ed.), *Stevens handbook of experimental psychology* (vol. 4). New York: Wiley.

Dahl, R.E. (2004). Adolescent brain development: A period of vulnerabilities and opportunities. *Annals of the New York Academy of Sciences, 1021,* 1-22.

Dahlen, H.G., Dowling, H., Tracy, M., Schmied, V., & Tracy, S. (2013). Maternal and perinatal outcomes amongst low risk women giving birth in water compared to six birth positions on land. A descriptive cross sectional study in a birth center over 12 years. *Midwifery, 29*(7), 759-764.

Damasio, A.R. (1994). Descartes' error and the future of human life. *Scientific American, 271,* 144.

Damon, W. (1988). *The moral child.* New York: Free Press.

Damon, W. (2008). *The path to purpose.* New York: The Free Press.

Danial, F.N.M., Cade, J.E., Greenwood, D.C., & Burley, V.J. (2018). Breastfeeding is associated with the risk of ovarian cancer in the UK Women's Cohort Study. *Proceedings of the Nutrition Society, 77,* e224.

Daniels, H. (2017). *Introduction to Vygotsky* (3rd ed.). New York: Routledge.

Darling-Hammond, L. (2018). *Education and the path to one nation, indivisible.* Washington, DC: Learning Policy Institute.

Darrah.J., & Bartlett, D.J. (2013). Infant rolling abilities—the same or different 20 years after the back to sleep campaign? *Early Human Development, 89*(5), 311-314.

Darsareh, F., Nourbakhsh, S., & Dabiri, F. (2018). Effect of water immersion on labor outcomes: A randomized clinical trial. *Nursing and Midwifery Studies, 7*(3), 111-115.

Darwin, C. (1859). *On the origin of species.* London: John Murray.

Davidson, M.R., & others (2015). *Olds' maternal-newborn nursing & women's health across the lifespan* (10th ed.). Upper Saddle River, NJ: Pearson.

Davies, P.T., & others (2019, in press). Emotional insecurity as a mediator of the moderating role of dopamine genes in the association between interparental conflict and youth externalizing problems. *Development and Psychopathology.*

Davies, P.T., Martin, M.J., & Cummings, E.M. (2018). Interparental conflict and children's social problems: Insecurity and friendship affiliation as cascading mediators. *Developmental Psychology, 54*(1), 83-97.

Davis, B.E., Moon, R.Y., Sachs, H.C., & Ottolini, M.C. (1998). Effects of sleep position on infant motor development. *Pediatrics, 102,* 1135-1140.

Davis, E.L., & Buss, K.A. (2012). Moderators of the relation between shyness and behavior with peers: Cortisol dysregulation and maternal emotional socialization. *Social Development, 21,* 801-820.

Davis, L., & Keyser, J. (1997). *Becoming the parent you want to be.* New York: Broadway Books.

Davis, T.N., & Rispoli, M. (2018). Introduction to the special issue: Interventions to reduce challenging behavior among individuals with autism spectrum disorder. *Behavior Modification, 42,* 307-313.

Davoodi, T., Nelson, L.J., & Blake, P.R. (2018). Children's conceptions of ownership for self and other: categorical ownership versus strength of claim. *Child Development.* doi:10.1111/cdev.13163

Dawson, P., & Guare, R. (2018). *Executive skills in children and adolescents: A practical guide to assessment and intervention* (3rd ed.). New York: Guilford.

Day, E., & Dotterer, A.M. (2018). Parental involvement and adolescent academic outcomes: Exploring differences in beneficial strategies across racial/ethnic groups. *Journal of Youth and Adolescence, 47*(6), 1332-1349.

Day, K.L., & Smith, C.L. (2019). Maternal behaviors in toddlerhood as predictors of children's private speech in preschool. *Journal of Experimental Child Psychology, 177,* 132-140.

Day, K.L., Smith, C.L., Neal, A., & Dunsmore, J.C. (2018). Private speech moderates the effects of effortful control on emotionality. *Early Education and Development, 29,* 161-177.

Dayton, C.J., & Malone, J.C. (2017). Development and socialization of physical aggression in very young boys. *Infant Mental Health, 38,* 150-165.

de Boer, H., Donker, A.S., Kostons, D.D., & van der Werf, G.P. (2018). Long-term effects of metacognitive strategy instruction on student academic performance: A meta-analysis. *Educational Research Review, 24,* 98-115.

De Brigard, F., & Parikh, N. (2018). Episodic counterfactual thinking. *Current Directions in Psychological Science, 28*(1), 59-66.

de Brigard, F., Szpunar, K.K., & Schacter, D.L. (2013). Coming to grips with the past: Effect of repeated stimulation on the perceived plausibility of episodic counterfactual thoughts. *Psychological Science, 24*(7), 1329-1334.

de Bruin, W.B., & Fischhoff, B. (2017). Eliciting probabilistic expectations: Collaborations between psychologists and economists. *Proceedings of the National Academy of Sciences, 114,* 3297-3304.

de Giambattista, C., & others (2019). Subtyping the autism spectrum disorder: Comparison of children with high-functioning autism and Asperger syndrome. *Journal of Autism and Developmental Disorders, 49,* 138-150.

De Meyer, S., & others (2017). "Boys should have the courage to ask a girl out": Gender norms in early adolescent romantic relationships. *Journal of Adolescent Health, 61*(4), S42-S47.

Deák, G.O., Krasno, A.M., Jasso, H., & Triesch, J. (2018). What leads to shared attention? Maternal cues and infant responses during object play. *Infancy, 23*(1), 4-28.

Deamen, S., & others. (2012). Identity and perceived peer relationship quality in emerging adulthood: The mediating role of attachment-related emotions. *Journal of Adolescence, 35,* 1417–1425.

Deans, C.L. (2018). Maternal sensitivity, its relationship with child outcomes, and interventions that address it: A systematic literature review. *Early Child Development and Care.* doi: 10.1080/03004430.2018.1465415

Dearing, E., & Zachrisson, H.D. (2017). Concern over internal, external, and incidence validity in studies of child-care quantity and externalizing behavior problems. *Child Development Perspectives, 11,* 133–138.

Deater-Deckard, K., & others (2018). Within- and between-person and group variance in behavior and beliefs in cross-cultural longitudinal data. *Journal of Adolescence, 62,* 207–217.

Deater-Deckard, K., & others (2019). Chaos, danger, and maternal parenting in families: Links with adolescent adjustment in low- and middle-income countries. *Developmental Science, 22,* e12855.

Deater-Deckard, K., & Sturge-Apple, M. (2017). Mind and matter: New insights on the role of parental cognitive and neurobiological functioning in process models of parenting. *Journal of Family Psychology, 31*(1), 5–7.

Deater-Deckard, K., Dodge, K.A., & Sorbring, E. (2005). Cultural differences in the effects of physical punishment. In M. Rutter & M. Tienda (Eds.), *Ethnicity and causal mechanisms* (pp. 205–226). Cambridge, UK: Cambridge University Press.

DeCasper, A.J., & Spence, M.J. (1986). Prenatal maternal speech influences newborn's perception of speech sounds. *Infant Behavior and Development, 9,* 133–150.

Decety, J., & Cowell, J. (2016). Developmental social neuroscience. In D. Cicchetti (Ed.), *Developmental psychopathology* (3rd ed.). New York: Wiley.

Decety, J., Meidenbauer, K.L., & Cowell, J.M. (2018). The development of cognitive empathy and concern in preschool children: A behavioral neuroscience investigation. *Developmental Science, 21*(3), e12570.

Deci, E.L., & Ryan, R.M. (2000). The "what" and "why" of goal pursuits: Human needs and the self-determination of behavior. *Psychological Inquiry, 11,* 227–268.

Degol, J.L., Wang, M.T., Ye, F., & Zhang, C. (2017). Who makes the cut? Parental involvement and math trajectories predicting college enrollment. *Journal of Applied Developmental Psychology, 50,* 60–70.

Dehaene-Lambertz, G. (2017). The human infant brain: A neural architecture able to learn language. *Psychonomic Bulletin & Review, 24,* 48–55.

DeKeyser, R.M. (2018). Age in learning and teaching grammar. In J.I. Liontas (Ed.), *The TESOL encyclopedia of English language teaching.*

Del Giudice, M. (2014). Middle childhood: An evolutionary-developmental synthesis. *Child Development Perspectives, 8,* 193–200.

DeLoache, J.S. (2011). Early development of the understanding and use of symbolic artifacts. In U. Goswami (Ed.), *Wiley-Blackwell handbook of childhood cognitive development* (2nd ed.). New York: Wiley.

Demetriou, A., & others (2018). Mapping dimensions of general intelligence: An integrated differential-developmental theory. *Human Development, 61,* 4–42.

Demetriou, A., & Spanoudis, G. (2018). *Growing minds: A developmental theory of intelligence, brain, and education.* New York: Routledge.

Demetriou, A., Makris, N., Kazi, S., Spanoudis, G., & Shayer, M. (2018). The developmental trinity of mind: Cognizance, executive control, and reasoning. *Wiley Interdisciplinary Reviews: Cognitive Science,* e1461.

Deming, D.M., & others (2017). Cross-sectional analysis of eating patterns and snacking in the US Feeding Infants and Toddlers Study 2008. *Public Health Nutrition, 20,* 1584–1592.

Demir-Lira, O.E., Applebaum, L.R., Goldin-Meadow, S., & Levine, S.C. (2019, in press). Parents' early book reading to children: Relation to children's later language and literacy outcomes controlling for other parent language input. *Developmental Science, 22*(3), 12764. doi:10.1111/desc.12764

Dempster, F.N. (1981). Memory span: Sources of individual and developmental differences. *Psychological Bulletin, 80,* 63–100.

Deng, Y., Chang, L., Yang, M., Huo, M., & Zhou, R. (2016). Gender differences in emotional response: Inconsistency between experience and expressivity. *PloS One, 11*(6), e0158666.

Denham, S.A., & Bassett, H.H. (2019, in press). 'You hit me! That's not nice and it makes me sad!': Relations of young children's social information processing and early school success. *Early Child Development and Care.*

Deoni, S., Dean III, D., Joelson, S., O'Regan, J., & Schneider, N. (2018). Early nutrition influences developmental myelination and cognition in infants and young children. *Neuroimage, 178,* 649–659.

DePasquale, C.E., Handley, E.D., & Cicchetti, D. (2018). Investigating multilevel pathways of developmental consequences of maltreatment. *Development and Psychopathology.* doi:10.1017/S0954579418000834

DeQuinzio, J.A., Poulson, C.L., Townsend, D.B., & Taylor, B.A. (2016). Social referencing and children with autism. *The Behavior Analyst, 39,* 319–331.

Dereymaeker, A., & others. (2017). Review of sleep-EEG in preterm and term neonates. *Early Human Development, 113,* 87–103.

Derlan, C.L., & Umaña-Taylor, A.J. (2015). Brief report: Contextual predictors of African American adolescents' ethnic-racial identity affirmation-belonging and resistance to peer pressure. *Journal of Adolescence, 41,* 1–6.

Desai, M., Beall, M., & Ross, M.G. (2013, in press). Developmental origins of obesity: Programmed adipogenesis. *Current Diabetes Reports.*

DeSisto, C.L., Hirai, A.H., Collins Jr., J.W., & Rankin, K.M. (2018). Deconstructing a disparity: Explaining excess preterm birth among US-born black women. *Annals of Epidemiology, 28*(4), 225–230.

Desmet, K., Ortuño-Ortín, I., & Wacziarg, R. (2017). Culture, ethnicity, and diversity. *American Economic Review, 107*(9), 2479–2513.

Dessì, A., Corona, L., Pintus, R., & Fanos, V. (2018). Exposure to tobacco smoke and low birth weight: From epidemiology to metabolomics. *Expert Review of Proteomics, 15*(8), 647–656.

Deutsch, A.R., Crockett, L.J., Wolf, J.M., & Russell, S.T. (2012). Parent and peer pathways to adolescent delinquency: Variations by ethnicity and neighborhood context. *Journal of Youth and Adolescence, 41,* 1078–1094.

Deutsch, A.R., Wood, P.K., & Slutske, W.S. (2016, June). Developmental etiologies of alcohol use and their relations to parent and peer influences over adolescence and young adulthood: A genetically informed approach. *Alcoholism: Clinical and Experimental Research, 40,* 2151–2162.

Deutsch, R., & Pruett, M.K. (2009). Child adjustment and high conflict divorce. In R. M. Galatzer-Levy and L. Kraus (Eds.), *The scientific basis of custody decisions* (2nd ed.). New York: Wiley.

Devaney, S.A., Palomaki, G.E., Scott, J.A., & Bianchi, D.W. (2011). Noninvasive fetal sex determination using cell-free DNA: A systematic review and meta-analysis. *Journal of the American Medical Association, 306,* 627–636.

Dever, B.V., & others. (2013). Predicting risk-taking with and without substance use: The effects of parental monitoring, school bonding, and sports participation. *Prevention Science, 13*(6), 605–615.

Dew, J., & Wilcox, W.B. (2011). "If momma ain't happy": Explaining declines in marital satisfaction among new mothers. *Journal of Marriage and the Family, 73,* 1–12.

DeWall, C.N., Anderson, C.A., & Bushman, B.J. (2013). Aggression. In I. B. Weiner & others (Eds.), *Handbook of psychology* (2nd ed., Vol. 5). New York: Wiley.

Dewey, J. (1933). *How we think.* Lexington, MA: D. C. Heath.

DeZolt, D.M., & Hull, S.H. (2001). Classroom and schools climate. In J. Worell (Ed.), *Encyclopedia of women and gender.* San Diego: Academic Press.

Di Giunta, L., & others (2017). Measurement invariance and convergent validity of anger and sadness self-regulation scales among youth from six cultural groups. *Assessment, 24,* 484–502.

Di Giunta, L., & others (2018). Parents' and early adolescents' self-efficacy about anger regulation and early adolescents' internalizing and externalizing problems: A longitudinal study in three countries. *Journal of Adolescence, 64,* 124–135.

Diamond, A., & Lee, K. (2011). Interventions shown to aid executive function development in children 4 to 12 years old. *Science, 333,* 959–964.

Diamond, A. (2013). Executive functioning. *Annual Review of Psychology* (Vol. 64). Palo Alto, CA: Annual Reviews.

Diamond, L.M. (2013a). Gender and same-sex sexuality. In D. T. Tolman & L. M. Diamond (Eds.), *APA handbook on sexuality and psychology.* Washington, DC: American Psychological Association.

Diamond, L.M. (2013b). Sexuality and same-sex sexuality in relationships. In J. Simpson & J. Davidio (Eds.), *Handbook of personality and social psychology.* Washington, DC: American Psychological Association.

Diamond, M., & Sigmundson, H.K. (1997). Sex reassignment at birth: Long-term review and clinical implications. *Archives of Pediatric and Adolescent Medicine, 151,* 298-304.

Diamond, L.M., & Savin-Williams, R.C. (2013). Same-sex activity in adolescence: Multiple meanings and implications. In R. F. Fassinger & S. L. Morrow (Eds.), *Sex in the margins.* Washington, DC: American Psychological Association.

Diaz, A., & Bell, M.A. (2012). Frontal EEG asymmetry and fear reactivity in different contexts at 10 months. *Developmental Psychobiology, 54,* 536-545.

DiBenedetto, M.K., & Schunk, D.H. (2018). Self-efficacy in education revisited through a sociocultural lens. In G.A.D. Liem & D.M. McInerney (Eds.), *Big theories revisited 2.* Charlotte, NC: Information Age Publishing.

Dickerson, A., & Popli, G.K. (2016). Persistent poverty and children's cognitive development: Evidence from the UK Millennium Cohort Study. *Journal of the Royal Statistical Society, 179,* 535-558.

Dickinson, D.K., & others (2019). Effects of teacher-delivered book reading and play on vocabulary learning and self-regulation among low-income preschool children. *Journal of Cognition and Development, 20*(2), 136-164.

Dijkstra, J.K., & Gest, S.D. (2015). Peer norm salience for academic achievement, prosocial behavior, and bullying: Implications for adolescent school experiences. *The Journal of Early Adolescence, 35*(1), 79-96.

Dilworth-Bart, J.E., & others (2018). Longitudinal associations between self-regulation and the academic and behavioral adjustment of young children born preterm. *Early Childhood Research Quarterly, 42,* 193-204.

Dimmitt, C., & McCormick, C.B. (2012). Metacognition in education. In K. R. Harris, S. Graham, & T. Urdan (Eds.), *Handbook of educational psychology.* Washington, DC: American Psychological Association.

Dineva, E., & Schöner, G. (2018). How infants' reaches reveal principles of sensorimotor decision making. *Connection Science, 30*(1), 53-80.

Dionne, J.M. (2017). Updated guideline may improve the recognition and diagnosis of hypertension in children and adolescents: Review of the 2017 AAP blood pressure clinical practice guideline. *Current Hypertension Reports, 19,* 84.

DiPerna, J.C., Lei, P., Cheng, W., Hart, S.C., & Bellinger, J. (2018). A cluster randomized trial of the Social Skills Improvement System-Classwide Intervention Program (SSIS-CIP) in first grade. *Journal of Educational Psychology, 110*(1), 1-16.

Dishion, T.J., & Tipsord, J.M. (2011). Peer contagion in child and adolescent social and emotional development. *Annual Review of Psychology* (Vol. 62). Palo Alto, CA: Annual Reviews.

Dishion, T.J., & Snyder, J.J. (Eds.). (2016). *The Oxford handbook of coercive relationship dynamics.* Oxford, UK: Oxford University Press.

DiTrapani, J., Jeon, M., De Boeck, P., & Partchev, I. (2016). Attempting to differentiate fast and slow intelligence: Using generalized item response trees to examine the role of speed on intelligence tests. *Intelligence, 56,* 82-92.

Divecha, D., & Brackett, M. (2019, in press). Rethinking school-based bullying prevention through the lens of social and emotional learning: A bioecological perspective. *International Journal of Bullying Prevention,* 1-21. doi:10.1007/s42380-019-00019-5

Dixon, R.A., McFall, G.P., Whitehead, B.P., & Dolcos, S. (2013). Cognitive development in adulthood and aging. In I. B. Weiner & others (2nd ed., Vol. 6). New York: Wiley.

Dlugonski, D., DuBose, K.D., & Rider, P. (2017). Accelerometer-measured patterns of shared physical activity among mother–young child dyads. *Journal of Physical Activity and Health, 14,* 808-814.

Dobson, K.G., Chow, C.H.T., Morrison, K.M., & Van Lieshout, R.J. (2017). Associations between childhood cognition and cardiovascular events in adulthood: A systematic review and meta-analysis. *Canadian Journal of Cardiology, 33,* 232-242.

Dodge, K.A. (1993). Social cognitive mechanisms in the development of conduct disorder and depression. *Annual Review of Psychology* (Vol. 44, pp. 559-584). Palo Alto, CA: Annual Reviews.

Dodge, K.A. (2011a). Context matters in child and family policy. *Child Development, 82,* 433-442.

Dodge, K.A. (2011b). Social information processing models of aggressive behavior. In M. Mikulincer & P. R. Shaver (Eds.), *Understanding and reducing aggression, violence, and their consequences.* Washington, DC: American Psychological Association.

Dodge, K.A., & others (2014). Implementation and randomized controlled trial evaluation of universal postnatal nurse home visiting. *American Journal of Public Health, 104*(S1), S136-S143.

Dodge, K.A., & others (2015). Hostile attributional bias and aggressive behavior in global context. *Proceedings of the National Academy of Sciences, 112*(30), 9310-9315.

Dodge, K.A., & others (2015). Impact of early intervention on psychopathology, crime, and well-being at age 25. *American Journal of Psychiatry, 172*(1), 59-70.

Doebel, S., & Zelazo, P.D. (2015). A meta-analysis of the Dimensional Change Card Sort: Implications for developmental theories and the measurement of executive function in children. *Developmental Review, 38,* 241-268.

Dollar, J.M., Perry, N.B., Calkins, S.D., Keane, S.P., & Shanahan, L. (2018). Temperamental anger and positive reactivity and the development of social skills: Implications for academic competence during preadolescence. *Early Education and Development, 29*(5), 747-761.

Dong, S.S., & others. (2018). Comprehensive review and annotation of susceptibility SNPs associated with obesity-related traits. *Obesity Reviews, 19,* 917-930.

Donnelly, K., & Twenge, J.M. (2017). Masculine and feminine traits on the Bem Sex-Role Inventory, 1993-2012: A cross-temporal meta-analysis. *Sex Roles, 76,* 556-565.

Doob, C.B. (2015). *Social inequality and social stratification in U.S. society.* New York: Routledge.

Doom, J.R., & others (2018). Family conflict, chaos, and negative life events predict cortisol activity in low-income children. *Developmental Psychobiology, 60*(4), 364-379.

Dopp, P.R., Mooney, A.J., Armitage, R., & King, C. (2012). Exercise for adolescents with depressive disorders: A feasibility study. *Depression Research and Treatment.* Article ID: 257472.

Dorsch, T.E., & others (2014). *Parent guide: Evidence-based strategies for parenting in organized youth sport.* Logan, UT: Utah State University Families in Sport Lab.

Dorsey, S., & others (2017). Evidence base update for psychosocial treatments for children and adolescents exposed to traumatic events. *Journal of Clinical Child & Adolescent Psychology, 46,* 303-330.

dos Santos, J.F., & others (2018). Maternal, fetal and neonatal consequences associated with the use of crack cocaine during the gestational period: A systematic review and meta-analysis. *Archives of Gynecology and Obstetrics, 298*(3), 487-503.

Dotti Sani, G.M., & Quaranta, M. (2017). The best is yet to come? Attitudes toward gender roles among adolescents in 36 countries. *Sex Roles, 77,* 30-45.

Dozier, M., Stovall-McClough, K.C., & Albus, K.E. (2009). Attachment and psychopathology in adulthood. In J. Cassidy & P. R. Shaver (Eds.), *Handbook of attachment* (2nd ed.). New York: Guilford.

DPIC (Death Penalty Information Center) (2019). *Execution of juveniles in the U.S. and other countries.* Retrieved from https://deathpenaltyinfo.org/execution-juveniles-us-and-other-countries

Draganova, R., & others (2018). Fetal auditory evoked responses to onset of amplitude modulated sounds. A fetal magnetoencephalography (fMEG) study. *Hearing Research, 363,* 70-77.

Duckworth, A.L., Taxer, J.L., Eskreis-Winkler, L., Galla, B.M., & Gross, J.J. (2019). Self-control and academic achievement. *Annual Review of Psychology, 70,* 373-399.

Dugas, C., & others (2017). Postnatal prevention of childhood obesity in offspring prenatally exposed to gestational diabetes mellitus: Where are we now. *Obesity Facts, 10*(4), 396-406.

Dunbar, R.I.M. (2018). The anatomy of friendship. *Trends in Cognitive Sciences, 22*(1), 32-51.

Duncan, G.J. (2012). Give us this day our daily breadth. *Child Development, 83,* 6-15.

Duncan, G., Magnuson, K., Kalil, A., & Ziol-Guest, K. (2012). The importance of early childhood poverty. *Social Indicators Research, 108,* 87-98.

Duncan, G.J., & others (2013). Early childhood poverty and adult achievement, employment and health. *Child Development, 81*(1), 306-325.

Duncan, G.J., Kalil, A., & Ziol-Guest, K.M. (2017). Increasing inequality in parent incomes and children's schooling. *Demography, 54*(5), 1603-1626.

Duncan, G.J., Magnuson, K., & Votruba-Drzal, E. (2017). Moving beyond correlations in assessing the consequences of poverty. *Annual Review of Psychology, 68,* 413–434.

Duncombe, M.E., Havighurst, S.S., Holland, K.A., & Frankling, E.J. (2012). The contribution of parenting practice and parent emotion factors in children at risk for disruptive behavior disorders. *Child Psychiatry and Human Development, 43,* 715–733.

Dunkel Schetter, C. (2011). Psychological science in the study of pregnancy and birth. *Annual Review of Psychology* (Vol. 62). Palo Alto, CA: Annual Reviews.

Dunn, J. (2007). Siblings and socialization. In J. E. Grusec & P. D. Hastings (Eds.), *Handbook of socialization.* New York: Guilford.

Dunn, J. (2010). Commentary and challenges to Grusec and Davidov's domain-specific approach. *Child Development, 81,* 710–714.

Dunn, J. (2013). Moral development in early childhood and social interaction in the family. In M. Killen & J. G. Smetana (Eds.), *Handbook of moral development* (2nd ed.). New York: Routledge.

Dunn, J., & Kendrick, C. (1982). *Siblings.* Cambridge, MA: Harvard University Press.

Dunne, T., Bishop, L., Avery, S., & Darcy, S. (2017). A review of effective youth engagement strategies for mental health and substance use interventions. *Journal of Adolescent Health, 60,* 487–512.

Dunphy, D.C. (1963). The social structure of urban adolescent peer groups. *Society, 26,* 230–246.

Dunst, C.J. (2017). Research foundations for evidence-informed early childhood intervention performance checklists. *Education Sciences, 7*(4), 78.

Dupéré, V., & others (2018). High school dropout in proximal context: The triggering role of stressful life events. *Child Development, 89,* e107–e122.

Durrant, J.E. (2008). Physical punishment, culture, and rights: Current issues for professionals. *Journal of Developmental and Behavioral Pediatrics, 29,* 55–66.

Durrant, R., & Ellis, B.J. (2013). Evolutionary psychology. In I. B. Weiner & others (Eds.), *Handbook of psychology* (2nd ed., Vol. 3). New York: Wiley.

Durston, S., & others (2006). A shift from diffuse to focal cortical activity with development. *Developmental Science, 9,* 1–8.

Dutil, C., & others (2018). Influence of sleep on developing brain functions and structures in children and adolescents: A systematic review. *Sleep Medicine Reviews, 42,* 184–201.

Dutton, E., & others (2018). A Flynn effect in Khartoum, the Sudanese capital, 2004–2016. *Intelligence, 68,* 82–86.

Dvornyk, V., & Waqar-ul-Haq, H. (2012). Genetics of age at menarche: A systematic review. *Human Reproduction Update, 18,* 198–210.

Dweck, C.S., & Master, A. (2009). Self-theories and motivation: Students' beliefs about intelligence. In K. R. Wentzel & A. Wigfield (Eds.), *Handbook of motivation at school.* New York: Routledge.

Dweck, C.S. (2006). *Mindset.* New York: Random House.

Dweck, C.S. (2012). Mindsets and human nature: Promoting change in the Middle East, the school

yard, the racial divide, and willpower. *American Psychologist, 67,* 614–622.

Dweck, C.S. (2013). Social development. In P. Zelazo (Ed.), *Oxford handbook of developmental psychology.* New York: Oxford University Press.

Dweck, C.S., & Yeager, D.S. (2018). Mindsets change the imagined and actual future. In G. Oettingen, A.T. Sevincer, & P.M. Gollwitzer (Eds.), *The psychology of thinking about the future.* New York: Guilford.

E

Eagleton, S.G., Williams, A.L., & Merten, M.J. (2016). Perceived behavioral autonomy and trajectories of depressive symptoms from adolescence to adulthood. *Journal of Child and Family Studies, 25*(1), 198–211.

Eagly, A.H., & Crowley, M. (1986). Gender and helping behavior: A meta-analytic review of the social psychological literature. *Psychological Bulletin, 100,* 283–308.

Eagly, A.H. (2013). Women as leaders: Paths through the labryrinth. In M. C. Bligh & R. Riggio (Eds.), *When near is far and far is near: Exploring distance in leader-follower relationships.* New York: Wiley Blackwell.

Eagly, A.H., & Wood, W. (2016). Social role theory of sex differences. In N. Naples (Ed.-in-Chief), R.C. Hoogland, M. Wickramasinghe, & W.C.A. Wong (Assoc. Eds.), *Wiley Blackwell encyclopedia of gender and sexuality studies.* New York: Wiley-Blackwell.

Eason, A.D., & Parris, B.A. (2018). Clinical applications of self-hypnosis: A systematic review and meta-analysis of randomized controlled trials. *Psychology of Consciousness: Theory, Research, and Practice.* doi:10.1037/cns0000173

East, P. (2009). Adolescent relationships with siblings. In R. M. Lerner & L. Steinberg (Eds.), *Handbook of adolescent psychology* (3rd ed.). New York: Wiley.

Easterbrooks, M.A., Bartlett, J.D., Beeghly, M., & Thompson, R.A. (2013). Social and emotional development in infancy. In R. M. Lerner, M. A. Easterbrooks, & J. Mistry (Eds.), *Handbook of psychology* (2nd ed., Vol. 6). New York: Wiley.

Eaton, D.K., & others. (2012). Youth risk behavior surveillance—United States, 2011. *MMWR Surveillance Summaries, 8, 61*(4), 1–162.

Ebbert, A.M., Kumar, N.L., & Luthar, S.S. (2019). Complexities in adjustment patterns among the "best and the brightest": Risk and resilience in the context of high-achieving schools. *Research in Human Development, 16*(1), 21–34.

Eccles, J.S., & Roeser, R.W. (2011). Schools as developmental contexts during adolescence. *Journal of Research on Adolescence, 21,* 225–241.

Eccles, J.S., & Roeser, R.W. (2013). Schools as developmental contexts during adolescence. In I. B. Weiner & others (Eds.), *Handbook of psychology* (2nd ed., Vol. 6). New York: Wiley.

Ecker-Lyster, M., & Niileksela, C. (2017). Enhancing gifted education for underrepresented students: Promising recruitment and programming strategies. *Journal for the Education of the Gifted, 40,* 79–95.

Edelman, M.W. (2017). Foreword: The state of America's children: We must keep moving forward.

In *The state of America's children, 2017.* Washington DC: Children's Defense Fund.

Eden-Friedman, Y., & others (2018). Delivery outcomes in subsequent pregnancy following primary breech cesarean delivery: A retrospective cohort study. *The Journal of Maternal-Fetal & Neonatal Medicine,* 1–11. doi:10.1080/14767058.2018.1523388

Ednick, M., & others. (2010). Sleep-related respiratory abnormalities and arousal pattern in achondroplasia during early infancy. *Journal of Pediatrics, 155,* 510–515.

Edwards, C.P., & Liu, W. (2002). Parenting toddlers. In M. H. Bornstein (Ed.), *Handbook of parenting* (2nd ed., Vol. 1). Mahwah, NJ: Erlbaum.

Edwards, C.P., & Gandini, L. (2018). The Reggio Emilia approach to early childhood education. In J.L. Roopnarine & others (Eds.), *Handbook of international perspectives on early childhood education.* New York: Routledge.

Edwards, M. (2013). *Every child, every day: A digital conversion model for student achievement.* Upper Saddle River, NJ: Pearson.

Eggum-Wilkens, N.D., Reichenberg, R.E., Eisenberg, N., & Spinrad, T.L. (2016). Components of effortful control and their relations to children's shyness. *International Journal of Behavioral Development, 40,* 544–554.

Ehrlich, K.B., Dykas, M.J., & Cassidy, J. (2012). Tipping points in adolescent adjustment: Predicting social functioning from adolescents' conflict with parents and friends. *Journal of Family Psychology, 26,* 776–783.

Eisenberg, N., & others (2001). Mothers' emotional expressivity and children's behavior problems and social competence: Mediation through children's regulation. *Developmental Psychology, 37*(4), 475–490.

Eisenberg, N., & Spinrad, T.L. (2016). Multidimensionality of prosocial behavior: Rethinking the conceptualization and development of prosocial behavior. In L. Padilla-Walker & G. Carlo (Eds.), *Prosocial development: A multidimensional approach* (2nd ed.). New York: Oxford University Press.

Eisenberg, N., Morris, A.S., McDaniel, B., & Spinrad, T.L. (2009). Moral cognitions and prosocial responding in adolescence. In R. M. Lerner & L. Steinberg (Eds.), *Handbook of adolescent psychology* (3rd ed.). New York: Wiley.

Eisenberg, N., Spinrad, T., & Sadovsky, A. (2014). Empathy-related responding in children. In M. Killen & J.G. Smetana (Eds.), *Handbook of moral development* (2nd ed.) (pp. 184–207). New York: Routledge.

Eisenberg, N., Spinrad, T.L., & Knafo-Noam, A. (2015). Prosocial development. In R.M. Lerner (Ed.), *Handbook of child psychology and developmental science* (7th ed.). New York: Wiley.

Eisenberg, N., & Valiente, C. (2002). Parenting and children's prosocial and moral development. In M. H. Bornstein (Ed.), *Handbook of parenting* (2nd ed.). Mahwah, NJ: Erlbaum.

El-Hajj, N., & others (2013). Metabolic programming of MEST DNA methylation by intrauterine exposure to gestational diabetes mellitus. *Diabetes, 62*(4), 1320-1328.

El-Sheikh, M., & others (2013). Economic adversity and children's sleep problems: Multiple indicators and moderation of health. *Health Psychology, 32*(8), 849-859.

El-Sheikh, M., & Kelly, R.J. (2017). Family functioning and children's sleep. *Child Development Perspectives, 11,* 264-269.

Elder, G.H., & Shanahan, M.J. (2006). The life course and human development. In W. Damon & R. Lerner (Eds.), *Handbook of child psychology* (6th ed.). New York: Wiley.

Elkind, D. (1978). Understanding the young adolescent. *Adolescence, 13,* 127-134.

Ellis, B.J., & Boyce, W.T. (2008). Biological sensitivity to context. *Current Directions in Psychological Science, 17,* 183-187.

Ellis, C.T., & Turk-Browne, N.B. (2018). Infant fMRI: A model system for cognitive neuroscience. *Trends in Cognitive Sciences, 22,* 375-387.

Ellis, W.E., & Zarbatany, L. (2017). Understanding processes of peer clique influence in late childhood and early adolescence. *Child Development Perspectives, 11*(4), 227-232.

Eme, R. (2015). Greater male exposure to prenatal testosterone. *Violence and Gender, 2,* 19-23.

Emery, R.E. (1994). *Renegotiating family relationships.* New York: Guilford Press.

Endendijk, J.J., Groeneveld, M.G., Bakermans-Kranenburg, M.J., & Mesman, J. (2016). Gender-differentiated parenting revisited: Meta-analysis reveals very few differences in parental control of boys and girls. *PLoS One, 11*(7), e0159193.

Enfield, A., & Collins, D. (2008). The relationship of service-learning, social justice, multicultural competence, and civic engagement. *Journal of College Student Development, 49,* 95-109.

Engberg, E., & others (2018). A randomized lifestyle intervention preventing gestational diabetes: Effects on self-rated health from pregnancy to postpartum. *Journal of Psychosomatic Obstetrics & Gynecology, 39*(1), 1-6.

England, L.J., & others (2017). Developmental toxicity of nicotine: A transdisciplinary synthesis and implications for emerging tobacco products. *Neuroscience & Biobehavioral Reviews, 72,* 176-189.

Erdogan, S.U., Yanikkerem, E., & Goker, A. (2017). Effects of low back massage on perceived birth pain and satisfaction. *Complementary Therapies in Clinical Practice, 28,* 169-175.

Erikson, E.H. (1950). *Childhood and society.* New York: W. W. Norton.

Erikson, E.H. (1968). *Identity: Youth and crisis.* New York. W. W. Norton.

Eriksson, U.J. (2009). Congenital malformations in diabetic pregnancy. *Seminar in Fetal and Neonatal Medicine, 14,* 85-93.

Ericsson, K.A., & others (2018). *The Cambridge handbook of expertise and expert performance* (2nd ed.). Cambridge UK: Cambridge University Press.

Ericsson, K.A., Krampe, R., & Tesch-Romer, C. (1993). The role of deliberate practice in the acquisition of expert performance. *Psychological Review, 100,* 363-406.

Ertem, I.O., & others (2018). Similarities and differences in child development from birth to age 3 years by sex and across four countries: A cross-sectional, observational study. *The Lancet Global Health, 6*(3), e279-e291.

Eruyar, S., Maltby, J., & Vostanis, P. (2018). Mental health problems of Syrian refugee children: The role of parental factors. *European Child & Adolescent Psychiatry, 27,* 401-409.

Escobar-Chaves, S.L., & Anderson, C.A. (2008). Media and risky behavior. *Future of Children, 18*(1), 147-180.

Eskin, M., & others (2019). The role of religion in suicidal behavior, attitudes and psychological distress among university students: A multinational study. *Transcultural Psychiatry.* doi:10.1177/1363461518823933

Espelage, D.L., & Holt, M.K. (2012). Understanding and preventing bullying and sexual harassment in school. In K. R. Harris & others (Eds.), *APA handbook of educational psychology.* Washington, DC: American Psychological Association.

Esposito, G., Nakazawa, J., Venuti, P., & Bornstein, M.H. (2015). Judgment of infant cry: The roles of acoustic characteristics and sociodemographic characteristics. *Japanese Psychological Research, 57,* 126-134.

Esposito, G., Setoh, P., Shinohara, K., & Bornstein, M.H. (2017). The development of attachment: Integrating genes, brain, behavior, and environment. *Behavioural Brain Research, 325,* 87-89.

Etaugh, C., & Bridges, J.S. (2017). *Women's lives* (4th ed.). New York: Routledge.

Evans, G.W. (2004). The environment of childhood poverty. *American Psychologist, 59,* 77-92.

Evans, G.W., & English, K. (2002). The environment of poverty: Multiple stressor exposure, psychophysiological stress, and socioemotional adjustment. *Child Development, 73,* 1238-1248.

Evenson, K.R., & others (2014). Guidelines for physical activity during pregnancy: Comparisons from around the world. *American Journal of Lifestyle Medicine, 8*(2), 102-121.

Eviatar, Z., Taha, H., Cohen, V., & Schwartz, M. (2018). Word learning by young sequential bilinguals: Fast mapping in Arabic and Hebrew. *Applied Psycholinguistics, 39,* 649-674.

Extremera, N., Quintana-Orts, C., Mérida-López, S., & Rey, L. (2018). Cyberbullying victimization, self-esteem and suicidal ideation in adolescence: Does emotional intelligence play a buffering role? *Frontiers in Psychology, 9,* 367.

Eydal, G.B., & Rostgaard, T. (Eds.). (2016). *Fatherhood in the Nordic welfare states: Comparing care policies and practice.* Bristol, UK: Policy Press.

F

Faas, S., Wu, S.C., & Geiger, S. (2017). The importance of play in early childhood education: A critical perspective on current policies and practices in Germany and Hong Kong. *Global Education Review, 4,* 75-91.

Fabricius, W.V., Braver, S.L., Diaz, P., & Schenck, C. (2010). Custody and parenting time: Links to family relationships and well-being after divorce. In M. E. Lamb (Ed.), *The role of the father in child development* (5th ed.). New York: Wiley.

Fair, D., & Schlaggar, B.L. (2008). Brain development. In M. M. Haith & J. B. Benson (Eds.), *Encyclopedia of infant and early childhood development.* London, UK: Elsevier.

Fair, M.L., Reed, J.A., Hughey, S.M., Powers, A.R., & King, S. (2017). The association between aerobic fitness and academic achievement among elementary school youth. *Translational Journal of the American College of Sports Medicine, 2,* 44-50.

Falbo, T., & Poston, D.L. (1993). The academic, personality, and physical outcomes of only children in China. *Child Development, 64,* 18-35.

Falck-Ytter, T., & others (2012). Gaze performance in children with autism spectrum disorder when observing communicative actions. *Journal of Autism and Developmental Disorders, 42*(10), 2236-2245.

Fantz, R.L. (1963). Pattern vision in newborn infants. *Science, 140,* 296-297.

Fardouly, J., & Vartanian, L.R. (2016). Social media and body image concerns: Current research and future directions. *Current Opinion in Psychology, 9,* 1-5.

Fardouly, J., Magson, N.R., Johnco, C.J., Oar, E.L., & Rapee, R.M. (2018). Parental control of the time preadolescents spend on social media: Links with preadolescents' social media appearance comparisons and mental health. *Journal of Youth and Adolescence, 47*(7), 1456-1468.

Farrar, S., & Tapper, K. (2018). The effect of mindfulness on rational thinking. *Appetite, 123,* 468.

Farrington, D.P. (2009). Conduct disorder, aggression, and delinquency. In R. M. Lerner & L. Steinberg (Eds.), *Handbook of adolescent psychology* (3rd ed.). New York: Wiley.

Fatima, Y., Doi, S.A., Najman, J.M., & Al Mamun, A. (2017). Continuity of sleep problems from adolescence to young adulthood: Results from a longitudinal study. *Sleep Health, 3,* 290-295.

Fearon, R.P., & others (2010). The significance of insecure attachment and disorganization in the development of children's externalizing behavior: A meta-analytic study. *Child Development, 81,* 435-456.

Fearon, R.M.P., & Roisman, G.I. (2017). Attachment theory: Progress and future directions. *Current Opinion in Psychology, 15,* 131-136.

Fedock, G.L., & Alvarez, C. (2018). Differences in screening and treatment for antepartum versus postpartum patients: Are providers implementing the guidelines of care for perinatal depression? *Journal of Women's Health, 27.* doi:10.1089/jwh.2017.6765

Feeney, S., Moravcik, E., & Nolte, S. (2018). *Who am I in the lives of children?* (11th ed.). Upper Saddle River, NJ: Pearson.

Feil, R., & Fraga, M.F. (2012). Epigenetics and the environment: Emerging patterns and implications. *Nature Reviews: Genetics, 1,* 97–109.

Feinstein, B.A., & others (2018). Gay and bisexual adolescent boys' perspectives on parent–adolescent relationships and parenting practices related to teen sex and dating. *Archives of Sexual Behavior, 47*(6), 1825–1837.

Feldgus, E., Cardonick, I., & Gentry, R. (2017). *Kid writing in the 21st century.* Los Angeles: Hameray Publishing Group.

Feliciano, C., & Lanuza, Y.R. (2017). An immigrant paradox? Contextual attainment and intergenerational educational mobility. *American Sociological Review, 82*(1), 211–241.

Feliciano, C., & Rumbaut, R.G. (2018). The evolution of ethnic identity from adolescence to middle adulthood: The case of the immigrant second generation. *Emerging Adulthood, 7*(2), 85–96.

Ferguson, B., & Waxman, S. (2017). Linking language and categorization in infancy. *Journal of child language, 44*(3), 527–552.

Ferguson, C.J. (2015). Do angry birds make for angry children? A meta-analysis of video game influences on children's and adolescents' aggression, mental health, prosocial behavior, and academic performance. *Perspectives on Psychological Science, 10*(5), 646–666.

Fernald, A., Marchman, V.A., & Weisleder, A. (2013). SES differences in language processing skill and vocabulary are evident at 18 months. *Developmental Science, 16,* 234–248.

Fernandes, C., & others (2018). Mothers, fathers, sons, and daughters: Are there sex differences in the organization of secure base behavior during early childhood? *Infant Behavior and Development, 50,* 213–223.

Field, T., Figueiredo, B., Hernandez-Reif, M., Deeds, O., & Ascencio, A. (2008). Massage therapy reduces pain in pregnant women, alleviates prenatal depression in both parents and improves their relationships. *Journal of Bodywork and Movement Therapies, 12,* 146–150.

Field, T. (2010). Postpartum depression effects on early interactions, parenting, and safety practices: A review. *Infant Behavior and Development, 33,* 1–6.

Field, T. (2016). Massage therapy research review. *Complementary Therapies in Clinical Practice, 24,* 19–31.

Field, T.M., & Hernandez-Reif, M. (2013). Touch and pain perception in infants. In D. Narvaez & others (Eds.), *Evolution, early experience, and development.* New York: Oxford University Press.

Field, T.M., & others. (2012). Yoga and massage therapy reduce prenatal depression and prematurity. *Journal of Bodywork and Movement Therapies, 16,* 204–209.

Fiese, B., Jones, B., & Saltsman, J. (2018). Systems unify family psychology. In B. Fiese and others (Eds.), *APA handbook of contemporary family psychology.* Washington, DC: American Psychological Association.

Fiese, B. (Ed.) (2018). *APA handbook of contemporary family psychology.* Washington, DC: American Psychological Association.

Filippetti, M.L., & Tsakiris, M. (2018). Just before I recognize myself: the role of featural and multisensory cues leading up to explicit mirror self-recognition. *Infancy, 23*(4), 577–590.

Finelli, J., Zeanah, C.H., & Smyke, A.T. (2019). Attachment disorders in early childhood. In C.H. Zeanah (Ed.), *Handbook of infant mental health* (4th ed.). New York: Guilford.

Fingerman, K.L., Pillemer, K.A., Silverstein, M., & Suitor, J.J. (2012). The Baby Boomers' intergenerational relationships. *Gerontologist, 52,* 199–209.

Fingerman, K.L., Sechrest, J., & Birditt, K.S. (2013). Intergenerational relationships in a changing world. *Gerontology, 59*(1), 64–70.

Fiori, M., & Vesely-Maillefer, A.K. (2018). Emotional intelligence as an ability: Theory, challenges, and new directions. In K. Keefer, J. Parker, & D. Saklofske (Eds.), *Emotional intelligence in education* (pp. 23–47). Dordrecht, the Netherlands: Springer.

Firk, C., Dahmen, B., Lehmann, C., Herpertz-Dahlmann, B., & Konrad, K. (2018). Down-regulation of amygdala response to infant crying: A role for distraction in maternal emotion regulation. *Emotion, 18,* 412–423.

Fisher, C.B., Busch-Rossnagel, N.A., Jopp, D.S., & Brown, J.L. (2013). Applied developmental science: Contributions and challenges for the 21st century. In I. B. Weiner & others (Eds.), *Handbook of psychology* (2nd ed., Vol. 6). New York: Wiley.

Fisher, H.L., & others (2012). Bullying victimization and risk of self-harm in early adolescence: Longitudinal cohort study. *British Medical Journal, 344,* e2683.

Fisher, P.A. (2005, April). *Translational research on underlying mechanisms of risk among foster children: Implications for prevention science.* Paper presented at the meeting of the Society for Research in Child Development, Washington, DC.

Fite, P., Frazer, A., DiPierro, M., & Abel, M. (2019). Youth perceptions of what is helpful during the middle school transition and correlates of transition difficulty. *Children and Schools, 41,* 55–64.

FitzGerald, T.L., & others (2018). Body structure, function, activity, and participation in 3- to 6-year-old children born very preterm: An ICF-based systematic review and meta-analysis. *Physical Therapy, 98*(8), 691–704.

Fivush, R. (2019). *Family narratives and the development of an autobiographical self: Social and cultural perspectives on autobiographical memory.* New York: Routledge.

Fizke, E., & others (2017). Are there signature limits in early theory of mind? *Journal of Experimental Child Psychology, 162,* 209–224.

Fizke, E., Butterfill, S., van de Loo, L., Reindl, E., & Rakoczy, H. (2017). Are there signature limits in early theory of mind? *Journal of Experimental Child Psychology, 162,* 209–224.

Flanagan, C.A., Kim, T., Collura, J., & Kopish, M.A. (2015). Community service and adolescents' social capital. *Journal of Research on Adolescence, 25*(2), 295–309.

Flanagan, D.P., & McDonough, E.M. (Eds.). (2018). *Contemporary intellectual assessment: Theories, tests, and issues* (4th ed.). New York: Guilford.

Flanigan, A.E., & Kiewra, K.A. (2018). What college instructors can do about student cyber-slacking. *Educational Psychology Review, 30*(2), 585–597.

Flavell, J.H., Friedrichs, A., & Hoyt, J. (1970). Developmental changes in memorization processes. *Cognitive Psychology, 1,* 324–340.

Flavell, J.H. (2004). Theory-of-mind development: Retrospect and prospect. *Merrill-Palmer Quarterly, 50,* 274–290.

Fletcher-Watson, S., & Happé, F. (2019). *Autism: A new introduction to psychological theory and current debate.* New York: Routledge.

Fletcher, B.R., & Rapp, P.R. (2013). Normal neurocognitive aging. In I. B. Weiner & others (Eds.), *Handbook of psychology* (2nd ed., Vol. 3). New York: Wiley.

Fletcher, J.M., Lyon, G.R., Fuchs, L.S., & Barnes, M.A. (2018). *Learning disabilities: From identification to intervention.* New York: Guilford.

Flores, D., Docherty, S.L., Relf, M.V., McKinney, R.E., & Barroso, J.V. (2018). "It's almost like gay sex doesn't exist": Parent-child sex communication according to gay, bisexual, and queer male adolescents. *Journal of Adolescent Research,* 0743558418757464.

Florin, T., & Ludwig, S. (2011). *Netter's Pediatrics.* New York: Elsevier.

Flouri, E., & Buchanan, A. (2004). Early father's and mother's involvement and child's later educational outcomes. *British Journal of Educational Psychology, 74,* 141–153.

Flynn, H.K., Felmlee, D.H., & Conger, R.D. (2017). The social context of adolescent friendships: Parents, peers, and romantic partners. *Youth & Society, 49*(5), 679–705.

Flynn, H.K. (2018). Friendships of adolescence. *The Blackwell encyclopedia of sociology.* New York: Wiley.

Flynn, J.R. (2013). *Are we getting smarter?* New York: Cambridge University Press.

Flynn, J.R. (2018). Reflections about intelligence over 40 years. *Intelligence, 70,* 73–83.

Foley, J.E., & Weinraub, M. (2017). Sleep, affect, and social competence from preschool to preadolescence: Distinct pathways to emotional and social adjustment for boys and for girls. *Frontiers in Psychology, 8,* 711.

Fonagy, P., Luyten, P., Allison, E., & Campbell, C. (2016). Reconciling psychoanalytic ideas with attachment theory. In J. Cassidy & P. Shaver (Eds.), *Handbook of attachment theory* (3rd ed., pp. 780–804). New York: Guilford Press.

Fong, C.J., Patall, E.A., Vasquez, A.C., & Stautberg, S. (2019). A meta-analysis of negative feedback on intrinsic motivation. *Educational Psychology Review, 31,* 121–162.

Ford, D.Y. (2012). Gifted and talented education: History, issues, and recommendations. In K. R. Harris, S. Graham, & T. Urdan (Eds.), *APA handbook of educational psychology.* Washington, DC: American Psychological Association.

Forgatch, M.S., Patterson, G.R., Degarmo, D.S., & Beldavs, Z.G. (2009). Testing the Oregon delinquency model with 9-year follow-up of the Oregon Divorce Study. *Development and Psychopathology, 21,* 637–660.

Foss, K.D.B., Thomas, S., Khoury, J.C., Myer, G.D., & Hewett, T.E. (2018). A school-based neuromuscular training program and sport-related injury incidence: A prospective randomized controlled clinical trial. *Journal of Athletic Training, 53*(1), 20–28.

Foulkes, L., & Blakemore, S.J. (2018). Studying individual differences in human adolescent brain development. *Nature Neuroscience, 21,* 315–323.

Fox, B.J. (2012). *Word identification strategies* (5th ed.). Boston: Allyn & Bacon.

Fox, E.L., & others (2018). Who knows what: An exploration of the infant feeding message environment and intracultural differences in Port-au-Prince, Haiti. *Maternal & Child Nutrition, 14*(2), e12537.

Fox, S.E., Levitt, P., & Nelson, C.A. (2010). How the timing and quality of early experiences influence the development of brain architecture. *Child Development, 81,* 28–40.

Fraley, R.C., Roisman, G.I., & Haltigan, J.D. (2013). The legacy of early experiences in development: Formalizing alternative models of how early experiences are carried forward over time. *Developmental Psychology.*

Franchak, J.M., Kretch, K.S., Soska, K.C., & Adolph, K.E. (2011). Head-mounted eye-tracking: A new method to describe the visual ecology of infants. *Child Development, 82,* 1738–1750.

Franchak, J.M. (2018). Changing opportunities for learning in everyday life: Infant body position over the first year. *Infancy.* doi:10.1111/infa.12272

Frank, M.C., Vul, E., & Johnson, S.P. (2009). Development of infants' attention to faces during the first year. *Cognition, 110,* 160–170.

Franke, B., & Buitelaar, J.K. (2018). Gene-environment interactions. In T. Banaschewski, D. Coghill, & A. Zuddas (Eds.), *Oxford textbook of attention deficit hyperactivity disorder.* Oxford: Oxford University Press.

Frankenhuis, W.E., & Fraley, R.C. (2017). What do evolutionary models teach us about sensitive periods in psychological development? *European Psychologist, 22,* 141–150.

Franklin, A., Bevis, L., Ling, Y., & Hulbert, A. (2010). Biological components of color preference in infancy. *Developmental Science, 13,* 346–354.

Franz, C.E. (1996). The implications of preschool tempo and motoric activity level for personality decades later. Reported in A. Caspi (1998), Personality development across the life course. In W. Damon (Ed.), *Handbook of child psychology* (Vol. 3, p. 337). New York: Wiley.

Freemark, M. (2018). Childhood obesity in the modern age: Global trends, determinants, complications, and costs. In M.S. Freemark (Ed.), *Pediatric obesity: Etiology, pathogenesis, and treatment* (pp. 3–24). Humana Press, Cham.

Freitag, C.M., & others (2018). Focused issue on conduct disorder and aggressive behavior. *European Child & Adolescent Psychiatry, 27,* 1231–1234.

Freitas-Vilela, A.A., & others. (2018). Maternal dietary patterns during pregnancy and intelligence quotients in the offspring at 8 years of age: Findings from the ALSPAC cohort. *Maternal and Child Nutrition, 14*(1), e12431.

Freud, S. (1917). *A general introduction to psychoanalysis.* New York: Washington Square Press.

Frey, W.H. (2018). *Diversity explosion: How new racial demographics are remaking America.* Washington, DC: Brookings Institution Press.

Frey, W.H. (2019). *America's not full. Its future rests with young immigrants.* Washington, DC: Brookings Institution. Retrieved May 4, 2019, from https://www.brookings.edu/blog/the-avenue/2019/04/10/america-is-not-full-its-future-rests-with-young-immigrants/

Frick, M.A., & others (2018). The role of sustained attention, maternal sensitivity, and infant temperament in the development of early self-regulation. *British Journal of Psychology, 109,* 277–298.

Friedman, N.P., & Miyake, A. (2017). Unity and diversity of executive functions: Individual differences as a window on cognitive structure. *Cortex, 86,* 186–204.

Friedman, S.L., Melhuish, E., & Hill, C. (2010). Childcare research at the dawn of a new millennium: An update. In G. Bremner & T. Wachs (Eds.), *Wiley-Blackwell handbook of infant development* (2nd ed.). Oxford, UK: Wiley-Blackwell.

Friend, M., & Bursuck, W.D. (2018). *Including students with special needs* (8th ed.). Upper Saddle River, NJ: Pearson.

Friend, M. (2018). *Special education* (5th ed.). Upper Saddle River, NJ: Pearson.

Frisen, A., Hasselblad, T., & Holmqvist, K. (2012). What actually makes bullying stop? Reports from former victims. *Journal of Adolescence, 35,* 981–990.

Fromberg, D., & Bergen, D. (2015). *Play from birth to twelve* (3rd ed.). New York: Routledge.

Fuchs, L.S., & others. (2013). Instructional intervention for students with mathematical learning disabilities. In H. L. Swanson & others (Eds.), *Handbook of learning disabilities* (2nd ed.). New York: Guilford.

Fuligni, A.J. (2012). Gaps, conflicts, and arguments between adolescents and their parents. *New Directions for Child and Adolescent Development, 135,* 105–110.

Fuligni, A.J., Arruda, E.H., Krull, J.L., & Gonzales, N.A. (2018). Adolescent sleep duration, variability, and peak levels of achievement and mental health. *Child Development, 89,* e18–e28.

Fuligni, A.J. (2019). The need to contribute during adolescence. *Perspectives on Psychological Science, 14*(3), 331–343.

Fung, C., & others (2012). From "best practice" to "next practice": The effectiveness of school-based health promotion in improving healthy eating and physical activity and preventing childhood obesity. *International Journal of Behavioral Nutrition and Physical Activity, 9,* 27.

Fung, H., Li, J., & Lam, C.K. (2017). Multi-faceted discipline strategies of Chinese parenting. *International Journal of Behavioral Development, 41,* 472–481.

Fung, H. (2011). Cultural psychological perspectives on social development. In P. K. Smith & C. H. Hart (Eds.), *Wiley-Blackwell handbook of childhood social development* (2nd ed.). New York: Wiley.

Furth, H.G., & Wachs, H. (1975). *Thinking goes to school.* New York: Oxford University Press.

G

Gámez, P.B., Griskell, H.L., Sobrevilla, Y.N., & Vazquez, M. (2019). Dual language and English-only learners' expressive and receptive language skills and exposure to peers' language. *Child Development, 90*(2), 471–479.

Galambos, N.L., Berenbaum, S.A., & McHale, S.M. (2009). Gender development in adolescence. In R. M. Lerner & L. Steinberg (Eds.), *Handbook of adolescent psychology.* New York: Wiley.

Galinsky, E. (2010). *Mind in the making.* New York: Harper Collins.

Galinsky, E., & David, J. (1988). *The preschool years: Family strategies that work—from experts and parents.* New York: Times Books.

Galland, B.C., Taylor, B.J., Edler, D.E., & Herbison, P. (2012). Normal sleep patterns in infants and children: A systematic review of observational studies. *Sleep Medicine Review, 16,* 213–222.

Galloway, A.T., Watson, P., Pitama, S., & Farrow, C.V. (2018). Socioeconomic position and picky eating behavior predict disparate weight trajectories in infancy. *Frontiers in Endocrinology, 9,* 528.

Ganong, L., & Coleman, M. (Eds.) (2017). *Stepfamily relationships: Development, dynamics, and interventions.* New York: Springer.

Ganong, L., Coleman, M., & Jamison, T. (2011). Patterns of stepchild-stepparent relationship development. *Journal of Marriage and the Family, 73,* 396–413.

Garcia Coll, C., & Pachter, L.M. (2002). Ethnic and minority parenting. In M. H. Bornstein (Ed.), *Handbook of parenting* (2nd ed., Vol. 4). Mahwah, NJ: Erlbaum.

Garcia, E.P., McKee, L.G., & Forehand, R. (2012). Discipline. In J. R. Levesque (Ed.), *Encyclopedia of adolescence.* New York: Springer.

Gardner, H. (1983). *Frames of mind.* New York: Basic Books.

Gardner, M., & Steinberg, L. (2005). Peer influence on risk taking, risk preference, and risky decision making in adolescence and adulthood: An experimental study. *Developmental Psychology, 41,* 625–635.

Gardner, M., Brooks-Gunn, J., & Chase-Lansdale, P.L. (2016). The two-generation approach to building human capital: Past, present, and future. In E. Votruba-Drzal & E. Dearing (Eds.), *Handbook of early childhood development programs, practices, and policies.* New York: Wiley.

Gareth, T. (2017). *Decision-making by expectant parents: NIPT, NIPD, and current methods of prenatal screening for Down's Syndrome (Evidence Review).*

[Project Report]. Nuffield Council on Bioethics. Retrieved from http://nuffieldbioethics.org/wp-content/uploads/Gareth-Thomas-evidence-review-decision-making-NIPT.pdf

Garg, N., Schiebinger, L., Jurafsky, D., & Zou, J. (2018). Word embeddings quantify 100 years of gender and ethnic stereotypes. *Proceedings of the National Academy of Sciences, 115*(16), E3635–E3644.

Gariépy, G., Janssen, I., Sentenac, M., & Elgar, F.J. (2017). School start time and sleep in Canadian adolescents. *Journal of Sleep Research, 26,* 195–201.

Garrett, G.S., & Bailey, L.B. (2018). A public health approach for preventing neural tube defects: Folic acid fortification and beyond. *Annals of the New York Academy of Sciences, 1414*(1), 47–58.

Garthe, R.C., Sullivan, T.N., & Behrhorst, K.L. (2018). A latent class analysis of early adolescent peer and dating violence: Associations with symptoms of depression and anxiety. *Journal of Interpersonal Violence,* 0886260518759654.

Gartstein, M.A., & Skinner, M.K. (2018). Prenatal influences on temperament development: The role of environmental epigenetics. *Development and Psychopathology, 30,* 1269–1303.

Gasparini, C., Sette, S., Baumgartner, E., Martin, C.L., & Fabes, R.A. (2015). Gender-biased attitudes and attributions among young Italian children: Relation to peer dyadic interaction. *Sex Roles, 73,* 427–441.

Gasser, L., & Keller, M. (2009). Are the competent morally good? Perspective taking and moral motivation of children involved in bullying. *Social Development, 18*(4), 798–816.

Gassman-Pines, A., & Skinner, A. (2018). Psychological acculturation and parenting behaviors in Mexican American families. *Journal of Family Issues, 39*(5), 1139–1164.

Gates, G.J. (2013). *LGBT parenting in the United States.* Los Angeles: The Williams Institute.

Gates, W. (1998, July 20). Charity begins when I'm ready (interview). *Fortune.*

Gauvain, M. (2013). Sociocultural contexts of development. In P. D. Zelazo (Ed.), *Oxford handbook of developmental psychology.* New York: Oxford University Press.

Gauvain, M. (2018). Collaborative problem solving: Social and developmental considerations. *Psychological Science in the Public Interest, 19,* 53–58.

Gazelle, H., & Faldowski, R.A. (2019, in press). Multiple trajectories in anxious solitary youths: The middle school transition as a turning point in development. *Journal of Abnormal Child Psychology.*

Geary, D.C., Nicholas, A., Li, Y., & Sun, J. (2017). Developmental change in the influence of domain-general abilities and domain-specific knowledge on mathematics achievement: An eight-year longitudinal study. *Journal of Educational Psychology, 109*(5), 680–693.

Gee, C.L., & Heyman, G.D. (2007). Children's evaluations of other people's self-descriptions. *Social Development, 16*(4), 800–818.

Gelbar, N.W., Bray, M., Kehle, T.J., Madaus, J.W., & Makel, C. (2018). Exploring the nature of compensation strategies in individuals with dyslexia. *Canadian Journal of School Psychology, 33,* 110–124.

Gelman, R. (1969). Conservation acquisition: A problem of learning to attend to relevant attributes. *Journal of Experimental Child Psychology, 7,* 67–87.

Gelman, S.A. (2013). Concepts in development. In P. D. Zelazo (Ed.), *Oxford handbook of developmental psychology.* New York: Oxford University Press.

Gelman, S.A., & Kalish, C.W. (2006). Conceptual development. In W. Damon & R. Lerner (Eds.), *Handbook of child psychology* (6th ed.). New York: Wiley.

Gelman, S.A., Taylor, M.G., & Nguyen, S.P. (2004). Mother-child conversations about gender. *Monographs of the Society for Research in Child Development, 69* (1, Serial No. 275).

Geniole, S.N., & Carré, J.M. (2018). Human social neuroendocrinology: Review of the rapid effects of testosterone. *Hormones and Behavior, 104,* 192–205.

Gennetian, L.A., & Miller, C. (2002). Children and welfare reform: A view from an experimental welfare reform program in Minnesota. *Child Development, 73,* 601–620.

Germeroth, C., & others (2019, in press). Play it high, play it low: Examining the reliability and validity of a new observation tool to measure children's make-believe play. *American Journal of Play, 11*(2).

Gershoff, E.T., & others. (2010). Parent discipline practices in an international sample: Associations with child behaviors and moderation by perceived normativeness. *Child Development, 81,* 487–502.

Gershoff, E.T. (2002). Corporal punishment by parents and associated child behaviors and experiences: A meta-analysis and theoretical review. *Psychological Bulletin, 128,* 539–579.

Gershoff, E.T., Lansford, J.E., Sexton, H.R., Davis-Kean, P., & Sameroff, A. (2012). Longitudinal links between spanking and children's externalizing behaviors in a national sample of White, Black, Hispanic, and Asian American families. *Child Development, 83,* 838–843.

Gershoff, E.T., & Grogan-Kaylor, A. (2016). Race as a moderator of associations between spanking and child outcomes. *Family Relations, 65,* 490–501.

Gertner, Y., & Fisher, C. (2012). Predicted errors in children's early sentence comprehension. *Cognition, 124*(1), 85–94.

Gesell, A.L. (1934b). *Infancy and human growth.* New York: MacMillan.

Gesell, A. (1934a). *An atlas of human behavior.* New Haven, CT: Macmillan.

Geurten, M., Meulemans, T., & Lemaire, P. (2018). From domain-specific to domain-general? The developmental path of metacognition for strategy selection. *Cognitive Development, 48,* 62–81.

Ghazarian, S.R., & Roche, K.M. (2010). Social support and low-income, urban mothers: Longitudinal associations with delinquency. *Journal of Youth and Adolescence, 39,* 1097–1108.

Gibbons, J., & Poelker, K. (2019). Adolescent development in cross-cultural perspective. In K. Keith (Ed.), *Cross-cultural psychology: Contemporary themes and perspectives* (2nd ed.). New York: Wiley.

Gibbons, L., & others (2013). Inequities in the use of cesarean section deliveries in the world. *American Journal of Obstetrics and Gynecology, 206*(4), 331.

Gibbs, B.G., Forste, R., & Lybbert, E. (2018). Breastfeeding, parenting, and infant attachment behaviors. *Maternal and Child Health Journal, 22,* 579–588.

Gibbs, J. (2019). *Moral development and reality: Beyond the theories of Kohlberg, Hoffman, and Haidt* (4th ed.). New York: Oxford University Press.

Gibson, E.J. (1989). Exploratory behavior in the development of perceiving, acting, and the acquiring of knowledge. *Annual Review of Psychology* (Vol. 39). Palo Alto, CA: Annual Reviews.

Gibson, E.J., & Walk, R.D. (1960). The "visual cliff." *Scientific American, 202,* 64–71.

Gibson, J.J. (2014). *The ecological approach to visual perception.* New York: Routledge.

Giedd, J.N. (2012). The digital revolution and the adolescent brain. *Journal of Adolescent Health, 51,* 101–105.

Giedd, J.N., & others (2012). Anatomic magnetic resonance imaging of the developing child and adolescent brain. In V. F. Reyna & others (Eds.), *The adolescent brain.* Washington, DC: American Psychological Association.

Gieysztor, E.Z., Choińska, A.M., & Paprocka-Borowicz, M. (2018). Persistence of primitive reflexes and associated motor problems in healthy preschool children. *Archives of Medical Science: AMS, 14*(1), 167–173.

Gilkerson, J., & others (2018). Language experience in the second year of life and language outcomes in late childhood. *Pediatrics, 142,* e20174276.

Gilkerson, J., Richards, J.A., & Topping, K.J. (2017). The impact of book reading in the early years on parent–child language interaction. *Journal of Early Childhood Literacy, 17,* 92–110.

Gilligan, C. (1992, May). *Joining the resistance: Girls' development in adolescence.* Paper presented at the symposium on development and vulnerability in close relationships, Montreal, Quebec.

Gilmore, J.H., Knickmeyer, R.C., & Gao, W. (2018). Imaging structural and functional brain development in early childhood. *Nature Reviews Neuroscience, 19,* 123–137.

Giménez-Dasí, M., Pons, F., & Bender, P.K. (2016). Imaginary companions, theory of mind and emotion understanding in young children. *European Early Childhood Education Research Journal, 24*(2), 186–197.

Giovannini, M., Verduci, E., Salvatici, E., Paci, S., & Riva, E. (2012). Phenylketonuria: Nutritional advances and challenges. *Nutrition and Metabolism, 9*(1), 7.

Glock, S., & Kleen, H. (2017). Gender and student misbehavior: Evidence from implicit and explicit measures. *Teaching and Teacher Education, 67,* 93–103.

Gobet, F. (2018). The future of expertise: The need for a multidisciplinary approach. *Journal of Expertise, 1*(2), 107–113.

Goffin, K.C., Boldt, L.J., & Kochanska, G. (2018). A secure base from which to cooperate: Security, child and parent willing stance, and adaptive and maladaptive outcomes in two longitudinal studies. *Journal of Abnormal Child Psychology, 46*(5), 1061–1075.

Goga, A.E., & others. (2012). Infant feeding practices at routine PMTCT site, South Africa: Results of a prospective observational study amongst HIV exposed and unexposed infants–birth to 9 months. *International Breastfeeding Journal, 7*(1), 4.

Gogtay, N., & Thompson, P.M. (2010). Mapping gray matter development: Implications for typical development and vulnerability to psychopathology. *Brain and Cognition, 72*, 6-15.

Goldberg, W.A., & Lucas-Thompson, R. (2008). Maternal and paternal employment, effects of. In M. M. Haith & J. B. Benson (Eds.), *Encyclopedia of infant and early childhood development.* Oxford, UK: Elsevier.

Golden, R.L., Furman, W., & Collibee, C. (2016). The risks and rewards of sexual debut. *Developmental Psychology, 52*(11), 1913-1925.

Goldenberg, R.L., & Culhane, J.F. (2007). Low birth weight in the United States. *American Journal of Clinical Nutrition, 85*(Suppl.), S584-S590.

Goldfield, G.S. (2011). Making access to TV contingent on physical activity: Effects on liking and relative reinforcing value of TV and physical activity in overweight and obese children. *Journal of Behavioral Medicine, 35*, 1-7.

Goldfield, G.S., Adamo, K.B., Rutherford, J., & Murray, M. (2012). The effects of aerobic exercise on psychosocial functioning of adolescents who are overweight or obese. *Journal of Pediatric and Adolescent Psychology, 37*, 1136-1147.

Goldin-Meadow, S. (2018). Taking a hands-on approach to learning. *Policy Insights from the Behavioral and Brain Sciences, 5*, 163-170.

Goldin-Meadow, S., & Alibali, M.W.A. (2013). Gesture's role in learning and development. In P. Zelazo (Ed.), *Oxford University handbook of developmental psychology.* New York: Oxford University Press.

Goldscheider, F., & Sassler, S. (2006). Creating stepfamilies: Integrating children into the study of union formation. *Journal of Marriage and the Family, 68*, 275-291.

Goldstein, M.H., King, A.P., & West, M.J. (2003). Social interaction shapes babbling: Testing parallels between birdsong and speech. *Proceedings of the National Academy of Sciences, 100*(13), 8030-8035.

Goleman, D. (1995). *Emotional intelligence.* New York: Basic Books.

Goliath, V., & Pretorius, B. (2016). Peer risk and protective factors in adolescence: Implications for drug use prevention. *Social Work, 52*(1), 113-129.

Golinkoff, R.M., Hoff, E., Rowe, M.L., Tamis-LeMonda, C.S., & Hirsh-Pasek, K. (2019). Language matters: Denying the existence of the 30-million-word gap has serious consequences. *Child Development, 90*(3), 985-992.

Gollnick, D.M., & Chinn, P.C. (2016). *Multicultural education in a pluralistic society* (10th ed.). Upper Saddle River, NJ: Pearson.

Golombok, S., & Tasker, F. (2010). Gay fathers. In M. E. Lamb (Ed.), *The role of the father in child development* (5th ed.). New York: Wiley.

Golombok, S. (2017). Parenting in new family forms. *Current Opinion in Psychology, 15*, 76-80.

Gomes, J.D.A., & others (2018). Genetic susceptibility to thalidomide embryopathy in humans: Study of candidate development genes. *Birth Defects Research, 110*(5), 456-461.

Gonzales, M., Jones, D.J., Kincaid, C.Y., & Cuellar, J. (2012). Neighborhood context and adjustment in African American youths from single mother homes: The intervening role of hopelessness. *Cultural Diversity and Ethnic Minority Psychology, 18*, 109-117.

González, J.M. (Ed.). (2009). *Encyclopedia of bilingual education.* Thousand Oaks, CA: Sage.

Gonzalez, C.L., & Sacrey, L.A.R. (2018). The development of the motor system. In R. Gibb & B. Kolb (Eds.), *The neurobiology of brain and behavioral development* (pp. 235-256). New York: Academic Press.

Good, C., Rattan, A., & Dweck, C.S. (2012). Why do women opt out? Sense of belonging and women's representation in mathematics. *Journal of Personality and Social Psychology, 102*, 700-717.

Good, M., & Willoughby, T. (2008). Adolescence as a sensitive period for spiritual development. *Child Development Perspectives, 2*, 32-37.

Good, T.L., & Lavigne, A.L. (2017). *Looking in classrooms.* New York: Routledge.

Goodkind, S. (2013). Single-sex public education for low-income youth of color: A critical theoretical review. *Sex Roles, 69*(7-8), 393-402.

Goodman, W.B., & others. (2011). Parental work stress and latent profiles of father-infant parenting quality. *Journal of Marriage and the Family, 73*, 588-604.

Goodwin, S., McPherson, J.D., & McCombie, W.R. (2016). Coming of age: Ten years of next-generation sequencing technologies. *Nature Reviews Genetics, 17*, 331-351.

Gopnik, A. (2010). Commentary. In E. Galinsky (2010). *Mind in the making.* New York: Harper Collins.

Gorrese, A., & Ruggieri, R. (2012). Peer attachment: A meta-analytic review of gender and age differences and associations with parent attachment. *Journal of Youth and Adolescence, 41*, 650-672.

Gottlieb, G. (2007). Probabilistic epigenesis. *Developmental Science, 10*, 1-11.

Gottlieb, G., Wahlsten, D., & Lickliter, R. (2006). The significance of biology for human development: A developmental psychobiological systems view. In W. Damon & R. Lerner (Eds.), *Handbook of child psychology* (6th ed.). New York: Wiley.

Gottman Relationship Institute. (2009). *Research on parenting.* Retrieved December 9, 2009, from www.gottman.com/parenting/research

Gottman, J.M., & DeClaire, J. (1997). *The heart of parenting: Raising an emotionally intelligent child.* New York: Simon & Schuster.

Gottman, J.M. (2012). *Emotion coaching.* Retrieved July 8, 2012, from www.gottman.com/parenting/

Gottman, J.M. (2013). *Research on parenting.* Retrieved January 10, 2013, from www.gottman.com/parenting/research

Gottman, J., Gottman, J., & Shapiro, A. (2009). A new couples approach to interventions for the transition to parenthood. In M. S. Schulz, P. K. Kerig, M. K. Pruett, & R. D. Parke (Eds.), *Feathering the nest.* Washington, DC: American Psychological Association.

Gottman, J.M., & Parker, J.G. (Eds.). (1987). *Conversations of friends.* New York: Cambridge University Press.

Gould, S.J. (1981). *The mismeasure of man.* New York: W. W. Norton.

Gradisar, M., Gardner, G., & Dohnt, H. (2011). Recent worldwide sleep patterns and problems during adolescence: A review and meta-analysis of age, region, and sleep. *Sleep Medicine, 12*, 110-118.

Graham, J., & Valdesolo, P. (2017). Morality. In K. Deaux & M. Snyder (Eds.), *Oxford handbook of personality and social psychology.* New York: Oxford University Press.

Graham, S., & Harris, K.R. (2018). An examination of the design principles underlying a self-regulated strategy development study. *Journal of Writing Research, 10*, 139-187.

Graham, S., & Perin, D. (2007). A metaanalysis of writing instruction for adolescent students. *Journal of Educational Psychology, 99*, 445-476.

Graham, S., Harris, K.R., & Chambers, A.B. (2016). Evidence-based practice and writing instruction: A review of reviews. In C.A. MacArthur, S. Graham, & J. Fitzgerald (Eds.), *Handbook of writing research* (2nd ed.). New York: Guilford.

Granqvist, P., & others (2017). Disorganized attachment in infancy: A review of the phenomenon and its implications for clinicians and policy-makers. *Attachment and Human Development, 19*, 534-558.

Grant, J.P. (1997). *The state of the world's children.* New York: UNICEF and Oxford University Press.

Grant, J.H., & others (2018). Implementing group prenatal care in southwest Georgia through public–private partnerships. *Maternal and Child Health Journal, 22*(11), 1535-1542.

Grard, A., & others (2018). Same-sex friendship, school gender composition, and substance use: a social network study of 50 European schools. *Substance use & misuse, 53*(6), 998-1007.

Gravetter, R.J., & Forzano, L.B. (2019). *Research methods for the behavioral sciences* (6th ed.). Boston: Cengage.

Gray, J. (1992). *Men are from Mars, women are from Venus.* New York: HarperCollins.

Gray, K., & Graham, J. (2018). *The atlas of moral psychology.* New York: Guilford.

Gray, S., & others (2017). The structure of working memory in young children and its relation to intelligence. *Journal of Memory and Language, 92*, 183-201.

Graziano, A.M., & Raulin, M.L. (2013). *Research methods* (8th ed,). Boston: Allyn & Bacon.

Green, R., Collingwood, A., & Ross, A. (2010). *Characteristics of bullying victims in schools.* London: National Centre for Social Research.

Green, T., Flash, S., & Reiss, A.L. (2019). Sex differences in psychiatric disorders: What we can learn from sex chromosome aneuploidies. *Neuropsychopharmacology, 44*, 9-21.

Greenberg, D.M., Warrier, V., Allison, C., & Baron-Cohen, S. (2018). Testing the empathizing-systemizing theory of sex differences and the extreme male brain theory of autism in half a million people. *Proceedings of the National Academy of Sciences, 115*(48), 12152-12157.

Greenberg, E.H. (2018). Public preferences for targeted and universal preschool. *AERA Open, 4*(1), 1-20.

Greenfield, P.M. (2018). Studying social change, culture, and human development: A theoretical framework and methodological guidelines. *Developmental Review, 50,* 16-30.

Greer, F.R., Sicherer, S.H., Burks, A.W., & Committee on Nutrition and Section on Allergy and Immunology (2008). Effects of early nutritional interventions on the development of atopic disease in infants and children: The role of maternal dietary restriction, breast feeding, timing of introduction of complementary foods, and hydrolyzed formulas. *Pediatrics, 121,* 183-191.

Gregorson, M., Kaufman, J.C., & Snyder, H. (Eds.). (2013). *Teaching creatively and teaching creativity.* New York: Springer.

Griffiths, J.D., Marslen-Wilson, W.D., Stamatakis, E.A., & Tyler, L.K. (2013). Functional organization of the neural language system: Dorsal and ventral pathways are critical for syntax. *Cerebral Cortex, 23*(1), 139-147.

Grigg, R., & Lewis, H. (2019). *Teaching creative and critical thinking in schools.* Thousand Oaks, CA: SAGE.

Grigorenko, E. (2000). Heritability and intelligence. In R. J. Sternberg (Ed.), *Handbook of intelligence.* New York: Cambridge University Press.

Grisaru-Granovsky, S., & others (2018). The mortality of very low birth weight infants: The benefit and relative impact of changes in population and therapeutic variables. *The Journal of Maternal-Fetal & Neonatal Medicine, 32*(15), 2443-2451.

Groh, A.M., & others (2019, in press). Mothers' physiological and affective responding to infant distress: Unique antecedents of avoidant and resistant attachments. *Child Development.*

Groh, A.M., Fearon, R.M.P., van IJzendoorn, M.H., Bakermans-Kranenburg, M.J., & Roisman, G.I. (2017). Attachment in the early life course: Meta-analytic evidence for its role in socioemotional development. *Child Development Perspectives, 11,* 70-76.

Gross, L.S. (2013). *Electronic media* (11th ed.). New York: McGraw-Hill.

Grossmann, K., Grossmann, K.E., Spangler, G., Suess, G., & Unzner, L. (1985). Maternal sensitivity and newborns' orientation responses as related to quality of attachment in northern Germany. In I. Bretherton & E. Waters (Eds.), Growing points of attachment theory and research. *Monographs of the Society for Research in Child Development, 50* (1-2, Serial No. 209).

Grotevant, H.D., & Cooper, C.R. (1998). Individuality and connectedness in adolescent development: Review and prospects for research on identity, relationship, and context. In E. Skoe & A. von der Lippe (Eds.), *Personality development in adolescence: A cross-national and life-span perspective.* London: Routledge.

Grusec, J.E., & Davidov, M. (2010). Integrating different perspectives on socialization theory and research: A domain-specific approach. *Child Development, 81,* 687-709.

Grusec, J.E. (2009). Unpublished review of J. W. Santrock's *Child Development,* 13th ed. (New York: McGraw-Hill).

Grusec, J.E. (2011). Human development: Development in the family. *Annual Review of Psychology* (Vol. 62). Palo Alto, CA: Annual Reviews.

Grusec, J.E. (2013). The development of moral behavior and conscience from a socialization perspective. In M. Killen & J. G. Smetana (Eds.), *Handbook of moral development* (2nd ed.). New York: Routledge.

Grusec, J.E., Chaparro, M.P., Johnston, M., & Sherman, A. (2013). Social development and social relationships in middle childhood. In I. B. Weiner & others (Eds.), *Handbook of psychology* (2nd ed., Vol. 6). New York: Wiley.

Grusec, J. (2017). A domains-of-socialization perspective on children's social development. In N. Budwig & others (Eds.), *New perspectives on human development.* Cambridge, UK: Cambridge University Press.

Grusec, J.E., & others (2014). The development of moral behavior from a socialization perspective. In M. Killen & J. Smetana (Eds.) *Handbook of moral development* (2nd ed., pp. 113-134). New York: Psychology Press.

Grych, J.H. (2002). Marital relationships and parenting. In M. H. Bornstein (Ed.), *Handbook of parenting.* Mahwah, NJ: Erlbaum.

Gryzwacz, J., & Demerouti, E. (Eds.). (2013). *New frontiers in work and family research.* New York: Routledge.

Gubbels, J., Segers, E., Keuning, J., & Verhoeven, L. (2016). The Aurora-a Battery as an assessment of triarchic intellectual abilities in upper primary grades. *Gifted Child Quarterly, 60,* 226-238.

Gui, D.Y., Gan, T., & Liu, C. (2016). Neural evidence for moral intuition and the temporal dynamics of interactions between emotional processes and moral cognition. *Social Neuroscience, 11,* 380-394.

Guild, D.J., Alto, M.E., & Toth, S.L. (2017). Preventing the intergenerational transmission of child maltreatment through relational interventions. In D. Teti (Ed.), *Parenting and family processes in child maltreatment and intervention* (pp. 127-137). New York: Springer.

Gunderson, E.A., Ramirez, G., Levine, S.C., & Beilock, S.L. (2012). The role of parents and teachers in the development of math attitudes. *Sex Roles, 66,* 153-166.

Gunderson, E.A., & others (2018). The specificity of parenting effects: Differential relations of parent praise and criticism to children's theories of intelligence and learning goals. *Journal of Experimental Child Psychology, 173,* 116-135.

Gunderson, E.A., Hamdan, N., Sorhagen, N.S., & D'Esterre, A.P. (2017). Who needs innate ability to succeed in math and literacy? Academic-domain-specific theories of intelligence about peers versus adults. *Developmental Psychology, 53,* 1188-1205.

Gunnar, M.R., Fisher, P.A., & The Early Experience, Stress, and Prevention Network (2006). Bringing basic research on early experience and stress neurobiology to bear on preventive interventions for neglected and maltreated children. *Development and Psychopathology, 18,* 651-677.

Gunnar, M.R., & Quevado, K. (2007). The neurobiology of stress and development. *Annual Review of Psychology* (Vol. 58). Palo Alto, CA: Annual Reviews.

Gunnar, M.R., & Hostinar, C.E. (2015). The social buffering of the hypothalamic-pituitary-adrenocortical axis in humans: Developmental and experiential determinants. *Social Neuroscience, 10,* 479-488.

Guo, S., & Wong, L. (2019). *Immigration, racial and ethnic studies in 150 years of Canada.* Leiden, The Netherlands: Brill.

Guo, S. (2018). A model of religious involvement, family processes, self-control, and juvenile delinquency in two-parent families. *Journal of Adolescence, 63,* 175-190.

Gurwitch, R.H., Silovsky, J.F., Schultz, S., Kees, M., & Burlingame, S. (2001). *Reactions and guidelines for children following trauma/disaster.* Norman, OK: Department of Pediatrics, University of Oklahoma Health Sciences Center.

H

Höchli, B., Brügger, A., & Messner, C. (2018). How focusing on superordinate goals motivates broad, long-term goal pursuit: A theoretical perspective. *Frontiers in Psychology, 9,* 1879.

Hadad, B.S., Maurer, D., & Lewis, T.L. (2017). The role of early visual input in the development of contour interpolation: The case of subjective contours. *Developmental Science, 20*(3), e12379.

Hadd, A.R., & Rodgers, J.L. (2017). Intelligence, income, and education as potential influences on a child's home environment: A (maternal) sibling-comparison design. *Developmental Psychology, 53,* 1286-1299.

Hadders-Algra, M. (2018). Early human brain development: Starring the subplate. *Neuroscience & Biobehavioral Reviews, 92,* 276-290.

Hadders-Algra, M. (2018). Early human motor development: From variation to the ability to vary and adapt. *Neuroscience & Biobehavioral Reviews, 90,* 411-427.

Hadley, K., & Sheiner, E. (2017). The significance of gender in perinatal medicine. In M.J. Legato (Ed.), *Principles of gender-specific medicine* (3rd ed., pp. 219-236). New York: Academic Press.

Hafen, C.A., & others (2012). The pivotal role of adolescent autonomy in secondary school classrooms. *Journal of Youth and Adolescence, 41,* 245-255.

Haga, M., & others (2018). Cross-cultural aspects: exploring motor competence among 7- to 8-year-old children from Greece, Italy, and Norway. *Sage Open, 8*(2), 2158244018768381.

Haidt, J. (2013). *The righteous mind.* New York: Random House.

Haidt, J. (2017). *Three stories about capitalism.* New York: Pantheon.

Haier, R.J. (2017). *The neuroscience of intelligence.* Cambridge, UK: Cambridge University Press.

Haines, E.L., Deaux, K., & Lofaro, N. (2016). The times they are a-changing . . . or are they not? A comparison of gender stereotypes, 1983–2014. *Psychology of Women Quarterly, 40,* 353–363.

Hakala, M., & others (2017). The realization of BFHI Step 4 in Finland: Initial breastfeeding and skin-to-skin contact according to mothers and midwives. *Midwifery, 50,* 27–35.

Hakuno, Y., Pirazzoli, L., Blasi, A., Johnson, M.H., & Lloyd-Fox, S. (2018). Optical imaging during toddlerhood: brain responses during naturalistic social interactions. *Neurophotonics, 5*(1), 011020.

Halfon, N., & Forrest, C.B. (2018). The emerging theoretical framework of life course health development. In N. Halfon & others (Eds.), *Handbook of life course health development* (pp. 19–43). London: Springer.

Halim, M.L.D., & others (2018). The roles of self-socialization and parent socialization in toddlers' gender-typed appearance. *Archives of Sexual Behavior, 47,* 2277–2285.

Hall, G.N. (2018). *Multicultural psychology* (3rd ed.). New York: Routledge.

Hall, J.A. (2011). Sex differences in friendship expectations: A meta-analysis. *Journal of Social and Personal Relationships, 28*(6), 723–747.

Halldorsdottir, T., & Binder, E.B. (2017). Gene × environment interactions: From molecular mechanisms to behavior. *Annual Review of Psychology, 68,* 215–241.

Hallemans, A., & others (2018). Developmental changes in spatial margin of stability in typically developing children relate to the mechanics of gait. *Gait & Posture, 63,* 33–38.

Halpern, D.F., Beninger, A.S., & Straight, C.A. (2011). Sex differences in intelligence. In R. J. Sternberg & S. B. Kaufman (Eds.), *Handbook of intelligence.* New York: Cambridge University Press.

Han, A., Fu, A., Cobley, S., & Sanders, R.H. (2017). Effectiveness of exercise intervention on improving fundamental movement skills and motor coordination in overweight/obese children and adolescents: A systematic review. *Journal of Science and Medicine in Sport, 21,* 89–102.

Han, W-J. (2009). Maternal employment. In D. Carr (Ed.). *Encyclopedia of the life course and human development.* Boston: Gale Cengage.

Hanford, L.C., & others (2018). The impact of caregiving on the association between infant emotional behavior and resting state neural network functional topology. *Frontiers in Psychology, 9,* 1968.

Hannigan, S. (2018). A theoretical and practice-informed reflection on the value of failure in art. *Thinking Skills and Creativity, 30,* 171–179.

Hannon, E.E., Schachner, A., & Nave-Blodgett, J.E. (2017). Babies know bad dancing when they see it: Older but not younger infants discriminate between synchronous and asynchronous audiovisual musical displays. *Journal of Experimental Child Psychology, 159,* 159–174.

Hanushek, E.A., Kain, J.F., & Rivkin, S.G. (2004). Disruption versus Tiebout improvement: The costs and benefits of switching schools. *Journal of Public Economics, 88*(9–10), 1721–1746.

Harakeh, Z., & others (2012). Individual and environmental predictors of health risk behaviors among Dutch adolescents: The HBSC study. *Public Health, 126,* 566–573.

Hare, B.R., & Castenell, L.A. (1985). No place to run, no place to hide: Comparative status and future prospects of Black boys. In M. B. Spencer, G. K. Brookins, & W. R. Allen (Eds.), *Beginnings: The social and affective development of Black children.* Hillsdale, NJ: Erlbaum.

Hare, B.D., & others (2018). Two weeks of variable stress increases Gamma-H2AX levels in the mouse bed nucleus of the stria terminalis. *Neuroscience, 373,* 137–144.

Harkness, S., & Super, B.M. (1995). Culture and parenting. In M. H. Bornstein (Ed.), *Handbook of parenting* (Vol. 3). Hillsdale, NJ: Erlbaum.

Harlen, W., & Qualter, A. (2018). *The teaching of science in primary schools* (7th ed.). New York: Routledge.

Harlow, H.F. (1958). The nature of love. *American Psychologist, 13,* 673–685.

Harlow, H.F., & Suomi, S.J. (1970). Nature of love: Simplified. *American Psychologist, 25,* 161–168.

Harper, J.M., Padilla-Walker, L.M., & Jensen, A.C. (2016). Do siblings matter independent of both parents and friends? Sympathy as a mediator between sibling relationship quality and adolescent outcomes. *Journal of Research in Adolescence, 26,* 101–114.

Harrington, B., & O'Connell, M. (2016). Video games as virtual teachers: Prosocial video game use by children and adolescents from different socioeconomic groups is associated with increased empathy and prosocial behaviour. *Computers in Human Behavior, 63,* 650–658.

Harris, J., Golinkoff, R.M., & Hirsh-Pasek, K. (2012). Lessons from the crib for the classroom: How children really learn vocabulary. In S. B. Neuman & D. K. Dickinson (Eds.), *Handbook of early literacy research.* New York: Guilford.

Harris, R.J., Schoen, L.M., & Hensley, D.L. (1992). A cross-cultural study of story memory. *Journal of Cross-Cultural Psychology, 23,* 133–147.

Harrison-Hale, A.O., McLoyd, V.C., & Smedley, B. (2004). Racial and ethnic status: Risk and protective processes among African-American families. In K. L. Maton, C. J. Schellenbach, B. J. Leadbetter, & A. L. Solarz (Eds.), *Investing in children, families, and communities.* Washington, DC: American Psychological Association.

Hart, B., & Risley, T.R. (1995). *Meaningful differences.* Baltimore, MD: Paul Brookes.

Hart, S., & Wandeler, C. (2018). The impact of action civics service-learning on eighth-grade students' civic outcomes. *International Journal of Research on Service-Learning and Community Engagement, 6*(1), Article 11.

Hart, S., & Carrington, H. (2002). Jealousy in 6-month-old infants. *Infancy, 3,* 395–402.

Hart, S.L. (2018). Jealousy and attachment: Adaptations to threat posed by the birth of a sibling. *Evolutionary Behavioral Sciences, 12,* 263–275.

Hartanto, A., Toh, W.X., & Yang, H. (2018). Bilingualism narrows socioeconomic disparities in executive functions and self-regulatory behaviors during early childhood: Evidence from the Early Childhood Longitudinal Study. *Child Development.* doi:10.1111/cdev.13032

Harter, S. (1985). *Self-Perception Profile for Children.* Denver: University of Denver. Department of Psychology.

Harter, S. (1989). *Self-Perception Profile for Adolescents.* Denver: University of Denver. Department of Psychology.

Harter, S. (2012). *The construction of the self* (2nd ed.). New York: Wiley.

Harter, S. (2015). Self-processes and developmental psychopathology. In D. Cicchetti & D. Cohen (Eds.), *Developmental psychopathology* (2nd ed., pp. 370–418). New York: Wiley.

Hartley, C.A., & Somerville, L.H. (2015). The neuroscience of adolescent decision-making. *Current Opinion in Behavioral Sciences, 5,* 108–115.

Hartshorne, H., & May, M.S. (1928–1930). *Moral studies in the nature of character: Studies in deceit* (Vol. 1); *Studies in self-control* (Vol. 2). *Studies in the organization of character* (Vol. 3). New York: Macmillan.

Hartup, W.W. (1983). The peer system. In P. H. Mussen (Ed.), *Handbook of child psychology* (4th ed., Vol. 4). New York: Wiley.

Hartup, W.W. (2005). Peer interaction: What causes what? *Journal of Abnormal Child Psychology, 33,* 387–394.

Harwood, R., Leyendecker, B., Carlson, V., Asencio, M., & Miller, A. (2002). Parenting among Latino families in the U.S. In M. H. Bornstein (Ed.), *Handbook of parenting* (2nd ed.). Mahwah, NJ: Erlbaum.

Hassan, B., Vignoles, V.L., & Schwartz, S.J. (2018). Reconciling social norms with personal interests: Indigenous styles of identity formation among Pakistani youth. *Emerging Adulthood.* doi:10.1177/2167696817754004

Hatano, K., & Sugimura, K. (2017). Is adolescence a period of identity formation for all youth? Insights from a four-wave longitudinal study of identity dynamics in Japan. *Developmental Psychology, 53*(11), 2113–2126.

Hatton, H., & others (2008). Family and individual difference predictors of trait aspects of negative interpersonal behaviors during emerging adulthood. *Journal of Family Psychology, 22,* 448–455.

Hauptman, M., Bruccoleri, R., & Woolf, A.D. (2017). An update on childhood lead poisoning. *Clinical Pediatric Emergency Medicine, 18,* 181–192.

Havighurst, S.S., & others (2013). "Tuning into Kids": Reducing young children's behavior problems using an emotion coaching parenting program. *Child Psychiatry and Human Development, 44*(2), 247–264.

Hawes, Z., Moss, J., Caswell, B., Naqvi, S., & MacKinnon, S. (2017). Enhancing children's spatial and numerical skills through a dynamic spatial approach to early geometry instruction: Effects of a 32-week intervention. *Cognition and Instruction, 35,* 236–264.

Hawkes, K. (2017). Grandmothering and human evolution: Some updates. Anthropology Colloquium. University of Toronto. Invited talk/keynote, presented 11/05/2017.

Hay, D., Kaplan, M., & Nash, A. (2018). The beginnings of peer relations. In W. Bukowski & others (Eds.), *Handbook of peer interactions, relationships, and groups* (2nd ed.). New York: Guilford.

Hay, D.F., Caplan, M., & Nash, A. (2018). The beginnings of peer relations. In W.M. Bukowski, B. Laursen, & K.H. Rubin (Eds.), *Handbook of peer interactions, relationships, and groups*. New York: Guilford.

Hayes, J.R., & Berninger, V. (2013). Cognitive processes in writing: A framework. In B. Arte, J. Dockrell, & V. Berninger (Eds.), *Writing development and instruction in children with hearing, speech, and language disorders*. New York: Oxford University Press.

Hayes, N., O'Toole, L., & Halpenny, A. (2017). *Introducing Bronfenbrenner*. London: Routledge.

Haynes, R.L., & others (2017). High serum serotonin in sudden infant death syndrome. *Proceedings of the National Academy of Sciences, 114,* 7695-7700.

Hayslip, B., Fruhauf, C.A., & Dolbin-MacNab, M.L. (2017, June 28). Grandparents raising grandchildren: What have we learned over the past decade? *The Gerontologist, 57*(6), 1196-1207.

He, Y., Chen, J., Zhu, L.H., Hua, L.L., & Ke, F.F. (2017). Maternal smoking during pregnancy and ADHD: Results from a systematic review and meta-analysis of prospective cohort studies. *Journal of Attention Disorders.* doi:10.1177/1087054717696766

Hein, S., Röder, M., & Fingerle, M. (2018). The role of emotion regulation in situational empathy-related responding and prosocial behaviour in the presence of negative affect. *International Journal of Psychology, 53*(6), 477-485.

Heinze, J.E., Cook, S.H., Wood, E.P., Dumadag, A.C., & Zimmerman, M.A. (2018). Friendship attachment style moderates the effect of adolescent exposure to violence on emerging adult depression and anxiety trajectories. *Journal of Youth and Adolescence, 47*(1), 177-193.

Hek, K., & others (2013). A genome-wide association study of depression symptoms. *Biological Psychiatry, 73*(7), 667-678.

Helgeson, V. (2016). *Psychology of gender* (5th ed.). Upper Saddle River, NJ: Prentice Hall.

Helwig, C.C. (2017). Identifying universal developmental processes amid contextual variations in moral judgment and reasoning. *Human Development, 60,* 342-349.

Henderson, A., Brown, S.D., & Pancer, S.M. (2019, in press). Curriculum requirements and subsequent civic engagement: Is there a difference between 'forced' and 'free' community service? *The British Journal of Sociology.*

Henderson, C.E., Hogue, A., & Dauber, S. (2019). Family therapy techniques and one-year clinical outcomes among adolescents in usual care for behavior problems. *Journal of Consulting and Clinical Psychology, 87*(3), 308-312.

Hendry, J. (1995). *Understanding Japanese society.* London: Routledge.

Herman, J.L., Flores, A.R., Brown, T.N.T., Wilson, B.D.M., & Conron, K.J. (2017). *Age of individuals who identify as transgender in the United States.* Los Angeles, CA: The Williams Institute.

Herman-Giddens, M.E. (2007). The decline in the age of menarche in the United States: Should we be concerned? *Journal of Adolescent Health, 40,* 201-203.

Herman-Giddens, M.E., & others (2012). Secondary sex characteristics in boys: Data from the pediatric research in office settings network. *Pediatrics, 130,* e1058-e1068.

Hernández, M.M., & others (2017). Observed emotions as predictors of quality of kindergartners' social relationships. *Social Development, 26,* 21-39.

Hernandez-Reif, M., Diego, M., & Field, T. (2007). Preterm infants show reduced stress behaviors and activity after 5 days of massage therapy. *Infant Behavior and Development, 30,* 557-561.

Hertz, S.G., & Krettenauer, T. (2016). Does moral identity effectively predict moral behavior?: A meta-analysis. *Review of General Psychology, 20*(2), 129-140.

Hespos, S.J., Ferry, A.L., Anderson, E.M., Hollenbeck, E.N., & Rips, L.J. (2016). Five-month-old infants have general knowledge of how nonsolid substances behave and interact. *Psychological Science, 27,* 244-256.

Hetherington, E.M. (2005). Divorce and the adjustment of children. *Pediatrics in Review, 26,* 163-169.

Hetherington, E.M. (2006). The influence of conflict, marital problem solving, and parenting on children's adjustment in nondivorced, divorced, and remarried families. In A. Clarke-Stewart & J. Dunn (eds.), *Families count.* New York: Oxford University Press.

Hetherington, E.M., & Kelly, J. (2002). *For better or for worse: Divorce reconsidered.* New York: Norton.

Hetherington, E.M., & Stanley-Hagan, M. (2002). Parenting in divorced and remarried families. In M. H. Bornstein (Ed.), *Handbook of parenting* (2nd ed., Vol. 3). Mahwah, NJ: Erlbaum.

Hetherington, E., McDonald, S., Williamson, T., Patten, S.B., & Tough, S.C. (2018). Social support and maternal mental health at 4 months and 1 year postpartum: Analysis from the All Our Families cohort. *Journal of Epidemiology and Community Health, 72*(10). doi:10.1136/jech-2017-210274

Hewlett, B.S., & MacFarlan, S.J. (2010). Fathers' roles in hunter-gatherer and other small-scale cultures. In M. E. Lamb (Ed.), *The role of the father in child development* (5th ed.). New York: Wiley.

Heyman, G.D., & Legare, C.H. (2005). Children's evaluation of source of information about traits. *Developmental Psychology, 41,* 636-647.

Heyman, G.D., & others (2016). Children's evaluation of public and private generosity and its relation to behavior: Evidence from China. *Journal of Experimental Child Psychology, 150,* 16-30.

Hill, W.D., & others (2018). A combined analysis of genetically correlated traits identifies 187 loci and a role for neurogenesis and myelination in intelligence. *Molecular Psychiatry.* doi:10.1038/s41380-017-0001-5

Hillman, C.H., Erickson, K.I., & Hatfield, B.D. (2017). Run for your life! Childhood physical activity effects on brain and cognition. *Kinesiology Review, 6*(1), 12-21.

Hine, B., England, D., Lopreore, K., Horgan, E.S., & Hartwell, L. (2018). The rise of the androgynous princess: Examining representations of gender in prince and princess characters of Disney movies released 2009-2016. *Social Sciences, 7*(12), 245.

Hirschfield, P.J. (2018). Schools and crime. *Annual Review of Criminology, 1,* 149-169.

Hirsh-Pasek, K., & Golinkoff, R.M. (2013). Early language and literacy: Six principles. In S. Gilford (Ed.), *Head Start teacher's guide.* New York: Teacher's College Press.

Hitokoto, H., & Uchida, Y. (2018). Interdependent happiness: Progress and implications. In M. Demir & N. Sümer (Eds.), *Close relationships and happiness across cultures* (pp. 19-39). London: Springer.

Hoch, J.E., O'Grady, S.M., & Adolph, K.E. (2018). It's the journey, not the destination: Locomotor exploration in infants. *Developmental Science, 22,* e12740.

Hockenberry, S. (2019). *Juvenile justice statistics: National report series fact sheet.* Washington, DC: U.S. Department of Justice. Retrieved April 9, 2019, from https://www.ojjdp.gov/pubs/252473.pdf

Hodapp, R.M. (2016). Blurring boundaries, continuing change: Fifty years of research in intellectual and developmental disabilities. *International Review of Research in Developmental Disabilities, 50,* 1-31.

Hodel, A.S. (2018). Rapid infant prefrontal cortex development and sensitivity to early environmental experience. *Developmental Review, 48,* 113-144.

Hoefnagels, M. (2013). *Biology: The essentials.* New York: McGraw-Hill.

Hoehl, S., & Striano, T. (2018). Social referencing. In M.H. Bornstein (Ed.) & M. Arterberry, K. Fingerman, & J.E. Lansford (Assoc. Eds.), *The SAGE encyclopedia of lifespan human development.* Thousand Oaks, CA: SAGE.

Hoff, E., Laursen, B., & Tardif, T. (2002). Socioeconomic status and parenting. In M. H. Bornstein (Ed.), *Handbook of parenting* (2nd ed.). Mahwah, NJ: Erlbaum.

Hoff, E., Quinn, J.M., & Giguere, D. (2018). What explains the correlation between growth in vocabulary and grammar? New evidence from latent change score analyses of simultaneous bilingual development. *Developmental Science, 21*(2), e12536.

Holden, G.W., Vittrup, B., & Rosen, L.H. (2011). Families, parenting, and discipline. In M. K. Underwood & L. H. Rosen (Eds.), *Social development.* New York: Guilford.

Holder, M.D., & Coleman, B. (2015). Children's friendships and positive well-being. In M. Demir (Ed.), *Friendship and happiness: Across the lifespan and cultures* (pp. 81-97). Dordrecht: Springer.

Holliday, R.E., Brainerd, C.J., & Reyna, V.F. (2011). Developmental reversals in false memory: Now you see them, now you don't! *Developmental Psychology, 47,* 442-449.

Hollifield, C.R., & Conger, K.J. (2015). The role of siblings and psychological needs in predicting life satisfaction during emerging adulthood. *Emerging Adulthood, 3*(3), 143-153.

Holsen, I., Carlson Jones, D., & Skogbrott Birkeland, M. (2012). Body image satisfaction among Norwegian adolescents and young adults: A longitudinal study of interpersonal relationships and BMI. *Body Image, 9,* 201-208.

Hood, B.M. (1995). Gravity rules for 2- to 4-year-olds? *Cognitive Development, 10,* 577-598.

Hooper, S.R., & others (2018). Developmental trajectories of executive functions in young males with fragile X syndrome. *Research in Developmental Disabilities, 81,* 73-88.

Hoover, J., & others (2018). Into the wild: Building value through moral pluralism. In K. Gray & J. Graham (Eds.), *Atlas of moral psychology.* New York: Guilford.

Hopkins, E.J., Smith, E.D., Weisberg, D.S., & Lillard, A.S. (2016). The development of substitute object pretense: The differential importance of form and function. *Journal of Cognition and Development, 17*(2), 197-220.

Horne, R.S., Franco, P., Adamson, T.M., Groswasser, J., & Kahn, A. (2002). Effects of body position on sleep and arousal characteristics in infants. *Early Human Development, 69,* 25-33.

Houde, O., & others (2011). Functional magnetic resonance imaging study of Piaget's conservation-of-number task in preschool and school-age children: A neo-Piagetian approach. *Journal of Experimental Child Psychology, 110,* 332-346.

Howe, M.L., Courage, M.L., & Rooksby, M. (2009). The genesis and development of autobiographical memory. In M. Courage & N. Cowan (Eds.), *The development of memory in infancy and childhood.* New York: Psychology Press.

Howell, J.C., & Griffiths, E. (2019). *Gangs in America's communities* (3rd ed.). Thousand Oaks, CA: SAGE.

Howerton, C.L., & Bale, T.L. (2012). Prenatal programming: At the intersection of maternal stress and immune activation. *Hormones and Behavior, 62*(3), 237-242.

Howes, C. (1985, April). *Predicting preschool sociometric status from toddler peer interaction.* Paper presented at the meeting of the Society for Research in Child Development, Toronto.

Howes, C. (2009). Friendship in early childhood. In K. H. Rubin, W. M. Bukowski, & B. Laursen (Eds.), *Handbook of peer interactions, relationships, and groups.* New York: Guilford.

Howlin, P., Magiati, I., & Charman, T. (2009). Systematic review of early intensive behavioral interventions with autism. *American Journal on Intellectual and Developmental Disabilities, 114,* 23-41.

Hoyt, L.T., Craske, M.G., Mineka, S., & Adam, E.K. (2015). Positive and negative affect and arousal: cross-sectional and longitudinal associations with adolescent cortisol diurnal rhythms. *Psychosomatic Medicine, 77*(4), 392.

Hrdy, S.B. (2009). *Mothers and others: The evolutionary origins of mutual understanding.* Cambridge: Harvard University Press.

Huang, F.L., Moon, T.R., & Boren, R. (2014). Are the reading rich getting richer? Testing for the presence of the Matthew effect. *Reading & Writing Quarterly, 30*(2), 95-115.

Huang, H.Y., Chen, H.L., & Feng, L.P. (2017). Maternal obesity and the risk of neural tube defects in offspring: A meta-analysis. *Obesity Research & Clinical Practice, 11*(2), 188-197.

Huang, L.N., and Ying, Y. (1989). Chinese American children and adolescents. In J. T. Gibbs and L. N. Huang (Eds.), *Children of color.* San Francisco: Jossey-Bass.

Huang, P.-S., Peng, S.-L., Chen, H.-C., Tseng, L.-C., & Hsu, L.-C. (2017). The relative influences of domain knowledge and domain-general divergent thinking on scientific creativity and mathematical creativity. *Thinking Skills and Creativity, 25,* 1-9.

Huang, X., & others (2019, in press). LPHN3 gene variations and susceptibility to ADHD in Chinese Han population: A two-stage case-control association study and gene–environment interactions. *European Child & Adolescent Psychiatry.*

Huang, Y., Espelage, D.L., Polanin, J.R., & Hong, J.S. (2019). A meta-analytic review of school-based anti-bullying programs with a parent component. *International Journal of Bullying Prevention, 1*(1), 32-44.

Huebner, A.M., & Garrod, A.C. (1993). Moral reasoning among Tibetan monks: A study of Buddhist adolescents and young adults in Nepal. *Journal of Cross-Cultural Psychology, 24,* 167-185.

Hughes, C., & Dunn, J. (2007). Children's relationships with other children. In C. A. Brownell & C. B. Kopp (Eds.), *Socioemotional development in the toddler years.* New York: Guilford.

Hughes, C., McHarg, G., & White, N. (2018). Sibling influences on prosocial behavior. *Current Opinion in Psychology, 20,* 96-101.

Hughes, D., Del Toro, J., Harding, J.F., Way, N., & Rarick, J.R. (2016). Trajectories of discrimination across adolescence: Associations with academic, psychological, and behavioral outcomes. *Child Development, 87*(5), 1337-1351.

Hughes, J.N., & Cao, Q. (2018). Trajectories of teacher-student warmth and conflict at the transition to middle school: Effects on academic engagement and achievement. *Journal of School Psychology, 67,* 148-162.

Hughson, J.A., & others (2018). Health professionals' views on health literacy issues for culturally and linguistically diverse women in maternity care: Barriers, enablers and the need for an integrated approach. *Australian Health Review, 42*(1), 10-20.

Huijsmans, T., Eichelsheim, V.I., Weerman, F., Branje, S.J., & Meeus, W. (2018). The role of siblings in adolescent delinquency next to parents, school, and peers: Do gender and age matter? *Journal of Developmental and Life-Course Criminology.* doi:10.1007/s40865-018-0094-9

Hummel, A.C., & Kiel, E.J. (2015). Maternal depressive symptoms, maternal behavior, and toddler internalizing outcomes: A moderated mediation model. *Child Psychiatry & Human Development, 46,* 21-33.

Huppert, E., & others (2019). The development of children's preferences for equality and equity across 13 individualistic and collectivist cultures. *Developmental Science, 22*(2), e12729.

Hurley, K.M., Black, M.M., Merry, B.C., & Caulfield, L.E. (2013). Maternal mental health and infant dietary patterns in a statewide sample of Maryland WIC participants. *Maternal and Child Nutrition, 11*(2), 229-239.

Hurst, C.E., Gibbon, H.M.F., & Nurse, A.M. (2016). *Social inequality: Forms, causes, and consequences.* New York: Routledge.

Huston, A.C., & Ripke, M.N. (2006). Experiences in middle childhood and children's development: A summary and integration of research. In A. C. Huston & M. N. Ripke (Eds.), *Developmental contexts in middle childhood.* New York: Cambridge University Press.

Huston, A.C., & others (2008). *New Hope's effects on social behavior, parenting, and activities at eight years.* New York: MDRC.

Hutson, J.R., & others. (2013). Adverse placental effect of formic acid on hCG secretion is mitigated by folic acid. *Alcohol and Alcoholism, 48*(3), 283-287.

Huttenlocher, J., Haight, W., Bruk, A., Seltzer, M., & Lyons, T. (1991). Early vocabulary growth: Relation to language input and gender. *Developmental Psychology, 27,* 236-248.

Huttenlocher, P.R., & Dabholkar, A.S. (1997). Regional differences in synaptogenesis in human cerebral cortex. *Journal of Comparative Neurology, 37*(2), 167-178.

Huynh, Q.L., Benet-Martinez, V., & Nguyen, A.M.D. (2018). Measuring variations in bicultural identity across US ethnic and generational groups: Development and validation of the Bicultural Identity Integration Scale–Version 2 (BIIS-2). *Psychological Assessment, 30*(12), 1581.

Hwang, S.H., Hwang, J.H., Moon, J.S., & Lee, D.H. (2012). Environmental tobacco smoke and children's health. *Korean Journal of Pediatrics, 55,* 35-41.

Hyde, D.C., & Spelke, E.S. (2012). Spatio-temporal dynamics of numerical processing: An ERP source localization study. *Human Brain Mapping, 33*(9), 2189-2203.

Hyde, J.S. (2005). The gender similarities hypothesis. *American Psychologist, 60,* 581-592.

Hyde, J.S., & DeLamater, J.D. (2013). *Understanding human sexuality* (13th ed.). New York: McGraw-Hill.

Hyde, J. (2014). Gender similarities and differences. *Annual Review of Psychology, 65,* 373-398.

Hyde, J.S., & Else-Quest, N. (2018). *The psychology of women and gender: Half the human experience* (9th ed.). Thousand Oaks, CA: SAGE.

Hyde, J.S., Bigler, R.S., Joel, D., Tate, C.C., & van Anders, S.M. (2019). The future of sex and gender in psychology: Five challenges to the gender binary. *American Psychologist, 74,* 171–193.

Hyman, I., & others (2006). Bullying: Theory, research, and interventions. In C. M. Evertson & C. S. Weinstein (Eds.), *Handbook of classroom management: Research, practice, and contemporary issues.* Mahwah, NJ: Erlbaum.

Hymel, S., & Espelage, D.L. (2018). Preventing aggression and youth violence in schools. In T. Malti & K. Rubin (Eds.), *Handbook of child and adolescent aggression.* New York: Guilford.

Hymel, S., Closson, L.M., Caravita, C.S., & Vaillancourt, T. (2011). Social status among peers: From sociometric attraction to peer acceptance to perceived popularity. In P. K. Smith & C. H. Hart (Eds.), *Wiley-Blackwell handbook of childhood social development* (2nd ed.). New York: Wiley.

Hyson, M.C., Copple, C., & Jones, J. (2006). Early childhood development and education. In W. Damon & R. Lerner (Eds.), *Handbook of child psychology* (6th ed.). New York: Wiley.

I

"I Have a Dream" Foundation (2019). Our impact. Retrieved from https://www.ihaveadreamfoundation.org/our-impact/

Ibernon, L., Touchet, C., & Pochon, R. (2018). Emotion recognition as a real strength in Williams syndrome: Evidence from a dynamic non-verbal task. *Frontiers in Psychology, 9,* 463.

Ibrahim, R., & Eviatar, Z. (2013). The contribution of two hemispheres to lexical decision in different languages. *Behavioral and Brain Functions, 8*(1), 3.

Ige, F., & Shelton, D. (2004). Reducing risk of sudden infant death syndrome (SIDS) in African-American communities. *Journal of Pediatric Nursing, 19,* 290–292.

Ikeda, A., Kobayashi, T., & Itakura, S. (2018). Sensitivity to linguistic register in 20-month-olds: Understanding the register-listener relationship and its abstract rules. *PLOS One, 13*(4), e0195214.

Ikenouye, D., & Clarke, V.B. (2018). An integral analysis of teachers' attitudes and perspectives on the integration of technology in teaching. In *Handbook of research on digital content, mobile learning, and technology integration models in teacher education* (pp. 88–114). Hershey, PA: IGI Global.

Imada, T., & others (2007). Infant speech perception activates Broca's area: A developmental magnetoencephalography study. *Neuroreport, 17,* 957–962.

International Montessori Council (2006). Larry Page and Sergey Brin, founders of Google.com, credit their Montessori education for much of their success on prime-time television. Retrieved June 24, 2010, from www.Montessori.org/enews/barbara_walters.html

Ip, P., & others (2017). Impact of nutritional supplements on cognitive development of children in developing countries: A meta-analysis. *Scientific Reports, 7,* 10611.

Ip, S., Chung, M., Raman, G., Trikalinos, T.A., & Lau, J. (2009). A summary of the Agency for Healthcare Research and Quality's evidence report on breastfeeding in developed countries. *Breastfeeding Medicine, 4*(Suppl. 1), S17–S30.

Isaacs, J., Healy, O., & Peters, H.E. (2017). *Paid family leave in the United States: Time for a new national policy.* Washington, DC: Urban Institute.

Isbell, E., & others (2017). Neuroplasticity of selective attention: Research foundations and preliminary evidence for a gene by intervention interaction. *Proceedings of the National Academy of Sciences, 114*(35), 9247–9254.

Ivanova, K., Veenstra, R., & Mills, M. (2012). Who dates? The effects of temperament, puberty, and parenting on early adolescent experiences with dating. *Journal of Early Adolescence, 42,* 340–363.

Izard, C.E. (2009). Emotion theory and research: Highlights, unanswered questions, and emerging issues. *Annual Review of Psychology* (Vol. 60). Palo Alto, CA: Annual Reviews.

J

Järvelä, S., Hadwin, A., Malmberg, J., & Miller, M. (2018). Contemporary perspectives of regulated learning in collaboration. In F. Fischer & others (Eds.), *International handbook of the learning sciences.* New York: Routledge.

Jónsdóttir, S.R. (2017). Narratives of creativity: How eight teachers on four school levels integrate creativity into teaching and learning. *Thinking Skills and Creativity, 24,* 127–139.

Jabès, A., & Nelson, C.A. (2015). 20 years after "The ontogeny of human memory: A cognitive neuroscience perspective," where are we? *International Journal of Behavioral Development, 39*(4), 293–303.

Jaccard, J., Blanton, H., & Dodge, T. (2005). Peer influences on risk behavior: An analysis of the effects of a close friend. *Developmental Psychology, 41*(1), 135–147.

Jaciw, A.P., & others (2016). Assessing impacts of *Math in Focus,* a "Singapore Math" program. *Journal of Research on Educational Effectiveness, 9,* 473–502.

Jacobs, W., Goodson, P., Barry, A.E., & McLeroy, K.R. (2016). The role of gender in adolescents' social networks and alcohol, tobacco, and drug use: A systematic review. *Journal of School Health, 86*(5), 322–333.

Jaffee, S., & Hyde, J.S. (2000). Gender differences in moral orientation: A meta-analysis. *Psychological Bulletin, 126,* 703–726.

Jaffee, S. (2017). Child maltreatment and risk for psychopathology in childhood and adulthood. *Annual Review of Clinical Psychology, 19*(3–4), 135–144.

Jagger-Rickels, A.C., Kibby, M.Y., & Constance, J.M. (2018). Global gray matter morphometry differences between children with reading disability, ADHD, and comorbid reading disability/ADHD. *Brain and Language, 185,* 54–66.

Jambon, M., & Smetana, J.G. (2018). Individual differences in prototypical moral and conventional judgments and children's proactive and reactive aggression. *Child Development, 89*(4), 1343–1359.

James, J., Thomas, P., Cavan, D., & Kerr, D. (2004). Preventing childhood obesity by reducing consumption of carbonated drinks. *British Medical Journal, 328,* 1237.

James, W. (1890/1950). *The principles of psychology.* New York: Dover.

Jamieson, J.P., & Mendes, W.B. (2016). Social stress facilitates risk in youths. *Journal of Experimental Psychology: General, 145*(4), 467–485.

Jamshidifarsani, H., Garbaya, S., Lim, T., Blazevic, P., & Ritchie, J.M. (2019). Technology-based reading intervention programs for elementary grades: An analytical review. *Computers & Education, 128,* 427–451.

Jansen, J., de Weerth, C., & Riksen-Walraven, J.M. (2008). Breastfeeding and the mother-infant relationship—A review. *Developmental Review, 28,* 503–521.

Jaszczolt, K.M. (2016). *Meaning in linguistic interaction: Semantics, metasemantics, philosophy of language.* Oxford, UK: Oxford University Press.

Jenkins, L.N., & Nickerson, A.B. (2019). Bystander intervention in bullying: Role of social skills and gender. *Journal of Early Adolescence, 39,* 141–166.

Jensen, A.R. (2008). Book review. *Intelligence, 36,* 96–97.

Jeynes, W.H. (2017). A meta-analysis: The relationship between parental involvement and Latino student outcomes. *Education and Urban Society, 49*(1), 4–28.

Ji, B.T., & others (1997). Paternal cigarette smoking and the risk of childhood cancer among offspring of nonsmoking mothers. *Journal of the National Cancer Institute, 89,* 238–244.

Jia, R., & Schoppe-Sullivan, S.J. (2011). Relations between coparenting and father involvement in families with preschool-age children. *Developmental Psychology, 47,* 106–118.

Jiang, P., & others (2018). Functional connectivity of intrinsic cognitive networks during resting state and task performance in preadolescent children. *PLoS One, 13*(10), e0205690.

Jiao, S., Ji, G., & Jing, Q. (1996). Cognitive development of Chinese urban only children and children with siblings. *Child Development, 67,* 387–395.

Jin, K.-S., Houston, J.L., Baillargeon, R., Groh, A.M., & Roisman, G.I. (2018). Young infants expect an unfamiliar adult to comfort a crying baby: Evidence from a standard violation-of-expectation task and a novel infant-triggered-video task. *Cognitive Psychology, 102,* 1–20.

Jin, K., Houston, J.L., Baillargeon, R., Groh, A.M., & Roisman, G.I. (2018). Young infants expect an unfamiliar adult to comfort a crying baby: Evidence from a standard violation-of-expectation task and a novel infant-triggered-video task. *Cognitive Development, 102,* 1–20.

Jin, K.S., & Baillargeon, R. (2017). Infants possess an abstract expectation of ingroup support. *Proceedings of the National Academy of Sciences, 114,* 8199–8204.

Johansson, J.V., Segerdahl, P., Ugander, U.H., Hansson, M.G., & Langenskiöld, S. (2018). Making sense of genetic risk: A qualitative focus-group study of healthy participants in genomic research. *Patient Education & Counseling, 101,* 422–427.

Johns Hopkins University (2006). *Research: Tribal connections.* Retrieved January 31, 2008, from http://www.krieger.jhu.edu/research/spotlight/prabhakar.html

Johnson, A.D., Finch, J.E., & Phillips, D.A. (2019). Associations between publicly funded preschool and low-income children's kindergarten readiness: The moderating role of child temperament. *Developmental Psychology, 55,* 623–636.

Johnson, C.M., & others (2018). Observed parent-child feeding dynamics in relation to child body mass index and adiposity. *Pediatric Obesity, 13,* 222–231.

Johnson, J.S., & Newport, E.L. (1991). Critical period effects on universal properties of language: The status of subjacency in the acquisition of a second language. *Cognition, 39,* 215–258.

Johnson, J.A., & others (2018). *Foundations of American education* (17th ed.). Upper Saddle River, NJ: Pearson.

Johnson, L., Giordano, P.C., Manning, W.D., & Longmore, M.A. (2011). Parent-child relations and offending in young adulthood. *Journal of Youth and Adolescence, 40,* 786–799.

Johnson, M.D. (2017). *Human biology* (8th ed.). Upper Saddle River, NJ: Pearson.

Johnson, M.H., Grossmann, T., & Cohen-Kadosh, K. (2009), Mapping functional brain development: Building a social brain through Interactive Specialization. *Developmental Psychology, 45,* 151–159.

Johnson, M.H., & de Haan, M. (2015). *Developmental cognitive neuroscience* (4th ed.). New York: Wiley-Blackwell.

Johnson, S.B., Dariotis, J.K., & Wang, C. (2012). Adolescent risk taking under stressed and nonstressed conditions: Conservative, calculating, and impulsive types. *Journal of Adolescent Health, 51*(Suppl. 2), S34–S40.

Johnson, S.P. (2004). Development of perceptual completion in infancy. *Psychological Science, 15,* 769–775.

Johnson, S.P. (2013). Object perception. In P. D. Zelazo (Ed.), *Handbook of developmental psychology.* New York: Oxford University Press.

Johnson, S., & Marlow, N. (2017). Early and long-term outcome of infants born extremely preterm. *Archives of Disease in Childhood, 102*(1), 97–102.

Johnson, S.P., & Hannon, E.E. (2015). Perceptual development. In R. Lerner & others (Eds.), *Handbook of child psychology and developmental science,* (7th ed., pp. 63–112). Hoboken, NJ: Wiley.

Johnson, S.P. (2019, in press). Development of visual-spatial attention. In M.A. Geyer & others (Eds.), *Current topics in behavioral neurosciences.* Berlin: Springer.

Johnston, M. (2008, April 30). Commentary on R. Highfield, *Harvard's baby brain research lab.* Retrieved January 24, 2008, from www.telegraph.co.uk/scienceandtechnology/science/sciencenews/3341166/

Jones-Mason, K., Alkon, A., Coccia, M., & Bush, N.R. (2018). Autonomic nervous system functioning assessed during the still-face paradigm: A meta-analysis and systematic review of methods, approach and findings. *Developmental Review, 50,* 113–139.

Jones, C.R., & others (2018). The association between theory of mind, executive function, and the symptoms of autism spectrum disorder. *Autism Research, 11*(1), 95–109.

Jones, H.W. (2007). Iatrogenic multiple births: A 2003 checkup: *Fertility and Sterility, 87,* 453–455.

Jones, J., & Placek, P. (2017). *Adoption: By the numbers.* Alexandria, VA: National Council for Adoption.

Jones, M.C. (1965). Psychological correlates of somatic development. *Child Development, 36,* 899–911.

Jones, T.H. (2018). Testosterone. In M.H. Bornstein (Ed.), & M. Arterberry, K. Fingerman, & J. E. Lansford (Assoc. Eds.), *The SAGE encyclopedia of lifespan human development.* Thousand Oaks, CA: SAGE.

Jonkman, L.M., Hurks, P.P., & Schleepen, T.M. (2016). Effects of memory strategy training on performance and event-related brain potentials of children with ADHD in an episodic memory task. *Neuropsychological Rehabilitation, 26*(5–6), 910–941.

Jonson-Reid, M., Kohl, P.L., & Drake, B. (2012). Child and adolescent outcomes of chronic child maltreatment. *Pediatrics, 129,* 839–845.

Joos, C.M., Wodzinski, A.M., Wadsworth, M.E., & Dorn, L.D. (2018). Neither antecedent nor consequence: Developmental integration of chronic stress, pubertal timing, and conditionally adapted stress response. *Developmental Review, 48,* 1–23.

Jordan, J.W., & others (2019). Peer crowd identification and adolescent health behaviors: Results from a statewide representative study. *Health Education & Behavior, 46*(1), 40–52.

Jorgensen, G. (2007). Kohlberg and Gilligan: Duet or duel? *Journal of Moral Education, 35*(2), 179–196.

Joseph, J. (2006). *The missing gene.* New York: Algora.

Josephson Institute of Ethics (2008). *The ethics of American youth 2008.* Los Angeles: Josephson Institute.

Juang, L.P., & Umana-Taylor, A.J. (2012). Family conflict among Chinese- and Mexican-origin adolescents and their parents in the U.S.: An introduction. *New Directions in Child and Adolescent Development, 135,* 1–12.

Juffer, F., & van IJzendoorn, M.H. (2007). Adoptees do not lack self-esteem: A meta-analysis of studies on self-esteem of transracial, international, and domestic adoptees, *Psychological Bulletin, 133,* 1067–1083.

K

Körük, S. (2017). The effect of self-esteem on student achievement. In E. Keradag (Ed.), The factors affecting student achievement (pp. 247–257). Berlin: Springer.

Kachel, U., & Tomasello, M. (2019, in press). 3- and 5-year-old children's adherence to explicit and implicit joint commitments. *Developmental Psychology.*

Kadir, M.S., Yeung, A.S., & Diallo, T.M. (2017). Simultaneous testing of four decades of academic self-concept models. *Contemporary Educational Psychology, 51,* 429–446.

Kaestle, C.E. (2019, in press). Sexual orientation trajectories based on sexual attractions, partners, and identity: A longitudinal investigation from adolescence through young adulthood using a US representative sample. *The Journal of Sex Research,* 1–16. doi: 10.1080/00224499.2019.1577351

Kaffashi, F., Scher, M.S., Ludington-Hoe, S.M., & Loparo, K.A. (2013). An analysis of kangaroo care intervention using neonatal EEG complexity: A preliminary study. *Clinical Neurophysiology, 124,* 238–246.

Kagan, J. (2002). Behavioral inhibition as a temperamental category. In R. J. Davidson, K. R. Scherer, & H. H. Goldsmith (Eds.), *Handbook of affective sciences.* New York: Oxford University Press.

Kagan, J. (2003). Biology, context, and development. *Annual Review of Psychology* (Vol. 54). Palo Alto, CA: Annual Reviews.

Kagan, J. (2008). Fear and wariness. In M. M. Haith & J. B. Benson (Eds.), *Encyclopedia of infant and early childhood development.* Oxford, UK: Elsevier.

Kagan, J. (2010). Emotions and temperament. In M. H. Bornstein (Ed.), *Handbook of cultural developmental science.* New York: Psychology Press.

Kagan, J. (2013). Temperamental contributions to inhibited and uninhibited profiles. In P. D. Zelazo (Ed.), *Oxford handbook of developmental psychology.* New York: Oxford University Press.

Kagan, J. (2018). Three unresolved issues in human morality. *Perspectives on Psychological Science, 13,* 346–358.

Kagan, J.J., Kearsley, R.B., & Zelazo, P.R. (1978). *Infancy: Its place in human development.* Cambridge, MA: Harvard University Press.

Kagan, J., & Snidman, N. (1991). Infant predictors of inhibited and uninhibited behavioral profiles. *Psychological Science, 2,* 40–44.

Kail, R.V., Lervåg, A., & Hulme, C. (2016). Longitudinal evidence linking processing speed to the development of reasoning. *Developmental Science, 19*(6), 1067–1074.

Kalaitzopoulos, D.R., Chatzistergiou, K., Amylidi, A.L., Kokkinidis, D.G., & Goulis, D.G. (2018). Effect of methamphetamine hydrochloride on pregnancy outcome: A systematic review and meta-analysis. *Journal of Addiction Medicine, 12*(3), 220–226.

Kalak, N., & others (2012). Daily morning running for 3 weeks improved sleep and psychological functioning in health of adolescents compared to controls. *Journal of Adolescent Health, 51,* 615–622.

Kalisch-Smith, J.I., & Moritz, K.M. (2018). Detrimental effects of alcohol exposure around conception: Putative mechanisms. *Biochemistry and Cell Biology, 96*(2), 107–116.

Kallol, S., Huang, X., Müller, S., Ontsouka, C., & Albrecht, C. (2018). Novel insights into concepts and directionality of maternal-fetal cholesterol transfer across the human placenta. *International Journal of Molecular Sciences, 19*(8), 2334.

Kanakis, G.A., & Nieschlag, E. (2018). Klinefelter syndrome: more than hypogonadism. *Pediatric Reproductive Endocrinology, 86,* 135-144.

Kang, J. (2019, in press). Do co-ethnic concentrated neighborhoods protect children with undocumented parents? Focusing on child behavioral functioning. *Social Science Research.*

Kania-Richmond, A., & others (2017). The impact of introducing Centering Pregnancy in a community health setting: A qualitative study of experiences and perspectives of health center clinical and support staff. *Maternal and Child Health Journal, 21*(6), 1327–1335.

Kanji, A., Khoza-Shangase, K., & Moroe, N. (2018). Newborn hearing screening protocols and their outcomes: A systematic review. *International Journal of Pediatric Otorhinolaryngology, 115,* 104–109.

Kanoy, K., Ulku-Steiner, B., Cox, M., & Burchinal, M. (2003). Marital relationship and individual psychological characteristics that predict physical punishment of children. *Journal of Family Psychology, 17,* 20–28.

Kaplan, J.S. (2012). The effects of shared environment on adult intelligence: A critical review of adoption, twin, and MZA studies. *Developmental Psychology, 48,* 1292–1298.

Kapur, B.M., & Baber, M. (2017). FASD: Folic acid and formic acid—an unholy alliance in the alcohol abusing mother. *Biochemistry and Cell Biology, 96*(2), 189–197.

Karaman, F., & Hay, J.F. (2018). The longevity of statistical learning: When infant memory decays, isolated words come to the rescue. *Journal of Experimental Psychology: Learning, Memory, and Cognition, 44,* 221–232.

Karg, K., & Sen, S. (2012). Gene × environment interaction models in psychiatry. *Current Topics in Behavioral Neuroscience.*

Karle, K.N., & others (2018). Neurobiological correlates of emotional intelligence in voice and face perception networks. *Social Cognitive and Affective Neuroscience, 13,* 233–244.

Karlsson, J., & others (2018). Four evolutionary trajectories underlie genetic intratumoral variation in childhood cancer. *Nature Genetics, 50,* 944–950.

Karreman, A., van Tuijl, C., van Aken, M.A.G., & Dekovic, M. (2008). Parenting, coparenting, and effortful control in preschoolers. *Journal of Family Psychology, 22,* 30–40.

Kassai, R., Futo, J., Demetrovics, Z., & Takacs, Z.K. (2019). A meta-analysis of the experimental evidence on the near- and far-transfer effects among children's executive function skills. *Psychological Bulletin, 145*(2), 165–188.

Kauchak, D., & Eggen, P. (2017). *Introduction to teaching* (6th ed.). Upper Saddle River, NJ: Pearson.

Kauffman, J.M., McGee, K., & Brigham, M. (2004). Enabling or disabling? Observations on changes in special education. *Phi Delta Kappan, 85,* 613–620.

Kaufman-Parks, A., & others (2017). Intimate partner violence perpetration from adolescence to young adulthood: Trajectories and the role of familial factors. *Journal of Family Violence, 33*(1), 27–41.

Kaufman, J.C., & Sternberg, R.J. (2012). The creative mind. In C. Jones, M. Lorenzen, & J. Sapsed (Eds.), *Oxford handbook of creative industries.* New York: Oxford University Press.

Kaufman, J.C., & Sternberg, R.J. (2013). The creative mind. In C. Jones, M. Lorenzen, &

R. F. Proctor (Eds.), *Handbook of psychology: Experimental psychology,* Vol. 4. New York: Wiley.

Kaur, A., & Phadke, S.R. (2012). Analysis of short stature cases referred for genetic evaluation. *Indian Journal of Pediatrics, 79*(12), 1597–1600.

Kavsek, M. (2013). The comparator model of infant visual habituation and dishabituation: Recent insights. *Developmental Psychobiology, 55*(8), 793–808.

Kawabata, Y., Tseng, W.L., Murray-Close, D., & Crick, N.R. (2012). Developmental trajectories of Chinese children's relational and physical aggression: Associations with social-psychological adjustment problems. *Journal of Abnormal Child Psychology, 40*(7), 1087–1097.

Kawwass, J.F., & Badell, M.L. (2018). Maternal and fetal risk associated with assisted reproductive technology. *Obstetrics and Gynecology, 132,* 763–772.

Keag, O.E., Norman, J.E., & Stock, S.J. (2018). Long-term risks and benefits associated with cesarean delivery for mother, baby, and subsequent pregnancies: Systematic review and meta-analysis. *PLoS Medicine, 15*(1), e1002494.

Keefer, K.V., Parker, J.D., & Saklofske, D.H. (2018). Three decades of emotional intelligence research: Perennial issues, emerging trends, and lessons learned in education: Introduction to emotional intelligence in education. In K. Keefer, J. Parker, & D. Saklofske (Eds.), *Emotional intelligence in education* (pp. 1–19). Dordrecht, the Netherlands: Springer.

Keen, R. (2011). The development of problem solving in young children: A critical cognitive skill. *Annual Review of Psychology* (Vol. 62). Palo Alto, CA: Annual Reviews.

Keeton, C.P., Schleider, J.L., & Walkup, J.T. (2017). Separation anxiety, generalized anxiety, and social anxiety. In B.J. Sadock, V.A. Sadock, & P. Ruiz (Eds.), *Kaplan & Sadock's comprehensive textbook of psychiatry* (10th ed.). Philadelphia: Wolters Kluwer.

Kellman, P.J., & Arterberry, M.E. (2006). Infant visual perception. In W. Damon & R. Lerner (Eds.), *Handbook of child psychology* (6th ed.). New York: Wiley.

Kelly, K.M., & others (2013). Children's Oncology Group's 2013 blueprint for research on Hodgkin's lymphoma. *Pediatric and Blood Cancer, 60*(6), 1009–1015.

Kelmanson, I.A. (2010). Sleep disturbances in two-month-old infants sharing the bed with parent(s). *Minerva Pediatrica, 62,* 162–169.

Kelty, E., & Hulse, G. (2017). A retrospective cohort study of birth outcomes in neonates exposed to naltrexone in utero: A comparison with methadone-, buprenorphine-and non-opioid-exposed neonates. *Drugs, 77*(11), 1211–1219.

Kendler, K.S., & others (2012). Genetic and familial environmental influences on the risk for drug abuse: A national Swedish adoption study. *Archives of General Psychiatry, 69*(7), 690–697.

Kendler, K.S., Ohlsson, H., Sundquist, K., & Sundquist, J. (2018). Sources of parent-offspring resemblance for major depression in a national Swedish extended adoption study. *JAMA Psychiatry, 75,* 194–200.

Kendrick, K., Jutengren, G., & Stattin, H. (2012). The protective role of supportive friends against bullying perpetration and victimization. *Journal of Adolescence, 35,* 1069–1080.

Kennell, J.H. (2006). Randomized controlled trial of skin-to-skin contact from birth versus conventional incubator for physiological stabilization in 1200 g to 2199 g newborns. *Acta Paediatrica (Sweden), 95,* 15–16.

Kern, P., & Tague, D.B. (2017). Music therapy practice status and trends worldwide: An international survey study. *The Journal of Music Therapy, 54*(3), 255–286.

Kerpelman, J.L., & Pittman, J.F. (2018). Erikson and the relational context of identity: Strengthening connections with attachment theory. *Identity, 18*(4), 306–314.

Kessen, W., Haith, M.M., & Salapatek, P. (1970). Human infancy. In P. H. Mussen (Ed.), *Manual of child psychology* (3rd ed., Vol. 1). New York: Wiley.

Kezuka, E., Amano, S., & Reddy, V. (2017). Developmental changes in locating voice and sound in space. *Frontiers in Psychology, 8,* 1574.

Khatun, M., & others (2017). Do children born to teenage parents have lower adult intelligence? A prospective birth cohort study. *PloS One, 12*(3), e0167395.

Khodaverdi, M., & others (2013). Hearing 25 years after surgical treatment of otitis media with effusion in early childhood. *International Journal of Otorhinolaryngology, 77*(2), 241–247.

Khuc, K., & others (2013). Adolescent metabolic syndrome risk is increased with higher infancy weight gain and decreased with longer breast feeding. *Indian Journal of Pediatrics, 2012,* 478610.

Khundrakpam, B.S., & others (2017). Imaging structural covariance in the development of intelligence. *NeuroImage, 144,* 227–240.

Kidd, C., Piantadosi, S.T., & Aslin, R.N. (2012). The Goldilocks effect: Human infants allocate attention to visual sequences that are neither too simple nor too complex. *PLoS One, 7*(5), e36399.

Kilic, S., & others (2012). Environmental tobacco smoke exposure during intrauterine period promotes granulosa cell apoptosis: A prospective, randomized study. *Journal Maternal-Fetal and Neonatal Medicine, 25*(10), 1904–1908.

Killen, M., & Dahl, A. (2018). Moral judgment: Reflective, interactive, spontaneous, challenging, and always evolving. In K. Gray & J. Graham (Eds.), *Atlas of moral psychology* (pp. 20–30). New York: Guilford.

Killen, M., Rutland, A., & Yip, T. (2016). Equity and justice in developmental science: Discrimination, social exclusion, and intergroup attitudes. *Child Development, 87,* 1317–1336.

Kim-Spoon, J., Deater-Deckard, K., Calkins, S.D., King-Casas, B., & Bell, M.A. (2019). Commonality between executive functioning and effortful control related to adjustment. *Journal of Applied Developmental Psychology, 60,* 47–55.

Kim, J., & Morgül, K. (2017). Long-term consequences of youth volunteering: Voluntary versus involuntary service. *Social Science Research, 67,* 160–175.

Kim, J., & others (2006). Trends in overweight from 1980 through 2001 among preschool-aged children enrolled in a health maintenance organization. *Obesity, 14,* 1107-1112.

Kim, J., Kim, H., Kim, N., Kwon, J.H., & Park, M. (2017). Effects of radiofrequency field exposure on glutamate-induced oxidative stress in mouse hippocampal HT22 cells. *International Journal of Radiation Biology, 93,* 249-256.

Kim, K.H. (2010, July 10). Interview. *Newsweek,* pp. 42-48.

Kim, P., Evans, G.W., Chen, E., Miller, G., & Seeman, T. (2018). How socioeconomic disadvantages get under the skin and into the brain to influence health development across the lifespan. In N. Halfon & others (Eds.), *Handbook of life course health development* (pp. 463-497). London: Springer.

Kim, S.Y., Chen, Q., Wang, Y., Shen, Y., & Orozco-Lapray, D. (2012). Longitudinal linkages among parent-child acculturation discrepancy, parenting, parent-child sense of alienation, and adolescent adjustment in Chinese immigrant families. *Developmental Psychology, 49*(5), 900-912.

Kim, S., & Kochanska, G. (2017). Relational antecedents and social implications of the emotion of empathy: Evidence from three studies. *Emotion, 17*(6), 981-992.

Kim, Y., Park, I., & Kang, S. (2018). Age and gender differences in health risk perception. *Central European Journal of Public Health, 26*(1).

Kim-Spoon, J., Cicchetti, D., & Rogosch, F.A. (2013). A longitudinal study of emotion regulation, emotion lability-negativity, and internalizing symptomatology in maltreated and nonmaltreated children. *Child Development, 84*(2), 512-527.

Kinard, J.L., & Watson, L.R. (2015). Joint attention during infancy and early childhood across cultures. In *International encyclopedia of the social and behavioral sciences* (2nd ed., pp. 844-850). London: Elsevier.

King, K.A., Topalian, A., & Vidourek, R.A. (2019, in press). Religiosity and adolescent major depressive episodes among 12-17-year-olds. *Journal of Religion and Health.*

King, P.E., Ramos, J.S., & Clardy, C.E. (2012). Searching for the sacred: Religious and spiritual development among adolescents. In K. I. Pargament, J. Exline, & J. Jones (Eds.), *APA handbook of psychology, religion, and spirituality.* Washington, DC: American Psychological Association.

King, P.E., Kim, S.H., Furrow, J.L., & Clardy, C.E. (2017). Preliminary exploration of the Measurement of Diverse Adolescent Spirituality (MDAS) among Mexican youth. *Applied Developmental Science, 21*(4), 235-250.

Kingsmore, S.F., & others. (2013). Next-generation community genetics for low- and middle-income countries. *Genomic Medicine, 4*(3), 25.

Kingston, M.H. (1976). *The woman warrior: Memoirs of a girlhood among ghosts.* New York: Vintage Books.

Kini, S., & others (2010). Lack of impact of semen quality on fertilization in assisted conception. *Scottish Medicine, 55,* 20-23.

Kiraly, I., Takacs, S., Kaldy, Z., & Blaser, E. (2017). Preschoolers have better long-term memory for rhyming text than adults. *Developmental Science, 20*(3), e12398.

Kirk, R.E. (2013). Experimental design. In I. B. Weiner & others (Eds.), *Handbook of psychology* (2nd ed., Vol. 2). New York: Wiley.

Kirkorian, H.L., Anderson, D.R., & Keen, R. (2012). Age differences in online processing of video: An eye movement study. *Child Development, 83,* 497-507.

Kirkorian, H.L., Wartella, E.A., & Anderson, D.A. (2008). Media and young children's learning. *Future of Children, 18*(1), 39-61.

Kirova, A., & Jamison, N.M. (2018). Peer scaffolding techniques and approaches in preschool children's multiliteracy practices with iPads. *Journal of Early Childhood Research, 16,* 245-257.

Kitsantas, P., & Gaffney, K.F. (2010). Racial/ethnic disparities in infant mortality. *Journal of Perinatal Medicine, 38,* 87-94.

Kjelgaard, H.H., Holstein, B.E., Due, P., Brixval, C.S., & Rasmussen, M. (2017). Adolescent weight status: Associations with structural and functional dimensions of social relations. *Journal of Adolescent Health, 60,* 460-468.

Klausen, T., Hansen, K.J., Munk-Jørgensen, P., & Mohr-Jensen, C. (2017). Are assisted reproductive technologies associated with categorical or dimensional aspects of psychopathology in childhood, adolescence or early adulthood? Results from a Danish prospective nationwide cohort study. *European Child and Adolescent Psychiatry, 26,* 771-778.

Kleiman, E.M., & Riskand, J.H. (2013). Utilized social support and self-esteem mediate the relationship between perceived social support and suicide ideation. *Crisis, 34,* 42-49.

Kleiman, K., & Wenzel, A. (2017). Principles of supportive psychotherapy for perinatal distress. *Journal of Obstetric, Gynecologic & Neonatal Nursing, 46*(6), 895-903.

Kleinsorge, C., & Covitz, L.M. (2012). Impact of divorce on children: Developmental considerations. *Pediatrics in Review, 33,* 147-154.

Klemfuss, J.Z., & Olaguez, A.P. (2018). Individual differences in children's suggestibility: An updated review. *Journal of Child Sexual Abuse,* 1-25. doi:10.1 080/10538712.2018.1508108

Klimstra, T.A., Hale, W.W., Raaijmakers, Q.A., Branje, S.J.T., & Meeus, W.H. (2010). Identity formation in adolescence: Change or stability? *Journal of Youth and Adolescence, 39,* 150-162.

Klinger, L.G., & Dudley, K.M. (2019). Autism spectrum disorder. In M.J. Prinstein & others (Eds.), *Treatment of disorders in childhood and adolescence.* New York: Guilford.

Klopp-Dutote, N., Kolski, C., Strunski, V., & Page, C. (2018). Tympanostomy tubes for serous otitis media and risk of recurrences. *International Journal of Pediatric Otorhinolaryngology, 106,* 105-109.

Knifsend, C.A., Camacho-Thompson, D.E., Juvonen, J., & Graham, S. (2018). Friends in activities, school-related affect, and academic outcomes in diverse middle schools. *Journal of Youth and Adolescence, 47,* 1208-1220.

Knopik, V.S., Neiderhiser, J.M., DeFries, J.C., & Plomin, R. (2016). *Behavioral genetics.* New York: Macmillan.

Knopp, K., & others (2017). Within- and between-family associations of marital functioning and child well-being. *Family Relations, 79,* 451-461.

Knopp, K.A. (2019). The Children's Social Comprehension Scale (CSCS): Construct validity of a new social intelligence measure for elementary school children. *International Journal of Behavioral Development, 43*(1), 90-96.

Knox, M. (2010). On hitting children: A review of corporal punishment in the United States. *Journal of Pediatric Health Care, 24,* 103-107.

Ko, C.H., & others (2015). Bidirectional associations between family factors and Internet addiction among adolescents in a prospective investigation. *Psychiatry and Clinical Neurosciences, 69*(4), 192-200.

Kochanska, G., Barry, R.A., Jimenez, N.B., Hollatz, A.L., & Woodard, J. (2009). Guilt and effortful control: Two mechanisms that prevent disruptive developmental trajectories. *Journal of Personality and Social Psychology, 97,* 322-333.

Kochanska, G., Barry, R.A., Stellern, S.A., & O'Bleness, J.J. (2010). Early attachment organization moderates the parent-child mutually coercive pathway to children's antisocial conduct. *Child Development, 80,* 1288-1300.

Kochanska, G., Gross, J.N., Lin, M., & Nichols, K.E. (2002). Guilt in young children: Development, determinants, and relations with a broader set of standards. *Child Development, 73,* 461-482.

Kochanska, G., & Kim, S. (2013). Early attachment organization with both parents and future behavior problems: From infancy to middle childhood. *Child Development, 84*(1), 283-296.

Koeblinger, C., & others. (2013). Fetal magnetic resonance imaging of lymphangiomas. *Journal of Perinatal Medicine, 41*(4), 437-443.

Koehn, A.J., & Kerns, K.A. (2017). Parent-child attachment: Meta-analysis of associations with parenting behaviors in middle childhood and adolescence. *Attachment & Human Development,* 1-28.

Koenig, L.B., McGue, M., & Iacono, W.G. (2008). Stability and change in religiousness during emerging adulthood. *Developmental Psychology, 44,* 523-543.

Kofler, M.J., & others (2019). Do working memory deficits underlie reading problems in attention-deficit/hyperactivity disorder (ADHD)? *Journal of Abnormal Child Psychology, 47,* 433-446.

Kohlberg, L. (1958). *The development of modes of moral thinking and choice in the years 10 to 16.* Unpublished doctoral dissertation, University of Chicago.

Kohlberg, L. (1969). Stage and sequence: The cognitive-developmental approach to socialization. In D. A. Goslin (Ed.), *Handbook of socialization theory and research.* Chicago: Rand McNally.

Kohlberg, L. (1986). A current statement on some theoretical issues. In S. Modgil & C. Modgil (Eds.), *Lawrence Kohlberg.* Philadelphia: Falmer.

Kohlhoff, J., & others (2017). Oxytocin in the postnatal period: Associations with attachment and maternal caregiving. *Comprehensive Psychiatry, 76,* 56-68.

Kokkinaki, T.S., Vasdekis, V.G.S., Koufaki, Z.E., & Trevarthen, C.B. (2017). Coordination of emotions in mother–infant dialogues. *Infant and Child Development, 26*, e1973.

Koleilat, M., Whaley, S.E., Esguerra, K.B., & Sekhobo, J.P. (2017). The role of WIC in obesity prevention. *Current Pediatrics Reports, 5*, 132–141.

Kondo-Ikemura, K., Behrens, K.Y., Umemura, T., & Nakano, S. (2018). Japanese mothers' prebirth Adult Attachment Interview predicts their infants' response to the Strange Situation Procedure: The strange situation in Japan revisited three decades later. *Developmental Psychology, 54*, 2007–2015.

Kong, A., & others (2012). Rate of *de novo* mutations and the importance of father's age to disease risk. *Nature, 488*, 471–475.

Kopp, C.B., & Neufeld, S.J. (2002). Emotional development in infancy. In R. Davidson & K. Scherer (Eds.), *Handbook of affective sciences.* New York: Oxford University Press.

Kopp, F., & Lindenberger, U. (2012). Effects of joint attention on long-term memory in 9-month-old infants: An event-related potentials study. *Developmental Science, 15*, 540–556.

Koppleman, K.L. (2017). *Understanding human differences* (5th ed.). Upper Saddle River, NJ: Pearson.

Kosik-Bogacka, D., & others (2018). Concentrations of mercury (Hg) and selenium (Se) in afterbirth and their relations with various factors. *Environmental Geochemistry and Health, 40*(4), 1683–1695.

Kotovsky, L., & Baillargeon, R. (1994). Calibration-based reasoning about collision events in 11-month-old infants. *Cognition, 51*, 107–129.

Kotte, E.M., Winkler, A.M., & Takken, T. (2013). Fitkids exercise therapy program in the Netherlands. *Pediatric Physical Therapy, 25*(1), 7–13.

Kozol, J. (2005). *The shame of the nation: The restoration of apartheid schooling in America.* New York: Three Rivers Press.

Kramer, L., & Radey, C. (1997). Improving sibling relationships among young children: A social skills training model. *Family Relations, 46*, 237–246.

Kramer, L. (2006, July 10). Commentary in "How your siblings make you who you are" by J. Kluger. *Time*, pp. 46–55.

Krafft, C., Davis, E.E., & Tout, K. (2017). Child care subsidies and the stability and quality of child care arrangements. *Early Childhood Research Quarterly, 39*, 14–34.

Kramer, L., & Perozynski, L. (1999). Parental beliefs about managing sibling conflict. *Developmental Psychology, 35*, 489–499.

Krassner, A.M., & others (2017). East–west, collectivist-individualist: A cross-cultural examination of temperament in toddlers from Chile, Poland, South Korea, and the US. *European Journal of Developmental Psychology, 14*, 449–464.

Krauss, R.A., & Glucksberg, S. (1969). The development of communication: Competence as a function of age. *Child Development, 40*, 255–266.

Kreutzer, L.C., & Flavell, J.H. (1975). An interview study of children's knowledge about memory. *Monographs of the Society for Research in Child Development, 40*(1), Serial No. 159.

Kring, A.M. (2000). Gender and anger. In A. H. Fischer (Ed.), *Gender and emotion: Social psychological perspectives.* New York: Cambridge University Press.

Krist, H., Atlas, C., Fischer, H., & Wiese, C. (2018). Development of basic intuitions about physical support during early childhood: Evidence from a novel eye-tracking paradigm. *Quarterly Journal of Experimental Psychology, 71*, 1988–2004.

Kroesbergen, E.H., van 't Noordende, J.E., & Kolkman, M.E. (2014). Training working memory in kindergarten children: Effects on working memory and early numeracy. *Child Neuropsychology.*

Kubarych, T.S., & others. (2012). A multivariate twin study of hippocampal volume, self-esteem, and well-being in middle-aged men. *Genes, Brain, and Behavior, 11*, 539–544.

Kuchirko, Y., Tafuro, L., & Tamis-LeMonda, C.S. (2018). Becoming a communicative partner: Infant contingent responsiveness to maternal language and gestures. *Infancy, 23*(4), 558–576.

Kuhl, P.K. (2017). Big surprises from little brains. *Early Childhood Matters, 126*, 20–25.

Kuhn, D. (2009). Adolescent thinking. In R. M. Lerner & L. Steinberg (Eds.), *Handbook of adolescent psychology* (3rd ed.). New York: Wiley.

Kuhn, D. (2013). Reasoning. In P. D. Zelazo (Ed.), *Oxford handbook of developmental psychology.* New York: Oxford University Press.

Kuhn, D., & Franklin, S. (2006). The second decade: What develops (and how)? In W. Damon & R. Lerner (Eds.), *Handbook of child psychology* (6th ed.). New York: Wiley.

Kuhns, C., & Cabrera, N. (2018). Fathering. In M.H. Bornstein (Ed.) & M. Arterberry, K. Fingerman, & J.E. Lansford (Assoc. Eds.), *The SAGE encyclopedia of lifespan human development.* Thousand Oaks, CA: SAGE.

Kulig, T.C., Cullen, F.T., Wilcox, P., & Chouhy, C. (2019). Personality and adolescent school-based victimization: Do the big five matter? *Journal of School Violence, 18*(2), 176–199.

Kuo, L.J., Ramirez, G., de Marin, S., Kim, T.J., & Unal-Gezer, M. (2017). Bilingualism and morphological awareness: A study with children from general education and Spanish-English dual language programs. *Educational Psychology, 37*, 94–111.

Kupán, K., Király, I., Kupán, K., Krekó, K., Miklósi, A., & Topál, J. (2017). Interacting effect of two social factors on 18-month-old infants' imitative behavior: Communicative cues and demonstrator presence. *Journal of Experimental Child Psychology, 161*, 186–194.

Kupersmidt, J.B., & Coie, J.D. (1990). Preadolescent peer status, aggression, and school adjustment as predictors of externalizing problems in adolescence. *Child Development, 61*, 1350–1363.

Kurkul, K.E., & Corriveau, K.H. (2018). Question, explanation, follow-up: A mechanism for learning from others? *Child Development, 89*, 280–294.

Kwiatkowski, M.A., & others (2018). Cognitive outcomes in prenatal methamphetamine exposed children aged six to seven years. *Comprehensive Psychiatry, 80*, 24–33.

L

La Rooy, D.J., Brown. D., & Lamb, M.E. (2013). Suggestibility and witness interviewing. In A. Ridley, F. Gabber, & D. J. La Rooy (Eds.), *Investigative suggestibility.* New York: Wiley.

La Salle, T., George, H.P., McCoach, D.B., Polk, T., & Ivanovich, L.L. (2018). An examination of school climate, victimization, and mental health problems among middle school students self-identifying with emotional and behavioral disorders. *Behavioral Disorders, 43*, 383–392.

Labella, M.H. (2018). The sociocultural context of emotion socialization in African American families. *Clinical Psychology Review, 59*, 1–15.

Lacelle, C., Hebert, M., Lavoie, F., Vitaro, F., & Tremblay, R.E. (2012). Sexual health in women reporting a history of child sexual abuse. *Child Abuse and Neglect, 36*, 247–259.

Ladd, G.W., Ettekal, I., & Kochenderfer-Ladd, B. (2017). Peer victimization trajectories from kindergarten through high school: Differential pathways for children's school engagement and achievement? *Journal of Educational Psychology, 109*(6), 826–841.

Ladd, H.C. (2017). No Child Left Behind: A deeply flawed federal policy. *Journal of Policy Analysis and Management, 36*, 461–469.

LaFontana, K.M., & Cillessen, A.H.N. (2010). Developmental changes in the priority of perceived status in childhood and adolescence. *Social Development, 19*, 130–147.

Lagattuta, K.H., & others (2015). Beyond Sally's missing marble: Further development in children's understanding of mind and emotion in middle childhood. *Advances in Child Development and Behavior, 48*, 185–217.

Lagattuta, K.H., Elrod, N.M., & Kramer, H.J. (2016). How do thoughts, emotions, and decisions align? A new way to examine theory of mind during middle childhood and beyond. *Journal of Experimental Child Psychology, 149*, 116–133.

Laird, R.D., & Marrero, M.D. (2011). Mothers' knowledge of early adolescents' activities following the middle school transition and pubertal maturation. *Journal of Early Adolescence, 31*, 209–233.

Lamb, M.E. (2013a). Commentary: Early experience, neurobiology, plasticity, vulnerability, and resilience. In D. Narvaez & others (Eds.), *Evolution, early experience, and human development.* New York: Oxford University Press.

Lamb, M.E. (2013b). Non-parental care and emotional development. In S. Pauen & M. Bornstein (Eds.), *Early childhood development and later outcomes.* New York: Cambridge University Press.

Lamb, M.E., & Lewis, C. (2013). Father-child relationships. In C. S. Tamis-LeMonda & N. Cabrera (Eds.), *Handbook of father involvement* (2nd ed.). New York: Psychology Press.

Lamb, M.E., & Malloy, L.C. (2013). Child development and the law. In I. B. Weiner & others (Eds.), *Handbook of psychology* (2nd ed., Vol. 6). New York: Wiley.

Lampi, K.M., & others. (2012). Risk of autism spectrum disorders in low birth weight and small for gestational age infants. *Journal of Pediatrics, 161*(5), 830–836.

Lampl, M. (2008). Physical growth. In M. M. Hath & J. B. Benson (Eds.), *Encyclopedia of infant and early childhood development.* Oxford, UK: Elsevier.

Langer, E.J. (2005). *On becoming an artist.* New York: Ballantine.

Laninga-Wijnen, L., & others (2019). The role of academic status norms in friendship selection and influence processes related to academic achievement. *Developmental Psychology, 55*(2), 337–350.

Lansford, J.E. (2009). Parental divorce and children's adjustment. *Perspectives on Psychological Science, 4,* 140–152.

Lansford, J.E. (2012). Divorce. In R. J. R. Levesque (Ed.), *Encyclopedia of adolescence.* New York: Springer.

Lansford, J.E., & Deater-Deckard, K. (2012). Childrearing discipline and violence in developing countries. *Child Development, 83*(1), 62–75.

Lansford, J.E., Wager, L.B., Bates, J.E., Pettit, G.S., & Dodge, K.A. (2013). Forms of spanking and children's externalizing problems. *Family Relations, 61*(2), 224–236.

Lansford, J.E., & others. (2005). Cultural normativeness as a moderator of the link between physical discipline and children's adjustment: A comparison of China, India, Italy, Kenya, Philippines, and Thailand. *Child Development, 76,* 1234–1246.

Lansford, J.E., & others (2011). Reciprocal relations between parents' physical discipline and children's externalizing behavior during middle childhood and adolescence. *Development and Psychopathology, 23,* 225–238.

Lansford, J.E., & others (2016). How international research on parenting advances understanding of child development. *Child Development Perspectives, 10*(3), 202–207.

Lansford, J.E., & others (2017). Change over time in parents' beliefs about and reported use of corporal punishment in eight countries with and without legal bans. *Child Abuse & Neglect, 71,* 44–55.

Lansford, J.E., & others (2018). Bidirectional relations between parenting and behavior problems from age 8 to 13 in nine countries. *Journal of Research on Adolescence, 28,* 571–590.

Lantagne, A., & Furman, W. (2017). Romantic relationship development: The interplay between age and relationship length. *Developmental Psychology, 53*(9), 1738.

Lapsley, D.K., & Yeager, D. (2013). Moral-character education. In I. B. Weiner & others (Eds.), *Handbook of psychology* (2nd ed., Vol. 7). New York: Wiley.

Lapsley, D., & Woodbury, R.D. (2015). Social cognitive development in emerging adulthood. In J.J. Arnett (Ed.), *The Oxford handbook of emerging adulthood.* New York: Oxford University Press.

Larzelere, R.E., & Kuhn, B.R. (2005). Comparing child outcomes of physical punishment and alternative disciplinary tactics: A meta-analysis. *Clinical Child and Family Psychology Review, 8,* 1–37.

Larzelere, R.E., Morris, A.S., & Harrist, A.W. (Eds.) (2013). *Authoritative parenting.* Washington, DC: American Psychological Association.

Laslett, A.M., Room, R., Dietze, P., & Ferris, J. (2012). Alcohol's involvement in recurrent child abuse and neglect cases. *Addiction, 107*(10), 1786–1793.

Laslett, A.M., & others (2017). A multi-country study of harms to children because of others' drinking. *Journal of Studies on Alcohol and Drugs, 78*(2), 195–202.

Lauer, R.H., & Lauer, J.C. (2019). *Marriage and family* (9th ed.). New York: McGraw-Hill.

Laurent, G., Hecht, H.K., Ensink, K., & Borelli, J.L. (2018). Emotional understanding, aggression, and social functioning among preschoolers. *American Journal of Orthopsychiatry.* doi:10.1037/ort0000377

Laursen, B., & Collins, W.A. (2009). Parent-child relationships during adolescence. In R. M. Lerner & L. Steinberg (Eds.), *Handbook of adolescent psychology* (3rd ed.). New York: Wiley.

Lavelli, M., & others (2018). Communication dynamics between mothers and their children with cochlear implants: Effects of maternal support for language production. *Journal of Communication Disorders, 73,* 1–14.

Lawton, C.A. (2018). Sex and gender in geographic behavior and cognition. In D.R. Montello (Ed.), *Handbook of behavioral and cognitive geography.* Northampton, MA: Edward Elgar Publishing.

Leach, P. (2010). *Your baby and child: From birth to age five* (rev. ed.) New York: Knopf.

Lean, R.E., Smyser, C.D., & Rogers, C.E. (2017). Assessment: The newborn. *Child and Adolescent Psychiatric Clinics, 26*(3), 427–440.

Leaper, C. (2013). Gender development during childhood. In P. D. Zelazo (Ed.), *Oxford handbook of developmental psychology.* New York: Oxford University Press.

Leaper, C. (2018). Gender, dispositions, peer relations, and identity: Toward an integrative developmental model. In N.K. Dess, J. Marecek, & L.C. Bell (Eds.), *Gender, sex, and sexualities: Psychological perspectives.* New York: Oxford University Press.

Leaper, C. (2019, in press). Young adults' conversational strategies during negotiation and self-disclosure in same-gender and mixed-gender friendships. *Sex Roles.*

LeBourgeois, M.K., & others (2017). Digital media and sleep in childhood and adolescence. *Pediatrics, 140*(Suppl. 2), S92.

Lebrun-Harris, L.A., Sherman, L.J., Limber, S.P., Miller, B.D., & Edgerton, E.A. (2018). Bullying victimization and perpetration among US children and adolescents: 2016 National Survey of Children's Health. *Journal of Child and Family Studies,* 1–15.

Lee-St.John, T.J., & others (2018). The long-term impact of systemic student support in elementary school: Reducing high school dropout. *AERA Open, 4*(4).

Lee, B., Jeong, S., & Roh, M. (2018). Association between body mass index and health outcomes among adolescents: The mediating role of traditional and cyber bullying victimization. *BMC Public Health, 18*(1), 674.

Lee, B.R., Kobulsky, J.M., Brodzinsky, D., & Barth, R.P. (2018). Parent perspectives on adoption preparation: Findings from the Modern Adoptive Families project. *Children and Youth Services Review, 85,* 63–71.

Lee, C.C., Jhang, Y., Chen, L.M., Relyea, G., & Oller, D.K. (2017). Subtlety of ambient-language effects in babbling: A study of English- and Chinese-learning infants at 8, 10, and 12 months. *Language Learning and Development, 13,* 100–126.

Lee, D.K., Cole, W.G., Golenia, L., & Adolph, K.E. (2018). The cost of simplifying complex developmental phenomena: A new perspective on learning to walk. *Developmental Science, 21*(4), e12615. doi:10.1111/desc.12615

Lee, G.Y., & Kisilevsky, B.S. (2014). Fetuses respond to father's voice but prefer mother's voice after birth. *Developmental Psychobiology, 56*(1), 1–11.

Lee, J.E., Pope, Z., & Gao, Z. (2018). The role of youth sports in promoting children's physical activity and preventing pediatric obesity: A systematic review. *Behavioral Medicine, 44*(1), 62–76.

Lee, K., Quinn, P.C., & Pascalis, O. (2017). Face race processing and racial bias in early development: A perceptual-social linkage. *Current Directions in Psychological Science, 26*(3), 256–262.

Lee, N.C., Hollarek, M., & Krabbendam, L. (2018). Neurocognitive development during adolescence. In J.E. Lansford & P. Banati (Eds.), *Handbook of adolescent development research and its impact on global policy.* New York: Oxford University Press.

Lee, Y.Y. (2018). Integrative ethical education: Narvaez's project and Xunzi's insight. *Educational Philosophy and Theory, 50*(13), 1203–1213.

Leedy, P.D., & Ormrod, J.E. (2018). *Practical research* (12th ed.). Upper Saddle River, NJ: Pearson.

Leerkes, E.M., & Zhou, N. (2018). Maternal sensitivity to distress and attachment outcomes: Interactions with sensitivity to nondistress and infant temperament. *Journal of Family Psychology, 32,* 753–761.

Leerkes, E.M., Su, J., Calkins, S.D., O'Brien, M., & Supple, A.J. (2017). Maternal physiological dysregulation while parenting poses risk for infant attachment disorganization and behavior problems. *Development and Psychopathology, 29,* 245–257.

Legare, C.H., & Harris, P.L. (2016). The ontogeny of cultural learning. *Child Development, 87*(3), 633–642.

Legare, C.H., Sobel, D.M., & Callanan, M. (2017). Causal learning is collaborative: Examining explanation and exploration in social contexts. *Psychonomic Bulletin & Review, 24,* 1548–1554.

Leger, D., Beck, F., Richard, J.B., & Godeau, E. (2012). Total sleep time severely drops in adolescence. *PLoS One, 7*(10), e45204.

Legerstee, M. (1997). Contingency effects of people and objects on subsequent cognitive functioning in 3-month-old infants. *Social Development, 6,* 307–321.

Legette, K. (2018). School tracking and youth self-perceptions: Implications for academic and racial identity. *Child Development, 89,* 1311–1327.

Lehrer, R., & Schauble, L. (2015). The development of scientific thinking. In R.M. Lerner & others (Eds.), *Handbook of child psychology and* developmental science (7th ed., pp. 671–714). New York: Wiley.

Leith, G., Yuill, N., & Pike, A. (2018). Scaffolding under the microscope: Applying self-regulation and other-regulation perspectives to a scaffolded task. *British Journal of Educational Psychology, 88*(2), 174–191.

Lemaire, P. (Ed). (2017). *Cognitive development from a strategy perspective.* New York: Routledge.

Lennon, E.M., Gardner, J.M., Karmel, B.Z., & Flory, M.J. (2008). Bayley Scales of Infant Development. In M. M. Haith & J. B. Benson (Eds.), *Encyclopedia of infant and early childhood development.* Oxford, UK: Elsevier.

Leonardi-Bee, J.A., Smyth, A.R., Britton, J., & Coleman. T. (2008). Environmental tobacco smoke and fetal health: Systematic review and analysis. *Archives of Disease in Childhood. Fetal and Neonatal Edition, 93,* F351–F361.

Leong, V., & others (2017). Speaker gaze increases information coupling between infant and adult brains. *Proceedings of the National Academy of Sciences, 114* (50), 13290–13295.

Lerner, J.V., & others (2013). Positive youth development: Processes, philosophies, and programs. In I. B. Weiner & others (Eds.), *Handbook of psychology* (2nd ed., Vol. 6). New York: Wiley.

Lerner, R.M., Boyd, M., & Du, D. (2009). Adolescent development. In I. B. Weiner & C. B. Craighead (Eds.), *Encyclopedia of psychology* (4th ed.). Hoboken, NJ: Wiley.

Lerner, R.M., Roeser, R.W., & Phelps, E. (Eds.). (2009). *Positive youth development and spirituality: From theory to research.* West Conshohocken, PA: Templeton Foundation Press.

Lerner, R.M. (2017). Commentary: Studying and testing the positive youth development model: A tale of two approaches. *Child Development, 88*(4), 1183–1185.

Lessard, L.M., & Juvonen, J. (2018). Losing and gaining friends: Does friendship instability compromise academic functioning in middle school? *Journal of School Psychology, 69,* 143–153.

Levett, K.M., & others (2016). Complementary therapies for labour and birth study: A randomised controlled trial of antenatal integrative medicine for pain management in labour. *BMJ Open, 6*(7), e010691.

Levitan, R.D., & others (2017). A DRD 4 gene by maternal sensitivity interaction predicts risk for overweight or obesity in two independent cohorts of preschool children. *Journal of Child Psychology and Psychiatry, 58,* 180–188.

Leviton, A. (2018). Biases inherent in studies of coffee consumption in early pregnancy and the risks of subsequent events. *Nutrients, 10.*

Levy, G.D., Sadovsky, A.L., & Troseth, G.L. (2000). Aspects of young children's perceptions of gender-typed occupations. *Sex Roles, 42,* 993–1006.

Lew, C.H., Brown, C., Bellugi, U., & Semendeferi, K. (2017). Neuron density is decreased in the prefrontal cortex in Williams syndrome. *Autism Research, 10,* 99–112.

Lewald, J. (2012). Exceptional ability of blind humans to hear sound motion: Implications for the emergence of auditory space. *Neuropsychologia, 51,* 181–186.

Lewis, A.C. (2007). Looking beyond NCLB. *Phi Delta Kappan, 88,* 483–484.

Lewis, C., Hill, M., Skirton, H., & Chitty, L.S. (2012). Non-invasive prenatal diagnosis for fetal sex determination: Benefits and disadvantages from the service users' perspective. *European Journal of Genetics, 20,* 1127–1133.

Lewis, F.C., Reeve, R.A., Kelly, S.P., & Johnson, K.A. (2017). Sustained attention to a predictable, unengaging Go/No-Go task shows ongoing development between 6 and 11 years. *Attention, Perception, & Psychophysics, 79*(6), 1726–1741.

Lewis, M., & Brooks-Gunn, J. (1979). *Social cognition and the acquisition of the self.* New York: Plenum.

Lewis, M. (2014). *The rise of consciousness and the development of emotional life.* New York: Guilford.

Lewis, R. (2017). *Human genetics* (12th ed.). New York: McGraw-Hill.

Li, B.J., Jiang, Y.J., Yuan, F., & Ye, H.X. (2010). Exchange transfusion of least incompatible blood for severe hemolytic disease of the newborn due to anti-Rh17. *Transfusion Medicine, 20,* 66–69.

Li, C., Goran, M.I., Kaur, H., Nollen, N., & Ahluwalia, J.S. (2007). Developmental trajectories of overweight during childhood: Role of early life factors. *Obesity, 15,* 760–761.

Li, D., Zhang, W., Li, X., Li, N., & Ye, B. (2012). Gratitude and suicidal ideation and suicide attempts among Chinese adolescents: Direct, mediated, and moderated effects. *Journal of Adolescence, 35,* 55–66.

Li, G., Kung, K.T., & Hines, M. (2017). Childhood gender-typed behavior and adolescent sexual orientation: A longitudinal population-based study. *Developmental Psychology, 53,* 764–777.

Li, J., & others (2017). VarCards: An integrated genetic and clinical database for coding variants in the human genome. *Nucleic Acids Research, 46,* D1029–D1048.

Li, J., Deng, M., Wang, X., & Tang, Y. (2018). Teachers' and parents' autonomy support and psychological control perceived in junior-high school: Extending the dual-process model of self-determination theory. *Learning and Individual Differences, 68,* 20–29.

Li, L., & others (2018). Texting/emailing while driving among high school students in 35 states, United States, 2015. *Journal of Adolescent Health, 63*(6), 701–708.

Li, M., Fiese, B., & Deater-Deckard, K. (2019, in press). An overview of biological methods in family science. In B. Fiese (Ed.), *Handbook of contemporary family psychology.* Washington, DC: American Psychological Association.

Li, W., Cao, B., Hu, L., & Li, F. (2017). Developmental trajectory of rule detection in four-to six-year-old children. *International Journal of Behavioral Development, 41*(2), 238–244.

Li, W., Christiansen, L., Hjelmborg, J., Baumbach, J., & Tan, Q. (2018). On the power of epigenome-wide association studies using a disease-discordant twin design. *Bioinformatics, 34,* 4073–4078.

Li, W., Farkas, G., Duncan, G.J., Burchinal, M.R., & Vandell, D.L. (2013). Timing of high-quality child care and cognitive, language, and preacademic development. *Developmental Psychology, 49*(8), 1440–1451.

Liben, L.S. (2017). Gender development: A constructivist-ecological perspective. In N. Budwig, E. Turiel, & P.D. Zelazo (Eds.), *New perspectives on human development.* New York: Cambridge University Press.

Libertus, K., & Needham, A. (2011). Teach to reach: The effects of active versus passive reaching experiences on action and perception. *Vision Research, 50,* 2750–2757.

Lickliter, R. (2013). Biological development: Theoretical approaches, techniques, and key findings. In P. D. Zelazo (Ed.), *Handbook of developmental psychology.* New York: Oxford University Press.

Lickliter, R., & Witherington, D.C. (2017). Towards a truly developmental epigenetics. *Human Development, 60,* 124–138.

Liddle, M.J.E., Bradley, B.S., & McGrath, A. (2015). Baby empathy: Infant distress and peer prosocial responses. *Infant Mental Health Journal, 36*(4), 446–458.

Lieb, W., & Vasan, R.S. (2018). Scientific contributions of population-based studies to cardiovascular epidemiology in the GWAS era. *Frontiers in Cardiovascular Medicine, 5,* 57.

Lieberman, O.J., McGuirt, A.F., Tang, G., & Sulzer, D. (2019). Roles for neuronal and glial autophagy in synaptic pruning during development. *Neurobiology of Disease, 122,* 149–163.

Liem, D.G. (2017). Infants' and children's salt taste perception and liking: A review. *Nutrients, 9*(9), 1011.

Lightbody, T.K., & Williamson, D.L. (2017). The timing and intensity of maternal employment in early childhood: Implications for Canadian children. *Journal of Child and Family Studies, 26*(5), 1409–1421.

Lilgendahl, J.P., & others (2018). "So now, I wonder, what am I?": A narrative approach to bicultural identity integration. *Journal of Cross-Cultural Psychology, 49*(10), 1596–1624.

Lillard, A.S., & Taggart, J. (2019). Pretend play and fantasy: What if Montessori was right? *Child Development Perspectives, 13*(2), 85–90.

Lillard, A.S., Li, H., & Boguszewski, K. (2015). Television and children's executive function. *Advances in Child Development and Behavior, 48,* 219–248.

Lillard, A.S. (2016). *Montessori: The science behind the genius.* New York: Oxford University Press.

Lillard, A.S. (2018). Rethinking education: Montessori's approach. *Current Directions in Psychological Science, 27*(6), 395–400.

Lillis, T.A., & others (2018). Sleep quality buffers the effects of negative social interactions on maternal mood in the 3-6 month postpartum period: A daily diary study. *Journal of Behavioral Medicine, 41*(5), 733–746.

Limber, S.P. (2004). Implementation of the Olweus Bullying Prevention program in American schools: Lessons learned from the field. In D. L. Espelage &

S. M. Swearer (Eds.), *Bullying in American schools*. Mahwah, NJ: Erlbaum.

Lin, W.C., & others (2017). Postnatal paternal involvement and maternal emotional disturbances: The effect of maternal employment status. *Journal of Affective Disorders, 219*, 9–16.

Lin, Y.C., Latner, J.D., Fung, X.C., & Lin, C.Y. (2018). Poor health and experiences of being bullied in adolescents: Self-perceived overweight and frustration with appearance matter. *Obesity, 26*, 397–404.

Lindsay, A.C., Wasserman, M., Muñoz, M.A., Wallington, S.F., & Greaney, M.L. (2018). Examining influences of parenting styles and practices on physical activity and sedentary behaviors in Latino children in the United States: Integrative review. *JMIR Public Health and Surveillance, 4*(1), e14.

Lindsey, E.W. (2019). Frequency and intensity of emotional expressiveness and preschool children's peer competence. *The Journal of Genetic Psychology, 180*(1), 45–61.

Lippa, R.A. (2005). *Gender, nature, and nurture* (2nd ed.). Mahwah, NJ: Erlbaum.

Litman, C., & Greenleaf, C. (2018). Argumentation tasks in secondary English language arts, history, and science: Variations in instructional focus and inquiry space. *Reading Research Quarterly, 53*(1), 107–126.

Liu, J., & others (2010). Neonatal neurobehavior predicts medical and behavioral outcome. *Pediatrics, 125*(1), e90–e98.

Liu, R., Calkins, S.D., & Bell, M.A. (2018). Fearful inhibition, inhibitory control, and maternal negative behaviors during toddlerhood predict internalizing problems at age 6. *Journal of Abnormal Child Psychology, 46*, 1665–1675.

Liu, W., & others (2018). Bridging mechanisms in multiethnic communities: Place-based communication, neighborhood belonging, and intergroup relations. *Journal of International and Intercultural Communication, 11*(1), 58–80.

Liu, Y., Simpkins, S.D., & Lin, A.R. (2018). Ethnic cultural features in organized activities: relations to Latino adolescents' activity experiences and parental involvement. *Journal of Youth and Adolescence, 47*(10), 2243–2260.

Livas-Dlott, A., & others (2010). Commands, competence, and *Cariño:* Maternal socialization processes in Mexican American families. *Developmental Psychology, 46*, 566–578.

Livingston, G. (2014, November). *Four in ten couples are saying 'I do,' again.* Washington, DC: Pew Research Center.

Livingston, G. (2018). Stay-at-home moms and dads account for about one-in-five U.S. parents. Pew Research Center. Retrieved from http://www.pewresearch.org/fact-tank/2018/09/24/stay-at-home-moms-and-dads-account-for-about-one-in-five-u-s-parents/

Lo, C.C., Hopson, L.M., Simpson, G.M., & Cheng, T.C. (2017). Racial/ethnic differences in emotional health: A longitudinal study of immigrants' adolescent children. *Community Mental Health Journal, 53*(1), 92–101.

Lo, C.K., Hew, K.F., & Chen, G. (2017). Toward a set of design principles for mathematics flipped classrooms: A synthesis of research in mathematics education. *Educational Research Review, 22*, 50–73.

Lo, C.O., & Porath, M. (2017). Paradigm shifts in gifted education: An examination vis-à-vis its historical situatedness and pedagogical sensibilities. *Gifted Child Quarterly, 61*, 343–360.

Lobel, A., Engels, R.C., Stone, L.L., & Granic, I. (2019). Gaining a competitive edge: Longitudinal associations between children's competitive video game playing, conduct problems, peer relations, and prosocial behavior. *Psychology of Popular Media Culture, 8*(1), 76–87.

Lockhart, K.L., Goddu, M.K., & Keil, F.C. (2018). When saying "I'm best" is benign: Developmental shifts in perceptions of boasting. *Developmental Psychology, 54*(3), 521–535.

Loeffen, E.A.H., & others (2017). The importance of evidence-based supportive care practice guidelines in childhood cancer: A plea for their development and implementation. *Supportive Care in Cancer, 25*, 1121–1125.

Loftus, E.F. (2003). Make-believe memories. *American Psychologist, 58*(11), 867–873.

Lombardi, C.M., & Coley, R.L. (2017). Early maternal employment and children's academic and behavioral skills in Australia and the United Kingdom. *Child Development, 88*(1), 263–281.

Loos, R.J., & Janssens, A.C.J. (2017). Predicting polygenic obesity using genetic information. *Cell Metabolism, 25*, 535–543.

Loosli, S.V., Buschkuehl, M., Perrig, W.J., & Jaeggi, S.M. (2012). Working memory training improves reading processes in typically developing children. *Child Neuropsychology, 18*, 62–78.

Lorenz, K.Z. (1965). *Evolution and the modification of behavior.* Chicago: University of Chicago Press.

Lotto, R., Smith, L.K., & Armstrong, N. (2018). Diagnosis of a severe congenital anomaly: A qualitative analysis of parental decision making and the implications for healthcare encounters. *Health Expectations, 21*, 678–684.

Lovallo, W.R., & others (2017). Joint impact of early life adversity and COMT Val158Met (rs4680) genotypes on the adult cortisol response to psychological stress. *Psychosomatic Medicine, 79*, 631–637.

Low, J., Apperly, I.A., Butterfill, S.A., & Rakoczy, H. (2016). Cognitive architecture of belief reasoning in children and adults: A primer on the two-systems account. *Child Development Perspectives, 10*(3), 184–189.

Low, S., & Shortt, J.W. (2017). Family, peer, and pubertal determinants of dating involvement among adolescents. *Journal of Research on Adolescence, 27*(1), 78–87.

Low, S., Snyder, J., & Shortt, J.W. (2012). The drift toward problem behavior during the transition to adolescence: The contributions of youth disclosure, parenting, and older siblings. *Journal of Research on Adolescence, 22*, 65–79.

Lowe, J.R., & others (2016). Maternal touch and infant affect in the Still Face Paradigm: A cross-cultural examination. *Infant Behavior and Development, 44*, 110–120.

Lowell, A., & Mayes, L. (2019). Assessment and treatment of prenatally exposed infants and children. In A. Hauptman & J. Salpekar (Eds.), *Pediatric Neuropsychiatry*. New York: Springer.

Lu, J., Wang, Z., Cao, J., Chen, Y., & Dong, Y. (2018). A novel and compact review on the role of oxidative stress in female reproduction. *Reproductive Biology and Endocrinology, 16*(1), 80.

Lucca, K., & Wilbourn, M.P. (2019). The what and the how: Information-seeking pointing gestures facilitate learning labels and functions. *Journal of Experimental Child Psychology, 178*, 417–436.

Luizon, M.R., Pereira, D.A., & Sandrim, V.C. (2018). Pharmacogenomics of hypertension and preeclampsia: Focus on gene-gene interactions. *Frontiers in Pharmacology, 9*, 168.

Lund, T.J., & Dearing, E. (2013). Is growing up affluent risky for adolescents or is the problem growing up in an affluent neighborhood? *Journal of Research on Adolescence.*

Luthar, S.S., Small, P.J., & Ciciolla, L. (2018). Adolescents from upper middle class communities: Substance misuse and addiction across early adulthood. *Development and Psychopathology, 30*(1), 315–335.

Lye, P., & others (2018). Glucocorticoids modulate multidrug resistance transporters in the first trimester human placenta. *Journal of Cellular and Molecular Medicine, 22*, 3652–3660.

Lykken, D. (2001). *Happiness: What studies on twins show us about nature, nurture, and the happiness set point.* New York: Golden Books.

Lykken, E.A., Shyng, C., Edwards, R.J., Rozenberg, A., & Gray, S.J. (2018). Recent progress and considerations for AAV gene therapies targeting the central nervous system. *Journal of Neurodevelopmental Disorders, 10*, 16.

Lyman, E.L., & Luthar, S.S. (2014). Further evidence on the "costs of privilege": Perfectionism in high-achieving youth at socioeconomic extremes. *Psychology in the Schools, 51*(9), 913–930.

Lynn, M.G., Grych, J.H., & Fosco, G.M. (2016). Influences on father involvement: Testing for unique contributions of religion. *Journal of Child and Family Studies, 25*, 3247–3259.

Lyon, G.J., & Wang, K. (2013). Identifying disease mutations in genomic medicine settings: Current challenges and how to accelerate the process. *Genome Medicine, 4*(7), 58.

Lyon, T.D., & Flavell, J.H. (1993). Young children's understanding of forgetting over time. *Child Development, 64*, 789–800.

Lyovin, A.V., Kessler, B., & Leben, W.R. (2017). *An introduction to lanugages of the world.* Oxford, UK: Oxford University Press.

Lytle, L.A. (2012). Dealing with the childhood obesity epidemic: A public health approach. *Abdominal Imaging, 37*, 719–724.

M

Müller, E., Seiler, C.W., Perren, S., & Simoni, H. (2015). Young children's self-perceived ability: Development, factor structure and initial validation of a self-report instrument for preschoolers. *Journal of Psychopathology and Behavioral Assessment, 37*(2), 256–273.

Maag, J.W., Kauffman, J.M., & Simpson, R.L. (2019). The amalgamation of special education? On practices and policies that may render it unrecognizable. *Exceptionality, 27*(3), 185–200. doi:10.1080/09362835.2018.1425624

Maas, M.K., & others (2018). Division of labor and multiple domains of sexual satisfaction among first-time parents. *Journal of Family Issues, 39*(1), 104–127.

Mabbe, E., Soenens, B., De Muynck, G.J., & Vansteenkiste, M. (2018). The impact of feedback valence and communication style on intrinsic motivation in middle childhood: Experimental evidence and generalization across individual differences. *Journal of Experimental Child Psychology, 170,* 134–160.

Maccoby, E.E. (1984). Middle childhood in the context of the family. In W. A. Collins (Ed.), *Development during middle childhood.* Washington, DC: National Academy Press.

Maccoby, E.E. (2002). Gender and group process: A developmental perspective. *Current Directions in Psychological Science, 11,* 54–57.

Maccoby, E.E. (2007). Historical overview of socialization research and theory. In J. E. Grusec & P. D. Hastings (Eds.), *Handbook of socialization.* New York: Guilford.

Maccoby, E.E., & Mnookin, R.H. (1992). *Dividing the child: Social and legal dilemmas of custody.* Cambridge, MA: Harvard University Press.

MacFarlane, J.A. (1975). Olfaction in the development of social preferences in the human neonate. In *Parent-infant interaction.* Ciba Foundation Symposium No. 33. Amsterdam: Elsevier.

Mackie, F.L., Hemming, K., Allen, S., Morris, R.K., & Kilby, M.D. (2017). The accuracy of cell-free fetal DNA-based non-invasive prenatal testing in singleton pregnancies: A systematic review and bivariate meta-analysis. *British Journal of Obstetrics and Gynaecology, 124,* 32–46.

MacNeill, L.A., Ram, N., Bell, M.A., Fox, N.A., & Pérez-Edgar, K. (2018). Trajectories of infants' biobehavioral development: Timing and rate of A-not-B performance gains and EEG maturation. *Child Development, 89,* 711–724.

Macon, T.A., Tamis-LeMonda, C.S., Cabrera, N.J., & McFadden, K.E. (2017). Predictors of father investment of time and finances: The specificity of resources, relationships, and parenting beliefs. *Journal of Family Issues, 38,* 2642–2662.

MacSwan, J., Thompson, M.S., Rolstad, K., McAlister, K., & Lobo, G. (2017). Three theories of the effects of language education programs: An empirical evaluation of bilingual and English-only policies. *Annual Review of Applied Linguistics, 37,* 218–240.

Mader, S.S., & Windelspecht, M. (2013). *Biology* (11th ed.). New York: McGraw-Hill.

Mader, S.S., & Windelspecht, M. (2017). *Inquiry into life.* New York: McGraw-Hill.

Magid, R.W., Yan, P., Siegel, M.H., Tenenbaum, J.B., & Schulz, L.E. (2018). Changing minds: Children's inferences about third party belief revision. *Developmental Science, 21*(2), e12553.

Magno, C. (2010). The role of metacognitive skills in developing critical thinking. *Metacognition and Learning, 5,* 137–156.

Mahany, E.B., & Smith, Y.R. (2017) Assisted reproductive technology: Clinical aspects. In T. Falcone & W. Hurd (Eds.), *Clinical reproductive medicine and surgery.* Netherlands: Springer.

Mahrer, N.E., O'Hara, K.L., Sandler, I.N., & Wolchik, S.A. (2018). Does shared parenting help or hurt children in high-conflict divorced families? *Journal of Divorce & Remarriage, 59*(4), 324–347.

Mahmud, R.A., Sultana, M., & Sarker, A.R. (2017). Distribution and determinants of low birth weight in developing countries. *Journal of Preventive Medicine and Public Health, 50*(1), 18–28.

Major Depressive Disorder Working Group of the Psychiatric GWAS Consortium (2013). A mega-analysis of genome-wide association studies for major depressive disorder. *Molecular Psychiatry 18,* 497–511.

Makhlouf Obermeyer, C. (2015). Adolescents in Arab countries: Health statistics and social context. *DIFI Family Research and Proceedings, 1.* doi:10.5339/difi.2015.1

Malatesta-Muncher, R., & Mitsnefes, M.M. (2012). Management of blood pressure in children. *Current Opinion in Nephrology and Hypertension, 21,* 318–322.

Malik, M.A.R., & Butt, A.N. (2017). Rewards and creativity: Past, present, and future. *Applied Psychology, 66,* 290–325.

Malin, H., Ballard, P.J., & Damon, W. (2015). Civic purpose: An integrated construct for understanding civic development in adolescence. *Human Development, 58*(2), 103–130.

Malizia, B.A., Hacker, M.R., & Penzias, A.S. (2009). Cumulative live-birth rates after in vitro fertilization. *New England Journal of Medicine, 360,* 236–243.

Mallett, C.A., & Tedor, M.F. (2019). *Juvenile delinquency: Pathways and prevention.* Thousand Oaks, CA: SAGE.

Malloy, L.C., La Rooy, D.J., Lamb, M.A., & Katz, C. (2012). Developmentally sensitive interviewing for legal purposes. In M. E. Lamb, D. J. La Rooy, L. C. Malloy, & C. Katz (Eds.), *Children's testimony* (2nd ed.). New York: Wiley.

Maloy, R.W., & others (2015). *Transforming learning with new technologies* (2nd ed.). Upper Saddle River, NJ: Pearson.

Maloy, R.W., & others (2016). *Transforming learning with new technologies* (3rd ed.). Upper Saddle River, NJ: Pearson.

Malti, T., Dys, S., Colasante, T., & Peplak, J. (2017). Emotions and morality: New developmental perspectives. In C. Helwig (Ed.), *New perspectives on moral development.* New York: Psychology Press.

Malti, T. (2016). Toward an integrated clinical-developmental model of guilt. *Developmental Review, 39,* 16–36.

Mandara, J. (2006). The impact of family functioning on African American males' academic achievement: A review and clarification of the empirical literature. *Teachers College Record, 108,* 206–233.

Mandler, J.M., & DeLoache, J. (2013). The beginnings of conceptual development. In S. Pauen & M. Bornstein (Eds.), *Early child development and later outcome.* New York: Cambridge University Press.

Mandler, J.M., & McDonough, L. (1993). Concept formation in infancy. *Cognitive Development, 8,* 291–318.

Mandler, J.M. (2012). On the spatial foundations of the conceptual system and its enrichment. *Cognitive Science, 36*(3), 421–451.

Manduca, R., & Sampson, R.J. (2019). Punishing and toxic neighborhood environments independently predict the intergenerational social mobility of black and white children. *Proceedings of the National Academy of Sciences, 116*(16), 7772–7777.

Manganaro, L., & others (2018). Highlights on MRI of the fetal body. *La Radiologia Medica, 123,* 271–285.

Marchman, V.A., & Fernald, A. (2008). Speed of word recognition and vocabulary knowledge in infancy predict cognitive and language outcomes in later childhood. *Developmental Science, 11,* F9–16.

Marcia, J.E. (1994). The empirical study of ego identity. In H. A. Bosma, T. L. G. Graafsma, H. D. Grotevant, & D. J. DeLevita (Eds.), *Identity and development.* Newbury Park, CA: Sage.

Marcia, J.E. (1993). The ego identity status approach to ego identity. In J. Marcia & others (Eds.), *Ego identity* (pp. 3–21). New York: Springer.

Marengo, L., Farag, N.H., & Canfield, M. (2013). Body mass index and birth defects: Texas, 2005–2008. *Maternal and Child Health Journal, 17*(10), 1898–1907.

Marie, C., & Trainor, L.J. (2012). Development of simultaneous pitch encoding: Infants show a high voice superiority effect. *Cerebral Cortex, 23*(3), 660–669.

Marks, A.K., & Garcia-Coll, C. (2018). Education and developmental competencies of ethnic minority children: Recent theoretical and methodological advances. *Developmental Review, 50,* 90–98.

Marks, P.E., Babcock, B., van den Berg, Y.H., & Cillessen, A.H. (2019). Effects of including versus excluding nonparticipants as potential nominees in peer nomination measures. *International Journal of Behavioral Development, 43*(3), 255–262.

Markus, H.R., & Kitayama, S. (2012). Culture and the self. In K. Vohs & R. F. Baumeister (Eds.), *Self and identity.* Thousand Oaks, CA: Sage.

Marshall, C., & others (2013). WIC participation and breastfeeding among White and Black mothers: Data from Mississippi. *Maternal and Child Health Journal, 17*(10), 1784–1792.

Marshall, C. (2017). Montessori education: A review of the evidence base. *Science of Learning, 2*(1), 11.

Martínez, M.L., Cumsille, P., Loyola, I., & Castillo, J.C. (2019, in press). Patterns of civic and political commitment in early adolescence. *The Journal of Early Adolescence.* doi: 10.1177/0272431618824714

Martin, C.L., & Fabes, R.A. (2001). The stability and consequences of young children's same-sex peer interactions. *Development Psychology, 37,* 431–446.

Martin, C.L., Ruble, D.N., & Szkrybalo, J. (2002). Cognitive theories of early gender development. *Psychological Bulletin, 128,* 903–933.

Martin, C.L., & others (2013). The role of sex of peers and gender-typed activities in young children's peer affiliative networks: A longitudinal analysis of selection and influence. *Child Development, 84*(3), 921–937.

Martin, J.A., & others (2018). Births: Final data for 2016. *National Vital Statistics Reports, 67*(1). Hyattsville, MD: National Center for Health Statistics.

Martin, K.B., & Messinger, D.S. (2018). Smile. In M.H. Bornstein (Ed.) & M. Arterberry, K. Fingerman, & J.E. Lansford (Assoc. Eds.), *The SAGE encyclopedia of lifespan human development.* Thousand Oaks, CA: SAGE.

Martinez, G.M., & others (2018). Fertility of men and women aged 15–44 in the United States: National Survey of Family Growth, 2011–2015. *National Health Statistics Reports, 113.* Hyattsville, MD: National Center for Health Statistics.

Masarik, A.S., & others (2013). Romantic relationships in early adulthood: Influences of family, personality, and relationship cognitions. *Personal Relationships, 20*(2), 356–373.

Masselink, M., & others (2018). The longitudinal association between self-esteem and depressive symptoms in adolescents: Separating between-person effects from within-person effects. *European Journal of Personality, 32*(6), 653–671.

Masten, A.S. (2012). Faculty profile: Ann Masten. *The Institute of Child Development further developments.* Minneapolis: School of Education.

Masten, A.S. (2013). Risk and resilience in development. In P. D. Zelazo (Ed.), *Oxford handbook of developmental psychology.* New York: Oxford University Press.

Masten, A.S., & Cicchetti, D. (2016). Resilience in development: Progress and transformation. In D. Cicchetti (Ed.), *Developmental psychopathology* (pp. 271–333). New York: Wiley.

Masten, A.S., Fiat, A.E., Labella, M.H., & Strack, R.A. (2015). Educating homeless and highly mobile students: Implications of research on risk and resilience. *School Psychology Review, 44*(3), 315–330.

Masten, A.S. (2018). Resilience theory and research on children and families: Past, present and promise. *Journal of Family Theory & Review, 10*(1), 12–31.

Mateus, V., Martins, C., Osorio, A., Martins, E.C., & Soares, I. (2013). Attention at 10 months of age in infant-mother dyads: Contrasting free-toy play with semi-structured toy-play. *Infant Behavior and Development, 36*(1), 176–179.

Matheis, M., Matson, J.L., & Burns, C.O. (2018). Premature birth, low birth weight, and positive screening for autism spectrum disorder in an early intervention sample. *Journal of Developmental and Physical Disabilities, 30*(5), 689–705.

Mathew, L., Phillips, K.F., & Sandanapitchai, P. (2018). Interventions to reduce postpartum fatigue: An integrative review of the literature. *GJ Health Science Nursing, 1,* 112.

Mathews, T.J., & Hamilton, B.E. (2016). Mean age of mothers is on the rise: United States, 2000–2014. *NCHS Data Brief, 232.* Hyattsville, MD: National Center for Health Statistics.

Matlin, M.W. (2012). *The psychology of women* (7th ed.). Boston: Cengage.

Matlow, J.N., Jubetsky, A., Aleksa, K., Berger, H., & Koren, G. (2013). The transfer of ethyl

glucuronide across the dually perfused human placenta. *Placenta, 34*(4), 369–373.

Matsuba, M.K., Murazyn, T., & Hart, D. (2014). Moral identity and community. In M. Killen & J.G. Smetana (Eds.), *Handbook of moral development* (2nd ed.). New York: Psychology Press.

Matsumoto, D., & Juang, L. (2017). *Culture and psychology* (6th ed.). Boston: Cengage.

Mattson, S., & Smith, J.E. (2015). *Core curriculum for maternal-newborn nursing* (5th ed.). New York: Elsevier.

Mau, W.-C.J., & Li, J. (2018). Factors influencing STEM career aspirations of underrepresented high school students. *Career Development Quarterly, 66,* 246–258.

Maurer, D., & Lewis, T.L. (2018). Visual systems. In R. Gibb & B. Kolb (Eds.), *The neurobiology of brain and behavioral development* (pp. 213–233). New York: Routledge.

Maurer, D. (2017). Critical periods re-examined: Evidence from children treated for dense cataracts. *Cognitive Development, 42,* 27–36.

Maxson, S.C. (2013). Behavioral genetics. In I. B. Weiner & others (Eds.), *Handbook of psychology* (2nd ed., Vol. 3). New York: Wiley.

May, K.E., & Elder, A.D. (2018). Efficient, helpful, or distracting? A literature review of media multitasking in relation to academic performance. *International Journal of Educational Technology in Higher Education, 15*(1), 13.

Mayer, R.E. (2008). *Curriculum and instruction* (2nd ed.). Upper Saddle River, NJ: Prentice Hall.

Mazur, J.E. (2016). *Learning and behavior* (8th ed.). New York: Routledge.

McAdams, D.P., & McLean, K.C. (2013). Narrative identity. *Current Directions in Psychological Science, 22*(3), 233–238.

McAdoo, H.P. (2006). *Black families* (4th ed.). Thousand Oaks, CA: Sage.

McBride, C., Wang, Y., & Cheang, L.M.L. (2018). Dyslexia in Chinese. *Current Developmental Disorders Reports, 5,* 217–225.

McBride, C. (2016). *Children's literacy development: A cross-cultural perspective on learning to read and write* (2nd ed.). New York: Routledge.

McCabe, A., & Dinh, K.T. (2016). Agency and communion, ineffectiveness and alienation: Themes in the life stories of Latino and Southeast Asian adolescents. *Imagination, Cognition and Personality, 36*(2), 150–171.

McCabe, D. (2016). Cheating and honor: Lessons from a long-term research project. In T. Bretag (Ed.), *Handbook of academic integrity* (pp. 187–198). Singapore: Springer.

McCall, R.B., Appelbaum, M.I., & Hogarty, P.S. (1973). Developmental changes in mental performance. *Monographs of the Society for Research in Child Development, 38* (Serial No. 150).

McCall, R.B., & others (2019). Early caregiver–child interaction and children's development: Lessons from the St. Petersburg-USA Orphanage Intervention Research Project. *Clinical Child and Family Psychology Review, 22,* 208–224.

McCartney, K. (2003, July 16). Interview with Kathleen McCartney in A. Bucuvalas, Child care

and behavior, *HGSE News,* pp. 1–4. Cambridge, MA: Harvard Graduate School of Education.

McCarty, S., Teie, S., McCutchen, J., & Geller, E.S. (2016). Actively caring to prevent bullying in an elementary school: Prompting and rewarding prosocial behavior. *Journal of Prevention & Intervention in the Community, 44*(3), 164–176.

McClelland, K., Bowles, J., & Koopman, P. (2012). Male sex determination: Insights into molecular mechanisms. *Asian Journal of Andrology, 14,* 164–171.

McCluskey, K.W. (2017). Identification of the gifted redefined with ethics and equity in mind. *Roeper Review, 39,* 195–198.

McCombs, B.L. (2013). Educational psychology and educational transformation. In I. B. Weiner & others (Eds.), *Handbook of psychology* (2nd ed., Vol. 7). New York: Wiley.

McCormick, C.B., Dimmitt, C., & Sullivan, F.R. (2013). Metacognition, learning, and instruction. In I. B. Weiner & others (Eds.), *Handbook of psychology* (2nd ed., Vol. 7). New York: Wiley.

McCoy, S.S., Dimler, L.M., Samuels, D.V., & Natsuaki, M.N. (2019). Adolescent susceptibility to deviant peer pressure: Does gender matter? *Adolescent Research Review, 4*(1), 59–71.

McDermott, B.M., & Cobham, V.E. (2012). Family functioning in the aftermath of a disaster. *BMC Psychiatry, 12,* 55.

McDermott, E.R., Umaña-Taylor, A.J., & Martinez-Fuentes, S. (2018). Family ethnic socialization predicts better academic outcomes via proactive coping with discrimination and increased self-efficacy. *Journal of Adolescence, 65,* 189–195.

McDermott, J.M., & Fox, N.A. (2018). Emerging executive functions in early childhood. In C. Zeanah (Ed.), *Handbook of infant mental health* (4th ed., pp. 120–133). New York: Guilford.

McDonald, E.M., Mack, K., Shields, W.C., Lee, R.P., & Gielen, A.C. (2018). Primary care opportunities to prevent unintentional home injuries: A focus on children and older adults. *American Journal of Lifestyle Medicine, 12,* 96–106.

McDonald, K.L., & Asher, S.R. (2018). Peer acceptance, peer rejection, and popularity: Social-cognitive and behavioral perspectives. In W. Bukowski & others (Eds.), *Handbook of peer relationships, interactions, and groups* (2nd ed.). New York: Guilford.

McElhaney, K.B., & Allen, J.P. (2012). Sociocultural perspectives on adolescent autonomy. In P. K. Kerig, M. S. Schulz, & S. T. Hauser (Eds.), *Adolescence and beyond.* New York: Oxford University Press.

McEwen, B.S., & Milner, T.A. (2017). Understanding the broad influence of sex hormones and sex differences in the brain. *Journal of Neuroscience Research, 95,* 24–39.

McFarland, J., & others (2018). *The condition of education 2018* (NCES 2018-144). U.S. Department of Education. Washington, DC: National Center for Education Statistics.

McGee, T.R., & Moffitt, T. (2019). The developmental taxonomy. In D. Farrington & others (Eds.), *Oxford handbook of developmental and* life-course criminology (pp. 149-158). New York: Oxford University Press.

McGettigan, C., & others (2017). You talkin' to me? Communicative talker gaze activates left-lateralized superior temporal cortex during perception of degraded speech. *Neuropsychologia, 100,* 51-63.

McGloin, J.M., & Thomas, K.J. (2019). Peer influence and delinquency. *Annual Review of Criminology, 2,* 241-264.

McHale, J.P., & Sirotkin, Y. (2019). Coparenting in diverse family systems. In M.H. Bornstein (Ed.), *Handbook of parenting* (3rd ed.). New York: Taylor and Francis.

McHale, S.M., & Crouter, A.C. (2013). How do children exert an impact on family life? In A. C. Crouter & A. Booth (Eds.), *Children's influence on family dynamics.* New York: Routledge.

McHale, S.M., Updegraff, K.A., & Whiteman, S.D. (2011). Sibling relationships. In G. W. Peterson & K. R. Bush (Eds.), *Handbook of marriage and family* (3rd ed.). New York: Springer.

McKenney, S.J., & Bigler, R.S. (2016). Internalized sexualization and its relation to sexualized appearance, body surveillance, and body shame among early adolescent girls. *Journal of Early Adolescence, 36,* 171-197.

McKinney, C., & Renk, K. (2011). A multivariate model of parent-adolescent relationship variables in early adolescence. *Child Psychiatry and Human Development, 42*(4), 442-462.

McKinnon, C.J., & others (2019). Restricted and repetitive behavior and brain functional connectivity in infants at risk for developing autism spectrum disorder. *Biological Psychiatry, 4,* 50-61.

McLean, K.C., Breen, A.V., & Fournier, M.A. (2010). Constructing the self in early, middle, and late adolescent boys: Narrative identity, individuation, and well-being. *Journal of Research on Adolescence, 20,* 166-187.

McLean, K.C., & Syed, M. (Eds.). (2013). *Oxford handbook of identity development.* New York: Oxford University Press.

McLean, K.C., & Lilgendahl, J.P. (2019). Narrative identity in adolescence and adulthood. In D.P. McAdams, R.L. Shiner, & J.L. Tackett (Eds.), *Handbook of personality development.* New York: Guilford.

McLean, K.C., & others (2018). Identity development in cultural context: The role of deviating from master narratives. *Journal of Personality, 86*(4), 631-651.

McLeish, J., & Redshaw, M. (2018). A qualitative study of volunteer doulas working alongside midwives at births in England: Mothers' and doulas' experiences. *Midwifery, 56,* 53-60.

McLeod, G.F., Horwood, L.J., Boden, J.M., & Fergusson, D.M. (2018). Early childhood education and later educational attainment and socioeconomic wellbeing outcomes to age 30. *New Zealand Journal of Educational Studies,* 1-17.

McLeod, R.H., Hardy, J.K., & Kaiser, A.P. (2017). The effects of play-based intervention on vocabulary acquisition by preschoolers at risk for reading and language delays. *Journal of Early Intervention, 39,* 147-160.

McLeskey, J.M., Rosenberg, M.S., & Westling, D.L. (2018). *Inclusion* (3rd). Upper Saddle River, NJ: Pearson.

McLoyd, V.C., Kaplan, R., Purtell, K.M., & Huston, A.C. (2011). Assessing the effects of a work-based antipoverty program for parents on youth's future orientation and employment experiences. *Child Development, 82,* 113-132.

McLoyd, V.C., Kaplan, R., Purtell, K.M., Bagley, E., Hardaway, C.R., & Smalls, C. (2009). Poverty and socioeconomic disadvantage in adolescence. In R. M. Lerner & L. Steinberg (Eds.), *Handbook of adolescent psychology* (3rd ed.). New York: Wiley.

McLoyd, V.C., Jocson, R.M., & Williams, A.B. (2016). Linking poverty and children's development: Concepts, models, and debates. In D. Brady & L. Burton (Eds.), *The Oxford handbook of the social science of poverty.* Oxford, UK: Oxford University Press.

McLoyd, V.C. (2019). How children and adolescents think about, make sense of, and respond to economic inequality: Why does it matter? *Developmental Psychology, 55*(3), 592-600.

McMahon, M., & Stryjewski, G. (2011). *Pediatrics.* New York: Elsevier.

McMurray, B., Horst, J.S., & Samuelson, L.K. (2012). Word learning emerges from the interaction of online referent selection and slow associative learning. *Psychological Review, 119,* 831-877.

McNamara, F., & Sullivan, C.E. (2000). Obstructive sleep apnea in infants. *Journal of Pediatrics, 136,* 318-323.

McPhail, B.L. (2019). Religious heterogamy and the intergenerational transmission of religion: A cross-national analysis. *Religions, 10*(2), 109.

McWhorter, R.R., & Ellinger, A.D. (2018). Qualitative case study research: An initial primer. In *Handbook of research on innovative techniques, trends, and analysis for optimized research methods* (pp. 185-201). Hershey, PA: IGI Global.

Meaney, M.J. (2010). Epigenetics and the biological definition of gene × environment interactions. *Child Development, 81,* 41-79.

Medoff, N.J., & Kaye, B. (2017). *Electronic media: Then, now and later* (3rd ed.). New York: Routledge.

Meehan, C.L., Hagen, E.H., & Hewlett, B.S. (2017). Persistence of infant care patterns among Aka foragers. In V. Reyes-García & A. Pyhälä (Eds.), *Hunter-gatherers in a changing world.* Cham, Switzerland: Springer.

Meerlo, P., Sgoifo, A., & Suchecki, D. (2008). Restricted and disrupted sleep: Effects on autonomic function, neuroendocrine stress systems, and stress responsivity. *Sleep Medicine Review, 12,* 197-210.

Meeus, W. (2018). *Adolescent development: Longitudinal research into the self, personal relationships and psychopathology.* New York: Routledge.

Mehta, C.M., & Smith, K.R. (2019). "As you grow up the divide still tends to happen": A qualitative investigation of gender segregation in adulthood. *Gender Issues, 36*(2), 176-200.

Mehta, C.M., & Strough, J. (2009). Sex segregation in friendships and normative contexts across the life span. *Developmental Review, 29*(3), 201-220.

Mehta, P. (2017). "Steps to our culture": Cultural cultivation and teaching children about a culture "left behind." *Michigan Family Review, 21*(1).

Meier, A., & Musick, K. (2014). Variations in associations between family dinners and adolescent well-being. *Journal of Marriage and Family, 76*(1), 13-23.

Meindl, P., Jayawickreme, E., Furr, R.M., & Fleeson, W. (2015). A foundation beam for studying morality from a personological point of view: Are individual differences in moral behaviors and thoughts consistent? *Journal of Research in Personality, 59,* 81-92.

Meldrum, R.C., & Hay, C. (2012). Do peers matter in the development of self-control? Evidence from a longitudinal study of youth. *Journal of Youth and Adolescence, 41,* 691-703.

Mello, Z.R. (2009). Racial/ethnic group and socioeconomic status variation in educational and occupational expectations from adolescence to adulthood. *Journal of Applied Developmental Psychology, 30,* 494-504.

Meltzoff, A.N., & Marshall, P.J. (2018). Human infant imitation as a social survival circuit. *Current Opinion in Behavioral Sciences, 24,* 130-136.

Meltzoff, A.N., Saby, J.N., & Marshall, P.J. (2019). Neural representations of the body in 60-day-old human infants. *Developmental Science, 22*(1). e12698.

Melzi, G., Schick, A.R., & Kennedy, J.L. (2011). Narrative elaboration and participation: Two dimensions of maternal elicitation style. *Child Development, 82*(4), 1282-1296.

Mercy, E., & others (2013). Noninvasive detection of fetal trisomy 21: Systematic review and report of quality and outcomes of diagnostic accuracy studies performed between 1997 and 2012. *Human Reproduction Update, 19*(4), 318-329.

Merz, E.C., Landry, S.H., Johnson, U.Y., Williams, J.M., & Jung, K. (2016). Effects of a responsiveness-focused intervention in family child care homes on children's executive function. *Early Childhood Research Quarterly, 34,* 128-139.

Mesman, J., & others (2016). Is the ideal mother a sensitive mother? Beliefs about early childhood parenting in mothers across the globe. *International Journal of Behavioral Development, 40,* 385-397.

Mesman, J., van IJzendoorn, M.H., Bakermans-Kranenburg, M.J. (2009). The many faces of the still-face paradigm: A review and meta-analysis. *Developmental Review, 29,* 120-162.

Messenger, K., & Fisher, C. (2018). Mistakes weren't made: Three-year-olds' comprehension of novel-verb passives provides evidence for early abstract syntax. *Cognition, 178,* 118-132.

Mesurado, B., Richaud, M.C., & Rodriguez, L.M. (2018). The varying roles of parents and the cognitive-emotional variables regarding the different types of adolescent prosocial behavior. *Journal of Social and Personal Relationships.* doi: 10.1177/0265407518780365

Metzger, A., & others (2013). Information management strategies with conversations about cigarette smoking: Parenting correlates and longitudinal associations with teen smoking. *Developmental Psychology, 49*(8), 1565-1578.

Michalczyk, M., Torbé, D., & Torbé, A. (2018). Comparison of the effect of patient-controlled epidural anesthesia (PCEA) and parenteral use of opioid analgesics on the postpartum condition of the newborn. *Journal of Education, Health and Sport, 8*(9), 277–428.

Michalopoulos, C., Faucetta, K., Warren, A., & Mitchell, R. (2017). Evidence on the long-term effects of home visiting programs: Laying the groundwork for long-term follow-up in the Mother and Infant Home Visiting Program Evaluation (MIHOPE). *OPRE Report 2017-73.* U.S. Department of Health and Human Services.

Michikyan, M., Dennis, J., & Subrahmanyam, K. (2015). Can you guess who I am? Real, ideal, and false self-presentation on Facebook among emerging adults. *Emerging Adulthood, 3*(1), 55–64.

Micu, I., Plemel, J.R., Caprariello, A.V., Nave, K.A., & Stys, P.K. (2018). Axo-myelinic neurotransmission: A novel mode of cell signalling in the central nervous system. *Nature Reviews Neuroscience, 19,* 49–58.

Mihov, K.M., Denzler, M., & Forster, J. (2010). Hemispheric specialization and creative thinking: A meta-analytic review of lateralization of creativity. *Brain and Cognition, 72,* 442–448.

Miles, G., & Siega-Riz, A.M. (2017). Trends in food and beverage consumption among infants and toddlers: 2005–2012. *Pediatrics, 139,* e20163290.

Mileva-Seitz, V.R., Bakermans-Kranenburg, M.J., Battaini, C., & Luijk, M.P. (2017). Parent-child bed-sharing: The good, the bad, and the burden of evidence. *Sleep Medicine Reviews, 32,* 4–27.

Milevsky, A. (2011). *Sibling relations in childhood and adolescence.* New York: Columbia University Press.

Milledge, S.V., & others (2018). Peer relationships and prosocial behaviour differences across disruptive behaviours. *European Child & Adolescent Psychiatry,* 1–13. doi:10.1007/s00787-018-1249-2

Miller, C., Martin, C.L., Fabes, R., & Hanish, D. (2013). Bringing the cognitive and social together: How gender detectives and gender enforcers shape children's gender development. In M. Banaji & S. Gelman (Eds.), *Navigating the social world: A developmental perspectives.* New York: Oxford University Press.

Miller, D.I., Nolla, K.M., Eagly, A.H., & Uttal, D.H. (2018). The development of children's gender-science stereotypes: A meta-analysis of 5 decades of U.S. draw-a-scientist studies. *Child Development, 89,* 1943–1955.

Miller, M.B., Janssen, T., & Jackson, K.M. (2017). The prospective association between sleep and initiation of substance use in young adolescents. *Journal of Adolescent Health, 60,* 154–160.

Miller, P.J., & Cho, G.E. (2018). *Self-esteem in time and place: How American families imagine, enact, and personalize a cultural ideal.* New York: Oxford University Press.

Miller, S.E., & Marcovitch, S. (2015). Examining executive function in the second year of life: coherence, stability, and relations to joint attention and language. *Developmental Psychology, 51*(1), 101–114.

Miller-Perrin, C.L., Perrin, R.D., & Kocur, J.L. (2009). Parental physical and psychological aggression: Psychological symptoms in young adults. *Child Abuse and Neglect, 33,* 1–11.

Miller-Slough, R.L., Dunsmore, J.C., Zeman, J.L., Sanders, W.M., & Poon, J.A. (2018). Maternal and paternal reactions to child sadness predict children's psychosocial outcomes: A family-centered approach. *Social Development, 27,* 495–509.

Mills, C.M. (2013). Knowing when to doubt: Developing a critical stance when learning from others. *Developmental Psychology, 49*(3), 404–418.

Mills, K.L., Dumontheil, I., Speekenbrink, M., & Blakemore, S.J. (2015). Multitasking during social interactions in adolescence and early adulthood. *Royal Society Open Science, 2*(11), 150117.

Mills-Koonce, W.R., Propper, C.B., & Barnett, M. (2012). Poor infant soothability and later insecure-ambivalent attachment: Developmental change in phenotypic markers of risk or two measures of the same construct? *Infant Behavior and Development, 35,* 215–235.

Milot, T., Ethier, L.S., St-Laurent, D., & Provost, M.A. (2010). The role of trauma symptoms in the development of behavioral problems in maltreated preschoolers. *Child Abuse and Neglect, 34*(4), 225–234.

Milunsky, A., & Milunsky, J.M. (Eds.). (2016). *Genetic disorders and the fetus: Diagnosis, prevention, and treatment.* New York: Wiley.

Misra, S., Cheng, L., Genevie, J., & Yuan, M. (2016). The iPhone effect: The quality of in-person social interactions in the presence of mobile devices. *Environment and Behavior, 48*(2), 275–298.

Mistry, J., & Dutta, R. (2015). Human development and culture: Conceptual and methodological Issues. In W.F. Overton & P.C. Molenaar (Eds.), *Handbook of child psychology and developmental science: Theory and method* (7th ed., Vol. 1). Hoboken, NJ: Wiley.

Mistry, J., & Dutta, R. (2015). Culture and development. In R. Lerner (Ed.), *Handbook of child psychology and developmental science* (7th ed.). Hoboken, NJ: Wiley.

Mistry, J., Contreras, M., & Dutta, R. (2013). Culture and development. In I. B. Weiner & others (Eds.), *Handbook of psychology* (2nd ed., Vol. 6). New York: Wiley.

Misuraca, R., Miceli, S., & Teuscher, U. (2017). Three effective ways to nurture our brain. *European Psychologist, 22,* 101–120.

Mitanchez, D., & Chavatte-Palmer, P. (2018). Review shows that maternal obesity induces serious adverse neonatal effects and is associated with childhood obesity in their offspring. *Acta Paediatrica.* doi:10.1111/apa.14269

Mitchell, A.B., & Stewart, J.B. (2013). The efficacy of all-male academies: Insights from critical race theory (CRT). *Sex Roles, 69*(7–8), 382–392.

Mitchell, C., Harwin, A., Vara-Orta, F., & Sheehan, F. (2017). Single-gender public schools in 5 charts. *Education Week, 37,* 10.

Mitchell, E.A., Stewart, A.W., Crampton, P., & Salarnod, C. (2000). Deprivation and sudden infant death syndrome. *Social Science and Medicine, 51,* 147–150.

Miyakoshi, K., & others (2013). Perinatal outcomes: Intravenous patient-controlled fentanyl versus no analgesia in labor. *Journal of Obstetrics and Gynecology Research, 39*(4), 783–789.

Mize, K.D., & Jones, N.A. (2012). Infant physiological and behavioral responses to loss of maternal attention to a social-rival. *International Journal of Psychophysiology, 83,* 16–23.

Moberg, S.A., Ng, R., Johnson, D.E., & Kroupina, M.G. (2017). Impact of joint attention on social-communication skills in internationally adopted children. *Infant Mental Health Journal, 38,* 575–587.

Moffitt, T.E., & others. (2011). A gradient of childhood self-control predicts health, wealth, and public safety. *Proceedings of the National Academy of Sciences U.S.A., 108,* 2693–2698.

Mohan L., & Ray, S. (2019). Conduct disorder. In *StatPearls [Internet].* Treasure Island, FL: StatPearls Publishing. Retrieved from https://www.ncbi.nlm.nih.gov/books/NBK470238/

Moilanen, K.L., Padilla-Walker, L.M., & Blaacker, D.R. (2019, in press). Dimensions of short-term and long-term self-regulation in adolescence: Associations with maternal and paternal parenting and parent-child relationship quality. *Journal of Youth and Adolescence.*

Molitor, A., & Hsu, H.C. (2019). Child development across cultures. In K. Keith (Ed.), *Cross-cultural psychology: Contemporary themes and perspectives* (2nd ed., pp. 153–189). New York: Wiley.

Mollborn, S., & Lawrence, E. (2018). Family, peer, and school influences on children's developing health lifestyles. *Journal of Health and Social Behavior, 59,* 133–150.

Moller, A.B., Petzold, M., Chou, D., & Say, L. (2017). Early antenatal care visit: A systematic analysis of regional and global levels and trends of coverage from 1990 to 2013. *The Lancet Global Health, 5*(10), e977–e983.

Momany, A.M., Kamradt, J.M., & Nikolas, M.A. (2018). A meta-analysis of the association between birth weight and attention deficit hyperactivity disorder. *Journal of Abnormal Child Psychology, 46,* 1409–1426.

Money, J. (1975). Ablato penis: Normal male infant sex-reassigned as a girl. *Archives of Sexual Behavior, 4,* 65–71.

Montagna, P., & Chokroverty, S. (2011). *Sleep disorders.* New York: Elsevier.

Monti, J.M., Hillman, C.H., & Cohen, N.J. (2012). Aerobic fitness enhances relational memory in preadolescent children: The FITKids randomized control trial. *Hippocampus, 22*(9), 1876–1882.

Montoya Arizabaleta, A.V., & others (2010). Aerobic exercise during pregnancy improves health-related quality of life: A randomized trial. *Journal of Physiotherapy, 56,* 253–258.

Montroy, J.J., Bowles, R.P., Skibbe, L.E., McClelland, M.M., & Morrison, F.J. (2016). The development of self-regulation across early childhood. *Developmental Psychology, 52,* 1744–1762.

Moon, C. (2017). Prenatal experience with the maternal voice. In M. Filippa & others (Eds.), *Early vocal contact and preterm infant brain development* (pp. 25–37). Berlin: Springer.

Moon, R.Y., & Fu, L. (2012). Sudden infant death syndrome: An update. *Pediatric Reviews, 33,* 314–320.

Moon, R.Y., & Task Force on Sudden Infant Death Syndrome (2016). Recommendations for a safe infant sleeping environment. *Pediatrics, 138*, e20162940.

Moore, D. (2013). Behavioral genetics, genetics, and epigenetics. In P. D. Zelazo (Ed.), *Oxford handbook of developmental psychology.* New York: Oxford University Press.

Moore, D.S. (2018). Gene × environment interaction: What exactly are we talking about? *Research in Developmental Disabilities, 82*, 3–9.

Moore, T.J., Tank, K.M., & English, L. (2018) Engineering in the early grades: Harnessing children's natural ways of thinking. In L. English & T. Moore (Eds.), *Early mathematics learning and development.* Singapore: Springer.

Moran, M.B., Walker, M.W., Alexander, T.N., Jordan, J.W., & Wagner, D.E. (2017). Why peer crowds matter: Incorporating youth subcultures and values in health education campaigns. *American Journal of Public Health, 107*(3), 389–395.

Morasch, K.C., Raj, V.R., & Bell, M.A. (2013). The development of cognitive control from infancy through childhood. In D. Reisberg (Ed.), *Oxford handbook of cognitive psychology.* New York: Oxford University Press.

Morgan, H. (2019). Does high-quality preschool benefit children? What the research shows. *Education Science, 9*, 19.

Morra, S., & Panesi, S. (2017). From scribbling to drawing: The role of working memory. *Cognitive Development, 43*, 142–158.

Morris, A.S., Criss, M.M., Silk, J.S., & Houltberg, B.J. (2017). The impact of parenting on emotion regulation during childhood and adolescence. *Child Development Perspectives, 11*, 233–238.

Morris, A.S., Cui, L., & Steinberg, L. (2013). Parenting research and themes: What we have learned and where to go next. In R.E. Larzelere, A.S. Morris, & A.W. Harrist (Eds.), *Authoritative parenting.* Washington, DC: American Psychological Association.

Morris, P.A., & others (2018). New findings on impact variation from the Head Start Impact Study: Informing the scale-up of early childhood programs. *AERA Open, 4*(2), 2332858418769287.

Morrongiello, B.A., & Cox, A. (2016). Motor development as a context for understanding parent safety practices. *Developmental Psychobiology, 58*(7), 909–917.

Mortensen, O., Torsheim, T., Melkevik, O., & Thuen, F. (2012). Adding a baby to the equation. Married and cohabiting women's relationship satisfaction in the transition to parenthood. *Family Process, 51*, 122–139.

Moseley, R.L., & Pulvermueller, F. (2018). What can autism teach us about the role of sensorimotor systems in higher cognition? New clues from studies on language, action semantics, and abstract emotional concept processing. *Cortex, 100*, 149–190.

Moulson, M.C., & Nelson, C.A. (2008). Neurological development. In M. M. Haith & J. B. Benson (Eds.), *Encyclopedia of infancy and early childhood.* Oxford. UK: Elsevier.

Movahed Abtahi, M., & Kerns, K.A. (2017). Attachment and emotion regulation in middle

childhood: Changes in affect and vagal tone during a social stress task. *Attachment & Human Development, 19*, 221–242.

Mrug, S., & McCay, R. (2013). Parental and peer disapproval of alcohol use and its relationship to adolescent drinking: Age, gender, and racial differences. *Psychology of Addictive Behaviors, 27*(3), 604–614.

Mrug, S., Borch, C., & Cillessen, A.H.N. (2011). Other-sex friendships in late adolescence: Risky associations for substance abuse and sexual debut? *Journal of Youth and Adolescence, 40*, 875–888.

Muentener, P., Herrig, E., & Schulz, L. (2018). The efficiency of infants' exploratory play is related to longer-term cognitive development. *Frontiers in Psychology, 9*, 635.

Muhonen, H., Pakarinen, E., Poikkeus, A.-M., Lerkkanen, M.-K., & Rasku-Puttonen, H. (2018). Quality of educational dialogue and association with students' academic performance. *Learning and Instruction, 55*, 67–79.

Muller, C., Sampson, R.J., & Winter, A.S. (2018). Environmental inequality: The social causes and consequences of lead exposure. *Annual Review of Sociology, 44*, 263–282.

Mullola, S., & others (2012). Gender differences in teachers' perceptions of students' temperament, educational competence, and teachability. *British Journal of Educational Psychology, 82*(Pt 2), 185–206.

Mulvey, K.L., & Killen, M. (2015). Challenging gender stereotypes: Resistance and exclusion. *Child Development, 86*, 681–694.

Mundy, P. (2018). A review of joint attention and social-cognitive brain systems in typical development and autism spectrum disorder. *European Journal of Neuroscience, 47*(6), 497–514.

Murakami, M., Suzuki, M., & Yamaguchi, T. (2017). Presenting information on regulation values improves the public's sense of safety: Perceived mercury risk in fish and shellfish and its effects on consumption intention. *PloS One, 12*(12), e0188758.

Murdock-Perriera, L.A., & Sedlacek, Q.C. (2018). Questioning Pygmalion in the twenty-first century: The formation, transmission, and attributional influence of teacher expectancies. *Social Psychology of Education, 21*, 691–707.

Murray, J., & Arnett, J. (Eds.) (2019). *Emerging adulthood and higher education: A new student development paradigm.* New York: Routledge.

Murray-Close, D., Nelson, D.A., Ostrov, J.M., Casas, J.F., & Crick, N.R. (2016). Relational aggression: A developmental psychopathology perspective. In D. Cicchetti (Ed.), *Developmental psychopathology.* Hoboken, NJ: Wiley.

Muscatelli, F., & Bouret, S.G. (2018). Wired for eating: How is an active feeding circuitry established in the postnatal brain? *Current Opinion in Neurobiology, 52*, 165–171.

Mustafa, G., & Nazir, B. (2018). Trust in transformational leadership: Do followers' perceptions of leader femininity, masculinity, and androgyny matter? *Journal of Values-Based Leadership, 11*(2), 13.

Mutti, D.O., & others (2018). Ocular component development during infancy and early childhood. *Optometry and Vision Science, 95*(11), 976–985.

Myatchin, I., & Lagae, O. (2013). Developmental changes in visuo-spatial working memory in normally developing children: Event-related potentials study. *Brain Development, 35*(9), 853–864.

Myers, D.G. (2018). *Psychology* (12th). New York: Worth.

N

Na'Allah, R., & Griebel, C. (2017). Postpartum care. In P. Paulman & others (Eds.), *Family medicine.* New York: Springer.

Nader, P.R., & others (2006). Identifying risk for obesity in early childhood. *Pediatrics, 118*, e594–e601.

NAEYC (National Association for the Education of Young Children) (2009). *Developmentally appropriate practice in early childhood programs serving children from birth through age 8.* Washington, DC: Author.

Nagai, Y., Nomura, K., Nagata, M., Kaneko, T., & Uemura, O. (2018). Children's Perceived Competence Scale: Reevaluation in a population of Japanese elementary and junior high school students. *Child and Adolescent Psychiatry and Mental Health, 12*(1), 36.

Nagata, D.K. (1989). Japanese American children and adolescents. In J. T. Gibbs & L. N. Huang (Eds.), *Children of color.* San Francisco: Jossey-Bass.

Nakamoto, J., & Schwartz, D. (2010). Is peer victimization associated with academic achievement? A meta-analytic review. *Social Development, 19*, 221–242.

Nancarrow, A.F., Gilpin, A.T., Thibodeau, R.B., & Farrell, C.B. (2018). Knowing what others know: Linking deception detection, emotion knowledge, and Theory of Mind in preschool. *Infant and Child Development, 27*(5), e2097.

Nanni, V., Uher, R., & Danese, A. (2012). Childhood maltreatment predicts unfavorable course of illness and treatment outcome in depression: A meta-analysis. *American Journal of Psychiatry, 169*, 141–151.

Narváez, D. (2010). Moral complexity: The fatal attraction of truthiness and the importance of mature moral functioning. *Perspectives on Psychological Science, 5*(2), 163–181.

Narváez, D., & Hill, P.L. (2010). The relation of multicultural experiences to moral judgment and mindsets. *Journal of Diversity in Higher Education, 3*, 43–55.

Narváez, D., & Lapsley, D. (Eds.). (2009). *Moral personality, identity, and character: An interdisciplinary future.* New York: Cambridge University Press.

Narváez, D., Panksepp, J., Schore, A.N., & Gleason, T.R. (Eds.). (2013). *Evolution, early experience, and development.* New York: Oxford University Press.

Narváez, D. (2018). Ethogenesis: Evolution, early experience, and moral becoming. In J. Graham & K. Gray (Eds.), *The atlas of moral psychology.* New York: Guilford.

NASSPE (2012). *Single-sex schools/schools with single-sex classrooms/what's the difference?* Retrieved January 21, 2013, from http://www.singlesexschools.org/schools-schools.htm

National Assessment of Educational Progress (2000). *Reading achievement*. Washington, DC: National Center for Education Statistics.

National Assessment of Educational Progress (2018). *Reading performance*. Washington, DC: National Center for Education Statistics.

National Association for Gifted Children & The Council of State Directors of Programs for the Gifted (2015). *2014-2015 state of the states in gifted education: Policy and practice data*. Washington, DC: National Association for Gifted Children.

National Cancer Institute (2018). *Childhood cancers*. Retrieved from https://www.cancer.gov/types/childhood-cancers

National Center for Education Statistics (2018). *The condition of education 2018* (NCES 2018-144). Washington, DC: National Center for Education Statistics.

National Center for Education Statistics (2018). Status dropout rates. *Digest of Education Statistics*. Washington, DC: U.S. Department of Education.

National Center on Shaken Baby Syndrome. (2011). *Shaken baby syndrome*. Retrieved April 22, 2011, from www.dontshake.org

National Head Start Association (2016). *The Head Start Impact Study in 2016*. Retrieved from https://www.nhsa.org/files/resources/head_start_impact_study_2016_0.pdf

National Human Genome Research Institute (2012). *Genome-wide association method*. Washington, DC: Author.

National Institute of Child Health and Development (2013). *SIDS*. Rockville, MD: NICHD.

National Institute of Neurological Disorders and Stroke (2018). *Brain basics: Understanding sleep*. Retrieved from www.ninds.nih.gov/Disorders/Patient-Caregiver-Education/Understanding-Sleep

National Research Council (2004). *Engaging schools: Fostering high school students' motivation to learn*. Washington, DC: National Academic Press.

National Sleep Foundation (2006). *Sleep in America poll: Children and sleep*. Washington, DC: National Sleep Foundation.

National Sleep Foundation (2007). *Sleep in America poll 2007*. Washington, DC: Author.

Naumann, L.P., Benet-Martínez, V., & Espinoza, P. (2017). Correlates of political ideology among US-Born Mexican Americans: Cultural identification, acculturation attitudes, and socioeconomic status. *Social Psychological and Personality Science, 8*(1), 20-28.

NCES, National Center for Education Statistics (2018). *The condition of education 2018 (NCES 2018-144)*. Washington, DC: U.S. Department of Education.

Near, C.E. (2013). Selling gender: Associations of box art representation of female characters with sales for teen- and mature-rated video games. *Sex Roles, 68*(3-4), 252-269.

Neblett, E.W., Rivas-Drake, D., & Umana-Taylor, A.J. (2011). The promise of racial and ethnic protective factors in promoting ethnic minority youth development. *Child Development Perspectives, 6*, 295-303.

Needham, A., Barrett, T., & Peterman, K. (2002). A pick-me-up for infants' exploratory skills: Early simulated experiences reaching for objects using "sticky mittens" enhances young infants' object exploration skills. *Infant Behavior and Development, 25*, 279-295.

Negriff, S., Susman, E.J., & Trickett, P.K. (2011). The development pathway from pubertal timing to delinquency and sexual activity from early to late adolescence. *Journal of Youth and Adolescence, 40*, 1343-1356.

Negru-Subtirica, O., Pop, E.I., & Crocetti, E. (2017). A longitudinal integration of identity styles and educational identity processes in adolescence. *Developmental Psychology, 53*(11), 2127-2138.

Neitzel, C.L., Alexander, J.M., & Johnson, K.E. (2019, in press). The emergence of children's interest orientations during early childhood: When predisposition meets opportunity. *Learning, Culture and Social Interaction*. doi:10.1016/j.lcsi.2019.01.004

Nelson, C.A. (2003). Neural development and lifelong plasticity. In R. M. Lerner, F. Jacobs, & D. Wertlieb (Eds.), *Handbook of applied developmental science*. Thousand Oaks, CA: Sage.

Nelson, C.A. (2012). Brain development and behavior. In A. M. Rudolph, C. Rudolph, L. First, G. Lister, & A. A. Gershon (Eds.), *Rudolph's pediatrics* (22nd ed.). New York: McGraw-Hill.

Nelson, C.A. (2013a). The effects of early psychosocial deprivation. In M. Woodhead & J. Oates (Eds.), *Early childhood in focus 7: Developing brains*. Great Britain: The Open University.

Nelson, C.A. (2013b). Some thoughts on the development and neural bases of face processing. In M. Banaji & S. Gelman (Eds.), *The development of social cognition*. New York: Oxford University Press.

Nelson, S.C., Kling, J., Wängqvist, M., Frisén, A., & Syed, M. (2018). Identity and the body: Trajectories of body esteem from adolescence to emerging adulthood. *Developmental Psychology, 54*, 1159-1171.

Neubauer, J., & others (2017). Post-mortem whole-exome analysis in a large sudden infant death syndrome cohort with a focus on cardiovascular and metabolic genetic diseases. *European Journal of Human Genetics, 25*, 404-409.

Neuman, S.B. (2019). First steps toward literacy: what effective pre-K instruction looks like. *American Educator, 42*(4), 9-11.

Newcombe, N.S. (2007). Developmental psychology meets the mommy wars. *Journal of Applied Developmental Psychology, 28*, 553-555.

Newkirk, K., Perry-Jenkins, M., & Sayer, A.G. (2017). Division of household and childcare labor and relationship conflict among low-income new parents. *Sex Roles, 76*(5-6), 319-333.

Newland, R.P., & Crnic, K.A. (2017). Developmental risk and goodness of fit in the mother–child relationship: Links to parenting stress and children's behaviour problems. *Infant and Child Development, 26*, e1980.

Newton, A.W., & Vandeven, A.M. (2010). Child abuse and neglect: A worldwide concern. *Current Opinion in Pediatrics, 22*, 226-233.

Ng, R., & others (2018). Neuroanatomical correlates of emotion-processing in children with unilateral brain lesion: A preliminary study of limbic system organization. *Social Neuroscience, 13*, 688-700.

Ng, S.W., & others (2018). Federal nutrition program revisions impact low-income households' food purchases. *American Journal of Preventive Medicine, 54*, 403-412.

Nguyen, B., Jin, K., & Ding, D. (2017). Breastfeeding and maternal cardiovascular risk factors and outcomes: A systematic review. *PLoS ONE, 12*(11), e0187923.

Nguyen, V.T., & others (2017). Radiological studies of fetal alcohol spectrum disorders in humans and animal models: An updated comprehensive review. *Magnetic Resonance Imaging, 43*, 10-26.

NICHD Early Child Care Research Network (2000). Factors associated with fathers' caregiving activities and sensitivity with young children. *Developmental Psychology, 14*, 200-219.

NICHD Early Child Care Research Network (2001). Nonmaternal care and family factors in early development: An overview of the NICHD study of Early Child Care. *Journal of Applied Developmental Psychology, 22*, 457-492.

NICHD Early Child Care Research Network (2002). Structure→Process→Outcome: Direct and indirect effects of child care quality on young children's development. *Psychological Science, 13*, 199-206.

NICHD Early Child Care Research Network (2003). Does amount of time spent in child care predict socioemotional adjustment during the transition to kindergarten? *Child Development, 74*, 976-1005.

NICHD Early Child Care Research Network (2004). Type of child care and children's development at 54 months. *Early Childhood Research Quarterly, 19*, 203-230.

NICHD Early Child Care Research Network (2005a). *Child care and development*. New York: Guilford.

NICHD Early Child Care Research Network (2006). Infant-mother attachment classification: Risk and protection in relation to changing maternal caregiving quality. *Developmental Psychology, 42*, 38-58.

NICHD Early Child Care Research Network (2009). Family-peer linkages: The mediational role of attentional processes. *Social Development, 18*(4), 875-895.

NICHD Early Child Care Research Network (2010). Testing a series of causal propositions relating time spent in child care to children's externalizing behavior. *Developmental Psychology, 46*(1), 1-17.

Nieto, S., & Bode, P. (2018). *Affirming diversity* (8th ed.). Upper Saddle River, NJ: Pearson.

Nieuwenhuis, R., & Maldonado, L.C. (Eds). (2018). *The triple bind of single-parent families*. Bristol, UK: Policy Press.

Nikulina, V., & Widom, C.S. (2019). Higher levels of intelligence and executive functioning protect maltreated children against adult arrests: A prospective study. *Child Maltreatment, 24*(1), 3-16.

Nisbett, R.E., & others (2012). Intelligence: New findings and theoretical developments. *American Psychologist, 67*, 130-159.

Nkuba, M., Hermenau, K., & Hecker, T. (2019). The association of maltreatment and socially deviant behavior—Findings from a national study with adolescent students and their parents. *Mental Health & Prevention, 13*, 159-168.

Noll, J.G., & others (2017). Childhood sexual abuse and early timing of puberty. *Journal of Adolescent Health, 60,* 65-71.

Nomura, Y., & others (2017). Neurodevelopmental consequences in offspring of mothers with preeclampsia during pregnancy: Underlying biological mechanism via imprinting genes. *Archives of Gynecology and Obstetrics, 295,* 1319-1329.

Non, A.L., León-Pérez, G., Glass, H., Kelly, E., & Garrison, N.A. (2019). Stress across generations: A qualitative study of stress, coping, and caregiving among Mexican immigrant mothers. *Ethnicity & Health, 24*(4), 378-394.

Noor, S., & Milligan, E.D. (2018). Life-long impacts of moderate prenatal alcohol exposure (PAE) on neuro-immune function. *Frontiers in Immunology, 9,* 1107.

Norman, J.E., & others (2009). Progesterone for the prevention of preterm birth in twin pregnancy (STOPPIT): A randomized, double-blind, placebo-controlled study and meta-analysis. *Lancet, 373,* 2034-2040.

Nottleman, E.D., & others (1987). Gonadal and adrenal hormone correlates of adjustment in early adolescence. In R. M. Lerner & T. T. Foch (Eds.), *Biological-psychological interactions in early adolescence.* Hillsdale, NJ: Erlbaum.

Novak, A.M., & Treagust, D.F. (2018). Adjusting claims as new evidence emerges: Do students incorporate new evidence into their scientific explanations? *Journal of Research in Science Teaching, 55*(4), 526-549.

Nucci, L. (2014). The personal and the moral. In M. Killen & J.G. Smetana (Eds.), *Handbook of moral development* (2nd ed.). New York: Routledge.

Nyström, C.D., & others (2017). Does cardiorespiratory fitness attenuate the adverse effects of severe/morbid obesity on cardiometabolic risk and insulin resistance in children? A pooled analysis. *Diabetes Care, 40,* 1580-1587.

O

O'Brien, A.P., & others (2017). New fathers' perinatal depression and anxiety—Treatment options: An integrative review. *American Journal of Men's Health, 11*(4), 863-876.

O'Brien, M., & Moss, P. (2010). Fathers, work, and family policies in Europe. In M. E. Lamb (Ed.), *The role of the father in child development* (5th ed.). New York: Wiley.

O'Conner, A., Peterson, R.L., & Fluke, S. (2014). *Character education, Policy Q & A.* Lincoln, NE: Student Engagement Project, University of Nebraska-Lincoln and the Nebraska Department of Education. Retrieved from http://k12engagement.unl.edu/character-education-policy

O'Dea, R.E., Lagisz, M., Jennions, M.D., & Nakagawa, S. (2018). Gender differences in individual variation in academic grades fail to fit expected patterns for STEM. *Nature Communications, 9,* 3777.

O'Farrelly, C., Doyle, O., Victory, G., & Palamaro-Munsell, E. (2018). Shared reading in infancy and later development: Evidence from an early intervention. *Journal of Applied Developmental Psychology, 54,* 69-83.

O'Neill, S., & others. (2013). Cesarean section and subsequent ectopic pregnancy: A systematic review and meta-analysis. *BJOG, 120*(6), 671-680.

O'Roak, B.J., & others (2012). Sporadic autism exomes reveal a highly interconnected protein network of *de novo* mutations. *Nature, 485,* 246-250.

Oakes, L.M. (2017). Sample size, statistical power, and false conclusions in infant looking-time research. *Infancy, 22*(4), 436-469.

Oates, J., & Abraham, S. (2016). *Llewellyn-Jones fundamentals of obstetrics and gynecology* (10th ed.). New York: Elsevier.

Odic, D. (2018). Children's intuitive sense of number develops independently of their perception of area, density, length, and time. *Developmental Science, 21,* e12533.

OECD (2016). *SF3.1: Marriage and divorce rates.* Retrieved from https://www.oecd.org/els/family/SF_3_1_Marriage_and_divorce_rates.pdf

OECD (2017). *The pursuit of gender equality: An uphill battle.* Paris: OECD Publishing.

OECD (2018). *PISA 2015 results in focus.* Paris, France: OECD.

OECD (2018). C01.3, Low birth weight. Retrieved November 24, 2018, from https://www.oecd.org/els/family/CO_1_3_Low_birth_weight.pdf

OECD (2018). OECD family database. Paris: OECD Publishing. Retrieved August 24, 2018, from http://www.oecd.org/els/CO_2_2_Child_Poverty.pdf

Ojodu, J., & others (2017). NewSTEPs: The establishment of a national newborn screening technical assistance resource center. *International Journal of Neonatal Screening, 4*(1), 1.

Okun, M.L. (2015). Sleep and postpartum depression. *Current Opinion in Psychiatry, 28*(6), 490-496.

Oldehinkel, A.J., Ormel, J., Veenstra, R., De Winter, A., & Verhulst, F.C. (2008). Parental divorce and offspring depressive symptoms: Dutch developmental trends during early adolescence. *Journal of Marriage and the Family, 70,* 284-293.

Oldereid, N.B., & others (2018). The effect of paternal factors on perinatal and paediatric outcomes: A systematic review and meta-analysis. *Human Reproduction Update, 24*(3), 320-389.

Olds, D.L., & others (2004). Effects of home visits by paraprofessionals and nurses: Age four follow-up of a randomized trial. *Pediatrics, 114,* 1560-1568.

Olds, D.L., & others (2007). Effects of nurse home visiting on maternal and child functioning: Age-9 follow-up of a randomized trial. *Pediatrics, 120,* e832-e845.

Olin, S.C.S., & others (2017). Beyond screening: A stepped care pathway for managing postpartum depression in pediatric settings. *Journal of Women's Health, 26*(9), 966-975.

Oliver, B.R. (2017). Editorial: Genetically-informed approaches to the study of psychopathology. *Psychopathology Review, 4,* 1-3.

Oller, D.K., & Jarmulowicz, L. (2010). Language and literacy in bilingual children in the early school years. In E. Hoff & M. Shatz (Eds.), *Blackwell handbook of language development.* New York:

Olney, D.K., Leroy, J., Bliznashka, L., & Ruel, M.T. (2018). PROCOMIDA, a food-assisted maternal and child health and nutrition program, reduces child stunting in Guatemala: A cluster-randomized controlled intervention trial. *The Journal of Nutrition, 148,* 1493-1505.

Olson, B.H., Haider, S.J., Vangjel, L., Bolton, T.A., & Gold, J.G. (2010). A quasi-experimental evaluation of a breastfeeding support program for low-income women in Michigan. *Maternal and Child Health Journal, 14*(1), 86-93.

Olson, B.H., Horodynski, M.A., Brophy-Herb, H., & Iwanski, K.C. (2010). Health professionals' perspectives on the infant feeding practices of low-income mothers. *Maternal and Child Health Journal, 14*(1), 75-85.

Olson, K.R., & Enright, E.A. (2018). Do transgender children (gender) stereotype less than their peers and siblings? *Developmental Science, 21*(4), e12606.

Olson, K.R., & Gülgöz, S. (2018). Early findings from the TransYouth Project: Gender development in transgender children. *Child Development Perspectives, 12,* 93-97.

Olson, K.R., Durwood, L., DeMeules, M., & McLaughlin, K.A. (2016). Mental health of transgender children who are supported in their identities. *Pediatrics, 137,* e20153223.

Olson, K.R., Key, A.C., & Eaton, N.R. (2015). Gender cognition in transgender children. *Psychological Science, 26,* 467-474.

Olson, S.L., Lopez-Duran, N., Lunkenheimer, E.S., Chang, H., & Sameroff, A.J. (2011). Individual differences in the development of early peer aggression: Integration contributions of self-regulation, theory of mind, and parenting. *Development and Psychopathology, 23,* 253-266.

Olszewski-Kubilius, P., & Thomson, D. (2013). Gifted education programs and procedures. In I. B. Weiner & others (Eds.), *Handbook of psychology* (2nd ed., Vol. 7). New York: Wiley.

Olweus, D., Limber, S.P., & Breivik, K. (2019, in press). Addressing specific forms of bullying: A large-scale evaluation of the Olweus Bullying Prevention Program. *International Journal of Bullying Prevention,* 1-15.

Ones, D.S., Viswesvaran, C., & Dilchert, S. (2017). Cognitive ability in personnel selection decisions. In A. Evers, N. Anderson, & O. Voskuijl (Eds.), *The Blackwell handbook of personnel selection.* Hoboken, NJ: Wiley-Blackwell.

Ornaghi, V., Brazzelli, E., Grazzani, I., Agliati, A., & Lucarelli, M. (2017). Does training toddlers in emotion knowledge lead to changes in their prosocial and aggressive behavior toward peers at nursery? *Early Education and Development, 28,* 396-414.

Ornstein, P.A., Coffman, J.L., Grammer, J.K., San Souci, P.P., & McCall, L.E. (2010). Linking the classroom context and the development of children's memory skills. In J. Meece & J. Eccles (Eds.), *The handbook of research on schools, schooling, and human development.* New York: Routledge.

Orr, A.J. (2011). Gendered capital: Childhood socialization and the "boy crisis" in education. *Sex Roles, 65,* 271-284.

Orth, U., Erol, R.Y., & Luciano, E.C. (2018). Development of self-esteem from age 4 to 94 years:

A meta-analysis of longitudinal studies. *Psychological Bulletin, 144,* 1045-1080.

Osório, C., Probert, T., Jones, E., Young, A.H., & Robbins, I. (2017). Adapting to stress: Understanding the neurobiology of resilience. *Behavioral Medicine, 43,* 307-322.

Osterhaus, C., Koerber, S., & Sodian, B. (2017). Scientific thinking in elementary school: Children's social cognition and their epistemological understanding promote experimentation skills. *Developmental Psychology, 53*(3), 450-462.

Otgaar, H., Howe, M.L., Merckelbach, H., & Muris, P. (2018, in press). Who is the better eyewitness? Adults and children. *Current Directions in Psychological Science.*

Otsuka, Y. (2017). Development of recognition memory for faces during infancy. In T. Tsukiura & S. Umeda (Eds.), *Memory in a social context* (pp. 207-225). Tokyo: Springer.

Ouellette, G., & Sénéchal, M. (2017). Invented spelling in kindergarten as a predictor of reading and spelling in Grade 1: A new pathway to literacy, or just the same road, less known? *Developmental Psychology, 53,* 77-88.

Owens, A., & Candipan, J. (2019, in press). Social and spatial inequalities of educational opportunity: A portrait of schools serving high-and low-income neighbourhoods in U.S. metropolitan areas. *Urban Studies,* 0042098018815049.

Owens, D., Middleton, T.J., Rosemond, M.M., & Meniru, M.O. (2018). Underrepresentation of Black children in gifted education programs: Examining ethnocentric monoculturalism. In J. Cannaday (Ed.), *Curriculum development for gifted education programs.* Hershey, PA: IGI Global.

Owens, S., Galloway, R., & Gutin, B. (2017). The case for vigorous physical activity in youth. *American Journal of Lifestyle Medicine, 11,* 96-115.

Oyefiade, A.A., & others (2018). Development of short-range white matter in healthy children and adolescents. *Human Brain Mapping, 39*(1), 204-217.

Oyserman, D., Destin, M., & Novin, S. (2015). The context-sensitive future self: Possible selves motivate in context, not otherwise. *Self and Identity, 14*(2), 173-188.

Oyserman, D. (2017). Culture three ways: Culture and subcultures within countries. *Annual Review of Psychology, 68,* 435-463.

Özel, S., & others (2018). Maternal second trimester blood levels of selected heavy metals in pregnancies complicated with neural tube defects. *The Journal of Maternal-Fetal & Neonatal Medicine.* doi:10.1080/14767058.2018.1441280

P

Pace, A., Luo, R., Hirsh-Pasek, K., & Golinkoff, R.M. (2017). Identifying pathways between socioeconomic status and language development. *Annual Review of Linguistics, 3,* 285-308.

Packer, M., & Cole, M. (2016). Culture in development. In M. Bornstein & M. Lamb (Eds.), *Social and personality development: An advanced textbook* (7th ed., pp. 67-124). New York/London: Psychology Press.

Padilla, J., McHale, S.M., Rodríguez De Jesús, S.A., Updegraff, K.A., & Umaña-Taylor, A.J. (2017). Longitudinal course and correlates of parents' differential treatment of siblings in Mexican-origin families. *Family Process, 57*(4), 979-995.

Padilla-Walker, L.M., Carlo, G., Christensen, K.J., & Yorgason, J.B. (2012). Bidirectional relations between authoritative parenting and adolescents' prosocial behaviors. *Journal of Research on Adolescence, 22,* 400-408.

Padilla-Walker, L.M., & Coyne, S.M. (2011). "Turn that thing off!" Parent and adolescent predictors of proactive media monitoring. *Journal of Youth and Adolescence, 34*(4), 705-715.

Pahlke, E., Hyde, J., Shibley, A., & Carlie, M. (2014). The effects of single-sex compared with coeducational schooling on students' performance and attitudes: A meta-analysis. *Psychological Bulletin, 140,* 1042-1072.

Palczewski, C.H., DeFrancisco, V.P., & McGeough, D.D. (2017). *Gender in communication: A critical introduction.* Thousand Oaks, CA: SAGE.

Palmquist, C.M., Keen, R., & Jaswal, V.K. (2018). Visualization instructions enhance preschoolers' spatial problem-solving. *British Journal of Developmental Psychology, 36*(1), 37-46.

Palomaki, G.E., & Kloza, E.M. (2018). Prenatal cell-free DNA screening test failures: A systematic review of failure rates, risks of Down syndrome, and impact of repeat testing. *Genetics in Medicine, 20,* 1312-1323.

Pan, M., Stiles, B.L., Tempelmeyer, T.C., & Wong, N. (2019). A cross-cultural exploration of academic dishonesty: Current challenges, preventive measures, and future directions. In D. Velliaris (Ed.), *Prevention and detection of academic misconduct in higher education* (pp. 63-82). Hershey, PA: IGI Global.

Papadopoulos, N., & others (2019). The efficacy of a brief behavioral sleep intervention in school-aged children with ADHD and comorbid autism spectrum disorder. *Journal of Attention Disorders, 23,* 341-350.

Papafragou, A. (2018). Pragmatic development. *Language Learning and Development, 14,* 167-169.

Papasavva, T.E., & others (2013). A minimal set of SNPs for the noninvasive prenatal diagnosis of b-thalassaemia. *Annuals of Human Genetics, 77*(2), 115-124.

Park, C.L. (2012b). Meaning making in cancer survivorship. In P. T. P. Wong (Ed.), *Handbook of meaning* (2nd ed.). Thousand Oaks, CA: Sage.

Park, W., & Epstein, N.B. (2013). The longitudinal causal directionality between body image distress and self-esteem among Korean adolescents: The moderating effect of relationships with parents. *Journal of Adolescence, 36*(2), 403-411.

Parkay, F.W. (2016). *Becoming a teacher* (10th ed.). Upper Saddle River, NJ: Pearson.

Parke, R.D., & Buriel, R. (2006). Socialization in the family: Ethnic and ecological perspectives. In W. Damon & R. Lerner (Eds.), *Handbook of child psychology* (6th ed.). New York: Wiley.

Parke, R.D., & Clarke-Stewart, A.K. (2011). *Social development.* New York: Wiley.

Parke, R.D., & Cookston, J.T. (2019). Fathers and families. In M.H. Bornstein (Ed.), *Handbook of parenting* (3rd ed.). New York: Taylor and Francis.

Parlade, M.V., & others (2009). Anticipatory smiling: Linking early affective communication and social outcome. *Infant Behavior and Development, 32,* 33-43.

Paruthi, S., & others (2016). Recommended amount of sleep for pediatric populations: A consensus statement of the American Academy of Sleep Medicine. *Journal of Clinical Sleep Medicine, 12,* 785-786.

Paschall, K.W., Mastergeorge, A.M., & Ayoub, C.C. (2019). Associations between child physical abuse potential, observed maternal parenting, and young children's emotion regulation: Is participation in Early Head Start protective? *Infant Mental Health Journal, 40,* 169-185.

Pascoe, J.M., & others (2016). Mediators and adverse effects of child poverty in the United States. *Pediatrics, 137*(4), e20160340.

Pasterski, V., & others (2015). Increased cross-gender identification independent of gender role behavior in girls with congenital adrenal hyperplasia: Results from a standardized assessment of 4- to 11-year-old children. *Archives of Sexual Behavior, 44,* 1363-1375.

Pasterski, V., Golombok, S., & Hines, M. (2011). Sex differences in social behavior. In P. K. Smith & C. H. Hart (Eds.), *Wiley-Blackwell handbook of childhood social development* (2nd ed.). New York: Wiley.

Patall, E.A., & others (2018). Daily autonomy supporting or thwarting and students' motivation and engagement in the high school science classroom. *Journal of Educational Psychology, 110,* 269-288.

Pate, R.R., Pfeiffer, K.A., Trost, S.G., Ziegler, P., & Dowda, M. (2004). Physical activity among children attending preschools. *Pediatrics, 114,* 1258-1263.

Patrick, R.B., & Gibbs, J.C. (2012). Inductive discipline, parental expression of disappointed expectations, and moral identity in adolescence. *Journal of Youth and Adolescence, 41,* 973-983.

Pattaro, C. (2016). Character education: Themes and researches. An academic literature review. *Italian Journal of Sociology of Education, 8*(1), 6-30.

Patterson, C.J. (2004). What difference does a civil union make? Changing public policies and the experience of same-sex couples. Comment on Solomon, Rothblum, & Balsam (2004). *Journal of Family Psychology, 18,* 287-289.

Patterson, C.J., & Farr, R.H. (2012). Children of lesbian and gay parents: Reflections on the research-policy interface. In H. R. Schaeffer & K. Durkin (Eds.), *Wiley-Blackwell handbook of developmental psychology in action.* New York: Wiley.

Patterson, C.J. (2013). Sexual minority youth with sexual minority parents. In A. Ben-Arieh & others (Eds.), *Handbook child research.* Thousand Oaks, CA: Sage.

Patterson, C., &. D'Augelli, A.R. (Eds.). (2013). *The psychology of sexual orientation.* New York: Cambridge University Press.

Patterson, G.R. (2016). Coercion theory: The study of change. In T.J. Dishion & J.J. Snyder (Eds.), *The Oxford handbook of coercive relationship dynamics* (pp. 7–22). Oxford, UK: Oxford University Press.

Paulhus, D.L. (2008). Birth order. In M. M. Haith & J. B. Benson (Eds.), *Encyclopedia of infant and early childhood development*. Oxford, UK: Elsevier.

Paus, T., & others (2007). Morphological properties of the action-observation cortical network in adolescents with low and high resistance to peer influence. *Social Neuroscience, 3,* 303–316.

Pavelko, S.L., Lieberman, R.J., Schwartz, J., & Hahs-Vaughn, D. (2018). The contributions of phonological awareness, alphabet knowledge, and letter writing to name writing in children with specific language impairment and typically developing children. *American Journal of Speech-Language Pathology, 27,* 166–180.

Pavlov, I.P. (1927). In G. V. Anrep (Trans.), *Conditioned reflexes.* London: Oxford University Press.

Paxton, S.J., & Damiano, S.R. (2017). The development of body image and weight bias in childhood. In *Advances in Child Development and Behavior, 52,* 269–298.

Peña, J.B., Masyn, K.E., Thorpe, L.E., Peña, S.M., & Caine, E.D. (2016). A cross-national comparison of suicide attempts, drug use, and depressed mood among Dominican youth. *Suicide and Life-Threatening Behavior, 46*(3), 301–312.

Pearson, N., Braithwaite, R.E., Biddle, S.J., van Sluijs, E.M., & Atkin, A.J. (2014). Associations between sedentary behaviour and physical activity in children and adolescents: A meta-analysis. *Obesity Reviews, 15*(8), 666–675.

Pecker, L.H., & Little, J. (2018). Clinical manifestations of sickle cell disease across the lifespan. In E. Meier, A. Abraham, & R. Fasano (Eds.), *Sickle cell disease and hematopoietic stem cell transplantation.* Netherlands: Springer.

Peek, L., & Stough, L.M. (2010). Children with disabilities in the context of disaster: A social vulnerability perspective. *Child Development, 81,* 1260–1270.

Peeters, M.C.W., & others (2013). Consequences of combining work and family roles: A closer look at cross-domain versus within-domain relations. In J. Grzywacz & E. Demerouti (Eds.), *New frontiers in work and family research.* New York: Routledge.

Peets, K., & Hodges, E.V. (2018). Authenticity in friendships and well-being in adolescence. *Social Development, 27*(1), 140–153.

Peets, K., Hodges, E.V., & Salmivalli, C. (2013). Forgiveness and its determinants depending on the interpersonal context of hurt. *Journal of Experimental Child Psychology, 114*(1), 131–145.

Peets, K., Hodges, E.V., & Salmivalli, C. (2011). Actualization of social cognitions into aggressive behavior toward disliked targets. *Social Development, 20,* 233–250.

Pelaez, M., & Monlux, K. (2017). Operant conditioning methodologies to investigate infant learning. *European Journal of Behavior Analysis, 18*(2), 212–241.

Pelka, M., & Kellmann, M. (2017). Demands of youth sports. In J. Baker & others (Eds.), *Routledge handbook of talent identification and development in sport.* New York: Routledge.

Percy-Smith, L., & others (2018). Differences and similarities in early vocabulary development between children with hearing aids and children with cochlear implant enrolled in 3-year auditory verbal intervention. *International Journal of Pediatric Otorhinolaryngology, 108,* 67–72.

Perez-Febles, A.M. (1992). *Acculturation and interactional styles of Latina mothers and their infants.* Unpublished honors thesis, Brown University, Providence, RI.

Perlovsky, L., & Sakai, K.L. (2014). Language and cognition. *Frontiers in Behavioral Neuroscience, 8,* 436.

Perner, J., & Leahy, B. (2016). Mental files in development: Dual naming, false belief, identity and intentionality. *Review of Philosophy and Psychology, 7*(2), 491–508.

Perry, D.G., & Pauletti, R.E. (2011). Gender and adolescent development. *Journal of Research on Adolescence, 21,* 61–74.

Persike, M., & Seiffge-Krenke, I. (2016). Stress with parents and peers: How adolescents from 18 nations cope with relationship stress. *Anxiety, Stress, & Coping, 29*(1), 38–59.

Pertea, M., & others (2018). Thousands of large-scale RNA sequencing experiments yield a comprehensive new human gene list and reveal extensive transcriptional noise. *bioRxiv 332825.* doi:10.1101/332825

Peskin, H. (1967). Pubertal onset and ego functioning. *Journal of Abnormal Psychology, 72,* 1–15.

Peter, V., Kalashnikova, M., Santos, A., & Burnham, D. (2016). Mature neural responses to infant-directed speech but not adult-directed speech in pre-verbal infants. *Scientific Reports, 6,* 34273.

Peters, H., Whincup, P.H., Cook, D.G., Law, C., & Li, L. (2012). Trends in blood pressure in 9- to 11-year-old children in the United Kingdom, 1980–2008: The impact of obesity. *Journal of Hypertension, 30,* 1708–1717.

Petersen, A.C. (1979, January). Can puberty come any faster? *Psychology Today,* pp. 45–56.

Petersen, I.T., & others (2012). Interaction between serotonin transporter polymorphism (5-HTTLPR) and stressful life events in adolescents' trajectories of anxious/depressed symptoms. *Developmental Psychology, 48*(5), 1463–1475.

Peterson, J.A., McFarland, J.G., Curtis, B.R., & Aster, R.H. (2013). Neonatal alloimmune thrombocytopenia: Pathogenesis, diagnosis, and management. *British Journal of Hematology, 161*(1), 3–14.

Petrill, S.A., & Deater-Deckard, K. (2004). The heritability of general cognitive ability: A within-family adoption design. *Intelligence, 32,* 403–409.

Petruzzello, S.J., Greene, D.R., Chizewski, A., Rougeau, K.M., & Greenlee, T.A. (2018). Acute vs. chronic effects of exercise on mental health. In *The Exercise Effect on Mental Health: Neurobiological Mechanisms.* New York: Taylor & Francis.

Pew Research Center (2010). *Millennials: Confident, connected, open to change.* Washington, DC: Pew Research Center.

Pew Research Center (2015). *Table 40, Statistical portrait of Hispanics in the United States, 2013.* Washington, DC: Pew Research Center.

Pew Research Center (2016). *Religion and public life: The gender gap in religion around the world.* Retrieved April 28, 2019, from https://www.pewforum.org/2016/03/22/the-gender-gap-in-religion-around-the-world

Pew Research Center (2018). *Religion and public life: The age gap in religion around the world.* Retrieved April 28, 2019, from https://www.pewforum.org/2018/06/13/why-do-levels-of-religious-observance-vary-by-age-and-country/

Pew Research Center (2018a). *Teens, social media & technology 2018.* Retrieved May 5, 2019, from www.pewinternet.org/2018/05/31/teens-social-media-technology-2018/

Pew Research Center (2018b). *Smartphone ownership on the rise in emerging economies.* Retrieved May 5, 2019, from https://www.pewglobal.org/2018/06/19/2-smartphone-ownership-on-the-rise-in-emerging-economies/

Pew Research Center (2019). *Religious landscape study: Parent of children under 18.* Retrieved April 28, 2019, from https://www.pewforum.org/religious-landscape-study/parent-of-children-under-18/

Pfeifer, M., Goldsmith, H.H., Davidson, R.J., & Rickman, M. (2002). Continuity and change in inhibited and uninhibited children. *Child Development, 73,* 1474–1485.

Phillips, K., Healy, L., Smith, L., & Keenan, R. (2018). Hydroxyurea therapy in UK children with sickle cell anaemia: A single-centre experience. *Pediatric Blood & Cancer, 65.*

Phinney, J.S., & Alipuria, L.L. (1990). Ethnic identity in college students from four ethnic groups. *Journal of Adolescence, 13,* 171–183.

Phinney, J.S., & Ong, A.D. (2007). Conceptualization and measurement of ethnic identity: Current status and future directions. *Journal of Counseling Psychology, 54,* 271–281.

Phinney, J.S. (2006). Ethnic identity exploration in emerging adulthood. In J. J. Arnett & J. L. Tanner (Eds.), *Emerging adults in America.* Washington, DC: American Psychological Association.

Piaget, J., & Inhelder, B. (1969). *The child's conception of space* (F. J. Langdon & J. L. Lunger, Trans.). New York: W. W. Norton.

Piaget, J. (1932). *The moral judgment of the child.* New York: Harcourt Brace Jovanovich.

Piaget, J. (1952). *The origins of intelligence in children.* (M. Cook, Trans.). New York International Universities Press.

Piaget, J. (1954). *The construction of reality in the child.* New York: Basic Books.

Piaget, J. (1962). *Play, dreams, and imitation in childhood.* New York: W. W. Norton.

Pieterse, J.N. (2020). *Globalization and culture* (4th ed.). Lanham, MD: Rowman & Littlefield.

Pietraszewski, D., Wertz, A.E., Bryant, G.A., & Wynn, K. (2017). Three-month-old human infants use vocal cues of body size. *Proc. R. Soc. B, 284*(1856), 20170656.

Pineda-Alhucema, W., Aristizabal, E., Escudero-Cabarcas, J., Acosta-Lopez, J.E., & Vélez, J.I.

(2018). Executive function and theory of mind in children with ADHD: A systematic review. *Neuropsychology Review, 28,* 341–358.

Ping, H., & Hagopian, W. (2006). Environmental factors in the development of type 1 diabetes. *Review in Endocrine and Metabolic Disorders, 7,* 149–162.

Pinquart, M. (2017). Associations of parenting dimensions and styles with externalizing problems of children and adolescents: An updated meta-analysis. *Developmental Psychology, 53*(5), 873–932.

Pinto, A., Veríssimo, M., Gatinho, A., Santos, A.J., & Vaughn, B.E. (2015). Direct and indirect relations between parent–child attachments, peer acceptance, and self-esteem for preschool children. *Attachment & Human Development, 17*(6), 586–598.

Plancoulaine, S., & others (2018). Night sleep duration trajectories and associated factors among preschool children from the EDEN cohort. *Sleep Medicine, 48,* 194–201.

Pleck, J.H. (2018). The theory of male sex-role identity: Its rise and fall, 1936 to the present. In H. Brod (Ed.), *The making of masculinities.* New York: Routledge.

Plomin, R., & von Stumm, S. (2018). The new genetics of intelligence. *Nature Reviews Genetics, 19,* 148–159.

Plomin, R. (2004). Genetics and developmental psychology. *Merrill-Palmer Quarterly, 50,* 341–352.

Plucker, J. (2010, July 10). Interview. In P. Bronson & A. Merryman. The creativity crisis. *Newsweek,* pp. 42–48.

Plumert, J. (Ed.). (2018). Studying the perception-action system as a model system for understanding development. *Advances in Child Development and Behavior, 55,* 1–272.

Podzimek, Š., & others (2018). The evolution of taste and perinatal programming of taste preferences. *Physiological Research, 67,* S421–S429.

Poehner, M.E., Davin, K.J., & Lantolf, J.P. (2017). Dynamic assessment. In E. Shohamy, I. Or, & S. May (Eds.), Language testing and assessment. *Encyclopedia of language and education* (3rd ed.). Dordrecht, the Netherlands: Springer.

Pollastri, A.R., Raftery-Helmer, J.N., Cardemil, E.V., & Addis, M.E. (2018). Social context, emotional expressivity, and social adjustment in adolescent males. *Psychology of Men & Masculinity, 19*(1), 69–77.

Pomerantz, E.M., Kim, E.M., & Cheung, C.S. (2012). Parents' involvement in children's learning. In K. R. Harris & others (Eds.), *APA educational psychology handbook.* Washington, DC: American Psychological Association.

Pomerantz, H., Parent, J., Forehand, R., Breslend, N.L., & Winer, J.P. (2017). Pubertal timing and youth internalizing psychopathology: The role of relational aggression. *Journal of Child and Family Studies, 26,* 416–423.

Popham, W.J. (2017). *Classroom assessment* (8th ed.). Upper Saddle River, NJ: Pearson.

Posada, G., & others (2016). Maternal sensitivity and child secure base use in early childhood: Studies in different cultural contexts. *Child Development, 87,* 297–311.

Posner, M.I., & Rothbart, M.K. (2007). *Educating the human brain.* Washington, DC: American Psychological Association.

Posner, M.I., Rothbart, M.K., & Tang, Y.Y. (2015). Enhancing attention through training. *Current Opinion in Behavioral Sciences, 4,* 1–5.

Potard, C., Kubiszewski, V., Camus, G., Courtois, R., & Gaymard, S. (2018). Driving under the influence of alcohol and perceived invulnerability among young adults: An extension of the theory of planned behavior. *Transportation Research Part F: Traffic Psychology and Behaviour, 55,* 38–46.

Potter, M., Spence, J.C., Boulé, N., Stearns, J.A., & Carson, V. (2018). Behavior tracking and 3-year longitudinal associations between physical activity, screen time, and fitness among young children. *Pediatric Exercise Science, 30,* 132–141.

Poulain, T., Peschel, T., Vogel, M., Jurkutat, A., & Kiess, W. (2018). Cross-sectional and longitudinal associations of screen time and physical activity with school performance at different types of secondary schools. *BMC Public Health, 18*(1), 563.

Poulin-Dubois, D., & Pauen, S. (2017). The development of object categories: What, when, and how? In H. Cohen & C. Lefebvre (Eds.), *Handbook of categorization in cognitive science* (2nd ed., pp. 653–671). Amsterdam: Elsevier.

Poulin-Dubois, D. (2018). Animism. In M.H. Bornstein (Ed.) & M. Arterberry, K. Fingerman, & J.E. Lansford (Assoc. Eds.), *SAGE encyclopedia of lifespan human development* (pp. 126–128). Thousand Oaks, CA: SAGE.

Poulin, F., & Denault, A-S. (2012). Other-sex friendship as a mediator between parental monitoring and substance use in boys and girls. *Journal of Youth and Adolescence, 41,* 1488–1501.

Poulin, F., & Pedersen, S. (2007). Developmental changes in gender composition of friendship networks in adolescent girls and boys. *Developmental Psychology, 43,* 1484–1496.

Pouwels, J.L., Lansu, T.A., & Cillessen, A.H. (2018). A developmental perspective on popularity and the group process of bullying. *Aggression and Violent Behavior, 43,* 64–70.

Povell, P. (2017). Maria Montessori: Yesterday, today, and tomorrow. In L.E. Cohen & S. Waite-Stupiansky (Eds.), *Theories of early childhood education.* New York: Routledge.

Powellsbooks.blog (2006). *Interviews: Maxine Hong Kingston after the fire.* Retrieved March 27, 2019, from https://www.powells.com/post/interviews/maxine-hong-kingston-after-the-fire

Power, F.C., & Higgins-D'Alessandro, A. (2008). The Just Community Approach to moral education and moral atmosphere of the school. In L. Nucci & D. Narvaez (Eds.), *Handbook of moral and character education.* Clifton, NJ: Psychology Press.

Power, T.G., & Lee, S.Y. (2018). Coping. In M.H. Bornstein (Ed.) & M. Arterberry, K. Fingerman, & J.E. Lansford (Assoc. Eds.), *The SAGE encyclopedia of lifespan human development.* Thousand Oaks, CA: SAGE.

Prabhakar, H. (2007). Hopkins Interactive Guest Blog: *The public health experience at Johns Hopkins.* Retrieved January 31, 2008, from http://hopkins.typepad.com/guest/2007/03/the_public_heal.html.

Prameela, K.K. (2011). Breastfeeding—anti-viral potential and relevance to the influenza virus pandemic. *Medical Journal of Malaysia, 66,* 166–169.

Pratt, M.W., Norris, J.E., Hebblethwaite, S., & Arnold, M.L. (2008). Intergenerational transmission of values: Family generativity and adolescents' narratives of parent and grandparent value teaching. *Journal of Personality, 76,* 171–198.

Prelock, P.A., & Hutchins, T.L. (2018). An introduction to communication development. In P.A. Prelock & T.L Hutchins (Eds.), *Clinical guide to assessment and treatment of communication disorders.* Dordrecht: Springer.

Pressley, M., & Hilden, K. (2006). Cognitive strategies. In W. Damon & R. Lerner (Eds.), *Handbook of child psychology* (6th ed.). New York: Wiley.

Pressley, M., Mohan, L., Fingeret, L., Reffitt, K., & Raphael Bogaert, L.R. (2007). Writing instruction in engaging and effective elementary settings. In S. Graham, C. A. MacArthur, & J. Fitzgerald (Eds.), *Best practices in writing instruction.* New York: Guilford.

Pressley, M., Mohan, L., Raphael, L.M., & Fingeret, L. (2007). How does Bennett Woods Elementary School produce such high reading and writing achievement? *Journal of Educational Psychology, 99,* 221–240.

Pressley, M. (2007a). Achieving best practices. In L. B. Gambrell, L. M. Morrow, & M. Pressley (Eds.), *Best practices in literacy instruction.* New York: Guilford.

Pressley, M. (2007b). An interview with Michael Pressley by Terri Flowerday and Michael Shaughnessy. *Educational Psychology Review, 19,* 1–12.

Prevoo, M.J., & Tamis-LeMonda, C.S. (2017). Parenting and globalization in western countries: Explaining differences in parent–child interactions. *Current Opinion in Psychology, 15,* 33–39.

Prinstein, M.J., & Dodge, K.A. (2008). Current issues in peer influence. In M. J. Prinstein & K. A. Dodge (Eds.), *Understanding peer influence in children and adolescents.* New York: Guilford.

Proulx, M.J., Brown, D.J., Pasqualotto, A., & Meijer, P. (2013). Multisensory perceptual learning and sensory substitution. *Neuroscience and Behavioral Reviews, 41,* 16–25.

Provenzi, L., & others (2018). NICU Network Neurobehavioral Scale: 1-month normative data and variation from birth to 1 month. *Pediatric Research, 83,* 1104–1109.

Pryor, L., Strandberg-Larsen, K., Andersen, A.M.N., Rod, N.H., & Melchior, M. (2019). Trajectories of family poverty and children's mental health: Results from the Danish National Birth Cohort. *Social Science & Medicine, 220,* 371–378.

Pulgaron, E.R. (2013). Childhood obesity: A review of increased risk for physical and psychological morbidities. *Clinical Therapeutics, 35,* A18–A32.

Purtell, K.M., & McLoyd, V.C. (2013). Parents' participation in a work-based anti-poverty program can enhance their children's future orientation: Understanding pathways of influence. *Journal of Youth and Adolescence, 42*(6), 777–791.

Putnick, D., & others (2012). Agreement in mother and father acceptance-rejection, warmth, and hostility/rejection/neglect of children across nine countries. *Cross Cultural Research, 46,* 191–223.

Q

Qu, J., & Leerkes, E.M. (2018). Patterns of RSA and observed distress during the still-face paradigm predict later attachment, compliance and behavior problems: A person-centered approach. *Developmental Psychobiology, 60,* 707-721.

Qu, Y., Galván, A., Fuligni, A.J., & Telzer, E.H. (2018). A biopsychosocial approach to examine Mexican American adolescents' academic achievement and substance use. *Russell Sage Foundation Journal of the Social Sciences, 4,* 84-97.

Quinn, P.C., & others (2013). On the developmental origins of differential responding to social category information. In M. R. Banaji & S. A. Gelman (Eds.), *Navigating the social world.* New York: Oxford University Press.

Quinn, P.C. (2016). Establishing cognitive organization in infancy. *Child psychology: A handbook of contemporary issues* (3rd ed., pp. 79-104). New York: Routledge.

Quintanilla, L., Giménez-Dasí, M., & Gaviria, E. (2018). Children's perception of envy and modesty: Does depreciation serve as a mask for failure or success? *Current Psychology,* 1-13. doi:10.1007/s12144-018-0022-5

R

Rabbani, B., & others (2012). Next-generation sequencing: Impact of exome sequencing in Mendelian disorders. *Journal of Human Genetics, 57*(10), 621.

Radulescu, L., & others (2013). Multicenter evaluation of Neurelec Digisonic SP cochlear implant reliability. *European Archives of Oto-rhino-laryngology, 270*(4), 1507-1512.

Raikes, H.A., & Thompson, R.A. (2009). Attachment security and parenting quality predict children's problem-solving, attributions, and loneliness with peers. *Attachment and Human Development, 10,* 319-344.

Railton, P. (2016). Moral learning: Why learning? Why moral? And why now? *Cognition, 167.* doi:10.1016/j.cognition.2016.08.015.

Raipuria, H.D., Lovett, B., Lucas, L., & Hughes, V. (2018). A literature review of midwifery-led care in reducing labor and birth interventions. *Nursing for Women's Health, 22*(5), 387-400.

Rajaraman, P., & others (2011). Early life exposure to diagnostic radiation and ultrasound scans and risk of childhood cancer: Case-control study. *British Medical Journal, 342.*

Rajendran, G., & Mitchell, P. (2007). Cognitive theories of autism. *Developmental Review, 27,* 224-260.

Rakison, D.H., & Lawson, C.A. (2013). Categorization. In P. D. Zelazo (Ed.), *Oxford handbook of developmental psychology.* New York: Oxford University Press.

Ramberg, J., & Modin, B. (2019, in press). School effectiveness and student cheating: Do students' grades and moral standards matter for this relationship? *Social Psychology of Education.* doi:10.1007/s11218-019-09486-6

Ramdahl, M.E., & others (2018). Family wealth and parent-child relationships. *Journal of Child and Family Studies, 27,* 1534.

Ramey, C.T. (2018). The Abecedarian approach to social, educational, and health disparities. *Clinical Child and Family Psychology Review, 21,* 527-544.

Ramey, S.L. (2005). Human developmental science serving children and families: Contributions of the NICHD study of early child care. In NICHD Early Child Care Network (Eds.), *Child care and development.* New York: Guilford.

Rao, C., & Vaid, J. (2017). Morphology, orthography, and the two hemispheres: A divided visual field study with Hindi/Urdu biliterates. *Neuropsychologia, 98,* 46-55.

Raval, V.V., & Walker, B.L. (2019). Unpacking 'culture': Caregiver socialization of emotion and child functioning in diverse families. *Developmental Review, 51,* 146-174.

Raval, V.V., Walker, B.L., & Daga, S.S. (2018). Parental socialization of emotion and child functioning among Indian American families: Consideration of cultural factors and different modes of socialization. In S.S. Chuang & C.L. Costigan (Eds.), *Parental roles and relationships in immigrant families.* Cham, Switzerland: Springer.

Reader, J.M., Teti, D.M., & Cleveland, M.J. (2017). Cognitions about infant sleep: Interparental differences, trajectories across the first year, and coparenting quality. *Journal of Family Psychology, 31,* 453-463.

Reed-Fitzke, K. (2019, in press). The role of self-concepts in emerging adult depression: A systematic research synthesis. *Journal of Adult Development.* doi:10.1007/s10804-018-09324-7

Reed, J., Hirsh-Pasek, K., & Golinkoff, R.M. (2017). Learning on hold: Cell phones sidetrack parent-child interactions. *Developmental Psychology, 53,* 1428-1436.

Reese, E., Fivush, R., Merrill, N., Wang, Q., & McAnally, H. (2017). Adolescents' intergenerational narratives across cultures. *Developmental Psychology, 53*(6), 1142-1153.

Regalado, M., Sareen, H., Inkelas, M., Wissow, L.S., & Halfon, N. (2004). Parents' discipline of young children: Results from the National Survey of Early Childhood Health. *Pediatrics, 113,* 1952-1958.

Reid, P.T., & Zalk, S.R. (2001). Academic environments: Gender and ethnicity in U.S. higher education. In J. Worell (Ed.), *Encyclopedia of women and gender.* San Diego: Academic Press.

Reiner, W.G., & Gearhart, J.P. (2004). Discordant sexual identity in some genetic males with cloacal exstrophy assigned to female sex at birth. *New England Journal of Medicine, 350,* 333-341.

Reis, S.M., & Renzulli, J.S. (2011). Intellectual giftedness. In R. J. Sternberg & S. B. Kaufman (Eds.), *Cambridge handbook of intelligence.* New York: Cambridge.

Reiss, F., & others (2019). Socioeconomic status, stressful life situations and mental health problems in children and adolescents: Results of the German BELLA cohort-study. *PLoS ONE, 14*(3), e0213700.

Rende, R. (2013). Behavioral resilience in the post-genomic era: Emerging models linking genes with environment. *Frontiers in Human Neuroscience, 6,* 50.

Repacholi, B.M., & Gopnik, A. (1997). Early reasoning about desires: Evidence from 14- and 18-month-olds. *Developmental Psychology, 33,* 12-21.

Reutzel, D.R., & Cooter, R.B. (2013). *Essentials of teaching children to read* (3rd ed.). Boston: Allyn & Bacon.

Reutzel, D.R., & Cooter, R.B. (2018). *Teaching children to read* (8th ed.). Boston: Pearson.

Rey, L., Sánchez-Álvarez, N., & Extremera, N. (2018). Spanish Gratitude Questionnaire: Psychometric properties in adolescents and relationships with negative and positive psychological outcomes. *Personality and Individual Differences, 135,* 173-175.

Reyna, V.F., & Brainerd, C.J. (2011). Dual processes in decision making and developmental neuroscience: A fuzzy-trace model. *Developmental Review, 31,* 180-206.

Reyna, V.F., & Rivers, S.E. (2008). Current theories of risk and rational decision making. *Developmental Review, 28,* 1-11.

Reyna, V.F. (2018). Neurobiological models of risky decision-making and adolescent substance use. *Current Addiction Reports, 5*(2), 128-133.

Reynolds, G.D., & Richards, J.E. (2017). Infant visual attention and stimulus repetition effects on object recognition. *Child Development.* doi:10.1111/cdev.12982

Reynolds, G.D., & Romano, A.C. (2016). The development of attention systems and working memory in infancy. *Frontiers in Systems Neuroscience, 10,* 15.

Reznick, J.S. (2013). Research designs and methods: Toward a cumulative developmental science. In P. D. Zelazo (ed.), *Handbook of developmental psychology.* New York: Oxford University Press.

Richards, D.R. (2017). Children's first experiences in school. *International Journal for Innovation Education and Research, 5,* 169-177.

Richmond, A.D., Laursen, B., & Stattin, H. (2019). Homophily in delinquent behavior: The rise and fall of friend similarity across adolescence. *International Journal of Behavioral Development, 43*(1), 67-73.

Rideout, V.J., Foehr, U.G., & Roberts, D.F. (2010). *Generation M2: Media in the lives of 8- to 18-year-olds.* Menlo Park, CA: Kaiser Family Foundation.

Riede, F., Johannsen, N.N., Högberg, A., Nowell, A., & Lombard, M. (2018). The role of play objects and object play in human cognitive evolution and innovation. *Evolutionary Anthropology: Issues, News, and Reviews, 27*(1), 46-59.

Riggins, T., Geng, F., Blankenship, S.L., & Redcay, E. (2016). Hippocampal functional connectivity and episodic memory in early childhood. *Developmental Cognitive Neuroscience, 19,* 58-69.

Righi, G., & Nelson, C.A. (2013). The neural architecture and developmental course of face processing. In P. Rakic & J. Rubenstein (Eds.), *Comprehensive developmental neuroscience.* New York: Elsevier.

Riley, M., & Bluhm, B. (2012). High blood pressure in children and adolescents. *American Family Physician, 85,* 693-700.

Riley, T.N., Sullivan, T.N., Hinton, T.S., & Kliewer, W. (2019). Longitudinal relations between emotional awareness and expression, emotion regulation, and peer victimization among urban adolescents. *Journal of Adolescence, 72,* 42-51.

Rios-Castillo, I., Cerezo, S., Corvalan, C., Martinez, M., & Kain, J. (2013). Risk factors during the prenatal period and the first year of life associated with overweight in 7-year-old low-income Chilean children. *Maternal and Child Nutrition, 11*(4), 595-605.

Rita, T.H.S., Nobre, C.S., Jácomo, R.H., Nery, L.F.A., & Barra, G.B. (2018). Noninvasive fetal sex determination by analysis of cell-free fetal DNA in maternal capillary blood obtained by fingertip puncture. *Prenatal Diagnosis, 38,* 620-623.

Ritchie, M.D., & Van Steen, K. (2018). The search for gene-gene interactions in genome-wide association studies: Challenges in abundance of methods, practical considerations, and biological interpretation. *Annals of Translational Medicine, 6*(8), 157.

Ritchie, S.J., & Tucker-Drob, E.M. (2018). How much does education improve intelligence? A meta-analysis. *Psychological Science, 29,* 1358-1369.

Riumallo-Herl, C., & others (2018). Poverty reduction and equity benefits of introducing or scaling up measles, rotavirus and pneumococcal vaccines in low-income and middle-income countries: A modelling study. *BMJ Global Health, 3*(2), e000613.

Rivenbark, J.G., & others (2019). Perceived social status and mental health among young adolescents: Evidence from census data to cellphones. *Developmental Psychology, 55*(3), 574-585.

Rizzo, M.S. (1999, May 8). Genetic counseling combines science with a human touch. *Kansas City Star,* p. 3.

Roberge, S., Bujold, E., & Nicolaides, K.H. (2018). Meta-analysis on the effect of aspirin use for prevention of preeclampsia on placental abruption and antepartum hemorrhage. *American Journal of Obstetrics and Gynecology, 218*(5), 483-489.

Robins, R.W., Trzesniewski, K.H., Tracy, J.L., Gosling, S.D., & Potter, J. (2002). Global self-esteem across the life span. *Psychology and Aging, 17,* 423-434.

Robinson-Riegler, B., & Robinson-Riegler, G.L. (2016). *Cognitive psychology* (4th ed.). Upper Saddle River, NJ: Pearson.

Robinson, A.J., & Ederies, M.A. (2018). Fetal neuroimaging: An update on technical advances and clinical findings. *Pediatric Radiology, 48,* 471-485.

Roblyer, M.D. (2016). *Integrating educational technology into teaching* (7th ed.). Upper Saddle River, NJ: Pearson.

Rochat, P. (2013). Self-conceptualizing in development. In P. D. Zelazo (Ed.), *Oxford handbook of developmental psychology.* New York: Oxford University Press.

Rode, S.S., Chang, P., Fisch, R.O., & Sroufe, L.A. (1981). Attachment patterns of infants separated at birth. *Developmental Psychology, 17,* 188-191.

Roeser, R.W., & Zelazo, P.D. (2012). Contemplative science, education and child development. *Child Development Perspectives, 6,* 143-145.

Rogoff, B., & others (2017). Noticing learners' strengths through cultural research. *Perspectives on Psychological Science, 12,* 876-888.

Rogoff, B., Dahl, A., & Callanan, M. (2018). The importance of understanding children's lived experience. *Developmental Review, 50,* 5-15.

Rogoff, B. (2003). *The cultural nature of human development.* New York: Oxford University Press.

Rogoff, B. (2016). Culture and participation: A paradigm shift. *Current Opinion in Psychology, 8,* 182-189.

Rohner, R.P., & Rohner, E.C. (1981). Parental acceptance-rejection and parental control: Cross-cultural codes. *Ethnology, 20,* 245-260.

Rohrer, J.M., Egloff, B., & Schmukle, S.C. (2015). Examining the effects of birth order on personality. *PNAS, 112*(46), 14224-14229.

Romeo, R.D. (2017). The impact of stress on the structure of the adolescent brain: Implications for adolescent mental health. *Brain Research, 1654,* 185-191.

Romeo, R.R., & others (2018). Language exposure relates to structural neural connectivity in childhood. *Journal of Neuroscience, 38,* 7870-7877.

Romero, A., & Piña-Watson, B. (2017). Acculturative stress and bicultural stress: Psychological measurement and mental health. In S. Schwartz & J. Unger (Eds.), *The Oxford handbook of acculturation and health* (pp. 119-133). New York: Oxford University Press.

Romstad, C., & Xiong, Z.B. (2017). Measuring formal intelligence in the informal learner: A case study of Hmong American students and cognitive assessment. *Hmong Studies Journal, 18,* 1-31.

Ropars, S., Tessier, R., Charpak, N., & Uriza, L.F. (2018). The long-term effects of the Kangaroo Mother Care intervention on cognitive functioning: Results from a longitudinal study. *Developmental Neuropsychology, 43*(1), 82-91.

Roque, L.S., & Schieffelin, B.B. (2018). Learning how to know: Egophoricity and the grammar of Kaluli (Bosavi, Trans New Guinea), with special reference to child language. In S. Floyd, E. Norcliffe, & L.S. Roque (Eds.), *Egophoricity.* Amsterdam: John Benjamins.

Rosa, H., & others (2019). Automatic cyberbullying detection: A systematic review. *Computers in Human Behavior, 93,* 333-345.

Rosario, M. (2019, in press). Sexual orientation development of heterosexual, bisexual, lesbian, and gay individuals: Questions and hypotheses based on Kaestle's (2019) research. *Journal of Sex Research,* 1-5. doi:10.1080/00224499.2019

Rose, A.J., Carlson, W., & Waller, E.M. (2007). Prospective associations of co-rumination with friendship and emotional adjustment: Considering the socioemotional trade-offs of co-rumination. *Developmental Psychology, 43,* 1019-1031.

Rose, A.J., & others (2012). How girls and boys expect disclosure about problems will make them feel: Implications for friendship. *Child Development, 83,* 844-863.

Rose, A.J., & Smith, R.L. (2009). Sex differences in peer relationships. In K. H. Rubin, W. M. Bukowski, & B. Laursen (Eds.), *Handbook of peer interactions, relationships, and groups.* New York: Guilford.

Rose, A.J., Smith, R.L., Glick, G.C., & Schwartz-Mette, R.A. (2016). Girls' and boys' problem talk:

Implications for emotional closeness in friendships. *Developmental Psychology, 52*(4), 629-639.

Rose, S.A., Feldman, J.F., & Jankowski, J.J. (2009). A cognitive approach to the development of early language. *Child Development, 80,* 134-150.

Rosen, L.D., Cheever, N.A., & Carrier, L.M. (2008). The association of parenting style and child age with parental limit setting and adolescent MySpace behavior. *Journal of Applied Developmental Psychology, 29,* 459-471.

Rosenstein, D., & Oster, H. (1988). Differential facial responses to four basic tastes in newborns. *Child Development, 59,* 1555-1568.

Rosnow, R.L., & Rosenthal, R. (2013). *Beginning psychological research* (7th ed.). Boston: Cengage.

Ross, J., & others (2017). Cultural differences in self-recognition: The early development of autonomous and related selves? *Developmental Science, 20*(3), e12387.

Rossi, N.F., & Giacheti, C.M. (2017). Association between speech-language, general cognitive functioning and behaviour problems in individuals with Williams syndrome. *Journal of Intellectual Disability Research, 61,* 707-718.

Rostad, K., & Pexman, P.M. (2015). Preschool-aged children recognize ambivalence: Emerging identification of concurrent conflicting desires. *Frontiers in Psychology, 6,* 425.

Rote, W.M., Smetana, J.G., Campione-Barr, N., Villalobos, M., & Tasopouos-Chan, M. (2012). Associations between observed mother-adolescent interactions and adolescent information management. *Journal of Research on Adolescence, 22,* 206-214.

Rote, W.M., & Smetana, J.G. (2015). Parenting, adolescent-parent relationships, and social domain theory: Implications for identity development. In K. McLean & M. Syed (Eds.), *Oxford handbook of identity* (pp. 437-453). New York: Oxford University Press.

Rote, W.M., & Smetana, J.G. (2017). Situational and structural variation in youth perceptions of maternal guilt induction. *Developmental Psychology, 53*(10), 1940-1953.

Rothbart, M.K., & Bates, J.E. (2006). Temperament. In W. Damon & R. Lerner (Eds.), *Handbook of child psychology* (6th ed.). New York: Wiley.

Rothbart, M.K., & Gartstein, M.A. (2008). Temperament. In M. M. Haith & J. B. Benson (Eds.), *Encyclopedia of infant and early childhood development.* Oxford, UK: Elsevier.

Rothbart, M.K. (2004). Temperament and the pursuit of an integrated developmental psychology. *Merrill-Palmer Quarterly, 50,* 492-505.

Rothbart, M.K. (2011). *Becoming who we are.* New York: Guilford.

Rothbaum, F., & Trommsdorff, G. (2007). Do roots and wings complement or oppose one another?: The socialization of relatedness and autonomy in cultural context. In J. E. Grusec & P. D. Hastings (Eds.), *Handbook of socialization.* New York: Guilford.

Roundfield, K.D., Sánchez, B., & McMahon, S.D. (2018). An ecological analysis of school engagement among urban, low-income Latino adolescents. *Youth and Society, 50,* 905-925.

Rovee-Collier, C., & Barr, R. (2010). Infant learning and memory. In J. G. Bremner & T. D. Wachs (Ed.), *Wiley-Blackwell handbook of infant development* (2nd ed.). New York: Wiley.

Rowe, D.W. (2018). Pointing with a pen: The role of gesture in early childhood writing. *Reading Research Quarterly.* doi:10.1002/rrq.215

Royer-Pokora, B. (2012). Genetics of pediatric renal tumors. *Pediatric Nephrology, 28*(1), 13-23.

Ruan, Y., Georgiou, G.K., Song, S., Li, Y., & Shu, H. (2018). Does writing system influence the associations between phonological awareness, morphological awareness, and reading? A meta-analysis. *Journal of Educational Psychology, 110,* 180-202.

Rubie-Davies, C.M. (2007). Classroom interactions: Exploring the practices of high- and low-expectation teachers. *British Journal of Educational Psychology, 77,* 289-306.

Rubin, K.H., Bowker, J.C., McDonald, K.L., & Menzer, M. (2013). Peer relationships in childhood. In P. D. Zelazo (Ed.), *Oxford handbook of developmental psychology.* New York: Oxford University Press.

Rubin, K.H., Bukowski, W., & Parker, J. (2006). Peer interactions, relationships, and groups. In W. Damon & R. Lerner (Eds.), *Handbook of child psychology* (6th ed.). New York: Wiley.

Rubin, K.H., Mills, R.S.L., & Rose-Krasnor, L. (1989). Maternal beliefs and children's competence. In B. Schneider, G. Attili, J. Nadel, & R. Weissberg (Eds.), *Social competence in developmental perspective.* Amsterdam: Kluwer Academic.

Rubin, K.H., Bowker, J.C., Barstead, M.G., & Coplan, R.J. (2018). Avoiding and withdrawing from the peer group. In W. Bukowski & others (Eds.), *Handbook of peer relationships, interactions, and groups* (2nd ed.). New York: Guilford.

Rueda, M.R. (2018). Attention in the heart of intelligence. *Trends in Neuroscience and Education, 13,* 26-33.

Ruffman, T., & others (2018). Variety in parental use of "want" relates to subsequent growth in children's theory of mind. *Developmental Psychology, 54*(4), 677-688.

Ruffman, T., Puri, A., Galloway, O., Su, J., & Taumoepeau, M. (2018). Variety in parental use of "want" relates to subsequent growth in children's theory of mind. *Developmental Psychology, 54*(4), 677-688.

Ruigrok, A.N.V., & others (2014). A meta-analysis of sex differences in human brain structure. *Neuroscience & Biobehavioral Reviews, 39,* 34-50.

Ruiz-Hernández, J.A., Moral-Zafra, E., Llor-Esteban, B., & Jiménez-Barbero, J.A. (2019). Influence of parental styles and other psychosocial variables on the development of externalizing behaviors in adolescents: A systematic review. *European Journal of Psychology Applied to Legal Context, 11*(1), 9-21.

Rumberger, R.W. (1995). Dropping out of middle school: The influence of race, sex, and family background. *American Educational Research Journal, 3,* 583-625.

Rung, J.M., & Madden, G.J. (2018). Experimental reductions of delay discounting and impulsive

choice: A systematic review and meta-analysis. *Journal of Experimental Psychology: General, 147,* 1349-1381.

Russell, E.E. (2017). Children's label-learning experience within superordinate categories facilitates their generalization of labels for additional category members. *Psychology of Language and Communication, 21,* 51-83.

Russell, S.T., Crockett, L.J., & Chao, R.K. (2010). *Asian American parenting and parent-adolescent relationships.* New York: Springer.

Ryan, R.M., & Deci, E.L. (2009). Promoting self-determined school engagement: Motivation, learning, and well-being. In K. Wentzel & A. Wigfield (Eds.), *Handbook of motivation at school.* New York: Routledge.

Ryan, S.A., Ammerman, S.D., & O'Connor, M.E. (2018). Marijuana use during pregnancy and breastfeeding: Implications for neonatal and childhood outcomes. *Pediatrics, 142*(3), e20181889.

Rytioja, M., Lappalainen, K., & Savolainen, H. (2019, in press). Behavioural and emotional strengths of sociometrically popular, rejected, controversial, neglected, and average children. *European Journal of Special Needs Education.*

S

Sénat, M.V., & others (2018). Prevention and management of genital herpes simplex infection during pregnancy and delivery: Guidelines from the French College of Gynaecologists and Obstetricians (CNGOF). *European Journal of Obstetrics & Gynecology and Reproductive Biology, 224,* 93-101.

Saarni, C., Campos, J., Camras, L.A., & Witherington, D. (2006). Emotional development. In W. Damon & R. Lerner (Eds.), *Handbook of child psychology* (6th ed.). New York: Wiley.

Sadeh, A. (2008). Sleep. In M. M. Haith & J. B. Benson (Eds.), *Encyclopedia of infant and early childhood development.* Oxford, UK: Elsevier.

Sadker, M.P., & Zittleman, K. (2018). *Teachers, schools, and society* (5th ed.). New York: McGraw-Hill.

Sagiv, S.K., Epstein, J.N., Bellinger, D.C., & Korrick, S.A. (2013). Pre- and postnatal risk factors for ADHD in a nonclinical pediatric population. *Journal of Attention Disorders, 17*(1), 47-57.

Saint-Jacques, M.C., & others (2018). Researching children's adjustment in stepfamilies: How is it studied? What do we learn? *Child Indicators Research, 11*(6), 1831-1865.

Sala, G., Tatlidil, K.S., & Gobet, F. (2018). Video game training does not enhance cognitive ability: A comprehensive meta-analytic investigation. *Psychological Bulletin, 144*(2), 111.

Salley, B., Miller, A., & Bell, M.A. (2013). Associations between temperament and social responsiveness in young children. *Infant and Child Development, 22*(3), 270-288.

Salmivalli, C., & Peets, K. (2009). Bullies, victims, and bully-victim relationships in middle childhood and adolescence. In K. H. Rubin, W. M. Bukowski, & B. Laursen (Eds.), *Handbook of peer interactions, relationships, and groups.* New York: Guilford.

Salmon, K., O'Kearney, R., Reese, E., & Fortune, C.A. (2016). The role of language skill in child psychopathology: Implications for intervention in the early years. *Clinical Child and Family Psychology Review, 19,* 352-367.

Salo, V.C., Rowe, M.L., & Reeb-Sutherland, B.C. (2018). Exploring infant gesture and joint attention as related constructs and as predictors of later language. *Infancy, 23,* 432-452.

Salovey, P., & Mayer, J.D. (1990). Emotional intelligence. *Imagination, Cognition, and Personality, 9,* 185-211.

Salsa, A.M., & Gariboldi, M.B. (2018). Symbolic experience and young children's comprehension of drawings in different socioeconomic contexts. *Avances en Psicología Latinoamericana, 36,* 29-44.

Salvatore, J.E., Larsson Lönn, S., Sundquist, J., Sundquist, K., & Kendler, K.S. (2018). Genetics, the rearing environment, and the intergenerational transmission of divorce: A Swedish national adoption study. *Psychological Science, 29*(3), 370-378.

Salvy, S.-J., Feda, D.M., Epstein, L.H., & Roemmich, J.N. (2017). Friends and social contexts as unshared environments: A discordant sibling analysis of obesity- and health-related behaviors in young adolescents. *International Journal of Obesity, 41,* 569-575.

Sameroff, A.J. (2009). The transactional model. In A. J. Sameroff (Ed.), *The transactional model of development: How children and contexts shape each other.* Washington, DC: American Psychological Association.

Samhan, Y.M., El-Sabae, H.H., Khafagy, H.F., & Maher, M.A. (2013). A pilot study to compare epidural identification and catheterization using a saline-filled syringe versus a continuous hydrostatic pressure system. *Journal of Anesthesia, 27*(4), 607-610.

Sanchez, D., Whittaker, T.A., Hamilton, E., & Arango, S. (2017). Familial ethnic socialization, gender role attitudes, and ethnic identity development in Mexican-origin early adolescents. *Cultural Diversity and Ethnic Minority Psychology, 23,* 335-347.

Sanders, J., Munford, R., & Boden, J. (2017). Culture and context: The differential impact of culture, risks and resources on resilience among vulnerable adolescents. *Children and Youth Services Review, 79,* 517-526.

Sanders, K., & Farago, F. (2018). Developmentally appropriate practice in the twenty-first century. In M. Fleer & B. van Oers (Eds.), *International handbook of early childhood education.* Dordrecht: Springer.

Sanders, M.R. (2008). Triple P-Positive Parenting Program as a public health approach to strengthening parenting. *Journal of Family Psychology, 22*(3), 506-517.

Sanders, R.A. (2013). Adolescent psychosocial, social, and cognitive development. *Pediatrics in Review, 34*(8), 354-358.

Sandoval-Motta, S., Aldana, M., Martínez-Romero, E., & Frank, A. (2017). The human microbiome and the missing heritability problem. *Frontiers in Genetics, 8,* 80.

Sands, A., Thompson, E.J., & Gaysina, D. (2017). Long-term influences of parental divorce on offspring affective disorders: A systematic review and meta-analysis. *Journal of Affective Disorders, 218,* 105–114.

Sanson, A., & Rothbart, M.K. (1995). Child temperament and parenting. In M. H. Bornstein (Ed.), *Handbook of parenting* (Vol. 4). Hillsdale, NJ: Erlbaum.

Santi, K., & Reed, D. (Eds). (2015). *Improving reading comprehension of middle and high school students.* New York: Springer.

Santiago, C.D., Etter, E.M., Wadsworth, M.E., & Raviv, T. (2012). Predictors of responses to stress among families coping with poverty-related stress. *Anxiety, Stress, and Coping, 25*(3), 239–258.

Santrock, J.W., Sitterle, K.A., & Warshak, R.A. (1988). Parent-child relationships in stepfather families. In P. Bronstein & C. P. Cowan (Eds.), *Fatherhood today: Men's changing roles in the family.* New York: Wiley.

Santrock, J.W., & Warshak, R.A. (1979). Father custody and social development in boys and girls. *Journal of Social Issues, 35,* 112–125.

Saroglou, V. (2013). Religion, spirituality, and altruism. In K. I. Pargament, J. Exline, & J. Jones (Eds.), *Handbook of psychology, religion, and spirituality.* Washington, DC: American Psychological Association.

Sasson, N.J., & Elison, J.T. (2013). Eye tracking in young children with autism. *Journal of Visualized Experiments, 61,* e3675.

Sauce, B., & Matzel, L.D. (2018). The paradox of intelligence: Heritability and malleability coexist in hidden gene-environment interplay. *Psychological Bulletin, 144,* 26–47.

Saul, A., & others (2019). Polymorphism in the serotonin transporter gene polymorphisms (5-HTTLPR) modifies the association between significant life events and depression in people with multiple sclerosis. *Multiple Sclerosis Journal, 25,* 848–855.

Saunders, M.C., & others (2019). The associations between callous-unemotional traits and symptoms of conduct problems, hyperactivity and emotional problems: A study of adolescent twins screened for neurodevelopmental problems. *Journal of Abnormal Child Psychology, 47,* 447–457.

Saunders, N.R., Dziegielewska, K.M., Møllgård, K., & Habgood, M.D. (2018). Physiology and molecular biology of barrier mechanisms in the fetal and neonatal brain. *The Journal of Physiology, 596,* 5723–5756.

Savage, J.E., & others (2018). Early maturation and substance use across adolescence and young adulthood: A longitudinal study of Finnish twins. *Development and Psychopathology, 30,* 79–92.

Savin-Williams, R.C. (2013). The new sexual-minority teenager. In J. S. Kaufman & D. A. Powell (Eds.), *Sexual identities.* Thousand Oaks, CA: Sage.

Savina, E., & Wan, K.P. (2017). Cultural pathways to socio-emotional development and learning. *Journal of Relationships Research, 8,* e19.

Sawyer, J. (2017). I think I can: Preschoolers' private speech and motivation in playful versus non-playful contexts. *Early Childhood Research Quarterly, 38,* 84–96.

Saxbe, D., & others (2018). Longitudinal associations between family aggression, externalizing behavior, and the structure and function of the amygdala. *Journal of Research on Adolescence, 28,* 134–149.

Scarr, S. (1993). Biological and cultural diversity: The legacy of Darwin for development. *Child Development, 64,* 1333–1353.

Scarr, S., & Weinberg, R.A. (1983). The Minnesota adoption studies: Genetic differences and malleability. *Child Development, 54,* 182–259.

Schaal, B. (2017). Infants and children making sense of scents. In A. Buettner (Ed.), *Springer handbook of odor* (pp. 107–108). Berlin: Springer.

Schaefer, R.T. (2019). *Race and ethnicity in the United States* (9th ed.). Upper Saddle River, NJ: Pearson.

Schaffer, H.R. (1996). *Social development.* Cambridge, MA: Blackwell.

Schaie, K.W. (2012). *Developmental influences on adult intellectual development: The Seattle Longitudinal Study.* New York: Oxford University Press.

Schalkwijk, F., & others (2016). The conscience as a regulatory function: Empathy, shame, pride, guilt, and moral orientation in delinquent adolescents. *International Journal of Offender Therapy and Comparative Criminology, 60,* 675–693.

Scherrer, V., & Preckel, F. (2018). Development of motivational variables and self-esteem during the school career: A meta-analysis of longitudinal studies. *Review of Educational Research, 89*(2), 211–258.

Scherrer, V., & Preckel, F. (2019). Development of motivational variables and self-esteem during the school career: A meta-analysis of longitudinal studies. *Review of Educational Research, 89,* 211–258.

Schick, A.R., Melzi, G., & Obregon, J. (2017). The bidirectional nature of narrative scaffolding: Latino caregivers' elaboration while creating stories from a picture book. *First Language, 37*(3), 301–316.

Schiff, W.J. (2015). *Nutrition for healthy living* (5th ed.). New York: McGraw-Hill.

Schilder, A.G., & others (2017). Panel 7: Otitis media: treatment and complications. *Otolaryngology-Head and Neck Surgery, 156*(4 Suppl.), S88–S105.

Schlam, T.R., Wilson, N.L., Shoda, Y., Mischel, W., & Ayduk, O. (2013). Preschoolers' delay of gratification predicts their body mass 30 years later. *Journal of Pediatrics, 162*(1), 90–93.

Schmidt, J.A., Shumow, L., & Kackar, H.Z. (2012). Associations of participation in service activities with academic, behavioral, and civic outcomes of adolescents at varying risk levels. *Journal of Youth and Adolescence, 41,* 932–947.

Schmidt, J., Shumow, L., & Kackar, H. (2007). Adolescents' participation in service activities and its impact on academic, behavioral, and civic outcomes. *Journal of Youth and Adolescence. 36,* 127–140.

Schmutz, E.A., & others (2017). Correlates of preschool children's objectively measured physical activity and sedentary behavior: A cross-sectional analysis of the SPLASHY study. *International Journal of Behavioral Nutrition and Physical Activity, 14*(1), 1.

Schneider, B.H., & others (2011). Cooperation and competition. In P. K. Smith & C. H. Hart (Eds.), *Wiley-Blackwell handbook of childhood social development* (2nd ed.). New York: Wiley.

Schneider, W., & Ornstein, P.A. (2015). The development of children's memory. *Child Development Perspectives, 9*(3), 190–195.

Schneider, W. (2015). *Memory development from early childhood through emerging adulthood.* New York: Springer.

Schneider, W.J., & McGrew, K.S. (2018). The Cattell-horn-Carroll theory of cognitive abilities. In D.P. Flanagan & E.M. McDonough (Eds.), *Contemporary intellectual assessment: Theories, tests, and issues* (4th ed.). New York: Guilford.

Schoeler, T., Duncan, L., Cecil, C.M., Ploubidis, G.B., & Pingault, J.B. (2018). Quasi-experimental evidence on short-and long-term consequences of bullying victimization: A meta-analysis. *Psychological Bulletin, 144*(12), 1229–1246.

Schoon, I., Jones, E., Cheng, H., & Maughan, B. (2011). Family hardship, family instability, and cognitive development. *Journal of Epidemiology and Community Health, 66,* 718–722.

Schoppmann, J., Schneider, S., & Seehagen, S. (2019). Wait and see: Observational learning of distraction as an emotion regulation strategy in 22-month-old toddlers. *Journal of Abnormal Child Psychology, 47*(5), 851–863.

Schreiner, D., Savas, J.N., Herzog, E., Brose, N., & de Wit, J. (2017). Synapse biology in the 'circuit-age'—paths toward molecular connectomics. *Current Opinion in Neurobiology, 42,* 102–110.

Schubert, A.L., Hagemann, D., & Frischkorn, G.T. (2017). Is general intelligence little more than the speed of higher-order processing? *Journal of Experimental Psychology, 146,* 1498–1512.

Schunk, D.H., Pintrich, P.R., & Meece, J.L. (2014). *Motivation in education: Theory, research, and applications* (4th ed.). Upper Saddle River, NJ: Pearson.

Schunk, D.H. (2019). *Learning theories: An educational perspective* (8th ed.). Upper Saddle River, NJ: Pearson.

Schwalbe, C.S., Gearing, R.E., MacKenzie, M.J., Brewer, K.B., & Ibrahim, R. (2012). A meta-analysis of experimental studies of diversion programs for juvenile defenders. *Clinical Psychology Review, 32,* 26–33.

Schwartz-Mette, R.A., & Smith, R.L. (2018). When does co-rumination facilitate depression contagion in adolescent friendships? Investigating intrapersonal and interpersonal factors. *Journal of Clinical Child & Adolescent Psychology, 47*(6), 912–924.

Schwartz, D., Hopmeyer, A., Luo, T., Ross, A.C., & Fischer, J. (2017). Affiliation with antisocial crowds and psychosocial outcomes in a gang-impacted urban middle school. *Journal of Early Adolescence, 37*(4), 559–586.

Schwartz, S.J., & others (2019). Biculturalism dynamics: A daily diary study of bicultural identity and psychosocial functioning. *Journal of Applied Developmental Psychology, 62,* 26–37.

Schwartz, S.J., Luyckx, K., & Crocetti, E. (2015). What have we learned since Schwartz (2001)? A reappraisal of the field of identity development. In K. McLean & M. Syed (Eds.) *The Oxford handbook of identity development* (pp. 539–561).

Schwartz-Mette, R.A., & Rose, A.J. (2013). Co-rumination mediates contagion of internalizing symptoms within youths' friendships. *Developmental Psychology, 48*(5), 1355–1365.

Schwarz, S.P. (2004). A mother's story. Retrieved from http://www.makinglifeeasier.com

Schweinhart, L.J. (2019). Lessons on sustaining early gains from the life-course study of Perry Preschool. In A.J. Reynolds & J.A. Temple (Eds.), *Sustaining early childhood learning gains: Program, school, and family influences.* Cambridge, UK: Cambridge University Press.

Scott, R.M., & Baillargeon, R. (2013). Do infants really expect others to act efficiently? A critical test of the rationality principle. *Psychological Science, 24*(4), 466–474.

Sebastiani, G., & others (2018). The effects of alcohol and drugs of abuse on maternal nutritional profile during pregnancy. *Nutrients, 10*(8), 1008.

Segal, M., & others (2012). *All about child care and early education* (2nd ed.). Upper Saddle River, NJ: Pearson.

Seider, S., & others (2019). Black and Latinx adolescents' developing beliefs about poverty and associations with their awareness of racism. *Developmental Psychology, 55*(3), 509–524.

Selkie, E.M., Fales, J.L., & Moreno, M.A. (2016). Cyberbullying prevalence among U.S. middle and high school–aged adolescents: A systematic review and quality assessment. *Journal of Adolescent Health, 58*(2), 125–133.

Sellers, R.M., Linder, N.C., Martin, P.P., & Lewis, R.L. (2006). Racial identity matters: The relationship between racial discrimination and psychological functioning in African American adolescents. *Journal of Research on Adolescence, 16*(2), 187–216.

Selvam, S., & others (2018). Development of norms for executive functions in typically-developing Indian urban preschool children and its association with nutritional status. *Child Neuropsychology, 24,* 226–246.

Sempowicz, T., Howard, J., Tambyah, M., & Carrington, S. (2018). Identifying obstacles and opportunities for inclusion in the school curriculum for children adopted from overseas: Developmental and social constructionist perspectives. *International Journal of Inclusive Education, 22,* 606–621.

Senter, L., Sackoff, J., Landi, K., & Boyd, L. (2010). Studying sudden and unexpected deaths in a time of changing death certification and investigation practices: Evaluating sleep-related risk factors for infant death in New York City. *Maternal and Child Health, 15*(2), 242–248.

Sernau, S.R. (2013). *Global problems* (3rd ed.). Upper Saddle River, NJ: Pearson.

Sethi, V., & others (2013). Single ventricle anatomy predicts delayed microstructural brain development. *Pediatric Research, 73,* 661–667.

Sethna, V., Murray, L., & Ramchandani, P.G. (2012). Depressed fathers' speech to their 3-month-old infants: A study of cognitive and mentalizing features in paternal speech. *Psychological Medicine, 42*(11), 2361–2371.

Sethna, V., Murray, L., Edmondson, O., Iles, J., & Ramchandani, P.G. (2018). Depression and playfulness in fathers and young infants: A matched design comparison study. *Journal of Affective Disorders, 229,* 364–370.

Sette, S., Colasante, T., Zava, F., Baumgartner, E., & Malti, T. (2018). Preschoolers' anticipation of sadness for excluded peers, sympathy, and prosocial behavior. *The Journal of Genetic Psychology, 179,* 286–296.

Shanahan, L., & Sobolewski, J.M. (2013). Child effects on family processes. In A. C. Crouter & A. Booth (Eds.), *Children's influence on family dynamics.* New York: Routledge.

Shankaran, S., & others (2011). Risk for obesity in adolescence starts in childhood. *Journal of Perinatology, 31,* 711–716.

Shapiro, A.F., & Gottman, J.M. (2005). Effects on marriage of a psycho-education intervention with couples undergoing the transition to parenthood: Evaluation at 1-year post-intervention. *Journal of Family Communication, 5,* 1–24.

Shapiro, C.J., Prinz, R.J., & Sanders, M.R. (2012). Facilitators and barriers to implementation of an evidence-based parenting intervention to prevent child maltreatment: The Triple P–Positive Parenting Program. *Child Maltreatment, 17,* 86–95.

Shapiro, J.R. (2018). Stranger wariness. In M.H. Bornstein (Ed.) & M. Arterberry, K. Fingerman, & J.E. Lansford (Assoc. Eds.), *The SAGE encyclopedia of lifespan human development.* Thousand Oaks, CA: SAGE.

Sharma, D., Murki, S., & Pratap, O.T. (2016). The effect of kangaroo ward care in comparison with "intermediate intensive care" on the growth velocity in preterm infant with birth weight, 1100 g: Randomized control trial. *European Journal of Pediatrics, 175*(10), 1317–1324.

Sharma, N., Classen, J., & Cohen, L.G. (2013). Neural plasticity and its contribution to functional recovery. *Handbook of Clinical Psychology, 110,* 3–12.

Shaw, P., & others (2007). Attention-deficit/hyperactivity disorder is characterized by a delay in cortical maturation. *Proceedings of the National Academy of Sciences, 104*(49), 19649–19654.

Shaywitz, S.E., Gruen, J.R., & Shaywitz, B.A. (2007). Management of dyslexia, its rationale, and underlying neurobiology. *Pediatric Clinics of North America, 54,* 609–623.

Sheikh, M., & Anderson, J.R. (2018). Acculturation patterns and education of refugees and asylum seekers: A systematic literature review. *Learning and Individual Differences, 67,* 22–32.

Sheinman, N., Hadar, L.L., Gafni, D., & Milman, M. (2018). Preliminary investigation of whole-school mindfulness in education programs and children's mindfulness-based coping strategies. *Journal of Child and Family Studies, 27*(1), 1316–1328.

Shek, D.T. (2012). Spirituality as a positive youth development construct: A conceptual review. *Scientific World Journal, 2012,* 458953.

Shen, L.H., Liao, M.H., & Tseng, Y.C. (2013). Recent advances in imaging of dopaminergic neurons for evaluation of neuropsychiatric disorders. *Journal of Biomedicine and Biotechnology, 2012,* 259349.

Shen, Y., Kim, S.Y., & Benner, A.D. (2019). Burdened or efficacious? Subgroups of Chinese American language brokers, predictors, and long-term outcomes. *Journal of Youth and Adolescence, 48*(1), 154–169.

Shenhav, A., & Greene, J.D. (2014). Integrative moral judgment: Dissociating the roles of the amygdala and the ventromedial prefrontal cortex. *Journal of Neuroscience, 34,* 4741–4749.

Shenhav, S., Campos, B., & Goldberg, W.A. (2017). Dating out is intercultural: Experience and perceived parent disapproval by ethnicity and immigrant generation. *Journal of Social and Personal Relationships, 34*(3), 397–422.

Sher-Censor, E., Parke, R.D., & Coltrane, S. (2011). Parents' promotion of psychological autonomy, psychological control, and Mexican-American adolescents' adjustment. *Journal of Youth and Adolescence, 40,* 620–632.

Sherman, A., & Mitchell, T. (2017). Economic security programs help low-income children succeed long-term. *Challenge, 60*(6), 514–542.

Sherman, A., Grusec, J.E., & Almas, A.N. (2017). Mothers' knowledge of what reduces distress in their adolescents: Impact on the development of adolescent approach coping. *Parenting: Science and Practice, 17,* 187–199.

Shibata, Y., & others (2012). Extrachromosomal microDNAs and chromosomal microdeletions in normal tissues. *Science, 336,* 82–86.

Shiino, A., & others (2017). Sex-related difference in human white matter volumes studied: Inspection of the corpus callosum and other white matter by VBM. *Scientific Reports, 7,* 39818.

Shin, H. (2017). Friendship dynamics of adolescent aggression, prosocial behavior, and social status: The moderating role of gender. *Journal of Youth and Adolescence, 46,* 2305–2320.

Shin, S.H., Hong, H.G., & Hazen, A.L. (2010). Childhood sexual abuse and adolescence substance use: A latent class analysis. *Drug and Alcohol Dependence, 109*(1), 226–235.

Shiner, R.L. (2019). Negative emotionality and neuroticism from childhood to adulthood: A lifespan perspective. In D.P. McAdams, R.L. Shiner, & J.L. Tackett (Eds.), *Handbook of personality development.* New York: Guilford.

Shiraev, E., & Levy, D. (2016). *Cross-cultural psychology: Critical thinking and critical applications* (6th ed.). New York: Routledge.

Shockley, K.M., & others (2017). Disentangling the relationship between gender and work–family conflict: An integration of theoretical perspectives using meta-analytic methods. *Journal of Applied Psychology, 102*(12), 1601.

Shore, B., & Kauko, S. (2017). The landscape of family memory. In B. Wagoner (Ed.), *Handbook of culture and memory.* New York: Oxford University Press.

Short, M.A., Gradisar, M., Lack, L.C., Wright, H.R., & Dohnt, H. (2013). The sleep patterns and well-being of Australian adolescents. *Journal of Adolescence, 36*(1), 103–110.

Short, M.A., & Weber, N. (2018). Sleep duration and risk-taking in adolescents: A systematic review and meta-analysis. *Sleep Medicine Reviews, 41,* 185–196.

Short, S.J., & others (2013). Associations between white matter microstructure and infants' working memory. *NeuroImage, 64,* 156–166.

Shulman, S., Davila, J., & Shachar-Shapira, L. (2011). Assessing romantic competence among older adolescents. *Journal of Adolescence, 34,* 397–406.

Shulman, S., Zlotnik, A., Shachar-Shapira, L., Connolly, J., & Bohr, Y. (2012). Adolescent daughters' romantic competence: The role of divorce, quality of parenting, and maternal romantic history. *Journal of Youth and Adolescence, 41,* 593–606.

Shultz, S., Klin, A., & Jones, W. (2018). Neonatal transitions in social behavior and their implications for autism. *Trends in Cognitive Sciences, 22*(5), 452–469.

Shwalb, D.W., Shwalb, B.J., & Lamb, M.E. (2013). *Fathers in cultural context.* New York: Routledge.

Siegler, R.S. (1976). Three aspects of cognitive development. *Cognitive Psychology, 8,* 481–520.

Siegler, R.S. (2006). Microgenetic analysis of learning. In W. Damon & R. Lerner (Eds.). *Handbook of child psychology* (6th ed.). New York: Wiley.

Siegler, R.S. (2013). How do people become experts? In J. Staszewski (Ed.), *Experience and skill acquisition.* New York: Taylor & Francis.

Siegler, R.S. (2016). Continuity and change in the field of cognitive development and in the perspectives of one cognitive developmentalist. *Child Development Perspectives, 10*(2), 128–133.

Sigal, A., Sandler, I., Wolchik, S., & Braver, S. (2011). Do parent education programs promote healthy post-divorce parenting? Critical directions and distinctions and a review of the evidence. *Family Court Review, 49,* 120–129.

Silva, C. (2005, October 31). When teen dynamo talks, city listens. *Boston Globe,* pp. 81–84.

Silva, K., Chein, J., & Steinberg, L. (2016). Adolescents in peer groups make more prudent decisions when a slightly older adult is present. *Psychological Science, 27*(3), 322–330.

Silva, S., Canavarro, M.C., & Fonseca, A. (2018). Why women do not seek professional help for anxiety and depression symptoms during pregnancy or throughout the postpartum period: Barriers and facilitators of the help-seeking process. *The Psychologist: Practice & Research Journal, 1*(1). 47–58.

Simmonds, D.J., Hallquist, M.N., & Luna, B. (2017). Protracted development of executive and mnemonic brain systems underlying working memory in adolescence: A longitudinal fMRI study. *Neuroimage, 157,* 695–704.

Simon, E.J., Dickey, J.L., & Reece, J.B. (2019). *Campbell essential biology* (7th ed.). Upper Saddle River, NJ: Pearson.

Simon, F., & others (2018). International consensus (ICON) on management of otitis media with effusion in children. *European Annals of Otorhinolaryngology, Head and Neck Diseases, 135*(1), S33–S39.

Simonato, I., Janosz, M., Archambault, I., & Pagani, L.S. (2018). Prospective associations between toddler televiewing and subsequent lifestyle habits in adolescence. *Preventive Medicine, 110,* 24–30.

Simoncini, K., & Caltabiono, N. (2012). Young school-aged children's behaviour and their participation in extra-curricular activities. *Australasian Journal of Early Childhood, 37*(3), 35–42.

Singer, D., Golinkoff, R.M., & Hirsh-Pasek, K. (Eds.). (2006). *Play = learning: How play motivates and enhances children's cognitive and social-emotional growth.* New York: Oxford University Press.

Singer, T. (2012). The past, present, and future of social neuroscience: A European perspective. *Neuroimage, 61*(2), 437–449.

Sinha, C. (2017). Language as a biocultural niche and social institution. In *Ten lectures on language, culture and mind.* Leiden: Brill.

Sisson, S.B., Broyles, S.T., Baker, B.L., & Katzmarzyk, P.T. (2010). Screen time, physical activity, and overweight in U.S. youth: National Survey of Children's Health 2003. *Journal of Adolescent Health, 47,* 309–311.

Skinner, B.F. (1938). *The behavior of organisms: An experimental analysis.* New York: Appleton-Century-Crofts.

Skinner, B.F. (1957). *Verbal behavior.* New York: Appleton-Century-Crofts.

Skinner, E.A., & Zimmer-Gembeck, M.J. (2016). *The development of coping: Stress, neurophysiology, social relationships, and resilience during childhood and adolescence.* Cham, Switzerland: Springer.

Slagt, M., Dubas, J.S., Deković, M., & van Aken, M.A. (2016). Differences in sensitivity to parenting depending on child temperament: A meta-analysis. *Psychological Bulletin, 142,* 1068–1110.

Slater, A., Morison, V., & Somers, M. (1988). Orientation discrimination and cortical function in the human newborn. *Perception, 17,* 597–602.

Slaughter, V., Imuta, K., Peterson, C.C., & Henry, J.D. (2015). Meta-analysis of theory of mind and peer popularity in the preschool and early school years. *Child Development, 86*(4), 1159–1174.

Slaughter, V. (2015). Theory of mind in infants and young children: A review. *Australian Psychologist, 50*(3), 169–172.

Slobin, D. (1972, July). Children and language: They learn the same way around the world. *Psychology Today,* 71–76.

Slone, L.K., & others (2018). Gaze in action: Head-mounted eye tracking of children's dynamic visual attention during naturalistic behavior. *JoVE (Journal of Visualized Experiments), 141,* e58496.

Slone, L.K., & Sandhofer, C.M. (2017). Consider the category: The effect of spacing depends on individual learning histories. *Journal of Experimental Child Psychology, 159,* 34–49.

Slot, P.L., & von Suchodoletz, A. (2018). Bidirectionality in preschool children's executive functions and language skills: Is one developing skill the better predictor of the other? *Early Childhood Research Quarterly, 42,* 205–214.

Small, S.A., Ishida, I.M., & Stapells, D.R. (2017). Infant cortical auditory evoked potentials to lateralized noise shifts produced by changes in interaural time difference. *Ear and Hearing, 38*(1), 94–102.

Smetana, J.G. (2011a). *Adolescents, families, and social development: How adolescents construct their worlds.* New York: Wiley-Blackwell.

Smetana, J.G. (2011b). Adolescents' social reasoning and relationships with parents: Conflicts and coordinations within and across domains. In E. Amsel & J. Smetana (Eds.), *Adolescent vulnerabilities and opportunities: Constructivist and developmental perspectives.* New York: Cambridge University Press.

Smetana, J.G. (2013). Social-cognitive domain theory: Consistencies and variations in children's moral and social judgments. In M. Killen & J. Smetana (Eds.), *Handbook of moral development* (2nd ed.). New York: Routledge.

Smetana, J.G., Ball, C.L., Jambon, M., & Yoo, H.N. (2018). Are young children's preferences and evaluations of moral and conventional transgressors associated with domain distinctions in judgments? *Journal of Experimental Child Psychology, 173,* 284–303.

Smetana, J.G., Jambon, M., & Ball, C. (2014). The social domain approach to children's moral and social judgements. In M. Killen & J. Smetana (Eds.), *Handbook of moral development* (2nd ed., pp. 23–45). New York: Psychology Press.

Smith, J., & Ross, H. (2007). Training parents to mediate sibling disputes affects children's negotiation and conflict understanding. *Child Development, 78,* 790–805.

Smith, N.A., Folland, N.A., Martinez, D.M., & Trainor, L.J. (2017). Multisensory object perception in infancy: 4-month-olds perceive a mistuned harmonic as a separate auditory and visual object. *Cognition, 164,* 1–7.

Smith, P.K., Shu, S., & Madsen, K. (2001). Characteristics of victims of school bullying. In J. Jovonen & S. Graham (Eds.), *Peer harassment in school* (pp. 332–351). New York: Guilford.

Smith, P.K. (Ed.) (2019). *Making an impact on school bullying: Interventions and recommendations.* London: Routledge.

Smith, T., & Coffey, R. (2015). Two-generation strategies for expanding the middle class. In C. van Horn & others (Eds)., *Transforming U.S. workforce development policies for the 21st century.* Atlanta, GA: Federal Reserve Bank of Atlanta.

Smith, T.W., & Son, J. (2014). Measuring occupational prestige on the 2012 General Social Survey. *GSS Methodological Report No. 122.* Chicago: NORC of the University of Chicago.

Smorti, M., & Ponti, L. (2018). How does sibling relationship affect children's prosocial behaviors and best friend relationship quality? *Journal of Family Issues, 39*(8), 2413–2436.

Snarey, J. (1987, June). A question of morality. *Psychology Today,* pp. 6–8.

So, H.K., Li, A.M., Choi, K.C., Sung, R.Y., & Nelson, E.A. (2013). Regular exercise and a healthy dietary pattern are associated with lower resting blood pressure in non-obese adolescents: A population-based study. *Journal of Human Hypertension, 27,* 304–308.

Society of Health and Physical Educators (2018). *Active start.* Retrieved from https://www.shapeamerica.org/standards/guidelines/activestart.aspx

Solantaus, T., Leinonen, J., & Punamäki, R. (2004). Children's mental health in times of economic recession: Replication and extension of the family economic stress model in Finland. *Developmental Psychology, 40*(3), 412.

Somerville, L.H., & others (2018). The Lifespan Human Connectome Project in Development: A large-scale study of brain connectivity development in 5–21-year-olds. *NeuroImage, 183,* 456–468.

Sommer, T.E., & others (2018). A two-generation human capital approach to anti-poverty policy. *RSF: The Russell Sage Foundation Journal of the Social Sciences, 4*(3), 118–143.

Son, S.H.C., & Chang, Y.E. (2018). Childcare experiences and early school outcomes: The mediating role of executive functions and emotionality. *Infant and Child Development, 27,* e2087.

Sorensen, A., & others (2013). Changes in human placental oxygenation during maternal hyperoxia as estimated by BOLD MRI. *Ultrasound in Obstetrics and Gynecology, 42*(3), 310–314.

Sorensen, L.C., Dodge, K.A., & Conduct Problems Prevention Research Group (2016). How does the fast track intervention prevent adverse outcomes in young adulthood? *Child Development, 87*(2), 429–445.

Soubry, A., Hoyo, C., Jirtle, R.L., & Murphy, S.K. (2014). A paternal environmental legacy: Evidence for epigenetic inheritance through the male germ line. *Bioessays, 36*(4), 359–371.

Spector, L.G., & others (2013). Children's Oncology Group's 2013 blueprint for research: Epidemiology. *Pediatric and Blood Cancer, 60*(6), 1059–1062.

Spelke, E.S., & Owsley, C.J. (1979). Intermodal exploration and knowledge in infancy. *Infant Behavior and Development, 2,* 13–28.

Spelke, E.S., Bernier, E.P., & Snedeker, J. (2013). Core social cognition. In M. R. Banaji & S.A. Gelman (Eds.), *Navigating the social world: What infants, children, and other species can teach us.* New York: Oxford University Press.

Spence, J.T., & Helmreich, R. (1978). *Masculinity and femininity: Their psychological dimensions.* Austin: University of Texas Press.

Spencer, D., & others (2017). Prenatal androgen exposure and children's aggressive behavior and activity level. *Hormones and Behavior, 96,* 156–165.

Spencer, J.R., & Lamb, M.E. (Eds.). (2013). *Children and cross-examination: Time to change the rules.* Oxford, UK: Hart.

Sperry, E.D., Sperry, L.L., & Miller, P.J. (2018). Reexamining the verbal environments of children from different socioeconomic backgrounds. *Child Development.* doi:10.1111/cdev.13072

Spilman, S.K., Neppl, T.K., Donnellan, M.B., Schofield, T.J., & Conger, R.D. (2012). Incorporating religiosity into a developmental model

of positive family functioning across generations. *Developmental Psychology, 49*(4), 762–774.

Spilman, S.K., Neppl, T.K., Donnellan, M.B., Schofield, T.J., & Conger, R.D. (2013). Incorporating religiosity into a developmental model of positive family functioning across generations. *Developmental Psychology, 49*(4), 762–774.

Spinelli, M., Fasolo, M., & Mesman, J. (2017). Does prosody make the difference? A meta-analysis on relations between prosodic aspects of infant-directed speech and infant outcomes. *Developmental Review, 44,* 1–18.

Spinner, L., Cameron, L., & Calogero, R. (2018). Peer toy play as a gateway to children's gender flexibility: The effect of (counter) stereotypic portrayals of peers in children's magazines. *Sex Roles, 79,* 314–328.

Spring, J. (2016). *Deculturalization and the struggle for equality* (8th ed.). New York: Routledge.

Squires, J., Pribble, L., Chen, C-I., & Pomes, M. (2013). Early childhood education: Improving outcomes for young children and families. In I. B. Weiner & others (Eds.), *Handbook of psychology* (2nd ed., Vol. 7). New York: Wiley.

Sroufe, L.A., Coffino, B., & Carlson, E.A. (2010). Conceptualizing the role of early experience: Lessons from the Minnesota longitudinal study. *Developmental Review, 30,* 36–51.

Sroufe, L.A., Egeland, B., Carlson, E., & Collins, W.A. (2005b). The place of early attachment in developmental context. In K. E. Grossman, K. Grossman, & E. Waters (Eds.), *The power of longitudinal attachment research: From infancy and childhood to adulthood.* New York: Guilford.

Sroufe, L.A., Waters, E., & Matas, L. (1974). Contextual determinants of infant affectional response. In M. Lewis & L. Rosenblum (Eds.), *Origins of fear.* New York: Wiley.

Stadelmann, S., & others (2017). Self-esteem of 8–14-year-old children with psychiatric disorders: Disorder- and gender-specific effects. *Child Psychiatry & Human Development, 48*(1), 40–52.

Staiano, A.E., Abraham, A.A., & Calvert, S.L. (2012). Competitive versus cooperative exergame play for African American adolescents' executive functioning skills. *Developmental Psychology, 48,* 337–342.

Staiano, A.E., & others (2018). Home-based exergaming among children with overweight and obesity: A randomized clinical trial. *Pediatric Obesity, 13*(11), 724–733.

Standage, D., & Pare, M. (2018). Slot-like capacity and resource-like coding in a neural model of multiple-item working memory. *Journal of Neurophysiology, 120,* 1945–1961.

Stanovich, K.E. (2019). *How to think straight about psychology* (11th ed.). Upper Saddle River, NJ: Pearson.

Starmans, C. (2017). Children's theories of the self. *Child Development, 88*(6), 1774–1785.

Starr, C., Taggart, R., Evers, C., & Starr, L. (2016). *Evolution of life* (14th ed.). Boston: Cengage.

Starr, C.R., & Zurbriggen, E.L. (2017). Sandra Bem's gender schema theory after 34 years: A review of its reach and impact. *Sex Roles, 76,* 566–578.

Starr, L.R., & others (2013). Love hurts (in more ways than one): Specificity of psychological symptoms as predictors and consequences of romantic activity among early adolescent girls. *Journal of Clinical Psychology.*

Starr, L.R., & Davila, J. (2015). Social anxiety and romantic relationships. In K. Ranta & others (Eds.), *Social anxiety and phobia in adolescents* (pp. 183–199). London: Springer.

Staszewski, J. (Ed.). (2013). *Expertise and skill acquisition: The impact of William C. Chase.* New York: Taylor & Francis.

Stefansson, K.K., Gestsdottir, S., Birgisdottir, F., & Lerner, R.M. (2018). School engagement and intentional self-regulation: A reciprocal relation in adolescence. *Journal of Adolescence, 64,* 23–33.

Stein, G.L., & others (2015). The protective role of familism in the lives of Latino adolescents. *Journal of Family Issues, 36*(10), 1255–1273.

Stein, G.L., & others (2016). A longitudinal examination of perceived discrimination and depressive symptoms in ethnic minority youth: The roles of attributional style, positive ethnic/racial affect, and emotional reactivity. *Developmental Psychology, 52*(2), 259–271.

Stein, G.L., Coard, S.I., Kiang, L., Smith, R.K., & Mejia, Y.C. (2018). The intersection of racial–ethnic socialization and adolescence: A closer examination at stage-salient issues. *Journal of Research on Adolescence, 28*(3), 609–621.

Steinbeis, N., Crone, E., Blakemore, S.-J., & Kadosh, K.C. (2017). Development holds the key to understanding the interplay of nature versus nurture in shaping the individual. *Developmental Cognitive Neuroscience, 25,* 1–4.

Steinberg, L.D., & Silk, J.S. (2002). Parenting adolescents. In M. Bornstein (Ed.), *Handbook of parenting* (2nd ed., Vol. 1). Mahwah, NJ: Erlbaum.

Steinberg, L., & Monahan, K. (2007). Age differences in resistance to peer influence. *Developmental Psychology, 43,* 1531–1543.

Steinberg, L., & others (2018). Around the world, adolescence is a time of heightened sensation seeking and immature self-regulation. *Developmental Science, 21*(2), e12532.

Steinberg, L. (2009). Adolescent development and juvenile justice. *Annual Review of Clinical Psychology* (Vol. 5). Palo Alto, CA: Annual Reviews.

Steinberg, L. (2013). How should the science of adolescent brain development inform legal policy? In J. Bhabha (Ed.), *Coming of age: A new framework for adolescent rights.* Philadelphia: University of Pennsylvania Press.

Steinmayr, R., Weidinger, A.F., & Wigfield, A. (2018). Does students' grit predict their school achievement above and beyond their personality, motivation, and engagement? *Contemporary Educational Psychology, 53,* 106–122.

Sternberg, R.J., & Sternberg, K. (2013). Teaching cognitive science. In D. Dunn (Ed.), *Teaching psychology education.* New York: Oxford University Press.

Sternberg, R.J. (2013b). Personal wisdom in balance. In M. Ferrari & N. Westrate (Eds.), *Personal wisdom.* New York: Springer.

Sternberg, R.J. (2017). Some lessons from a symposium on cultural psychological science. *Perspectives on Psychological Science, 12,* 911–921.

Sternberg, R.J. (2018). Context-sensitive cognitive and educational testing. *Educational Psychology Review, 30,* 857–884.

Sternberg, R.J. (2018a). Creative giftedness is not just what creativity tests test: Implications of a triangular theory of creativity for understanding creative giftedness. *Roeper Review, 40,* 158–165.

Sternberg, R.J. (2018b). The triarchic theory of successful intelligence. In D.P. Flanagan & E.M. McDonough (Eds.), *Contemporary intellectual assessment: Theories, tests, and issues* (4th ed.). New York: Guilford.

Stetka, B. (2017). "Extended adolescence: When 25 is the new 18." *Scientific American.* Retrieved March 17, 2019, from https://www.scientificamerican.com/article/extended-adolescence-when-25-is-the-new-18l/

Stevenson, H.W., & Zusho, A. (2002). Adolescence in China and Japan: Adapting to a changing environment. In B. B. Brown, R. W. Larson, & T. S. Saraswathi (Eds.), *The world's youth.* New York: Cambridge University Press.

Stevenson, H.W., Lee, S., & Stigler, J.W. (1986). Mathematics achievement of Chinese, Japanese, and American children. *Science, 231,* 693–699.

Stevenson, H.W., Lee, S., Chen, C., Stigler, J.W., Hsu, C., & Kitamura, S. (1990). Contexts of achievement. *Monograph of the Society for Research in Child Development, 55* (Serial No. 221).

Stevenson, H.W. (1995). Mathematics achievement of American students: First in the world by the year 2000? In C. A. Nelson (Ed.), *Basic and applied perspectives on learning, cognition, and development.* Minneapolis: University of Minnesota Press.

Steward, D.J. (2015). The history of neonatal anesthesia. In J. Lerman (Ed.), *Neonatal anesthesia* (pp. 1–15). London: Springer.

Stiggins, R. (2008). *Introduction to student-involved assessment for learning* (5th ed.). Upper Saddle River. NJ: Prentice Hall.

Stipek, D.J. (2002). *Motivation to learn* (4th ed.). Boston: Allyn & Bacon.

Strauss, M.A., Sugarman, D.B., & Giles-Sims, J. (1997). Spanking by parents and subsequent anti-social behavior in children. *Archives of Pediatrics and Adolescent Medicine, 151,* 761–767.

Stright, A.D., Herr, M.Y., & Neitzel, C. (2009). Maternal scaffolding of children's problem solving and children's adjustment in kindergarten: Hmong families in the United States. *Journal of Educational Psychology, 101,* 207–218.

Strudwick-Alexander, M.A. (2017). Identity achievement as a predictor of intimacy in young urban Jamaican adults. In K. Carpenter (Ed.), *Interweaving tapestries of culture and sexuality in the Caribbean* (pp. 191–221). London: Palgrave Macmillan.

Stuebe, A.M., & Schwartz, E.G. (2010). The risks and benefits of infant feeding practices for women and their children. *Journal of Perinatology, 30,* 155–162.

Stuebe, A.M., & others (2017). An online calculator to estimate the impact of changes in breastfeeding rates on population health and costs. *Breastfeeding Medicine, 12*(10).

Stump, G. (2017). The nature and dimensions of complexity in morphology. *Annual Review of Linguistics, 3,* 65–83.

Suárez-Orozco, M.M., Suárez-Orozco, C., & Qin-Hilliard, D. (Eds.). (2014). *The new immigrant in the American economy: Interdisciplinary perspectives on the new immigration.* New York: Routledge.

Su, L., Meng, X., Ma, Q., Bai, T., & Liu, G. (2018). LPRP: A gene–gene interaction network construction algorithm and its application in breast cancer data analysis. *Interdisciplinary Sciences: Computational Life Sciences, 10,* 131–142.

Sucksdorff, M., & others (2018). Lower Apgar scores and Caesarean sections are related to attention-deficit/hyperactivity disorder. *Acta Paediatrica, 107*(10), 1750–1758.

Sue, D., Sue, D.W., Sue, D., & Sue, S. (2016). *Essentials of understanding abnormal behavior* (3rd ed.). Boston: Cengage.

Sue, D.W., Sue, D., Neville, H.A., & Smith, L. (2019). *Counseling the culturally diverse: Theory and practice* (8th ed.). New York: Wiley.

Sue, S., & Morishima, J.K. (1982). *The mental health of Asian Americans: Contemporary issues in identifying and treating mental problems.* San Francisco: Jossey-Bass.

Sugden, N.A., & Marquis, A.R. (2017). Meta-analytic review of the development of face discrimination in infancy: Face race, face gender, infant age, and methodology moderate face discrimination. *Psychological Bulletin, 143*(11), 1201.

Suggate, S., Schaughency, E., McAnally, H., & Reese, E. (2018). From infancy to adolescence: The longitudinal links between vocabulary, early literacy skills, oral narrative, and reading comprehension. *Cognitive Development, 47,* 82–95.

Sugimura, K., & others (2018). A cross-cultural perspective on the relationships between emotional separation, parental trust, and identity in adolescents. *Journal of Youth and Adolescence, 47*(4), 749–759.

Sugimura, K., Matsushima, K., Hihara, S., Takahashi, M., & Crocetti, E. (2019). A culturally sensitive approach to the relationships between identity formation and religious beliefs in youth. *Journal of Youth and Adolescence, 48*(8), 668–679.

Sugita, Y. (2004). Experience in early infancy is indispensable for color perception. *Current Biology, 14,* 1267–1271.

Sullivan, H.S. (1953). *The interpersonal theory of psychiatry.* New York: W. W. Norton.

Sullivan, K., & Sullivan, A. (1980). Adolescent-parent separation. *Developmental Psychology, 16,* 93–99.

Sultan, C., Gaspari, L., Kalfa, N., & Paris, F. (2017). Management of peripheral precocious puberty in girls. In C. Sultan & A. Genazzani (Eds.), *Frontiers in Gynecological Endocrinology* (Vol. 4, pp. 39–48). Netherlands: Springer.

Sumaroka, M., & Bornstein, M.H. (2008). Play. In M. M. Haith & J. B. Benson (Eds.), *Encyclopedia of infant and early childhood development.* Oxford, UK: Elsevier.

Sung, L., & others (2013). Children's oncology group's 2012 blueprint for research: Cancer control and supportive care. *Pediatric and Blood Cancer, 60*(6), 1027–1030.

Super, C.M., & Harkness, S. (2010). Culture and infancy. In J. G. Bremner & T. D. Wachs (Eds.), *Wiley-Blackwell handbook of infant development* (2nd ed.). New York: Wiley.

Susman, E.J., & Dorn, L.D. (2013). Puberty: Its role in development. In I. B. Weiner & others (Eds.), *Handbook of psychology* (2nd ed., Vol. 6). New York: Wiley.

Sutton, T.E. (2019). Review of attachment theory: Familial predictors, continuity and change, and intrapersonal and relational outcomes. *Marriage & Family Review, 55,* 1–22.

Swain, J.E., & others (2017). Parent–child intervention decreases stress and increases maternal brain activity and connectivity during own baby-cry: An exploratory study. *Development and Psychopathology, 29,* 535–553.

Swain, K.D., Leader-Janssen, E.M., & Conley, P. (2017). Effects of repeated reading and listening passage preview on oral reading fluency. *Reading Improvement, 54,* 105–111.

Swamy, G.K., Ostbye, T., & Skjaerven, R. (2008). Association of preterm birth with long-term survival, reproduction, and next generation preterm birth. *Journal of the American Medical Association, 299,* 1429–1436.

Swanson, H.L. (1999). What develops in working memory: A life-span perspective. *Developmental Psychology, 35,* 985–1000.

Swanson, H.L., & Berninger, V.W. (2018). Role of working memory in the language learning mechanism by ear, mouth, eye and hand in individuals with and without specific learning disabilities in written language. In T.P. Alloway (Ed.), *Working memory and clinical developmental disorders.* New York: Routledge.

Syed, M., & Mitchell, L.L. (2016). How race and ethnicity shape emerging adulthood. *The Oxford handbook of emerging adulthood* (pp. 87–101).

Syed, M. (2013). Assessment of ethnic identity and acculturation. In K. Geisinger (Ed.), *APA handbook of testing and assessment in psychology.* Washington, DC: American Psychological Association.

Szwedo, D.E., Mikami, A.Y., & Allen, J.P. (2011). Qualities of peer relations on social networking websites: Predictions from negative mother-teen interactions. *Journal of Research on Adolescence, 21,* 595–607.

Szwedo, D.E., & others (2017). Adolescent support seeking as a path to adult functional independence. *Developmental Psychology, 53*(5), 949.

T

Törmänen, S., & others (2017). Polymorphism in the gene encoding toll-like receptor 10 may be associated with asthma after bronchiolitis. *Scientific Reports, 7.*

Tager, M.B. (2017). *Challenging the school readiness agenda in early childhood education.* New York: Routledge.

Taggart, T., & others (2018). The role of religious socialization and religiosity in African American and Caribbean Black adolescents' sexual initiation. *Journal of Religion and Health, 57*(5), 1889-1904.

Taige, N.M., & others (2007). Antenatal maternal stress and long-term effects on child neurodevelopment: How and why? *Journal of Child Psychology and Psychiatry, 48,* 245-261.

Tamborini, C.R., Couch, K.A., & Reznik, G.L. (2015). Long-term impact of divorce on women's earnings across multiple divorce windows: A life course perspective. *Advances in Life Course Research, 26,* 44-59.

Tamir, M. (2016). Why do people regulate their emotions? A taxonomy of motives in emotion regulation. *Personality and Social Psychology Review, 20,* 199-222.

Tamis-LeMonda, C.S., & others (2008). Parents' goals for children: The dynamic coexistence of individualism and collectivism in cultures and individuals. *Social Development, 17,* 183-209.

Tamis-LeMonda, C.S., & Song, L. (2013). Parent-infant communicative interactions in cultural context. In R. M. Lerner (Ed.), *Handbook of psychology* (Vol. 6). New York: Wiley.

Tamis-LeMonda, C.S., Custode, S., Kuchirko, Y., Escobar, K., & Lo, T. (2018). Routine language: Speech directed to infants during home activities. *Child Development.* doi:10.1111/cdev.13089

Tamminga, S., Oepkes, D., Weijerman, M.E., & Cornel, M.C. (2018). Older mothers and increased impact of prenatal screening: Stable livebirth prevalence of trisomy 21 in the Netherlands for the period 2000-2013. *European Journal of Human Genetics, 26*(2), 157.

Tannen, D. (1990). *You just don't understand!* New York: Ballantine.

Tardif, T. (2016). Culture, language, and emotion: Explorations in development. In M.D. Sera, M. Maratsos, & S.M. Carlson (Eds.), *Minnesota Symposium on Child Psychology, Volume 38: Culture and developmental systems.* Hoboken, NJ: Wiley.

Tatangelo, G.L., & Ricciardelli, L.A. (2017). Children's body image and social comparisons with peers and the media. *Journal of Health Psychology, 22,* 776-787.

Taylor, C.A., Manganello, J.A., Lee, S.J., & Rice, J.C. (2010). Mothers' spanking of 3-year-old children and subsequent risk of children's aggressive behavior. *Pediatrics, 125,* e1057-e1065.

Taylor, N.A., Greenberg, D., & Terry, N.P. (2016). The relationship between parents' literacy skills and their preschool children's emergent literacy skills. *Journal of Research and Practice for Adult Literacy, Secondary, and Basic Education, 5,* 5-16.

Taylor, R.D., Oberle, E., Durlak, J.A., & Weissberg, R.P. (2017). Promoting positive youth development through school-based social and emotional learning interventions: A meta-analysis of follow-up effects. *Child Development, 88*(4), 1156-1171.

te Velde, S.J., & others (2012). Energy balance-related behaviors associated with overweight and obesity in preschool children: A systematic review of prospective studies. *Obesity Reviews, 13*(Suppl. 1), S56-S74.

Teery-McElrath, Y.M., O'Malley, P.M., & Johnston, L.D. (2012). Factors affecting sugar-sweetened beverage availability in competitive venues of U.S. secondary schools. *Journal of School Health, 82,* 44-55.

Telford, R.M., & others (2016). The influence of sport club participation on physical activity, fitness and body fat during childhood and adolescence: The LOOK longitudinal study. *Journal of Science and Medicine in Sport, 19*(5), 400-406.

Telzer, E.H., van Hoorn, J., Rogers, C.R., & Do, K.T. (2018). Social influence on positive youth development: A developmental neuroscience perspective. *Advances in Child Development and Behavior, 54,* 215-258.

Temple, C.A., & others (2018). *All children read: Teaching for literacy* (5th ed.). Upper Saddle River, NJ: Pearson.

Tenenbaum, H.R., Callahan, M., Alba-Speyer, C., & Sandoval, L. (2002). Parent-child science conversations in Mexican-descent families: Educational background, activity, and past experience as moderators. *Hispanic Journal of Behavioral Sciences, 24,* 225-248.

Teratology Society (2017). *Teratology primer* (3rd ed.). Reston, VA: The Teratology Society.

Terman, L. (1925). *Genetic studies of genius. Vol. 1: Mental and physical traits of a thousand gifted children.* Stanford, CA: Stanford University Press.

Teti, D. (2001). Retrospect and prospect in the psychological study of sibling relationships. In J. P. McHale & W. S. Grolnick (Eds.), *Retrospect and prospect in the psychological study of families.* Mahwah, NJ: Erlbaum.

Teunissen, H.A., & others (2012). Adolescents' conformity to their peers' pro-alcohol and anti-alcohol norms: The power of popularity. *Alcoholism: Clinical and Experimental Research, 36*(7), 1257-1267.

Thakur, N., & others (2017). Perceived discrimination associated with asthma and related outcomes in minority youth: The GALA II and SAGE II studies. *Chest, 151*(4), 804-812.

The Hospital for Sick Children & others (2010). *The Hospital for Sick Children's handbook of pediatrics* (11th ed.). London: Elsevier.

Thelen, E., & others (1993). The transition to reaching: Mapping intention and intrinsic dynamics. *Child Development, 64,* 1058-1098.

Thelen, E., & Smith, L.B. (2006). Dynamic development of action and thought. In W. Damon & R. Lerner (Eds.), *Handbook of child psychology* (6th ed.). New York: Wiley.

Theo, L.O., & Drake, E. (2017). Rooming-in: Creating a better experience. *The Journal of Perinatal Education, 26*(2), 79-84.

Theodotou, E. (2019). Examining literacy development holistically using the Play and Learn through the Arts (PLA) programme: A case study. *Early Child Development and Care, 189*(3), 488-499.

Thio, A., Taylor, J., & Schwartz, M. (2018). *Deviant behavior* (12th ed.). New York: Pearson.

Thomas, A., & Chess, S. (1991). Temperament in adolescence and its functional significance. In R. M. Lerner, A. C. Petersen, & J. Brooks-Gunn (Eds.), *Encyclopedia of adolescence* (Vol. 2). New York: Garland.

Thomas, B.L., Karl, J.M., & Whishaw, I.Q. (2015). Independent development of the Reach and the Grasp in spontaneous self-touching by human infants in the first 6 months. *Frontiers in Psychology, 5,* 1526.

Thomas, H.J., Connor, J.P., & Scott, J.G. (2018). Why do children and adolescents bully their peers? A critical review of key theoretical frameworks. *Social Psychiatry and Psychiatric Epidemiology, 53*(5), 437-451.

Thomas, M.S.C., & Johnson, M.H. (2008). New advances in understanding sensitive periods in brain development. *Current Directions in Psychological Science, 17,* 1-5.

Thompson, D.R., & others (2007). Childhood overweight and cardiovascular disease risk factors: The National Heart, Lung, and Blood Institute Growth and Health Study. *Journal of Pediatrics, 150,* 18-25.

Thompson, J.M.D., & others (2017). Duration of breastfeeding and risk of SIDS: An individual participant data (IPD) meta-analysis. *Pediatrics, 140*(5), e20171324.

Thompson, K.D. (2015). English learners' time to reclassification: An analysis. *Educational Policy, 31,* 330-363.

Thompson, R.A. (2006). The development of the person. In W. Damon & R. Lerner (Eds.), *Handbook of child psychology* (6th ed.). New York: Wiley.

Thompson, R.A. (2008). Unpublished review of J. W. Santrock's *Life-span development,* 2nd ed. (New York: McGraw-Hill).

Thompson, R.A. (2009). Early foundations: Conscience and the development of moral character. In D. Narváez & D. Lapsley (Eds.), *Moral personality, identity, and character: Prospects for a new field of study.* New York: Cambridge University Press.

Thompson, R.A. (2012). Whither the preoperational child? Toward a life-span moral development theory. *Child Development Perspectives, 6,* 423-429.

Thompson, R.A. (2013a). Attachment development: Precis and prospect. In P. Zelazo (Ed.), *Oxford handbook of developmental psychology.* New York: Oxford University Press.

Thompson, R.A. (2013b). Interpersonal relations. In A. Ben-Arieh, I. Frones, F. Cases, & J. Korbin (Eds.), *Handbook of child well-being.* New York: Springer.

Thompson, R.A. (2013c). Relationships, regulation, and development. In R. M. Lerner (Ed.), *Handbook of child psychology* (7th ed.). New York: Wiley.

Thompson, R.A. (2013d). Socialization of emotion regulation in the family. In J. Gross (Ed.), *Handbook of emotion regulation* (2nd ed.). New York: Guilford.

Thompson, R.A. (2014). Conscience development in early childhood. In M. Killen & J.G. Smetana (Eds.), *Handbook of moral development* (2nd ed., pp. 73-92). New York: Routledge.

Thompson, R.A. (2015a). Relationships, regulation, and early development. In R.M. Lerner (Ed.), *Handbook of child psychology and developmental science* (7th ed.). Hoboken, NJ: Wiley.

Thompson, R.A. (2015b). Socialization of emotion regulation in the family. In J. Gross (Ed.), *Handbook of emotion regulation* (2nd ed.). New York: Guilford.

Thompson, R.A. (2018). *Social-emotional development in the first three years: Establishing the foundations.* University Park, PA: Edna Bennett Pierce Prevention Research Center, Pennsylvania State University.

Thompson, R.A. (2019, in press). Emotion dysregulation: A theme in search of definition. *Development and Psychopathology.*

Thorisdottir, A., Gunnarsdottir, I., & Thorisdottir, I. (2013). Revised infant dietary recommendations: The impact of maternal education and other parental factors on adherence rates in Iceland. *Acta Pediatrica, 102*(2), 143-148.

Thurman, S.L., & Corbetta, D. (2017). Spatial exploration and changes in infant–mother dyads around transitions in infant locomotion. *Developmental Psychology, 53,* 1207-1221.

Tibi, S., & Kirby, J.R. (2018). Investigating phonological awareness and naming speed as predictors of reading in Arabic. *Scientific Studies of Reading, 22*(1), 70-84.

Tikotzky, L., & Shaashua, L. (2012). Infant sleep and early parental sleep-related cognitions predict sleep in pre-school children. *Sleep Medicine, 13,* 185-192.

Tincoff, R., & Jusczyk, P.W. (2012). Six-month-olds comprehend words that refer to parts of the body. *Infancy, 17*(4), 432-444.

Tincoff, R., Seidl, A., Buckley, L., Wojcik, C., & Cristia, A. (2019). Feeling the way to words: Parents' speech and touch cues highlight word-to-world mappings of body parts. *Language Learning and Development, 15,* 103-125.

Titzmann, P., & Gniewosz, B. (2017). With a little help from my child: A dyad approach to immigrant mothers' and adolescents' socio-cultural adaptation. *Journal of Adolescence, 62,* 198-206.

Titzmann, P.F., & Fuligni, A.J. (2015). Immigrants' adaptation to different cultural settings: A contextual perspective on acculturation: Introduction for the special section on immigration. *International Journal of Psychology, 50*(6), 407-412.

Tobin, J.J., Wu, D.Y.H., & Davidson, D.H. (1989). *Preschool in three cultures.* New Haven, CT: Yale University Press.

Tobler, A.L., & others (2013). Perceived racial/ethnic discrimination, problem behaviors, and mental health among minority urban youth. *Ethnicity and Health, 18*(4), 337-349.

Toh, S.H., Howie, E.K., Coenen, P., & Straker, L.M. (2019). "From the moment I wake up I will use it . . . every day, very hour": A qualitative study on the patterns of adolescents' mobile touch screen device use from adolescent and parent perspectives. *BMC Pediatrics, 19*(1), 30.

Toma, C., & others. (2013). Neurotransmitter systems and neurotrophic factors in autism: Association study of 37 genes suggests involvement of DDC. *World Journal of Biology, 14*(7), 516-527.

Tomasello, M., & Vaish, A. (2013). Origins of human cooperation and morality. *Annual Review of Psychology, 64,* 231-255.

Tomasello, M. (2009). *Why we cooperate.* Cambridge, MA: MIT Press.

Tomasello, M. (2011b). Language development. In U. Goswami (Ed.), *Wiley-Blackwell handbook of childhood cognitive development* (2nd ed.). New York: Wiley.

Tomasello, M. (2018). Great apes and human development: A personal history. *Child Development Perspectives, 12,* 189-193.

Tomasello, M. (2018). How children come to understand false beliefs: A shared intentionality account. *Proceedings of the National Academy of Sciences, 115*(34), 8491-8498.

Tompkins, V., Benigno, J.P., Lee, B.K., & Wright, B.M. (2018). The relation between parents' mental state talk and children's social understanding: A meta-analysis. *Social Development, 27,* 223-246.

Tortora, G.J., Funke, B.R., & Case, C.L. (2013). *Microbiology* (11th ed.). Upper Saddle River, NJ: Pearson.

Trafimow, D., Triandis, H.C., & Goto, S.G. (1991). Some tests of the distinction between the private and collective self. *Journal of Personality and Social Psychology, 60,* 649-655.

Trejos-Castillo, E., Bedore, S., & Trevino Schafer, N. (2013). Human capital development among immigrant youth. In E. Trejos-Castillo (Ed.), *Youth: Practices, perspectives, and challenges.* Hauppage, NY: Nova Science Publishers.

Tremblay, M.W., & Jiang, Y.H. (2019). DNA methylation and susceptibility to autism spectrum disorder. *Annual Review of Medicine, 70,* 151-166.

Trentacosta, C.J., & Fine, S.E. (2009). Emotion knowledge, social competence, and behavior problems in childhood and adolescence: A meta-analytic review. *Social Development, 19*(1), 1-29.

Triandis, H.C. (2007). Culture and psychology: A history of their relationship. In S. Kitayama & D. Cohen (Eds.), *Handbook of cultural psychology.* New York: Guilford.

Trimble, J.E., & Bhadra, M. (2013). Ethnic gloss. *The encyclopedia of cross-cultural psychology* (Vol. 2, pp. 500-504).

Troppe, P., & others (2017). Implementation of Title I and Title II-A program initiatives. Results from 2013-2014. NCEE 2017-4014. *ERIC,* ED572281.

Tsai, K.M., & others (2018). The roles of parental support and family stress in adolescent sleep. *Child Development, 89,* 1577-1588.

Tucker, C.J., & Finkelhor, D. (2017). The state of interventions for sibling conflict and aggression: A systematic review. *Trauma, Violence, & Abuse, 18*(4), 396-406.

Tucker, C.J., & Kazura, K. (2013). Parental responses to school-aged children's sibling conflict. *Journal of Child and Family Studies, 22*(5), 737-745.

Tudge, J., & Freitas, L. (2018). Developing gratitude: An introduction. In J. Tudge & L. Freitas (Eds.), *Developing gratitude in children and adolescents* (pp. 1-24). Cambridge, UK: Cambridge University Press.

Tunçgenç, B., & Cohen, E. (2018). Interpersonal movement synchrony facilitates pro-social behavior in children's peer-play. *Developmental Science, 21*(1), e12505.

Turiel, E., & Gingo, M. (2017). Development in the moral domain: Coordination and the need to consider other domains of social reasoning. In N. Budwig, E. Turiel, & P.D. Zelazo (Eds.), *New perspectives on human development.* New York: Cambridge University Press.

Turiel, E. (2015). Moral development. In R. Lerner (Ed.), *Handbook of child psychology and developmental science* (7th ed.). New York: Wiley.

Turoy-Smith, K.M., & Powell, M.B. (2017). Interviewing of children for family law matters: A review. *Australian Psychologist, 52*(3), 165-173.

Twenge, J.M., & Campbell, W.K. (2019, in press). Media use is linked to lower psychological well-being: Evidence from three datasets. *Psychiatric Quarterly,* 1-21.

Twenge, J.M., & Park, H. (2019). The decline in adult activities among US adolescents, 1976-2016. *Child Development, 90*(2), 638-654.

Twomey, C., O'Connell, H., Lillis, M., Tarpey, S.L., & O'Reilly, G. (2018). Utility of an abbreviated version of the Stanford-Binet intelligence scales (5th ed.) in estimating 'full scale' IQ for young children with autism spectrum disorder. *Autism Research, 11,* 503-508.

Tyrell, F.A., Wheeler, L.A., Gonzales, N.A., Dumka, L., & Millsap, R. (2016). Family influences on Mexican American adolescents' romantic relationships: Moderation by gender and culture. *Journal of Research on Adolescence, 26,* 142-158.

Tzourio-Mazoyer, N., Perrone-Bertolotti, M., Jobard, G., Mazoyer, B., & Baciu, M. (2017). Multi-factorial modulation of hemispheric specialization and plasticity for language in healthy and pathological conditions: A review. *Cortex, 86,* 314-339.

U

Ullman, T.D., Stuhlmüller, A., Goodman, N.D., & Tenenbaum, J.B. (2018). Learning physical parameters from dynamic scenes. *Cognitive Psychology, 104,* 57-82.

Umaña-Taylor, A.J., Kornienko, O., Bayless, S.D., & Updegraff, K.A. (2018). A universal intervention program increases ethnic-racial identity exploration and resolution to predict adolescent psychosocial functioning one year later. *Journal of Youth and Adolescence, 47*(1), 1-15.

Umaña-Taylor, A.J. (2016). A post-racial society in which ethnic-racial discrimination still exists and has significant consequences for youths' adjustment. *Current Directions in Psychological Science, 25*(2), 111-118.

Umana-Taylor, A.J., Wong, J.J., Gonzalez, N.A., & Dumka, L.E. (2012). Ethnic identity and gender as moderators of the association between discrimination and academic adjustment among Mexican-origin adolescents. *Journal of Adolescence, 35*(4), 773-786.

Unar-Munguía, M., Torres-Mejía, G., Colchero, M.A., & González de Cosío, T. (2017). Breastfeeding mode and risk of breast cancer: A dose–response meta-analysis. *Journal of Human Lactation, 33,* 422-434.

Underwood, M.K. (2011). Aggression. In M. K. Underwood & L. Rosen (Eds.), *Social development*. New York: Guilford.

UNESCO (2016). *Global education monitoring report: Gender review*. Paris: UNESCO.

UNICEF. (2004). *The state of the world's children: 2004*. Geneva, Switzerland: Author.

UNICEF. (2007). *The state of the world's children: 2007*. Geneva, Switzerland: Author.

UNICEF. (2012). *The state of the world's children: 2012*. Geneva, Switzerland: Author.

UNICEF (2014). Children of the Recession: The impact of the economic crisis on child well-being in rich countries. *Innocenti Report Card 12*. Florence, Italy: UNICEF Office of Research.

UNICEF (2017). *The state of the world's children, 2017*. Geneva, Switzerland: UNICEF.

UNICEF (2018). *HIV/AIDS and children*. Retrieved from https://www.unicef.org/aids/index_1.php

UNICEF (2018). *Nutrition*. Retrieved from https://www.unicef.org/nutrition/

UNICEF (2018). *The state of the world's children*. New York: UNICEF.

UNICEF (2019). *Early childhood education*. Retrieved from https://www.unicef.org/education/early-childhood-education

United Nations. (2002). *Improving the quality of life of girls*. Geneva: UNICEF.

United Nations (2019). Gender equality. Retrieved from http://www.un.org/en/sections/issues-depth/gender-equality/

Updegraff, K.A., Kim, J-Y, Killoren, S.E., & Thayer, S.M. (2010). Mexican American parents' involvement in adolescents' peer relationships: Exploring the role of culture and adolescents' peer experiences. *Journal of Research on Adolescence, 20*, 65–87.

Updegraff, K.A., Umana-Taylor, A.J., McHale, S.M., Wheeler, L.A., & Perez-Brena, J. (2012). Mexican-origin youths' cultural orientations and adjustment: Changes from early to late adolescence. *Child Development, 83*, 1655–1671.

Updegraff, K.A., & Umaña-Taylor, A.J. (2015). What can we learn from the study of Mexican-origin families in the United States? *Family Process, 54*(2), 205–216.

Urban, J.B., Lewin-Bizan, S., & Lerner, R.M. (2010). The role of intentional self-regulation, lower neighborhood ecological assets, and activity involvement in youth developmental outcomes. *Journal of Youth and Adolescence, 39*, 783–800.

Urdan, T. (2012). Factors affecting the motivation and achievement of immigrant students. In K. R. Harris, S. Graham, & T. Urdan (Eds.), *APA educational psychology handbook*. Washington, DC: American Psychological Association.

Ursache, A., Blair, C., & Raver, C.C. (2012). The promotion of self-regulation as a means of enhancing school readiness and early achievement in children at risk for school failure. *Child Development Perspectives, 6*, 122–128.

Ursache, A., Blair, C., Stifter, C., & Voegtline, K. (2013). Emotional reactivity and regulation in infancy interact to predict executive functioning in early childhood. *Developmental Psychology, 49*(1), 127–137.

Ursin, M. (2015). Geographies of sleep among Brazilian street youth. In K. Nairn & others (Eds.), *Space, Place and Environment*, 1–27. London: Springer.

U.S. Census Bureau (2017a). Income and poverty in the United States. *Current Population Reports*. Washington, DC: U.S. Department of Commerce.

U.S. Census Bureau (2015). *Millennials outnumber baby boomers and are far more diverse*. Washington DC: U.S. Department of Commerce. Retrieved September 15, 2018, from https://www.census.gov/newsroom/press-releases/2015/cb15-113.html

U.S. Census Bureau (2017b). The nation's older population is still growing. *Current Population Reports*, Release Number CB17-100. Washington DC: U.S. Department of Commerce.

U.S. Census Bureau (2018). *Current Population Survey, Annual Social and Economic Supplements 1968 to 2017* (Figure CH-2.3.4). Washington, DC: Author.

U.S. Department of Education, National Center for Education Statistics (2018). *Early childhood care arrangements: Choices and costs*. Retrieved from https://nces.ed.gov/programs/coe/indicator_tca.asp

U.S. Department of Education (2019). About IDEA. Retrieved from https://sites.ed.gov/idea/about-idea/

U.S. Department of Health and Human Services (2017). *Child maltreatment 2015*. Retrieved from www.acf.hhs.gov/programs/cb/research-data-technology/statistics-research/child-maltreatment

U.S. Department of Health and Human Services (2017). *Trends in foster care and adoption: FY 2007 - FY 2016*. Washington, DC: Author.

U.S. Department of Health and Human Services (2018). *Womenshealth.gov: Folic acid fact sheet*. https://www.womenshealth.gov/files/documents/fact-sheet-folic-acid.pdf

USA Today (2000, October 10). All-USA first teacher team. Retrieved November 15, 2004, from http://www.usatoday.com/life/teacher/teach/htm

Uwaezuoke, S.N., Eneh, C.I., & Ndu, I.K. (2017). Relationship between exclusive breastfeeding and lower risk of childhood obesity: A narrative review of published evidence. *Clinical Medicine Insights: Pediatrics, 11*, 1179556517690196.

V

Vacca, J.A., & others (2018). *Reading and learning to read* (10th ed.). Boston: Allyn & Bacon.

Vöhringer, I.A., & others (2018). The development of implicit memory from infancy to childhood: On average performance levels and interindividual differences. *Child Development, 89*, 370–382.

Valenzuela, C.F., Morton, R.A., Diaz, M.R., & Topper, L. (2012). Does moderate drinking harm the fetal brain? Insights from animal models. *Trends in Neuroscience, 35*(5), 284–292.

Van Boekel, M., & others (2016). Effects of participation in school sports on academic and social functioning. *Journal of Applied Developmental Psychology, 46*, 31–40.

van de Bongardt, D., Yu, R., Deković, M., & Meeus, W.H. (2015). Romantic relationships and sexuality in adolescence and young adulthood: The role of parents, peers, and partners. *European Journal of Developmental Psychology, 12*, 497–515.

Van den Akker, H., Van der Ploeg, R., & Scheepers, P. (2013). Disapproval of homosexuality: Comparative research on individual and national determinants of disapproval of homosexuality in 20 European countries. *International Journal of Public Opinion Research, 25*(1), 64–86.

Van den Bergh, B.R., Dahnke, R., & Mennes, M. (2018). Prenatal stress and the developing brain: Risks for neurodevelopmental disorders. *Development and Psychopathology, 30*, 743–762.

van den Boom, D.C. (1989). Neonatal irritability and the development of attachment. In G. A. Kohnstamm, J. E. Bates, & M. K. Rothbart (Eds.), *Temperament in childhood*. New York: Wiley.

Van der Graaff, J., Carlo, G., Crocetti, E., Koot, H.M., & Branje, S. (2018). Prosocial behavior in adolescence: Gender differences in development and links with empathy. *Journal of Youth and Adolescence, 47*(5), 1086–1099.

van der Stel, M., & Veenman, M.V.J. (2010). Development of metacognitive skillfulness: A longitudinal study. *Learning and Individual Differences, 20*, 220–224.

van der Wal, R.C., Karremans, J.C., & Cillessen, A.H. (2017). Causes and consequences of children's forgiveness. *Child Development Perspectives, 11*(2), 97–101.

van der Wilt, F., van der Veen, C., van Kruistum, C., & van Oers, B. (2018). Popular, rejected, neglected, controversial, or average: Do young children of different sociometric groups differ in their level of oral communicative competence? *Social Development, 27*(4), 793–807.

van Geel, M., & Vedder, P. (2011). The role of family obligations and school adjustment in explaining the immigrant paradox. *Journal of Youth and Adolescence, 40*(2), 187–196.

van Harmelen, A.L., & others (2010). Child abuse and negative explicit and automatic self-associations: The cognitive scars of emotional maltreatment. *Behavior Research and Therapy, 48*(6), 486–494.

van Hover, S., & Hicks, D. (2017). Social constructivism and student learning in social studies. *The Wiley Handbook of Social Studies Research, 5*, 270.

van Huizen, T., Dumhs, L., & Plantenga, J. (2019). The costs and benefits of investing in universal preschool: Evidence from a Spanish reform. *Child Development. 90*(3), e386–e406.

Van Iddekinge, C.H., Aguinis, H., Mackey, J.D., & DeOrtentiis, P.S. (2018). A meta-analysis of the interactive, additive, and relative effects of cognitive ability and motivation on performance. *Journal of Management, 44*, 249–279.

van IJzendoorn, M.H., & Kroonenberg, P.M. (1988). Cross-cultural patterns of attachment: A meta-analysis of the Strange Situation. *Child Development, 59*, 147–156.

van IJzendoorn, M.H., Kranenburg, M.J., Pannebakker, F., & Out, D. (2010). In defense of situational morality: Genetic, dispositional, and situational determinants of children's donating to charity. *Journal of Moral Education, 39*, 1–20.

Van Loo, K.J., & Boucher, K.L. (2017). Stereotype threat. In A.J. Elliot, C.S. Dweck, & D.S. Yeager (Eds.), *Handbook of competence and motivation: Theory and application*. New York: Guilford.

van Merendonk, E.J., & others (2017). Identification of prenatal behavioral patterns of the gross motor movements within the early stages of fetal development. *Infant and Child Development, 26*(5), e2012.

Van Petegem, S., de Ferrerre, E., Soenens, B., van Rooij, A.J., & Van Looy, J. (2019). Parents' degree and style of restrictive mediation of young children's digital gaming: Associations with parental attitudes and perceived child adjustment. *Journal of Child and Family Studies, 28*(5), 1379-1391.

Van Rijn, S., de Sonneville, L., & Swaab, H. (2018). The nature of social cognitive deficits in children and adults with Klinefelter syndrome (47,XXY). *Genes, Brain, and Behavior, 17*.

van Rijsewijk, L.G., Snijders, T.A., Dijkstra, J.K., Steglich, C., & Veenstra, R. (2019, in press). The interplay between adolescents' friendships and the exchange of help: A longitudinal multiplex social network study. *Journal of Research on Adolescence*.

Van Ryzin, M.J., Carlson, E.A., & Sroufe, L.A. (2011). Attachment discontinuity in a high-risk sample. *Attachment and Human Development, 13*, 381-401.

van Schaik, S.D., Oudgenoeg-Paz, O., & Atun-Einy, O. (2018). Cross-cultural differences in parental beliefs about infant motor development: A quantitative and qualitative report of middle-class Israeli and Dutch parents. *Developmental Psychology, 54*(6), 999-1010.

Vandell, D.L., & Wilson, K.S. (1988). Infants' interactions with mother, sibling, and peer: Contrasts and relations between interaction systems. *Child Development, 48*, 176-186.

Vandell, D.L., Burchinal, M., & Pierce, K.M. (2016). Early child care and adolescent functioning at the end of high school: Results from the NICHD Study of Early Child Care and Youth Development. *Developmental Psychology, 52*, 1634-1645.

Vandenbroucke, L., Verschueren, K., & Baeyens, D. (2017). The development of executive functioning across the transition to first grade and its predictive value for academic achievement. *Learning and Instruction, 49*, 103-112.

Vansteenkiste, M., Sierens, E., Soenens, B., Luyckx, K., & Lens, W. (2009). Motivational profiles from a self-determination perspective: The quality of motivation matters. *Journal of Educational Psychology, 101*(3), 671-688.

Vanwesenbeeck, I., Ponnet, K., Walrave, M., & Van Ouytsel, J. (2018). Parents' role in adolescents' sexting behaviour. In M. Walrave & others (Eds.), *Sexting* (pp. 63-80). London: Palgrave Macmillan.

Vargas-Terrones, M., Barakat, R., Santacruz, B., Fernandez-Buhigas, I., & Mottola, M.F. (2018). Physical exercise programme during pregnancy decreases perinatal depression risk: A randomised controlled trial. *British Journal of Sports Medicine, 53*(6). doi:10.1136/bjsports-2017-098926

Vaughn, A.R., Tannhauser, P., Sivamani, R.K., & Shi, V.Y. (2017). Mother nature in eczema: Maternal factors influencing atopic dermatitis. *Pediatric Dermatology, 34*, 240-246.

Veenstra, R., Lindenberg, S., Munniksma, A., & Dijkstra, J.K. (2010). The complex relationship between bullying, victimization, acceptance, and rejection: Giving special attention to status, affection, and sex differences. *Child Development, 81*(2), 480-486.

Velez, C.E., Wolchik, S.A., Tein, J.Y., & Sandler, I. (2011). Protecting children from the consequences of divorce: A longitudinal study of the effects of parenting on children's coping responses. *Child Development, 82*, 244-257.

Veraksa, N., & Sheridan, S. (Eds.) (2018). *Vygotsky's theory in early childhood education and research*. New York: Routledge.

Verkuyten, M. (2018). *The social psychology of ethnic identity* (2nd ed.). New York: Routledge.

Verriotis, M., & others (2018). The distribution of pain activity across the human neonatal brain is sex dependent. *NeuroImage, 178*, 69-77.

Verschuren, O., Gorter, J.W., & Pritchard-Wiart, L. (2017). Sleep: An underemphasized aspect of health and development in neurorehabilitation. *Early Human Development, 113*, 120-128.

Vida, M., & Maurer, D. (2012). The development of fine-grained sensitivity to eye contact after 6 years of age. *Journal of Experimental Child Psychology, 112*, 243-256.

Viejo, C., Monks, C.P., Sánchez-Rosa, M., & Ortega-Ruiz, R. (2018). Attachment hierarchies for Spanish adolescents: Family, peers and romantic partner figures. *Attachment & human development*. doi:10.1080/14616734.2018.1466182

Vietze, J., Juang, L., Schachner, M.K., & Werneck, H. (2018). Feeling half-half? Exploring relational variation of Turkish-heritage young adults' cultural identity compatibility and conflict in Austria. *Identity, 18*(1), 60-76.

Vignoles, V.L., & others (2016). Beyond the 'east-west' dichotomy: Global variation in cultural models of selfhood. *Journal of Experimental Psychology: General, 145*(8), 966.

Vijayakumar, N., de Macks, Z.O., Shirtcliff, E.A., & Pfeifer, J.H. (2018). Puberty and the human brain: Insights into adolescent development. *Neuroscience & Biobehavioral Reviews, 92*, 417-436.

Villar, J., & others (2014). International standards for newborn weight, length, and head circumference by gestational age and sex: The Newborn Cross-Sectional Study of the INTERGROWTH-21st Project. *The Lancet, 384*(9946), 857-868.

Villegas, R., & others (2008). Duration of breast-feeding and the incidence of type 2 diabetes mellitus in the Shanghai Women's Health Study. *Diabetologia, 51*, 258-266.

Vink, J., & Quinn, M. (2018). Chorionic villus sampling. In *Obstetric imaging: Fetal diagnosis and care* (2nd ed.). Philadelphia: Elsevier.

Virk, J., & others (2018). Pre-conceptual and prenatal supplementary folic acid and multivitamin intake, behavioral problems, and hyperkinetic disorders: A study based on the Danish National Birth Cohort (DNBC). *Nutritional Neuroscience, 21*(5), 352-360.

Vishkaie, R., Shively, K., & Powell, C.W. (2018). Perceptions of digital tools and creativity in the classroom. *International Journal of Digital Literacy and Digital Competence (IJDLDC), 9*(4), 1-18.

Vitaro, F., Boivin, M., & Poulin, F. (2018). The interface of aggression and peer relations in childhood and adolescence. In W. Bukowski & others (Eds.), *Handbook of peer relationships, interactions, and groups* (2nd ed.). New York: Guilford.

Vitaro, F., Pedersen, S., & Brendgen, M. (2007). Children's disruptiveness, peer rejection, friends' deviancy, and delinquent behaviors: A process-oriented approach. *Development and Psychopathology, 19*, 433-453.

Viteri, O.A., & others (2015). Fetal anomalies and long-term effects associated with substance abuse in pregnancy: A literature review. *American Journal of Perinatology, 32*(05), 405-416.

Vittrup, B., Holden, G.W., & Buck, M. (2006). Attitudes predict the use of physical punishment: A prospective study of the emergence of disciplinary practices. *Pediatrics, 117*, 2055-2064.

Vixner, L., Schytt, E., & Mårtensson, L.B. (2017). Associations between maternal characteristics and women's responses to acupuncture during labour. *Acupuncture in Medicine, 35*(3), 180-188.

Voepel-Lewis, T., & others (2018). Deliberative prescription opioid misuse among adolescents and emerging adults: Opportunities for targeted interventions. *Journal of Adolescent Health, 63*, 594-600.

Vogelsang, L., & others (2018). Potential downside of high initial visual acuity. *Proceedings of the National Academy of Sciences, 115*(44), 11333-11338.

Vogelsang, M., & Tomasello, M. (2016). Giving is nicer than taking: Preschoolers reciprocate based on the social intentions of the distributor. *PloS One, 11*(1), e0147539.

Voltmer, K., & von Salisch, M. (2017). Three meta-analyses of children's emotion knowledge and their school success. *Learning and Individual Differences, 59*, 107-118.

von Soest, T., Wichstrøm, L., & Kvalem, I.L. (2016). The development of global and domain-specific self-esteem from age 13 to 31. *Journal of Personality and Social Psychology, 110*(4), 592.

Vos, P.H. (2018). *Journal of Beliefs & Values, 39*(1), 17-28.

Vygotsky, L.S. (1962). *Thought and language*. Cambridge, MA: MIT Press.

W

Wachs, T.D. (1994). Fit, context and the transition between temperament and personality. In C. Halverson, G. Kohnstamm, & R. Martin (Eds.), *The developing structure of personality from infancy to adulthood*. Hillsdale, NJ: Erlbaum.

Wachs, T.D. (2000). *Necessary but not sufficient*. Washington, DC: American Psychological Association.

Wade, M., & others (2018). On the relation between theory of mind and executive functioning: A developmental cognitive neuroscience perspective. *Psychonomic Bulletin & Review, 25*(6), 2119-2149.

Wade, M., Jenkins, J.M., Venkadasalam, V.P., Binnoon-Erez, N., & Ganea, P.A. (2018). The role of maternal responsiveness and linguistic input in pre-academic skill development: A longitudinal analysis of pathways. *Cognitive Development, 45,* 125–140.

Wadsworth, M.E., & others (2013). A longitudinal examination of the adaptation to poverty-related stress model: Predicting child and adolescent adjustment over time. *Journal of Clinical Child and Adolescent Psychology, 42*(5), 713–725.

Wadsworth, M.E., Evans, G.W., Grant, K., Carter, J.S., & Duffy, S. (2016). Poverty and the development of psychopathology. In D. Cicchetti (Ed.), *Developmental psychopathology.* New York: Wiley.

Wagner, J.B., Luyster, R.J., Moustapha, H., Tager-Flusberg, H., & Nelson, C.A. (2018). Differential attention to faces in infant siblings of children with autism spectrum disorder and associations with later social and language ability. *International Journal of Behavioral Development, 42*(1), 83–92.

Wagner, L., & Hoff, E. (2013). Language development. In I. B. Weiner & others (Eds.), *Handbook of psychology* (2nd ed.). New York: Wiley.

Wagoner, B. (Ed.). (2017). *Handbook of culture and memory.* Oxford, UK: Oxford University Press.

Wainryb, C., & Recchia, H. (2017). Mother–child conversations about children's moral wrongdoing: A constructivist perspective on moral socialization. In N. Budwig & others (Eds.), *New perspectives on human development.* Cambridge, UK: Cambridge University Press.

Wainryb, C., & Recchia, H.E. (Eds.). (2014). *Talking about right and wrong: Parent-child conversations as contexts for moral development.* Cambridge, UK: Cambridge University Press.

Waite-Stupiansky, S. (2017). Jean Piaget's constructivist theory of learning. In L.E. Cohen & S. Waite-Stupiansky (Eds.), *Theories of early childhood education.* New York: Routledge.

Waldron, J.C., Scarpa, A., & Kim-Spoon, J. (2018). Religiosity and interpersonal problems explain individual differences in self-esteem among young adults with child maltreatment experiences. *Child Abuse & Neglect, 80,* 277–284.

Walker, L.J., & Hennig, K.H. (2004). Differing conceptions of moral exemplars: Just, brave, and caring. *Journal of Personality and Social Psychology, 86,* 629–647.

Walker, L.J., Hennig, K.H., & Krettenauer, T. (2000). Parent and peer contexts for children's moral development. *Child Development, 71,* 1033–1048.

Walker, L.J. (2002). Moral exemplarity. In W. Damon (Ed.), *Bringing in a new era of character education.* Stanford, CA: Hoover Press.

Walker, L.J. (2013). Moral personality, motivation, and identity. In M. Killen & J. G. Smetana (Eds.), *Handbook of moral development* (2nd ed.). New York: Routledge.

Walker, L. (1982). The sequentiality of Kohlberg's stages of moral development. *Child Development, 53,* 1130–1136.

Walker, L. (2006). Gender and morality. In M. Killen & J. G. Smetana (Eds.), *Handbook of moral development.* Mahwah, NJ: Erlbaum.

Walker, L.J., & Taylor, J.H. (1991). Family interactions and the development of moral reasoning. *Child Development, 62*(2), 264–283.

Walker, L.J. (2014). Moral personality, motivation, and identity. In M. Killen & J.G. Smetana (Eds.), *Handbook of moral development* (2nd ed.). New York: Routledge.

Walle, E.A., Reschke, P.J., & Knothe, J.M. (2017). Social referencing: Defining and delineating a basic process of emotion. *Emotion Review, 9,* 245–252.

Walle, E.A., Reschke, P.J., Camras, L.A., & Campos, J.J. (2017). Infant differential behavioral responding to discrete emotions. *Emotion, 17,* 1078–1091.

Wallerstein, J.S. (2008). Divorce. In M. M. Haith & J. B. Benson (Eds.), *Encyclopedia of infant and early childhood development.* Oxford, UK: Elsevier.

Walters, G.D. (2019). Are the effects of parental control/support and peer delinquency on future offending cumulative or interactive? A multiple group analysis of 10 longitudinal studies. *Journal of Criminal Justice, 60,* 13–24.

Walton-Fisette, J., & Wuest, D. (2018). *Foundations of physical education, exercise science and sport* (19th ed.). New York: McGraw-Hill.

Wan, Q., & Wen, F.Y. (2018). Effects of acupressure and music therapy on reducing labor pain. *International Journal of Clinical and Experimental Medicine, 11*(2), 898–903.

Wang, A.Y., & others (2018). Neonatal outcomes among twins following assisted reproductive technology: An Australian population-based retrospective cohort study. *BMC Pregnancy and Childbirth, 18,* 320.

Wang, E.T., & others (2017). Fertility treatment is associated with stay in the neonatal intensive care unit and respiratory support in late preterm infants. *Journal of Pediatrics, 187,* 309–312.

Wang, F., & others (2018). A novel *TSC2* missense variant associated with a variable phenotype of tuberous sclerosis complex: Case report of a Chinese family. *BMC Medical Genetics, 19,* 90.

Wang, H.Y., Sigerson, L., & Cheng, C. (2019). Digital nativity and information technology addiction: Age cohort versus individual difference approaches. *Computers in Human Behavior, 90,* 1–9.

Wang, L., & others (2018). Paternal smoking and spontaneous abortion: A population-based retrospective cohort study among non-smoking women aged 20–49 years in rural China. *Journal of Epidemiology and Community Health, 72*(9), 783–789.

Wang, M.L., & others (2013). Dietary and physical activity factors related to eating disorder symptoms among middle school youth. *Journal of School Health, 83,* 14–20.

Wang, Z., Deater-Deckard, K., Petrill, S.A., & Thompson, L. (2012). Externalizing problems, attention regulation, and household chaos: A longitudinal behavioral genetic study. *Development and Psychopathology, 24,* 755–769.

Ward, D.S., & others (2017). Strength of obesity prevention interventions in early care and education settings: A systematic review. *Preventive Medicine, 95,* S37–S52.

Ward, L.M. (2016). Media and sexualization: State of empirical research, 1995–2015. *The Journal of Sex Research, 53,* 560–577.

Ware, E.A. (2017). Individual and developmental differences in preschoolers' categorization biases and vocabulary across tasks. *Journal of Experimental Child Psychology, 153,* 35–56.

Warembourg, C., Cordier, S., & Garlantézec, R. (2017). An update systematic review of fetal death, congenital anomalies, and fertility disorders among health care workers. *American Journal of Industrial Medicine, 60*(6), 578–590.

Warneken, F. (2018). How children solve the two challenges of cooperation. *Annual Review of Psychology, 69,* 205–229.

Warton, F.L., & others (2018). Prenatal methamphetamine exposure is associated with reduced subcortical volumes in neonates. *Neurotoxicology and Teratology, 65,* 51–59.

Wasserberg, M.J. (2017). High-achieving African American elementary students' perspectives on standardized testing and stereotypes. *The Journal of Negro Education, 86,* 40–51.

Wasserman, J.D. (2018). A history of intelligence assessment: The unfinished tapestry. In D.P. Flanagan & E.M. McDonough (Eds.), *Contemporary intellectual assessment: Theories, tests, and issues* (4th ed.). New York: Guilford.

Watamura, S.E., Phillips, D.A., Morrissey, D.A., McCartney, T.W., & Bub, K. (2011). Double jeopardy: Poorer social-emotional outcomes for children in the NICHD SECCYD who experience home and child-care environments that convey risk. *Child Development, 82,* 48–65.

Watkins, M.K., & Waldron, M. (2017). Timing of remarriage among divorced and widowed parents. *Journal of Divorce & Remarriage, 58*(4), 244–262.

Watson, D. (2012). Objective tests as instruments of psychological theory and research. In H. Cooper (Ed.), *APA handbook of research methods in psychology.* Washington, DC: American Psychological Association.

Watson, J.B. (1928). *Psychological care of infant and child.* New York: W. W. Norton.

Watson, J.B., & Rayner, R. (1920). Conditioned emotional reactions. *Journal of Experimental Psychology, 3,* 1–14.

Watson, N.F., & others (2017). Delaying middle school and high school start times promotes student health and performance: An American Academy of Sleep Medicine position statement. *Journal of Clinical Sleep Medicine, 13,* 623–625.

Waugh, W.E., & Brownell, C.A. (2015). Development of body-part vocabulary in toddlers in relation to self-understanding. *Early Child Development and Care, 185*(7), 1166–1179.

Way, N., & Silverman, L.R. (2012). The quality of friendships during adolescence: Patterns across context, culture, and age. In P. K. Kerig, M. S. Shulz, & S. T. Hauser (Eds.), *Adolescence and beyond.* New York: Oxford University Press.

Wayne, A. (2011). Commentary in interview: Childhood cancers in transition. Retrieved April 12, 2011, from http://home.ccr.cancer.gov/connections/2010/Vol4_No2/clinic2.asp

Weedon, B.D., & others (2018). The relationship of gross upper and lower limb motor competence to measures of health and fitness in adolescents aged 13-14 years. *BMJ Open Sport–Exercise Medicine, 4*(1), e000288. doi: 10.1136/bmjsem-2017-000288

Weger Jr., H., Cole, M., & Akbulut, V. (2019). Relationship maintenance across platonic and non-platonic cross-sex friendships in emerging adults. *The Journal of Social Psychology, 159*(1), 15-29.

Wei, J., & others (2019). Why does parents' involvement in youth's learning vary across elementary, middle, and high school? *Contemporary Educational Psychology, 56,* 262-274.

Wei, J. (2015). Prediction of English-speaking children's Chinese spoken word learning: Contributions of phonological short-term memory. *The Arizona Working Papers in Second Language Acquisition and Teaching, 22,* 101-129.

Wei, R., & others (2013). Dynamic expression of microRNAs during the differentiation of human embryonic stem cells into insulin-producing cells. *Gene, 518*(2), 246-255.

Weinraub, M., & others (2012). Patterns of developmental change in infants' nighttime sleep awakenings from 6 through 36 months of age. *Developmental Psychology, 48*(6), 1511-1528.

Weisband, Y.L., Gallo, M.F., Klebanoff, M., Shoben, A., & Norris, A.H. (2018). Who uses a midwife for prenatal care and for birth in the United States? A secondary analysis of Listening to Mothers III. *Women's Health Issues, 28*(1), 89-96.

Welker, K.M., Roy, A.R., Geniole, S., Kitayama, S., & Carré, J.M. (2019). Taking risks for personal gain: An investigation of self-construal and testosterone responses to competition. *Social Neuroscience, 14,* 99-113.

Weller, D., & Lagattuta, K. (2013). Helping the in-group feels better: Children's judgments and emotion attributions in response to prosocial dilemmas. *Child Development, 84*(1), 253-268.

Weller, D., & Lagattuta, K.H. (2013). Helping the in-group feels better: Children's judgments and emotion attributions in response to prosocial dilemmas. *Child Development, 84*(1), 253-268.

Wellman, H.M. (2011). Developing a theory of mind. In U. Goswami (Ed.), *The Blackwell handbook of childhood cognitive development* (2nd ed.). New York: Wiley.

Wentzel, K. (1997). Student motivation in middle school: The role of perceived pedagogical caring. *Journal of Educational Psychology, 89,* 411-419.

Wentzel, K.R. (2013). School adjustment. In I. B. Weiner & others (Eds.), *Handbook of psychology* (2nd ed., Vol. 7). New York: Wiley.

Wentzel, K.R., & Asher, S.R. (1995). The academic lives of neglected, rejected, popular, and controversial children. *Child Development, 66,* 754-763.

Wentzel, K. (2018). A competence-in-context approach to understanding motivation at school. In G. Liem & D. McInerney (Eds.), *Big theories revisited* (2nd ed.). Charlotte, NC: Information Age Publishing.

Werner, B., Berg, M., & Höhr, R. (2019). "Math, I don't get it": An exploratory study on verbalizing mathematical content by students with speech and language impairment, students with learning disability, and students without special educational needs. In D. Kollosche & others (Eds.), *Inclusive mathematics education.* Cham, Switzerland: Springer.

Wertz, J., & others (2018). Genetics and crime: Integrating new genomic discoveries into psychological research about antisocial behavior. *Psychological Science, 29,* 791-803.

Whaley, A.L. (2018). Advances in stereotype threat research on African Americans: Continuing challenges to the validity of its role in the achievement gap. *Social Psychology of Education, 21,* 111-137.

Whaley, L. (2013). Syntactic typology. In J. J. Song (Ed.), *Oxford handbook of linguistic typology.* New York: Oxford University Press.

Whaley, S.E., Jiang, L., Gomez, J., & Jenks, E. (2011). Literacy promotion for families participating in the Women, Infants, and Children program. *Pediatrics, 127,* 454-461.

Whisman, M.A. (2017). Interpersonal perspectives on depression. In R. DeRubeis & D. Strunk (Eds.), *The Oxford handbook of mood disorders* (pp. 167-178). New York: Oxford University Press.

Whitaker, K.J., Vendetti, M.S., Wendelken, C., & Bunge, S.A. (2018). Neuroscientific insights into the development of analogical reasoning. *Developmental Science, 21*(2), e12531.

White, C.N., & Poldrack, R.A. (2018). Methods for fMRI Analysis. *Stevens' handbook of experimental psychology and cognitive neuroscience, 5.*

White, R., Nair, R.L., & Bradley, R.H. (2018). Theorizing the benefits and costs of adaptive cultures for development. *American Psychologist, 73*(6), 727-739.

White, R.M., Knight, G.P., Jensen, M., & Gonzales, N.A. (2018). Ethnic socialization in neighborhood contexts: Implications for ethnic attitude and identity development among Mexican-origin adolescents. *Child Development, 89*(3), 1004-1021.

Whiteman, S.D., Jensen, A., & Bernard, J.M. (2012). Sibling influences. In J. R. Levesque (Ed.), *Encyclopedia of adolescence.* New York: Springer.

Whitesell, C.J., Crosby, B., Anders, T.F., & Teti, D.M. (2018). Household chaos and family sleep during infants' first year. *Journal of Family Psychology, 32,* 622-631.

Wichers, M., & others (2013). Genetic innovation and stability in externalizing problem behavior across development: A multi-informant twin study. *Behavioral Genetics, 43*(3), 191-201.

Wichstrøm, L., & von Soest, T. (2016). Reciprocal relations between body satisfaction and self-esteem: A large 13-year prospective study of adolescents. *Journal of Adolescence, 47,* 16-27.

Widom, C.S., Czaja, S.J., Bentley, T., & Johnson, M.S. (2012). A prospective investigation of physical health outcomes in abused and neglected children: New findings from a 30-year follow-up. *American Journal of Public Health, 102,* 1135-1144.

Wiers, C., & others (2018). Methylation of the dopamine transporter gene in blood is associated with striatal dopamine transporter availability in ADHD. *Biological Psychiatry, 83,* S258-S259.

Wigfield, A., & Gladstone, J.R. (2019). What does expectancy-value theory have to say about motivation and achievement in times of change and uncertainty? In E.N. Gonida & M.S. Lemos (Eds.), *Motivation in education at a time of global change.* Bingley, UK: Emerald Publishing Limited.

Wigfield, A., Eccles, J.S., Schiefele, U., Roeser, R., & Davis-Kean, P. (2006). Development of achievement motivation. In W. Damon & R. Lerner (Eds.), *Handbook of child psychology* (6th ed.). New York: Wiley.

Wille, B., Mouvet, K., Vermeerbergen, M., & Van Herreweghe, M. (2018). Flemish sign language development: A case study on deaf mother–deaf child interactions. *Functions of Language, 25,* 289-322.

Willfors, C., Tammimies, K., & Bölte, S. (2017). Twin research in autism spectrum disorder. In M.F. Casanova, A.S. El-Baz, & J.S. Suri (Eds.), *Autism imaging and devices.* New York: Taylor & Francis.

Williams, E.P., Wyatt, S.B., & Winters, K. (2013). Framing body size among African American women and girls. *Journal of Child Health Care, 17*(3), 219-229.

Williams, J.E., & Best, D.L. (1982). *Measuring sex stereotypes: A thirty-nation study.* Newbury Park, CA: Sage.

Williams, K.E., Berthelsen, D., Walker, S., & Nicholson, J.M. (2017). A developmental cascade model of behavioral sleep problems and emotional and attentional self-regulation across early childhood. *Behavioral Sleep Medicine, 15,* 1-21.

Williams, S.T., Ontai, L.L., & Mastergeorge, A.M. (2010). The development of peer interaction in infancy: Exploring the dyadic process. *Social Development, 19,* 348-368.

Wilson, B.J. (2008). Media and children's aggression, fear, and altruism. *Future of Children, 18*(1), 87-118.

Wilson, D.K., Sweeney, A.M., Kitzman-Ulrich, H., Gause, H., & George, S.M.S. (2017). Promoting social nurturance and positive social environments to reduce obesity in high-risk youth. *Clinical Child and Family Psychology Review, 20,* 64-77.

Wilson, T.M., & Jamison, R. (2019). Perceptions of same-sex and cross-sex peers: Behavioral correlates of perceived coolness during middle childhood. *Merrill-Palmer Quarterly, 65*(1), 1-27.

Winne, P.H. (2017). Cognition and metacognition within self-regulated learning. In B.J. Zimmerman & D.H. Schunk (Eds.), *Handbook of self-regulation of learning and performance.* New York: Routledge.

Winne, P.H. (2018). Theorizing and researching levels of processing in self-regulated learning. *British Journal of Educational Psychology, 88,* 9-20.

Winner, E., & Drake, J.E. (2018). Giftedness and expertise: The case for genetic potential. *Journal of Expertise, 1*(2).

Winner, E. (2000). The origins and ends of giftedness. *American Psychologist, 55,* 159-169.

Winsper, C., Lereya, T., Zanarini, M., & Wolke, D. (2012). Involvement in bullying and suicide-related behavior at 11 years: A prospective birth cohort study. *Journal of the Academy of Child and Adolescent Psychiatry, 51,* 271-282.

Wit, J.M., Kiess, W., & Mullis, P. (2011). Genetic evaluation of short stature. *Best Practices & Research: Clinical Endocrinology and Metabolism, 25,* 1–17.

Witelson, S.F., Kigar, D.L., & Harvey, T. (1999). The exceptional brain of Albert Einstein. *The Lancet, 353,* 2149–2153.

Witherington, D.C., Campos, J.J., Harriger, J.A., Bryan, C., & Margett, T.E. (2010). Emotion and its development in infancy. In J. G. Bremner & T. D. Wachs (Eds.), *Wiley-Blackwell handbook of infant development* (2nd ed.). New York: Wiley.

Witkin, H.A., & others. (1976). Criminality in XYY and XXY men. *Science, 193,* 547–555.

Wolfinger, N.H. (2011). More evidence for trends in the intergenerational transmission of divorce: A completed cohort approach using data from the general social survey. *Demography, 48,* 581–592.

Wolke, D., Schreier, A., Zanarini, M.C., & Winsper, C. (2012). Bullied by peers in childhood and borderline personality symptoms at 11 years of age: A prospective study. *Journal of Child Psychology and Psychiatry, 53,* 846–855.

Women's Sports Foundation (2009). *GoGirlGo! Parents' guide.* New York: Women's Sports Foundation.

Won, S., Wolters, C.A., & Mueller, S.A. (2018). Sense of belonging and self-regulated learning: Testing achievement goals as mediators. *Journal of Experimental Education, 86,* 402–418.

Wong, M.-L., & others (2017). The *PHF21B* gene is associated with major depression and modulates the stress response. *Molecular Psychiatry, 22,* 1015–1025.

Wood, C., Fitton, L., & Rodriguez, E. (2018). Home literacy of kindergarten Spanish-English speaking children from rural low SES backgrounds. *AERA Open, 4,* 1–14.

Wood, W., & Eagly, A.H. (2015). Two traditions of research on gender identity. *Sex Roles, 73*(11–12), 461–473.

Woodhouse, S.S. (2018). Attachment-based interventions for families with young children. *Journal of Clinical Psychology, 74,* 1296–1299.

Woods, R.J., & Schuler, J. (2014). Experience with malleable objects influences shape-based object individuation by infants. *Infant Behavior and Development, 37*(2), 178–186.

World Health Organization (2018). *Breastfeeding.* Retrieved from http://www.who.int/topics/breastfeeding/en/

World Health Organization (2018). *Childhood overweight and obesity.* Retrieved from http://www.who.int/dietphysicalactivity/childhood/en/

Worrell, F.C., Subotnik, R.F., Olszewski-Kubilius, P., & Dixson, D.D. (2019). Gifted students. *Annual Review of Psychology, 70.*

Wray, N.R., & others (2018). Genome-wide association analyses identify 44 risk variants and refine the genetic architecture of major depression. *Nature Genetics, 50,* 668–681.

Wright, R.H., Mindel, C.H., Tran, T.V., & Habenstein, R.W. (2012). *Ethnic families in America* (5th ed.). Upper Saddle River, NJ: Pearson.

Wright, V. (2018). Vygotsky and a global perspective on scaffolding in learning mathematics. In J. Zajda (Ed.), *Globalisation and education reforms.* Dordrecht, the Netherlands: Springer.

Wu, P., & others (2002). Similarities and differences in mothers' parenting of preschoolers in China and the United States. *International Journal of Behavioural Development, 6,* 481–491.

Wu, T.W., Lien, R.I., Seri, I., & Noori, S. (2017). Changes in cardiac output and cerebral oxygenation during prone and supine sleep positioning in healthy term infants. *Archives of Disease in Childhood: Fetal and Neonatal Edition, 102*(6), F483–F489.

Wu, Y., Muentener, P., & Schulz, L.E. (2017). One- to four-year-olds connect diverse positive emotional vocalizations to their probable causes. *Proceedings of the National Academy of Sciences,* 201707715.

Wynn, K. (1992). Addition and subtraction by human infants. *Nature, 358,* 749–570.

X

Xia, Q., & Grant, S.F. (2013). The genetics of human obesity. *Annals of the New York Academy of Sciences, 1281*(1), 178–190.

Xiao, Y., & others (2012). Systematic identification of functional modules related to heart failure with different etiologies. *Gene, 499*(2), 332–338.

Xie, W., Mallin, B.M., & Richards, J.E. (2018). Development of infant sustained attention and its relation to EEG oscillations: An EEG and cortical source analysis study. *Developmental Science, 21*(3), e12562.

Xie, W., Mallin, B.M., & Richards, J.E. (2019). Development of brain functional connectivity and its relation to infant sustained attention in the first year of life. *Developmental Science, 22,* e12703.

Xu, L., & others (2011). Parental overweight/obesity, social factors, and child overweight/obesity at 7 years of age. *Pediatric International, 53,* 826–831.

Y

Yackobovitch-Gavan, M., & others (2018). Intervention for childhood obesity based on parents only or parents and child compared with follow-up alone. *Pediatric Obesity, 13*(11), 647–655.

Yang, C.L., & Chen, C.H. (2018). Effectiveness of aerobic gymnastic exercise on stress, fatigue, and sleep quality during postpartum: A pilot randomized controlled trial. *International Journal of Nursing Studies, 77,* 1–7.

Yang, J., & others (2017). Only-child and non-only-child exhibit differences in creativity and agreeableness: Evidence from behavioral and anatomical structural studies. *Brain Imaging and Behavior, 11*(2), 493–502.

Yang, P., & others (2014). Developmental profile of neurogenesis in prenatal human hippocampus: An immunohistochemical study. *International Journal of Developmental Neuroscience, 38,* 1–9.

Yang, Y.H., Marslen-Wilson, W.D., & Bozic, M. (2017). Syntactic complexity and frequency in the neurocognitive language system. *Journal of Cognitive Neuroscience, 29,* 1605–1620.

Yasui, M., Dishion, T.J., Stormshak, E., & Ball, A. (2015). Socialization of culture and coping with discrimination among American Indian families: Examining cultural correlates of youth outcomes. *Journal of the Society for Social Work and Research, 6*(3), 317–341.

Yates, D. (2013). Neurogenetics: Unraveling the genetics of autism. *Nature Reviews: Neuroscience, 13*(6), 359.

Yau, J.C., & Reich, S.M. (2019). "It's just a lot of work": Adolescents' self-presentation norms and practices on Facebook and Instagram. *Journal of Research on Adolescence, 29*(1), 196–209.

Yazejian, N., & others (2017). Child and parenting outcomes after 1 year of Educare. *Child Development, 88,* 1671–1688.

Yeager, D.S., Dahl, R.E., & Dweck, C.S. (2018). Why interventions to influence adolescent behavior often fail but could succeed. *Perspectives on Psychological Science, 13*(1), 101–122.

Yeager, D.S., Dahl, R.E., & Dweck, C.S. (2018). Why interventions to influence adolescent behavior often fail but could succeed. *Perspectives on Psychological Science, 13,* 101–122.

Yearwood, K., Vliegen, N., Chau, C., Corveleyn, J., & Luyten, P. (2019). When do peers matter? The moderating role of peer support in the relationship between environmental adversity, complex trauma, and adolescent psychopathology in socially disadvantaged adolescents. *Journal of Adolescence, 72,* 14–22.

Yi, O., & others (2012). Association between environmental tobacco smoke exposure of children and parental socioeconomic status: A cross-sectional study in Korea. *Nicotine and Tobacco Research, 14,* 607–615.

Yip, T. (2018). Ethnic/racial identity—A double-edged sword? Associations with discrimination and psychological outcomes. *Current Directions in Psychological Science, 27*(3), 170–175.

Yogman, M., & others (2018). The power of play: A pediatric role in enhancing development in young children. *Pediatrics, 142*(3), e20182058.

Yonker, J.E., Schnabelrauch, C.A., & DeHaan, L.G. (2012). The relationship between spirituality and religiosity on psychological outcomes in adolescents and emerging adults: A meta-analytic review. *Journal of Adolescence, 35,* 299–314.

Yoshikawa, H. (2011). *Immigrants raising citizens: Undocumented parents and their young children.* New York: Russell Sage.

Young, M., Riggs, S., & Kaminski, P. (2017), Role of marital adjustment in associations between romantic attachment and coparenting. *Family Relations, 66,* 331–345.

Yousafzai, A.K., Aboud, F.E., Nores, M., & Britto, P.R. (Eds.). (2018). *Implementation research and practice for early childhood development.* New York: Wiley.

Yu, B., & others (2013). Association of genome-wide variation with highly sensitive cardiac tropin-T (hs-cTnT) levels in European- and African-Americans: A meta-analysis from the Atherosclerosis Risk in Communities and the Cardiovascular Health studies. *Circulation: Cardiovascular Genetics, 6*(1), 82–88.

Yu, H., & others (2016). Lack of association between polymorphisms in Dopa decarboxylase and dopamine receptor-1 genes with childhood autism in

Chinese Han population. *Journal of Child Neurology, 31,* 560-564.

Yu, H., McCoach, D.B., Gottfried, A.W., & Gottfried, A.E. (2017). *Using longitudinal structural equation modeling to study the development of intelligence and its relation to academic achievement.* Thousand Oaks, CA: SAGE.

Yu, H., McCoach, D.B., Gottfried, A.W., & Gottfried, A.E. (2018). Stability of intelligence from infancy through adolescence: An autoregressive latent variable model. *Intelligence, 69,* 8-15.

Yuan, F., Gu, X., Huang, X., Zhong, Y., & Wu, J. (2017). SLC6A1 gene involvement in susceptibility to attention-deficit/hyperactivity disorder: A case-control study and gene-environment interaction. *Progress in Neuro-Psychopharmacology and Biological Psychiatry, 77,* 202-208.

Yuan, L., Uttal, D., & Gentner, D. (2017). Analogical processes in children's understanding of spatial representations. *Developmental Psychology, 53*(6), 1098-1114.

Yuen, R., Chen, B., Blair, J.D., Robinson, W.P., & Nelson, D.M. (2013). Hypoxia alters the epigenetic profile in cultured human placental trophoblasts, *Epigenetics, 8*(2), 192-202.

Z

Zaboski, B.A., Kranzler, J.H., & Gage, N.A. (2018). Meta-analysis of the relationship between academic achievement and broad abilities of the Cattell-horn-Carroll theory. *Journal of School Psychology, 71,* 42-56.

Zaccaro, A., & Freda, M.F. (2014). Making sense of risk diagnosis in case of prenatal and reproductive genetic counseling for neuromuscular diseases. *Journal of Health Psychology, 19*(3), 344-357.

Zachary, C., Jones, D.J., McKee, L.G., Baucom, D.H., & Forehand, R.L. (2019). The role of emotion regulation and socialization in behavioral parent training: A proof-of-concept study. *Behavior Modification, 43,* 3-25.

Zeanah, C.H., Fox, N.A., & Nelson, C.A. (2012). Case study in ethical issues in research: The Bucharest Early Intervention Project. *Journal of Nervous and Mental Disease, 200,* 243-247.

Zeiders, K.H., Roosa, M.W., & Tein, J.Y. (2011). Family structure and family processes in Mexican-American families. *Family Process, 50,* 77-91.

Zeiders, K.H., Umana-Taylor, A.J., & Derlan, C.L. (2013). Trajectories of depressive symptoms and self-esteem in Latino youths: Examining the role of gender and perceived discrimination. *Developmental Psychology, 49*(5), 951-963.

Zelazo, P.D. (2015). Executive function: Reflection, iterative reprocessing, complexity, and the developing brain. *Developmental Review, 38,* 55-68.

Zell, E., Krizan, Z., & Teeter, S.R. (2015). Evaluating gender similarities and differences using metasynthesis. *American Psychologist, 70,* 10-20.

Zembal-Saul, C.L., McNeill, K.L., & Hershberger, K. (2013). *What's your evidence?* Upper Saddle River, NJ: Pearson.

Zhang, J., Shim, G., de Toledo, S.M., & Azzam, E.I. (2017). The translationally controlled tumor protein and the cellular response to ionizing radiation-induced DNA damage. *Results and Problems in Cell Differentiation, 64,* 227-253.

Zhang, L-F., & Sternberg, R.J. (2013). Learning in cross-cultural perspective. In T. Husen & T. N. Postlethwaite (Eds.), *International encyclopedia of education* (3rd ed.). New York: Elsevier.

Zhang, W., Xing, W., Li, L., Chen, L., & Deater-Deckard, K. (2017). Reconsidering parenting in Chinese culture: Subtypes, stability, and change of maternal parenting style during early adolescence. *Journal of Adolescence, 46*(5), 1117-1136.

Zhang, X., & others (2018). Characteristics of likability, perceived popularity, and admiration in the early adolescent peer system in the United States and China. *Developmental Psychology, 54*(8), 1568-1581.

Zhang, X., Hashimoto, J.G., & Guizzetti, M. (2018). Developmental neurotoxicity of alcohol: Effects and mechanisms of ethanol on the developing brain. *Advances in Neurotoxicology, 2,* 115-144.

Zhou, H., Wang, B., Sun, H., Xu, X., & Wang, Y. (2018). Epigenetic regulations in neural stem cells and neurological diseases. *Stem Cells International.* doi:10.1155/2018/6087143

Zhou, M., & Gonzales, R.G. (2019, in press). Divergent destinies: Children of immigrants growing up in the United States. *Annual Review of Sociology, 45.*

Zhu, M., Urhahne, D., & Rubie-Davies, C.M. (2018). The longitudinal effects of teacher judgement and different teacher treatment on students' academic outcomes. *Educational Psychology, 38,* 648-668.

Zhu, P., Wang, W., Zuo, R., & Sun, K. (2018). Mechanisms for establishment of the placental glucocorticoid barrier, a guard for life. *Cellular and Molecular Life Sciences, 76*(1), 13-26.

Zill, N. (2017). *The changing face of adoption in the United States.* Charlottesville, VA: Institute for Family Studies.

Zimmer-Gembeck, M.J., & others (2017). Is parent-child attachment a correlate of children's emotion regulation and coping? *International Journal of Behavioral Development, 41,* 74-93.

Zimmerman, B.J. (2002). Becoming a self-regulated learner: An overview. *Theory into Practice, 41,* 64-70.

Zimmerman, B.J. (2012). Motivational sources and outcomes of self-regulated learning and performance. In B. J. Zimmerman & D. H. Schunk (Eds.), *Handbook of self-regulation of learning and performance.* New York: Routledge.

Zimmerman, B.J., Bonner, S., & Kovach, R. (1996). *Developing self-regulated learners.* Washington, DC: American Psychological Association.

Zimmerman, B.J., & Kitsantas, A. (1997). Developmental phases in self-regulation: Shifting from process goals to outcome goals. *Journal of Educational Psychology, 89,* 29-36.

Zimmerman, B.J., & Labuhn, A.S. (2012). Self-regulation of learning: Process approaches to personal development. In K. R. Harris & others (Eds.), *APA handbook of educational psychology.* Washington, DC: American Psychological Association.

Zimmerman, F.J., Christakis, D.A., & Meltzoff, A.N. (2007). Associations between media viewing and language development in children under age 2 years. *Journal of Pediatrics, 151,* 364-368.

Ziol-Guest, K.M. (2009). Child custody and support. In D. Carr (Ed.), *Encyclopedia of the life course and human development.* Boston: Cengage.

Zotter, H., & Pichler, G. (2012). Breast feeding is associated with decreased risk of sudden infant death syndrome. *Evidence Based Medicine, 17,* 126-127.

Zsakai, A., Karkus, Z., Utczas, K., & Bodzsar, E.B. (2017). Body structure and physical self-concept in early adolescence. *The Journal of Early Adolescence, 37,* 316-338.

Zuckerman, M. (1999). *Vulnerability to psychopathology: A biosocial model.* Washington, DC: American Psychological Association.

Zych, I., Farrington, D.P., & Ttofi, M.M. (2018). Protective factors against bullying and cyberbullying: A systematic review of meta-analyses. *Aggression and Violent Behavior, 45,* 4-19.

name index

Kalish, C. W., 252
Kallol, S., 71
Kalutskaya, I., 285
Kaminski, P., 395
Kamradt, J. M., 458
Kan, M. L., 388
Kanacri, B. P. L., 367
Kanakis, G. A., 53
Kaneko, T., 315
Kang, J., 484
Kang, S., 172
Kania-Richmond, A., 81
Kanji, A., 150
Kannass, K. N., 236
Kanoy, K., 394
Kaplan, J. S., 61
Kaplan, R., 410, 481
Kapplinger, J. D., 113
Kapur, B. M., 71
Karaman, F., 249
Karasik, L. B., 139
Karkus, Z., 102
Karl, J. M., 141
Karle, K. N., 226
Karlsson, J., 116
Karmel, B. Z., 233
Kárpáti, A., 239
Karpyk, P., 207
Karreman, A., 395
Karremans, J. C., 369
Kassai, R., 192, 204
Katz, C., 201
Katzmarzyk, P. T., 127
Kauchak, D., 443
Kauffman, J. M., 461
Kaufman, J. C., 238
Kaufman-Parks, A., 397
Kauko, S., 399
Kaur, H., 119
Kavsek, M., 190
Kawwass, J. F., 58
Kaye, B., 13
Kazak, A. E., 4
Kazi, S., 175, 188
Kazura, K., 401
Ke, F. F., 458
Keag, O. E., 86
Keane, S. P., 418
Kearney, R., 280
Kearsley, R. B., 278
Keefer, K. V., 226
Keen, R., 142, 146, 149, 154
Keenan, R., 54
Kees, M., 282
Keeton, C. P., 278
Kehle, T. J., 457
Keil, F. C., 312
Keller, H., 244, 245
Keller, M., 358, 425
Kellman, P. J., 143, 147
Kellmann, M., 141
Kelly, E., 485
Kelly, J., 408
Kelly, K. M., 117
Kelly, R. J., 112, 113, 114
Kelly, S. P., 190
Kelmanson, I. A., 113
Kelty, E., 77

Kendler, K. S., 62, 438
Kendrick, C., 402
Kendrick, K., 424, 430
Kenko, Y., 273
Kennedy, J. F., 475
Kennedy, J. L., 382
Kennell, J. H., 93
Kenny, S., 148
Kern, M. L., 370
Kern, P., 85
Kerns, K. A., 296, 389
Kerpelman, J. L., 323
Kerr, D., 125
Kessen, W., 135
Kessler, B., 246
Keuning, J., 235
Key, A. C., 345
Keyser, J., 390
Kezuka, E., 150
Khatun, M., 88
Khoury, B., 205
Khoury, J. C., 140, 141
Khoza-Shangase, K., 150
Khundrakpam, B. S., 227
Kiang, L., 324, 438
Kibby, M. Y., 457
Kidd, C., 189
Kiel, E. J., 286
Kiess, W., 99, 492
Kiewra, K. A., 493
Kigar, D. L., 227
Kilby, M. D., 57
Killen, M., 309, 338, 355, 361, 362
Killoren, S. E., 398, 420
Kim, E. M., 470
Kim, H., 50
Kim, J., 50, 118, 366
Kim, J. M., 336
Kim, K. H., 238
Kim, N., 50
Kim, P., 480
Kim, S., 294, 359
Kim, S. H., 374, 375
Kim, S. Y., 484
Kim, T., 366
Kim, T. J., 260
Kim, T. Y., 485
Kim, Y., 172
Kim-Spoon, J., 193, 376, 396
Kinard, J. L., 191
Kincaid, C. Y., 485
King, A. P., 263
King, C., 127
King, K. A., 376
King, P. E., 374, 375
King, S., 127
King-Casas, B., 193
Kingston, M. H., 306, 324
Kini, S., 58
Király, I., 196, 290
Kirby, J. R., 187
Kirkby, J., 112
Kirkebøen, L. J., 404
Kirkorian, H. L., 146, 491
Kirova, A., 178
Kisilevsky, B. S., 150
Kitamura, S., 469
Kitayama, S., 102, 310

Kitsantas, A., 467
Kitsantas, P., 113
Kitzman-Ulrich, H., 124
Kjelgaard, H. H., 124
Klausen, T., 58
Klebanoff, M., 83
Kleen, H., 334
Kleiman, K., 92
Kleinsorge, C., 405
Klemfuss, J. Z., 200
Kliewer, W., 422
Klimek, B., 213
Klimstra, T. A., 320
Klin, A., 146
Kling, J., 103, 316
Klinger, L. G., 459
Klopp-Dutote, N., 151
Kloza, E. M., 57
Knafo-Noam, A., 356
Knickmeyer, R. C., 105
Knifsend, C. A., 453
Knight, G. P., 324, 369
Knopik, V. S., 286
Knopp, K., 383
Knopp, K. A., 421
Knox, M., 393
Ko, C. H., 493
Kobayashi, T., 254
Kobulsky, J. M., 60
Kochanska, G., 294, 359, 363
Kochenderfer-Ladd, B., 422
Kocur, J. L., 397
Koehn, A. J., 389
Koenig, L. B., 375
Koerber, S., 214
Kofler, M. J., 459
Kohl, P. L., 397
Kohlberg, L., 353–355
Kohlhoff, J., 296
Kokkinaki, T. S., 276
Kokkinidis, D. G., 77
Koleilat, M., 122
Kolkman, M. E., 195
Kolko, D. J., 4
Kolski, C., 151
Kondo-Ikemura, K., 294
Kong, A., 80
Konrad, K., 278
Koopman, P., 51
Koot, H. M., 368
Kopish, M. A., 366
Kopp, C. B., 278
Kopp, F., 191
Koppleman, K. L., 454, 455
Kornienko, O., 324
Körük, S., 316
Kosik-Bogacka, D., 79
Kostons, D. D., 188, 212
Kotovsky, L., 165
Kotte, E. M., 125
Koufaki, Z. E., 276
Kouros, C. D., 405
Kovach, R., 467
Kozbelt, A., 196, 236
Kozol, J., 454
Krabbendam, L., 273
Kraemer, H. C., 124
Krafft, C., 299

Kramer, H. J., 214, 310
Kramer, L., 401
Krampe, R., 236
Kranenburg, M. J., 358
Kranzler, J. H., 227
Krasno, A. M., 190
Krassner, A. M., 274, 287
Krauss, R. A., 421
Krekó, K., 290
Kretch, K. S., 146, 149
Krettenauer, T., 358, 361, 363
Kreutzer, L. C., 215
Kreye, M., 278
Kring, A. M., 342
Krist, H., 164
Kristjánsson, K., 365
Krizan, Z., 339, 342
Kroesbergen, E. H., 195
Kroger, J., 322
Kroonenberg, P. M., 294
Kroupina, M. G., 263, 267
Krowitz, A., 149
Krull, J. L., 114
Kruse, A., 401
Kubarych, T. S., 61
Kubiszewski, V., 172
Kuchirko, Y., 255, 382, 477
Kuhl, P. K., 245, 249, 263
Kuhn, B. R., 394
Kuhn, D., 110, 187, 188, 205, 209,
    210, 211, 215, 216
Kuhns, C., 297
Kulig, T. C., 418
Kumar, N. L., 479
Kung, K. T., 330
Kuo, L. J., 260
Kupán, K., 290
Kupersmidt, J. B., 422
Kurjak, A., 56
Kurkul, K. E., 168
Kurland, D. M., 199
Kvalem, I. L., 315
Kwiatkowski, M. A., 77
Kwon, J. H., 50

L

Labella, M. H., 204, 274
Labuhn, A. S., 467
Lacelle, C., 397
Lack, L. C., 114
Ladd, G. W., 422
Ladd, H. C., 444, 445
LaFontana, K. M., 422
Lagattuta, K. H., 214, 310, 311, 368
Laird, R. D., 390
Lam, C. K., 279
Lamaze, F., 84
Lamb, M. A., 201
Lamb, M. E., 108, 200, 291, 297
Lampl, M., 99
Landesman-Dwyer, S., 76
Landi, K., 113
Landry, S. H., 280
Lane, D. M., 236
Lang, E., 453
Langenskiöld, S., 55
Langer, A., 149

subject index

A

Abecedarian Project, 230
abstract, of journal articles, 32
abstract thinking, in adolescents, 171-172, 309
abuse. *See* child maltreatment
academic cheating, 366-367
accelerometer, 126
accent, 258
accommodation, 160-161
accountability, from schools, 444-445
acculturation, 324, 399, 411
achievement, 462-470
  cognitive processes and, 463-468
  cultural diversity and, 468
  electronic media and, 491-492
  ethnicity and, 468
  gender differences in, 343
  intelligence quotient and, 224
  motivation and, 462-463
  purpose and, 467-468
  screen time and, 492
  self-esteem and, 316
  socioeconomic status and, 479
achievement identity, 318
acquired immune deficiency syndrome (AIDS), 78, 118
active dimension, 308
active genotype-environment correlations, 62, 63
acupuncture, 85
adaptation, 160
adaptive behavior, 45
Adderall, 459
ADHD. *See* attention deficit hyperactivity disorder
adolescents
  adoption of, 60
  from affluent families, 479
  alcohol's impact on, 28
  antisocial behavior in, 369-373
  and attachment, 398, 420
  attention in, 193, 215-216
  autonomy and, 397-398
  brain development in, 110-111
  brain imaging of, 28, 110
  cognitive development in, 171-173, 480
  conflict with parents, 398-399
  dating and romantic relationships among, 435-438
  decision making in, 210-211
  definition of, 12
  of divorced parents, 405
  education of, 449-453
  egocentrism in, 172-173
  emotional development in, 273
  emotional intelligence in, 226
  Erikson's psychosocial theory on, 17-19
  ethnicity of, 483

exercise in, 127
friendships of, 430-431, 432, 433
gender development in, 334, 335
gender identity in, 344-345
gratitude in, 369
identity development in, 17, 18, 19, 319-321
intelligence in, 234
Internet use by, 492-493
language development in, 260-261
media use by, 489, 490, 492
memory in, 199, 201
metacognition in, 215-216
moral development in, 354
as mothers, 80, 88, 384
parental monitoring of, 390-391, 493
parents and, 397-399
peer relationships of, 419, 434-438
physical growth in, 100-103
Piaget's theory on, 20
in poverty, 480, 481
pregnancy in, 80, 88, 384
problem solving in, 207-208
prosocial behavior in, 368, 369
puberty in, 100-103
religious development in, 375-376
role of attachment for, 398
self-esteem in, 315, 316, 317
self-regulation in, 467
self-understanding in, 309-310
service learning for, 365-366
and sibling relationships, 401-402
sleep in, 114-115
social cognition in, 312-313
television's effects on, 490, 492
temperament in, 287
thinking in, 208-211
video game use of, 490-491
adoption, 59-61
adoption study, 61, 228, 286
affection, in friendship, 430
affordances, 143-144
Africa
  breast and bottle feeding in, 121
  childbirth in, 83
  female access to education in, 7
  infant massage in, 89, 139
  self-esteem in, 317
African Americans
  antipoverty programs for, 481-482
  child care decisions of, 411
  dating, 438
  discrimination against, 487
  education and, 455
  exercise rates for, 127
  gifted children, 238
  height of, 99
  intelligence test scores of, 231, 232
  overweight children, 124
  and parent-adolescent conflict, 399
  parental monitoring of, 390
  parenting styles of, 392

in poverty, 8, 479
preterm infants, 87
school dropout rate for, 452
self-esteem of, 486
in service learning programs, 366
sickle-cell anemia in, 54
single-parent families, 410
single-sex education for, 335
social cognition in, 312
sudden infant death syndrome in, 113
term used for, 34-35
afterbirth, 82
age
  chronological, 223
  and having children, 384, 387
  maternal, 80
  mental, 223
  paternal, 80
aggression
  discouraging, 343
  and friendship, 431
  gender differences in, 340-341, 342
  observation of, 26
  in peer relationships, 422, 423
  physical punishment and, 393
  social cognitive theory on, 23
  television and, 490
  testosterone and, 332
AIDS, 78, 118
Aka pygmy culture, 297
alcohol
  and adolescents, 28
  prenatal exposure to, 76
Algonquin people, 139
allergies, 119
alphabetic principle, 255
altruism, 368
ambiguous line drawing, 213-214
American Psychological Association (APA), 33
amnesia, infantile, 198
amniocentesis, 56-57
amnion, 71
amniotic fluid, 71, 72
amygdala, 105, 110, 286, 296
analgesia, 83
analogies, problem solving using, 208
anal stage, 16
analytical intelligence, 224-225
androgen-insensitive males, 331
androgens, 101, 331, 339
androgyny, 344
anemia, sickle-cell, 54
anencephaly, 74
anesthesia, 83
anger cry, 277
animism, 168
A-not-B error, 164
anticipatory smiling, 277
antidepressants, in postpartum period, 92
antipoverty programs, 480-482

antisocial behavior, 360, 369-373, 431
anxiety
  in postpartum period, 91
  during pregnancy, 80
  stranger, 278
Apgar Scale, 86
aphasia, 262
art prodigy, 236
Ascend (Aspen Institute), 9
ASD. *See* autism spectrum disorders
Asian Americans
  acculturation in, 411
  adolescents, 483
  discrimination against, 487
  diversity of, 487
  education and, 455
  overweight children, 124
  parental expectations of, 474
  parenting styles of, 392
  school dropout rate for, 452
Asperger syndrome, 459
assimilation, 160-161, 172
assisted reproductive technologies (ART), 58
asthma
  breast feeding protecting against, 119
  in children born at low birth weight, 88
  parental smoking and, 116
atopic dermatitis, 119
attachment, 292-296
  as adaptive behavior, 45
  in adolescence, 398, 420, 437
  adoption and, 60
  breast feeding and, 120
  child care and, 297
  child maltreatment and, 396
  definition of, 292
  developmental social neuroscience and, 296
  development of, 292-293
  divorce and, 405
  importance of, 292
  individual differences in, 293-294
  interpreting differences in, 294-296
  in middle and late childhood, 296
  and moral development, 363
  negative, 24, 293, 296
  parents responding to infant crying and, 279
  and peer relationships, 420
  positive, 24, 293, 295-296
  theories of, 292-293
attention, 189-193
  in adolescents, 193, 215-216
  in children, 191-192
  cognitive control of, 192, 193
  definition of, 189
  divided, 190, 193 (*See also* multitasking)
  executive, 190, 192, 193, 203
  improving, 192

effortful control, 285
egg, 50, 70
egocentrism, 167-168
    adolescent, 172-173
    definition of, 167
    in early childhood, 167-168, 311
    recent research on, 311, 352
ego support, in friendship, 430
Eisenhower Foundation, 482
elaboration, and memory, 199
electroencephalogram (EEG), 106
electronic media, 491-492
elementary school, 449
elementary school teacher, 39, 179
ELLs. See English Language Learners
embryo, 70
embryonic period, 70-72, 73, 75
emotional abuse, 396
emotional and behavioral disorders, 459
emotional competence, 274-275
emotional development, 275-282
    in adolescents, 274
    in early childhood, 279-281
    gender and, 339-343
    in infants, 273, 274, 276-279
    in middle and late childhood,
        281-282
    parents and, 280, 384
emotional expression, 276-278
emotional intelligence, 226, 274
emotional knowledge, 226
emotional neglect, 396
emotional regulation
    caregivers and, 274
    child maltreatment and, 396
    in early childhood, 280
    encouraging, 343
    gender differences in, 342, 343
    in infants, 278-279
    in middle and late childhood, 281
    peer relations and, 280-281, 421-422
emotional security theory, 405
emotion-coaching approach, 280, 384
emotion-dismissing approach, 280, 384
emotions
    biological foundation of, 273
    cultural variations in, 274
    and decision making, 210
    definition of, 273
    expressing, 279
    in family processes, 383-384
    functionalist view of, 274
    gender differences in, 342
    and moral reasoning, 356, 360
    negative, 273, 285
    other-conscious, 276
    play and, 429
    positive, 273, 285, 342
    in postpartum period, 91-93
    during pregnancy, 80
    primary, 276
    self-conscious, 276, 279
    in sibling relationships, 401
    and theory of mind, 212
    understanding, 279-280
empathy
    in adolescents, 312, 360
    capacity for, 281, 359

definition of, 359
development of, 359-360
    in early childhood, 359
    in infants, 359
    in middle and late childhood, 281,
        311, 359-360
empiricist view, 152, 153
encoding, 188
endoderm, 70
English Language Learners (ELLs),
    259, 260
entity theories of intelligence, 225-227
environmental experiences. See also
        nature-nurture issue
    and aggression, 340
    and attention deficit hyperactivity
        disorder, 458
    and autism, 460
    and brain development, 107-108
    and conduct disorder, 370
    and emotions, 273
    and growth, 99
    heredity and (See heredity-
        environment correlations)
    and intelligence, 228-229
    and language development, 262-264
    nonshared, 63
    and overweight, 124
    and puberty, 101
    shared, 63
environmental hazards, prenatal
        exposure to, 78
epigenetic view, 64
equality, 368
equilibration, 161
Erikson's psychosocial theory, 17-19
    on attachment, 292
    definition of, 17
    early-later experience issue and, 17
    on identity, 17-19, 319, 320
    life-span stages in, 17-19
    strategies based on, 18
Eskimo infants, sudden infant death
        syndrome in, 113
estradiol, 101, 331
estrogens, 101, 331, 339
ethical issues, in research, 33
ethnic bias, in research, 34-35
ethnic gloss, 34-35
ethnic identity, 318, 323-324, 325
ethnicity/ethnic groups, 483-488
    and achievement, 468
    of adolescents, 483
    and adoption, 59
    and autonomy-granting, 398
    and child care, 411
    definition of, 6, 483
    differences and diversity within,
        486-487
    and exercise, 127
    and family variations, 409-410
    and gender roles, 346
    and identity development, 323-324
    and intelligence tests, 231-232
    and overweight children, 124
    and parent-adolescent conflict, 399
    and parental monitoring, 390
    and parenting styles, 392

and poverty, 479
prejudice toward, 487
and preterm infants, 87
and school dropout rates,
    451-452, 484
in schools, 455-456
and service learning programs, 366
and social cognition, 312
and socioeconomic status, 485-486
ethnocentrism, 475
ethological theory, 23-24
    child development issues and, 26
    criticisms of, 24
    overview of, 23-24
ethology, definition of, 23
Every Student Succeeds Act (2015), 444
evocative genotype-environment
        correlations, 62-63
evolution, and brain development, 262
evolutionary psychology, 45-47
    criticisms of, 332
    definition of, 45
    on development, 46-47
    evaluating, 47
    on gender, 332
exceptional children teacher, 39
executive attention, 190, 192, 193, 203
executive function
    in adolescents, 208-209
    autism and, 214
    in children, 203-204
    definition of, 203
    and theory of mind, 215
exercise
    in adolescents, 127
    in early childhood, 125-126
    influences on, 127-128
    in middle and late childhood,
        126-127
    organized sports as, 140-141
    in postpartum period, 92
    during pregnancy, 30, 81
    video games requiring, 491
exergames, 491
exosystem, 24, 25
expanding, 263
expectations
    mutual interpersonal, 353
    of parents, 466, 469, 474, 478
    perceptual development and,
        164-166
    and performance, 465-466
    socioeconomic status and, 486
    of teachers, 466
experience, early or later, 14, 15, 17
experimental groups, 30
experimental research, 30, 31
experiments
    children designing, 205-206
    definition of, 30
expertise, 196
explicit memory, 197, 198
expressive traits, 337
extraversion/surgency, 284
extremely low birth weight newborns, 87
extrinsic motivation, 462-463
eye tracking equipment, 146
eyewitnesses, 200-201

face perception, 147
face-to-face play, 290
fairness, 368
false beliefs, 213
families/family influences, 380-412.
        See also fathers; mothers;
        parents/parenting; siblings
    child care and, 301
    child development careers
        involving, 41
    on coping with stress, 281
    on emotions, 273
    on identity development, 322
    intergenerational relationships in,
        399-400
    on juvenile delinquency, 371
    on language development, 254
    on moral development, 352,
        356-357, 363-364
    recently immigrated, 324, 399, 484
    of transgender children, 345
family and consumer science
        educator, 40
family intervention experiments,
    372, 373
family processes
    cognition and emotion in,
        383-384
    divorce and, 405-406
    domain-specific socialization in,
        384-385
    interactions in, 382-383
    multiple developmental trajectories
        in, 384
    sociocultural and historical changes
        in, 385-386
family therapist, 41, 395
family therapy, 371
family trends
    children in divorced families,
        404-406
    cultural and ethnic variations in,
        409-410
    gay and lesbian parents, 408-409
    socioeconomic variations in,
        410-411
    stepfamilies, 406-408
    working parents, 403-404
fast food, 123
fast mapping, 252, 253
Fast Track intervention program, 373
fathers. See also parents/parenting
    attachment to, 294, 297
    as caregivers, 272, 297
    depression in, 297
    fetus recognizing voice of, 150
    and gender development, 333
    involvement of, after divorce, 406
    in postpartum period, 92-93
    and prenatal development, 80
    and shaken baby syndrome, 106
    smoking, 80
fear
    amygdala and, 286
    classically conditioned, 22
    in infants, 277-278

postpartum expert, 92
postpartum period, 90–93
  definition of, 90
  emotional and psychological
    adjustments in, 91–93
  physical adjustments in, 91
post-traumatic stress disorder
  (PTSD), 282
posture, 136
poverty, 479–482
  and child-care quality, 299, 300–301
  and education, 454
  educational programs for children
    in, 446–448
  and health, 117–118
  and intelligence, 229, 230
  interventions to counter effects of,
    480–482
  and juvenile delinquency, 372–373
  and lead poisoning, 116
  and nutrition, 122
  and parenting style, 478, 480
  and prenatal care, 81
  and preterm and low birth weight
    infants, 88
  psychological ramifications of, 480
  risks to children living in, 481
  and self-esteem, 486
  social policy and, 8–10
  and stress, 8–9, 481, 486
  and sudden infant death
    syndrome, 113
  and vocabulary development, 254
power assertion, 363
practical intelligence, 225, 226
practical knowledge, 225
practice play, 427–428
pragmatics, 247, 253–254
praise
  inflated, 317
  and intrinsic motivation, 462
precocious puberty, 101
precocity, 236, 238
preconventional reasoning, 353, 354
prefrontal cortex, 108, 109–110, 111
prefrontal lobes, 198, 286
pregnancy. See also prenatal
    development
  in adolescents, 80, 88, 384
  alcohol use during, 76
  caffeine use during, 76
  diagnostic tests during, 56–57
  diet and nutrition during, 79
  exercise during, 30, 81
  maternal age and, 80
  maternal diseases during, 78–79
  maternal weight gain and, 118–119
  medications during, 76
  prenatal care during, 80–81
  psychoactive drugs during, 76–77
  smoking during, 71, 76–77, 99, 113
  trimesters of, 73, 74
prejudice, 487
prenatal care, 80–81
prenatal development, 70–81
  of brain, 74
  definition of, 11
  embryonic period of, 70–72, 73, 75

fetal period of, 72–74, 75
of gender, 331
germinal period of, 70, 71, 73, 75
hazards to, 74–80
of hearing, 149–150
normal, 81–82
paternal factors in, 80
teratogens and, 75–76
trimesters of, 73, 74
prenatal diagnostic tests, 56–57
preoperational stage, 166–169
  centration in, 168–169
  definition of, 167
  description of, 19, 20, 167
  intuitive thought substage of, 168
  symbolic function of, 167–168
preoperational thought, 167, 168–169
prepared childbirth, 84
preschool children. See also early
    childhood
  exercise in, 125–126
  games of, 429
  gender development in, 334
  language development in, 251,
    252, 253
  motor development in, 138–141
  peer relationships of, 418–419
  play by, 427, 428, 429
  self-understanding in, 308, 309
  sex-typed play in, 330
  temperament in, 285
  universal education for, 449
preschool teacher, 40
pretense/symbolic play, 428
preterm infants, 87–89
  assessment of, 87
  definition of, 87
  issues affecting, 87–88
  massage for, 89–90
  nurturing, 88–89
primary circular reactions, 162
primary emotions, 276
primates, brain sizes of, 46–47
princess movies, 329, 338
principle of persistence, 165
private speech, 177, 178
proactive parenting strategies, 364
problem solving, 206–208
  using analogies for, 208
  using rules for, 206–208
  using strategies for, 208
progestin, 87
Program for International Student
    Assessment (PISA), 445
Project Head Start, 446–448
prosocial behavior
  in adolescents, 368
  capacity for, 359
  development of, 368
  emotional regulation and, 311
  encouraging, 343
  and friendship, 431
  gender differences in, 342, 368
  and moral development, 368–369
  moral motivation of, 425
  types of, 369
  video games and, 491
protection, in parenting, 384

protest, separation, 278
proximodistal pattern, 99
psychiatrist, 40, 456
psychoactive drugs, prenatal exposure
    to, 76–77
psychoanalytic theories, 16–19. See
    also Erikson's psychosocial
    theory; Freudian theory
  child development issues and, 26
  definition of, 16, 17
  evaluating, 19
psychological invulnerability, 172
psychosocial moratorium, 319
psychotherapy, in postpartum
    period, 92
Psy.D. degree, 40
PTSD. See post-traumatic stress
    disorder
puberty
  body image in, 102–103, 451
  and dating, 435
  definition of, 100
  determinants of, 100–102
  early and late maturation in, 103
  growth spurt in, 102
  precocious, 101
  school transition in, 451
  sexual maturation in, 102, 103
Pukapukan culture, 83
punishments
  effectiveness of, 358
  marital conflict and use of, 394
  and moral development, 353
  operant conditioning and, 22
  physical, 392, 393–394
  socioeconomic status and, 478
purpose, and achievement, 467–468

Q

Quantum Opportunities Program, 482
questionnaire. See survey

R

random assignment, in research, 30
rapport talk, 341
reaching, in infants, 141–142
reaction-time task, 187
reading
  gender differences in, 340
  international comparisons of, 468
  in learning disabilities, 457
  shared, 264
reading comprehension, 257
reading development, 254–255
  in adolescents, 261
  fluency in, 257
  phonics approach to, 257
  stages of, 256–257
  strategy instruction in, 209
  whole-language approach to, 257
reading problems, 252
real self, 309, 310
reasoning
  vs. automatic responses, 356
  conventional, 353–354
  hypothetical-deductive, 171
  postconventional, 354

preconventional, 353, 354
  social conventional, 361–362
recasting, 263
receptive vocabulary, 249
receptors, 143
recessive gene, 51
reciprocal interactions, 277, 382
reciprocal socialization, 382, 383
reciprocity
  in parenting, 385
  in peer relationships, 419
reconstructive memory, 200–201
references, in journal articles, 32
referral bias, 457
reflexes, 134–135
  definition of, 134
  simple, 162
reflexive smile, 277
reframing, 281
Reggio Emilia approach, 442, 445
rejected children, 422
relational aggression, 340–341
relationship communication, 341
relationship identity, 318
relationships. See also families/family
    influences; parents/parenting;
    peer relationships; romantic
    relationships
  child development careers
    involving, 41
religion, definition of, 374
religious development, 374–376
religious identity, 318
religiousness, definition of, 374
remarriage, 406–408
REM sleep, 112
report talk, 341
reproductive technology, 57–58
research
  bias in, 34–35
  careers in, 39–40
  correlational, 29
  data collection methods for, 25–28
  descriptive, 29
  ethical issues in, 33
  experimental, 30, 31
  importance of, 15–16
  journal publication of, 32
  scientific method in, 16
  time span of, 30–31
researcher, 39, 206
research journals, 32
resilience, 6–8, 295, 479
results, in journal articles, 32
rewards
  effectiveness of, 358
  operant conditioning and, 22
Rh-factor, 78
RhoGAM, 78
risk/risk perception
  in adolescents, 172
  and decision making, 211
  intellectual, 239
Ritalin, 459
romantic relationships, 435–438
  adjustment and, 436–437
  heterosexual, 435–436
  and identity development, 322–323

romantic relationships—*Cont.*
  parent-adolescent relationships and, 437–438
  same-sex, 436
  sociocultural contexts of, 438
rooming-in arrangement, in hospitals, 93
rooting reflex, 134, 135
Rothbart and Bates' classification of temperament, 284–286
rubella, 78
rules
  in games, 429
  problem solving using, 206–208

S

same-sex education. *See* single-sex education
same-sex marriage, 408–409
same-sex play groups, 334
same-sex romantic relationships, 436
satire, 260
scaffolding, 176, 180, 382–383
schemas
  definition of, 195, 336
  gender, 336
schema theory, 195, 197
schemes, 160
  behavioral, 160
  coordination of, 163
  internalization of, 163
  mental, 160
school counselor, 40, 325
school dropout rate, 451–452
  in children born at low birth weight, 87, 88
  ethnicity and, 451–452, 484
  gender differences in, 340
  programs aimed at decreasing, 482
school psychologist, 40
school readiness, 192, 204
schools. *See also* education; teachers
  accountability from, 444–445
  elementary, 449
  ethnicity in, 455–456
  exercise in, 127
  extracurricular activities at, 453
  and gender development, 334–335
  high, 451–453
  middle and junior high, 449–451
  mindfulness training in, 205
  and moral development, 364–367
  recess eliminated in, 429
  scientific thinking taught in, 206
  socioeconomic variations in, 454
school segregation, 455
scientific method, 16, 17
scientific thinking, 205–206
screen time
  and achievement, 492
  and attention regulation, 192
  in early childhood, 491
  and exercise, 126, 127–128
  in infancy, 491
  negative effects of, 489, 491
  play time reduced due to, 427
scripts, 197

secondary circular reactions, 162–163, 164
second-generation immigrants, 324
secondhand smoke, 80, 116
second-language learning, 258–259
securely attached babies, 293, 295–296
security, 292
selective attention, 189
self
  contradictions with, 310
  definition of, 307
  fluctuating, 310
  ideal, 309, 310
  looking glass, 310
  possible, 310
  real, 309, 310
self-assertiveness, 343
self-awareness, 276
self-competence, 343
self-concept, 313–318
  assessment of, 314–315
  culture and, 477
  definition of, 313
self-conscious emotions, 276, 279
self-consciousness, 309
self-control. *See* self-regulation
self-determination, 462
self-efficacy, 239, 465
self-esteem, 313–318
  in adolescents, 315, 316, 317
  assessment of, 314–315, 316
  culture and, 317
  definition of, 313
  development of, 315–316
  high, 314, 316
  increasing, 317
  inflated, 317
  low, 313, 316, 317
  in middle and late childhood, 313, 315
  positive, 314, 316
  poverty and, 486
  variations in, 316–317
self-integration, 310
self-modification, 188
self-monitoring, 466–467
Self-Perception Profile for Adolescents, 314
Self-Perception Profile for Children, 314
self-preoccupation, 309
self-reflection, 467
self-regulation
  in adolescents, 467
  executive function and, 203, 204
  gender differences in, 342
  intentional, 467
  joint attention and, 191
  and juvenile delinquency, 373
  and moral development, 358
  parenting and, 29, 389
  in peer relationships, 422
  poverty and, 481
  private speech and, 177
  and temperament, 285, 286
self-responsibility, 463
self-understanding, 307–310
  in adolescents, 309–310
  definition of, 307

in early childhood, 308–309
in infants, 307–308
in middle and late childhood, 309
self-worth, 359
semantics, 246, 247, 251–253
sensation, 143
sensitive period of child development, 24
sensorimotor play, 427
sensorimotor stage, 161–166
  A-not-B error and, 164
  definition of, 161
  description of, 19, 20, 161
  evaluation of, 164–166
  nature-nurture issue and, 166
  object permanence in, 164, 165
  substages of, 161–163
sensory development
  ecological view of, 143–144
  patterns of, 99
separation, 407
separation-individuation process, 172–173
separation protest, 278
seriation, 171
service learning, 365–366
SES. *See* socioeconomic status
sex chromosomes, 331
sex-linked chromosomal abnormalities, 53
sex-linked genes, 51
sex-typed play, 330
sexual abuse, 396
sexual identity, 318
sexuality, gender differences in, 342
sexual maturation, 102, 103
shaken baby syndrome, 106
shame, 17, 279
The Shame of the Nation (Kozol), 454
shape constancy, 148
shared environmental experiences, 63
shared reading, 264
shared sleeping, 112–113
sharing, 368
short-term memory, 194, 195, 198–199
shy children, 287, 422
siblings, 400–403. *See also* twins
  birth order of, 402
  and juvenile delinquency, 372, 402
  relationship between, 400–402
sickle-cell anemia, 54
SIDS. *See* sudden infant death syndrome
sight. *See* visual perception
sign language, 244, 248
similarity, in friendship, 431–432
Singapore, 445, 468
single-parent families, 403, 410
single-sex education, 335
size constancy, 148
skepticism, 312
Skinner's operant conditioning, 22
sleep, 111–115
  in adolescents, 114–115
  in children, 113–114
  function of, 111
  in infants, 111–113

non-REM, 112
REM, 112
sleep apnea, 113
sleep debt, 114
slow-to-warm-up child, 283
small for date infants, 87
smartphones, 492
smart toys, 206
smell, 151
smiling, in infants, 277
smoking
  paternal, 80
  during pregnancy, 71, 76–77, 99, 113
  secondhand, 80, 116
Snellen chart, 147
social cognition, 310–313
  in adolescents, 312–313
  definition of, 310
  in early childhood, 310–311
  in middle and late childhood, 311–312
  and peer relationships, 420–422
social-cognitive domain theory, 351, 361–362
social cognitive monitoring, 312–313
social cognitive theory
  child development issues and, 26
  definition of, 23
  evaluating, 23
  of gender, 332, 333
  overview of, 23
social comparison
  in friendship, 430
  in self-evaluation, 308, 310
social competence, parents and, 383, 384, 385
social constructivist approach, 179
social context, and decision making, 211
social contract, 354
social conventional reasoning, 361–362
social descriptions, 309
social information-processing skills, 421
social intelligence, 421
social interactions
  in autism, 214
  and babbling, 263
  and emotional development, 273
  and emotional expression, 276–278
  and gender, 332–336
social isolation, 417
socialization
  domain-specific, 384–385
  reciprocal, 382, 383
social knowledge, 421
social media
  and body image, 335
  children engaging in, 386
  popularity of, 492
social orientation
  in early childhood, 290–291
  evolutionary psychology on, 46
  in infants, 290–291
social play, 428
social policy, 8–10
social referencing, 291
social role theory, 332–333
social skills, improving, 423
social smile, 277

social systems morality, 354
social worker, 40
sociocultural changes, in family processes, 385–386
sociocultural cognitive theory. *See* Vygotsky's theory
sociocultural contexts, and diversity, 6
socioeconomic processes, 11
socioeconomic status (SES). *See also* poverty
  and dating, 438
  definition of, 6, 478
  divorce and, 406
  and education, 411, 454
  ethnicity and, 485–486
  and expectations, 486
  and families, 410–411
  and intelligence, 229, 230
  and juvenile delinquency, 372–373, 479
  and language development, 254
  and sudden infant death syndrome, 113
  variations in, 478–479
socioemotional development, gender and, 339–343
sociometric status, 422
sole custody, 406
sounds, recognition of, 249
spanking, 388, 389, 391, 393, 394
spatial skills, 225, 339–340
spatial thinking, 46
special education teacher, 39
specificity of learning, 137
speech
  child-directed, 263
  inner, 178
  private, 177, 178
  telegraphic, 250
speech pathologist, 252
speech problems, 251
speech therapist, 41
spelling
  children inventing, 258
  in learning disabilities, 457
sperm, 50, 70
spina bifida, 54, 74, 79
spiritual development, 374–376
spirituality, definition of, 374
spoken vocabulary, 249
sports, 140–141. *See also* exercise
stagnation, 17, 19
standardized tests, 27–28, 31, 444–445
Stanford-Binet intelligence test, 27, 223, 229, 236
startle reflex. *See* Moro reflex
The State of the World's Children (UNICEF), 117
status offenses, 370
stepfamilies, 406–408
stepfather families, 408
stepmother families, 408
stepping reflex, 135
stereotype threat, 232
Sternberg's triarchic theory, 224–225
stimulation, in friendship, 430

stranger anxiety, 278
Strange Situation, 293–294
strategies, problem solving using, 208
strategy construction, 188
stress
  acculturation and, 324
  coping with, 281–282
  and decision making, 211
  and onset of puberty, 101
  poverty and, 8–9, 481, 486
  during pregnancy, 80
stress hormones, 50, 396–397
sucking behavior
  accommodation of, 161
  habituation in, 144–145
  high-amplitude, 145–146
sucking reflex, 134, 135, 162
sudden infant death syndrome (SIDS), 76, 112, 113, 119
suffering, prevention of, 356
suggestion, susceptibility to, 200
suicide attempts, bullying and, 424
summarizing strategies, 209
supervisor of gifted and talented education, 237
support, in friendship, 430, 431, 432
surrogate mothers, 292
survey, as data collection method, 27, 31
"survival of the fittest," 45
susceptibility, 200
sustained attention, 190, 192, 193, 373, 463
swaddling, 139
Sweden
  child-care policy in, 298
  reading and math scores in, 468
  single-parent families in, 403
swimming reflex, 135
symbol, 163, 168
symbolic function substage, 167–168
symbolic play, 428
synapses, 105, 108, 109
synchronous interactions, 277
syntax, 246, 247, 251
syphilis, 78

T

task persistence, 463
taste, 151
Tay-Sachs disease, 54
teachers. *See also* schools
  autonomy-supportive, 462
  career opportunities for, 39–40
  critical thinking taught by, 205
  effective, 173, 221, 444
  elementary school, 39
  of ethnically diverse students, 455–456
  of exceptional children, 39
  expectations of, 466
  and gender development, 334–335
  guiding creativity, 239
  improving attention, 192
  and intrinsic motivation, 462–463
  Montessori, 445
  and moral development, 365

more-skilled peers as, 178
  promoting industry, 18
  reading instruction by, 257
  scientific thinking taught by, 206
  strategy instruction by, 209
  writing instruction by, 258
teaching strategies
  based on Piaget's theory, 173–174
  based on Vygotsky's theory, 178–179, 180
  for learning, 209
  for memory, 199–200
technology, 489–493
  digital devices and Internet, 492–493
  electronic media, 491–492
  and family processes, 386
  media use and screen time and, 489–490
  millenials and, 13
  television, 490, 491, 492
  video games, 386, 490–491
teen pregnancy, 80, 88, 384
telegraphic speech, 250
television, 490, 491, 492
temperament, 283–289
  biological influences on, 286
  classification of, 283–286
  culture and, 286–287
  definition of, 283
  developmental connections to, 287
  developmental contexts of, 287
  gender and, 286
temporal lobes, 105, 109
teratogens
  definition of, 74
  environmental, 78
  exposure to, 74–75
  medications as, 76
  and prenatal development, 75–76
  psychoactive drugs as, 76–77
teratology, 74–80
  behavioral, 75
  principles of, 74–76
terrorist attacks, 282
tertiary circular reactions, 163
testosterone
  and aggression, 332
  definition of, 101
  functions of, 101
  production of, 331
tests, standardized, 27–28, 31, 444–445
Thailand
  collectivist culture in, 476
  physical punishment in, 394
theory, definition of, 16, 17
theory of mind, child's, 212–215
thinking, 202–211
  abstract, idealistic, and logical, 171–172, 309
  in adolescents, 208–211
  in children, 203–208
  convergent, 238
  creative, 238, 239
  critical, 204–205, 209–210
  and decision making, 210
  definition of, 202
  divergent, 238

flexibility in, 239
  in infants, 202–203
  information-processing theory on, 21
  and problem solving, 206–208
  scientific, 205–206
  spatial, 46
third-generation immigrants, 324
thought
  intuitive, 168
  language and, 177–178
  moral (*See* moral thought)
  preoperational, 167, 168–169
  unconscious, 17
three-mountains task, 167–168
time out, 393
tobacco. *See* smoking
toddlers. *See also* early childhood
  emotional development in, 279
  emotional regulation in, 278
  emotions in, 273
  fine motor skills in, 142
  gross motor skills in, 138
  independence in, 291
  language development in, 265
  metacognition in, 213
  parenting, 389–390
  reading to, 264
  self-understanding in, 308
  smiling in, 277
  temperament in, 285
  thinking in, 203
  visual perception in, 149
tomboy, 333–334
tonic neck reflex, 135
Tools of the Mind curriculum, 180
top-dog phenomenon, 451
touch, in newborns, 151
Touch Research Institute, 89
toy designer, 206
transactional interactions, 383
transgender children, 344–345
transitivity, 171
Trends in International Math and Science Study (TIMSS), 445
triarchic theory of intelligence, 224–225
Tribal India Health Foundation, 467
triple screen, 57
trophoblast, 70
trust *vs.* mistrust stage, 17, 292
Turner syndrome, 52, 53
turn-taking, 341, 383, 428
twins, 44, 50–51, 58, 60–61
twin studies, 44, 60–61, 228, 286, 460
two-word utterances, 250

U

ultrasound sonography, 56
umbilical arteries, 71, 72
umbilical cord, 71, 72
umbilical vein, 71, 72
unconscious thought, 17
underextension, of words, 250
understanding
  others (*See* social cognition)
  self (*See* self-understanding)